AN ILLUSTRATED TEXTBOOK OF DERMATOLOGY & Sexually Transmitted Diseases

(With Cells, Signs and Syndromes)

Editor-in-Chief

U S AGARWAL, MD, FIAD
Pro Vice-Chancellor and Head of Department of Dermatology
Venereology and Leprosy, National Institute of Medical Sciences and Research Institute
Jaipur, Rajasthan

Associate Editors

Bhumesh Kumar Katakam, MD, DCH
Associate Professor, Department of Dermatology, Venereology and Leprosy
Gandhi Medical College and Hospital, Hyderabad, Telangana

Puneet Agarwal, MD
Associate Professor, Department of Dermatology, Venereology and Leprosy
Sawai Man Singh Medical College, Jaipur, Rajasthan

Assistant Editors

Rajendra Devanda, MD, DNB
Assistant Professor, Department of Dermatology, Venereology and Leprosy
National Institute of Medical Sciences and Research Institute, Jaipur, Rajasthan.

Navneet Randhawa, MD
Assistant Professor, Department of Dermatology, Venereology and Leprosy
National Institute of Medical Sciences and Research Institute, Jaipur, Rajasthan.

Rachita Mathur, MD
Assistant Professor, Department of Dermatology, Venereology and Leprosy
Pandit Deen Dayal Upadhyay Medical College, Churu, Rajasthan

Shivi Nijhawan, MD
Assistant Professor, Department of Dermatology, Venereology and Leprosy
Mahatma Gandhi Medical College and Research Institute, Jaipur, Rajasthan.

Peepee Publishers and Distributors Private Limited®

AN ILLUSTRATED TEXTBOOK OF

DERMATOLOGY

& Sexually Transmitted Diseases
(With Cells, Signs and Syndromes)

Published by
Pawaninder P. Vij and Anupam Vij

Peepee Publishers and Distributors Private Limited
Head Office: 160, Shakti Vihar, Pitam Pura, Delhi-110 034 (India)

Correspondence Address:
7/31, First Floor, Ansari Road, Daryaganj
New Delhi-110 002 (India)
Ph: 41512412, 9811156083
e-mail: peepee160@yahoo.co.in
e-mail: peepee160@gmail.com
www.peepeepub.com
join us on facebook.com/pp.publishers

First Edition: 2025

ISBN: 978-81-9833-661-3

DEDICATED TO

My father
Whom I miss and who was a great driving force behind achieving this milestone.

My wife
A charming lady, who understands my dreams and endeavours and has supported me with utmost sincerity and dedication.

My teachers and patients
Who have been the guiding light throughout my journey.

FOREWORD

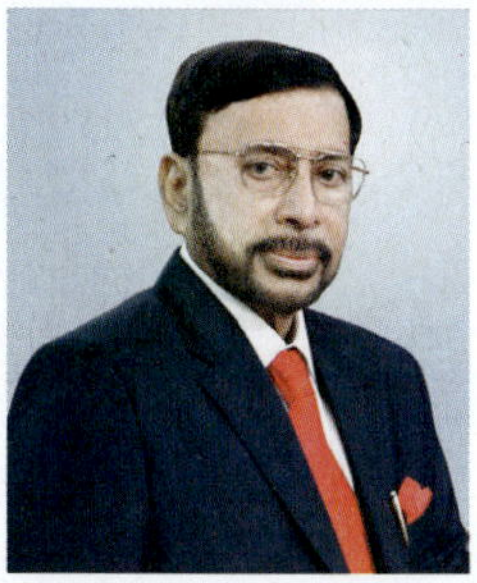

I feel privileged to pen the foreword of 'AN ILLUSTRATED TEXTBOOK OF DERMATOLOGY AND SEXUALLY TRANSMITTED DISEASES, with Cells and Signs and Syndromes', a remarkable schorlarly work by Dr. U.S. Agarwal, the esteemed Prof & Head of Department of DERMATOLOGY, VENEREOLOGY and LEPROSY at NATIONAL INSTITUTE OF MEDICAL SCIENCES Hospital.

The field of dermatology occupies a unique and essential place in medicine, bridging the gap between our external appearance and our internal health. Dermatology is a field that is constantly growing, combining clinical competence with technological and research advances.

In recent years, the field has seen tremendous growth, with innovative therapies and groundbreaking technologies revolutionizing our approach to diagnosing and treating skin conditions. This book serves as a beacon of knowledge in this dynamic field, offering a thorough exploration of dermatological science and practice as it encapsulates the latest findings and practices, providing insights that are crucial for effective patient care.

The book offers a detailed overview of common dermatological conditions, enriched with clinical photographs, cellular analyses and management strategies. Its structure and content makes it an invaluable resource for undergraduate and postgraduate students of dermatology. Through its meticulous descriptions and practical guidance, it is sure to become a trusted reference for learners and practitioners alike.

Dr. Agarwal has utilized his vast experience, deep expertise and an exceptional ability to distill complex concepts into accessible and practical knowledge to bring out this work. With a comprehensive description of each dermatosis, clinical pictures and approach to management, it becomes a 'go-to-book' for all students. I am sure that this book will not only enhance the understanding but also inspire a continued passion for learning and discovery in dermatology.

I extend my heartfelt congratulations to Dr. U.S. Agarwal for this brilliant initiative and wish him immense success with this publication.

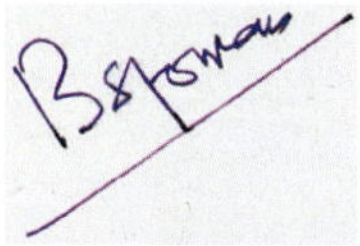

Prof. (Dr.) Balvir S. Tomar

M.B.B.S., M.D., M.C.H. (USA), M.I.A.P., M.A.H.T. (England)
F.I.A.P., F.A.A.P., (USA), F.I.C.A. (USA), F.A.C.U. (London)

Pediatric Hepatology: Kings College Hospital
School of Medicine, University of London, London (England)

Pediatric Gastroenterology, Harvard University (USA)
W.H.O. Fellow: Child Health in United States of America
Commonwealth: Medical Fellow in London (England)

Founder & Chancellor
NIMS University

FOREWORD

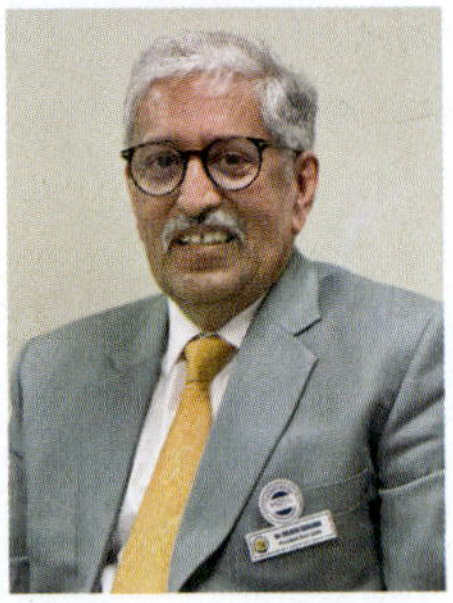

I feel honoured and pleased to pen the forward of **An Illustrated Textbook of Dermatology and Sexually Transmitted Diseases**, by an outstanding and distinguished academician Dr. U.S. Agarwal, a very senior and distinguished teacher and currently the Prof & Head of Department of Dermatology, Venereology and Leprosy at National Institute of Medical Sciences and its Hospitals.

Dermatology as a field, holds a distinctive and vital position within the medical field, serving as a connection between internal medicine and external medicine.

Dermatology is an evolving discipline of medicine that integrates clinical expertise with advancements in research and technology. The field has experienced a significant expansion in recent years, marked by introduction of innovative therapies and cutting-edge technologies that are transforming our diagnostic and therapeutic techniques.

This publication stands as a significant source of knowledge in the ever-evolving field of dermatology, providing an in-depth examination of dermatological science and practice. It incorporates the most recent research and methodologies, delivering essential insights for optimal patient care.

The book presents a comprehensive review of prevalent dermatological disorders, enhanced by clinical images, cellular evaluations, and treatment approaches. Its organization and content render it an indispensable tool for both undergraduate and postgraduate dermatology students. With its detailed explanations and practical advice, it is poised to be a reliable reference for both learners and professionals in the field.

Dr. U.S. Agarwal with his team of contributors has leveraged his extensive experience and profound expertise, along with a remarkable talent for simplifying intricate concepts into practical knowledge, to produce this remarkable work. Featuring detailed descriptions of various dermatoses, accompanied by clinical images and management strategies, this book serves as an essential resource for all students. I am confident that it will not only deepen understanding but also foster a lasting enthusiasm for learning and exploration in the field of dermatology.

I offer my sincere congratulations to Dr. U.S. Agarwal for this outstanding initiative and wish him great success with this publication.

Rajeev Sharma

Rajeev Sharma
President
Indian Association of Dermatology, Venereology and Leprosy (IADVL 2025)

Consultant Dermatologist
Aligarh, U.P.

PREFACE

Within the dynamic field of dermatology, the skin—the largest organ in the body—offers a wide and complex canvas of opportunities as well as challenges. The desire to explore the intricacies of skin health and shed light on the subtleties of dermatological science and practice served as the impetus for this book.

Dermatology comprises a vast range of illnesses, treatments, and advancements that reflect not only the variety of skin disorders but also their tremendous influence on patients' lives. Over time, advances in technology and research have substantially revolutionized our understanding and management of skin problems, providing fresh hope and answers where there were previously few.

The goal of this book is to bridge the gap between developing research and practical application by providing a complete resource for both experienced practitioners and newcomers to the area. It aims to improve the reader's knowledge and skills by providing extensive discussions, case studies, and current material, encouraging a greater appreciation for the art and science of dermatology.

This volume is designed in a way that it will be easily retained by both undergraduates and postgraduates and it strives to simplify the intricacies of dermatology. It contains a plethora of high-quality photos depicting various dermatological symptoms, as well as useful mnemonics and therapeutic applications to aid learning and recall during exams.

This book features beautifully articulated sections on cells, signs and syndromes in dermatology. Furthermore, the explanation of 'Immunology' is straightforward and easy to understand.

As you embark on this trip into the world of dermatology, I hope you will find not only useful insights and practical advice, but also motivation to continue studying and growing in this vibrant and gratifying specialty. Welcome to the vast and interesting world of dermatology.

U S AGARWAL, MD, FIAD

ACKNOWLEDGEMENTS

The editorial team is sincerely thankful to the following veteran dermatologists for their valuable advice and important clinical photographs.

Dr Amit Tiwari MD
Associate Professor
Department of Dermatology, Venereology and Leprosy
Sawai Man Singh Medical College
Jaipur, Rajasthan

Dr Archana Singhal MD, FAMS, MNAMS
Head of Department and Professor
Department of Dermatology, Venereology and Leprosy
University College of Medical Sciences and
Guru Teg Bahadur Hospital
New Delhi

Dr Asit Mittal MD
Senior Professor
Department of Dermatology
Venereology and Leprosy
Rabindranath Tagore Medical College
Jaipur, Rajasthan

Dr Bela Shah MD
Head of Department and Professor
Department of Dermatology, Venereology and Leprosy
BJ Medical College, Ahmedabad, Gujarat

Dr Deepak Mathur MD
Head of Department and Senior Professor
Department of Dermatology, Venereology and Leprosy
Sawai Man Singh Medical College, Jaipur, Rajasthan

Dr Dinesh Mathur MD, Medicine, MD, DVL
Former Head of Department and Senior Professor
Department of Dermatology, Venereology and Leprosy
Sawai Man Singh Medical College and Pro Vice-Chancellor
Rajasthan University of Health Sciences, Jaipur, Rajasthan

Dr Khushboo Gupta MD
Associate Professor
Department of Dermatology, Venereology and Leprosy
National Institute of Medical Sciences and Research Institute
Jaipur, Rajasthan

Dr Kishor Singh MD
Former Head of Department and Professor
Department of Dermatology, Venereology and Leprosy
National Institute of Medical Sciences and Research Institute
Jaipur, Rajasthan

Dr Lalit Gupta MD
Senior Professor
Department of Dermatology, Venereology and Leprosy
Rabindranath Tagore Medical College, Jaipur, Rajasthan

Dr Rashmi Sarkar MD, MNAMS
Director Professor
Department of Dermatology, Venereology and Leprosy
Lady Hardinge Medical College, New Delhi

Dr Nausheen Aara MD
Associate Professor
Department of Dermatology, Venereology and Leprosy
Sawai Man Singh Medical College, Jaipur, Rajasthan

Dr Ramsingh Meena MD
Senior Professor
Department of Dermatology, Venereology and Leprosy
Sawai Man Singh Medical College, Jaipur, Rajasthan

Dr Sanjay Sakarwal MD
Professor
Department of Dermatology, Venereology and Leprosy
National Institute of Medical Sciences and Research Institute
Jaipur, Rajasthan

Dr Saroj Purohit MD
Senior Professor
Department of Dermatology, Venereology and Leprosy
Sawai Man Singh Medical College, Jaipur, Rajasthan

Dr Sonal Jain MD, DNB
Assistant Professor
Department of Dermatology, Venereology and Leprosy
IIMSAR Medical College & Hospital, Haldia

Dr Surendra Thalor MD
Professor
Department of Dermatology, Venereology and Leprosy
Sawai Man Singh Medical College, Jaipur, Rajasthan

Dr Vijay Paliwal MD
Professor
Department of Dermatology, Venereology and Leprosy
Sawai Man Singh Medical College, Jaipur, Rajasthan

Our department postgraduates, **Dr Vishal Patel, Dr Rutva Amlani, Dr Hardik Shah, Dr Asmeen Chawla, Dr Prabhleen Grewal, Dr Ananya Choudhary, Dr Mohit Saini, Dr Sheetal, Dr Ayushi Tyagi, Dr Nancy Garg, Dr Moni Kashyap, Dr Ankita, Dr Apoorva Shekhawat, Dr Maharshi, Dr Juhi Tomar** for giving final shape to the manuscript and for time to time valuable suggestions.

CONTENTS

1 CHAPTER Structure and Function of the Skin

Contents

The core of the human beauty, skin, is the most fascinating and largest organ of the body with an average of 1.7 sq. meter surface area and about 5 million hairs on it. It constitutes 15% to 20% of body weight. It develops from both ectoderm (epidermis) and mesoderm (dermis). Neonatal skin is relatively immature compared to adult skin.

Human skin is of two types: Hairy and non-hairy.

Non-hairy (glabrous) skin, present on the palms and soles, is thicker and devoid of hair and sebaceous glands. It has alternating ridges and grooves arranged in patterns, which are unique to an individual. In addition, glabrous skin has special encapsulated sensory organs. **Hairy skin** is present on rest of the body, has hair and sebaceous glands but lacks encapsulated sensory organs. Skin has three layers (Figure 1.1):

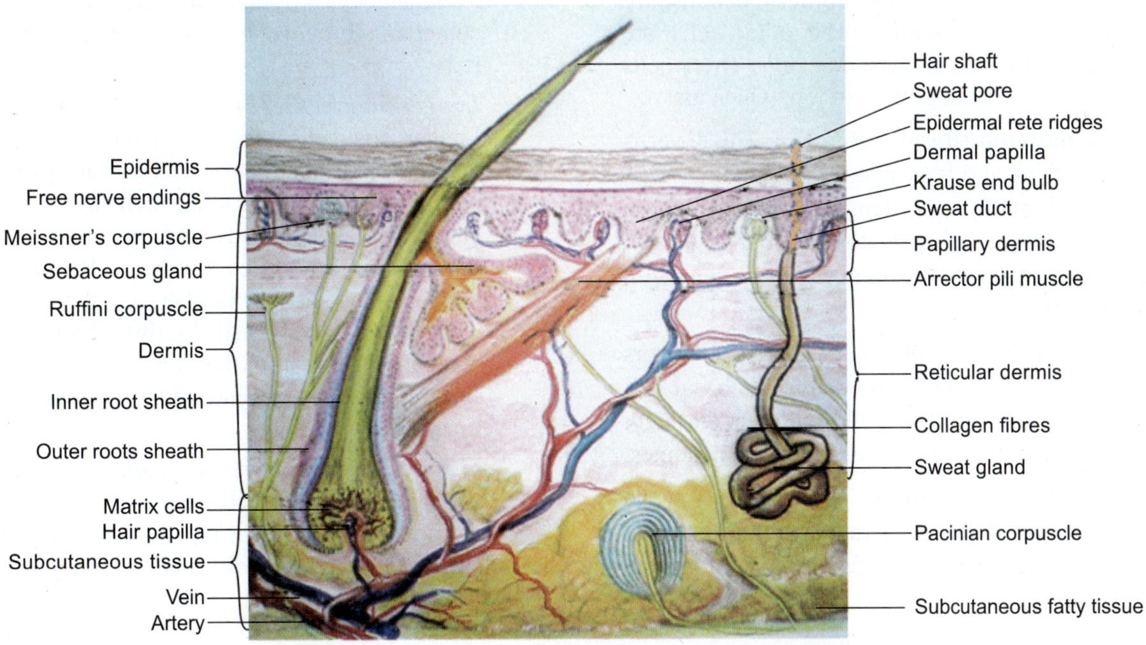

Figure 1.1: Structure of skin with its blood and nerve supply

- Epidermis.
- Dermis.
- Hypodermis (subcutis).

EMBRYOLOGICAL DEVELOPMENT OF SKIN

The juxtaposition of two major embryological elements, the prospective epidermis originating from the early gastrula, and the prospective mesoderm coming in contact with it, leads to the development of skin at about the third week of fetal life. The mesoderm forms the dermis and helps in differentiation of various epidermal structures. The neural crest contributes the pigment cells to the skin. The embryonic events occur as follows:

- 3rd month – Non-functioning melanocytes.
- 4th month – Hair pegs, nail, active melanocytes, Langerhans cells, Merkel cells.
- 5th month – Exposed hair, sebaceous glands, epidermal keratinization.
- 6th month – Apocrine gland, eccrine gland, follicular keratinization

EPIDERMIS

Epidermis, the outermost layer of skin, is mainly composed of epidermal cells known as **keratinocytes**. The thickness of the epidermis varies from 0.05 mm to 0.1 mm, being thinnest on the eyelids and thickest on palms and soles. The ratio of epidermis to dermis is 1:20. Epidermis is thrown into folds in the dermis as downward projections known as rete ridges. Areas of dermis enclosed between **rete ridges** are known as **dermal papillae**.

Cells of epidermis: 95% of the epidermal cells are keratinocytes which produce keratin. The other cells are ***melanocytes, Langerhans cells and Merkel cells***. These cells are arranged in four layers, from bottom to top, which are:

1. **Stratum germinativum (Basal cell layer):** This layer is one or two cells thick and is composed of columnar cells with dark-stained nuclei and dense cytoplasm. These cells divide and move upwards to the skin's surface. Melanocytes are lodged in between the basal cells in a ratio of about 1:10.
2. **Stratum spinosum (Prickle cell layer):** It is 8 to 10 layers thick consisting of polygonal cells above the basal cell layer. These cells are connected with each other and with the basal cells by intercellular bridges called desmosomes.
3. **Stratum granulosum (Granular cell layer):** As the keratinocytes ascend from the stratum spinosum, they lose their prickles, become flat and fusiform, and form the stratum granulosum, which is 1-3 layers thick. These cells contain keratohyaline granules, which include proteins such as keratin, loricrin, trichohyalin, and filaggrin. These proteins are essential for epidermal cornification or keratinization. The cells also contain lamellar granules, also known as keratinosomes or Odland bodies, which discharge their lipid components into the intercellular space, playing a crucial role in barrier function and intercellular cohesion within the stratum corneum.
4. **Stratum corneum (Horny layer):** This is the outermost layer of skin, consisting of flattened, dead cells that lack nuclei. These cells are constantly shed from the skin surface and are regularly replaced by a new crop of keratinized cells from the deeper layers. The stratum corneum is about 15-25 layers thick, with significantly greater thickness on the palms and soles. The cells are composed of a tough, fibrous protein known as keratin. In the palms and soles, there is an additional layer beneath the stratum corneum known as the stratum lucidum, which is a homogeneous layer of flattened cells.
   - ***Melanocytes (Figure 1.2):*** They are dendritic cells of neural crest origin, located in the basal layer of the epidermis. They synthesize melanin, which imparts color to the skin. One melanocyte supplies melanin to 36 keratinocytes through its dendrites, forming what is known as the epidermal melanin unit. Melanocytes are round to oval, clear cells with dark-stained nuclei and cytoplasmic organelles called melanosomes, which synthesize melanin with the help of an enzyme known as tyrosinase via a process called the Raper-Mason pathway. Melanosomes are transferred to keratinocytes through the dendrites. The color of an individual's skin is determined by the size, number, and density of melanosomes, not by the number of melanocytes. There are two types of melanin: eumelanin (brown or black) and pheomelanin (yellow-red).
   - ***Langerhans cells (Figure 1.2):*** Like melanocytes, Langerhans cells are also dendritic cells and are derived from bone marrow. They are present in the basal, spinous, and granular cell layers. These cells have a folded nucleus and tennis racquet-shaped cytoplasmic organelles known as Birbeck granules. They display distinct markers on their cell surface, CD1a and CD207 (Langerin). Langerhans cells present antigens from the skin surface to the immune system and carry out important immune surveillance functions.
   - ***Merkel cells (Haascheiben cell, Figure 1.2):*** They are regarded as the nerve cells of the epidermis and are abundantly present on the fingertips, lips, outer hair sheath, and gingival mucosa. They reside in the

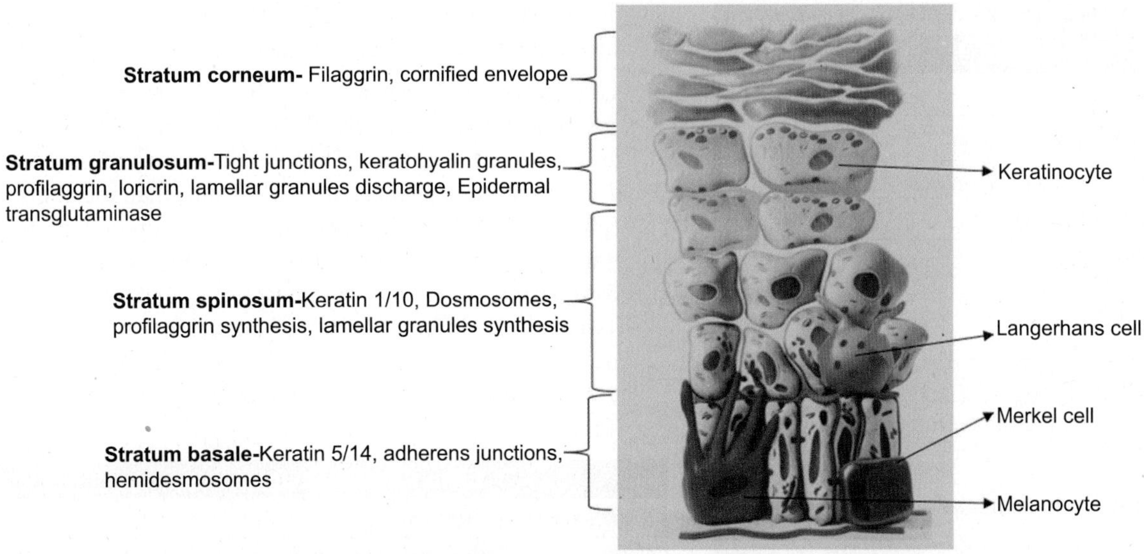

Figure 1.2: Showing different epidermal cells and process of keratinization

basal layer and are connected to keratinocytes through desmosomes. *These cells assist in the slow-adapting touch sensory function. They express neuroendocrine markers such as synaptophysin, chromogranin A, and cytokeratin 20. Cytokeratin 20 is a sensitive and specific marker for Merkel cell carcinoma.*

KERATINIZATION

Keratinization, also known as cornification, is a process of cytodifferentiation in which keratinocytes undergo successive changes from their post-germinative state (stratum basale) to fully differentiated, mechanically resistant, and toughened cornified cells (stratum corneum). The cornified cells forming the stratum corneum are larger and flatter than those of the stratum granulosum. All organelles, such as the nucleus, ribosomes, mitochondria, and keratohyalin granules, disappear. Ultrastructurally, the cells of the cornified layer are composed of densely packed filaments developed from tonofilaments, altered and coated by the basic protein of the keratohyalin granule, filaggrin. The cell membrane of these cells is replaced by a proteinaceous cornified envelope that is covalently cross-linked to the keratin filaments, providing a highly insoluble yet flexible structure that protects the underlying epithelial cells. These cells eventually desquamate. Various factors affecting keratinocyte differentiation include metabolites of Vitamin D3, epidermal growth factor (EGF), keratinocyte growth factor (KGF), fibroblast growth factor (FGF), interleukins 1-β and 6, hepatocyte growth factor (HGF), transforming growth factor (TGF-β), vitamin A, and calcium. The entire process of maturation from basal cells to stratum corneum is known as keratinization and is completed in about 30 days.

Classification of keratins

A. Based on the preferential synthesis:

1. Primary keratins – keratins which are always synthesized by the epithelial cells on a regular basis e.g. K 8/18 in simple epithelia and K 5/14 in the stratified epithelia.
2. Secondary keratins – Produced by epithelial cells in addition to primary keratins, K 7/19 in the simple epithelia and 6/16 in the stratified epithelia.

B. Based on biochemical properties (pki value):

- Type I: Acidic (pki= 4.9-5.4)- K9–28, K31-40
- Type II: Basic (pki= 6.5-8.5)- K1–8, K71-80, K81-86

To form functional intermediate filaments keratin molecules must form heterodimers by specific pairing of one acidic and one basic keratin e.g. K5 (II)-K14 or 15 (I).

Distribution of different keratin protein in epidermis are shown in Table 1.1 and associated disorders are described in Table 1.2.

Table 1.1: Showing distribution of keratins in different epithelial cells	
K5/14	Basal cell layer of both the keratinized and non-keratinized stratified epithelium
K1/10	Keratinized epidermis
K6/16	Spinous cell layer of keratinized mucosa
K4/13	Intermediate layer of non-keratinized epithelium
K19	Basal layer of non-keratinized epithelium
K9	Suprabasal cells of palmar and plantar epidermis

Table 1.2: Showing defects of different keratin associated disorders

Disorder	*Defect*
Epidermolysis bullosa simplex	K5/K14
Epidermolytic ichthyosis	K1/K10
Superficial epidermolytic ichthyosis	K2
Pachyonychia congenita	
• Jadassohn-lewandowsky type	K6a or K16
• Jackson Lawler type	K6b or K17
Epidermolytic palmoplantar keratoderma	K1/K9
Non epidermolytic palmoplantar keratoderma	K1
White sponge nevus	K4 and K13
Genodermatoses with reticulate pigmentation	
• Dowling Degos disease	K5
• Dermatopathia pigmentosa reticularis	K14
• Naegeli Francesschetti Jadassohn syndrome	K14
Steatocystoma multiplex	K17
Pseudo folliculitis barbae	K75
Monilethrix	K81, K83, K86
"Pure" hair-nail type ectodermal dysplasia	K85

CELL JUNCTIONS

These are multiprotein complexes that form connections either between cells or from cells to the extracellular matrix. The function of these junctions is to coordinate activity between cells, respond to external stimuli, and maintain homeostasis in tissue. Four main types of cell junctions are present in the skin:

1. **Tight junction (Zona occludens)**
2. **Adhering junction (Zonula adherens)**
3. **Gap junction**
4. **Desmosomes (macula adherens)**

1. **Tight junction (Zona occludens):** Tight junctions are composed of transmembrane claudin and occludin proteins which bind intracellularly to zonula occludens protein, ZO-1, ZO-2, ZO-3. They are important for maintaining barrier function and cell polarity.
2. **Adhering junction (Zonula adherens):** They are electron dense transmembrane structure composed of two components:
   - Transmembrane component: Cadherins, Nectin
   - Plaque component: Catenin, Afadin

   They initiate and stabilize cell to cell adhesion, regulate actin cytoskeleton, intracellular signaling and are also involved in transcriptional regulation.
3. **Gap junction:** These are specialized areas of the plasma membrane where intercellular channels (connexons) are clustered together. They transfer ions (Ca+, K+), secondary messengers (cAMP, IP3) and small metabolites (glucose, siRNA). Each connexin is composed of four transmembrane domains, two extracellular loops, one cytoplasmic loop and cytoplasmic C and N terminal. Twenty one different types of connexin isoforms have been identified. Abnormalities in connexin proteins lead to many diseases, some of them have been enumerated in Table 1.3.

Table 1.3: Connexinopathies

Connexin	*Disease*
Cx26	Vohwinkel's syndrome Bart Pumphrey syndrome Keratitis Ichthyosis Deafness syndrome (KID) Hysterix like ichthyosis deafness syndrome Palmoplantar keratoderma with deafness
Cx30	Clouston syndrome
Cx30.3	Erythrokeratoderma variabilis (EKV)
Cx31	Erythrokeratoderma variabilis
Cx43	Oculo dento digital dysplasia (ODDS)

4. **Desmosomes (macula adherens):** They are adhesion sites which link adjacent cytoskeleton of the keratinocytes. They have two major components (A and B), formed by three superfamily proteins:
   - Transmembrane component:
     - o Desmosomal cadherins (superfamily 1): Desmoglein and desmocollin
   - Plaque component:
     - o Plakin (superfamily 2): Desmoplakin, envoplakin and periplakin.
     - o Armadillo family proteins (superfamily 3): Plakoglobin and plakophilin

There are four types of desmoglein (Dsg 1 to 4) and three types of desmocollin (Dsc 1 to 3) and defects in these proteins are implicated in various vesiculobullous disorders.

The overview of basement membrane, hemidesmosomes and desmosomes given in Figure 1.3.

DERMOEPIDERMAL JUNCTION (Figure 1.4)

The epidermis is attached to the dermis by an interface called the basement membrane zone, which consists of the

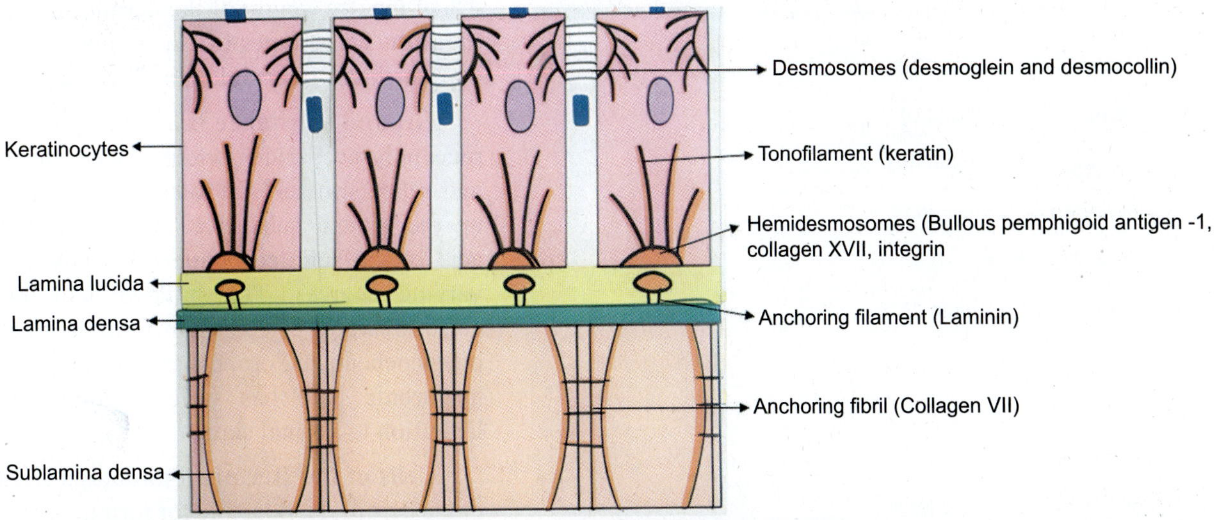

Figure 1.3: Overview of basement membrane, hemidesmosomes and desmosomes

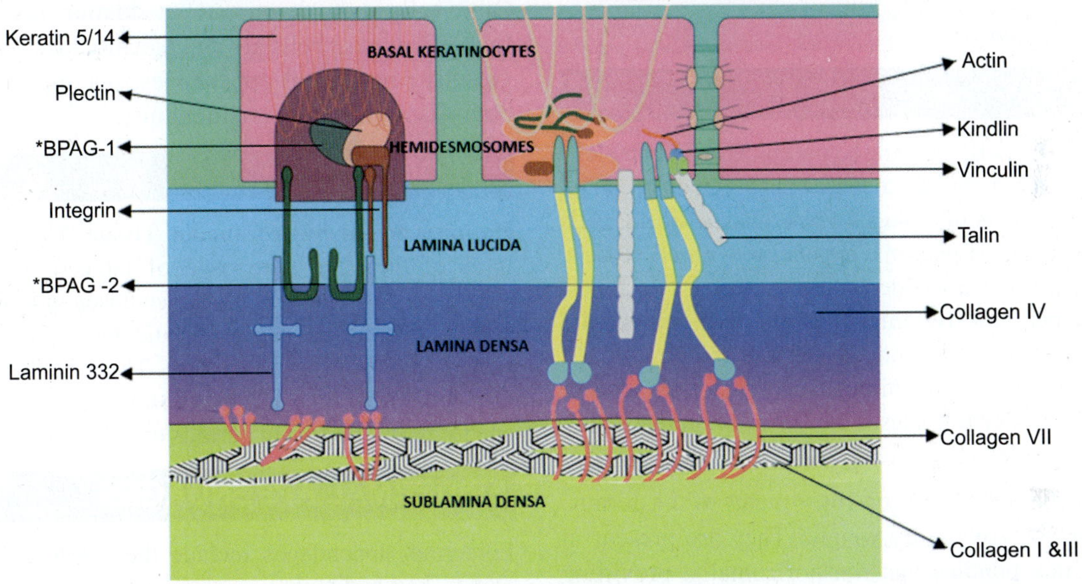

Figure 1.4: Showing ultrastructure of dermoepidermal junction (*BPAG-1–Bullous pemphigoid antigen-1, *BPAG-2 - Bullous pemphigoid antigen-2)

plasma membrane of basal keratinocytes, lamina lucida, lamina densa, and anchoring fibrils, as observed through an electron microscope. On PAS-stained sections, it appears as a homogeneous band with a thickness of 200 µm. This zone provides integrity to the skin and acts as a filter between the epidermis and dermis for various cells and molecules. The molecular components of the dermalepidermal junction (DEJ) are:

1. Intermediate filament (IF) components
   - Keratin 5
   - Keratin 14

Contd.

2. Hemidesmosomal plaque components
   - 230 kDa bullous pemphigoid antigen (BP230/BPAG1)
   - Plectin
3. Transmembrane components
   - α6β4 integrin
   - Type XVII collagen (180 kDa bullous pemphigoid antigen/BPAG2)
   - α3β1 integrin
     - Type XIII collagen
     - Syndecans 1 and 4

Contd.

4. Lamina lucida/lamina densa components
   - Laminin 332 (laminin 5)
   - Laminin 311 (laminin 6)
   - Laminin 511 (laminin 10)
5. Lamina densa components
   - Type IV collagen
   - Laminin 111 (laminin 1)
   - Nidogen
   - BM-40/SPARC
   - Perlecan
6. Anchoring fibril components
   - Type VII collagen
   - GDA-J/F3 antigen

DERMIS

Dermis is a connective tissue lying below epidermis, variable in thickness from 0.5 mm on face to more than 5 mm on back and thighs. Dermis consists of collagen fibers, elastic fibers, cells and ground substance. Epidermal appendages, blood vessels, nerves and muscles are embedded in it. Dermis has two zones: **papillary dermis and reticular dermis**. The **superficial papillary dermis** is a thin zone below the epidermis. It is highly vascular and contains thin collagen fibers. The deeper zone, **the reticular dermis** is less vascular and is composed of thick collagen bundles.

Collagen fibers are the main constituents of the dermis, forming about 70% of its dry weight. They are present in the form of thick bundles that run horizontally, providing structural support to the skin. There are 29 different types of collagen. In the dermis, 80% to 90% of collagen fibers are of type 1. These are composed of protein molecules having three polypeptide chains. Type 1 collagen associates with type 3 collagen to form broad extracellular fibers in the dermis. Biochemically, the papillary dermis is primarily composed of type 3 collagen, while the reticular dermis primarily contains type 1 collagen. **Reticular fibers** represent a special type of thin collagen that measures from 0.2 μm to 1 μm in diameter; they are the first formed fibers during embryonic life.

Elastic fibers are thin fibers arranged in bundles that extend from the dermoepidermal junction to the stroma of the subcutis. They are interspersed among the collagen fibers, with bundles being thicker in the lower dermis and thinner near the epidermis. These fibers constitute about 4% of the dry weight of the dermis and provide elasticity to the skin. Three types of elastic fibers found in the skin are mature elastic fibers, elaunin fibers, and oxytalan fibers.

Ground substance is a gelatinous material made up of mucopolysaccharides, which embeds the dermal fibrils, cells and other structures. Proteoglycan-GAG complexes make up the ground substance. The simplest GAG, hyaluronic acid is non sulfated, while other GAGs show sulfation of varying degrees. The sulfated acid mucopolysaccharide consists largely of chondroitin sulfate. It provides important physicochemical properties to the skin, most notably, hyaluronic acid has water binding capacity, providing hydration to normal skin.

Cells of the Dermis: Fibroblasts are the principal cells of the dermis, responsible for forming collagen fibers, elastic fibers, and ground substance. They are spindle-shaped. Other cells in the dermis include **histiocytes** and **mast cells**. In the skin, mast cells are strategically located close to blood vessels, nerves, and appendages, playing a critical role in both adaptive and innate immunity.

HYPODERMIS

Hypodermis or Subcutaneous Tissue: This is the innermost layer of the skin, composed of fat cells (adipocytes) that synthesize fat. The fat cells are enclosed in lobules, which are separated by fibrous septa. Through these septa, blood vessels, nerves, and lymphatics traverse. The subcutaneous fat serves as a shock absorber and heat insulator, and it also acts as an energy reservoir during periods of starvation.

EPIDERMAL APPENDAGES

Epidermal appendages include the sweat glands, sebaceous glands, hair and nails.

Sweat glands: They are of two types: **Eccrine glands and apocrine glands**.

Eccrine Glands: These are coiled tubular glands that open directly onto the skin surface. Humans have between 2 to 4 million eccrine sweat glands distributed throughout the body, except at mucocutaneous junctions, such as the nail bed, lips, and glans penis. They are especially abundant on the palms, soles, forehead, and axillae. The eccrine gland is composed of three parts (Figure 1.1).

1. **Coiled secretory part at the junction of dermis and subcutis.**
2. **Straight intradermal duct.**
3. **Spiral intraepidermal duct.**

The secretory portion of the eccrine gland contains three types of cells: clear (secretory), dark (mucoid), and myoepithelial. Eccrine sweat glands secrete sweat which helps regulate body temperature by cooling the body through evaporation. Additionally, they moisten the palms and soles to enhance grip and facilitate the excretion of certain drugs. These glands are innervated by cholinergic fibers.

Apocrine Sweat Glands: These glands are located in the axillae, areolae, and perineum. They open into the hair follicle above the sebaceous glands or directly onto the skin surface. Apocrine glands become functional only at puberty and are regulated by sex hormones. Although they produce an odor, this serves no function in humans. These glands are innervated by sympathetic adrenergic nerve fibers. Modified apocrine glands include the mammary glands, ceruminous glands of the external auditory canal, and Moll glands of the eyelids.

Sebaceous Glands: Sebaceous glands are either unilocular or multilocular holocrine glands that are associated with hair follicles, forming the pilosebaceous unit (Figure 1.5). They are found all over the body, except on the palms and soles, but are particularly abundant on the face, scalp, and upper chest. The glands consist of lipid-producing cells called sebocytes, which form acini. Sebum, the product of these glands, contains squalene, cholesterol, cholesterol esters, wax esters, and triglycerides. Sebum secretion helps prevent water loss from the skin and possesses antibacterial and antifungal properties. The secretion of sebum is regulated by androgens.

HAIR

Hair is a keratinous fiber coming out from hair follicle, which is an inward growth of epidermis in the dermis. There are three types of hair depending on their thickness.

1. **Lanugo hair:** They are present on fetal skin and are shed after birth.
2. **Terminal hair:** They are more than 60 μm in diameter, long, pigmented, medullated and are present on scalp, eyebrows, beard, axillae and pubic region.
3. **Vellus hair:** They are less than 30 μm in diameter, short, non-pigmented and non-medullated and are present on rest of the body.

The hair follicle has four parts:

1. **Hair bulb:** The lowermost portion of the hair follicle is broad, known as hair bulb, which encloses a small stud of dermis known as dermal papilla.
2. **Supra-bulbar part:** It extends from the bulb to insertion of arrector pili muscle.
3. **Isthmus:** It extends from insertion of arrector pili muscle to the opening of sebaceous glands in the follicle.
4. **Infundibulum:** It extends from sebaceous gland opening point to the follicular orifice on skin surface.

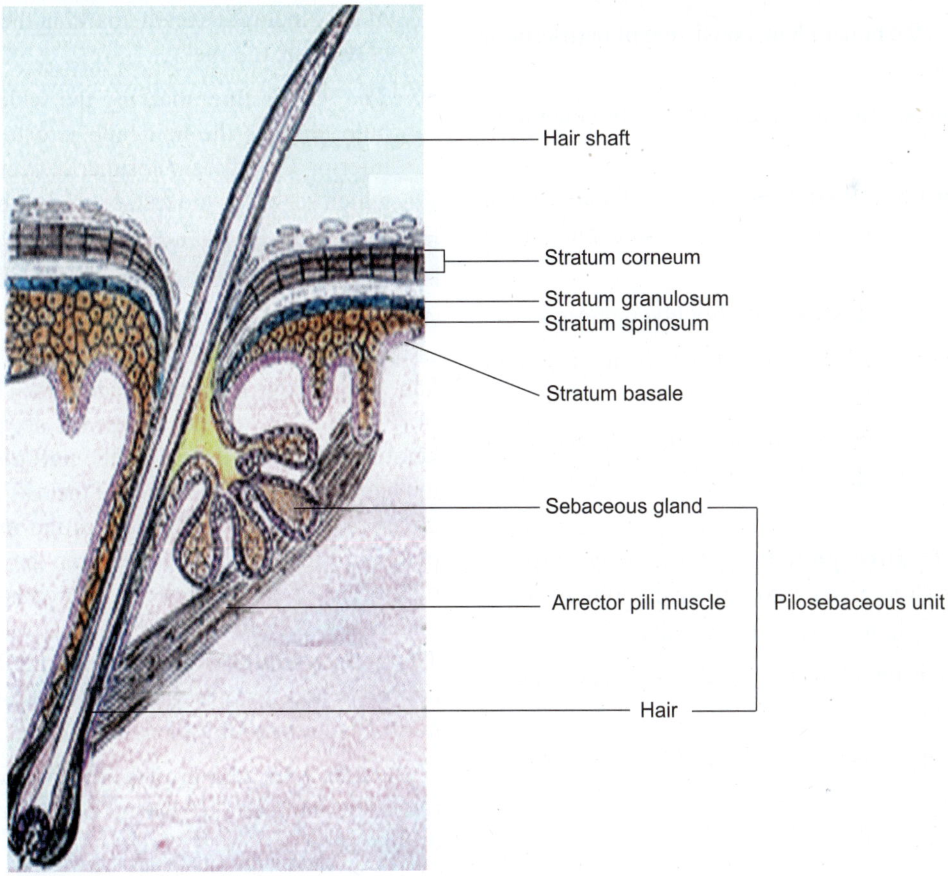

Figure 1.5: Structure of hair with pilosebaceous unit

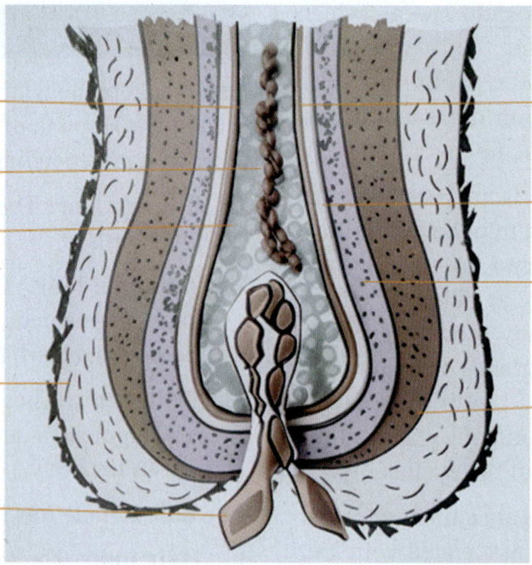

Figure 1.6: Showing layers of hair follicle

- The upper part of the follicle is permanent while the lower part undergoes repeated regression and regeneration during hair growth. The various layers of the anagen hair that can be recognized are (from inside to outside, Figure 1.6):

1. **Medulla:** It is the innermost part with two to three layers of soft keratin.
2. **Cortex:** It forms the bulk of hair, consisting of hard keratin containing cells.
3. **Cuticle:** It is the outermost single layer of cells containing hard keratin.
4. **Inner root sheath (IRS):** IRS consists of cuticle, the Huxley and the Henley layers. The IRS disintegrates at the isthmus.
5. **Outer root sheath (ORS):** It is highly glycogenated.
6. **Connective tissue sheath:** It is also known as dermal sheath or fibrous root sheath.

Hair growth varies with sex and part of the body but on an average, it is 0.4 mm per day. Hair growth is cyclical having following phases:

- **Anagen (Proliferative phase):** It is the active growth phase lasting for 3 to 5 years. At any given point of time, 80% to 85% of scalp hair are in anagen phase.
- **Catagen (Transition phase):** It is the regressing phase lasting for 3 weeks.
- **Telogen (Resting phase):** It is the resting phase lasting for 3 months.
- **Exogen:** Shedding of the hair.
- **Kenogen:** Hair follicles may remain in a state of latency after the club hair is shed known as kenogen.
- **Adamson's Fringe** is located at the upper part of the hair bulb where complete keratinization of the hair shaft occurs, resulting in the transformation into hard, anucleated keratin. This area is also characterized by the complete keratinization of the cuticle and the Henle layer of the inner root sheath, marking the beginning of the stem of the hair follicle.
- **The Auber line**, marking the widest portion of the hair bulb, divides the hair bulb into two parts: superior and inferior. Cell division primarily occurs in the inferior part, which serves as the true matrix of the hair.

NAILS

Apart from cosmetic purposes, nails also play a crucial role in protecting the distal phalanges of the fingers and toes. Like hair, nails grow from the epidermis. The nail unit, depicted in (Figure 1.7A and B), comprises six parts. The hard, pink, keratinized part of the nail is the **nail plate**. The skin folds on the lateral and posterior sides of the nail are the **nail folds**. Just under the proximal nail fold lies the **matrix**, where the nail plate is formed. The space between the nail folds and the nail plate is filled by the **cuticle**. The opaque, semilunar portion underlying the proximal part of the nail is called the **lunula**. The **hyponychium** is located underneath the free edge of the nail plate and denotes the transition from the nail bed to the normal epidermis of the fingers and toes.

Unlike hair, nail growth is continuous and grows at the rate of 0.1mm per day. Toe nails grow at one third of the rate of finger nails.

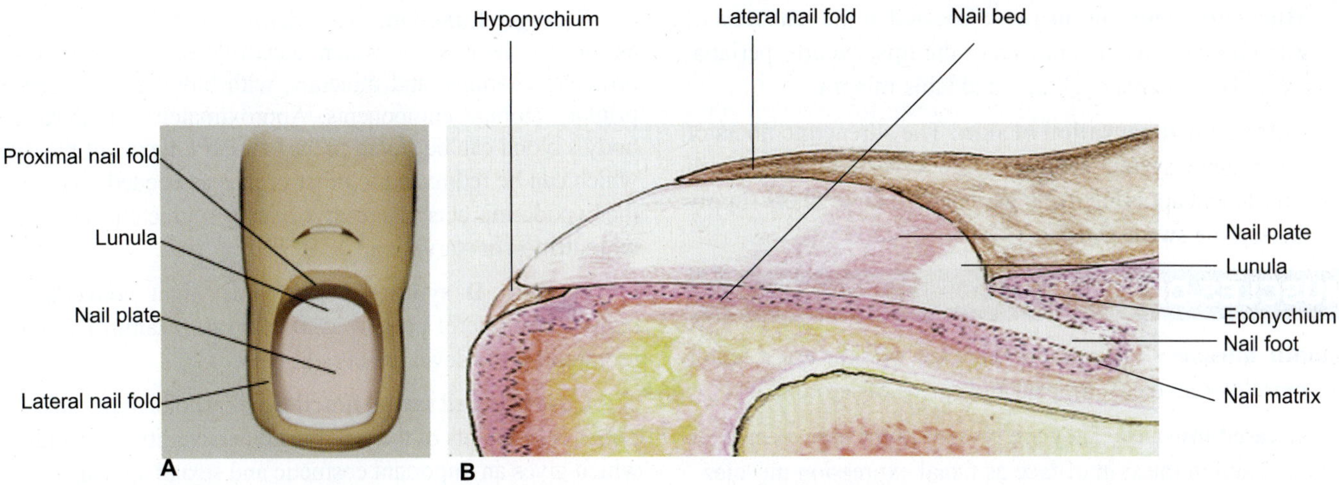

Figure 1.7A and B: Structure of nail unit

Blood Supply of Skin (Figure 1.8)

The blood supply of the skin is facilitated by two vascular plexuses: the superficial vascular plexus and the deep vascular plexus. The deep plexus, consisting of arterioles and venules, is located in the lower part of the reticular dermis. From there, arterioles ascend to form the superficial plexus just below the papillary dermis. Terminal arterioles arising from this plexus create capillary loops within the dermal papillae, which then drain into venules. Lymphatics run parallel to these plexuses.

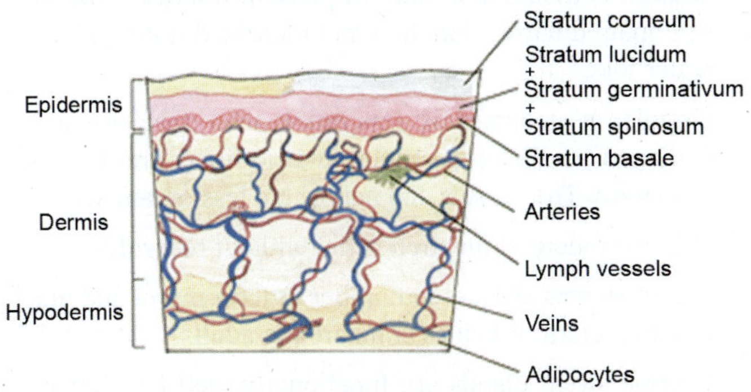

Figure 1.8: Blood supply of skin

NERVE SUPPLY OF SKIN

The sensory innervation of the skin, similar to its blood supply, originates from two nerve plexuses: superficial and deep. Large, myelinated cutaneous branches of the musculocutaneous nerves form a deep plexus in the reticular dermis. Nerves from this deep plexus ascend to form a superficial nerve plexus. Nerves from these plexuses innervate various skin structures either as free nerve endings or specialized sensory or corpuscular receptors. These nerve endings transmit sensations of pain, touch, temperature, itch, pressure, and vibration

Sensory Receptors of the Skin (Figure 1.9):

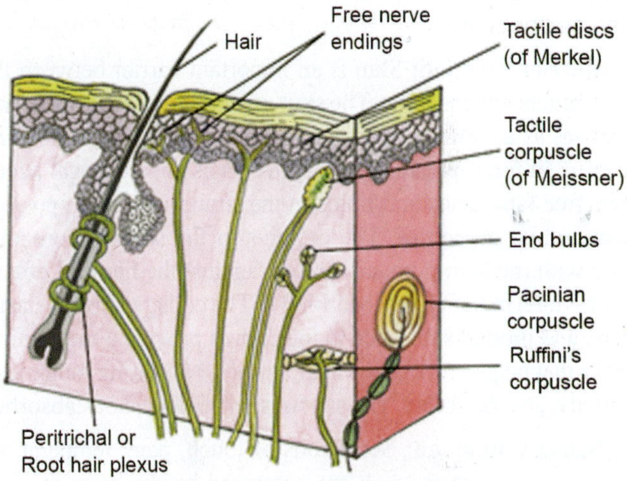

Figure 1.9: Sensory receptors of skin

- **Free nerve endings:** Penicillate nerve endings are located in the hair bearing skin in subepidermal location. They perceive pain, touch, temperature and itch. Papillary nerve endings are found at the follicular orifices and are receptive to cold sensation.
- **Pacinian corpuscle:** These occur in the deep dermis and subcutaneous tissue and are mechanoreceptors responding to vibratory stimuli.
- **Meissner's corpuscle:** These are elongated mechanoreceptors that occur in the dermal papillae of the digital skin.
- **Ruffini corpuscles:** These are nerve terminals present in human digits, the endings are directly related to collagen fibril.
- **Krause end bulb:** These are encapsulated swelling of myelinated fibers situated in the superficial layers of the dermis.

- **Mucocutaneous end organs:** Located at the junctions of skin and mucous membranes of the lips, eyelids, perianal area, glans, prepuce, clitoris and labia minora.
- **Autonomic innervation of skin:** The adrenergic fibers of sympathetic system supply the blood vessels, arrector pili muscle and apocrine ducts while cholinergic fibers supply the eccrine sweat glands.

MUSCLES OF THE SKIN

Smooth muscles: The smooth muscles of skin are arrector pili, muscle of areola of nipples and dartos of scrotum.

Striated muscles: They are present in the skin of neck as platysma and in the skin of face as facial expression muscles.

FUNCTIONS OF THE SKIN

Skin performs several vital functions for the body. Some of the important ones are:

Barrier function: Skin is an important barrier between the environment and the body. The stratum corneum of the epidermis functions as a water barrier, preventing water loss and blocking the entry of microorganisms. Sebum acts as an antifungal agent, while free fatty acids and lipids in the stratum corneum possess antimicrobial properties. The proteins in the stratum corneum, along with melanin pigment, protect against the harmful effects of ultraviolet radiation by absorbing it. The collagen fibers, elastic fibers, and ground substance in the dermis provide a mechanical barrier that helps prevent physical injuries by offering toughness, elasticity, and flexibility. The subcutis serves as a shock absorber.

Sensory function: Sensations of touch, pain, temperature, vibration, pressure and itch are perceived by the body through various sensory receptors in the skin. Many neuropeptides present in the skin act as neurotransmitters.

Thermoregulation: Skin plays a vital role in maintaining constant body temperature through its rich dermal vascularity and the process of sweating. In cold environments, heat is conserved via the constriction of arterioles in the dermis. Conversely, when the environmental temperature rises, heat loss is facilitated by the dilatation of arterioles and the evaporation of sweat from the skin surface. Thermoreceptors for heat and cold are located in the dermis; when stimulated, they send signals to the hypothalamus to initiate vaso-constriction or vasodilation and sweating.

Immunological function: Langerhans cells and keratinocytes in the epidermis and T cells in the dermis perform the immunological functions by presenting the antigen and initiating immune response.

Absorption: Skin can absorb substances dissolved in fatty substances. Percutaneous absorption mainly occurs through pilosebaceous canals.

Storage Function: The dermis and hypodermis serve as storage houses for water, electrolytes, carbohydrates, fat, proteins, vitamins, and minerals, with blood and fat being the primary storage components. Approximately one-third of the body's blood can be stored in the capillary plexus of the dermis, which can be redirected to other organs as needed. Fat stored in the hypodermis acts as a reserve energy source during periods of malnutrition or starvation.

Vitamin D synthesis: Ultraviolet light converts the 7-dehydrocholesterol present in the skin to Vitamin D3 which is required for the development of bones.

Cosmetic and sexual function: Skin color, hair, nails are the prime constituents of the beauty and personality of an individual which gives an important cosmetic and sexual appeal.

DIFFERENCES BETWEEN NEONATAL AND ADULT SKIN

Neonatal skin is similar to adult skin in structure and function except that:

1. Surface area to body mass ratio is five times more in term infants than in adults and seven times more in preterm infants.
2. The epidermal thickness in term infant is same as of adult but in preterm infant it is just half of the adult. The stratum corneum is thinner in preterm infants. This leads to impaired barrier function and increased transepidermal water loss.
3. Dermis in neonates is less thick than that of adults. Collagen bundles are smaller, elastic fibers are finer and immature. The vessels and nerves are less organized.
4. Dermo epidermal junction is flat without rete ridges.
5. Melanosomes are less in number in term infant and much less in preterm infant as compared to adults.
6. Eccrine sweat glands are functionally well developed in term infants but in preterm infants they are immature, resulting in poor thermal response on forehead and poor emotional sweating in palms and soles.
7. Thermoregulation is poor in preterm infants due to less fat, poor autonomic control of blood vessels and large surface area-body mass ratio.
8. Sebum secretion rate is higher in neonates under the influence of maternal hormones. It decreases by the end of first month and becomes stable at the end of first year.
9. Skin is more fragile in preterm infants leading to increased chances of infection and sepsis.
10. Neonatal skin is less hairy. In preterm infants lanugo hair persist.

2 Clinical Diagnosis

CHAPTER

Contents

Diagnosis of skin diseases is an art which can be mastered by the clinician through knowledge of basic skin lesions, their patterns and analyzing them with relevant history. Dermatology is a visual specialty where physician is tempted to make a diagnosis at a glance just by looking at the lesions but this is likely to result in wrong diagnosis in many cases. Therefore, the proper approach for the correct diagnosis is to proceed in a systematic manner of history taking and detailed physical examination.

HISTORY TAKING

It is customary to take history first and then to proceed for physical examination but in dermatology the usual practice is to perform a brief examination first followed by detailed history later. This will avoid unnecessary and irrelevant questions put to the patient. The important points to be charted out in the history are:

1. **Demographic data:** Name, age, sex, address, occupation, income, marital status and religion.
2. **Complaints with duration:** Presenting complaints like itching, burning, pain, rash with their duration.
3. **Systemic complaints with duration:** Like fever, cough, joint pain, breathlessness etc.
4. **History of present illness:** It should include:
   a. Onset of lesion–sudden or gradual.
   b. Type and site of lesion.
   c. Evolution of the lesion.

  d. Relation with season, food, drug, sun exposure, occupation, menstruation, pregnancy.
  e. Precipitating, aggravating, relieving factors.
  f. Previous therapy for the existing or other illness including ayurvedic or homeopathic drugs.

5. **Past history:** History of similar or other skin disease or related systemic disease should be taken.
6. **Family history:** It is important for genodermatoses, infective disorders like scabies, allergic, metabolic diseases.
7. **Personal history:** Details of occupation, hobbies, dietary habits, use of cosmetics, sexual exposure/abuse in case of suspected STDs are to be inquired into.
8. **Obstetric history:** In case of neonates and infants obstetric history including gestational and birth history is important. Gestational history should include exposure to viral infections like varicella, sexually transmitted diseases (STDs) and drugs during pregnancy.

PHYSICAL EXAMINATION

Physical examination should be conducted in bright light or natural light. Patient should be exposed fully from head to toe, so that no skin lesion is missed. Genitalia should also be examined whenever required. Infant is to be examined very thoroughly including creases, body folds and diaper region. Physical examination includes **general examination** and **cutaneous examination**.

General examination: It should contain information on pulse, temperature, blood pressure, respiratory rate, built, nutritional status, anemia, cyanosis, jaundice, edema, lymphadenopathy, teeth and tonsil.

Cutaneous examination: It includes examination of skin, mucosae, nails and hair. Anything which looks abnormal on skin, is the skin lesion. Depending upon the underlying pathology, skin lesions take different shape, size, color and texture. They are given different names accordingly. A good practice of identifying these lesions is essential for the diagnosis of skin diseases. Magnifying glass which is a binocular loupe (3X to 4X magnification) is a very simple and useful tool. Description of skin lesions is to be arranged under three heads: **Morphology**, **distribution** and **configuration**. A good description of lesions conveys the diagnosis to a great extent.

Morphology of Lesions

Skin lesions are classified as primary, secondary and special lesions. Primary lesions are initial lesions which have not been altered by trauma, scratching or rubbing. Secondary lesions are created by infection, scratching or rubbing. Special lesions are specific to some diseases or conditions.

Primary Lesions

The term primary refers to the most representative, but not necessarily the earliest, lesions; it is distinguished from the cutaneous features of secondary changes such as excoriation, eczematization, infection, or results of previous therapy.

Macule (Figure 2.1): It is a flat circumscribed lesion showing a change in skin color without any change in its consistency. Macules are non-palpable. They may be of any

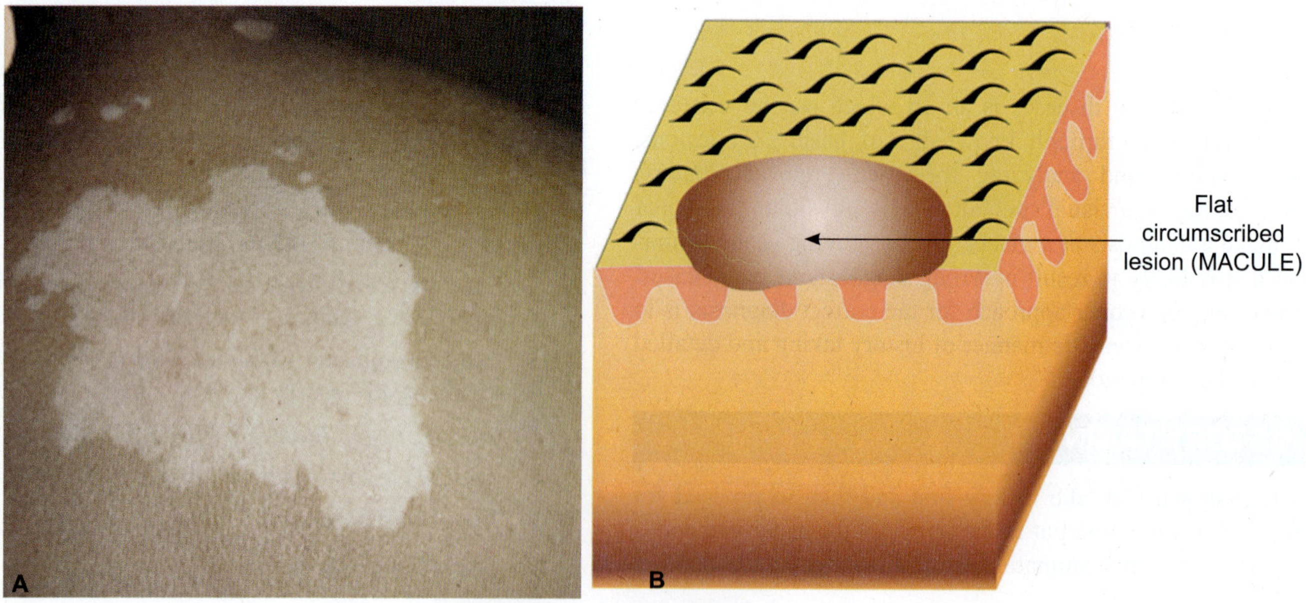

Figure 2.1: A. Vitiligo, B. Macule

shape and size. However, a larger macule is called an area or a patch. Depending upon its color, the macule can be described as (Figure 2.2):

Hypopigmented macule, when the color is lighter than the surrounding normal skin as in pityriasis versicolor and leprosy.

Depigmented macule, when there is total loss of skin color as in vitiligo.

Hyperpigmented macule, when the color is darker than normal skin color as in post-inflammatory hyperpigmentation and chloasma. These hyperpigmented macules can be due to dermal epidermal pigmentation or dermal pigmentation (Table 2.1)

Erythematous macule is red or pink colored lesion due to vasodilatation as in viral rash and drug rash.

Table 2.1: Differences between epidermal and dermal pigmentation

	Epidermal pigmentation	*Dermal pigmentation*
Colour	Brown	Slate -grey to blue
Wood's lamp	Epidermal pigmentation enhancement	No enhancement
Treatment	Brown pigment fade in few days by treatment	Poor response to therapy
Pathogenesis	Increase epidermal melanin	Melanin in dermis

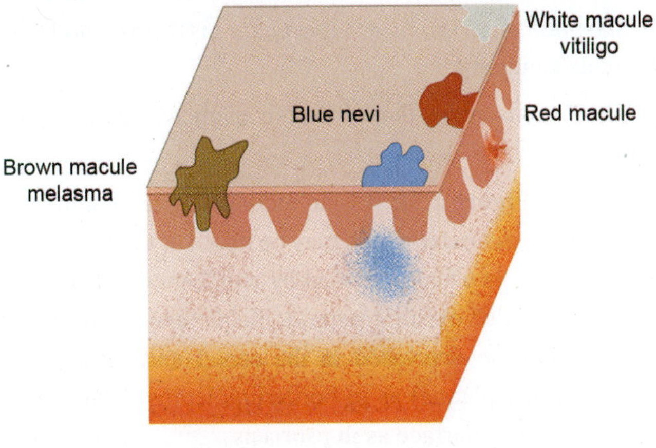

Figure 2.2: Different type of macules depending upon its color

Papule (Figure 2.3): Papule is a solid elevation of skin less than 0.5 cm in diameter. It is raised from the skin surface. Shape, size, surface and color of the papule depends upon the underlying pathological process and thus signify different skin diseases as follows (Table 2.2). Small sized papules about 1-2 mm in diameter are known as micro-papules such as in lichen nitidus while papules associated with hair follicles such as in pityriasis rubra pilaris, phrynoderma are known as follicular papules.

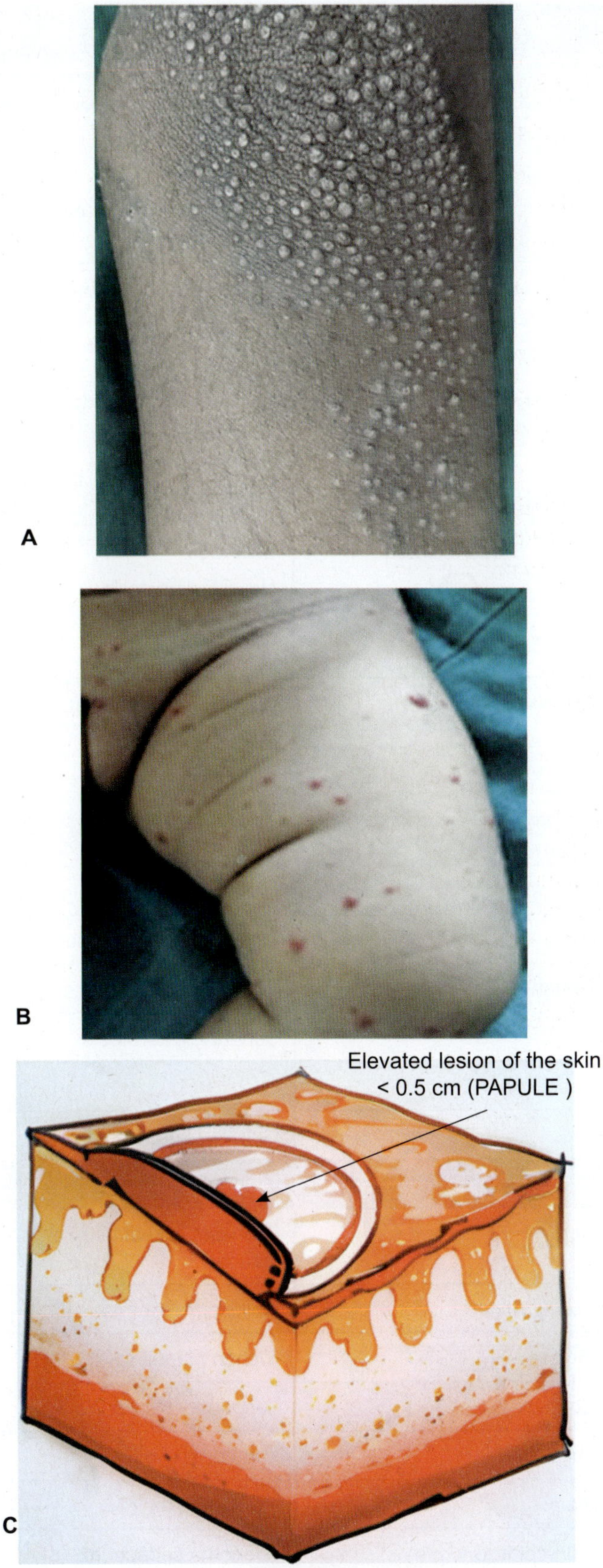

Figure 2.3: A. Phrynoderma B. Hemangioma C. Papule

Table 2.2:	
Shape of Papule	
Acuminate (pointed) 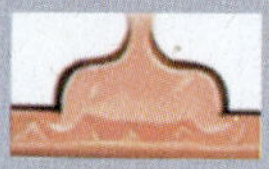	Acne Scabies Pityriasis Rubra Pilaris (PRP)
Dome-shaped 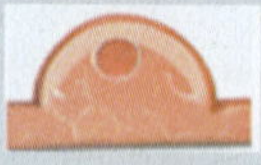	Molluscum contagiosum Pigmented moles
Flat-topped 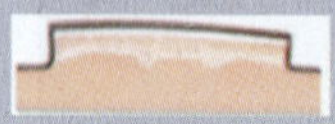	Lichen planus Xanthelasma Plane warts
Pedunculated 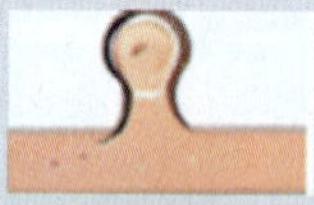	Skin tags Neurofibromatosis
Umbilicated 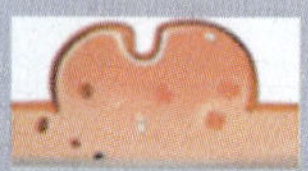	Molluscum contagiosum
Surface of Papule	
Smooth	Lichen planus
	Molluscum contagiosum
Rough	Warts
	Seborrheic keratosis
Scaly	Syphilis
	Guttate psoriasis.
Color of Papule	
Red	Psoriasis, insect bite, rosacea
Pearly white	Molluscum contagiosum
Violaceous	Lichen planus
Coppery	Secondary syphilis
Yellowish	Xanthoma
Black	Pigmented mole
Skin-colored	Adenoma sebaceum Amyloidosis

Nodule (Figure 2.4): It is a solid palpable lesion in the dermis or subcutis, which can be observed as an elevation or can be palpated, round or ellipsoidal more than 0.5 cm in diameter. It can be epidermal, dermal or subcutaneous. It is the size and the depth of involvement that differentiates a nodule from a large papule. Examples of nodule:

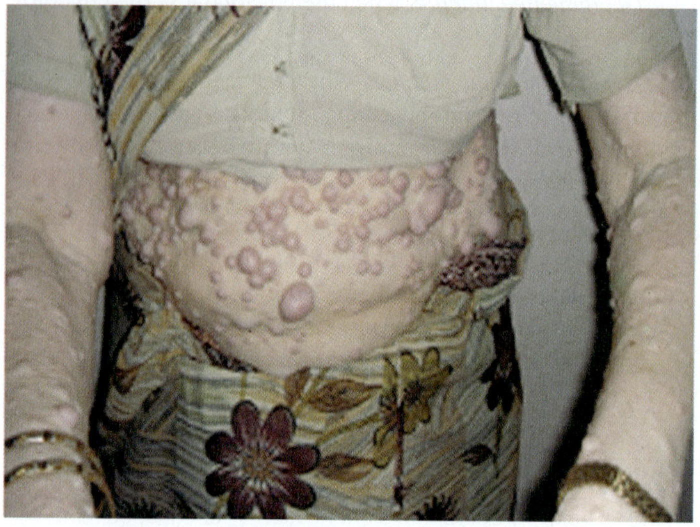

Figure 2.4: Nodules

Epidermal nodule: Keratoacanthoma, nodular basal cell carcinoma.

Dermal nodule: Histoid leprosy, dermatofibroma.

Subcutaneous nodule: Lipoma, erythema nodosum, tendinous xanthoma.

The lesions more than 1 cm in diameter are known as **tumours**.

Plaque (Figure 2.5): It is an indurated area of skin larger than 0.5 cm in diameter which may be raised or depressed from skin surface. It is usually formed by confluence of papules or by enlargement of existing papule. Plaque may be uniformly raised or may be depressed in the center and raised at the border (annular plaque) as in borderline leprosy. Plaque may have scales on its surface as in psoriasis.

Vesicle and bulla (Figures 2.6 and 2.7): Vesicle is a raised circumscribed lesion containing fluid, less than 0.5 cm in diameter. A vesicle bigger than 0.5 cm in diameter is called bulla. Vesicles and bullae are formed due to cleavage in the epidermis or just below epidermis and collection of fluid in the cavities so formed. The fluid may be clear or haemorrhagic. Depending upon the quantity of fluid the bulla may be flaccid as in pemphigus vulgaris or tense as in bullous pemphigoid. Vesicles are seen in chicken pox, herpes simplex, herpes zoster and dermatitis herpetiformis.

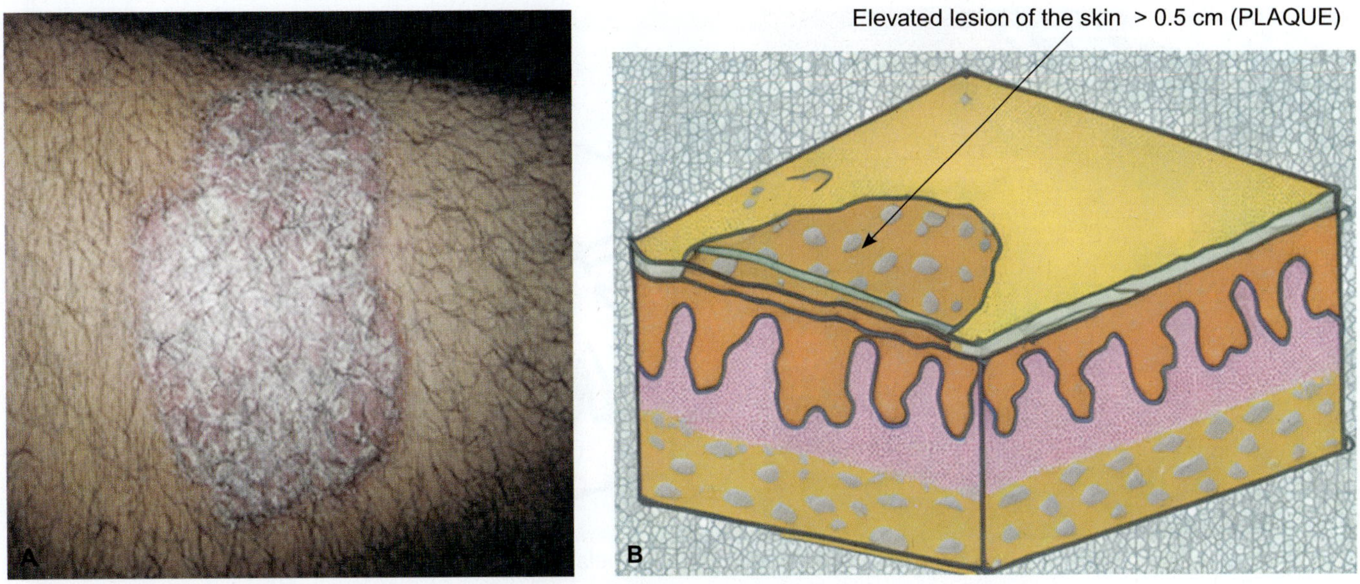

Figure 2.5: A. Psoriasis B. Plaque

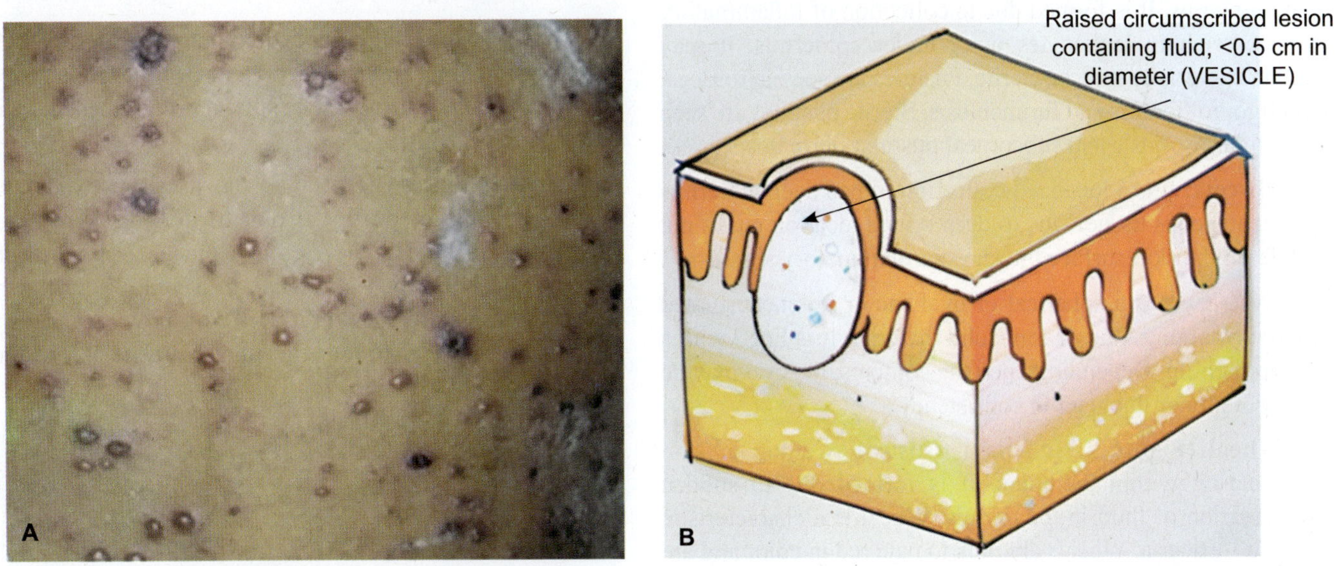

Figure 2.6: A. Varicella, B. Vesicle

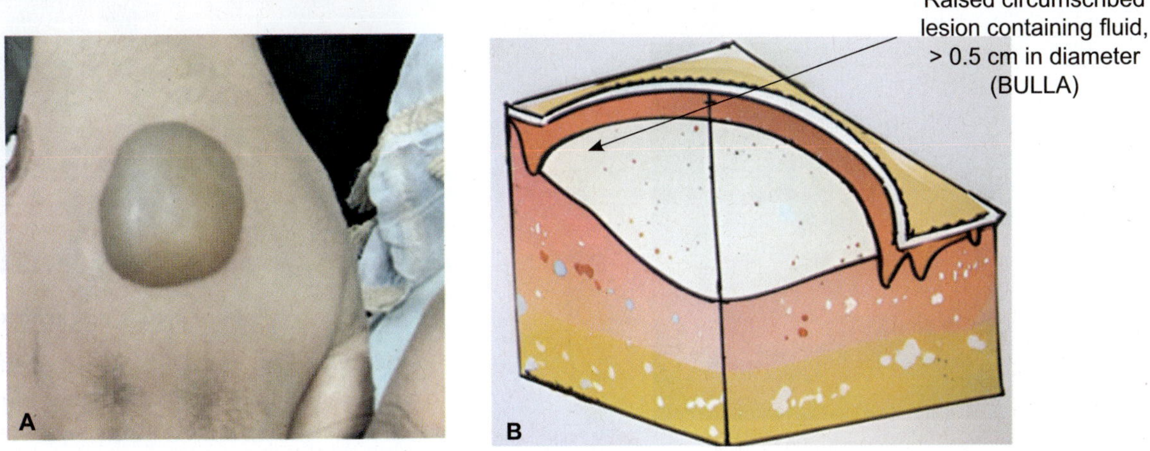

Figure 2.7: A. Burn, B. Bulla

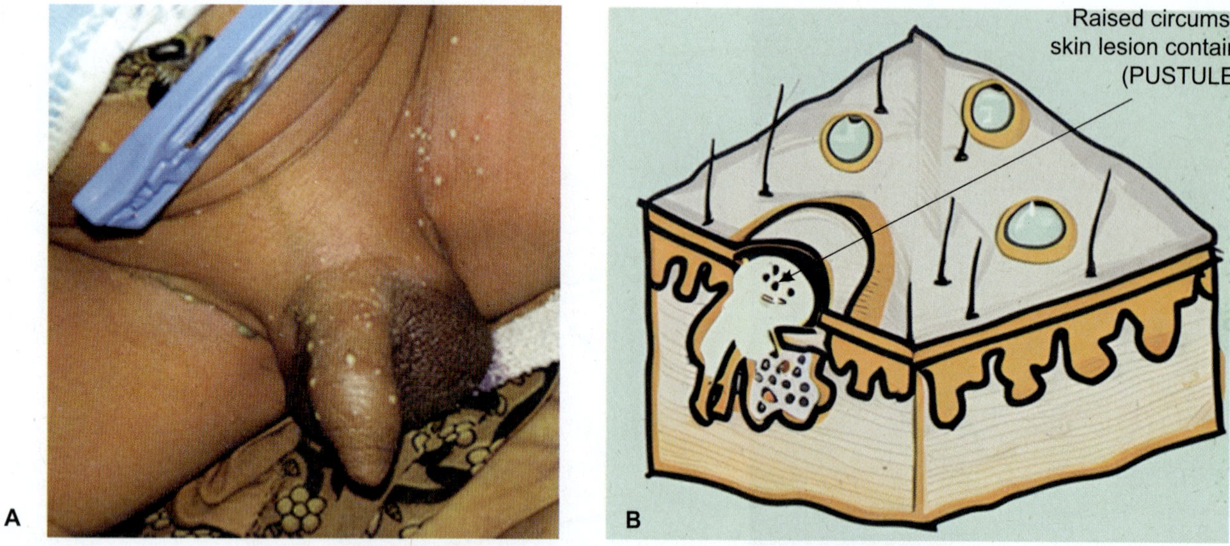

Figure 2.8: A. Transient pustular melanosis, B. Pustule

Pustule (Figure 2.8): It is raised circumscribed skin lesion containing pus. It is formed due to collection of inflammatory exudates rich in leukocytes in or under epidermis. It may contain bacteria or may be sterile. Pustules are seen in rosacea, impetigo, folliculitis and furunculosis. Sterile pustules are seen in pustular psoriasis and subcorneal pustular dermatosis.

Abscess: It is a localized collection of pus deep in dermis or subcutaneous tissue. Due to deep seated location pus is not visible on the skin surface but shows inflammatory signs.

Cyst: Cyst is a spherical or oval sac or an encapsulated cavity containing fluid or semisolid material. It is lined with a true epithelium. Depending upon the contents, the cyst may be hard, doughy or fluctuant in consistency.

Wheal (Figure 2.9): It is a transient swelling of skin disappearing within 24 hours. It is formed due to sudden extravasation of fluid in the dermis. Wheal is a characteristic lesion of urticaria. Wheals are pink to pale red in color and are surrounded by erythema. They may be very small to giant in size.

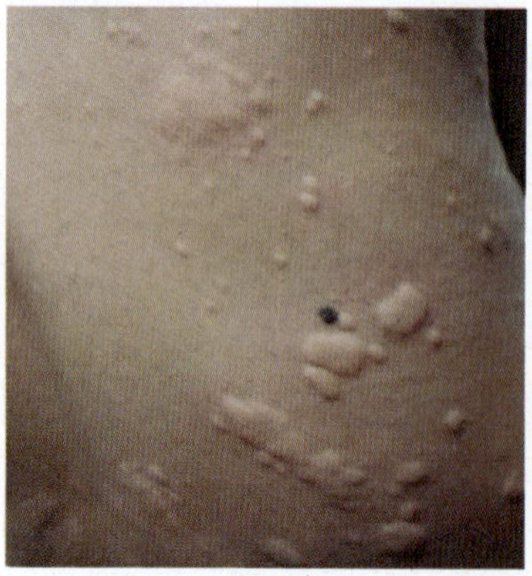

Figure 2.9: Urticaria (Wheals)

Secondary Lesions

Secondary lesions represent evolutionary changes that develop due to scratching, rubbing or infection of the primary lesions. They may also be formed normally in primary lesions with the passage of time.

Crust (Figure 2.10): It is the dried-up exudates from a vesicle, bulla or pustule. Color of the crust depends upon the nature of the exudate. Serous exudate forms a creamy or dirty white crust; pus gives rise to a yellow crust, whereas the hemorrhagic exudate produces dark brown or black crust. Yellow crust is seen in impetigo and chocolate colored crust is seen in ecthyma.

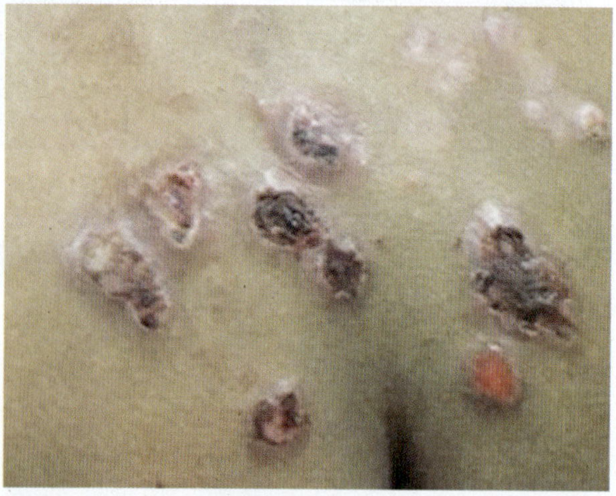

Figure 2.10: Crust in impetigo

Scale (Figure 2.11): Scale is flake-like lesion due to abnormal shedding of the skin. Normally skin is shed continuously in invisible form but when there is excessive production of stratum corneum it becomes visible as scale.

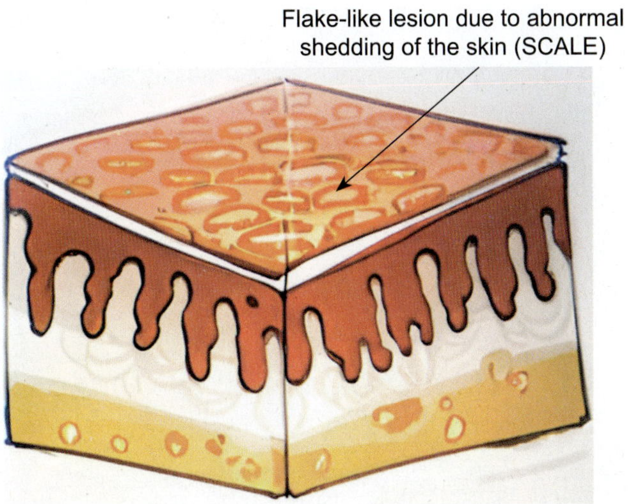

Figure 2.11: Scales

Scales vary in size and color which signify different diseases as follows (Table 2.3):

Table 2.3: Different types of scales and related diseases

Collarette scale	Pityriasis rosea (Figure 2.12 D).
Furfuraceous scale	Pityriasis versicolor (Figure 2.12 F).
Ichthyosiform scale	Ichthyosis vulgaris (Figure 2.12 E).
Micaceous scale or Silvery scales	Psoriasis (Figure 2.12 A).
Limpet like	Reiter's syndrome
Greasy scale	Seborrheic dermatitis (Figure 2.12 C)
Trailing scale	Erythema annulare centrifugum
Cornflake scale	Pemphigus foliaceous
Double-edged scale	Ichthyosis linearis circumflexa (Netherton syndrome)
Hystrix like scale	Ichthyosis hystrix
Sand paper like scale	Actinic keratosis
Bran like scales	Chronic erythroderma stage (Figure 2.12G)
Wafer or mica like scale	Pityriasis lichenoides chronica (Figure 2.12B)

Differentiation of scale from crust: Scaling is seen in dry lesions whereas crust is associated with some exudate.

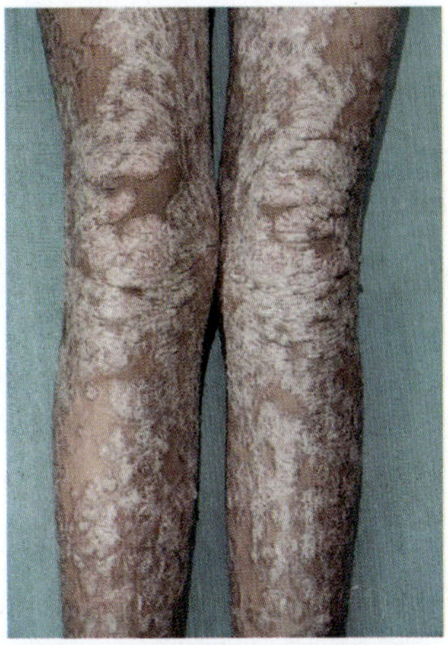

Figure 2.12A: Silvery scales in psoriasis

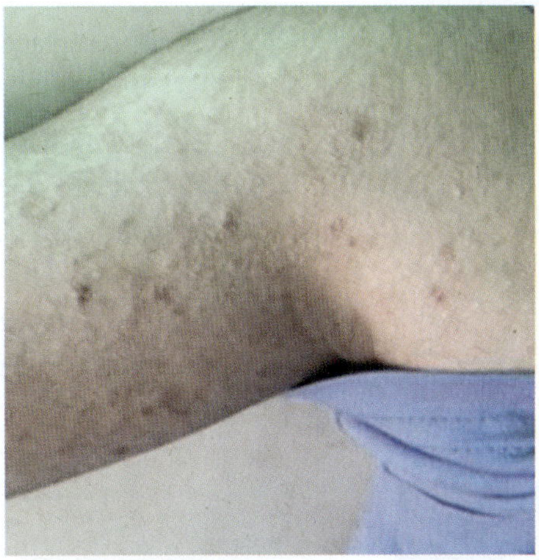

Figure 2.12B: Mica like scales in Pityriasis lichenoides chronica

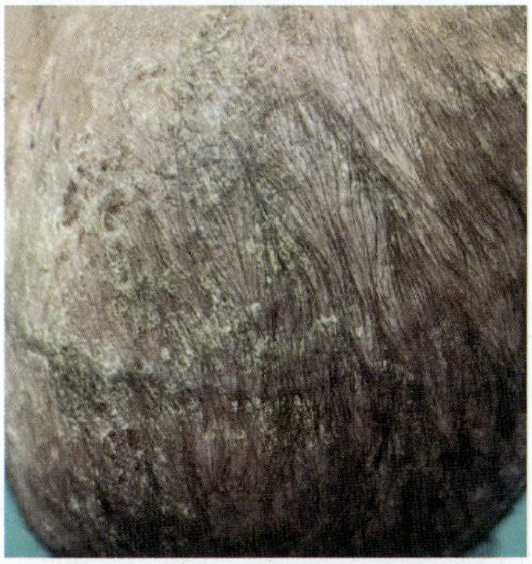

Figure 2.12C: Greasy scales in Seborrheic dermatitis

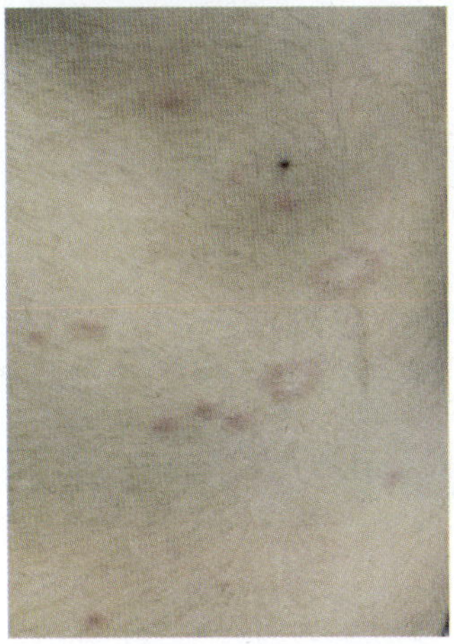

Figure 2.12D: Collarette scale in Pityriasis rosea

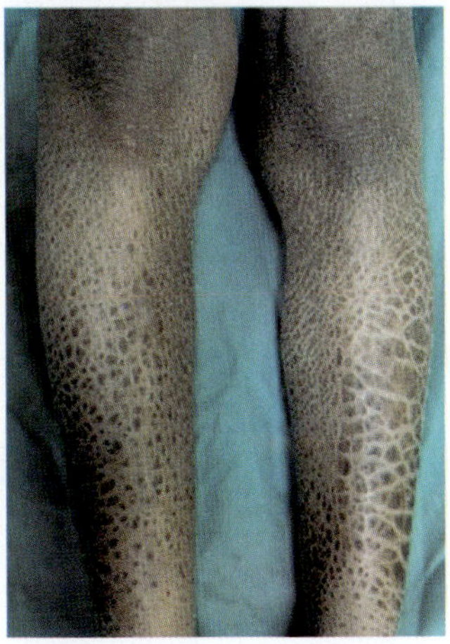

Figure 2.12E: Icthyosiform scales in Ichthyosis vulgaris

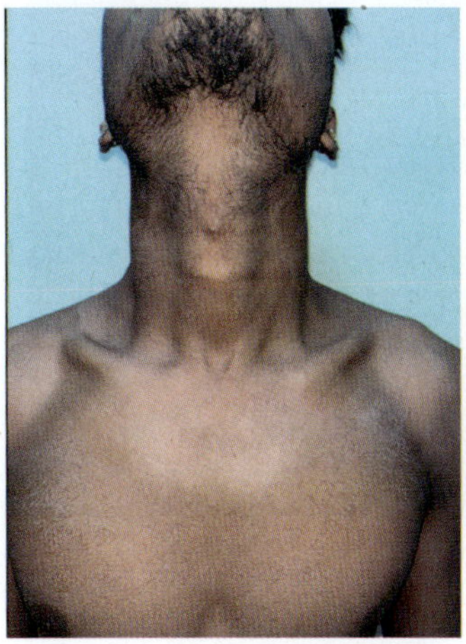

Figure 2.12F: Furfuraceous scales in Pityriasis versicolor

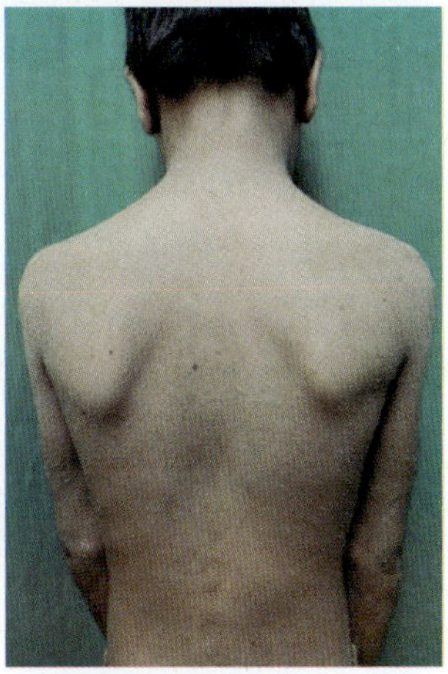

Figure 2.12G: Bran-like scale in erythroderma (Chronic stage)

Figure 2.12

Atrophy (Figure 2.13): It is reduction in the size and number of skin cells. Atrophy may be limited to epidermis, dermis or subcutis.

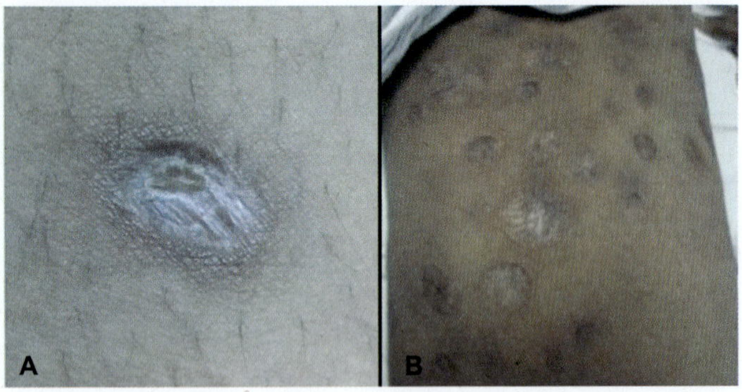

Figure 2.13: Cutaneous atrophy (A and B)

Epidermal atrophy is seen as shiny and wrinkled skin as in leprosy. Dermal atrophy manifests as an area of depression in the skin. In subcutaneous atrophy, the skin shows deep depression as in lipoatrophy and lupus profundus.

Ulcer (Figure 2.14): Ulcer is an area of skin or mucous membrane where epidermis and upper dermis have been lost. It may heal with scarring. Description of ulcer should include its site, size, shape, surface (floor), surrounding skin, base and border which helps in determining the cause of ulcer.

Erosion: It is the partial or complete loss of epidermis at a place. Healing occurs without scarring. Erosions are seen in epidermal bullous diseases such as pemphigus vulgaris and epidermolysis bullosa (Figure 2.15).

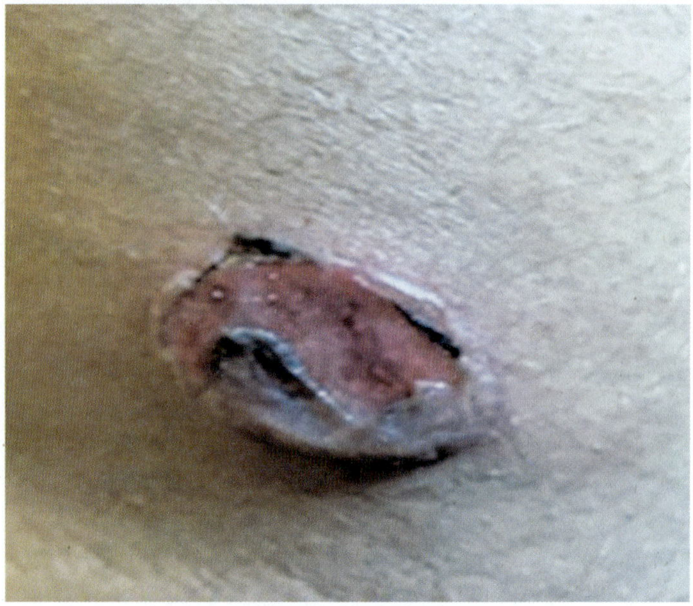

Figure 2.15: Erosion

Scar: It is replacement of normal skin by fibrous tissue in the process of healing of damaged skin. Scars are of two types:

Hypertrophic scar: Fibrous tissue formed is more than the destroyed tissue, e.g., scar of herpes zoster.

Atrophic scar: It is thin and depressed from the skin surface as in acne and smallpox scarring.

Keloid: Scar continues to grow in normal skin beyond the damaged area limit. Hypertrophic scar does not grow beyond the limit.

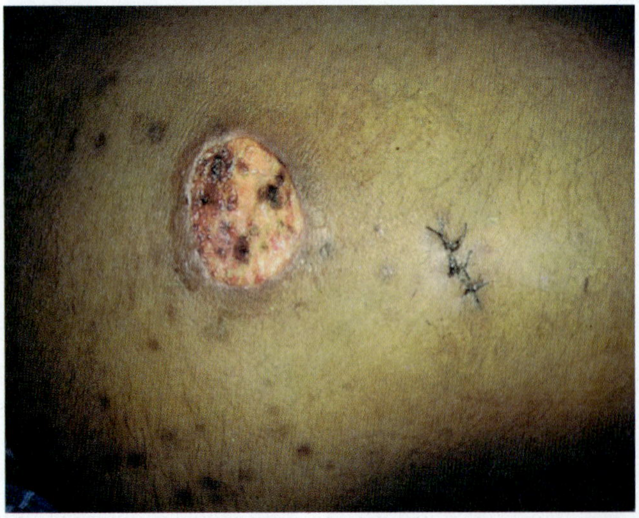

A

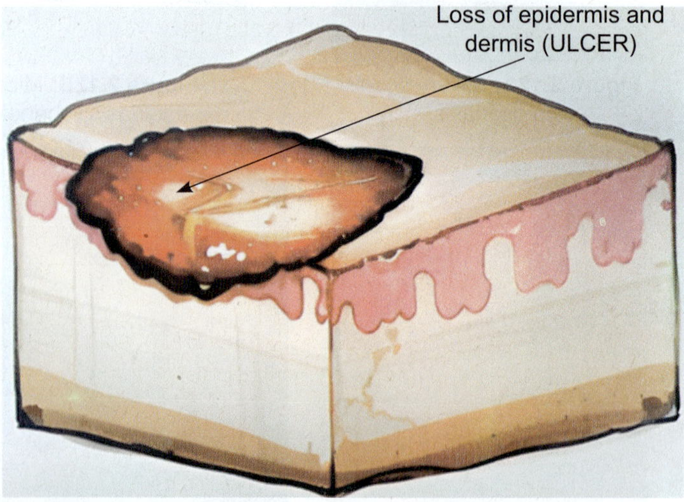

B

Figure 2.14: Ulcer (A & B)

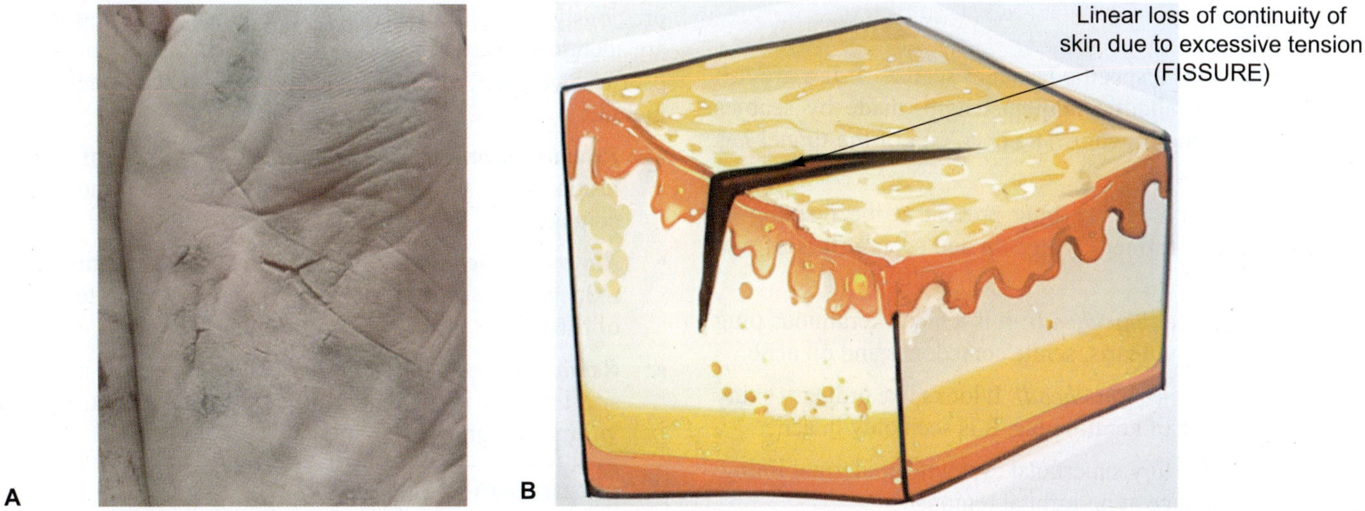

Figure 2.16: Fissure (A and B)

Fissure (Figure 2.16): It is a linear loss of continuity of skin due to excessive tension. It usually occurs in palms and soles and in folds of skin. *Clinical examples:* Psoriasis, keratoderma.

Excoriation (Figure 2.17): It is linear or oval erosion of epidermis due to scratching as seen in intense pruritic conditions like scabies and atopic dermatitis.

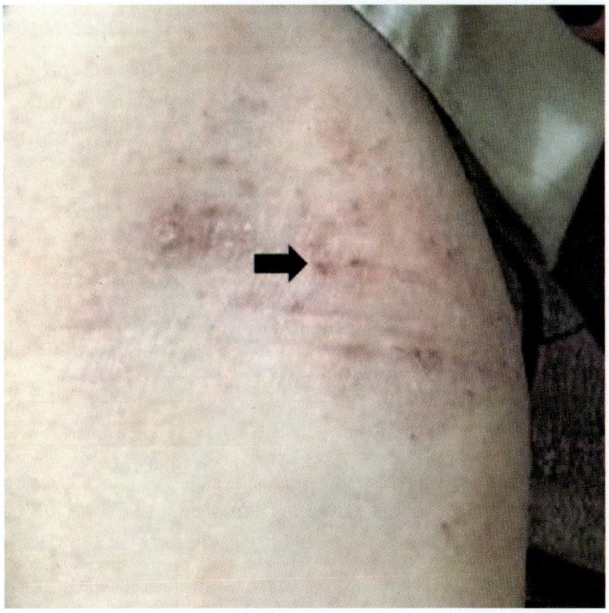

Figure 2.17: Excoriation

Lichenification (Figure 2.18): Repeated rubbing of skin results in thickening and hyperpigmentation of skin. The skin markings become prominent. It is seen in conditions associated with intense pruritus as in lichen simplex chronicus and atopic dermatitis.

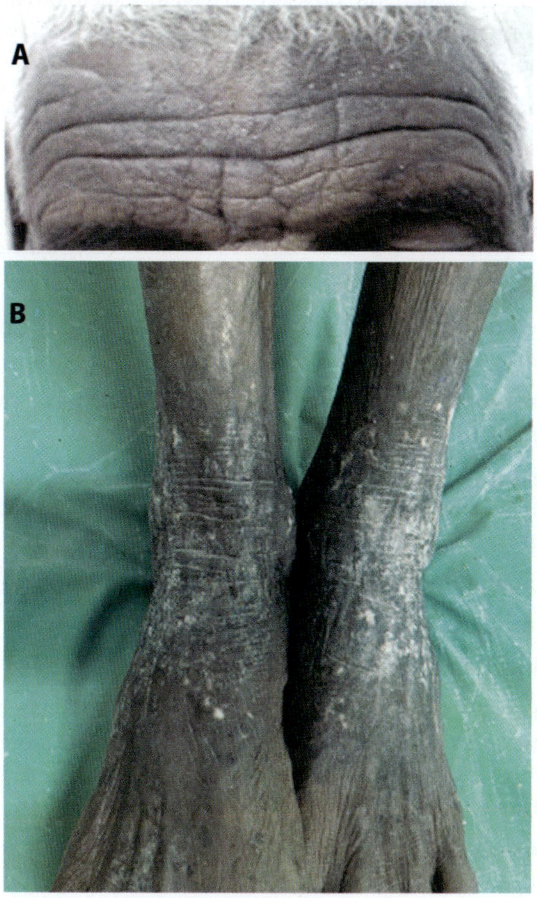

Figure 2.18: Lichenification

Sclerosis: It is a localized or diffuse area of induration or hardening of skin due to dermal fibrosis. It is better felt than seen. Clinical examples include morphoea and lichen sclerosis et atrophicus.

Special Lesions

Burrow: Burrow is a specific lesion of scabies. It is a greyish serpentine tunnel, about 5 mm in length, made by scabies mite in the stratum corneum. The open end of the tunnel has a papule.

Comedone: It is a tiny plug present at the opening of vellus hair follicle formed by keratin and sebum. It is of two types:

Open comedone (blackhead): It is a black keratinous plug and is seen in acne vulgaris, senile comedones and oil acne.

Closed comedone (whitehead): It looks like ordinary shiny papule and is made of keratin plug. It is seen only in acne.

Milium: It is a tiny superficial cyst with epidermal lining. Milia are seen on face at periorbital region.

Telangiectasia: It is visible dilatation of capillaries of skin which blanch on pressure. They are seen on the face in chronic sun exposure, lupus erythematosus, rosacea, dermatomyositis and systemic sclerosis.

Poikiloderma: It is a combination of reticulate telangiectasia, pigmentation, atrophy. It is seen in dermatomyositis and mycosis fungoides.

Other Terms Used in Dermatology

Callus: A localized hyperplasia of stratum corneum.

Cellulitis: Purulent inflammation of the deep dermis and subcutaneous tissue.

Erythema: Redness of the skin produced by vascular congestion or increased perfusion.

Fistula: An abnormal passage from a deep structure, such as a hollow viscus, to the skin surface or between two structures. It is often lined by epithelial tissue.

Haematoma: A localized tumour like collection of blood.

Keratoderma: A horny thickening of the skin.

Sinus: A cavity or track with a blind ending.

Target lesions: These are less than 3 cm in diameter and have three or more zones, usually a central area of dusky erythema or purpura, a middle paler zone of edema, and an outer ring of erythema with a well defined edge.

Purpura: Extravasation of red blood cells into skin results in formation of purpura. Erythema and purpura can be differentiated by using glass slide (diascopy). Erythema disappears while purpura remains unchanged. Purpura can be palpable (due to vasculitis) or nonpalpable (due to thrombocytopenia). Purpura can be small pin point macule (1-2 mm), known as petechiae or large bruise like patches (> 2mm) known as ecchymoses.

Koebner's phenomena /Isomorphic phenomena: Koebner phenomena is the appearance of new lesion on previously normal skin secondary to trauma. These new lesions are identical to existing skin disease. Seen in lichen planus, psoriasis vulgaris, vitiligo. Other type of koebner phenomena include:

- ***Pseudo-koebner's phenomena:*** Appearance of similar lesion due to autoinoculation, seen in molluscum contagiosum, verruca
- ***Reverse koebner's phenomena:*** Disappearance or reduction in size of lesion after trauma, seen in few cases of psoriasis.
- ***Remote reverse koebner's phenomena:*** Trauma at distant site leads to reduction in size or improvement, seen in vitiligo and granuloma annulare.

Configuration of Lesions

Arrangement of lesions with each other provides an important clue to the diagnosis of skin disease. Various configurations seen in different conditions are given in Table 2.4.

Table 2.4: Configuration and pattern of lesions

Pattern	*Diseases*
Linear (lesions along line)	Epidermal naevi, lichen striatus
Grouped (Figure 2.19)	Herpes simplex, herpes zoster
Annular (round or oval) (Figure 2.20)	Tinea corporis, granuloma annulare, borderline leprosy
Reticular (net like)	Livedo reticularis, oral lichen planus
Dermatomal/zosteriform	Herpes zoster
Arcuate	Erythema annulare centrifugum
Circinate	Circinate balanitis
Discoid	Discoid eczema, discoid lupus erythematosus
Confluent	Psoriasis
Iris or target	Erythema multiforme
Serpiginous	Larva migrans, snail track ulcer, elastosis perforans serpiginosa
Telangiectatic	Ataxia telangiectasia, hereditary hemorrhagic telangiectasia
Sporotrichoid (nodular lymphangitis)	Sporotrichosis (Sporothrix schenkii), atypical mycobacterial infection like fish tank granuloma or swimming pool granuloma (mycobacterium marinarum), cutaneous leishmaniasis (leishmania brasiliensis), nocardiosis and tularemia.

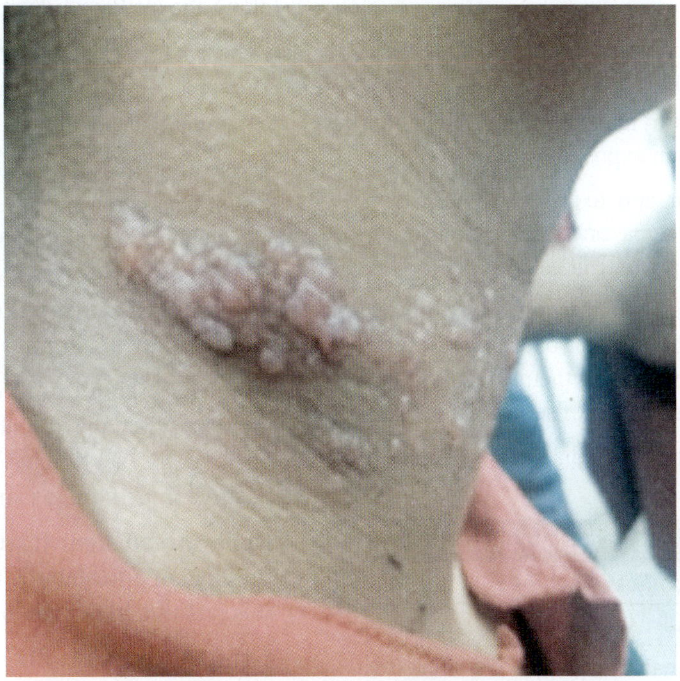

Figure 2.19: Grouped lesions

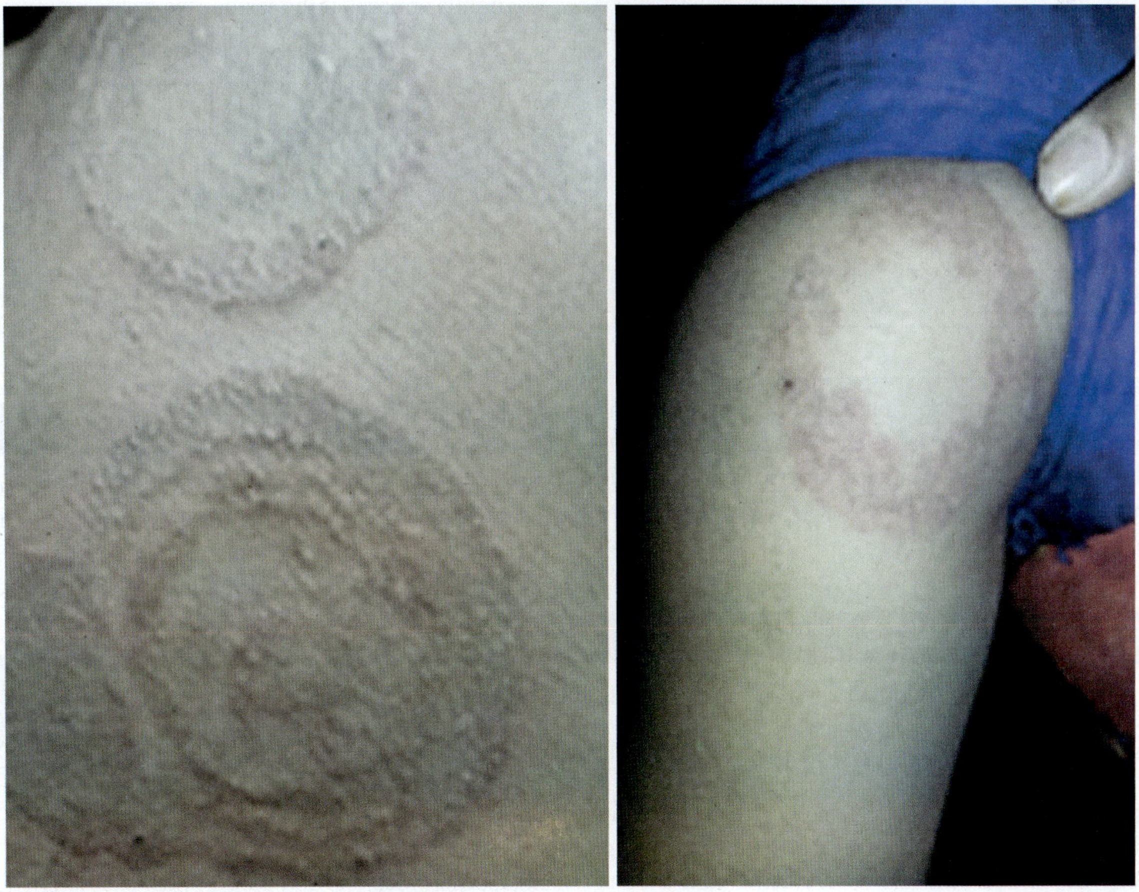

Figure 2.20: Annular lesions

Distribution of Lesions

Distribution of lesions depends upon:

1. Exposure of a particular site to etiological agent for example photodermatitis in sun exposed areas.
2. Susceptibility of a particular site to disease, e.g., acne lesions on face, infantile eczema on cheeks, nummular eczema on extensor surface of extremities.
3. **Ear sign:** Presence of erythematous papules, scaling or plaques over helix, antihelix, and retroauricular region in case of tinea capitis, whereas erythema, scaling, or fissuring in retroauricular fold in case of seborrhea capitis.

Distribution of lesions in some of the diseases is shown in Table 2.5.

Table 2.5: Distribution of lesions in certain diseases

Disease	*Distribution of Lesions*
Psoriasis	Extensor aspects of body, scalp
Seborrheic dermatitis	Scalp, nasolabial folds, retroauricular folds, sternal and interscapular region
Acne	Face, upper trunk, deltoid region
Photodermatoses	Face, upper portions of ear, V of neck, extensors of forearms
Scabies	Interdigital spaces, front of wrist, ulnar border of forearm, lower trunk, genitalia, sparing of face in adults
Pityriasis versicolor	Trunk
Hidradenitis suppurativa	Axillae, anogenital area

Symmetry of Lesions

If the lesions are identically distributed on both sides of the body, they are called symmetrical. Generally, diseases having hematogenous spread have symmetrical lesions as in drug eruptions and atopic dermatitis. Diseases in which agent acts on skin from outside the body, lesions are asymmetrical as in warts and pyoderma.

BEDSIDE CLINICAL TESTS

During physical examination one can perform some simple clinical tests relevant to particular diseases for reaching a conclusion. Some of the important tests are as follows:

- **Dermographism (Figure 11.3):** It is elicited by stroking the skin firmly with a blunt object like key or tongue depressor. A positive test shows erythema and edema along the striking line within 2-3 minutes. It is indicative of dermographic urticaria.
- **Darier's sign:** It is dermographism elicited in lesions of cutaneous mastocytosis.
- **Diascopy:** It is done to differentiate an erythematous lesion from a purpuric lesion. A glass slide is used to press a lesion, erythematous lesion blanches while purpuric does not. **Diascopy sarcoidosis, lupus vulgaris, cutaneous leishmaniasis, granuloma faciale shows yellowish nodule known as apple jelly nodule.**
- **Nikolsky's sign:** It is elicited by putting a tangential pressure with the thumb on normal skin. If the test is positive the superficial skin will peel off. This sign is positive in pemphigus and toxic epidermal necrolysis.
- **Bulla spread sign:** If we apply pressure with a finger on the edge of a fresh bulla it will extend into adjoining skin. It is positive in pemphigus.
- **Grattage test (Auspitz sign):** It It is positive in psoriasis. To elicit this test, the lesion is scraped with the edge of a glass slide. On repeated scraping, if minute bleeding points appear on the lesion, the test is positive.
- **Pathergy test:** State of altered tissue response which develops in response to minor trauma is known as pathergy phenomenon. Pathergy test is performed by pricking with 20 gauge disposable needle or intradermal injection of saline on volar aspect of forearm. Examination is done after 48 hours of the needle injury. Palpable papule and pustule formation are indicative of positive pathergy and only erythema without induration is interpreted as negative result. Alternative evaluation can be done by using histological examination of the site after 48 hrs.

SYSTEMIC EXAMINATION

Examination of the various systems like cardiovascular system, respiratory system, central nervous system, gastrointestinal system and the musculoskeletal system should be done in diseases like leprosy, autoimmune diseases like SLE, systemic sclerosis, etc.

DIAGNOSTIC METHODS AND INVESTIGATIONS

Magnifying Lens (Figure 2.21)

It is a binocular loop with magnification of 3X to 4X used to enhance skin lesions and their optical characteristics.

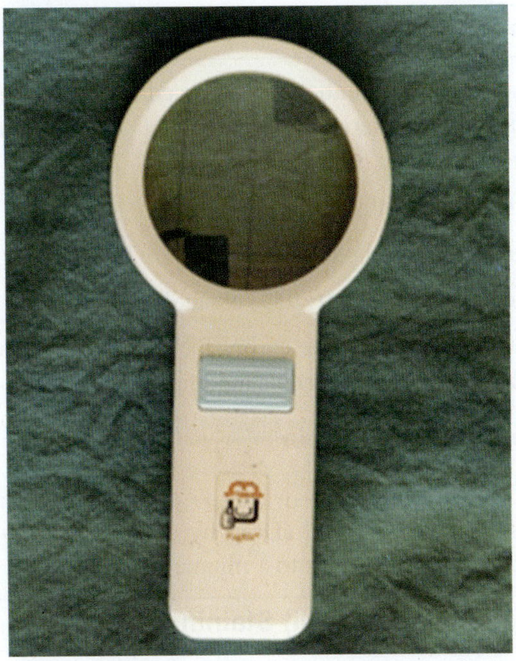

Figure 2.21: Magnifying lens

Wood's Lamp Examination

Wood's lamp (Figure 2.22) is a source of ultraviolet light with a filter (made of barium silicate with 9% nickel oxide) emitting rays above 365 nm. It is helpful in identifying disease by fluorescence on wood's lamp examination (Table 2.6).

Table 2.6: Various diseases and their fluorescence under wood's lamp	
Tinea capitis	Yellow green/blue green due to, Microsporum species, T. schoenleinii
Pityriasis versicolor	Yellow
Erythrasma	Coral pink
Vitiligo	Ivory white
Porphyria	Pink fluorescence (urine, feces, blister fluid)
Differentiating epidermal pigmentation from dermal pigmentation as in melasma	Under Wood's light the epidermal pigmentation becomes more prominent while dermal pigmentation shows no change
Ash leaf macule	Becomes more prominent on wood's lamp

Dermatoscopy

A dermatoscope (Figure 2.23) is a noninvasive tool that visualizes the subtle clinical patterns of clinical lesions and subsurface skin structures not visible to naked eye. In principle, it is similar magnifying lens with the ability of assessing structures as deep as the reticular dermis.

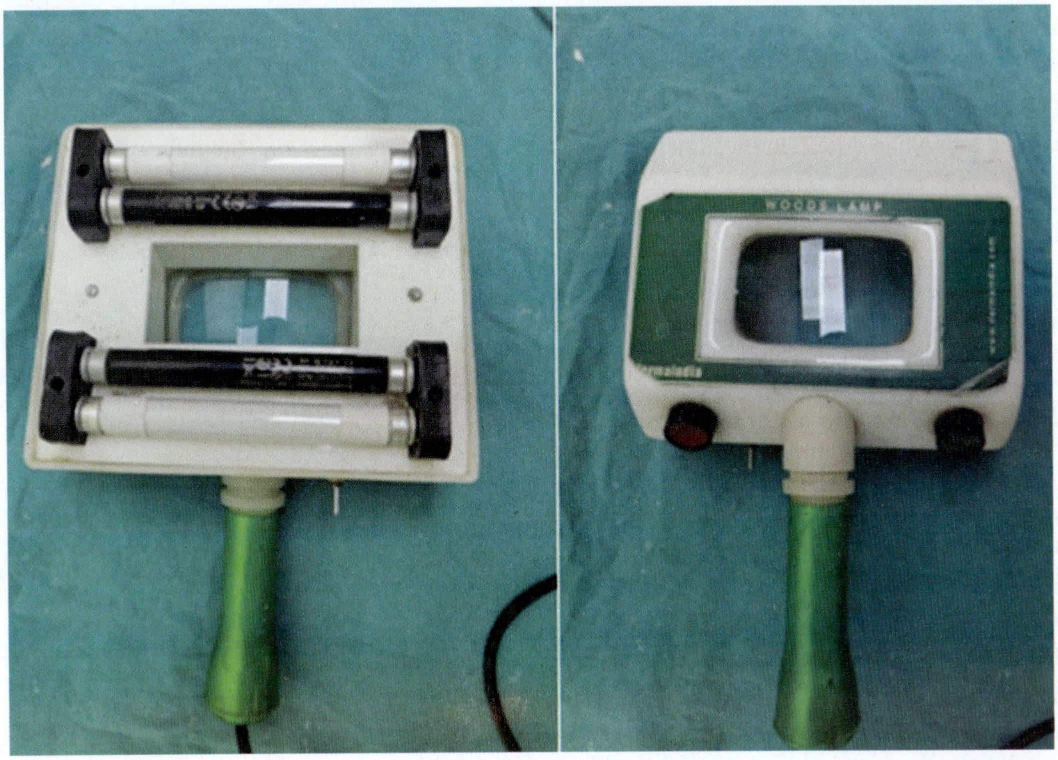

Figure 2.22: Wood's lamp

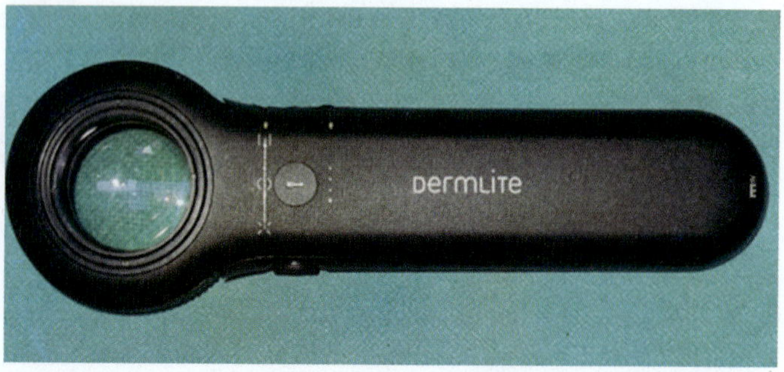

Figure 2.23: Dermatoscope

KOH Mount

This test confirms the diagnosis of dermatophytosis in the lesion. The lesion is scraped by the sharp edge of a surgical knife and the scraped material is placed on a glass slide. 1-2 drops of 20% potassium hydroxide solution is placed on slide and covered with a coverslip. After 10-15 minutes slide is examined under the microscope in low power. KOH mount is also useful in diagnosis of bacterial vaginosis, scabies, deep mycosis etc. Different microscopic findings are enumerated below:

- *Pityriasis versicolor:* Rounded yeast in small clusters which look like bunch of grapes or meat balls and short hyphae which resemble banana or spaghetti.
- *Dermatophytosis of skin:* Hyphae and spores.
- *Dermatophytosis of hair:* Fungal spores outside the hair shaft (ectothrix) and inside the hair shaft (endothrix).
- *Candida:* Yeast and hyphae.
- *Skin mount:* Used for scabies mite identification (Sarcoptes scabiei).

Tzanck Test

It is an examination of smear taken from the base of unroofed blister to see the type of cells. The blister is ruptured and the base of the blister is scraped with the blunt edge of scalpel and the material obtained is gently and evenly smeared onto a clean glass slide, allowed to air dry and fixed. It is then stained with Giemsa or Leishman stain and examined under low power. It shows acantholytic cells in pemphigus and multinucleated giant cells in herpes simplex and herpes zoster. **It shows inclusion bodies in molluscum (Henderson-Patterson bodies), leishmaniasis (LD bodies)**.

GIEMSA STAIN

Giemsa stain contains methylene blue, eosin and azure B. Giemsa stain powder (0.3 gm) mixed with 25 ml of glycerin and make stock solution. Working solution made by adding distilled water at 1:4 dilution. Giemsa staining slide should be fix with methanol then stain with Giemsa for 15 minutes.

Gram Stain

Gram stain is a differential staining used in gram positive and gram negative bacterial differentiation. Reagents used for gram stain are:

- **Basic dye:** Methyl violet
- **Mordant:** Gram's iodine
- **Decolourising agent:** 95% ethanol
- **Counter stain:** Dilute carbol fuchsin or 1% safranine or weak neutral red (Jensen's modification)

Method of Grams Stain

Methyl violet (1 minute) ---wash → Gram's iodine (1 minute) -----wash → 95% alcohol (Drop by drop)---wash → Dilute carbol fuchsin (30 seconds to 1 minute)-----wash.

AFB (Acid Fast Bacilli) Staining

AFB is a differential type of staining developed by Franz Ziehl and Friedrich Neelson. The basic principle of staining is the presence of unsaponifiable wax fraction mycolic acid in bacterial cell wall.

Reagents use for staining are:

- *Primary stain:* Strong carbol fuchsin.
- *Decolourising agent:* 20% sulphuric acid or 3% acid-alcohol (5% sulphuric acid or 1% acid-alcohol in modified acid-fast staining).
- *Counter stain:* Methylene blue.
- Fixation with methanol for 2-3 minutes.

Steps of Acid Fast Staining

STEP 1: Strong carbol fuchsin (5 minutes with intermittent heating)

↓

STEP 2: 20% sulphuric acid or 3% acid alcohol for 10 minutes

↓

STEP 3: Methylene blue for 15-20 second

For detection of mycobacterium leprae in tissue needs 10^4 bacilli/gram of tissue.

- Ridley's logarithmic scale on slit skin smear or acid fast bacilli staining for mycobacterium leprae:
    - 1 to 10 bacilli in 100 fields – 1 (+)
    - 1 to 10 bacilli in 10 fields – 2 (+)
    - 1 to 10 bacilli in an average field – 3 (+)
    - 10 to 100 bacilli in an average field – 4 (+)
    - 100 to 1000 bacilli in an average field – 5 (+)
    - Clumps and globi in an average field – 6 (+)

Intradermal Test

They are used frequently as an aid for the diagnosis of skin diseases and are based either on type I (immediate type of hypersensitivity reaction) or on type IV (delayed type hypersensitivity reaction) against exogenous or endogenous antigen. They are performed by injecting 0.1 ml agent intradermally with a 26 G needle and are read between 12 h to 4 days. Few intradermal tests are described in Table 2.7:

Table 2.7: Various intradermal test for infectious and non infectious diseases

Infectious diseases	*Non infectious diseases*
Tuberculin test / Pirquet's test- Tuberculosis	Autologous serum skin test – Autoimmune urticaria
Frei's test – Lymphogranuloma venereum	Kveim-Siltzbach test -Sarcoidosis
Ito Reenstierna test - Chancroid	Pathergy test- Pyoderma gangrenosum, Behcet's disease
Montenegro test – Leishmaniasis	Auto erythrocyte sensitivity test- Gardner diamond syndrome
Lepromin test – Leprosy	
Early response (Fernandez reaction) – seen after 48 -72 h. It is more prominent with Dharmendra antigen Late response (Mitsuda reaction) – seen after 3-4 week. It is more prominent with mitsuda antigen	Pilocarpine test – Leprosy
Candidin test- Candidiasis	Histamine test – Leprosy

Dark Ground Microscopy (DGM)

Dark ground microscopy is most specific and sensitive method to detect treponema when lesions are active, primary (chancre), secondary syphilis (condyloma lata) and early congenital syphilis. In this object appears bright in dark background due to use of condenser which blocks direct light and permits oblique scattered light to be transmitted to the specimen.

- **Steps:**
    - Remove crust and scab from the lesion
    - Wipe away blood stained exudate with dry gauze and apply pressure till clear serum exudates
    - Collect on glass slide or cover slip
    - Cover the edges of the cover slip with Vaseline
    - Examine under DGM

Patch test: They are performed to detect the antigens responsible for causing allergic contact dermatitis. The suspected antigens in standardized solution is applied on the back and covered with gauze and adhesive tape. The patches are removed after 48 hours. If the patch site shows erythema, papules, edema or vesicles the test is positive.

Skin Biopsy and Histopathology of Skin

It is an important tool to confirm the clinical diagnosis.

Procedure: Biopsy should be taken from the active edge of the lesion including surrounding normal skin. Area should be first cleaned with alcohol. To anaesthetize the area 2% lignocaine is to be injected locally below the lesion. If the area is highly vascular adrenaline can be added to lignocaine. Skin biopsy can be taken in three ways:

1. **Punch biopsy:** Skin biopsy punch of adequate size usually 4 mm is pressed down and rotated over the area till it cuts the skin of required depth. Punch is then withdrawn and skin piece is cut by scissors. If wound is bigger in size one stitch can be applied and cover it with a bandage.
2. **Shave biopsy:** It is done for raised lesions that separate easily from deeper skin, e.g., seborrheic keratosis.
3. **Scalpel biopsy:** An elliptical incision is made around the lesion parallel to the skin creases. Skin is excised upto the desired depth and wound is stitched and sealed with bandage. Suture is removed after 7 days.

The excised tissue is transferred to a vial containing 10% formalin and processed for histopathological examination. Clinical details should always be supplied to pathologist. Tissue reaction pattern are important morphological pattern.

Major Tissue Reaction Patterns

Majority of inflammatory dermatoses can be categorized in six different type of patterns known as major tissue reaction pattern.

1. **Lichenoid:** It presents with epidermal basal cell damage (interface dermatitis). A band like infiltrate of inflammatory cells in superficial dermis, pigment incontinence; Civatte bodies (shrunken, eosinophilic, degenerating basal cells)

are also seen. Lichenoid tissue reaction pattern is seen in Lichen planus, Lichen nitidus.

2. **Psoriasiform:** It presents with epidermal hyperplasia, uniform rete ridge elongation and regular acanthosis (squirting dermal papilla). This pattern is seen in psoriasis, Lichen simplex chronicus, Mycosis fungoides and Pityriasis rosea.
3. **Spongiotic:** It presents with Intraepidermal intercellular edema. Spongiotic tissue reaction has 5 patterns namely, Neutrophilic, Eosinophilic, Miliarial (acrosyringial), Follicular and Haphazard. Pityriasis rosea, Bullous pemphigus, Atopic dermatitis and Contact dermatitis all show spongiotic tissue reaction.
4. **Vesiculobullous:** It shows blistering within or beneath epidermis or at de junction. it can be further assessed by the level of split, underlying mechanism and the nature of inflammatory cells in the dermis. This pattern is seen in pemphigus vulgaris, impetigo and epidermolysis bullosa.
5. **Granulomatous:** It presents with chronic granulomatous inflammation and an aggregate of histiocytes. granulomatous tissue reaction pattern has 3 types;
   - Epithelioid, divided into sarcoidal and tuberculoid.
   - Palisading – Necrobiotic granuloma
   - Mixed cells which can be suppurative or foreign body.

   Granuloma annulare and tuberculosis are some of the examples of granulomatous tissue reaction pattern.
6. **Vasculopathic:** It shows pathological changes in cutaneous blood vessels. vasculitis presents with an infiltrate in vessel wall, fibrin deposition and endothelial necrosis. vasculopathic tissue reaction pattern is seen in leukocytoclastic vasculitis, granuloma faciale, TTP, sweet's syndrome and herpes zoster.

Minor Tissue Reaction Patterns

Less common diagnostic reaction pattern in inflammatory dermatoses know a minor reaction pattern. Important minor tissue reaction patterns in inflammatory reaction pattern are given below:

1. **Epidermolytic hyperkeratosis:** It shows compact hyperkeratosis with degeneration in granular cell and upper spinous layer of epidermis. Seen in epidermolytic hyperkeratosis, bullous and nonbullous ichthyosiform erythroderma and palmar-plantar keratoderma.
2. **Acantholytic dyskeratosis:** It shows epidermal hyperkeratosis, suprabasal clefts with acantholytic/dyskeratotic cells. Seen in Darier's disease, Grover's disease, Solar keratosis etc.
3. **Cornoid lamellation:** In porokeratosis, keratin filled invagination in epidermis occurs. In the center of invagination, a parakeratotic column of cells known as coronoid lamella is seen. Below parakeratotic layer granular cell layer is usually absent.
4. **Papillomatosis:** It shows undulations and protrusions of epidermis with a fibrovascular core. Epidermal hyperkeratosis and acanthosis may be associated with papillomatosis. Clinical examples include seborrheic keratosis, acrokeratosis verruciformis and solar keratosis.
5. **Angiofibromas:** Increased dermal vessels with surrounding coarse concentric fibrosis is seen. Periungual fibroma, pearly penile papules and adenoma sebaceum are examples of this tissue reaction pattern.
6. **Eosinophilic cellulitis with "FLAME FIGURES":** It shows intense and diffuse dermal eosinophilic infiltration and degranulation of eosinophils, resulting deposition of eosinophilic material adherent to collagen bundles. Clinical examples include wells syndrome, arthropod reaction, parasitic infection and bullous pemphigoid.
7. **Transepithelial elimination:** Elimination of altered dermal material or foreign component via the epidermis or hair follicles is seen. Clinical examples include "Black heel" (calcaneal petechiae or talon noir) and necrobiotic xanthogranuloma.

Various Histological Features In Skin

Different Epidermal Changes on Histopathology

1. **Acanthosis:** The stratum spinosum of the epidermis becomes thickened with the presence of enlarged cells, resulting in papules/plaques.
2. **Hyperkeratosis:** The stratum corneum becomes thickened, either due to accelerated epidermopoiesis or due to faulty maturation of keratocytes. It is of 2 types:
   (a) Orthokeratosis- nuclei are not visible in the cornified cells.
   (b) Parakeratosis- retention of nuclei in the cornified cells.
3. **Abscess:** It can be clinically defined as a circumscribed collection of pus and histopathologically defined as a localized collection of neutrophils.
4. **Hypergranulosis:** The stratum granulosum becomes thickened.
5. **Hypogranulosis:** Decreased number of cells containing keratohyalin granules results in thinning of the granular zone.

6. **Dyskeratosis:** Abnormal cornification of the keratocytes within the epidermis and epithelial structures of adnexa. Dyskeratotic cells have an eosinophilic cytoplasm and a pyknotic nucleus.
7. **Acantholysis:** Loss of coherence between the epidermal cells due to breakdown of their intercellular bridges. Acantholysis can be primary or secondary.
   (a) *Primary:* Actual damage to the intercellular adhesions takes place. Clinical examples include Pemphigus, Hailey-Hailey disease.
   (b) *Secondary:* Direct damage occurs to the cell. Clinical examples include SCC, herpes infections, warty dyskeratoma.
8. **Spongiosis:** Edema of the epidermis takes place along with exocytosis of the inflammatory cells.

Different Dermal Changes on Histopathology

1. **Grenz zone:** Narrow area of uninvolved dermis between the epidermis and a dermal inflammatory or neoplastic infiltrate, or adjacent to a hair follicle. Clinical examples include leprosy and granuloma faciale.
2. **Solar elastosis:** Chronic sun exposure results in basophilic change in the collagen.
3. **Fibrosis:** Increased number of collagen fibers results in thickening of the dermis. Clinical examples include morphea and scleroderma.
4. **Atrophy:** Thinning of the dermis.

Mediums for Skin Specimens

1. **Histopathology:** Formalin
2. **Tissue culture:** Normal saline
3. **Immunofluorescence:** Michel's medium

   Michel's medium is composed of a buffer (0.81 g potassium citrate), 0.0625 g N-ethylmaleimide, 0.123 g magnesium sulphate in 100 ml of distilled water. Before use 55 g ammonium sulphate is added and pH is adjusted between 7 to 7.2 with the use of KOH. Ideal fixation time for immunofluorescence by Michel's medium is 24-48 hrs. The samples can be stored for up to 1 month in the refrigerator at 4 °C in this medium (never freeze the sample in Michel's medium). Shelf life of the medium is upto 6 months.
4. **Electron microscopy:** 2.5% Glutaraldehyde

Special Stain In Dermatology

There are wide variety of special stains use to demonstrate pathologic processes in dermatology. Few special stain are highlighted in Table 2.8:

Table 2.8: Showing special stains in dermatology

Haematoxylin- eosin stain	*Routine histopathology stain*
Masson trichrome	Collagen
Verhoeff -van stain	Elastic fibers
Orcein stain	Elastic fibers
Martius scarlet blue (MSB)	Fibrin
Meson fontana stain	Melanin
Alcian blue pH 2.5	Acid mucopolysaccharides
Alcian blue pH	Sulfated mucopolysacharides
Toluidine blue stain	Acid mucopolysaccharide
Colloidal iron stain	Acid mucopolysaccharide
Mucicarmine stain	Epithelial mucin
Periodic Acid Schiff (PAS) stain	Glycogen, fungi
Perl's Prussian blue	Hemosiderin
Von Kossa stain	Calcium
Alizarin red	Calcium
Chloroacetate esterase stain or Leder stain	Mast cell
Congo red stain	Amyloid
Crystal violet	Amyloid & Acid mucopolysaccharide
Thioflavin T	Amyloid
Pagoda	Amyloid
Oil red O stain	Lipid
Brown - Brenn stain	Modified tissue gram stain
Grocott methenamine silver stain	Fungus
Ziehl -Neelsen /Fite faraco stain	Mycobacterium leprae

Immunofluorescence

In clinical immunodermatology there are two basic types of immunofluorescence staining methods: (1) Direct immunofluorescence staining in which the primary antibody is labeled with fluorescence dye to recognize in vivo antibody bound to an antigen; and (2) While in indirect immunofluorescence in which a secondary antibody labeled with fluorochrome is used to recognize circulating antibodies. These techniques are simple to perform, they are both reliable and reproducible and have allowed major advances in the diagnosis of autoimmune diseases.

Reflectance Confocal Microscopy (RCM)

It allows non invasive imaging of the epidermis and superficial dermis to a depth of 250 micrometer. These images may provide an alternative to histopathology.

Radiological and Imaging Examinations

Ultrasound, MRI, radioisotope scans and even positron emission tomography (PET), are all used in clinical dermatological practice, to detect lymphadenopathy or other metastatic skin cancer, and in the identification of occult malignancy in paraneoplastic conditions such as dermatomyositis.

ELISA (Enzyme linked immunosorbent assay), salt split technique, immunohistochemistry and polymerase chain reaction (PCR) are other diagnostic tools used in dermatology.

CHAPTER 3 Bacterial Infections

Contents

Skin is normally inhabited by non pathogenic bacteria known as normal skin flora, which are of two types: **resident flora and transient flora**. Resident flora are present permanently and multiply on the surface of the skin while transient flora are derived from exogenous source and do not multiply on skin. These flora are useful for the maintenance of normal environment on the skin surface by competing for nutrition with the pathogenic bacteria, thereby preventing their growth. They also produce antibiotics and chemicals inhibiting the growth of pathogenic bacteria. By modifying the secretions of skin, they further prevent the growth of unwanted bacteria. Resident flora do not cause disease.

Certain pathogenic bacteria like *Staphylococcus aureus* are present in nostrils, axilla and perineum as carriage in some people, especially in hospital born babies and may be an important cause of infections in the community. Pathogenic bacteria usually spread by direct contact in children but transmission by vectors, fomites and sometimes by airborne route may be important. Trauma, insect bites, thorn pricks, eczemas, immunocompromised state, fungal and other parasitic infections like scabies are all predisposing factors for bacterial infections.

S. aureus and Streptococci (Group A) are the most common pathogens implicated in cutaneous diseases. Diseases caused by staphylococcus and streptococcus described in Table 3.1 and toxin medicated diseases in Table 3.2.

Common bacterial infections of the skin, which will be discussed here are:

- **Impetigo**
  - Impetigo contagiosa.
  - Bullous impetigo.
- **Ecthyma.**
- **Folliculitis:**
  - Superficial folliculitis.
  - Deep folliculitis.
- **Furuncle.**
- **Carbuncle.**
- **Cellulitis and erysipelas.**

- **Toxic syndromes**
  - Staphylococcal scalded skin syndrome or SSSS
  - Staphylococcal toxic shock syndrome or TSS
  - Scarlet fever
  - Kawasaki disease
- **Corynebacterium infection**
  - Erythrasma
  - Trichomycosis axillaris
  - Pitted keratolysis
- **Miscellaneous**
  - Pseudomonas aeruginosa infection.
  - MRSA (Methicillin Resistant Staphylococcus Aureus)
  - Botryomycosis.
  - Cutaneous anthrax.
  - Bacillary angiomatosis.
  - Erysipeloid

Table 3.1: List of diseases caused by staphylococcus and streptococcus

Diseases caused by Staphylococcus		*Diseases caused by Streptococcus*	
1. Direct infection	Impetigo Ecthyma Folliculitis Furunculosis Carbuncle Sycosis Cellulitis	**1. Direct infection**	Impetigo Ecthyma Erysipelas Cellulitis Vulvovaginitis Perianal infection Streptococcal ulcers Blistering distal dactylitis Necrotizing fasciitis
2. Bacterial toxins	Staphylococcal scalded skin syndrome Toxic shock syndrome Staphylococcal scarlatina Recurrent toxin mediated perineal erythema	**2. Bacterial toxins**	Scarlet fever Toxic shock like syndrome Recurrent toxin mediated perineal erythema
3. Secondary infection	Eczema Infestations Ulcers	**3. Allergic hypersensitivity to streptococcal antigens**	Erythema nodosum, Vasculitis Psoriasis (guttate) Kawasaki disease
–	–	**4. Secondary infection**	Eczema Infestations Ulcers

Table 3.2: Toxin mediated diseases by staphylococcus and streptococcus

Staphylococcus aureus	Exfoliative type A & B	Epidermolytic	Bullous impetigo, Staphylococcal Skin Scalded Syndrome (SSSS) Recalcitrant erythematous desquamating disorders (REDD syndrome)
	Toxic shock syndrome toxin 1 (TSST-1)	Superantigen	Toxic shock syndrome (TSS) and food poisoning
	Staphylococcal enterotoxin A to C	Superantigen	TSS and food poisoning
Streptococcus pyogenes	Streptococcal pyrogenic exotoxins A and C	Superantigen	TSS (Non-menstrual female) and Scarlet fever

- Meningococcemia.
- Actinomycosis.
- Gram negative folliculitis.
- Melioidosis.

IMPETIGO

Impetigo is most common superficial bacterial infection of skin characterized by infection and inflammation in the epidermis.

Two major clinical forms of impetigo are:

1. **Impetigo contagiosa or non-bullous impetigo.**
2. **Bullous impetigo.**

Etiopathogenesis

Impetigo contagiosa is caused by *Staphylococcus aureus* (*S. aureus*) or *Streptococcus pyogenes* (*S. pyogenes*), or both, whereas bullous impetigo is caused by *S. aureus* only. It is commonly seen in infants and young children. Minor cutaneous trauma, insect bites or scratches cause breakdown of skin barrier, increasing the chances of acquiring infection. Impetigo is more prevalent under conditions of overcrowding, poor hygiene, low socioeconomic class and hot and humid climate. Epidemics of impetigo may occur in newborn nurseries or day care centers.

Pathogenesis includes interaction of host immunity with bacterial virulence factors. *S. aureus* produces many cellular components and toxins, which inhibit the host immune response. In bullous impetigo *S. aureus* produces epidermolytic toxin which targets extracellular amino terminal domain of desmoglein 1 (Dsg1), leading to cleavage in epidermis, forming bullous lesions.

Host factors such as immunosuppression, prolonged steroid therapy and atopy play an important role in the pathogenesis of impetigo.

Histopathology

Epidermis shows intraepidermal superficial bulla filled with neutrophils and cocci, as well as cellular edema.

Clinical Features

Impetigo contagiosa or non-bullous impetigo (Figure 3.1) starts as an erythematous macule over which a thin walled vesiculopustular develops which ruptures soon. The exuding seropurulent discharge forms a characteristic honey colored (yellowish brown) crust. Small satellite lesions appear around the main lesion. Lesions may coalesce to form a larger crusted area. Common site is face, especially perioral and perinasal region. Other sites are extremities and scalp. Itching, lymphadenopathy, fever and other constitutional symptoms may be seen sometimes.

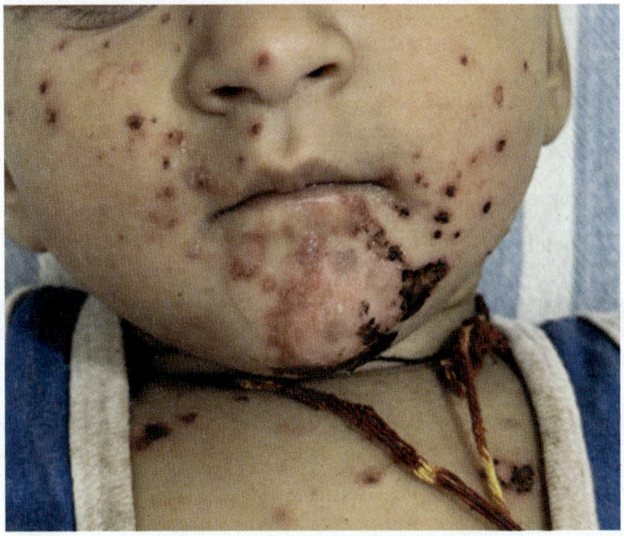

Figure 3.1: Impetigo contagiosa

Bullous Impetigo (Figure 3.2)

- Superficial blisters with surrounding erythema, seen commonly on face; other parts of body like palms and soles may be involved.

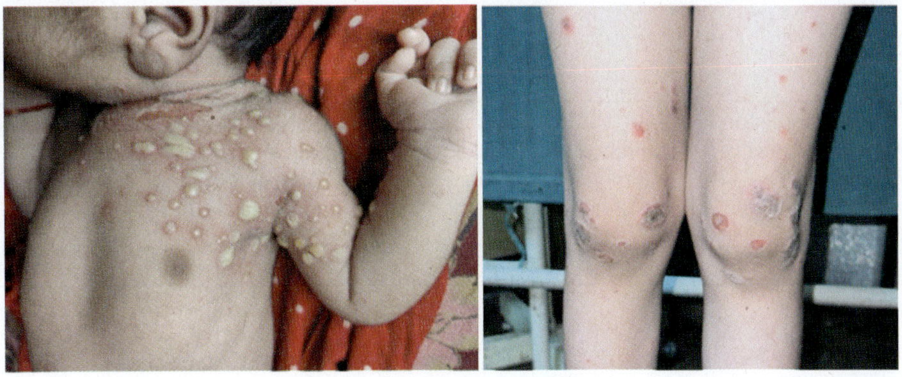

Figure 3.2: Bullous impetigo

- Bullous lesions may persist for a couple of days and rupture to form erosions with yellowish brown crusts.
- "Collarette of scale" is the pathognomonic finding which surrounds the blister roof at the periphery of ruptured lesion.

Complications

- Septic arthritis.
- Sepsis.
- Staphylococcal osteomyelitis.
- Pneumonia.
- Toxic shock syndrome (rare).
- Post-streptococcal glomerulonephritis (PSGN) (occurs after a period of 2-3 weeks).

Differential Diagnosis

- Herpes simplex.
- Varicella zoster infection.
- Atopic dermatitis.
- Tinea capitis (scalp lesions).
- Eczematous dermatitis.
- Immunobullous disease.

Disease Course and Prognosis

Impetigo is usually self-limiting and resolves within days to weeks with appropriate use of topical cleansers and antibiotics.

Treatment

- General measures like avoidance of insect bites, improvement of hygiene and correction of malnourishment help in treatment as well as in prevention of recurrence. Mupirocin ointment 2% in nasal vestibule decreases carriages.
- Removal of crust, topical antibiotics like fusidic acid and nadifloxacin are required for mild cases. Neomycin is also an effective topical agent. Mupirocin exerts a high level of bactericidal activity against a broad spectrum of gram-positive organisms and is being widely used now a days. Retapamulin (1%) ointment has been approved for impetigo.
- Extensive lesions require systemic antibiotics (Table 3.3 and Table 3.4) like azithromycin, cephalexin, amoxicillin-clavulanic acid, cloxacillin/dicloxacillin or erythromycin.

Table 3.3: Practical guidelines for treatment of pyoderma in children

S. No.	*Bacterial infection*	*Mild*		*Moderate*			*Severe*
		Topical antibiotics	*Systemic antibiotic*	*Topical antibiotics*	*Systemic antibiotic*	*Topical antibiotics*	*Systemic antibiotic*
1.	Impetigo	Mupirocin or fusidic acid cream	Oral azithromycin 5-10 mg/kg/ day 12 hourly for 7-10 days	Mupirocin or fusidic acid cream	Oral amoxicillin-clavulanic acid 50 mg/kg/day in 2-3 divided doses for 7 days or Oral cephalexin 25 mg/kg/dose TID for 7 days	Mupirocin or fusidic acid cream	Oral/IV amoxicillin-clavulanic acid 50 mg/kg/day in 2-3 divided doses for 7 days or IV cloxacillin 100-200 mg/kg 6 hourly for 7 days or dicloxacillin 25 mg/ kg/day 6 hourly for 7 days
2.	Ecthyma	Mupirocin or fusidic acid cream	Oral azithromycin 5-10 mg/kg/ day 12 hourly for 7-10 days	Mupirocin or fusidic acid cream	Oral amoxicillin-clavulanic acid 50 mg/kg/day in 2-3 divided doses for 7 days	Mupirocin or fusidic acid cream	Oral/IV amoxicillin-clavulanic acid 50 mg/kg/day in 2-3 divided doses for 7 days

Contd.

Contd.

3.	Folliculitis	–	Oral azithromycin 5-10 mg/kg/ day 12 hourly for 7-10 days	–	Oral azithromycin 5-10 mg/kg/ day 12 hourly or ciprofloxacin* 10 mg/kg/day 12 hourly for 7-10 days Or Oral cephalexin 25 mg/kg/dose TID for 7 days	–	Oral/IV amoxicillin-clavulanic acid 50 mg/kg/day in 2-3 divided doses for 7 days In MRSA infections: IV Vancomycin or linezolid (10 mg/ kg BD)
4.	Furuncle	–	Oral azithromycin 5-10 mg/kg/ day 12 hourly for 7-10 days	–	Oral amoxicillin-clavulanic acid 50 mg/kg/day in 2-3 divided doses for 7 days Or Oral cephalexin 25 mg/kg/dose TID for 7 days	–	Oral/IV amoxicillin-clavulanic acid 50 mg/kg/day in 2-3 divided doses for 7 days Or IV clindamycin 15-40 mg/kg 8 hourly Or IV/IM cephazolin 25-150 mg/kg 8 hourly. In MRSA, Vancomycin or linezolid
5.	Carbuncle	–	Oral azithromycin 5-10 mg/kg/ day 12 hourly for 7-10 days	–	Oral amoxicillin-clavulanic acid 50 mg/kg/day in 2-3 divided doses for 7 days Or Oral cephalexin 25 mg/kg/dose TID for 7 days	–	Oral/IV amoxicillin-clavulanic acid 50 mg/kg/day in 2-3 divided doses for 7 days or IV clindamycin 15-40 mg/kg 8 hourly for 7 days Or IV/IM cephazolin 25-150 mg/kg 8 hourly for 7 days. In MRSA, Vancomycin or linezolid
6.	Cellulitis and erysipelas	–	Oral azithromycin 5-10 mg/kg/ day 12 hourly for 7-10 days	–	Oral/IV amoxicillin-clavulanic acid 50 mg/kg/day in 2-3 divided doses for 7 days Or Oral cephalexin 25 mg/kg/dose TID for 7 days	–	IV amoxicillin-clavulanic acid 50 mg/kg/day Or piperacillin-tazobactam 80 mg/ kg 8 hourly with metronidazole 7.5 mg/kg 8 hourly for 7 days Or IV clindamycin 15-40 mg/kg 8 hourly for 7 days Or IV/IM cephazolin 25-150 mg/kg 8 hourly for 7 days. In MRSA, Vancomycin or linezolid

* Contraindicated in children less than 5 years of age.

- Azithromycin has good efficacy with dosage convenience and is used as the first line drug for treatment of impetigo. In cases where azithromycin cannot be given, cephalexin should be considered. For **severe** infections, amoxicillin-clavulanic acid is useful. Intravenous administration of amoxicillin-clavulanic acid, cloxacillin or dicloxacillin may be needed in severe cases. Second line antibiotics include macrolides such as erythromycin, clarithromycin (macrolide resistance can be quite high) and cotrimoxazole.

Table 3.4: Antibiotic doses for adults (Pyoderma)

Topical treatment	***Systemic treatment***
Fusidic acid cream twice a day Mupirocin ointment twice a day	**Flucloxacillin (dicloxacillin)** - 125 mg - 500 mg 6 hourly **Cephalexin** - 250-500 mg 6 hourly **Amoxicillin** - 250-500 mg 6 hourly **Amoxicillin/clavulanic acid** - 250-500/125 mg 8 hourly **Clindamycin** - 150-300 mg 12 hourly **Azithromycin** - 500 mg once daily for 3-5 days In severe cases intravenous antibiotics may be required e.g. Intravenous Amoxicillin/clavulanic acid 1.2 gm three time a day or piperacillin/ tazobactam 4.5 gm three time a day plus metronidazole 500 mg twice daily

- In methicillin resistant *Staphylococcus aureus* (MRSA) infection, clindamycin, vancomycin, linezolid or cotrimoxazole should be given.
- Recurrent infection should be investigated for carriage of staphylococci. Antibiotic creams can be applied to carriage sites.

ECTHYMA

Ecthyma is a deeper variety of pyoderma characterized by adherent crust and underlying purulent ulcer.

Etiopathogenesis

Group A beta hemolyticus Streptococcus pyogenes is the most common causative organism. *Staphylococcus aureus* and *pseudomonas aeruginosa* have also been isolated from lesions of ecthyma.

Predisposing factors include poor hygiene, malnutrition, skin trauma and co-existence of other skin conditions like eczema, scabies and insect bites.

Age

Extremes of age are most commonly affected.

Clinical Features

Initially lesions appear as small bullae/pustules with surrounding erythema. Later, a crust comprising the dried exudate is formed on the lesion (Figure 3.3). Removal of the crust reveals a purulent ulcer. The lesion eventually heals with scarring. Lower extremities are the most commonly affected sites.

Treatment

Removal of predisposing factors like improving hygiene and malnutrition as well as treatment of underlying skin disorders should be done.

Warm compresses are effective along with antibiotic cover.

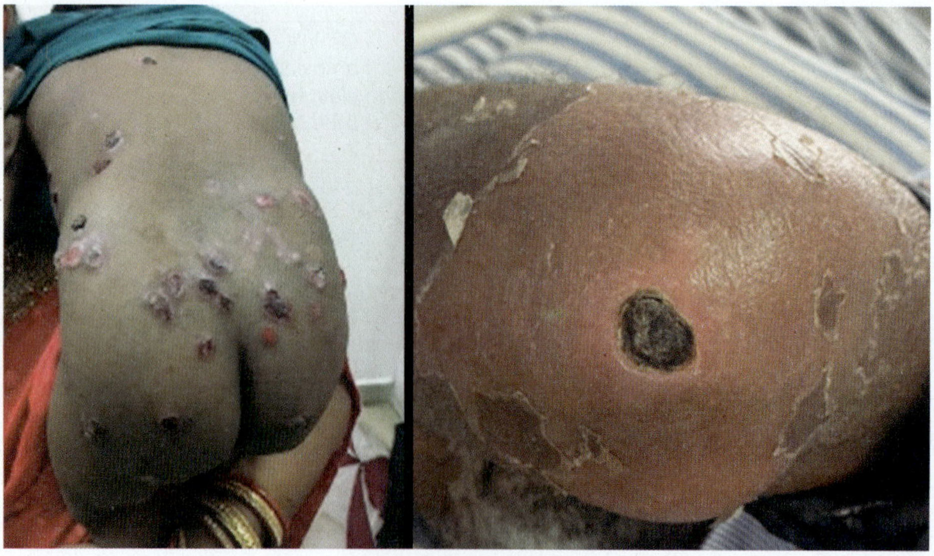

Figure 3.3: Ecthyma

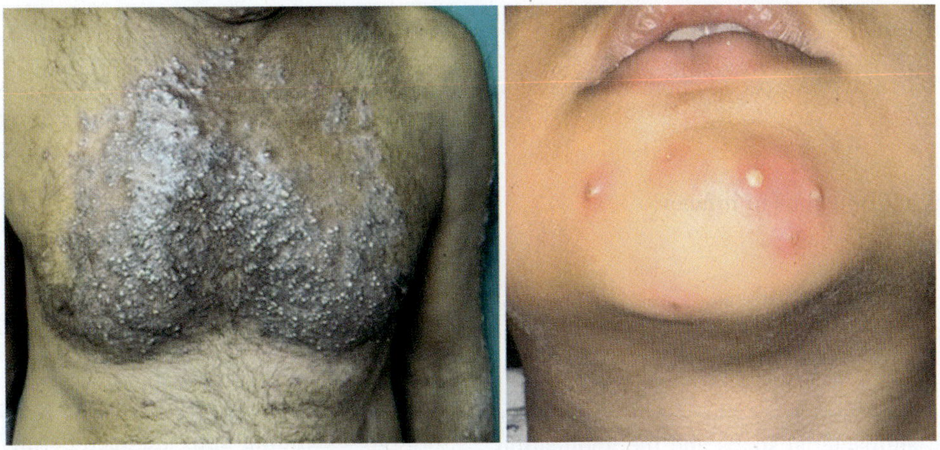

Figure 3.4: Superficial folliculitis

Systemic antibiotics active against gram-positive organisms like *Staphylococcus* and *Streptococcus* should be used, e.g., amoxicillin, azithromycin or erythromycin.

Topical antibiotic creams like mupirocin or fusidic acid can be applied.

Antipseudomonal therapy (e.g. ciprofloxacin, aminoglycoside andantipseudomonal penicillin) should be instituted in ecthyma gangrenosum.

FOLLICULITIS

Folliculitis is a bacterial infection of skin anatomically confined to hair follicle and perifollicular structures. Superficial folliculitis is the inflammation of the terminal part or ostium of hair follicle.

Deep folliculitis involves the whole depth of the hair follicle. When it presents with extensive perifollicular inflammation and abscess formation, it is termed as a furuncle.

Etiopathogenesis

- *Staphylococcus aureus* is by far the most common organism causing folliculitis.
- *Gram-negative bacteria can also cause folliculitis in acne patients receiving long term antibiotic therapy.*
- Factors that tend to increase the number of surface skin bacteria like occlusion, over hydration, maceration, excessive application of mineral oil, use of topical steroids etc. can lead to superficial folliculitis.
- Deep folliculitis is more often seen in immunocompromised patients and children with neutrophilic disorders like Job syndrome.
- Non-infective causes of folliculitis include contact with mineral oil, occlusive dressing, adhesive tapes or after waxing.

Histopathology

- Neutrophilic pustules are seen within the hair follicle, usually around the follicular opening.
- Perifollicular infiltrate of lymphocytes and histiocytes may be seen.
- Deep folliculitis is associated with a more dense dermal infiltration and involves the whole depth of the follicle.

Clinical Features

Superficial folliculitis (Figure 3.4): It is also known as **Bockhart impetigo**. Yellow dome shaped follicular pustules appear in crops on forehead, scalp hair margin and extremities. They heal in about a week without scarring.

Deep folliculitis (Figure 3.5): It is seen in beard area as **sycosis barbae** and on nape of the neck as **sycosis nuchae**. Lesions are erythematous papules or pustules which become crusted and heal with scarring.

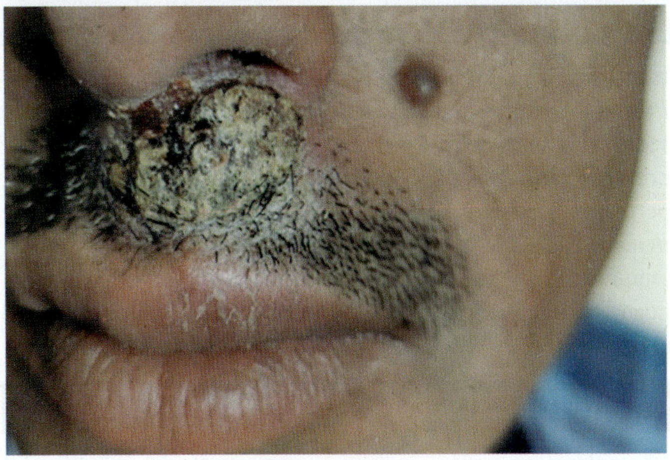

Figure 3.5: Deep folliculitis

Differential Diagnosis

- Other bacterial folliculitis like pseudomonas folliculitis, fungal/yeast folliculitis.
- Irritant folliculitis.
- Eosinophilic pustular folliculitis of infancy.
- Miliaria/periporitis.
- Tinea.
- Hidradenitis suppurativa.

Treatment

Gentle cleansing with antibacterial soaps and the application of topical antibiotics like mupirocin, fusidic acid, clindamycin or erythromycin alone may be sufficient in localized cases. In those with widespread lesions, systemic antibiotic such as azithromycin, ciprofloxacin or cephalexin should be given. For severe cases amoxicillin-clavulanic acid is given and vancomycin and linezolid should be reserved for MRSA infections. In such instances, bacterial culture should be obtained before the initiation of systemic therapy. Hand washing is the single most important behavioural modification in the prevention of spread. Other preventive measures may include avoidance of tight fitting clothing and loss of weight.

Deep folliculitis requires treatment with systemic antibiotics. Oral tetracyclines can be given in cases of chronic folliculitis due to their anti-inflammatory and anti-microbial activity but they should not be used in children below 8 years of age.

Periporitis

It is a staphylococcal sweat gland abscess. Mostly involves face of young children and occurs commonly during summer season.

GRAM NEGATIVE FOLLICULITIS

It is caused by gram negative bacilli like *E. coli, Klebsiella, Proteus, Serratia* and *Pseudomonas aeruginosa*. It is usually seen in patients with long term use of antibiotics in acne. It presents with pustules, with few papules around perioral, perinasal area and cheek area. Poor response to antibiotic in acne is a strong suspicion for gram negative folliculitis. Diagnosis can be done by grams stain, which shows gram negative bacilli. Treatment includes use of isotretinoin and antibiotics.

FURUNCLE (BOIL)

Furuncle is an acute, *usually necrotic* bacterial infection of the hair follicle which extends to perifollicular region and subcutaneous tissue.

Etiopathogenesis

Uncommon in early childhood, it is usually seen around puberty and early adulthood. *Staphylococcus aureus* is the most common causative agent and increase in skin surface colonization by *Staphylococcus*, or its nasal or perineum carriage may be responsible for most of the infections. Diabetes, malnutrition or immunocompromised state may be predisposing factors.

Pathology

There is formation of abscess in hair follicle with inflammatory infiltrate extending upto the deep dermis. This is followed by necrosis and destruction of follicle.

Clinical Features

Furuncle begins as a small tender, erythematous follicular nodule (Figure 3.6), which soon develops into indurated pustular lesion. The lesion becomes necrotic with discharge of pus from the follicular opening and ultimately heals with a scar. Lesions may be single or multiple and may appear in crops. Mild fever, pain and tenderness may be seen. Face, axillae, buttocks and perineal region are the common sites involved.

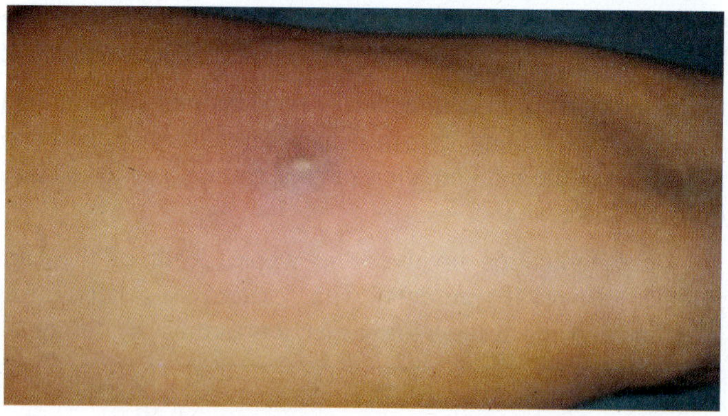

Figure 3.6: Furuncle with cellulitis

Complications

Cavernous sinus thrombosis may occur rarely in lesions on upper lip or cheek. Pyaemia or septicemia may result in untreated cases.

Differential Diagnosis

- Pustular acne.
- Vesiculopustular lesions of herpes simplex.

Treatment

The mainstay of therapy is systemic anti-staphylococcal antibiotics (azithromycin, cephalexin, amoxicillin-clavulanic acid and vancomycin, linezolid, clindamycin for MRSA infections) with incision and drainage of fluctuant lesions. Cultures should be done to rule out MRSA. Analgesics and antipyretics may be given for symptomatic relief.

The triple regime of chlorhexidine skin disinfection (21 days), mupirocin applied to the nares (5 days), and oral clindamycin (21 days) has been found to be effective with a prolonged remission. Many practitioners recommend sodium hypochlorite baths or washes for patients with recurrent disease. Topical and systemic antibiotics are required. Deep lesions respond to amoxicillin-clavulanic acid combination. Management of nasal carriage of *S. aureus* in patient and other household members is advised.

CARBUNCLE

Carbuncle is a deep bacterial infection of group of contiguous hair follicles with associated inflammation in subcutaneous tissue.

Etiopathogenesis

S. aureus is the most common agent. It occurs predominantly in adult men, and is rarely seen in children. It is commonly associated with diabetes, drug addiction, prolonged steroid therapy or any other immunocompromised condition.

Clinical Features

Disease starts as a red, painful, nodular lesion which increases in size over a week and eventually suppuration occurs through multiple follicular openings leading to sieve like appearance (Figure 3.7). Intervening skin is involved resulting in necrosis. Constitutional symptoms like fever, malaise may be severe. Commonly affected sites include back of neck, shoulders, lumbar region, hips and thighs. Lesions generally heal with scarring.

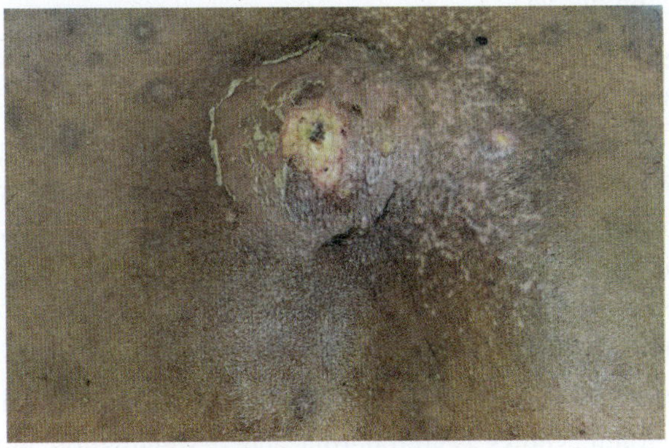

Figure 3.7: Carbuncle

Differential Diagnosis

- Cutaneous anthrax.
- Cutaneous ulcers caused by *Pseudomonas.*

Treatment

Treatment of underlying conditions like diabetes, immunosuppression etc. should be done.

Systemic antibiotics against *Staphylococcus,* e.g., azithromycin, amoxicillin-clavulanic acid, combination or flucloxacillin should be used. Surgical management in the form of saucerization and incision and drainage (I&D).

CELLULITIS AND ERYSIPELAS

- Cellulitis is an acute, bacterial infection with spreading inflammation involving mainly deeper subcutaneous tissue.
- Erysipelas is a bacterial infection primarily involving the dermis, upper subcutaneous fat and lymphatic vessels.
- These two disorders may coexist making a distinction difficult.

Etiopathogenesis

Streptococcus (Group A predominantly) is the most common organism responsible for erysipelas. Cellulitis may be due to *Streptococcus*, *Staphylococcus aureus*, *Hemophilus influenzae* type B, *Acinetobacter, Staphylococcus epidermidis, Bacteroides fragilis* or gram-negative bacteria.

Cellulitis and erysipelas usually occur after cutaneous trauma that precedes the infection by 1-2 days.

Clinical Features

Localized, but spreading erythema with warmth and edema are the presenting features (Figure 3.8). The borders of the lesion are well defined in erysipelas, but diffuse in cellulitis.

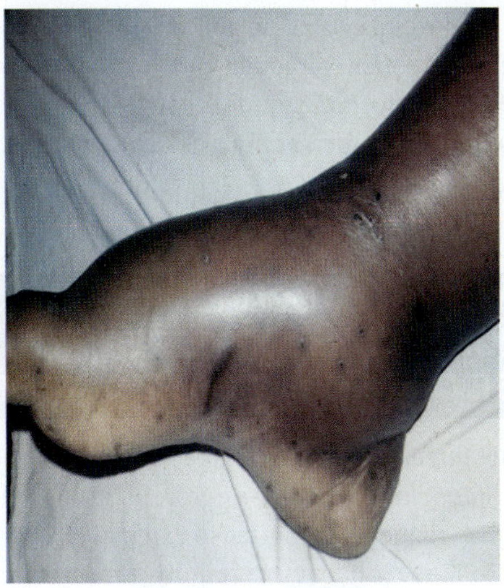

Figure 3.8: Cellulitis

Pain, tenderness, fever and other constitutional symptoms are frequently associated. Legs and face are the most common sites in children and abdominal wall in infants. Recurrent erysipelas may be caused by defective lymphatic drainage.

Ear involvement is called Milian's ear sign. It is distinguishing feature of erysipelas of face, because pinna has no deeper dermis and subcutaneous tissue, therefore it is spared in cellulitis.

Differential Diagnosis

- Necrotizing fasciitis
- Lymphedema
- Deep vein thrombosis is to be distinguished from cellulitis of leg.

Complications

- Subcutaneous abscess, fasciitis, myositis or septicemia may be seen without appropriate treatment.
- Post streptococcal glomerulonephritis (PSGN) may be seen with streptococcal infection.

Diagnosis

Diagnosis can be done clinically in most cases. History of trauma, morphology and constitutional symptoms helps in making the diagnosis.

Swabs, aspiration of tissue fluid or skin biopsy for bacteriological examination and culture can be taken from the lesions, but are not routinely recommended.

Treatment

Supportive treatment, analgesics and antipyretics are required for the constitutional symptoms.

There is no consensus on the choice between oral and intravenous antibiotics, although blood cultures, intravenous antibiotics and hospitalization have traditionally been recommended for children at high risk for cellulitis.

Systemic antibiotic therapy should be given in most of the cases (Table 3.3).

STAPHYLOCOCCAL SCALDED SKIN SYNDROME (SSSS) OR RITTER'S DISEASE OR PEMPHIGUS NEONATORUM

SSSS is a life threatening but treatable, toxin-mediated infection caused by *Staphylococcus aureus* group II phage 71 type. The syndrome may range from limited to extensive cutaneous and systemic disease characterized by tenderness, blistering and superficial denudation of skin. It results from exfoliative toxins (ETs) ET-A and ET-B released by staphylococci.

Etiopathogenesis

SSSS is predominantly a disease of infancy and early childhood with most cases seen before the age of six years. Lack of immunity to toxins, renal immaturity and decreased toxin clearance may be the possible reasons.

Outbreaks in newborn nurseries or neonatal ICUs may be because of nursing staff who are infected or colonized with ET-producing *Staphylococcus.*

Bullous impetigo is considered a localized form of SSSS and results after staphylococcal infection with toxin production having local effects. When the toxin diffuses from the infected focus, and there is absence of specific antibody, SSSS results. ETs have specificity for desmoglein 1, a desmosomal cadherin, therefore binding of the toxin results in formation of intra epidermal blisters below stratum corneum (splitting occurs between the granular and spinous layers which usually contain inflammatory cells).

Pathology

Acantholytic, intraepidermal blisters are seen, with clefts in granular layer or just below it.

Histopathological differentiation should be done from other disorders that cause superficial intraepidermal cleavage like pemphigus foliaceus, bullous impetigo and subcorneal pustular dermatosis.

Clinical Features

- Infections leading to SSSS typically originate in nasopharynx and go unrecognized. Other foci of infection include umbilicus, urinary tract and conjunctiva.
- Sudden onset of fever, irritability, cutaneous tenderness and erythema occur initially. Erythema is more in flexures.
- Blisters and erosions develop within 24-48 hours followed by desquamation. Skin peels off in sheets within a week leaving raw erythematous areas (Figure 3.9). Recovery from SSSS is common but sepsis or electrolyte abnormalities may lead to mortality.
- An abortive form of SSSS known as the scarlatiniform variant, shows erythroderma and desquamation without bullous lesions.
- SSSS may begin as bullous impetigo and progress to regionally limited bullae and denuded areas.

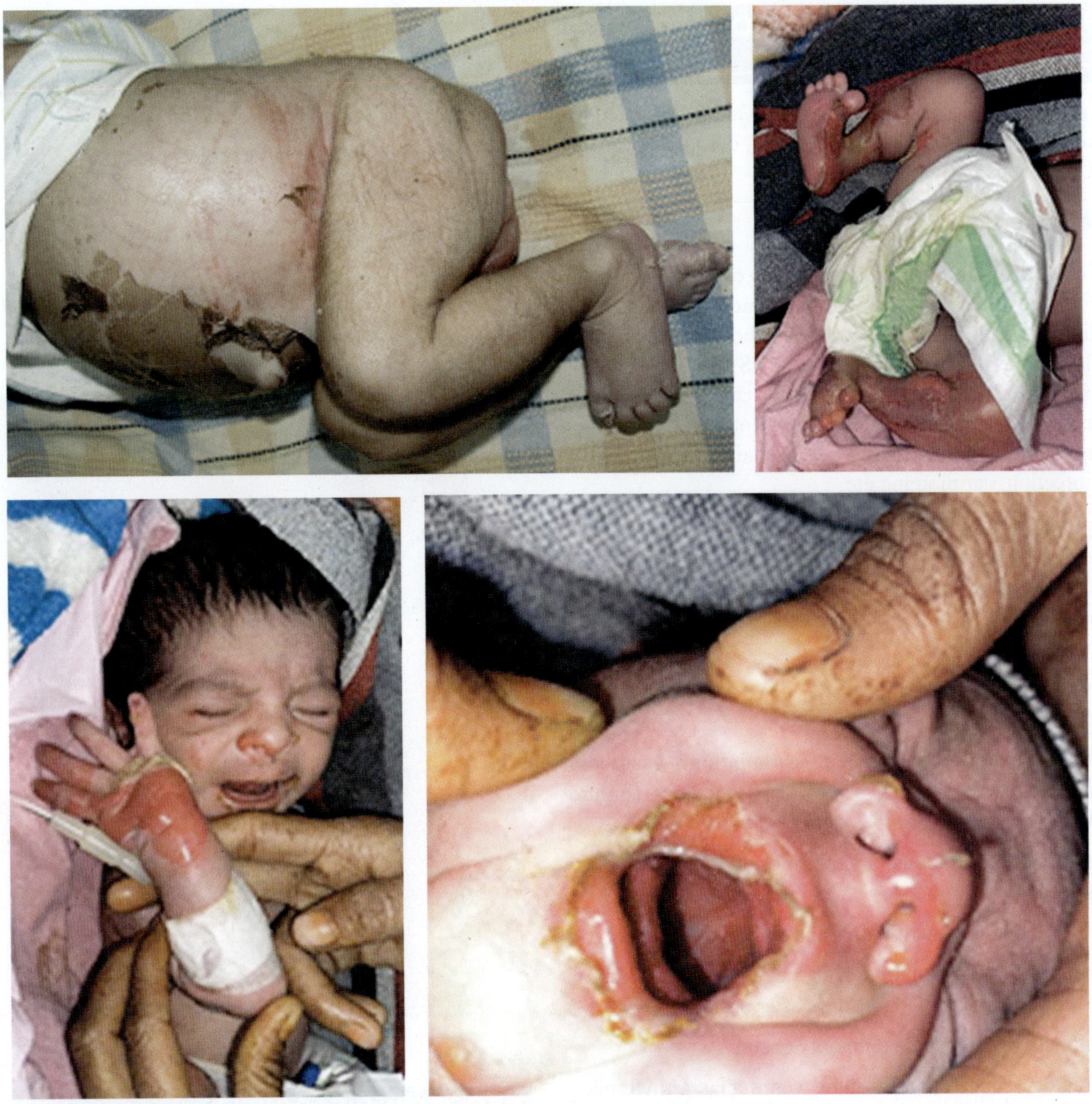

Figure 3.9: Staphylococcal scalded skin syndrome

Differential Diagnosis

- Toxic epidermal necrolysis is a rare but life threatening disease. It produces full thickness epidermal necrosis and dermoepidermal separation.
- Scarlatiniform variant of SSSS may be confused with TSS or exanthems.

Treatment

- Eradication of *Staphylococci* from focus of infection, by penicillinase resistant anti-staphylococcal antibiotics such as flucloxacillin, clindamycin, temocillin, tigecycline or daptomycin should be used as first line therapy, preferably parenterally.
- Widespread exfoliative lesions require hospital admission and broad-spectrum IV antibiotic coverage.
- Supportive skin care by topical antibiotics.
- Appropriate fluid, electrolyte management.
- Identification of nasal carriage in hospital staff and adequate management (chlorhexidine hand washing, oral antibiotic therapy, topical mupirocin ointment for nasal colonization).

STAPHYLOCOCCAL TOXIC SHOCK SYNDROME (TSS)

It is an acute multi organ illness caused by toxins liberated by *S. aureus*. It is characterized by fever, rash, desquamation and shock.

Etiopathogenesis

TSS is caused by toxin producing strains of *Staphylococcus aureus* phage group II in patients lacking protective antibodies at the time of infection. Newborns usually have passively acquired immunity against TSST-1 (Toxic shock syndrome toxin-1). The source of infection can be due to use of tampons in menstruation or other staphylococcal infections like empyema, osteomyelitis, peritonsillar abscess, surgical wound infection, ear piercing etc.

Clinical Features

- Sudden onset of fever with vomiting, diarrhea, headache, pharyngitis, myalgia and hypotension may be seen.
- Rash appears on the first day as macular or maculopapular rash.
- Diffuse, flexurally accentuated scarlatiniform exanthem over trunk which progresses to arms and legs (Figure 3.10) may also be seen.
- Erythema of mucous membranes with strawberry tongue.
- Erythema and edema of palms and soles may occur.
- Generalized desquamation with peeling of the skin of hands and feet occurs 10-21 days after onset of fever.
- Conjunctival erythema commonly occurs.
- Refractory shock, renal failure, ventricular arrhythmias, disseminated intravascular coagulation (DIC) and respiratory distress syndrome may occur.

Differential Diagnosis

- Kawasaki disease.
- Erythema multiforme.
- Rubeola, leptospirosis, enteroviral infections, rocky mountain spotted fever (intense conjunctival erythema).

Treatment

- Management of shock and multisystem involvement is of prime importance. Many experts recommend combination antibiotic therapy that includes clindamycin, which has effect on protein (i.e., toxin) synthesis inhibition, although clindamycin should not be used alone.
- Removal of foreign bodies, drainage of infected sites and antibiotics for eradication of infection.
- Circulating fluid volume replacement.
- Cardiovascular support, ventilator support.
- Correction of electrolyte disturbance and acid-base abnormalities.
- Systemic steroids in cases of severely affected patients.
- Immunoglobulin administration to provide specific neutralizing antibody against TSST-1.

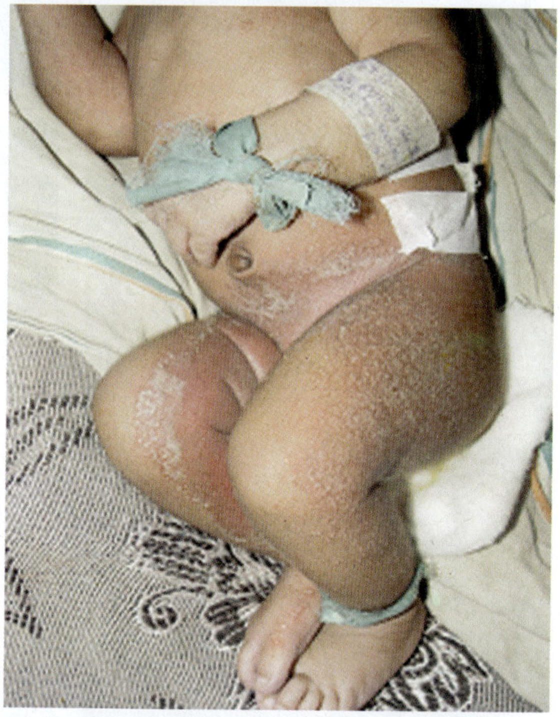

Figure 3.10: Toxic shock syndrome

NEROTIZING FASCIITIS

It is a rapidly progressive necrotizing infection of the skin and subcutaneous tissues which is potentially fatal. It is commonly associated with severe systemic toxicity.

Etiopathogenesis

Necrotizing fasciitis may be polymicrobial in nature and has been reported with Streptococci, *P. aeruginosa, S. aureus, Klebsiella* species, *E. coli,* Enterobacter cloacae, Serratia species, Proteus species, *Enterococcus, Clostridium, Bacteroides* and *Vibrio* species. It occurs in individuals with decreased local resistance, malnutrition or chronic disease. Although rare in children, in neonates it has been observed with omphalitis, balanitis, mastitis and fetal scalp monitoring.

Clinical Features

- Pain, edema and erythema with tenderness appears most commonly on extremities.
- Subsequently ecchymosis, bullae, necrosis and gangrene develop (Figure 3.11). In next 48 hours fever, shock and altered mental status typically develop.
- The most serious complication of necrotizing fasciitis is streptococcal toxic shock syndrome (TSS), which is characterized by hypotension, renal impairment, coagulopathy, liver abnormalities, respiratory distress and a diffuse erythematous cutaneous eruption.

Diagnosis

Confirmation of infection can be done by gram stain and culture of blister fluid, discharge or biopsy material, blood culture and polymerase chain reaction (PCR) analysis for pyrogenic exotoxin B. Imaging studies may be useful in confirming the diagnosis.

Treatment

- Surgical debridement of necrotic tissue is the most important treatment option to prevent mortality.
- Antimicrobial therapy should be started immediately, and it should have activity against gram positive, gram negative as well as anaerobic organisms. Clindamycin is quite effective as part of this antimicrobial regimen.
- Hyperbaric oxygen therapy and intravenous immunoglobulin (IVIG) have also been tried.

ACTINOMYCOSIS

Etiology

Actinomycosis is a chronic suppurative infection, which is caused by Actinomyces israelii (an anaerobic gram-positive saprophyte residing in tonsillar crypts, carious teeth and female genital tract).

Clinical Features

It tends to occur commonly in four areas: the cervicofacial region (most common), lungs, intestinal tract and genitourinary tract. Some patients present with mixed organ involvement that may include the skin, brain, pericardium and extremities.

Clinically it often presents as a soft tissue swelling, which increases to form a brawny, erythematous nodule that discharges serosanguineous or purulent material through multiple sinus tracts, from which the characteristic sulfur yellow granules consisting of masses of organisms can be demonstrated. Periostitis and osteomyelitis may occur. Regional lymph nodes are not involved.

Diagnosis

It is diagnosed by isolation and identification of the causative organism in anaerobic culture. Observation of the highly characteristic sulfur granules in purulent or biopsied material clinically suggest the diagnosis. Isolation and identification of causative organism in anaerobic culture will confirm diagnosis.

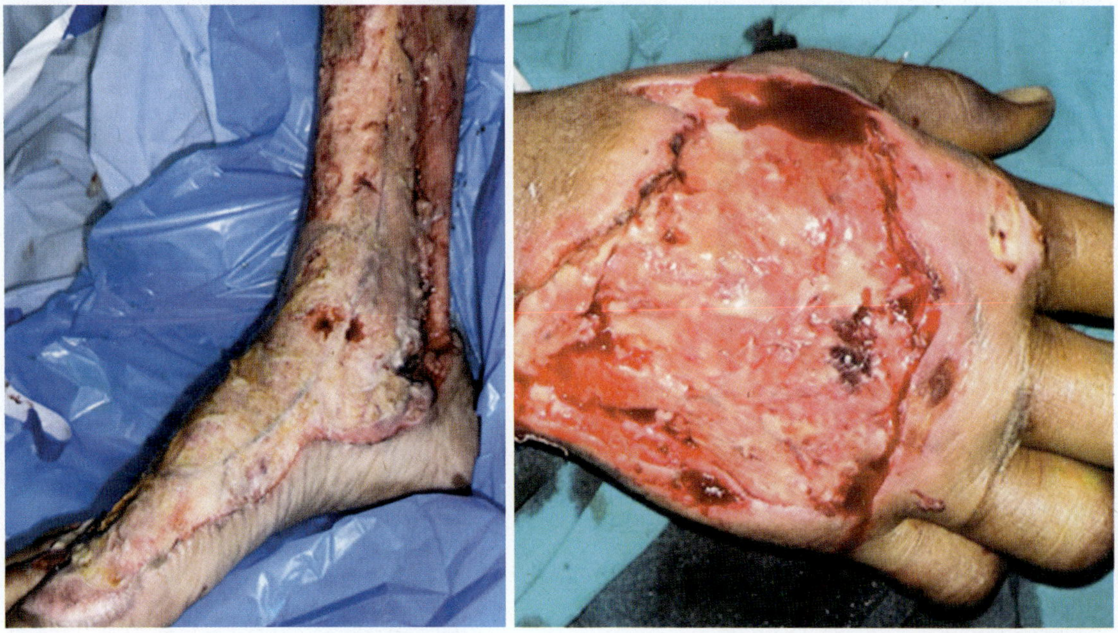

Figure 3.11: Necrotizing fasciitis

Treatment

Intravenous or oral penicillin as well as antibiotics like tetracyclines, erythromycin or clindamycin can treat this infection.

SCARLET FEVER

Scarlet fever is caused by group A streptococcus (GAS). The rash is diffuse, erythematous, blanchable and papular initially appearing around neck and then spreading over trunk and extremities, sparing the face. It fades with desquamation after 3-4 days. Strawberry tongue is also seen.

Pastia lines or Thompson's sign are pink or red lines seen in skin creases particularly in antecubital fossa due to capillary fragility. It occurs before the appearance of rash and persist as pigmented lines after desquamation (**details in chapter viral exanthems**).

CORYNEFORM BACTERIAL INFECTION

These are gram positive spore forming bacilli. Diseases caused by coryneform bacteria are:

1. **Erythrasma**
2. **Pitted keratolysis**
3. **Trichomycosis axillaris**

1. Erythrasma

It is caused by Corynebacterium minutissimum. Clinically it presents as well-defined or well marginated brown macules and patches in intertriginous areas like axilla, groin, inframammary and interdigital space (Figure 3.12). It is more prevalent in warm and humid climate.

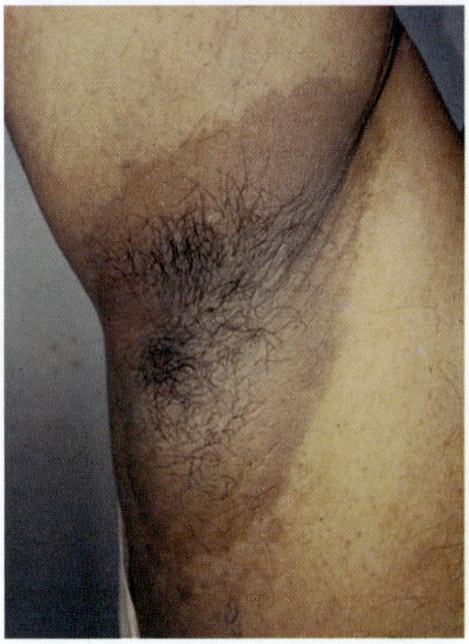

Figure 3.12: Erythrasma

These lesions produce coral red fluorescence under woods lamp examination due to presence to coproporphyrin III in bacteria (Figure 3.13). Localized disease can be treated by topical azoles, (clotrimazole, miconazole), fusidic acid, clindamycin, benzoyl peroxide etc. Extensive disease required oral clarithromycin, erythromycin or tetracycline.

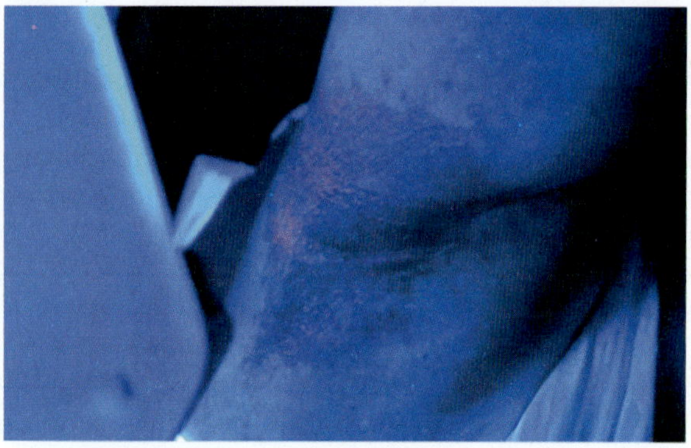

Figure 3.13: Coral red fluorescence on woods lamp in erythrasma

2. Pitted Keratolysis (Keratosis Plantare sulcatum/ring Keratolysis)

It is a superficial bacterial infection characterized by small discrete crater like pits over soles (Figure 3.14) and is caused by *Corynebacterium* species, *Micrococcus sedentarius (Kytococcus sedentarius), Dermatophilus congolensis, Actinomyces* and *Streptomyces.* It is more commonly seen in farmers, industrial workers, military personnel and athletes. Predisposing factor includes hyperhidrosis, keratoderma and immunodeficiency. Treatment includes

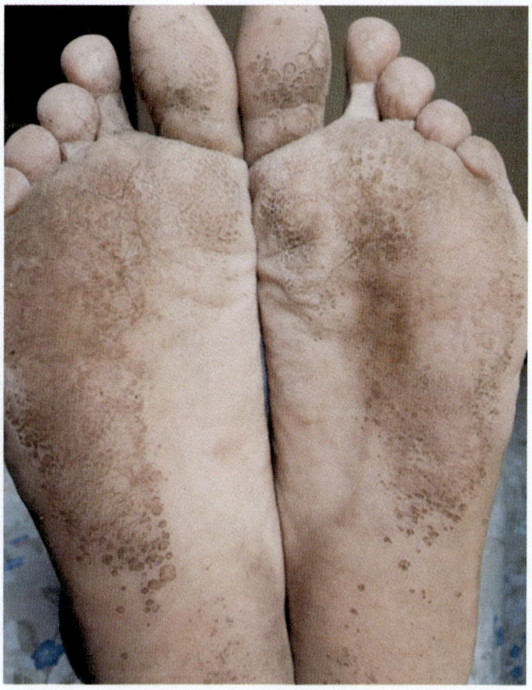

Figure 3.14: Pitted keratolysis

aluminium chloride, potassium permanganate soaks, topical antibiotics (fusidic acid ointment) and topical azoles (clotrimazole and miconazole).

3. *Trichomycosis Axillaris*

It is a corynebacterial infection (Corynebacterium tenuis, C. flavescens) of hair shaft of axilla, pubic region and intergluteal area. It is characterized by presence of yellow, red or black nodular thickening or concretions on hair shaft with malodour and yellow-brown staining of clothes (Figure 3.15). Treatment includes shaving of hair, antiperspirants (aluminium chloride), antiseptic (benzoyl peroxide) and topical antibacterial (clindamycin, erythromycin, fusidic acid).

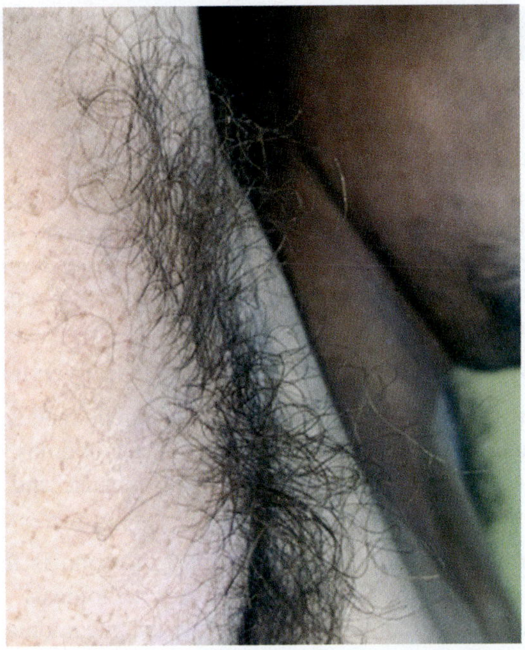

Figure 3.15: Trichomycosis axillaris

PSEUDOMONAS AERUGINOSA INFECTION

It is an aerobic gram negative bacilli commonly affecting immunocompromised patients. Following diseases occur due to Pseudomonas infection:

1. **Green nail syndrome:** Chronic paronychia, distal onycholysis and greenish discoloration of nail.
2. **Tropical immersion foot:** Pseudomonas toe web space infection, characterized by sharply marginated painful erosions of web space with maceration.
3. **Hot tub folliculitis:** Pseudomonas folliculitis is caused by *P. aeruginosa* and occurs after exposure to poorly chlorinated hot tubs, whirlpools or swimming pools. Clinical manifestations include erythematous, follicular pustules and vesiculo-pustules that occur commonly on the trunk, buttocks, and legs and develop within 1 to 2 days after exposure. Mild constitutional symptoms may be present. Urinary tract infection and pneumonia are serious complications that can occur. Lesions generally subside spontaneously over 7 to 10days. Antipseudomonal antibiotic therapy (i.e. ciprofloxacin, aminoglycoside and antipseudomonal penicillin) may be necessary in severe cases.
4. **Ecthyma gangrenosum:** It usually occurs in neutropenic patients and presents as erythematous ulcerated lesion with blackish discoloration in skin folds. Treatment includes antipseudomonal antibiotics (ceftazidime, cefepime, ciprofloxacin, penicillin, gentamycin, tobramycin and carbapenem) and 1% acetic acid dressing.

MRSA (Methicillin Resistant Staphylococcus Aureus)

It is major nosocomial infection due to overuse and indiscriminate use of systemic antibiotics, causing significant morbidity and mortality in hospitals. The common reservoir sites are anterior nares, axilla, perineal and web spaces. Following standard protocols during care of patients including aseptic precautions during handling of indoor patients in ICUs and appropriate treatment may reduce MRSA related infection rate. Recommended antibiotics for MRSA are linezolid, cotrimoxazole, vancomycin, daptomycin, doxycycline and clindamycin.

CUTANEOUS BOTRYOMYCOSIS (Bacterial Pseudomycosis or pyoderma vegetans or actinophytosis)

It is commonly caused by *Staphylococcus aureus* and occasionally by *Streptococcus,* Pseudomonas and *E. coli.* It is a chronic granulomatous disease with sinuses draining granules, mimicking actinomycosis. The patient presents with subcutaneous nodules, abscesses, ulcers and sinuses discharging purulent material over genitals, hand and feet. Treatment includes antibiotics like flucloxacillin and erythromycin.

CUTANEOUS ANTHRAX (Hide porter disease)

It is the most common and least dangerous form of anthrax infection (zoonotic infection) caused by endospores of Bacillus anthracis. Bacillus anthracis is a gram positive, capsulated, spore forming organism. It has two toxins, oedema toxin, a calmodulin dependent adenylate cyclase (inhibitor of neutrophilic function) and lethal toxin, a zinc metalloproteinase (inhibitor of mitogen activated protein kinase). Clinical features include painless blister with central black eschar and erythema with swelling in surrounding area (Figure 3.16). In some patients, it may form a large necrotic ulcer with reginal lymphadenopathy. Gram stain shows gram positive bacilli arranged in linear chain arrangement. Treatment includes fluoroquinolones (ciprofloxacin), doxycycline, penicillin (amoxicillin or penicillin G) and clindamycin.

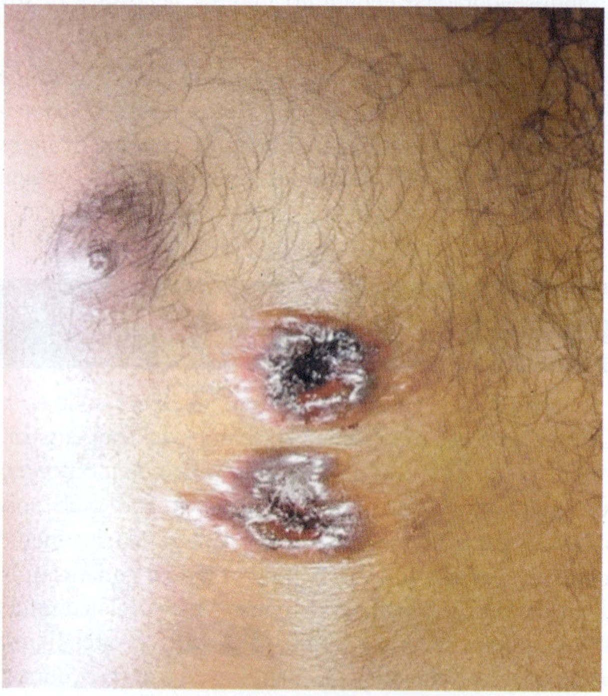

Figure 3.16: Cutaneous anthrax

BACILLARY ANGIOMATOSIS (Epithelioid angiomatosis)

It is caused by Bartonella henselae or Bartonella quintana, usually seen in immunocompromised individuals. Clinically it presents as pyogenic granuloma or haemangioma like papulonodular lesions due to vascular proliferation in skin, mucosa and internal organs.

Diagnosis can be done by histopathology which shows vascular proliferation surrounded with neutrophils. Bacilli can be demonstrated by Warthin-starry stain. Treatment includes erythromycin, tetracycline, ciprofloxacin and cotrimoxazole.

ERYSIPELOID

It is caused by Erysipelothrix rhusiopathiae due to direct contact with infected meat or bone of animals (poultry and sheep). It presents in three forms:

1. Localized cutaneous or erysipeloid of Rosenbach
2. Diffuse cutaneous form
3. Systemic form

Cutaneous lesions present with painful well demarcated bright dusky red edematous plaque, spreads centrifugally over hands which resolves leaving hyperpigmentation. Sometimes they present with vesicle and bulla formation. Treatment includes penicillin and cephalosporin.

MENINGOCOCCAEMIA

It is a severe form of a disseminated meningococcal infection characterized by fever, headache, nausea and vomiting with skin rash. Transient erythematous morbilliform rash, petechiae, haemorrhagic bulla, angular cutaneous infarcts and vasculitis are seen. Treatment includes, penicillin, ceftriaxone and cefotaxime. Two days of rifampicin prophylaxis is recommended for close contacts.

MELIOIDOSIS

Melioidosis (Whitmore disease) and glanders disease have similar clinical presentation and both are caused by Burkholderia species.

It is an endemic tropical disease caused by Burkholderia pseudomallei mainly seen in south east Asia and occurs in workers in paddy fields and travellers to endemic area, especially in immunocompromised patients. It presents in different clinical forms;

1. **Asymptomatic or asymptomatic seroconversion**
2. **Localized infection:** It is due to direct inoculation of organism resulting in formation of nodules, ulcers, abscesses. Patient may have fever, malaise and muscle pain.
3. **Pulmonary infection:** Pulmonary infection is the most common clinical presentation of melioidosis which presents with mild bronchitis to severe pneumonia. It may mimic tuberculosis in chronic cases.
4. **Disseminated infection:** It presents with abscesses in different organs like skin, lymph node, muscle, bone, brain, liver, spleen, lungs and may develop septicaemia.

Diagnosis: Diagnosis is made by culture.

Treatment: Ceftazidime is the drug of choice. Other treatment option includes cotrimoxazole and surgical drainage of abscesses.

Glanders disease is caused by Burkholderia mallei which is clinically similar to melioidosis and treatment option also same.

Clostridium	Yaws
Acinetobacter	Pinta
Glanders	Mycoplasma
Rhinoscleroma	Chlamydia

CHAPTER 4 Viral Infections

Contents

Virus is made up of either RNA or DNA enclosed in a protein shell called capsid. Viruses are classified based on their genome (DNA or RNA), the nature of their capsid and the presence of envelop. Accordingly they are grouped as poxviruses, herpesviruses, human papillomaviruses, myxoviruses etc. The common skin diseases caused by these viruses are herpes simplex, herpes zoster, Molluscum contagiosum, varicella and warts.

Classification of herpes family virus and related diseases are described in Table 4.1.

HERPES SIMPLEX

Introduction/Etiology/Epidemiology

Herpes simplex is caused by herpes simplex virus, which is a double stranded DNA virus having 2 antigenic types: HSV-1 and HSV-2.

HSV-1 causes facial/non-genital herpes while HSV-2 causes genital herpes, although there is considerable overlap in disease manifestations.

Table 4.1: Classification of herpes virus family affecting human beings

Family	*Virus*
Alpha herpesviridae	Human Simplex Virus 1 (HSV-1) • Orolabial herpes (cold sore) • Eczema herpeticum (Kaposi varicelliform eruption) • Herpetic whitlow • Genital herpes • Herpes gladiatorum • Herpetic keratitis • Herpes encephalitis • Eczema herpeticum
	Human Simplex Virus 2 (HSV-2) • Genital herpes
	Varicella Zoster Virus (VZV) • Varicella • Herpes zoster (Shingles)

Beta herpesviridae	Cytomegalovirus (CMV) • Chronic mucosal ulceration
	Human Herpes Virus 6 (HHV-6) • Roseola infantum/exanthem subitum/ sixth disease • Pityriasis rosea
	Human Herpes Virus 7 (HHV-7) • Pityriasis rosea
Gamma herpesviridae	Epstein Barr Virus (EBV) • Infectious mononucleosis (kissing disease, Glandular fever) • Oral Hairy Leukoplakia (OHL) • Lymphoma
	Human Herpes Virus 8 (HHV-8) • Kaposi sarcoma

- Primary infection is acquired when a non-immune child is exposed to contaminated saliva or secretions from the pharynx, genitalia or eyes from close personal contact.
- Source of infection may be clinical cases or asymptomatic virus shedders.
- Trauma facilitates transmission.
- Autoinoculation may also occur.
- Neonatal HSV infection occurs during child birth through an infected maternal genital tract.
- Congenital HSV infection can occur as a result of ascending infection in utero.
- HSV infections are uncommon under 6 months of age due to passive transfer of maternal antibodies.
- HSV-2 is mostly seen in sexually active adults.

Pathogenesis

After exposure, the virus causes primary infection and viral replication occurs at the site of infection. After recovery, the virus is transported by the nerve fibres to the dorsal root ganglion, where it remains latent.

On reactivation, the virus travels back down the sensory nerve and reinfects the epithelial cells at the nerve ending in epidermis.

Viral shedding may occur with no apparent lesion due to minimal viral replication in the epithelium.

Histopathology

Ballooning of cells, enlargement of nucleus, margination of chromatin, cytoplasmic vacuolation, multinucleated giant cells and eosinophilic viral inclusion bodies in the center of the nucleus which is surrounded by a halo are characteristic features which are seen in epithelial cells.

Clinical Features

Primary Infection

Herpetic Gingivostomatitis

- Infection is mostly due to HSV-1.
- Vesicles may occur on mucocutaneous junction, palate, gingiva, buccal mucosa, pharynx or perorally on the chin, nose and cheeks.
- Vesicles may rupture to form grouped shallow ulcers with exudative base and erythematous halo.
- Patient may have tender cervical lymphadenopathy, fever or halitosis.
- Dehydration may occur as oral intake is poor.

Herpes Genitalia (Primary)

- Most cases are seen in young sexually active individuals but possibility of child abuse should be considered in younger children.
- It is mostly caused by HSV-2 but sometimes by HSV-1.
- In male homosexuals, herpes simplex is common in the perianal area and may extend into the rectum.
- The lesions are more extensive in females due to larger surface area of skin and mucous membrane around genitals.
- Incubation period is 2-7 days.
- During primary attack erythematous papules are formed, which rapidly progress to vesicles. These vesicles rupture and form shallow, grouped, non-indurated ulcers.
- Painful shallow ulcers are seen on shaft, glans and prepuce of penis in males and on vulva, vagina and cervix in females.

Herpes Keratitis

- It may occur due to inoculation from digital lesions.
- Redness, watering, discharge, itching, swelling, pain and photophobia may be seen.
- Iridocyclitis, uveitis and corneal scarring may occur.

Neonatal Herpes Infection

- It is acquired either through birth passage or contact with infected person.

- Dissemination of infection may result in seizures, respiratory distress, hepatosplenomegaly with hepatitis and thrombocytopenia.

Herpetic Whitlow and Hand Lesions (Traumatic or Inoculation Herpes)

- Usually seen with herpetic gingivostomatitis due to autoinoculation from fingers or thumb sucking or nail biting.
- In teenage children and adults, hand infections may be secondary to primary genital infections.
- Finger (distal pulp) is the most commonly affected site.
- Vesicles in heavily keratinised tissue like palms may coalesce and resolve without breaking.
- It is important to distinguish herpes simplex viral infection from bacterial infections of hand to avoid unnecessary surgery.

Herpes Encephalitis

- Herpes encephalitis should be suspected in a febrile child with focal seizures, focal neurological signs and progressive decrease in level of consciousness.
- Skin lesions may not be prominently present.

Herpes Gladiatorum

- It is caused by HSV-1. It is common in rugby, football, and wrestling players.
- Clinically, it presents with painful blisters on neck, face, chest or legs with lymphadenopathy.

Disseminated HSV Infection

- Predisposing conditions include malnutrition, concomitant infections like measles, pertussis or *H. influenzae* and immunocompromised state or in neonates.
- Disseminated infection may involve liver, lungs, adrenals, pancreas, bowel, kidneys, bone marrow and central nervous system.

Recurrent Infection

- After primary infection, virus remains latent in the body and there may not be any lesion for the whole life. Recurrences may be observed in 30-50% cases of oral herpes, but are more frequent after genital herpes infection, developing in 95% of those with type 2 HSV compared with 50% in individuals with type 1 infection.
- Factors implicated in reactivation include emotional stress, local trauma, concurrent infections, dental or surgical procedures, pre menstruation period and UV radiation etc.

Herpes labialis (Recurrent)

- Prodrome of irritation, tingling, pain, numbness and itching occurs at the affected site before onset of lesions in recurrent herpes labialis (Figure 4.1).

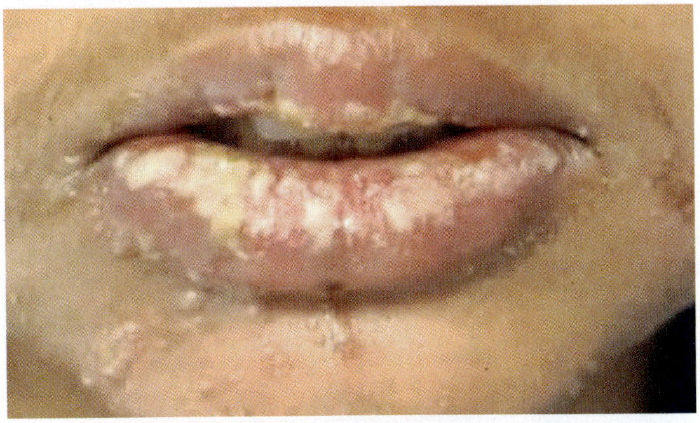

Figure 4.1: Herpes labialis

- There are closely grouped vesicles on an erythematous base, mostly on vermilion border of lips and around mouth.
- Recurrences of herpes labialis may be prevented or reduced in intensity by the use of topical sunscreen.
- Recurrent lesions are less severe, more localized and heal rapidly in 7-10 days.

Herpes Genitalis (Recurrent)

- Recurrences are fairly common occurring 2-6 times per year. Recurrent genital herpes presents as grouped small vesicles which form non-indurated ulcers on glans and shaft of penis in males and on labia, vagina and cervix in females.
- Pain, fever, itching, headache, malaise and myalgia may accompany the lesions.
- There is an increased risk of HIV and other sexually transmitted diseases (STDs) in patients, so a complete STD workup should be done.
- Recurrent infections occur for shorter duration, are less intense and without systemic manifestations.

Diagnosis

- The diagnosis is usually made clinically based on clinical morphology and distribution of lesions. Laboratory investigations are useful when the diagnosis is not certain.

- **Tzanck smear findings in herpes virus infection:** It is prepared after scrapping the base of active lesion. The typical features include characteristic multinucleated syncytial giant cells (Figure 4.2) and also the acantholytic cells. The cells appear inflated ("ballooning degeneration") and may grow tremendously, up to 60-80 microns in diameter. The giant cells have a tadpole, bipolar, or irregular teardrop shape with a smooth border as compared to the jagged configuration of abraded squamous epithelial cells. Syncytial giant cells contain multiple nuclei (many with 8 or more) and these nuclei have variable size and shape and fit together in a jigsaw puzzle like fashion. Intranuclear inclusion bodies surrounded by subtle clear halo are characteristic of herpetic infection, but are often difficult to locate.

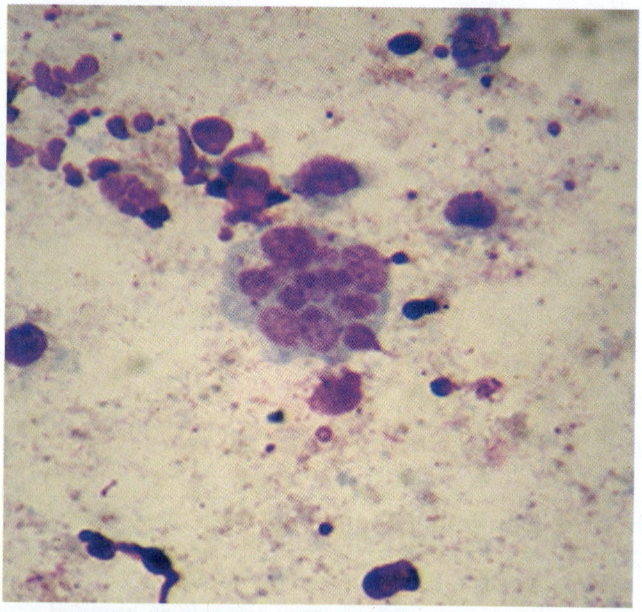

Figure 4.2: Tzanck smear showing multinucleated giant cell

- Electron microscopy and immunofluorescent antibody staining of the material obtained from the floor of the lesion is also helpful.
- PCR on scraping from the floor of the lesion may also be done.
- Viral isolation in cell culture.

Complications

- Secondary bacterial infection.
- Encephalitis.
- Meningism.
- Hepatitis.
- Radiculopathy.
- Erythema multiforme (Herpes-associated).
- Leukoderma.
- Atrophy and scarring.
- Phimosis.

Differential Diagnosis

- Aphthous stomatitis.
- Herpangina.
- Stevens-Johnson syndrome.
- Streptococcal infection.
- Infectious mononucleosis.
- Diphtheria.
- Oral candidiasis.
- Behçet's disease.
- Bullous impetigo.

Treatment

- Supportive therapy includes analgesics, local hygiene and antibiotics to prevent secondary infection.
- Specific treatment includes oral acyclovir, which is a nucleoside analogue and interferes with viral replication. Treatment should be started as early as possible because it acts only during active viral replication which peaks during the first 48 hours.
- It is given in a dose of 200 mg five times a day for children more than 2 years of age and 100 mg five times a day for children of less than 2 years of age for 5 days. Adult dose is 400 mg three times a day for 7 days.
- Dose should be modified in renal dysfunction.
- Valaciclovir and famciclovir have an advantage of twice/thrice daily dose regimen.
- Foscarnet and cidofovir have been used in cases of drug resistance especially in HIV positive patients.
- In recurrent infections which occur at monthly intervals or more frequently, acyclovir prophylaxis may be given as 200 mg four times a day in children and 400 mg three times a day in adults, gradually decreased to once a day. Therapy should be interrupted every 6 months to see if the frequency of recurrences has decreased.
- Intravenous acyclovir is indicated for mucocutaneous herpes simplex virus infections in immunocompromised patients in a dose of 5-10 mg/kg IV 8 hourly for 7 days.

Eczema Herpeticum (Kaposi varicelliform eruption)

- It is a severe, life threatening, disseminated form of herpes simplex virus 1 infection. It is usually seen in immunocompromised patient with underlying diseases like immune bullous disease, atopic dermatitis, erythroderma, Darier's disease or psoriasis.
- Typical lesions are sudden onset of monomorphic vesicles, angulated hemorrhagic crusts, punched out erosions with systemic symptoms like fever. It is a life threatening disease due to high mortality.

VARICELLA (CHICKENPOX)

Varicella is a common infectious disease of childhood. It is the primary infection with varicella zoster virus (VZV) that mainly affects young children and presents with a vesicular eruption.

Epidemiology

- Most cases of chickenpox are seen before 20 years of age, only 2% occur in adults.
- Over half of primary infections occur before the age of 5 and 85% cases occur before puberty.
- Complication rate is more when the infection occurs in adulthood.
- Substantial morbidity and mortality can occur when chickenpox occurs in immunocompromised patients, like those with HIV, leukemia, congenital immunodeficiency syndromes, patients on high dose of steroids and neonates.

Etiopathogenesis

- Causative agent is a DNA virus known as varicella zoster virus (human herpes virus 3).
- Incubation period is typically 14 to 16 days (range 10-21 days) from exposure to onset of symptoms.
- Transmission of infection occurs by respiratory droplets, which are shed by patients during prodrome of illness and early stage of the eruption. Few cases also occur by direct and indirect contact.
- Children are contagious from 2 days before to 5 days after the onset of eruption, a total of 6-7 days.
- The disease becomes non-contagious after scab formation.
- Completely dry scabs are not infectious.

Clinical Features

- Prodrome lasts for 2-3 days, may range from asymptomatic to severe illness with fever, cough, malaise or sore throat. In young children, prodrome is usually absent.
- Eruption consists of erythematous macules, which rapidly progress to papules and vesicles on an erythematous base (dew drop on rose petal) (Figure 4.3). Vesicles become cloudy and form umbilicated pustules, which dry and form crust.
- New crops of lesions continue to appear for upto 7 days and lesions in various stages of development are seen at the same time (pleomorphic eruption), which is a distinctive feature of chickenpox.

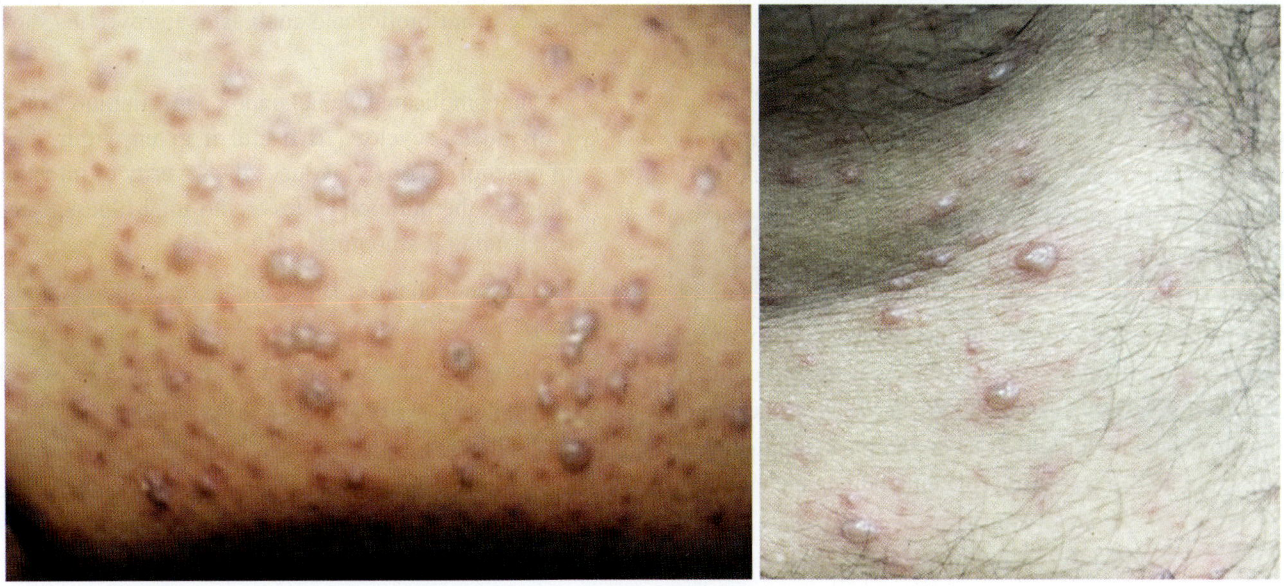

Figure 4.3: Chickenpox with umbilicated vesiculsar lesions

- Eventually all lesions undergo crusting, which takes anywhere between 2-12 days.
- Distribution of lesions is centripetal, i.e., mostly on the chest and proximal parts of limbs. Smaller numbers of lesions are seen on the distal extremities, face, scalp, palms, soles and in oral mucosa, chiefly over the palate. Sometimes few lesions may be seen in other mucosal areas like pharynx, conjunctiva, vagina etc.
- Pruritus varies from mild to severe.
- Second attack of varicella is rare, they may occur in immunocompromised individuals. In these instances, the lesions may be large and seen at the same stage of development.

Complications

- An immunocompetent child rarely develops complications.
- Secondary infection, usually by *Staphylococcus aureus* or *Streptococcus* group A.
- Eczematization.
- Pneumonitis.
- Purpura fulminans.
- Encephalitis, ataxia, Reye's syndrome and Guillain-Barré syndrome are rare, but more common in children than adults.
- Hemorrhagic chickenpox.
- Necrotizing fasciitis.
- Disseminated varicella, which may be fatal is seen in neonates born to mothers who have infection 5 days before to 2 days after delivery. When the mother has varicella more than 5 days before delivery, maternal antibodies are formed and provide some protection to the newborn.
- Rare complications are myocarditis, orchitis, nephritis, hepatitis, pancreatitis, appendicitis and ocular keratitis.

VARICELLA IN IMMUNOCOMPROMISED HOST

It is more severe and prolonged in such patients. There is risk of dissemination and involvement of internal organs like lungs, brain, liver and other viscera. There may be hemorrhagic complications leading to mild to severe purpura fulminans and DIC (disseminated intravascular coagulation) which may be fatal.

Diagnosis

Diagnosis is usually made clinically by history and morphology of the lesions.

- Tzanck smear made from scraping the base of the vesicle will show multinucleated giant cells and intranuclear eosinophilic inclusion bodies.
- Examination of vesicular fluid for viral particles under electron microscope.
- Polymerase chain reaction.
- Direct immunofluorescence.
- Viral isolation in cell cultures.
- Serological tests to detect IgG against VZV may be done, but are mainly used to document prior exposure and immunity.

Differential Diagnosis

- Insect bites.
- Rickettsial pox.
- Hand foot and mouth disease.
- Disseminated herpes simplex.
- Pityriasis lichenoides et varioliformis acuta.
- Neonatal syphilis.
- Kaposi's varicelliform eruption (Eczema herpeticum).

Treatment

The patient should be advised to take bed rest and children should not be allowed to go to the school for 7-10 days. Prophylactic antibiotics and analgesic, antipyretics should be given:

- In uncomplicated chickenpox in immunocompetent individuals, acyclovir is useful if given within 24 hours of onset of lesions. It reduces the severity of infection and shortens the duration of fever and total illness. Recovery and healing is smoother.
- Recommended dose: 10-20 mg/kg upto 800 mg orally five times a day for 5 days.
- In immunocompromised patients less than 12 years of age, IV acyclovir is given at 10-20 mg/kg/dose 8 hourly for 7 days.
- Acyclovir is quite useful when given in chickenpox in adults and in immunocompromised patients. The adult

dose consists of acyclovir 800 mg five times a day or valacyclovir 1 g three times a day for 7 days.

- Newer drugs like valaciclovir and famciclovir have better absorption and convenient dosage interval because of longer duration of action.

Prevention

- **Pre-exposure prophylaxis:** Live virus varicella vaccine is available as a monovalent vaccine (Oka strain) and is also available in combination with measles, mumps, rubella and varicella (MMRV) vaccine.
- MMRV vaccine may be given to children from 12 months to 12 years of age.
- Varicella vaccine is recommended for routine administration as two 0.5 ml doses administered subcutaneously to children at 12–15 months and at 4–6 years of age. It is recommended that MMR vaccine and varicella vaccine should be administered either at least 4 weeks apart or simultaneously at different sites.
- CDC recommends that MMR vaccine and varicella vaccine should be administered as separate injections for the first dose in children 12-47 months of age.
- Vaccination with 2 doses, separated by at least 4 weeks (preferably 3 months apart), is also recommended for children, adolescents and adults irrespective of immune status.
- Varicella vaccine is contraindicated in children with cell mediated immune deficiencies but may be given in humoral immune deficiencies. For HIV-infected children with CD4 T lymphocytes greater than 15% and in children with acute lymphoblastic leukemia (they should be in remission with a gap of at least 3 months from cancer chemotherapy), only monovalent varicella vaccine should be administered as 2 doses 3 months apart.
- Varicella vaccine is also recommended in adults (less than 50 years) who lack immunity against varicella virus.
- **Post-exposure prophylaxis:** Specific varicella zoster immune globulin (VZIG) if given within 10 days of contact can reduce the severity of varicella but cannot prevent it.
- Normally other susceptible members of the family should be isolated from the child having active varicella.

Dosage considerations of IV Acyclovir (preferred in immunocompromised patients) according to age is given in Table 4.2:

Table 4.2: Dosage considerations of IV Acyclovir according to age

	< 12 years	*> 12 years*
Mucocutaneous Herpes Simplex Virus Infection	5-10 mg/kg or 250-500 mg/m^2 IV 8 hourly for 7 days	5 mg/kg/day IV divided 8 hourly for 5-7 days
Herpes Zoster	10-20 mg/kg IV 8 hourly for 7 days (In infants 10 mg/kg)	10 mg/kg/day IV divided 8 hourly for 7-10 days
Varicella Zoster	10-20 mg/kg/dose or 500 mg/m^2 IV 8 hourly for 7 days (In infants 10 mg/kg)	10 mg/kg/dose IV 8 hourly for 7 days
Strengths	Injectable solution 50 mg/ml Injection, lyophilized powder for reconstitution 500 mg/vial 1000 mg/vial	
Adverse Effects	Inflammation or phlebitis at injection site (9%) Nausea (7%) Vomiting (7%) Rash or hives (2%) Elevated transaminase levels (1-2%)	

HERPES ZOSTER

Herpes zoster is caused by reactivation of varicella zoster virus (VZV), which remains latent in the sensory ganglia after previous primary infection of chickenpox. It is not very common in children.

Etiopathogenesis

- It is primarily a disease of the adults and elderly, but can occur in children who have had chickenpox early in life.
- It is more common in immunocompromised children.
- Although uncommonly reported in immunocompetent children, it may occur due to intrauterine VZV infection.
- It has been documented at as early as 3 months of age.
- Post herpetic neuralgia does not occur in children, its frequency increases with age.

Clinical Features

- Prodrome is unusual in children, adults have a dull aching pain upto a week preceding the symptoms, in severe cases patient may have fever, headache and malaise.

- Lesions occur as grouped vesicles (Figure 4.4) and sometimes bullae with an erythematous base.
- The striking feature is cut off at the midline.

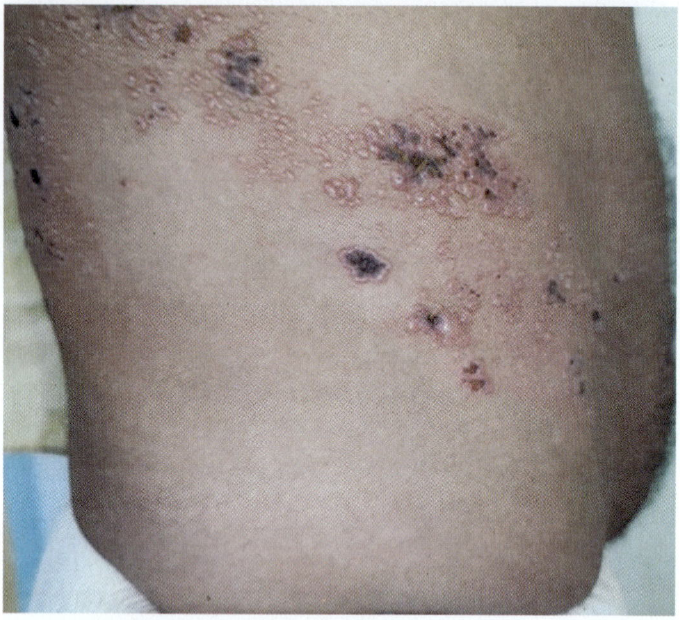

Figure 4.4: Herpes zoster

- Lesions are seen in dermatomal distribution, up to 50% have thoracic dermatome involvement.
- Lesions continue to appear for one week after the onset, the vesicles persist up to 7-10 days and usually heal without scarring in majority of cases in 2-3 weeks.
- The course of disease is milder in children.
- In immunocompromised individuals like HIV patients, malnourished individuals and patients with lymphomas, the lesions may be more severe, ulcerate, involve more than one dermatome and may be bilateral. There may be visceral dissemination too.
- Mucous membranes of the corresponding dermatome are also involved and the patient may have oral, genital or anal ulcers.
- Lymph nodes may be enlarged and tender.

Complications

- Chronic post herpetic neuralgia.
- Involvement of trigeminal nerve can lead to ophthalmoplegia, optic neuritis, corneal ulceration, uveitis, conjunctivitis, keratitis, scleritis and other ocular complications.
- Motor nerve involvement may lead to palsies of corresponding muscles, e.g., Bell's palsy in facial nerve involvement (Figure 4.5), ocular palsies, etc.
- Secondary infection.
- Scar, keloid formation.
- Encephalitis and meningoencephalitis.
- Guillain-Barré syndrome and transverse myelitis.

Diagnosis

- Diagnosis is mainly clinical, by history of pain and morphology of lesions.
- Electron microscopy, immunofluorescent antibody staining and PCR of scraping from the floor of lesion.

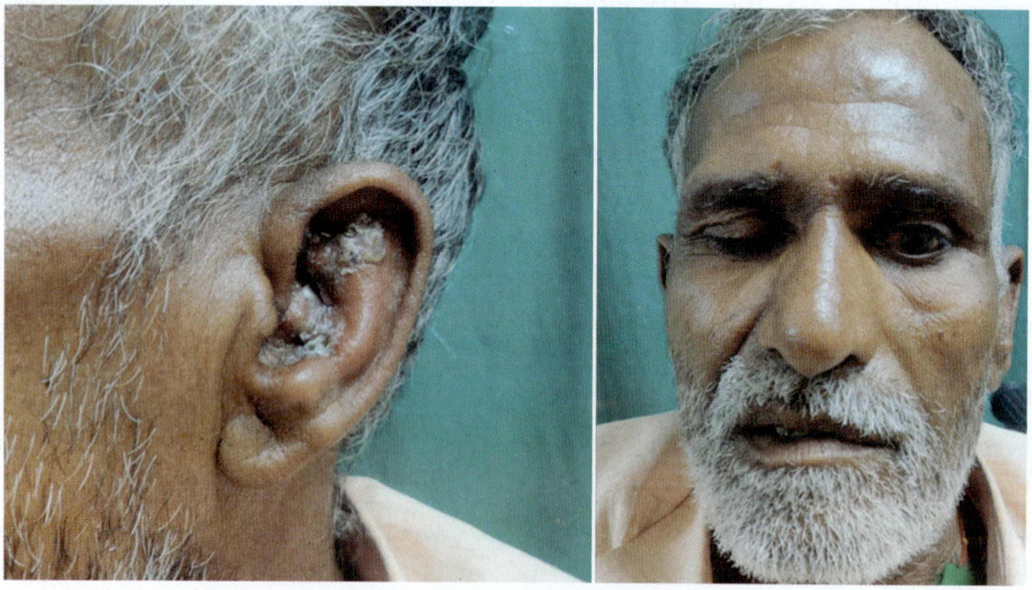

Figure 4.5: Herpes zoster oticus with bell's palsy

Differential Diagnosis

- HSV infection occurring in dermatomal distribution.
- Insect bites, blister beetle dermatitis.
- Allergic contact dermatitis.

Treatment

- In children between the age of 2 and 12 years, who are otherwise healthy, treatment with acyclovir is not required until they develop prodromal symptoms.
- The first line therapy is oral *acyclovir* 10-20 mg/kg upto a maximum dose of 800 mg, five times a day for 7-10 days.
- In immunocompromised patients with severe disease, drug can be given intravenously, in the dose of 10-20 mg/kg every 8 hours for 7-10 days.
- *Valaciclovir* (20 mg/kg three times a day) or *famciclovir* (10 mg/kg three times a day) for 7 days is an alternative choice.
- Use of acyclovir reduces pain, stops progression of the rash, fastens recovery, reduces risk of post herpetic neuralgia and prevents systemic complications and dissemination.
- Secondary infection should be prevented by giving oral antibiotics.
- Oral analgesics may be given for pain relief.
- Application of topical acyclovir or antibiotic cream does not have much role. Topically applied emollients containing aloe-vera and vitamin E are quiet effective in reducing pain and burning.

POST HERPETIC NEURALGIA (PHN)

PHN is persistent pain which occurs after resolution of lesions of herpes zoster. The incidence is 10%–15% of all patients with HZ. Pain associated with herpes zoster has three phases:

1. Acute herpetic neuralgia: Where the pain that accompanies the rash, lasts up to 30 days after the onset of rash.
2. Subacute herpetic neuralgia: Pain lasts for 30 to 120 days after the onset of rash.
3. Post herpetic neuralgia: Pain persists beyond 120 days after the onset of rash.

Most commonly thoracic or the trigeminal nerve, especially the ophthalmic branch is involved. Patient presents with complaints of continuous burning, aching and throbbing pain with hyperaesthesia. Spasmodic shooting or stabbing type of pain or a pruritic "crawling" paraesthesia may also occur. More than 90% of patients with PHN have allodynia (pain evoked by a normally non painful stimuli such as light touch). Sometimes patients with PHN demonstrate areas of anaesthesia as well as deficits of thermal, tactile, pinprick and vibration sensation within the affected dermatomes. PHN may cause sleep disturbances, depression and social isolation.

Pathophysiology

The reactivated virus replicates and migrates down the sensory nerve leading to inflammation, resulting in demyelination, wallerian degeneration and fibrosis of affected nerve. After healing, uninhibited and amplified activity in unmyelinated afferent nerve fibres leads to pain associated with post herpetic neuralgia. Central nerve system also plays a role by overall generalized augmentation in the excitability of spinal cord neurons, leading to enhanced response to any input from nociceptors.

At a cellular level, there is an increase in the number of voltage gated sodium channels, potassium voltage gated channel alterations and upregulation of receptors associated with pain such as transient receptor potential vanilloid 1 (TRPV1).

The factors that play a role in the development of PHN are sensitization and deafferentation. Risk factor for post herpetic neuralgia includes, advanced age, severe prodromal pain, extensive skin rash and immunosuppression.

Treatment

Most common protocol involves the use of gabapentin and a 5% lidocaine patch as first line treatment option and opioids and tricyclic antidepressants (TCA) as second line treatments for PHN.

Calcium Channel Modulators

- Gabapentin
- Pregabalin

They reduce pain by decreasing the calcium influx into the nerve endings and thereby inhibiting the release of excitatory neurotransmitters.

Tricyclic Antidepressants (TCA)

They block norepinephrine and serotonin uptake.

- Amitriptyline- Most widely used TCA in PHN.
- Nortriptyline
- Imipramine
- Desipramine

Amitriptyline is initially given at a dose of 10 to 25 mg orally at bedtime, which is increased by 25 mg every two to four weeks until response is adequate, or until a maximum dose of 150 mg per day is achieved. Adverse effects include - sedation, dry mouth, constipation, sweating, xerostomia, confusion, dysrhythmias, weight gain, dizziness etc.

Opioid

They affect μ receptors. They increase inhibition of norepinephrine and serotonin.

- Oxycodone - 10 – 40 mg every 12 hourly, titrated as required.
- Morphine - 5 – 50 mg every 12 hourly, titrated as required.
- Methadone - 2.5 mg – 10 mg three times a day.
- Tramadol - 50 mg per day, increased to a maximum of 400 mg per day.

Adverse effects include nausea, constipation, sedation, cognitive dysfunction, hormonal changes, skin irritation, vertigo etc.

Topical Agents

- Transdermal buprenorphine patch - 5 – 20 mcg / hour, changed after every three days.
- Transdermal fentanyl patch - 25 mcg / hour to 100 mcg / hour.
- Capsaicin cream 0.025%.
- 5% lidocaine gel.
- Transdermal 5% lidocaine patch.
- Eutectic mixture of local anaesthetics (2.5% lignocaine and 2.5% prilocaine).

Other Systemic Drugs Therapy

- N-methyl-D-aspartate (NMDA) antagonists: Dextromethorphan
- Intravenous lidocaine

Interventional Therapies

1. Epidural injection of a local anaesthetic either intermittently or via continuous catheter.
2. Paravertebral nerve block using repetitive injections of local anaesthetic mixture (bupivacaine 0.5% and clonidine) every 48 hours for three weeks, using a catheter inserted at the T2 -T3 level.
3. Jaipur block consisting of local subcutaneous infiltration of 2% xylocaine, 0.5% bupivacaine and dexamethasone.
4. Radiofrequency ablation using the heat lesioning protocol with temperature at 67 °C or higher.

Other block include sympathetic nerve blocks, intraspinal agents such as opioids and local anaesthetics, intrathecal methylprednisolone, pulsed radiofrequency lesioning and botulinum toxin.

Surgical Ablative Therapy

Surgical ablative therapy includes neurolytic nerve blocks, peripheral neurectomy, trans spinal ganglionectomy, dorsal root entry zone rhizotomy, prefrontal lobotomy and sympathectomy.

Other Therapies

Neuromodulation or spinal cord stimulation, acupuncture, Transcutaneous Electrical Nerve Stimulation (TENS), psychological intervention and vincristine iontophoresis.

FIRST TO SIX DISEASES

The diseases considered as first to sixth diseases which include measles, scarlet fever, rubella duke's disease, erythema infectiosum and roseola infantum are discussed in chapter 18.

POX VIRUS

It is a double stranded DNA virus. Major subtypes of pox virus are:

- Para pox virus ovis (PPOV)- Orf (Ecthyma contagiosum or Contagious pustular dermatitis).
- Para vaccinia virus – Milker's node.
- Molluscum contagiosum – Molluscum contagiosum 1-4.

ORF (Ecthyma Contagiosum or Contagious Pustular Dermatitis)

It is caused by para pox virus, which is primarily a disease of sheep and goats. Orf occurs in sheep handlers, veterinary surgeons. The incubation period is 5–6 days. Fingers and hands are commonly affected. Disease presents as a single, firm, tender, red papule which enlarges to form a haemorrhagic pustule or bulla with central umbilication and crusting (Figure 4.6). A fully developed lesion may show a greyish white ring around central crusting, further surrounded by erythema. Lesion spontaneously resolves in a few weeks.

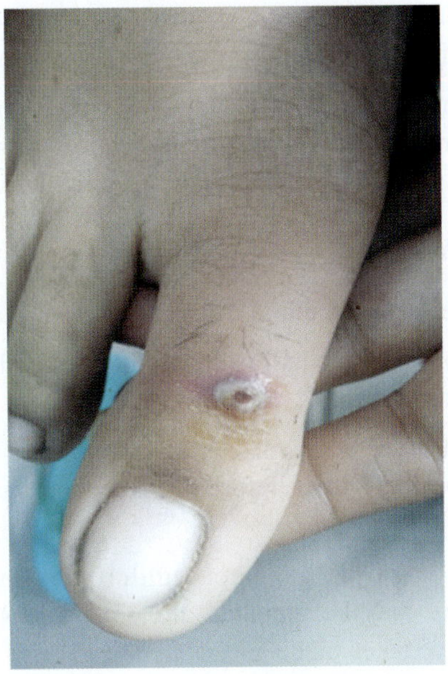

Figure 4.6: ORF (Ecthyma Contagiosum)

Milker's node/Para vaccinia virus

It is caused by parapox virus. Affected animals have sores and ulcers on the mouth. The incubation period is 1–2 weeks. They usually present with single or multiple, flat, red tender papules, usually on hands. As they enlarge, crusting occurs in the center with secondary erythema. Lymphangitis may occur. It is very vascular and are confused with pyogenic granuloma. The disease is self-limiting.

Molluscum Contagiosum

Molluscum contagiosum is a self-limiting viral infection of the skin characterized clinically by asymptomatic shiny, pearly white or skin colored, often umbilicated papules. It is caused by a virus of poxvirus family called molluscum contagiosum virus (MCV 1 to 4). Most infections are due to MCV1 while MCV 2 is seen in HIV infected individuals. The infection is specific to humans and this virus cannot be grown in tissue culture.

Epidemiology

The disease occurs throughout the world. It is rare below one year of age perhaps because of the presence of maternally transmitted immunity and long incubation period. The age of peak incidence is reported as between 2 and 5 years. Transmission occurs by direct skin to skin contact and also by contaminated fomites. Genital molluscum contagiosum may be sexually transmitted.

Pathology

- Cells infected by the virus are distorted and appear as large hyaline bodies (molluscum bodies) which are around 25 μm in diameter and contain cytoplasmic masses of viral material. They are present in large numbers in the centre of the lesion.
- Mild inflammatory infiltrate is seen in the adjacent dermis.

Clinical Features

- Incubation period is between 2 weeks to 6 months.
- Infection mostly occurs in late childhood in the age group of 8-12 years.
- The classical lesion is a shiny, pearly white, dome shaped, umbilicated papule (Figure 4.7A).
- Lesions vary in size from 1 to 10 mm, occasionally giant lesions are seen (Figure 4.7B).

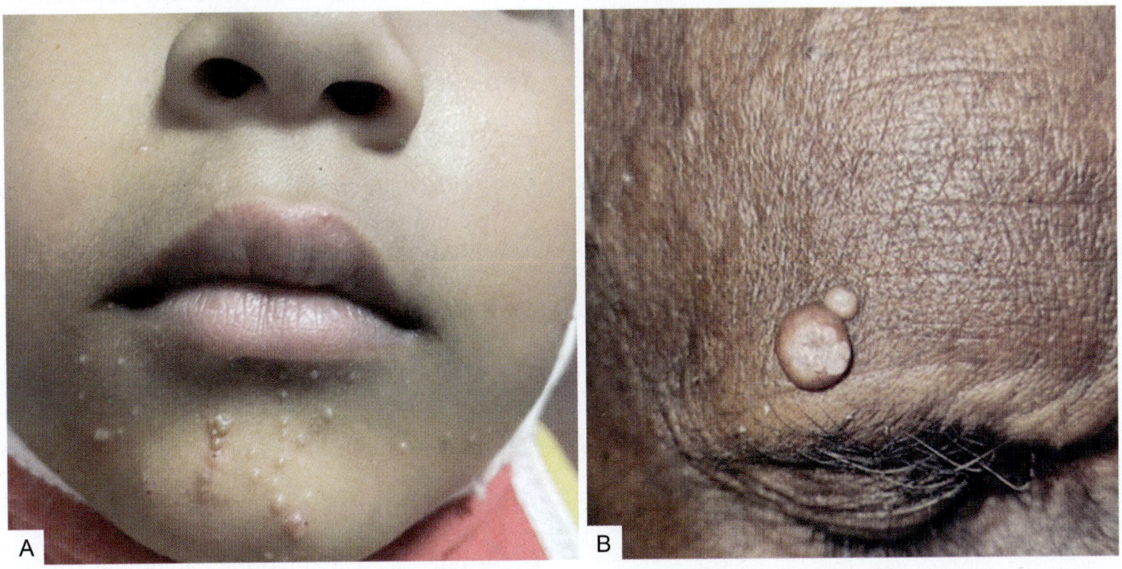

Figure 4.7: Molluscum contagiosum (A) and giant molluscum (B)

- Inflammation, suppuration, crusting and atrophy may be seen.
- Lesions are often distributed on face, trunk, limbs and sites of friction from clothing, e.g., around the neck, axilla.
- Rarely, they may be seen on the tongue, lips or buccal mucosa. Genitalia and perineum may be involved when it is sexually transmitted.
- Larger lesions >1 cm in size are known as giant molluscum and are more common in immunocompromised patients.
- Disseminated lesions (Figure 4.8) can also occur in immunosuppressed individuals.

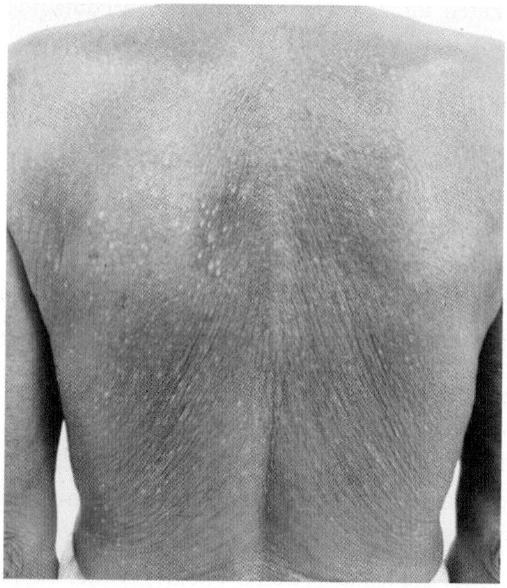

Figure 4.8: Disseminated molluscum contagiosum

- Involvement of limbs is more common in tropical climate, involvement of unusual sites like scalp and face and disseminated infection may be seen in HIV patients, atopics and in patients taking immunosuppressants.
- In most cases, lesions are self-limiting in 6-9 months but in some, they may persist for 3-4 years.

Diagnosis

- The typical skin colored, umbilicated papules are diagnostic clinically.
- Expressed material by a forceps from a lesion shows characteristic molluscum bodies under microscope.
- Large solitary lesions in adults may occasionally persist upto 3-4 years, and can be mistaken for basal cell carcinoma, keratoacanthoma or pyogenic granuloma.

Treatment

- Minor infections may have spontaneous resolution.
- Secondarily infected lesion may require topical antibiotic application.
- Active treatments for MC include destructive methods, e.g., cryotherapy and chemical cauterization, topical cytotoxic therapy, immunomodulators or antiviral preparations.

Cryotherapy

- It is an effective method of treatment.
- Induction of an ice ball is done in the lesion but not on the surrounding skin.
- Application of a cream containing mixture of prilocaine and lidocaine 1 hour before the procedure may be helpful in reducing pain.
- Patient should be kept under observation, and procedure may be repeated after 3-4 weeks if failure or recurrence takes place.

Chemical Cauterization

- Chemical cauterization with caustics like phenol, trichloroacetic acid (30-50%), KOH (10-20%) and silver nitrate (1%) are an effective and well-tolerated method.
- It is to be applied to each lesion individually with a pointed stick or with a 26-gauge needle.
- Care should be taken to remove excess of phenol by touching the stick at the rim of the container, before application to avoid spilling of phenol over the surrounding skin.
- Application should be repeated after 3-7 days.
- Parents of young children should be told that the procedure may require further application if failure or recurrence occurs.

Topical Cytotoxic Therapy

- It is done with 0.5% podophyllotoxin.
- Epidermal irritation disrupts the protein membrane around the molluscum, thereby facilitating an immune response.

Immunomodulators

- Imiquimod stimulates release of INF-α, TNF-α and IL-6, hence may be effective in clearing lesions.
- It can be applied twice or thrice weekly at home by parents.

Antiviral Agents

Cidofovir is a nucleotide analogue of deoxycytidine monophosphate. Topical formulation of cidofovir has been successfully used in molluscum contagiosum, but it is not available commercially due to its high cost.

Other methods include curettage, use of local tretinoin, etc.

PRACTICAL GUIDELINES FOR TREATMENT OF MOLLUSCUM INFECTION

Out of all the mentioned therapies, chemical cauterization by phenol is simple, inexpensive and most practical. Children are usually apprehensive for any procedure including the application of phenol, especially if done by medical personnel. If the parents are co-operative, they may be taught to apply phenol at home. They should be strictly told that phenol should be kept away from the reach of children. Care should be taken to avoid application around the eye, which should preferentially be done by a dermatologist.

INFECTIOUS MONONUCLEOSIS

Infectious mononucleosis is an acute febrile illness with sore throat and cervical lymphadenopathy. It is caused by Epstein-Barr virus. In developed communities, early childhood infection is less frequent and primary infection occurs commonly in early adult life, when kissing is the usual route of infection (kissing disease), though occasional droplet spread may occur. Primary infections in childhood are either asymptomatic or mild.

Clinical Features

It is characterized by fever, sore throat and lymphadenopathy. Malaise and fatigue is often present and splenomegaly is observed in acute cases.

An exanthem develops between the fourth and sixth day, which is commonly a macular or maculopapular eruption of the trunk or upper arms. It may also involve the face, forearms, thighs or legs occasionally. Morbilliform or scarlatiniform eruptions and acute urticaria may be occasionally seen. Skin lesions fade after a few days. With use of oral antimicrobials like amoxycillin, penicillin, tetracyclines and azithromycin, an extensive maculopapular or morbilliform eruption develops in over 90% of cases, 7-10 days after the start of treatment.

Management

- General measures include symptomatic treatment of fever and sore throat.
- An emollient and moderately potent topical steroid may be used for symptomatic skin lesions.

CYTOMEGALOVIRUS (CMV)

Cytomegalovirus infections are common throughout the world. There are several ways of transmitting CMV which are mostly age dependent.

- Intrauterine transmission occurs in 0.1-1.0% of births.
- Perinatal and neonatal infections arise as a result of exposure to infectious cervical secretions in the birth canal or from infected breast milk.
- Preschool children may acquire CMV from oral secretions or urine of other infected infants.
- At an older age, sexual transmission is important.
- Blood transfusion is also a source of CMV.

Clinical Features

Congenital CMV Infection

- Primary CMV infection can severely affect the fetus and manifest as hepatosplenomegaly, jaundice and purpura. Most cases die within 2 months and survivors are left with severe neurological damage and deafness. A characteristic cutaneous finding is presence of purple or red papules or nodules lasting 4-6 weeks ('blueberry muffin' lesions) which occur due to erythropoietic tissue in the dermis derived from undifferentiated dermal mesenchyme.

Primary Cytomegalovirus Mononucleosis

- In a healthy child, it manifests as fever, lymphocytosis and mildly deranged liver function, lymphadenopathy and splenomegaly. In upto a third of cases, a follicular, maculopapular or rubelliform eruption may develop over legs. Ampicillin may trigger widespread eruption similar to infectious mononucleosis.

Gianotti-Crosti syndrome, papular purpuric 'gloves and socks' syndrome and drug reaction with eosinophilia and systemic symptoms (DRESS) may occur together with CMV infection.

Investigations

Histologically, typical intranuclear inclusions surrounded by a clear halo in enlarged cells are seen. Virus culture from throat washings, urine, bronchoalveolar lavage fluid, blood or biopsy material is carried out in human embryo fibroblast cells. It produces cytopathic effect, seen as 'owl eye' nuclear inclusions. Rapid methods include viral DNA detection by PCR and detection of CMV antigenaemia. Primary infection show CMV IgM and IgG antibodies. Congenital CMV can be detected by PCR analysis of saliva in neonates and confirmed by virus isolation or the presence of CMV IgM antibody within 3 weeks of birth.

Management

In severe CMV infection or retinitis, ganciclovir and foscarnet have been used with some success. Valganciclovir, a prodrug of ganciclovir, is used as prophylactic in transplant recipients and has also been reported to be effective as treatment for acute or recurrent CMV disease.

WARTS (VERRUCA)

Warts are due to a benign epithelial hyperplasia of skin and mucosa, presenting as discrete hyperkeratotic, asymptomatic papules on skin and as soft pinkish lesions on mucosa.

Etiopathogenesis

Verruca is caused by an unenveloped, double stranded DNA virus known as human papilloma virus (HPV). Around more than 150 subtypes have been identified so far.

HPV subtypes associated with various clinical infections are:

Infection	*HPV Subtype*
Common warts	1, 2, 4, 7, 27, 57
Plantar/palmar warts	1, 4, 27, 57
Plane warts	3, 10, 28
Anogenital warts	6, 11, 16, 18
Epidermodysplasia verruciformis	3, 5, 8
Heck's disease	13, 37
Laryngeal papilloma	6, 11
Verrucous carcinoma	16, 18
Butcher's wart	8

Epidemiology

- HPV is distributed worldwide, affects all ages and both sexes, but it is less common in infants and young children. Incidence increases in school going children with peak in adolescence and early adulthood.
- It is more frequently seen in lower socioeconomic class.

Infectivity and Transmission

- Direct contact from person to person.
- Contact with contaminated surfaces and objects.
- Loss of the epidermal continuity by trauma or maceration is important for transmission.
- Autoinoculation (chewing or sucking the fingers in children causes perioral, subungual and periungual warts).
- Plantar warts are found more commonly in people involved in barefoot activities, including sharing of bath showers and swimming pools.

Latency and Incubation Period

- Incubation period varies from 3 weeks to 8 months. Virus has the ability to remain latent for long period of time.

Clinical Features

Clinical features vary with the type of warts.

Common Wart (Verruca Vulgaris)

- Common warts are mainly caused by HPV-2, other types like 1, 4, 27 and 57 may also be associated.
- Lesions are skin colored, single or multiple, firm, rough, papular lesions of variable sizes from less than 1mm to over 1cm (Figure 4.9).
- They are commonly seen on the backs of hands, fingers (Figure 4.10) and knees. They occur more commonly at the sites of injury (Pseudo-Koebner phenomenon) due to autoinoculation.
- Warts are more common in butchers, fish handlers and shaving may spread the warts in the beard region.

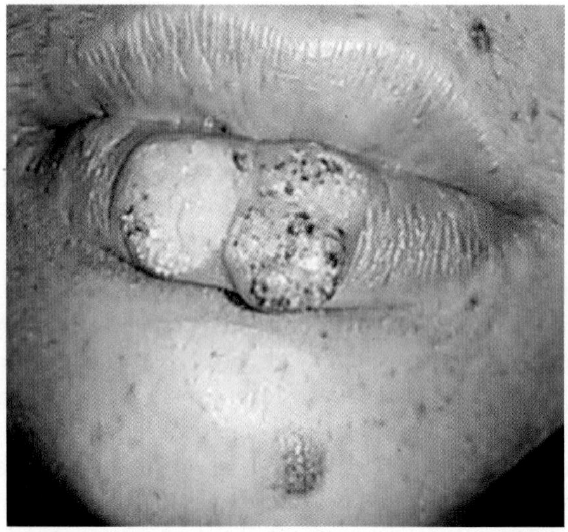

Figure 4.9: Common warts on lips

Plane Warts (Verruca Plana)

- Plane warts are mainly caused by HPV type 3 and 10.
- They are flat-topped, skin colored or slightly pigmented papules, with little hyperkeratosis, round to polygonal in shape and vary in size from 1-5 mm (Figure 4.11).
- Common sites include face and dorsum of hands, they may be few in number to hundreds.
- Koebner phenomenon is more commonly seen in plane warts.

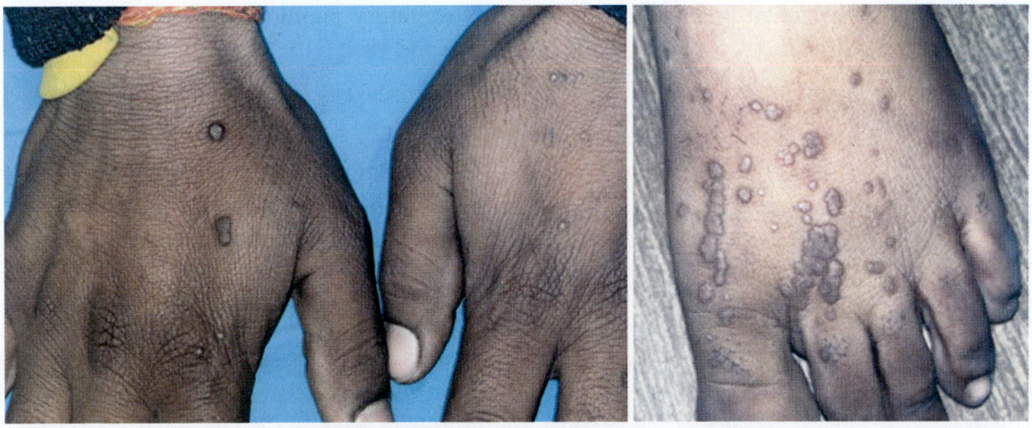

Figure 4.10: Verruca vulgaris on hand and feet

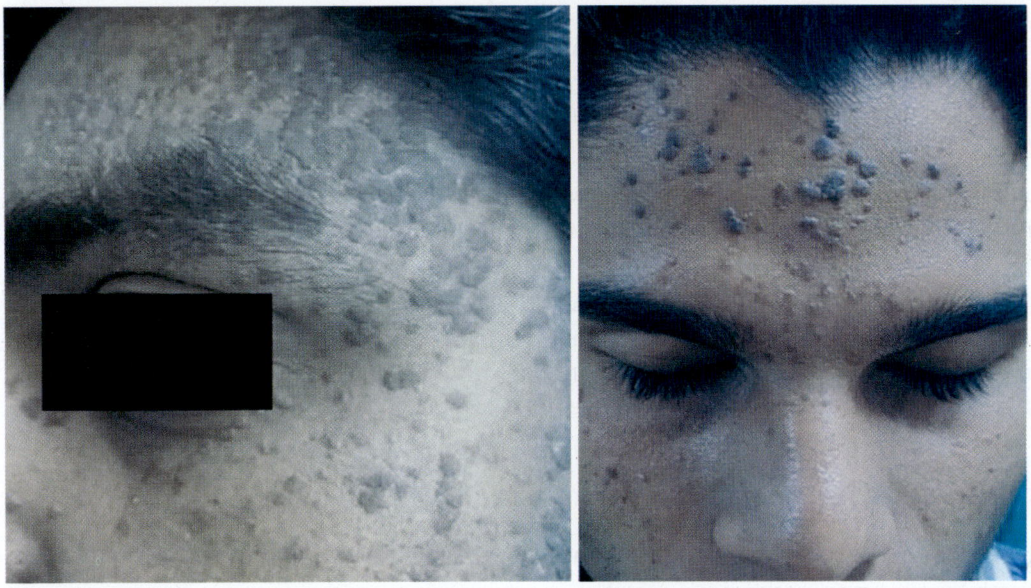

Figure 4.11: Plane warts

Plantar Warts (Figure 4.12)

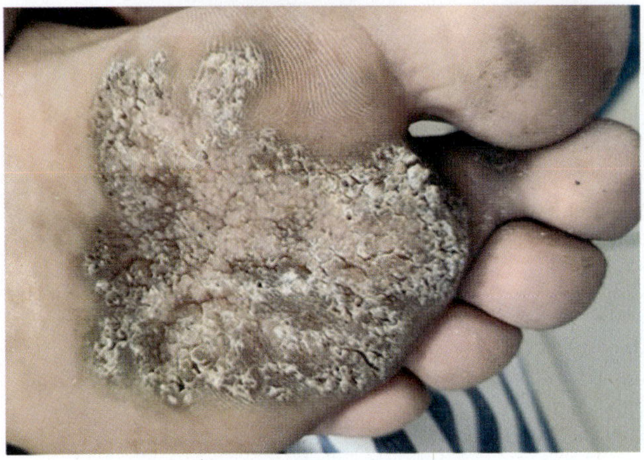

Figure 4.12: Plantar warts

- They are caused by HPV type 1, 2, 4, 27 or 57.
- Trauma is important for the transmission.
- They occur most frequently on weight bearing areas or pressure points, e.g., heels, under metatarsal heads etc.
- Plantar warts first appear as small sago grain like lesions which soon develop into hyperkeratotic, verrucous, rounded lesion surrounded by smooth collar of thickened horny tissue.
- They have to be differentiated from callosities. In warts, epithelial ridges from the surrounding skin are abruptly broken and are not continued on the surface of the wart, while in callosities they are continuous. Further, in warts, paring the surface with a scalpel will show bleeding points, which are tips of elongated dermal papillae. Also in plantar warts, there is pain on vertical pressure over the lesion

whereas; while in callosities, horizontal pressure causes pain.

- Two types of plantar warts are seen:
  - ***Myrmecia warts (HPV-1 MC)***: Deep seated, usually single and dome shaped.
  - ***Mosaic warts (HPV-2 MC)***: Superficial, multiple and confluent group of warts.

Anogenital Warts (Figure 4.13)

- They are uncommon in children and caused mainly by HPV type 6, 11, 16 and 18.
- Mode of transmission in adults is by sexual contact, but non-sexual transmission is also a possibility by inoculation from cutaneous warts or by sharing infected fomites, e.g. bath tubs, towels and door handles etc. if anogenital warts are present in children, personal or family history of warts should be taken, in addition to complete physical examination of the child.
- Perinatal transmission may lead to anogenital warts upto 2 years of age, beyond which sexual abuse should be considered.
- Clinically, flesh colored papules or verrucous lesions are seen at anal margin or situated some distance away from anal margin on buttocks in case of anal warts while in case of genital warts they are present on prepuce, glans or vulva.

Laryngeal Warts/ Laryngeal papillomatosis

- Laryngeal papillomatosis also known as recurrent respiratory papillomatosis is associated with HPV 6,11, 16 and 18.
- The disease is classified as childhood onset type and adult onset type.
- Laryngeal warts are rare in children. They may be caused due to infected maternal passage during vaginal delivery while in adults, the route of transmission in adults is sexual.

Treatment

Warts are self limiting, and do not necessarily require treatment. None of the current treatment are uniformly effective and it is important that patients/parents understand limitation of treatment.

Self Resolution

Warts show spontaneous resolution and 50-65% lesions would disappear without a trace in 6 months to 2 years duration.

Chemical Cauterization

It can be done by using the following:

- Salicylic acid (16.7%) and lactic acid (16.7%) with flexible collodion (Salicylic acid-lactic acid paint).
- Trichloroacetic acid (30%-80%).
- Glutaraldehyde (10%-20%).
- Podophyllotoxin (20%-30%).
- Formalin (2-3% formalin in water).
- Topical 5-fluorouracil (5-FU) 5%.
- Retinoic acid (0.05%).

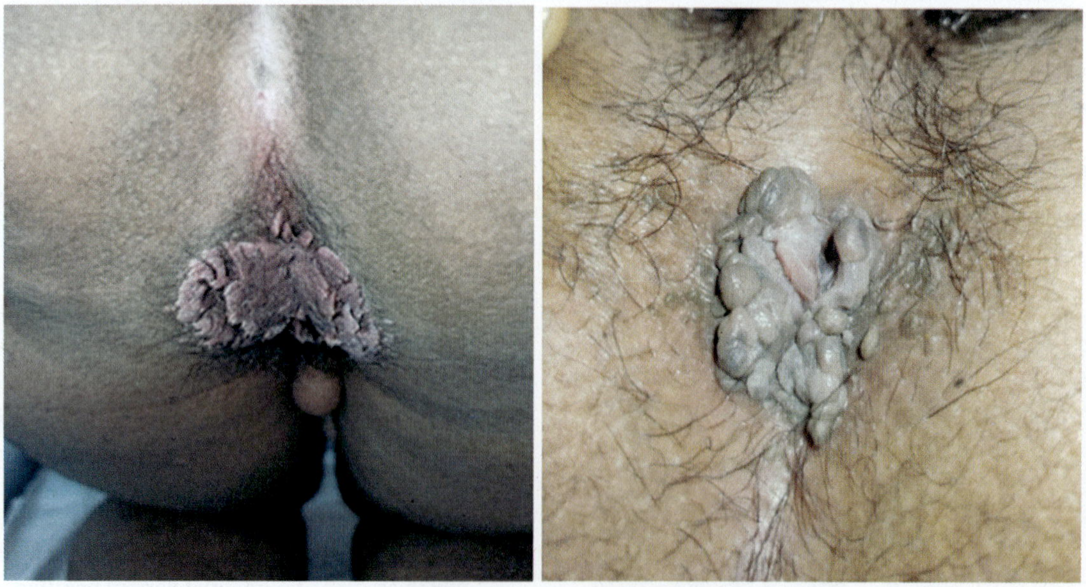

Figure 4.13: Peri-anal warts

Surgical Methods

- Excision.
- Electrocautery.
- Cryotherapy.
- Laser therapy.

Immunomodulators

- Stimulation of immune response against virus, e.g., by levamisole, zinc, TNF-α etc.

  Following procedures are commonly used:
  - Chemical cauterization.
  - Salicylic acid.
  - Keratolytic agent, it produces local irritant effect.
  - Available as 6%-40% ointments, creams or paints.
  - Application should be limited to the affected area only, to avoid maceration of surrounding skin.
  - The medicine should be applied over the surface of the wart by using a pointed stick, avoiding spilling over the surrounding normal skin.
  - It can be applied by parents at home, twice or thrice a week.

Podophyllin

- Available as 20%-30% podophyllin in tincture benzoin.
- It is a mixture of plant resins containing cytotoxic agents, with powerful irritant effects, hence extensive application should be avoided.
- It is teratogenic, so it is contraindicated in pregnancy.
- It is mainly used for anogenital and plantar warts.

Electrocauterization

- Pretreatment with subcutaneous injection of lignocaine (2%) or surface anaesthesia with EMLA (Eutectic mixture of local anesthetics) cream should be done.
- It is treatment of choice when warts are few in number.

Cryotherapy

- Cryotherapy is cheap and easy to perform.
- Mechanism of action is by cold injury which leads to formation of ice crystals and rupture of cell membranes and organelles, causing cell death.
- Liquid nitrogen (-196 °C) is mainly used.
- Simple cotton bud application or cryosprays or cryoprobes are used.
- Swelling or blistering of the skin may be seen.

Laser Therapy

- Carbon dioxide laser or pulsed dye lasers are used.
- Laser therapy is expensive, so it is reserved for recurrent cases, not as a first line treatment.

Imiquimod

- Produces TNF-α and other cytokines.
- Used as 5% cream in anogenital warts.

Practical guidelines (Warts)
Children are apprehensive to all procedures and simple methods like immunotherapy and use of salicylic acid should be the first line of therapy.
Following methods may be used according to the type of warts:
Common warts • Electrocauterization • Salicylic acid-lactic acid paint application • Cryotherapy
Plantar warts • Paring after local salicylic acid or salicylic acid-lactic acid paint application • Electrocauterization • Cryotherapy
Plane warts • Immunotherapy • Salicylic acid-lactic acid paint application • Tretinoin (0.05%) cream application • Cryotherapy • Electrocauterization

EPIDERMODYSPLASIA VERRUCIFORMIS (EV)

Epidermodysplasia verruciformis is an inherited disorder in which there is widespread and persistent infection with HPV, giving rise to a characteristic combination of plane warts, pityriasis versicolor like lesions and warty plaques. Malignant change is very common in adult life but metastasis is rare.

EV comprises flaking or hyperkeratotic skin lesions predominantly in sun-exposed sites presenting in childhood. A mild cell mediated immune deficiency and a high risk of development of cutaneous squamous cell carcinomas in early adult life may be seen. Those affected commonly have reduced numbers and function of T cells, although EV patients are not unusually susceptible to other infections. The increased NK cell activity in EV patients is interpreted as an appropriate response. There is no impairment of DNA repair, and no association with HLA-A or -B antigens.

Incidence and Prevalence

Classical congenital EV is very rare and most reported cases are identified among family members.

Pathology

The histological picture is similar in the different clinical types of lesion. As in ordinary plane warts, there are hyperkeratosis and acanthosis. However, vacuolation or ballooning in the perinuclear area of keratinocytes is more extensive, and may affect the upper half to three-quarters of the spinous layer. These classical 'clear cells' are not found in all lesions. Human papillomavirus DNA may be detected in these vacuolated cells by in situ hybridization, but the β human papillomaviruses will be more readily detected by PCR.

Causative Organisms

There are at least 20 HPV types characteristic of EV, most commonly found types are 5, 8, 9, 12, 14, 15, 17 and 19-25.

Genetics

The susceptibility to the virus is inherited, usually autosomal recessively, though autosomal dominant and probable X-linked dominant patterns have been reported. The mutations in EVER1 and EVER2 account for over 50% of the mutations responsible for inherited form of EV.

Clinical Features

Lesions on the face and neck are generally indistinguishable from verruca plana, but on the trunk and limbs they tend to be larger, and are of two main types. Scaly macular lesions resemble pityriasis versicolor, showing erythema, depigmentation or varying degrees of brown pigmentation. Thicker plaques are dull pink, violet or brown in colour and may resemble seborrhoeic keratoses or pigmented warts. The warts usually develop rapidly in childhood but may first appear at any age. They are most numerous on the face and neck and backs of the hands and feet, and may be restricted to these sites, but there are often scattered lesions elsewhere and the warts may be generalized over entire body surface.

Differential Diagnosis

Acrokeratosis verruciformis of Hopf.

Complication

Squamous cell carcinoma has ultimately developed in one or more lesions in about 20-30% of reported cases, even before the age of 20 and when the lesions have been present for more than 10 years. However, metastasis is rare.

Disease Course and Prognosis

Epidermodysplasia verruciformis is remarkably persistent and may remain unchanged for decades.

Management

If a diagnosis of EV is suspected or confirmed, avoidance of excessive sun exposure and UV-protective measures should be instigated. Monitoring for cutaneous malignancy is advisable. First line treatment includes imiquimod, photodynamic therapy and cryotherapy. More widespread and disfiguring lesions may warrant systemic therapy with oral retinoids including acitretin and isotretinoin.

HAND, FOOT AND MOUTH DISEASE (Figure 4.14)

It is the most distinctive enteroviral exanthem, an acute infection caused by coxsackie virus infection leading to mild malaise, oral ulcers and vesicular eruptions on hand and foot.

Age

Children aged below 10 years are those most commonly affected. Adults are also infrequently affected.

Pathology

Histology is not usually performed, but shows spongiosis, intraepidermal splits progressing to vesicle formation, mononuclear cells entering into the epidermis and necrosis of individual keratinocytes. There is a lymphocytic upper dermal and perivascular infiltrate. Viral particles are detectable with electron microscopy.

Causative Organisms

Outbreaks have most commonly been caused by Coxsackie virus -A16.

Clinical Features

The illness is usually mild, starting 5-7 days after infection and lasting a week. In children, the onset is with low grade fever, sore throat and malaise but in adults, painful stomatitis

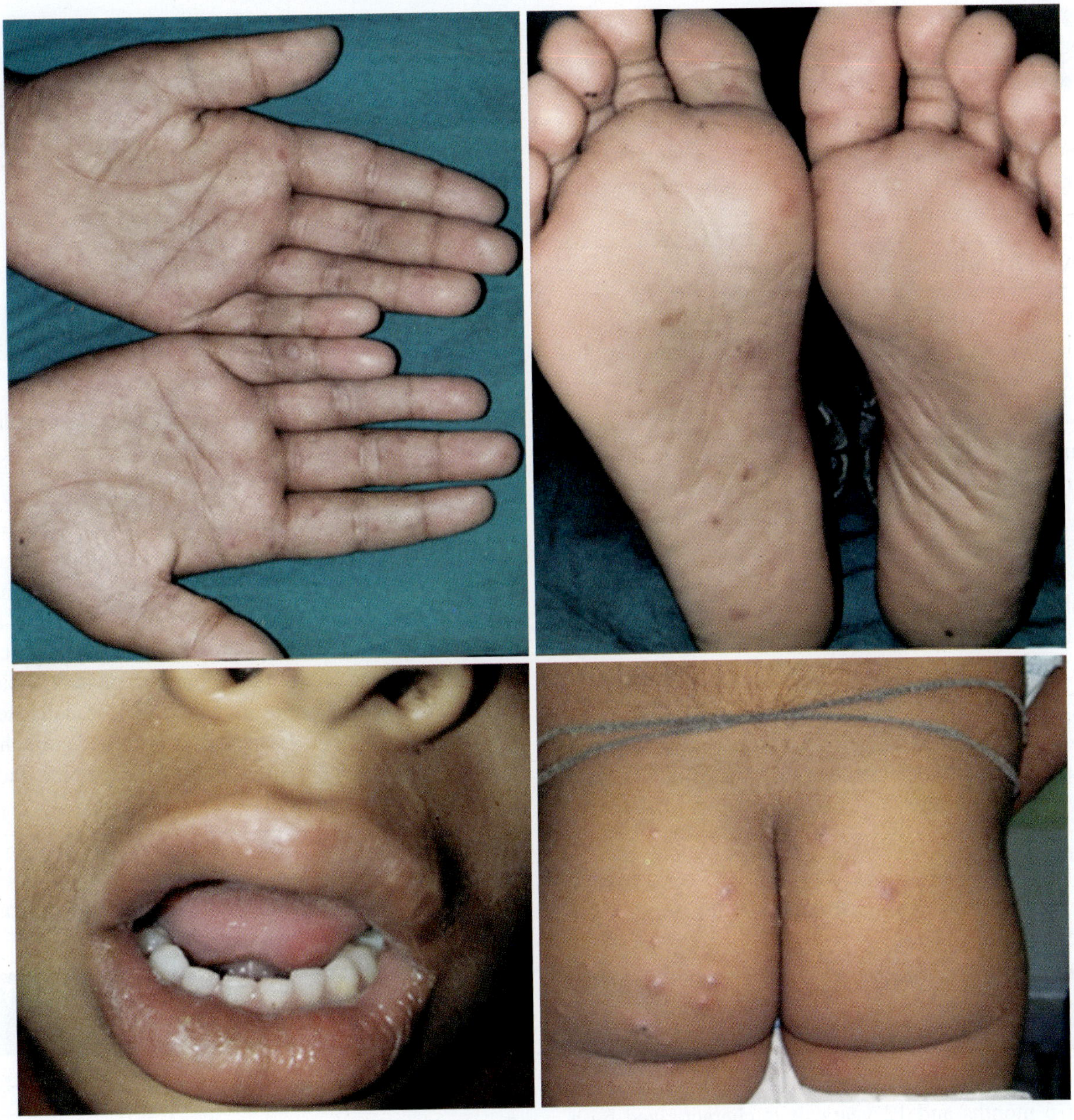

Figure 4.14: Hand, foot and mouth disease

is an early feature. Blisters in the mouth soon break down to form superficial ulcers. Children are more likely than adults to develop flaccid greyish 2-5 mm oval vesicles on the palms and less frequently on the soles. They occur on the sides or backs of the fingers and toes, especially around the nails, and around the margins of the heels, sometimes on buttocks. Cervical and submandibular adenopathy is sometimes observed.

Differential Diagnosis

- Herpes simplex.
- Stevens-Johnson syndrome.
- Aphthae.

Investigations

In majority of the patients, the diagnosis is clinical. However, in serious cases, samples are best collected from multiple sites: swabs from vesicle fluid, throat, rectum and skin, blood and cerebrospinal fluid when available for viral culture and PCR.

Management

Supportive measures (oral fluids, analgesics and antipyretics) are usually adequate. Severe cases with neurological symptoms may be treated with intravenous immunoglobulins. An inactivated monovalent enterovirus A71 (EV-A71) vaccine has been found to be effective.

PAPULAR PURPURIC GLOVES AND SOCKS SYNDROME

Papular purpuric gloves and socks syndrome presents as an acute acral dermatosis. It is regarded as an idiosyncratic reaction, usually to a viral infection. It is mainly seen in young adults and less commonly in children.

Causative Organisms

Parvovirus B19 infection is the most often associated infection. In children, EBV or CMV may be more common than in adults.

Clinical Features

Intense pruritus over hands, wrists, feet and ankles is observed with macular and papular erythema and associated oedema. Purpura and rarely petechiae may also be seen. There is often a distinct cutoff at wrists and ankles. Oral lesions and constitutional symptoms may accompany. The eruption can occasionally involve the perioral and perianal or other flexural skin. Clinical features settle within 1-2 weeks but in children, it may last a month.

Investigations

Antiviral IgM is usually detectable at the time of the eruption and IgG is detectable later.

Management

Supportive care with symptomatic treatment for pruritus. No specific therapy is available.

GIANOTTI-CROSTI SYNDROME (Figure 4.15)

Gianotti-Crosti syndrome is mainly seen in children between the ages of 6 months and 12 years. It is characterized by a self-limiting cutaneous reaction following a viral infection, in which erythematous papules appear on the extremities and face.

Causative Organisms

The majority of the cases reported have hepatitis B infection, but several other viral infections (like HSV, EBV, CMV, HHV6, coxsackie A16, coxsackie B4 and B5, poliovirus, hepatitis A, rotavirus, molluscum contagiosum, parvovirus B19, mumps, influenza, parainfluenza, HIV) and bacterial infections (Mycoplasma, Streptococcus A, Bartonella, Borrelia burgdorferi) have been associated.

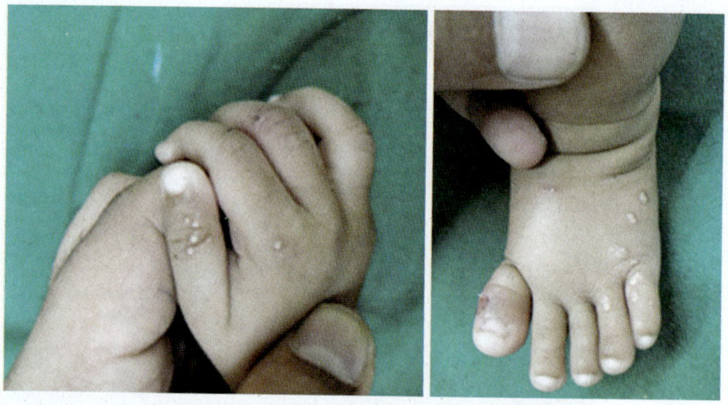

Figure 4.15: Gianotti-Crosti syndrome

Clinical Features

Multiple dull red, flat topped papules develop over a period of 3 to 4 days first on the thighs and buttocks, then may extend down to the legs, to the extensor aspects of the arms, and the face. Later the papules may develop purpuric staining, especially on the legs. Itching may be present, lesions range in size from 1 to 10 mm, but their size is consistent within an individual patient. Generalized lymphadenopathy, mostly axillary and inguinal, is common. The eruption fades in 2-8 weeks with mild desquamation.

Management

There is no specific treatment. Emollients or topical steroids can be used to give symptomatic relief.

ASYMMETRIC PERIFLEXURAL EXANTHEM OF CHILDHOOD

It is most commonly seen in young children aged 1-5 years.

Causative Organisms

There is no clear cut association but parainfluenza, adenovirus, parvovirus B19 or HHV7 infections have been associated with this condition.

Clinical Features

The eruption starts asymmetrically over axilla, groin or trunk and then spreads centrifugally. There are itchy small papules or macules often associated with lymphadenopathy.

After 2-4 weeks, the rash fades with desquamation.

CHAPTER 5 Fungal Infections

Contents

Fungi, once believed to be a part of plant kingdom, actually represent a distinct kingdom different from bacteria and plants. They can thrive on almost any organic matter in the environment. Many of them are capable of superficially invading the epidermis and its appendages (hair and nail) and cause superficial fungal infections of skin. Some of the fungi get inoculated into deeper parts of the skin resulting into chronic deep cutaneous infections. Systemic fungal infections mostly involve the lungs or gastrointestinal tract primarily and can disseminate into different organs of the body.

Fungal infections of skin are of two types:

1. **Superficial**
   - Dermatophytosis.
   - Pityriasis versicolor.
   - Candidiasis.
2. **Deep (divided into subcutaneous and systemic mycoses)**

   Subcutaneous mycoses include:

   - Mycetoma.
   - Sporotrichosis.
   - Chromoblastomycosis.
   - Lobomycosis
   - Rhinosporidiosis

- Subcutaneous Phaeohyphomycosis
- Subcutaneous Hyalohyphomycosis
- Subcutaneous zygomycosis

Systemic mycoses include:

Primary systemic mycosis

- Histoplasmosis.
- Blastomycosis.
- Coccidioidomycosis
- Paracoccidioidomycosis

Opportunistic mycosis

- Mucormycosis
- Cryptococcosis

SUPERFICIAL FUNGAL INFECTIONS

Superficial fungal infections are common in both temperate and tropical climates. They are often caused by overgrowth of transient or resident flora associated with a change in the microenvironment of the skin. Invasion by these fungi is restricted to skin, hair, nails and mucous membranes. In skin, they are usually found in the stratum corneum only.

Common superficial fungal infections and their causative agents are as follows:

1. **Dermatophytosis**	*Microsporum* species (11 species)
	Trichophyton species (16 species)
	Epidermophyton floccosum
	New genera of dermatophytes:
	• *Paraphyton*
	• *Lophophyton*
	• *Arthroderma*
	• *Nannizzia*
2. **Pityriasis versicolor**	*Malassezia* species
3. **Candidiasis**	*Candida* species

DERMATOPHYTOSIS

Dermatophytosis is an infection of skin caused by specialized group of fungi, the dermatophytes, which are able to invade and colonize stratum corneum of skin and keratinized tissue such as hair and nails. Severity of infection depends upon the dermatophyte species involved and the immunological response of the host. Clinical appearance of lesion varies according to the site of infection and the causative organism.

Etiopathogenesis

Dermatophytes are not a part of the normal skin flora and can be divided into 3 groups based on their natural habitat (Table 5.1). Microscopic identification of these species is also important (Table 5.2).

Table 5.1: Different species of dermatophytes

Dermatophytes	*Epidermophyton (E)*	*Microsporum (M)*	*Trichophyton (T)*
Geophilic (found in soil and are occasionally pathogenic for humans and animals)	None	*M. gypseum* *M. flavum*	None
Zoophilic (animals and humans both)	None	*M. canis* *M. equinum*	*T. verrucousum* *T. mentagrophytes* var. mentagrophytes
Anthrophilic (humans only)	*E. floccosum*	*M. audouinii* *M. ferrugineum*	*T. rubrum* *T. tonsurans* *T. violaceum* *T. schoenleinii* *T. concentricum* *T. mentagrophytes* var. interdigitale

Table 5.2: Microscopic identification of dermatophytes

Genera of dermatophytes	*Microscopic morphology*
Epidermophyton	Abundant broadly clavate, smooth walled, macroconidia, borne singly or in cluster. Microconidia are absent
Microsporum	Spindle shaped or fusiform rough walled macroconidia, usually numerous. Microconidia clavate and are arranged singly along sides of the hyphae
Trichophyton	Clavate to cylindrical smooth-walled macroconidia, which are often absent. Microconidia are numerous, pyriform to spherical usually arranged in clusters or singly along the coiled spiral hyphae

Dermatophytes are not able to infect intact and dry skin. Trauma and maceration due to sweating are predisposing factors for tinea cruris, tinea pedis and tinea corporis. Once they get a suitable environment, spores germinate and penetrate the stratum corneum either through horn cells or preferably making their way between horn cells. Keratinases and other proteolytic enzymes produced by dermatophytes may cause digestion of keratin.

Transmission and Source of Infection

Transmission is indirect, by infected scales and hair shed from hosts, spores (arthroconidia) in them may remain viable for many months. Clothings, towels, floor of showers and changing rooms are all possible sources of infections.

Scalp infections may be acquired through use of contaminated combs and hair brushes. In schools with outbreak of tinea capitis, many children in a classroom carry the causative fungus on their scalps. Scalp carriage is transient, but illustrates the widespread dissemination of fungal spores from children with scalp infections. Parents of children with tinea capitis are also likely to be asymptomatic carriers of the infecting fungus.

Clinical Features

Skin infections caused by dermatophytes are known as tinea infections. Different dermatophyte genera involve different cutaneous structures given in Table 5.3. Depending upon the site involved, they are called by different names like tinea capitis, tinea corporis, etc.

Table 5.3: Showing sites involved by different dermatophytes

Genera	*Site of infection*		
	Skin	**Hair**	**Nail**
Trichophyton	+	+	+
Microsporum	+	+	-
Epidermophyton	+	-	+

Tinea Capitis

Dermatophytes primarily affect the scalp of children. Tinea capitis accounts for more than 80% of fungal infections in children under 15 years of age. It is more common in boys than girls probably because of shorter hair, allowing easy access for fungal spores (Figure 5.1). Tinea capitis can be classified based on inflammation (Table 5.4) and according to localization of fungal spores in hair shaft (Table 5.5).

Table 5.4: Classification of tinea capitis based on inflammation

Non inflammatory tinea capitis	Grey patch type Black dot type Seborrheic type
Inflammatory tinea capitis	Kerion Favus Pustular

Table 5.5: Classification of tinea capitis according to location of spore

Ectothrix	*Endothrix*
Spore located outside hair shaft	Spore location inside hair shaft
Hair less breakable and break above scalp surface	Break easily and over surface
They give greenish fluorescence under wood's lamp	They don't give any fluorescence under wood's lamp
Microsporum species *Trichophyton verrucosum*	*Trichophyton tonsurans* *Trichophyton verrucosum*

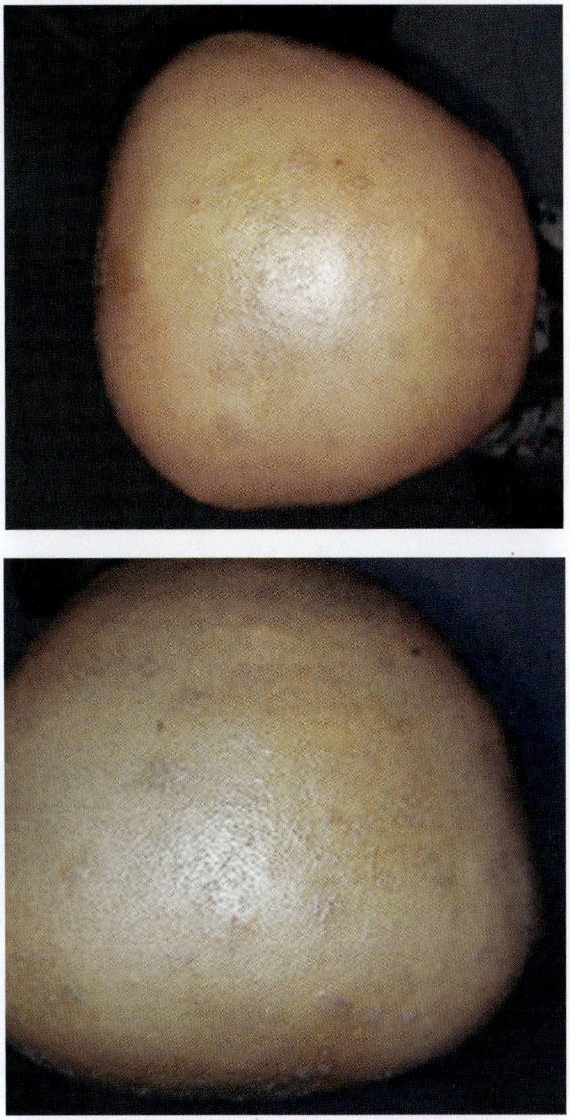

Figure 5.1: Tinea capitis

Patchy loss of hair and inflammatory changes (erythema, scaling, pustulation) are the cardinal signs for diagnosis of T. capitis, which differentiates it from alopecia areata, where the hair loss is patchy but non-inflammatory. In T. capitis, varying degree of inflammation results from immunological reaction to fungal antigens. The scaling is a result of increased epidermal replacement following inflammation. The following patterns are seen depending on the type of fungus and the degree of host response.

Grey Patch (Non-Inflammatory Type)

Grey patch tinea capitis is seen as erythematous papules, scaly plaques associated with partial or complete hair loss (Figure 5.2).

Hair may be dull grey and lusterless because of the presence of numerous arthrospores on the surface, hence called grey patch. This typical colour appearance is not seen commonly. The infection may be asymptomatic or associated with mild itching. It is most commonly caused by *M. audouinii.* Dermoscopy of lesion shows corkscrew hair or comma hairs (Figure 5.2).

Black Dot (Non-Inflammatory Type)

It is seen as patches of hair loss and mild scaling with black dot appearance (Figure 5.3). Signs of inflammation are minimum. Characteristic appearance is due to the hair left behind in infected follicle after breakage at the level of scalp. It is mostly caused by Trichophyton species. Dermoscopy of the lesion shows black dots (Figure 5.3).

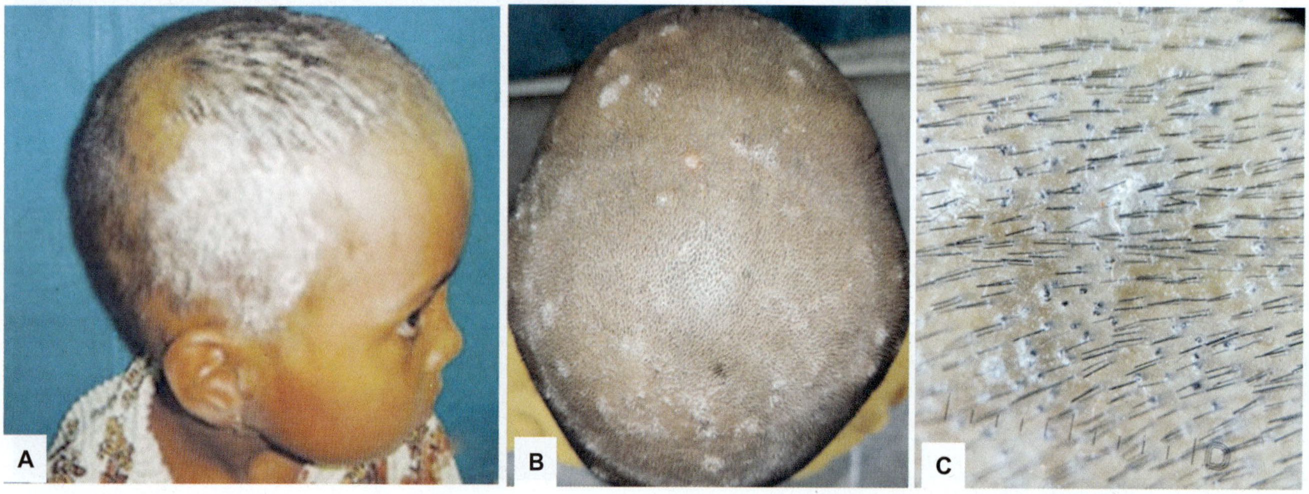

Figure 5.2: Grey patch tinea capitis with dermoscopy showing coma and cork screw hair

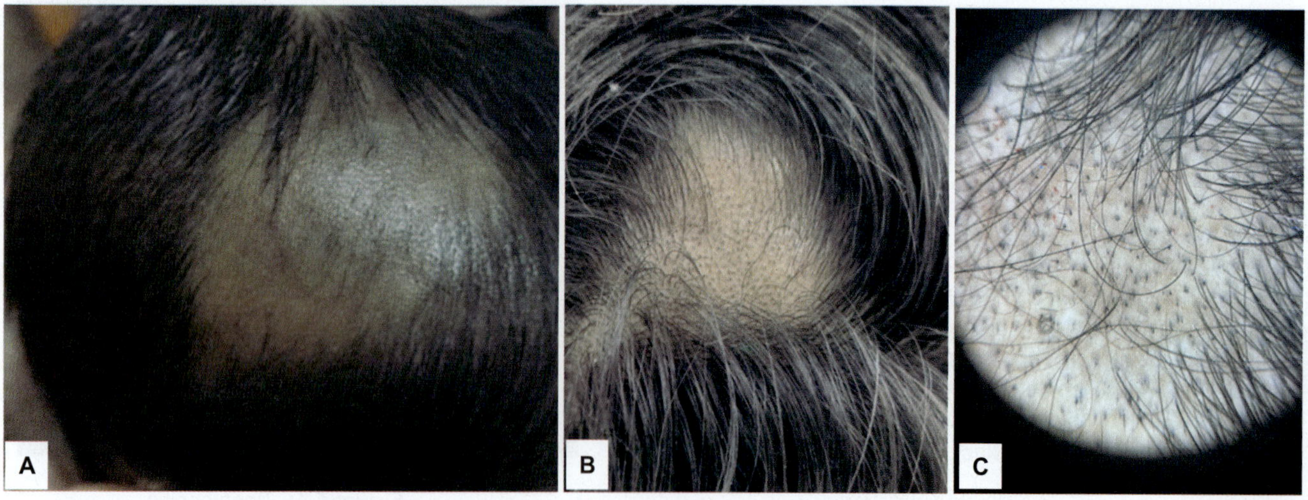

Figure 5.3: Black dot tinea capitis with dermoscopy showing black dots

Seborrheic Type (Non-inflammatory Type)

It is characterized by diffuse scaling with minimal hair loss (Figure 5.4), which can be easily confused with seborrheic capitis. Diagnosis may be confirmed by fungal culture or KOH mount and by presence of lesions elsewhere on the body. **Ear sign** if positive, can be very helpful.

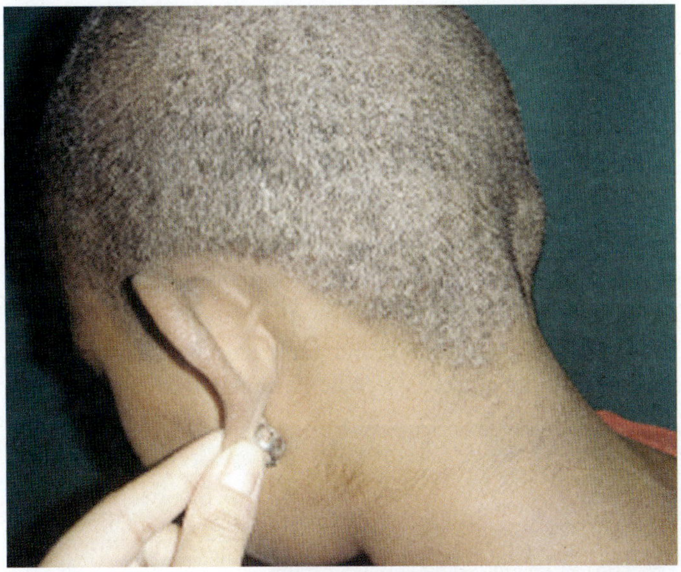

Figure 5.4: Seborrheic type of tinea capitis with multiple papular lesions over helix

Favus (Inflammatory Type)

Yellow, crusted, cup shaped lesions (called scutula) are seen at the follicular openings (Figure 5.5).

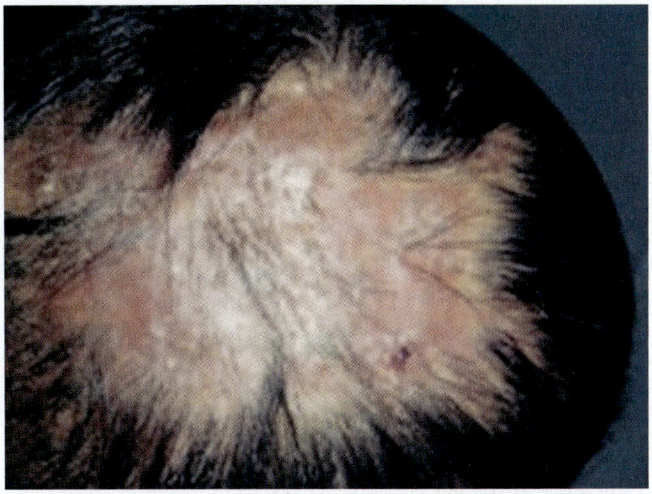

Figure 5.5: Favus showing scutula

It may be associated with characteristic mousy odor. Cicatricial alopecia may be seen later at the site of lesions. It is endemic in some families in Kashmir due to poor hygiene, frequent use of caps and less use of hair oil. Most common causative organism is *T. schoenleinii*.

Kerion (Inflammatory Type) (Figure 5.6)

It is caused by zoophilic or geophilic species and is characterized by inflammed, indurated and boggy swelling studded with broken hairs and pustules. Thick crusting and matting of hair is common. Lymphadenopathy and secondary infections are more common than other types. The lesions heal with scarring. It is mostly caused by infections due to *T. verrucosum, T. mentagrophytes, M. canis* or *M. gypseum*.

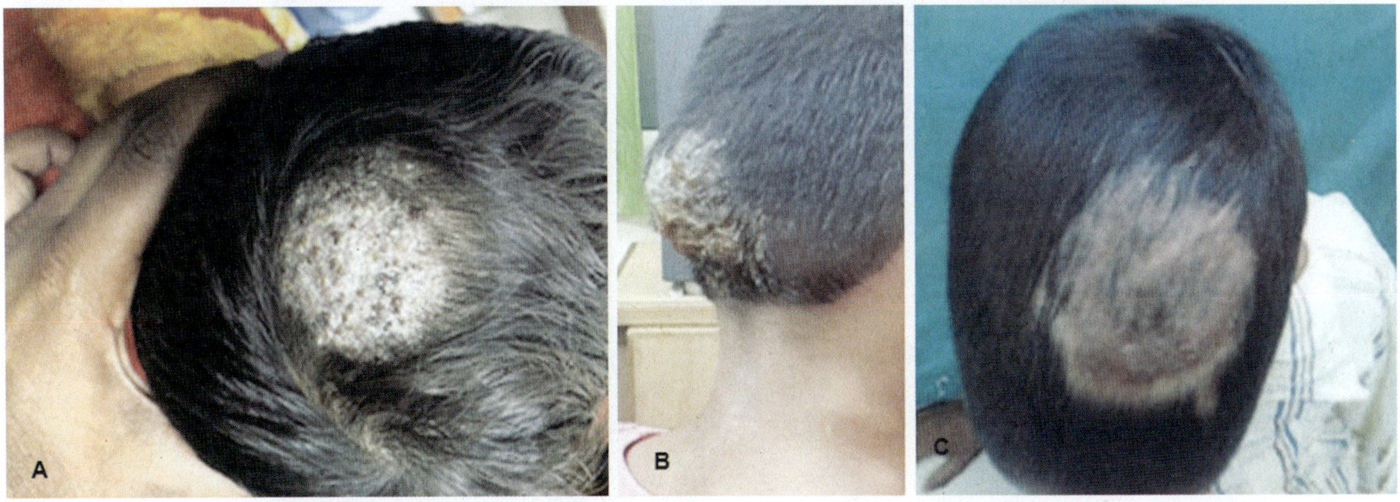

Figure 5.6: Kerion

Involvement of Other Body Sites

Non-inflammatory T. capitis, e.g., seborrheic type may show minimum hair loss and hence they may be confused with seborrheic capitis or psoriasis of scalp. Tinea capitis may be associated with tinea infections in other body sites in about one fourth of the children. Examining other body sites is very important in making the diagnosis. External ear is a common and important site which is frequently involved in tinea capitis. It may be involved in upto 40-50% of the cases.

Ear involvement in tinea capitis is seen more commonly as a scaly plaque, some cases show only papules, especially on the curvature of the helix (Figures 5.7 B and C). Such lesions may also be present over antihelix, near the tragus or on the back of the ear (Figure 5.7 D). In contrast, in seborrheic capitis, the retroauricular fold (Figure 5.7A), nasolabial folds, eyebrows, eyelashes, neck crease and inguinal fold in infants etc. are involved, which shows erythema, scaling and fissuring. **This finding which may be called as 'Ear sign', is helpful in differentiating T. capitis from seborrheic capitis.** Well-defined scaly plaques of tinea may also be seen on upper neck (posteriorly), cheeks, forehead and other body parts in association with tinea capitis. If present, they are also very helpful in substantiating the diagnosis of T. capitis in doubtful cases.

Repeated itching and poor hygiene may result in secondary scalp infection and lymphadenopathy. Such cases may show cicatricial alopecia after healing.

Tinea Faciei

It is the dermatophytic infection of non-beard area of the face. In children it is often caused by direct contact with pets. *T. mentagrophytes* and *T. rubrum* are the common species causing it. Burning, itching and photosensitivity are common symptoms. Lesions begin as erythematous, scaly macules which extend peripherally and form an annular lesion with raised border (Figure 5.8). When a unilateral lesion on face

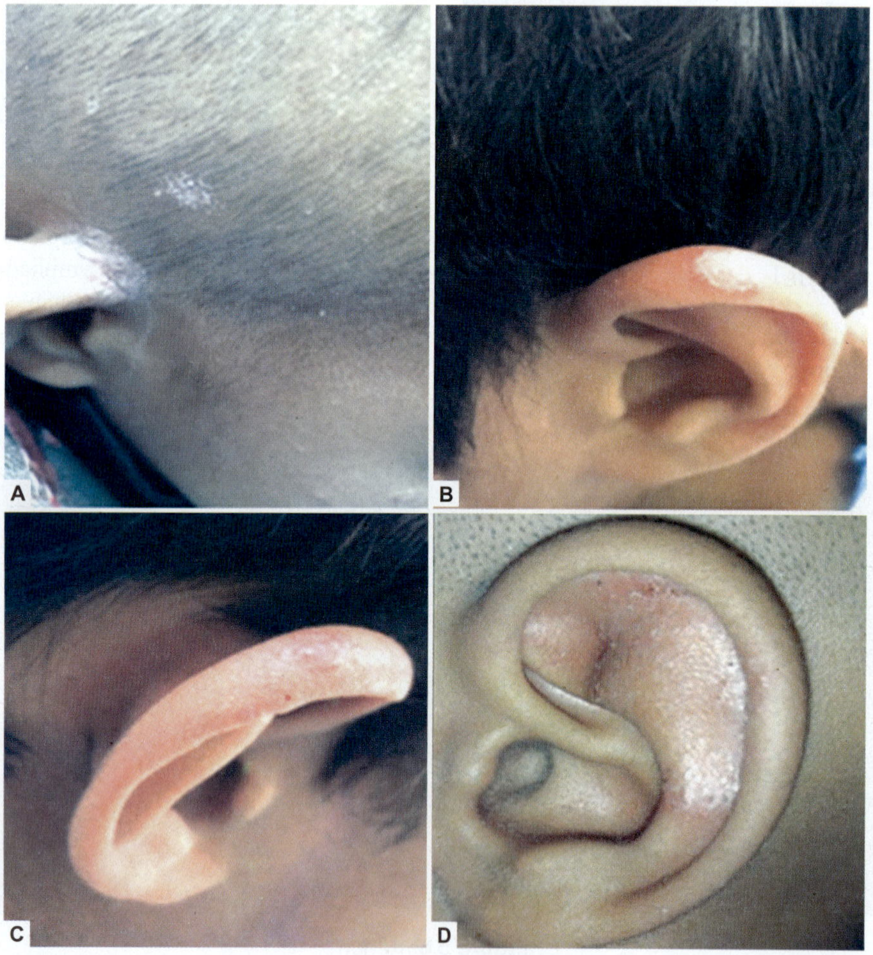

Figures 5.7: A, B,C,D: Ear sign in Tinea capitis (A–showing scaling and erythema and fissuring in retroauricular fold suggestive of seborrheic capitis, B–showing plaque over the helix, C–showing papules over the helix, D–showing lesion over antihelix)

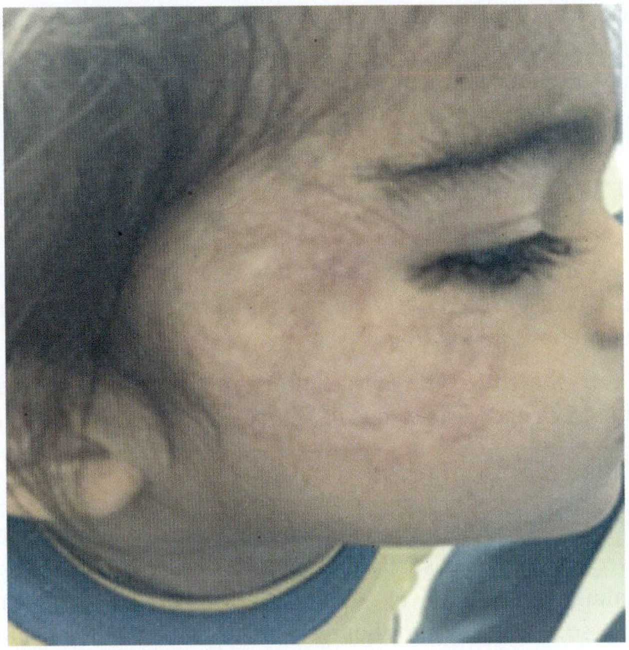

Figure 5.8: Tinea faciei in a child

also involves the ear, diagnosis of tinea faciei is more probable.

Tinea Corporis

It is a common dermatophytic infection and is caused by *T. rubrum, T. mentagrophytes* and *M. canis.* The typical lesion of tinea corporis is an erythematous, annular or polycyclic plaque with vesicular or scaly border (Figures 5.9 A, B and C). Lesions show central clearing and may be hyperpigmented. Exposed areas are commonly involved.

Tinea Incognito (Modified Tinea)

It is the infection in which usual signs of tinea are masked by application of potent topical steroids. Classical features of tinea like well-defined margins, erythema and scaling may be absent.

Pustular lesions, nodules and hyperpigmentation are commonly seen, especially in the groin.

Tinea Imbricata

It is a variant of tinea corporis, in which lesions are seen as multiple scaly concentric rings. It is caused by *T. concentricum* and is found only in Western Pacific area and South East Asia.

Tinea Pseudoimbricata (Figure 5.10)

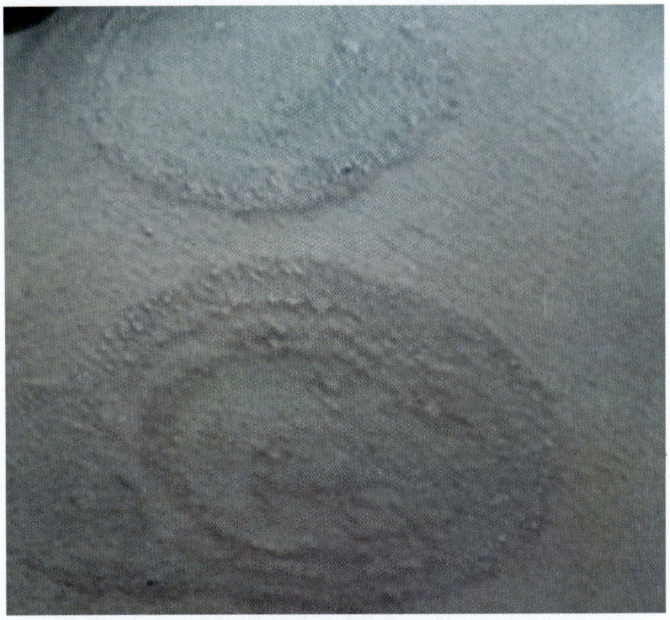

Figure 5.10: Tinea pseudoimbricata in a patient with steroid abuse

It is characterized by concentric scaly rings simulating *T. imbricata* and is caused by dermatophytes other than

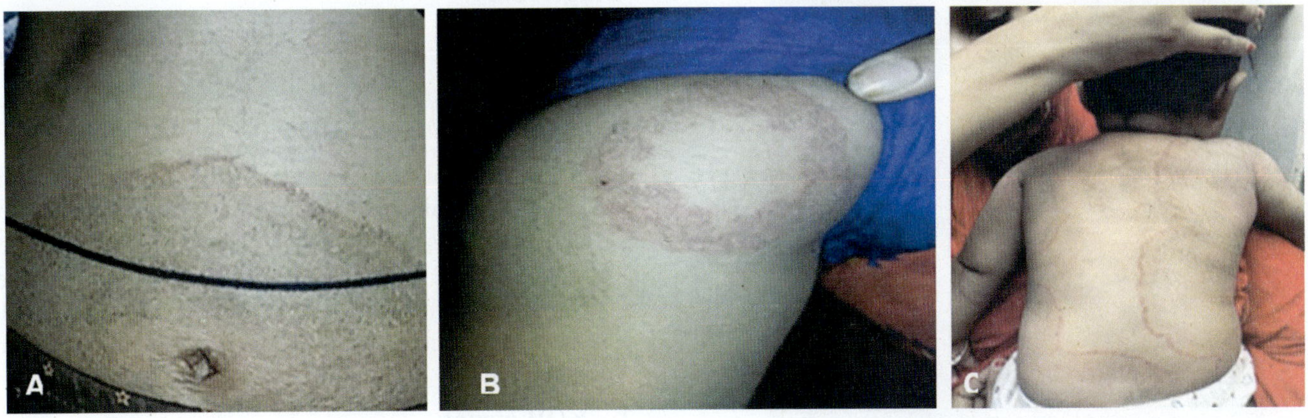

Figures 5.9A, B and C: Tinea corporis on lower abdomen, arm and back

Trichophyton concentricum. It is reported to occur in patients with steroid abuse and in immunocompromised individuals.

Tinea Cruris

Tinea cruris is infrequent before puberty and seen more commonly in adolescent males and adults, which may spread from thighs to perianal region and buttocks. Lesions are seen in groin as annular, scaly plaques with central clearing (Figure 5.11). *T. rubrum, T. interdigitale* or *E. floccosum* are the causative organisms. Humid climate, obesity and tight fitting clothes are the predisposing factors.

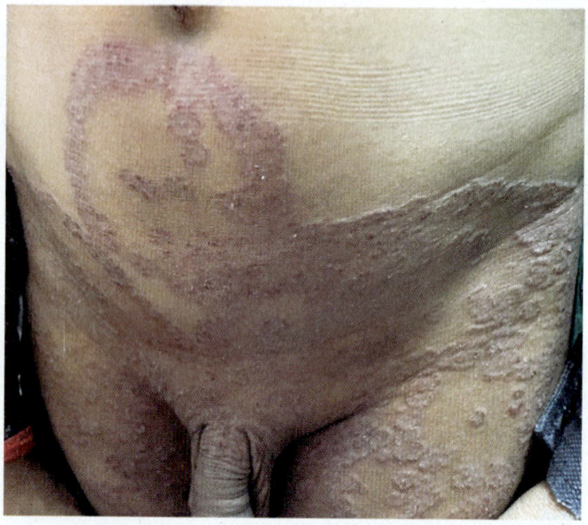

Figure 5.11: Tinea cruris et corporis

Tinea Pedis

It is uncommon in children below 15 years of age and occurs commonly in adults and elderly and is seen as peeling,

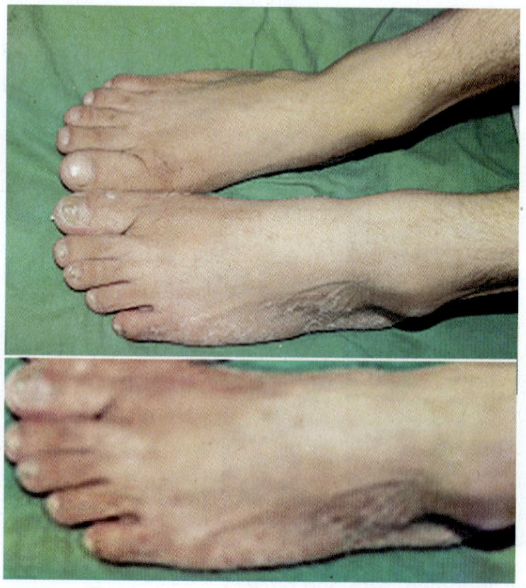

Figure 5.12: Tinea pedis (unilateral) with tinea unguium of left great toe

maceration and fissures between toe spaces. Sole and the side of foot may show hyperkeratosis and scaling (Figure 5.12). It may be associated with T. manuum concurrently. Clinically it is classified in different types:

Hyperkeratotic type or moccasin type: Usually caused by Trichophyton rubrum, which presents as well defined, fine scaly hyperkeratotic plaque over soles.

Chronic Interdigital type: It is the most common type of tinea pedis, caused by Trichophyton mentagrophyte. Scaling, maceration and fissuring is seen between web spaces.

Dyshidrotic type or vesicular type: Recurrent episodes of papules and vesicles occur over soles.

Tinea Manuum (Figure 5.13)

It is less common in children and usually follows foot infection. Lesions usually present with diffuse hyperkeratosis, scaling, with prominent palmar crease involvement and may be associated with onychomycosis. T. pedis and T. manuum are usually unilateral.

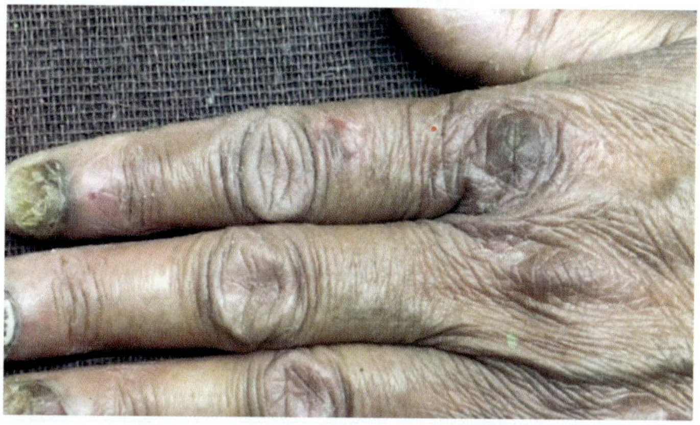

Figure 5.13: Tinea manuum

Diagnosis

Clinical diagnosis of tinea infection can be further confirmed by:

1. **Wood's lamp examination**

   It is helpful in screening the patients of tinea capitis. Examination is done in a dark room. Certain dermatophytes produce a characteristic fluorescence when exposed to ultraviolet rays (365-400 nm) filtered by Wood's filter. *M. canis* and *M. audouinii* produce brilliant green fluorescence. *T. schoenleinii* produces pale green fluorescence.

2. **KOH mount**

   Specimen from skin lesion is collected by blunt end of scalpel. In T. capitis, plucking of hair is done by forceps and scraping by scalpel. Nail scraping from subungual region and nail clipping is done by clippers or scalpel.

Sample is placed in a drop of 10% KOH in case of skin scrapings and 20-30% potassium hydroxide (KOH) in case of nail clippings on a slide. Softening of tissue may be done by heating or incorporation of dimethyl sulphoxide (DMSO) in KOH. Unstained preparations are usually examined.

Skin scrapings show branching hyphae with chains of arthroconidia (Figure 5.14). Size and arrangement of spores in infected hair in T. capitis helps in identification of species involved.

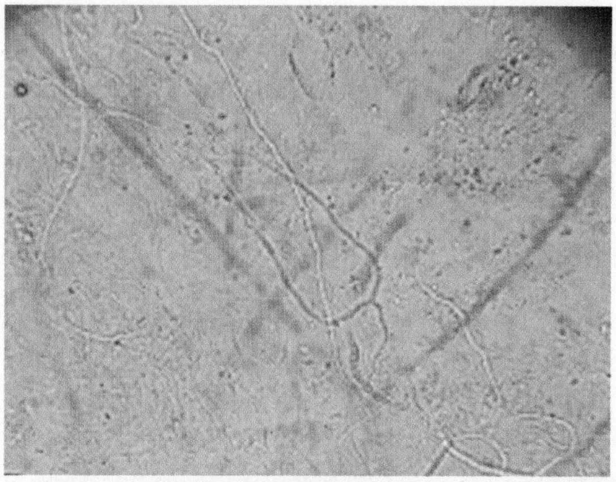

Figure 5.14: KOH mount showing branched hyphae

3. **Culture**

   Sabouraud's dextrose agar is the most common medium used.

   SDA (Sabouraud's dextrose agar): It is the standard media for fungal culture which contains peptone, agar and glucose.

   Modified SDA: It contains cycloheximide (inhibit saprophytic fungi) and chloramphenicol (inhibit bacteria) in addition to peptone, agar and glucose.

   Dermatophyte test media (DTM): It is made up of peptone, agar, glucose, cycloheximide, gentamycin and chlortetracycline with phenol red. Due to presence of phenol red, the media turns into red color by alkaline products of dermatophytes.

Differential Diagnosis

Depending Upon Clinical Presentation Tinea Capitis Can Mimic

- Alopecia areata.
- Trichotilomania.
- Bacterial folliculitis/abscess.
- Traction alopecia.
- Seborrheic capitis.
- Pityriasis amiantacea.
- Psoriasis.
- Pseudopelade of brocq.

Tinea Corporis

- Annular eczema.
- Granuloma annulare.
- Psoriasis.

Tinea Cruris

- Flexural psoriasis.
- Seborrheic dermatitis.
- Erythrasma.
- Candidal intertrigo.
- Napkin dermatitis in infants.

Tinea Pedis

- Candida infection.
- Pitted keratolysis.
- Hyperkeratotic eczema.

Tinea Manuum

- Eczema.
- Psoriasis.

Tinea Unguium

- Psoriasis.
- Eczema.
- Candida infection.

Treatment

Topical Therapy

Topical therapy is adequate to treat most of the localized tinea infections.

Topical antifungals include:

1. Imidazole derivatives like miconazole, clotrimazole, ketoconazole, sertaconazole and luliconazole.
2. Allylamines like terbinafine, butenafine.
3. Amorolfine is used as a lacquer in fungal infections of nail.

Table 5.6: Doses used for different antifungals

S. No.	Type	Ketaconazole*	Griseofulvin	Terbinafine	Itraconazole
1.	Tinea capitis	3-5 mg/kg for 4-6 weeks	10 mg/kg for at least 6-8 weeks	3-4 mg/kg daily for 4 weeks	3-5 mg/kg daily for 4 weeks
2.	Tinea corporis	3-5 mg/kg for 2-4 weeks	10 mg/kg for 4 weeks	3-4 mg/kg daily for 4 weeks	3-5 mg/kg daily for 2 weeks
3.	Tinea unguium	3-5 mg/kg for 3-6 months	10 mg/kg for 3-6 months	4 mg/kg daily for 6 weeks for fingernails and 12 weeks for toenails	3-5 mg/kg daily for 2 months for fingernails and 3 months for toenails

* Ketoconazole is usually the preferred agent due to wider spectrum of activity against all three fungal species such as dermatophytes, Pityrosporum ovale and Candida. It is a mildly hepatotoxic drug, so it should not be given in children below 5 years of age

Systemic Therapy (Table 5.6)

- Systemic therapy is required in the following cases:
  - Extensive tinea infections.
  - Tinea unguium.
  - Tinea capitis.
- Drugs used in systemic therapy includes:
  - Griseofulvin.
  - Azoles.
  - Allylamines.

Griseofulvin

It is a microtubular protein inhibitor and fungistatic in nature. It is given in a dose of 10 mg/kg in two divided doses daily. Griseofulvin is poorly absorbed orally, absorption is increased after a fatty meal. Ultra micronized and microcrystalline forms are absorbed better. Headache and gastrointestinal upset are common side effects. It is used infrequently nowadays.

Azoles

These drugs inhibit ergosterol biosynthesis. Ketoconazole and fluconazole are the most commonly used drugs.

Ketoconazole

It is well absorbed orally. Side effects include nausea, vomiting, headache, gynaecomastia, loss of libido and hepatitis.

Fluconazole

It has a longer half-life than ketoconazole, penetrates the CSF also. It is excreted by kidneys, hence can be given in patients with hepatic dysfunction. It is preferred in children below 5 years of age because it does not have much effect on liver profile. Its dose is 3-6 mg/kg daily or weekly.

Itraconazole

It is used for onychomycosis and tinea capitis. Side effects include dyspepsia, diarrhea, rash, headache, hepatic enzymes elevation.

Allylamines

These drugs block ergosterol formation in cell membrane by inhibition of squalene epoxidase. Terbinafine is the most common drug used in this group. Mild gastrointestinal upset and skin rash may be seen.

DERMATOPHYTID REACTIONS

This is a non-infective cutaneous eruption representing an allergic response to a distant focus of dermatophyte infection.

The essential criteria required for the diagnosis of an ID reaction to a dermatophyte infection are the following:

1. Proven dermatophyte infection, which usually becomes highly inflamed before the appearance of the secondary rash.
2. A distant eruption, which is demonstrably free of ringworm fungus.
3. Spontaneous disappearance of the rash when the ringworm infection settles, with or without treatment.
4. The morphology of the ID reaction should match one of the well-recognized types–widespread eruption of follicular papules grouped or scattered, a pompholyx like ID affecting web spaces and palmar surfaces of the fingers.

RECALCITRANT DERMATOPHYTOSIS

Various factors implicated are in recalcitrant dermatophytosis:

1. Host fungal immune response (Th1/17 being protective and Th2 causing chronicity of infection).
2. Virulence potential of the infecting strain or species.

3. Clinical type of dermatophytosis.
4. Barrier defect.
5. Local factors–heat, humidity, sweating, type of clothing.
6. Pharmacological factors–quality of drug, compliance, pharmacokinetics and absorption of the drug.
7. Reinfection from other sources.

MAJOCCHI'S GRANULOMA

Majocchi's granuloma is an inflammatory and granulomatous, rare fungal infection of the dermis and subcutaneous tissue that is mainly caused by dermatophytes, most frequently by T. rubrum. It is classified into two forms:

1. Perifollicular, papular form–seen in healthy individuals, induced by penetrating trauma mostly observed in lower limbs.
2. Granulomatous–seen in immunosuppressed, seen as a nodular form and usually appears on upper extremities.

Diagnosis: KOH examination is insufficient for diagnosis of invasive dermatophytoses. Therefore, histopathological examination is needed which shows perifollicular, granulomatous inflammation along with fungal hyphae and spores which stain with PAS.

Treatment: Topical and systemic antifungal drugs (Itraconazole, terbinafine, griseofulvin, voriconazole and Posaconazole).

TINEA NIGRA

Tinea nigra is an asymptomatic, superficial fungal infection caused by *Hortae werneckii*. It generally affects the skin of the palms.

The lesions are macular, sharply defined, non-scaly, brown or black in colour, mostly affecting the palms.

Treatment: Topical azole creams such as ketoconazole and econazole.

BLACK PIEDRA

This is a fungal infection confined to the hair shafts and resulting in the formation of hard, dark, superficial nodules. It is caused by Piedraia hortae.

The lesions are asymptomatic, characterized by firmly adherent, black, gritty, hard nodules on the hairs of the scalp, or less frequently of the beard, moustache or pubic area.

Treatment: Shaving or cutting the hairs is curative. To prevent recurrence, antifungal preparations such as benzoic acid ointment compound BPC can be applied. Terbinafine can also be used.

WHITE PIEDRA

This is a fungal infection confined to the hair shafts and resulting in the formation of soft, white, grey or brown superficial nodules caused by Trichosporon species. The infection is asymptomatic. More common on the hairs of the beard, moustache and genital areas than the scalp.

Treatment: Shaving or cutting the hair may lead to cure. Topical antifungals–azoles and allylamines can be used.

ONYCHOMYCOSIS OR TINEA UNGUIUM

It is the invasion of the nail plate by dermatophytes or non dermatophytic moulds or candida.

It is uncommon in children but can occur in association with tinea manuum or tinea pedis. T. unguium usually affects few nails only and is asymmetrical. Nail plate involvement starts from free edge and results in thickened yellow nail dystrophy, subungual hyperkeratosis and onycholysis (Figure 5.15).

Causative organisms: *T. rubrum, T. interdigitale* and *E. floccosum, T. tonsurans, Neoscytalidium, Candida.*

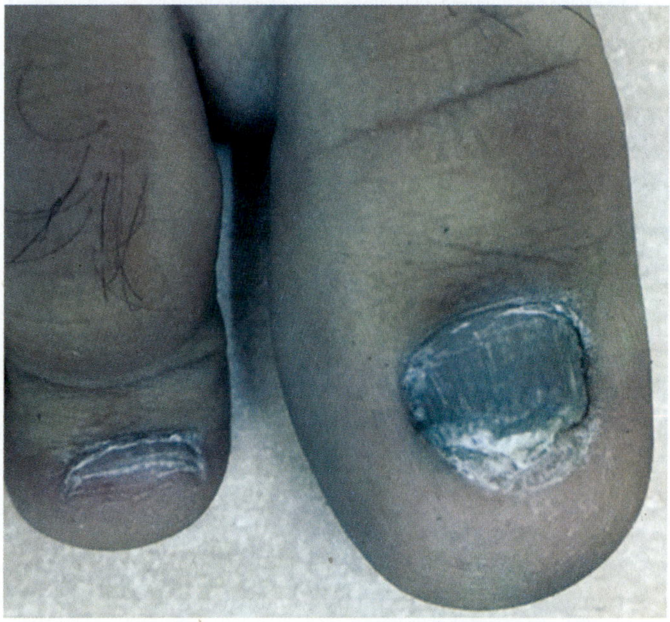

Figure 5.15: Tinea unguium of toenail

Fungal nail disease has been divided into seven main patterns:

1. **Distal and lateral subungual onychomycosis (DLSO):** This is the most common type of onychomycosis. Nail plate involvement starts from free edge and results in subungual hyperkeratosis, thickened and yellow nail plate, onychodystrophy, and onycholysis.
2. **Superficial white onychomycosis (SO):** Superficial patches of chalky white areas on nail plate are seen. Transverse and striate lines may also be seen.
3. **Proximal subungual onychomycosis (PSO):** The infection starts from proximal area of nail plate and leads to proximal onycholysis with leukonychia. It is usually seen in immunosuppressed individuals e.g. AIDS.
4. **Endonyx onychomycosis:** Diffuse leukonychia of nail plate without significant hyperkeratosis or onycholysis.
5. **Totally dystrophic onychomycosis:** Diffuse thickening, crumbling of nail plate and fragility of nail is the characteristic finding of total dystrophic onychomycosis.
6. **Mixed onychomycosis:** Here more than one subtype may be present simultaneously e.g., DLSO plus SO.
7. **Paronychia with onychomycosis or without onychomycosis:** It is caused by Candida species.

Treatment: Amorolfine nail lacquer to be applied once weekly or ciclopirox olamine lacquer to be applied daily and washed once a week, for 6-12 months.

Oral terbinafine 250 mg/day for 6 weeks for fingernails and for 3 months for toenails or itraconazole 400 mg/day for 1 week, monthly for 2-3 months for fingernails, for 3-4 months for toenails.

CANDIDIASIS

Candidiasis is an infection of the skin, mucous membranes or nails caused by a yeast known as *Candida*. *Candida* species are normal commensals in the mouth, vagina and gastrointestinal tract and infrequently on the skin also.

Etiopathogenesis (Table 5.7)

- *Candida albicans* is the major etiological agent for the superficial candida infections. Other candida species in humans include *C. tropicalis, C. glabrata* and *C. dubliniensis.*
- *Candida* cells show poor survival on dry surfaces, hence transmission of infection by fomites is unlikely.
- The most important source of *Candida* species in human disease is endogenous. Carriage rate of candida in mouths of healthy subjects is upto 40%. Vaginal carriage rate of candida species is less than 20%, which is more in pregnancy.
- Predisposing factors of candidiasis are given in Table 5.7:

Table 5.7: Predisposing factors of candidiasis
Local factors
Immature skin and low birth weight (invasive and systemic candidiasis)
Candida vaginitis in mother (neonatal oral thrush)
Premature labor in the presence of foreign body (congenital candidiasis)
Moist warm conditions (intertrigo)
Finger or thumb sucking (chronic paronychia)
Lip licking, dental malocclusion, orthodontic prosthesis (perleche)
Systemic factors
Endocrinal disorders
Diabetes mellitus
Hypothyroidism
Addison's disease
Cushing's syndrome
Genetic disorder
Chronic mucocutaneous candidiasis
Acrodermatitis enteropathica
Down syndrome
Immunological factors
HIV infection
Leukemia
Lymphoma
Drugs
Systemic antibiotics
Systemic or inhalational corticosteroids
Immunosuppressive drugs

- The change from a commensal status to pathogenic one is associated with underlying host factors like immunosuppressive therapy, immune deficiency disease, e.g., AIDS, pregnancy, endocrine diseases like diabetes, local occlusion, maceration and antibiotic therapy.
- Neonates, especially premature infants are more susceptible to candida infections, due to their immature immune mechanism. Occlusive effects of diapers and thumb sucking leading to maceration are important predisposing factors in infants.

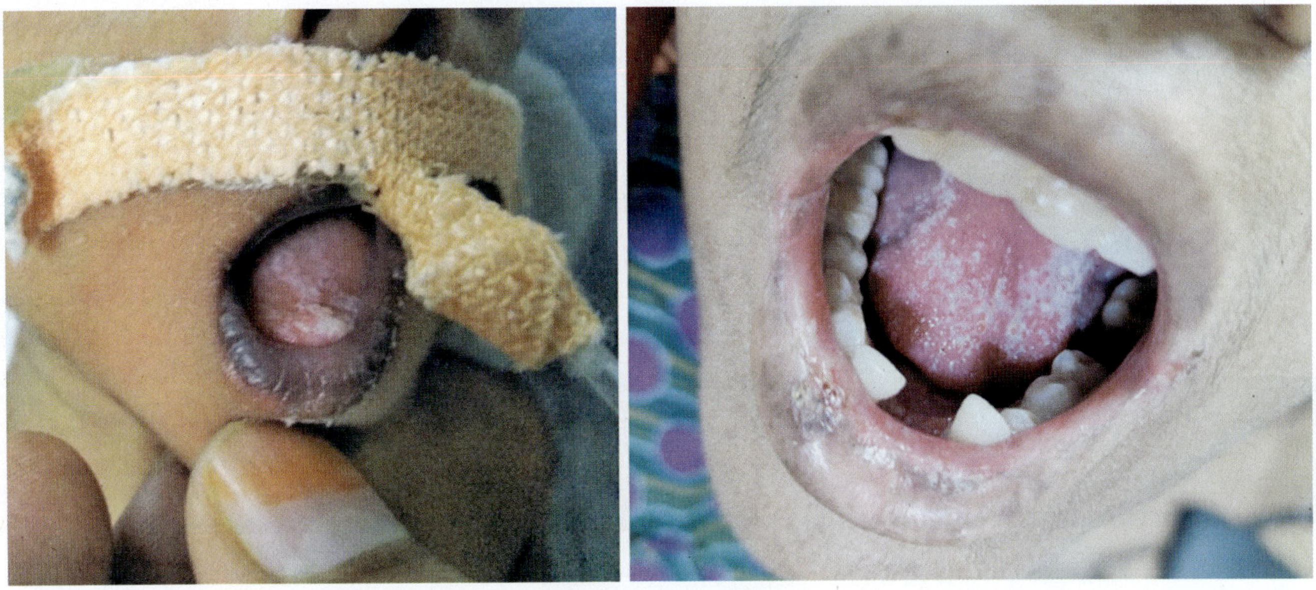

Figure 5.16: Oral thrush

Pathology

- The commensal organisms adhere to mucosal cells or keratinocytes, then germinates to produce germ tubes and hyphal elements, which can penetrate the host tissues.
- There is infiltration of epithelium by neutrophils with some hyperkeratosis and parakeratosis. This is accompanied by upper dermal infiltration by lymphocytes and plasma cells.

Clinical Features

Oral Candidiasis

Oral Thrush (Acute Pseudomembranous Candidiasis)

- It is seen as sharply defined curd-like or creamy white pseudomembranes on the buccal mucosa of cheeks, gums, palate (Figure 5.16) and on lateral borders of the tongue. Pseudomembrane consists of fungal hyphae, epithelial cells, fibrin and leucocytes. When scrapped, it leaves erythematous base. Oral plaques may coalesce and become confluent.
- Lesions may extend to the throat causing dysphagia.
- Oral candidiasis is seen commonly in the first few weeks of life. In older children, it is usually observed in neutropenic and immunocompromised patients.

Acute Erythematous Candidiasis (Acute Atrophic Oral Candidiasis)

- It is seen as atrophic lesions with erythematous base.
- Children on antibiotic therapy are usually affected.

Chronic Erythematous Candidiasis

- It is most common form of oral *Candida* infection associated with oral prostheses used in orthodontics.
- It presents as edema and erythema of the area in contact with the dentures.
- It is uncommon in children.

Chronic Plaque Like Candidiasis or Candidal Leukoplakia or Hyperplastic Candidiasis

- Lesions ranging from small white areas to large dense plaques are seen, which cannot be easily detached from the base.
- This is mainly seen in adults, and is associated with smoking.

Napkin or Diaper Dermatitis

- This type of candidal rash is seen on the buttocks and perianal region of babies, associated with wearing diapers.
- Typical erythema, scaling and satellite pustular lesions may be seen in some cases.
- In other cases, role of candida is doubtful.
- In cases of napkin rash who poorly respond to treatment, a trial of anti-candidal therapy may be given.

Candidal Vulvovaginitis

- It is common in adults but can occur in children and adolescents.
- It clinically presents as itching, burning in vulvar region or dysuria.

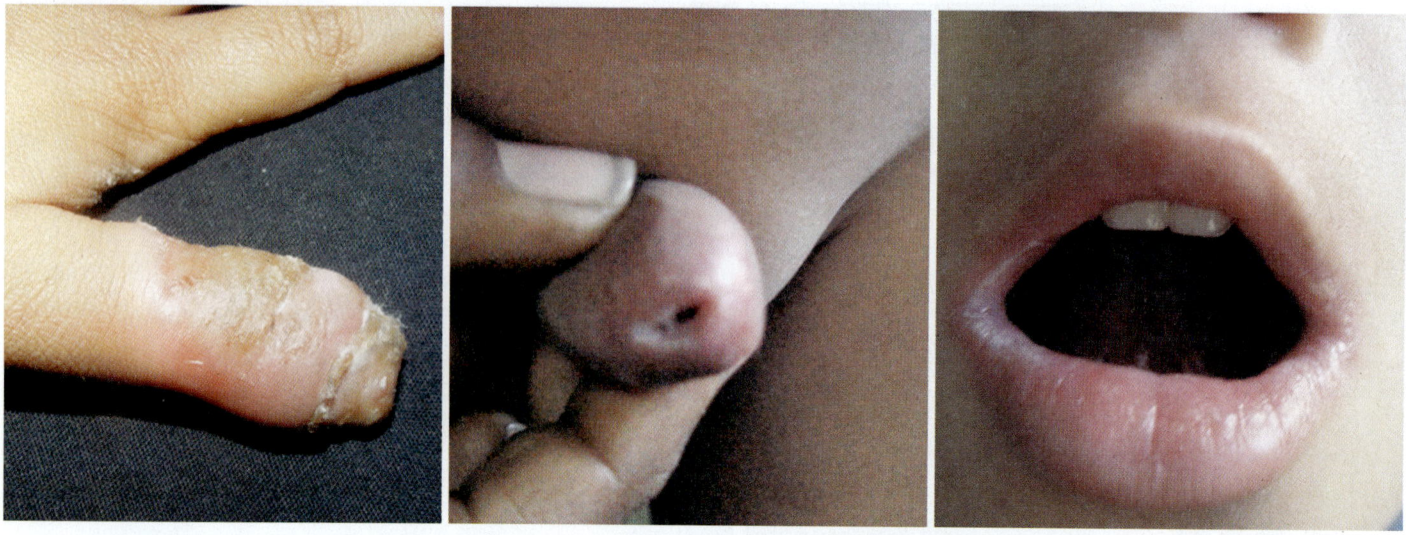

Figure 5.17: Chronic mucocutaneous candidiasis

- There is erythema and edema of vulva, white patches on vaginal mucosa and white curdy discharge.

Paronychia:

Etiology: The yeast is thought to play an etiological role, but bacteria and irritant or allergic contact dermatitis also play a part.

- Paronychia is acute or chronic infection of the nail folds and nails.
- Nail fold becomes erythematous, swollen and painful with pustular discharge.
- Nail plate invasion may occur which leads to discolored, ridged and thickened nails.
- Finally, the nail becomes friable and detached from the nail bed.
- Long history of finger sucking and maceration may be present.

Congenital Cutaneous Candidiasis (Chapter 32)

- It is rare condition in newborn infant whose mother has had intrauterine *Candida* infection prior to delivery.
- It is characterized by generalized eruption of multiple vesicles, pustules or papules on an erythematous base.
- Most cases are seen in pregnancy associated with foreign body in the uterus.

Neonatal Candidiasis

It occurs after the first week of life as oral thrush or diaper dermatitis. Infection is acquired during passage through birth canal or through nursery contacts.

Chronic mucocutaneous candidiasis (Figure 5.17)

- This is a rare syndrome that presents in infancy or childhood with recurrent oral, nail or cutaneous *Candida* infection which is resistant to treatment.
- It may be autosomal dominant type, autosomal recessive type or associated with autoimmune polyendocrinopathy.

Candidal Intertrigo

- Candidal intertrigo is candidal infections affecting skin folds (Figure 5.18) like gluteal region or axilla.

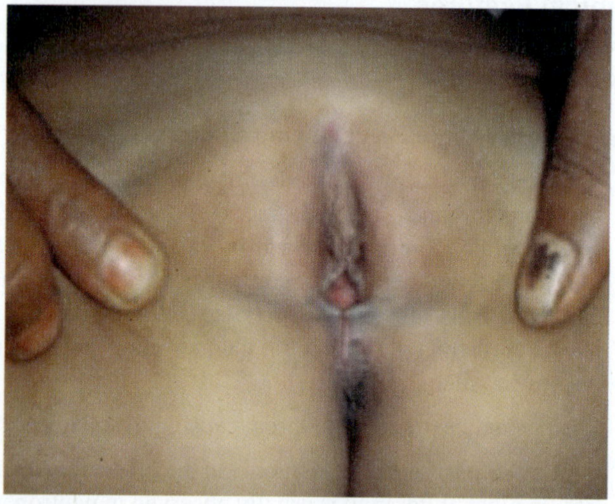

Figure 5.18: Candidal intertrigo

- The lesions are moist, erythematous patches with fringed irregular edges.
- Papular or pustular satellite lesions may be seen.

Candidal Allergy

Infection with *Candida* or gut carriage may be the cause of generalized pruritus or urticarial.

Angular cheilitis (perleche), median rhomboid glossitis are other morphological presentations which are found in adults and are not relevant in children.

Differential Diagnosis

Oral Lesions

- Lichen planus.
- Leukoplakia.
- Herpes stomatitis.
- Apthous stomatitis.
- Erythema multiforme.

Napkin Dermatitis

- Eczematous dermatitis.
- Psoriasis.

Paronychia

- Staphylococcal nail fold infections.
- Dermatophytosis.
- Psoriasis.

Congenital Cutaneous Candidiasis

- Neonatal staphylococcal infection.
- Transient neonatal pustulosis.
- Congenital syphilis.

Diagnosis

- Clinical picture is usually diagnostic, but microscopy and culture is confirmatory in all doubtful lesions.
- Mucosal smear can be examined under microscope as unstained wet KOH mounts, heat fixed specimens may be Gram stained or PAS (Periodic Acid Schiff) stained. Round or oval budding yeasts with long pseudohyphae are seen.
- Fungal culture can be done on sabouraud dextrose agar.

Treatment

Drugs used to treat dermatophytosis (except griseofulvin) are also effective for candida infections. In addition, polyene antifungals like amphotericin B, nystatin etc. are also effective.

Topical Therapy

- Imidazoles: Clotrimazole, miconazole, ketoconazole, luliconazole and eberconazole are highly effective.
- Amphotericin B and nystatin are also effective.
- For oral candidiasis oral solution of imidazoles or nystatin are used.

Systemic Therapy

- Systemic therapy is indicated for chronic cases, reinfection, extensive lesions and in unresponsive cases.
- Ketoconazole (3-5 mg/kg/day), fluconazole (3-6 mg/kg IV or orally per day), itraconazole (3-5 mg/kg/day) may be used orally in the dosage as used for dermatophytosis. Voriconazole (4-8 mg/kg) and posaconazole (200-800 mg/day) are newer alternatives and specially used in transplant patients. Amphotericin B (0.5-1mg/kg/day) can be used intravenously.

PITYRIASIS VERSICOLOR

It is a chronic, usually asymptomatic infection of stratum corneum, caused by the yeast *Malassezia* and is characterized by discrete or confluent, scaly, hypo or hyperpigmented macules or patches.

Epidemiology

- The disease is worldwide in distribution, but it is more prevalent in tropical areas.
- It occurs mostly in young adults and is comparatively less common in children.

Etiopathogenesis

Malassezia furfur or Pityrosporum ovale is a part of the normal flora of the human skin. In certain circumstances the normal skin organisms convert from yeast to mycelia phase, leading to pityriasis versicolor. Other *Malassezia* species are *Malassezia globosa, Malassezia sympodialis, Malassezia dermatis, Malassezia pachydermatis, Malassezia japonicum, Malassezia slooffiae, Malassezia restricta, Malassezia obtusa and Malassezia nana. Malassezia globosa* is the most common species causing pityriasis versicolor. *Malassezia* also responsible for other dermatosis either directly or as a triggering factor like *Malassezia* folliculitis, confluent and reticulate pigmentosus, paronychia, atopic dermatitis, seborrheic dermatitis, psoriasis, neonatal cephalic pustulosis and neonatal sepsis.

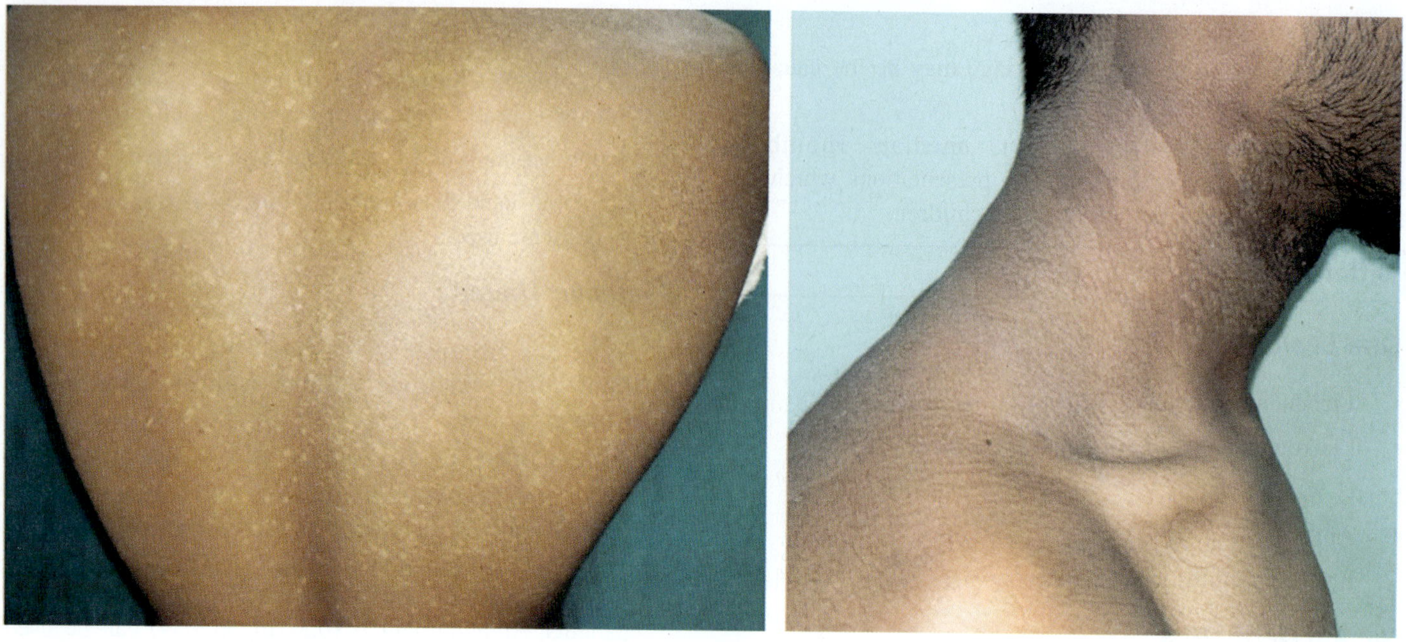

Figure 5.19: Pityriasis versicolor

The incidence is higher in warm and humid climate with sweating as a predisposing factor.

Changes in the skin lipids during puberty could increase the fungal pathogenicity, which might be a possible explanation for its common occurrence in young adults.

Pathology

- Yeast and hyphae are restricted to the outermost layer of stratum corneum.
- Hyphae invade between and inside the keratinocytes.
- Mild hyperkeratosis with few signs of inflammation are seen.

Clinical Features

Asymptomatic, scaly, hypo or hyperpigmented patches are seen, satellite lesions (Figure 5.19) may be present.

Few lesions may coalesce to form patches of various sizes and shapes. The pigmentary changes may be due to production of substances like azelaic acid by enzyme activity of the yeast, which suppresses pigment synthesis. Melanosomes are smaller in hypopigmented areas, while they are abnormally large in hyperpigmented areas (Figure 5.20).

Slight scratching of the lesions may lead to removal of superficial scales known as the scratch sign or coup d'ongle or Besnier's sign.

The disease occurs mainly on upper trunk and arms but face and neck may also be involved.

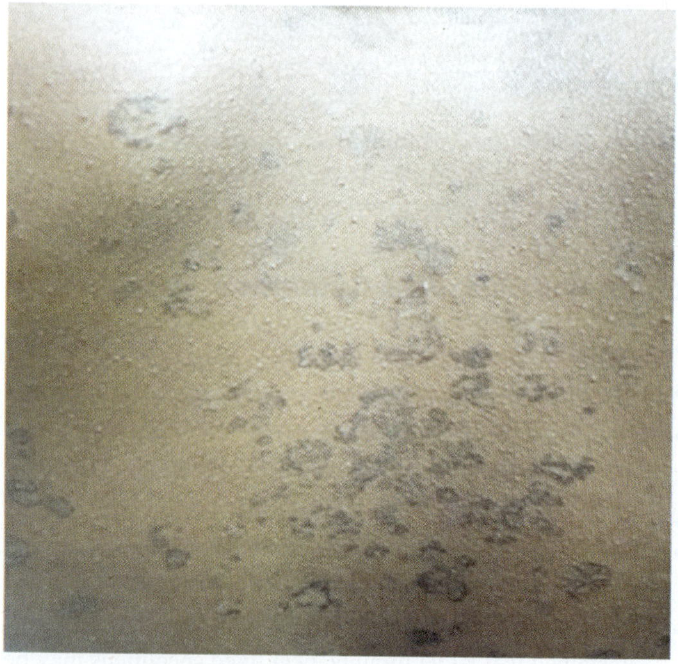

Figure 5.20: Pityriasis versicolor (hyperpigmented)

Differential Diagnosis

- Guttate psoriasis
- Erythrasma
- Pityriasis alba
- Confluent and reticulated papillomatosis

- Post inflammatory hypopigmentation and hyperpigmentation
- Pityriasis rosea

Diagnosis

- Clinical picture of asymptomatic, scaly patches over trunk and neck in young adults is usually diagnostic.
- Microscopic examination of scales mounted in 20-30% KOH may be done in doubtful cases. The mycelia are short, fragmented and wide, while the spores are spherical, thick walled, known as spaghetti and meatball appearance.
- Wood's lamp examination of the lesions shows golden yellow fluorescence.
- Culture is not very useful as *Malassezia* is a part of human skin flora.

Treatment

- Oral azole antifungals like ketoconazole 3-5 mg/kg once daily for 15-20 days or single dose of fluconazole 3-6 mg/kg once a week for 4-6 weeks are given.
- Systemic antifungals should be combined with topical antifungals like clotrimazole/ketoconazole cream/lotion.
- Topical selenium sulphide 2.5%/topical hypochlorite solution, previously used, are usually not used nowadays.
- Hypopigmentation may persist for months after cure of fungus, which leads to dissatisfaction of the patient. Patients should be explained about this, but highly concerned patients may be treated with night time application of topical psoralens for 2-3 weeks (10-15 drops of methoxsalen lotion should be mixed with 5 gm of aloe vera cream and applied on affected areas for 2-3 weeks).

SUBCUTANEOUS MYCOSES

Sporotrichosis

This is an acute or chronic fungal infection caused by Sporothrix schenckii and closely related species. The main clinical varieties are the cutaneous and systemic forms.

Cutaneous sporotrichosis is divided into two main types:

1. **Lymphangitic:** Patient presents with indurated and ulcerating nodules, which is characterized by involvement of the lymphatics from the draining area.
2. **Fixed variety,** where the pathogen remains more or less localized at the point of inoculation.

Diagnosis: Fungal culture on Sabouraud's Dextrose Agar (SDA), colonies are leathery, moist and initially white, which become progressively darker.

Microscopy: Slender hyphae bear small, oval to pyriform, hyaline conidia.

Treatment: Itraconazole 3-5 mg/kg/day or terbinafine 3-4 mg/kg/day until clinical recovery (at least 3 months). Potassium iodide can also be used.

Mycetoma (Figure 5.21)

Mycetoma is a localized chronic infection caused by various fungi or actinomycetes, and is characterized by the formation of aggregates of the causative organisms (grains) within abscesses.

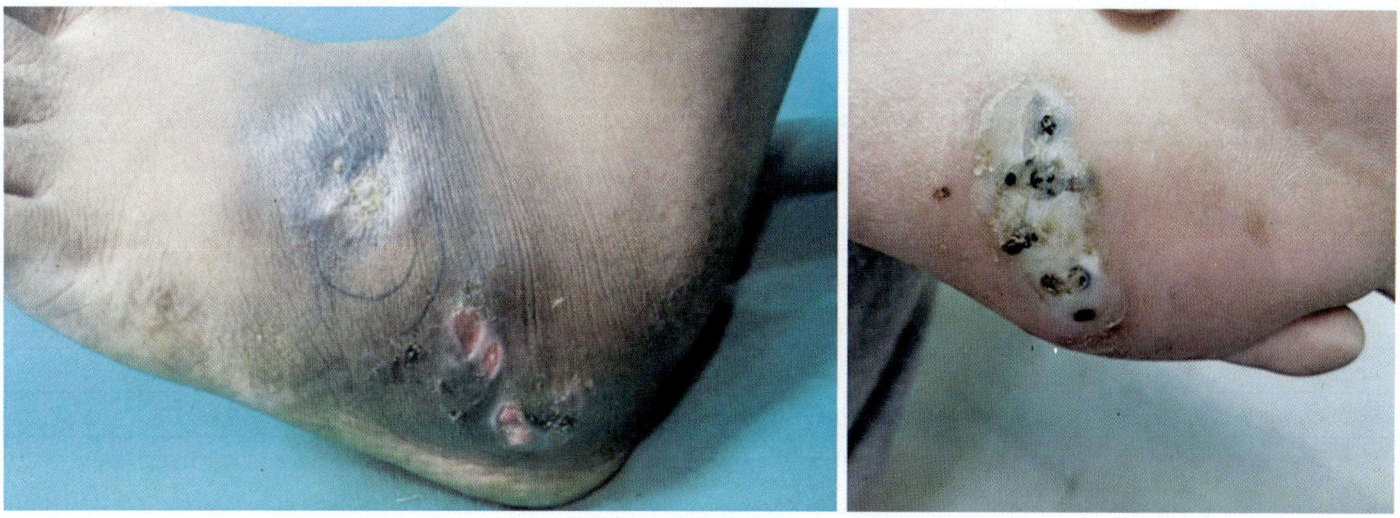

Figure 5.21: Mycetoma

Causative Organisms

1. **Fungi (dark grain)**
   - Madurella mycetomatis.
   - Madurella grisea.
   - Leptosphaeria senegalensis.
   - Curvularia lunata.
2. **Fungi (pale grain)**
   - Scedosporium apiospermum.
   - Neotestudina rosatii.
   - Acremonium.
   - Fusarium.
3. **Actinomycetes (yellow granules)**
   - Actinomadura madurae.
   - Actinomadura pelletieri.
   - Streptomyces somaliensis.
   - Nocardia brasiliensis.
   - Nocardia asteroides.
   - Nocardia otitidis-caviarum.

Clinical Presentation: History of trauma favours infection, most lesions are on the foot and lower leg but can occur anywhere. It is characterized by presence of (triad) a swelling, discharging sinuses and grains (Table 5.8).

Treatment

Eumycetoma

Complete surgical excision followed by antifungals form the 1st line of management.

Drugs Used

- Itraconazole (3-5 mg/kg/day).
- Ketoconazole (3-5 mg/kg/day.
- Terbinafine (250-500 mg/day).
- Voriconazole (4-8 mg/kg/day).
- Posaconazole (200-800 mg/day).
- Potassium iodide may also be used.

Actinomycetoma: Modified Welsh Regimen

Cyclical dosing of amikacin 15 mg/kg/day in 2 divided doses for 21 days. 3-6 cycles with intervals of 15 days in between each cycle is given depending on the severity and response of the patient. Trimethoprim-sulfamethoxazole (160 mg/800 mg) and rifampicin (600 mg) per day is administered continuously throughout the treatment period in the adults (doses in children may be modified as per their body weight).

Chromoblastomycosis (Figure 5.22)

This is a chronic fungal infection of the skin and subcutaneous tissue caused by pigmented fungi, which produce thick walled

Table 5.8: Difference between eumycetoma and actinomycetoma

Characteristics	*Eumycetoma*	*Actinomycetoma*
Etiology	Filamentous fungi	Fungus-like bacteria
Clinical course	Less aggresive	More aggresive
Progression of disease	Slow progression of disease	Rapid progression of disease
Swelling in the lesion	Seen in later stages	Swelling is less well defined and merges with surrounding tissue
Color of grains	Pale or black color	Yellow or red color
Tissue destruction	Appears in later stages	Involves bone early and extensively
Radiological features (bone cavities)	Bone cavities are less in number and are larger	More bone cavities, but smaller
Appearance of grains	Appears dark with coarse texture	Appears pale with fine texture
Filaments	Wide and septate	Slender and non septae
Response to management	Responds slowly, may require radical surgical excision	Responds early and in a better way

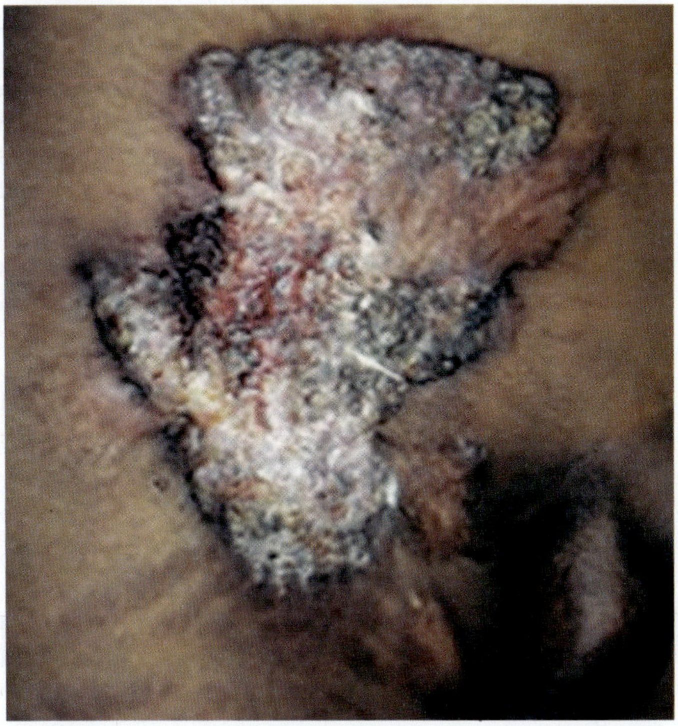

Figure 5.22: Chromoblastomycosis - warty hypertrophic plaque with scarring

single or multicelled clusters (sclerotic or muriform bodies) in tissue. Causative organisms: *Phialophora verrucosa, Fonsecaea pedrosoi, F. compacta and Cladophialophora carrionii.*

Clinical Presentation: Lesions are usually found on exposed sites like feet, legs, arms, face and neck. Warty papule slowly enlarges to form a hypertrophic plaque. Plaque is flat and expands slowly with central scarring.

Diagnosis: Biopsy and culture will establish the diagnosis.

Histopathology: The organized granuloma, mainly within foreign body giant cells, groups of fungal cells may be seen. Cells are chestnut or golden brown in colour, termed **muriform or sclerotic cells.**

Treatment: Itraconazole (3-5 mg/kg daily) or terbinafine (3-4 mg/kg daily) is often successful. Flucytosine and amphotericin B can also be used.

Lobomycosis (Keloidal blastomycosis)

- It is caused by Locazia loboi, which presents as painless keloidal, nodules and plaques with smooth surface over exposed parts of body. This disease is also known as keloidal blastomycosis.
- On PAS staining fungal spores are seen as rounded structures with a tip giving the organism a lemon like appearance. They may show single budding and often form single chain joined together by a small tubular bridge.
- Treatment includes clofazimine, itraconazole, posaconazole, surgical excision and cryotherapy.

Rhinosporidiosis

- It is a chronic granulomatous disease caused by Rhinosporidium seeberi. It is seen more in South India, South America and Srilanka.
- It commonly involves mucosal surfaces particularly the nasal mucosa and may also involve contiguous skin. The disease starts as a papule which enlarges to form a painless, erythematous, friable, polypoidal mass (raspberry like), obstructing nose and nasopharynx. A combination of pus, mucus and organism (tiny white dots) is discharged, which gives strawberry like appearance.
- On histopathological examination many globular cysts of varying shape representing sporangia are seen in different stages of development with a distinctive swiss cheese appearance.
- Surgical excision is required for treatment.

Subcutaneous Phaeohyphomycosis and Subcutaneous Hyalohyphomycosis

- **Subcutaneous Phaeohyphomycosis:** It is caused by moulds that form septate hyphae with darkly pigmented cell wall (dematiaceous fungi) like Bipolaris species, Cladophialophora species, Ochroconis species, Alternaria species, Wangiella species, Curvularia species etc.
- **Subcutaneous Hyalohyphomycosis:** It is caused by moulds that form septate hyphae with colourless cell wall like Fusarium species, Scedosporium species, Trichoderma species, Paecilomyces species etc.
- Both are opportunistic pathogens usually affecting compromised hosts. Usually, they present as chronic and slowly progressive painless nodules, plaques, cysts (Figure 5.23), abscess and verrucous lesions (rare).
- **Treatment:** Surgical excision followed by oral antifungals, mainly azoles (Itraconazole or voriconazole) can be used as co-adjunctive therapies.

Zygomycosis (Mucormycosis / Phycomycosis)

Moulds belonging to the Mucorales (opportunistic systemic infection) and Entomophthorales orders (subcutaneous infection) are the causative agents. These fungi are common saprophytes that are primitive in nature.

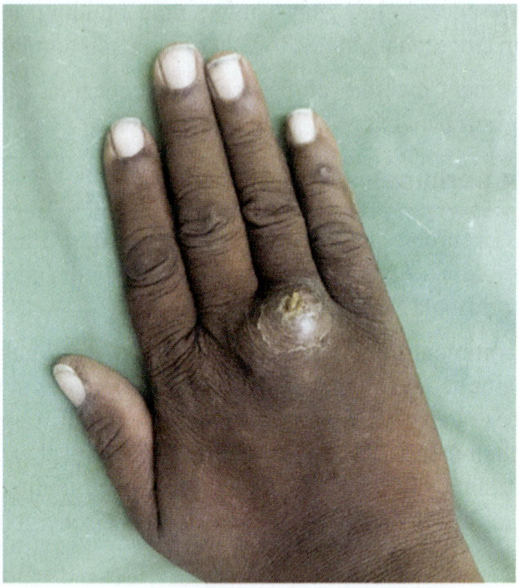

Figure 5.23: Subcutaneous Phaeohyphomycosis on hand.

1. *Mucorales*

Mucorales caused zygomycosis, also referred to as black fungus or mucormycosis, is characterised by a rapidly evolving course, angioinvasion, tissue necrosis, and fulminant systemic mycosis. It is especially common in immunocompromised hosts, such as those with diabetes, renal failure, iatrogenic immunosuppression, hematopoietic malignancy, AIDS, etc. Its rising frequency in patients with coronavirus infections has recently given it more attention. The most frequent species that causes mucormycosis is Rhizopus arrhizus (also known as Rhizopus oryzae). Direct implantation or haematogenous diffusion might cause cutaneous involvement. Among the cutaneous characteristics are necrotic ulcerated lesions, plaques, pustules, blisters, and abscesses. Other features include nasal discharge, eschar formation, mucocutaneous ulceration and swelling of the face. It has four different types:

- Rhinocerebral
- Pulmonary
- Gastrointestinal or abdomino-pelvis
- Cutaneous

Treatment includes liposomal amphotericin B (5-10 mg / kg /day for 3-6 weeks) and debridement.

2. *Entomophthorales*

The two pathogenic genera that constitute Entomophthorales are Conidiobolus and Basidiobolus. These cause the diseases known as conidiobolomycosis and basidiobolomycosis, respectively. The main risk factor for entomophthorales is trauma. Clinically, both manifest as persistent, gradually increasing, painless, hard, uniform, non pitting, disc shaped subcutaneous swellings or swellings with normal skin covering them. They can also manifest as single or numerous swellings. Fingers inserted underneath the lesion can elevate it, as it is not attached to any underlying structures. They do not invade the blood vessels; they are limited to subcutaneous tissue.

Conidiobolus mainly affects young males. It presents with nasal obstruction, nasal discharge, sinus pain and subcutaneous swelling around nose. Pulmonary and systemic infection has also been reported. **Basidiobolus** also commonly affects young children and presents with slowly progressive subcutaneous mass in the limb or limb girdle area.

Treatment includes saturated solution of potassium iodide (30 drops of saturated solution three times a day an adult), itraconazole etc.

SYSTEMIC MYCOSES

Histoplasmosis

This is a highly infectious mycosis caused by ***Histoplasma capsulatum*** and affects primarily the lungs, where it is generally asymptomatic.

Cutaneous involvement: Most skin lesions arise following dissemination from the primary pulmonary focus. Papules, ulcers, nodules, granulomas, abscesses, fistulae, scars and pigmentary changes may be seen.

Treatment: Itraconazole 3-5 mg/kg daily until clinical remission.

For patients who are severely ill, amphotericin B 0.5–1 mg/kg daily (or liposomal amphotericin B 3 mg/kg daily) for 2 weeks followed by Itraconazole (3-5 mg/kg) once or twice daily may then be used for a further period depending on clinical response.

Fluconazole 6-12 mg/kg daily for 3 months or until clinical remission may also be used.

Blastomycosis

Blastomycosis is a chronic granulomatous and suppurative mycosis caused by ***Blastomyces dermatitidis.*** It affects primarily the lungs but disseminated forms also affect the skin, bones, central nervous system and other sites.

Primary cutaneous blastomycosis is very rare and follows trauma to the skin and introduction of the fungus. It is characterized by an erythematous, indurated area followed by chancre appearing in 1–2 weeks with associated lymphangitis and lymphadenopathy.

Treatment: Itraconazole 3-5 mg/kg daily until clinical remission.

For patients who are severely ill, amphotericin B 0.5–1 mg/kg daily for 2 weeks followed by itraconazole for a further period depending on clinical response.

Coccidioidomycosis

This disease is also known as San Joaquin valley fever or desert rheumatism. It is primarily a disease of respiratory tract and lungs and is caused by a dimorphic fungi, Coccidioides immitis or Coccidioides posadasii.

Primary cutaneous coccidiodomycisis is very rare, which presents as tender, indurated ulcerated nodules which may enlarge to form a granulomatous, ulcerated plaque. They may spread in sporotrichoid pattern along the lymphatic vessels. Regional lymphadenopathy may also be present.

Itraconazole or posaconazole are used for the treatment.

Paracoccidioidomycosis

It is caused by the genus Paracoccidioides, which produce thick walled yeast cells with several buds on it. It causes chronic pulmonary or gastrointestinal infection, which may disseminate to skin and mucosa by lymphatics. It is seen as a rounded yeast with multiple budding yeast in steering wheel pattern on KOH preparation from bronchial secretions and histopathological examination.

Treatment includes itraconazole, posaconazole and amphotericin B.

Cryptococcosis

Cryptococcosis is an acute, subacute or chronic infection caused by the encapsulated yeast *Cryptococcus neoformans.* It is associated with AIDS, lymphomas, malignancies, collagen disease, systemic steroid therapy, immunosuppression in patients after renal transplant. Cutaneous and mucous membrane lesions may develop in about 10% and 3% of cases respectively but are seldom pathognomonic. The most frequent types of lesions seen are, firm or cystic, slow growing, subcutaneous, erythema nodosum like swellings. Acneiform papules or pustules are characteristic of widespread infection. Any of these lesions may ulcerate.

Treatment: Amphotericin B 0.5–1 mg/kg daily for 4-6 weeks or Amphotericin B 0.5–1 mg daily (or liposomal amphotericin B 3 mg/kg daily) for 2 weeks followed by fluconazole 6-12 mg/kg daily for 4 weeks or until remission.

Systemic and topical antifungals and their pregnancy categories are given in Table 5.9.

Table 5.9: Doses of systemic antifungals agents

Medication	*Dosage*	*Pregnancy category (FDA)*
Fluconazole (IV, PO)	6 mg/kg/day (continuous)	C
	8 mg/kg/once weekly (pulse)	
Griseofulvin (PO)	10-20 kg–125 mg/day OD	N/A
	20-40 kg–250 mg/day OD	
	>40 kg–500 mg/day OD	
	OR 10-30 mg/kg/day	
Itraconazole (IV, PO)	5 mg/kg/day	C
Ketoconazole (IV, PO)	200-400 mg OD	C
	OR	
	3-5 mg/kg/day	
Terbinafine (PO)	10-20 kg–62.5 mg/day	B
	21-40 kg–125 mg/day	
	>40 kg–250 mg/day	
	OR	
	3-4 mg/kg/day	
Voriconazole (IV, PO)	4-8 mg/kg/day	D
Amphotericin B (IV)	0.5 mg/kg/day	
Posaconazole (PO)	200-800 mg/kg/day (PO)	
	Topical antifungal agents	
Clotrimazole	1%, 2%	B
Miconazole	2%	C
Ciclopirox	1%, 1.5%, 8%	B
Ketoconazole	2%	C
Sertaconazole	2%, 5%	C
Luliconazole	1%	C
Terbinafine	1%	B
Amrolfine	0.25%, 5%	N/A
Eberconazole	1%	C
Bifonazole	1%	C
Fluconazole	0.5%, 1%, 2%	C

6 CHAPTER Arthropod, Protozoan and Parasite Borne Diseases

Contents

ARTHROPOD BORNE DISEASES

Arthropod borne diseases can pose major problem wherever outdoor activities bring arthropods and people into contact. Classification of arthropods causing diseases is given in Table 6.1.

<table>
<tr><th colspan="3">Table 6.1: Classification of important arthropods causing cutaneous diseases</th></tr>
<tr><td colspan="3">Class - Arachnida</td></tr>
<tr><td rowspan="3">Order</td><td>Araneae (spiders)</td><td>• Latrodectus (widow spider)
• Loxosceles (recluse or fiddle back spiders)
• Tegenaria (Hobo spider/ aggressive house spider)
• Tarantula</td></tr>
<tr><td>Acarina (ticks and mite)</td><td>Ticks:
• Ixodidae (Hard ticks)
• Argasidae (Soft ticks)
Mite:
• Sarcoptes scabiei var. hominis</td></tr>
<tr><td>Scorpiones</td><td>Scorpion</td></tr>
<tr><td colspan="3">Class - Insecta</td></tr>
<tr><td rowspan="7">Order</td><td>Anoplura (lice)</td><td>Species:
• Pediculosis humanus capitis (Head louse)
• Pediculosis humanus corporis (Body louse)
• Pthirus pubis (Crab louse)</td></tr>
<tr><td>Diptera (mosquitoes and flies)</td><td>Family:
• Culicidae: Mosquitoes
• Simuliidae: Black flies (Onchocerciasis and Tularemia)
• Tabanidae: Horse flies (Tularemia) and deer flies (Loa-Loa filariasis and Tularemia)
• Psychodidae: Subfamily: Phlebotominae (Sand flies): Species: Phlebotomus (Transmit old word leishamniasis) and Lutzomyia (New word leishmaniasis and Carrion disease or Bartonellosis)
• Glossinidae: Tsetse flies (African trypanosomiasis)</td></tr>
<tr><td>Coleoptera (beetles)</td><td>Family:
• Staphylinidae: Rove beetle contain pederin toxin (Paederus dermatitis)
• Meloidae: Cantheridin toxin (Blister beetle dermatitis)
• Oedemeridae: Cantharidin toxin (Blister beetle dermatitis)</td></tr>
<tr><td>Hemiptera (bedbugs or kissing bug)</td><td>Family:
• Cimicidae: Cimex lectularius (bed bug): Bed bug bite
• Reduviidae: Triatoma (Kissing bug): Chagas disease</td></tr>
<tr><td>Siphonaptera (fleas)</td><td>Family:
• Pulicidae:
○ Rat fleas (Xenopsylla cheosis and xenopsylla brasiliensis) – Plague
○ Cat fleas (Ctenocephalides felis) – Endemic typhus
○ Tungidae: Tunga penetrans – Tungiasis</td></tr>
<tr><td>Hymenoptera</td><td>• Ants
• Bees
• Wasps</td></tr>
<tr><td>Lepidoptera</td><td>• Butterflies
• Moths</td></tr>
</table>

CLASS: ARACHNIDA

Pathogenic organisms under this class comprises:

- **Mites.**
- **Ticks.**
- **Spiders.**
- **Scorpions.**

MITES (ACARI)

Scabies

Scabies is a common skin infestation caused by human scabies mite *Sarcoptes scabiei var hominis* (Figure 6.1) and is characterized by intense pruritus and eruptions.

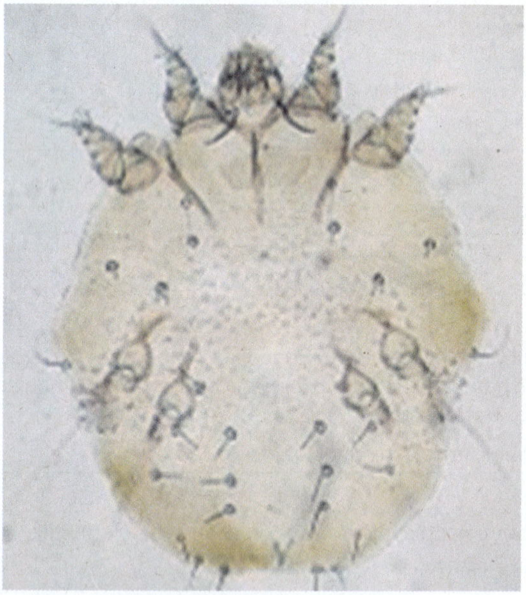

Figure 6.1: Sarcoptes scabiei

Epidemiology

Age: Scabies is essentially a disease of children but can occur at any age. Prevalence is highest below 5 years of age.

Sex: Both sexes are affected equally.

Geographical distribution: Scabies is distributed world-wide. It is endemic in developing countries of the world. Low socio-economic status, overcrowding and poor hygiene are predisposing factors for epidemics. It is more prevalent in urban areas than in rural areas.

Environmental factors: High humidity and low temperature favour the survival of the mite.

Etiopathogenesis

Adult mites have 4 pair of legs attached to the ventral surface and the anterior two pairs bear claws. Adult female mite measures 0.4 × 0.3 mm while the male is 0.2 × 0.15 mm in size.

Life Cycle

The gravid female creates a burrow within and beneath the stratum corneum by secreting a substance that dissolves skin scales. The mite lays an average of three eggs per day in the burrow. Eggs hatch in 2-3 days to produce three legged larvae. The larva undergoes moulting three times before the mite reaches adulthood and is capable of replication. Lifespan of female is 4-6 weeks, during which she lays upto 50 eggs. Patient with scabies on an average harbours 7-12 adult female mites.

In immunosuppressed or neurologically impaired patients, the mites on skin can multiply considerably, causing crusted (Norwegian) scabies which is characterized by minimal or no pruritus.

Transmission

Transmission via direct skin-to-skin contact, sharing bed is the primary mode of transmission. Infants and young children spread infestation to other children in day care facilities and schools.

In adults, transmission through sexual contact may be important.

Role of fomites is controversial.

True scabies infestation is not transmitted from animals to humans. The scabies mites responsible for animal scabies (i.e., sarcoptic mange) belong to distinct subspecies and typically cannot reproduce in humans. Reactions to such mites are usually self-limited and resolve if contact with the affected animal ceases.

Clinical Features

The cardinal symptom is pruritus all over the body except on face. In primary infestation, itching appears after about 4-6 weeks while re-infestation causes itching immediately. Pruritus is particularly severe at night. It results from a delayed-type hypersensitivity reaction to the mite, mite feces and eggs. Examination findings include burrows, erythematous papules, excoriations, nodules, vesiculopustular or bullous lesions, eczematization and secondary bacterial infection.

Burrows are the pathognomonic lesions of scabies.

Most common sites include hands, finger webs, flexor aspect of wrists, feet, axillary region, peri umbilical region, genitalia in males and areola and inframammary region in females. In infants and young children palms (Figure 6.2) and soles (Figure 6.3), lateral aspect of feet, scalp, face and post-auricular folds may be affected; and may show characteristic vesiculopustular lesions. Typical burrow is a serpiginous tract, about 1 cm in length with black dot at one end, which is the location of female mite. It may be obscured by excoriation or vesiculation, particularly in infants.

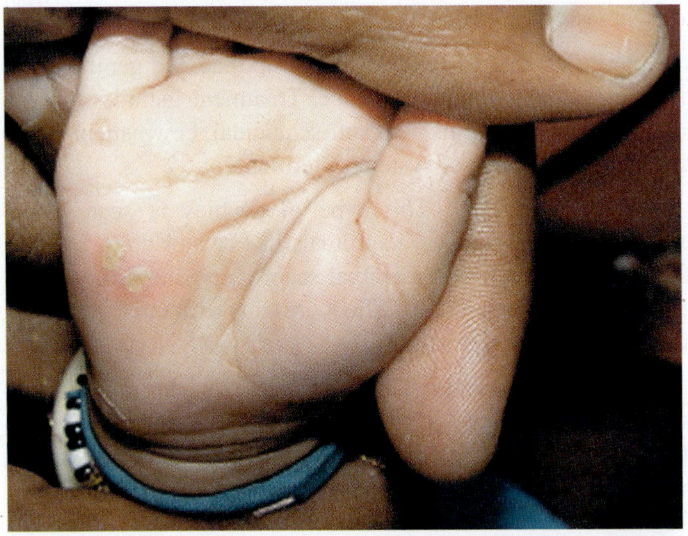

Figure 6.2: Lesions over palm of an infant

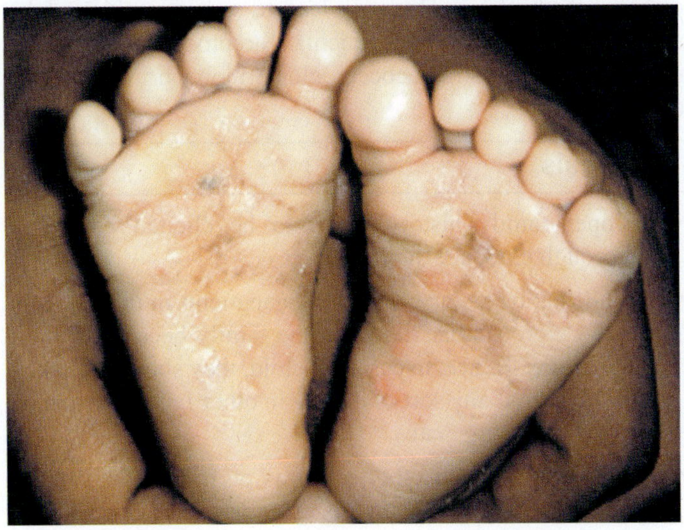

Figure 6.3: Lesions of scabies over soles

Non-specific erythematous papules and excoriations can be widespread.

Reddish-brown nodules of scabies may be seen in axillary and periumbilical regions (Figure 6.4) as well as around areola in females and on male genitalia (Figure 6.5).

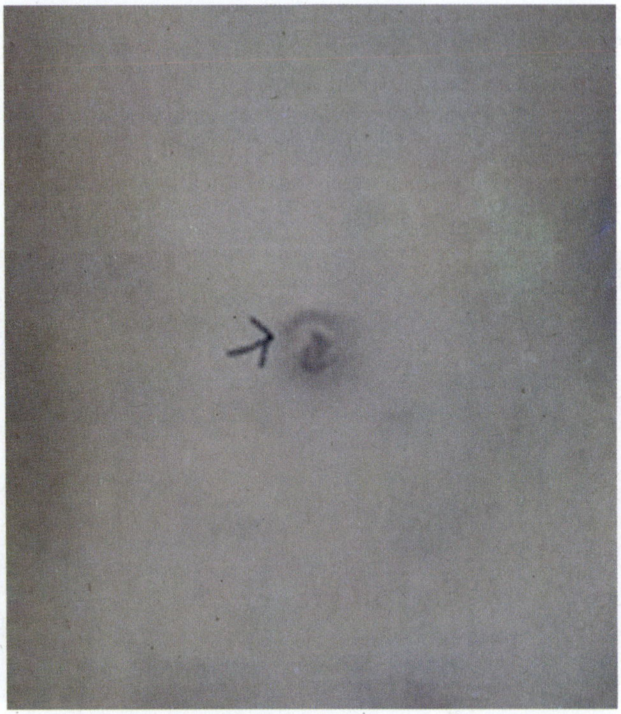

Figure 6.4: Lesions of scabies in periumbilical area

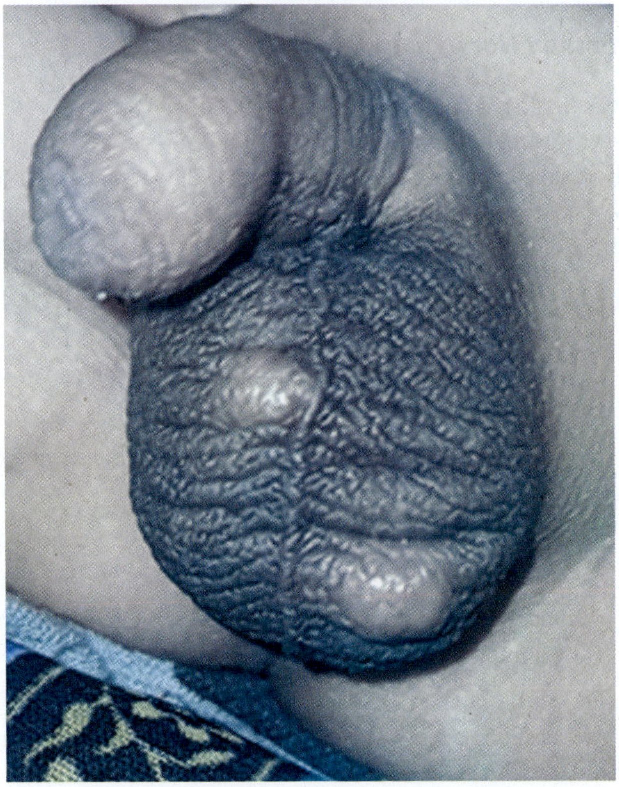

Figure 6.5: Nodular scabies on genitalia

Chronic scratching often results in extensive eczematization (Figure 6.6), patients may be misdiagnosed and treated for eczematous dermatitis.

Secondary infection with *Staphylococcus aureus* or group A *Streptococcus* is common in neglected cases of scabies and may present as pustules and impetigo. Infants as young as 9 days of age have shown evidence of scabies resulting from infestation shortly after birth. In infants and young children, vesiculopustular lesions are characteristically found on palms and soles, face, scalp and back.

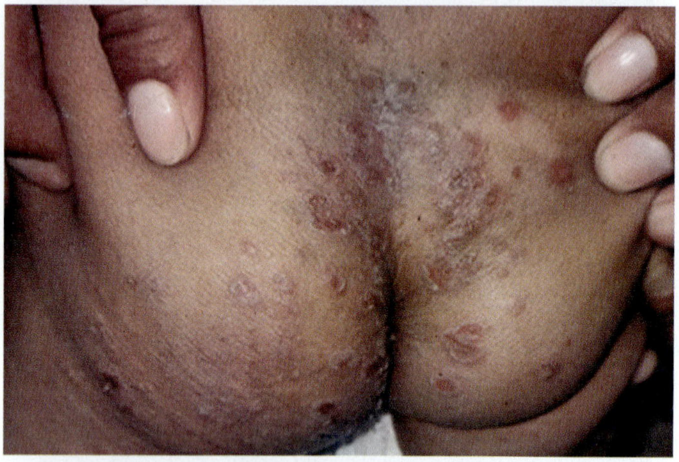

Figure 6.6: Infant with lesions on buttocks showing eczematization

Crusted / Norwegian Scabies

It was first described in leprosy patients in Norway in 1848. It is seen in immunocompromised and neurologically impaired individuals, occasionally in otherwise healthy subjects. Cases have been reported in association with HIV, Down's syndrome and organ transplant patients.

- Mites proliferate profusely and millions of mites are seen.
- Pruritus may be minimal or absent or host may be physically incapable of scratching. This protects mites from the destructive effect of excoriation.
- Diffuse hyperkeratosis associated with variable degree of underlying erythroderma may be seen.
- Crusting is seen on palms and soles, under fingernails, on ears, trunk and extremities.
- Secondary infection and generalized lymphadenopathy are common.
- Diagnosis can be established easily by mineral oil or KOH preparations of crust or skin scales which reveal numerous mites.
- Patients are highly contagious and it is a frequent cause of institutional outbreaks of scabies.
- Patients should be admitted in the ward with full precaution and isolation from other persons.

Other Type of Scabies

Scabies surrepticius: This term is used to describe all atypical clinical forms of scabies. In atypical forms of scabies, atypical lesions like bullous, urticarial, ecchymosis, rash resembling dermatomyositis, papulosquamous lesion resembling psoriasis, pityriasis rosea etc. may be seen.

Scabies incognito: Scabies incognito is seen in patients who maintain good hygiene or use topical or systemic steroids which results in complete masking of typical clinical features of scabies.

Nodular scabies: Nodules over axillae and genitalia are seen due to antigenic persistence. Treatment includes topical or intralesional steroids with anti-scabicidal. Few patients may require short course of systemic steroids.

Animal scabies: This type of scabies is seen when individual have exposure to animals like cats or dogs. Human is the accidental host for animal scabies and the mite cannot proliferate on human skin. Patient presents with intense pruritis on contact site to animal.

Ping pong scabies: This term is used when transmission of scabies occurs by symptomatic family member to other members. All family member should be treated simultaneously.

Complications

The fissures associated with crusted scabies provide a portal of entry for bacteria. This may lead to sepsis in older adults and immunocompromised patients. Streptococcal infections may lead to poststreptococcal glomerulonephritis or other complications.

Diagnosis

- Proper family history needs to be elicited besides a thorough clinical examination.
- While taking history, it is seen that patients or their parents may ignore similar illness in the family because of mild symptoms. Hence, in case of a child, they should be asked for history of any sort of itching in other family members, friends and classmates.
- History of visit to other relatives or friends who might have had some itching in the recent past may be found.
- Genitals should be examined to elicit nodular lesions in male patients.
- Itchy lesions at wrists, axillae, breast, umbilicus and buttocks may be a clue to the diagnosis of scabies in females.
- Scabies should be ruled out in case of infected and eczematous lesions in children.

- Microscopic identification of mite eggs, scybala (fecal pellets) is diagnostic.
- Specimen collection: Place a small drop of saline or mineral oil on the area to be sampled. Extract the female mite from the end of a burrow with the tip of a needle or by scraping the burrow with number 15 blade of scalpel. Specimen is placed in KOH or mineral oil on a glass slide and examined under low power of microscope.
- **Dermoscopic examination can identify sites of scabies mites or burrows and can facilitate placement of the scraping.**
  - The characteristic finding on dermoscopic examination is a dark, triangular shaped "delta wing"/hang glider/triangular head/delta jet sign, the anterior section of the mite including the head and the two anterior pairs of legs.
  - Contrail/curvilinear structure is a white S-shaped line (contrail) corresponds to the irregular burrow excavated by the mite. Delta jet with contrail sign is a mixture of the above two signs and is the colour of blood and thus has been historically associated with sacrifice, danger and courage.
  - "Mini-triangle sign" refers to the maturing scabies eggs that show the minute heads of the maturing mite within the egg.
  - "Noodle sign" is a recently defined dermoscopic sign in crusted scabies.

Laboratory abnormalities may include eosinophilia and increased immunoglobulin E (IgE) levels.

Definition criteria of scabies (Table 6.2).

Table 6.2: Definition of diagnostic criteria of scabies

A.	**Confirmed scabies**
	At least one of:
A1.	Mites, eggs or feces on light microscopy of skin samples
A2.	Mites, eggs or feces visualized on individual using high-powered imaging device
A3.	Mites visualized on individual using dermoscopy
B.	**Clinical scabies**
	At least one of:
B1.	Scabies burrows
B2.	Typical lesions affecting male genitalia
B3.	Typical lesions in a typical distribution and two history features
C.	**Suspected scabies**
	One of:
C1.	Typical lesions in a typical distribution and one history feature
C2.	Atypical lesions or atypical distribution and two history features
History features	
H1.	Itch
H2.	Close contact with an individual who has itch or typical lesions in a typical distribution

Differential Diagnosis

- Atopic dermatitis.
- Allergic contact dermatitis.
- Insect bites (Arthropod bites).
- Papular urticaria.
- Impetigo.
- Vesicular lesion on palms and soles in infants–infantile acropustulosis.
- Nodular scabies–Urticaria pigmentosa.
- On histology, nodules may be mistaken for lymphoma.
- Crusted/Norwegian scabies may be misdiagnosed as psoriasis or seborrhoeic dermatitis.

Treatment

Attention should be given to:

- Elimination of mite.
- Treatment of symptoms.
- Treatment of secondary infection, if present.

Antiscabietic Agents

- **Gamma-benzene hexachloride (lindane)**
  - To be applied as 1% lotion or cream to skin surface for 8-12 hours. Repeat application after one week is recommended.
  - It is neurotoxic to humans if ingested or excessive percutaneous absorption occurs, seizures may be seen.
  - Not recommended in infants less than 6 months of age, pregnant or nursing women or patients with severe underlying skin disorders.
- **Permethrin**
  - It is drug of choice in scabies, used as 5% cream.
  - Insignificant percutaneous systemic absorption occurs.
  - No serious adverse effects are seen, burning or stinging may be seen in few patients.

   - Not approved for use in infants less than 2 months of age. Guidelines recommend 7% sulphur preparation instead of permethrin.
   - Recommended to be applied twice to whole body below neck (to be applied on face also in infantile scabies) at the interval of one week. In chronic cases, repeat application twice daily below neck after 7 days may be necessary.
- **Crotamiton**
   - It is used as 10% cream or lotion.
   - Mode of action is unknown, it is an antipruritic agent also.
   - Daily application for 5 days is effective in children.
- **Benzyl benzoate**
   - It is used as 25% lotion.
   - Single application for 24 hours or 2-3 successive applications at 12 hours interval is recommended.
   - Irritant, less acceptable in children.
- **Ivermectin**
   - It is an oral antihelmenthic agent, macrocyclic lactone, structurally similar to macrolide antibiotics.
   - It acts by blocking GABA mediated neurotransmission in parasite.
   - Ivermectin as 200 μg/kg orally 2 doses at 2 weeks interval is recommended (Table 6.3).

Table 6.3: Weight-based guidelines for Ivermectin dose

Weight (kg)	*Dose (mg)*
15-24	3
25-35	6
36-50	9
51-65	12
66-79	15

- Two doses of ivermectin 7-10 days apart are as effective as single application of topical permethrin cream. Single dose is less effective than permethrin.
- Not approved for use in children of less than 15 kg of weight.
- Fever, pruritus, dizziness and oedema are uncommon side effects.

Treatment Guidelines

- Topical antiscabietic agent should be applied all over body except on face. Intra gluteal area, genitalia, umbilicus, flexures, fingernails and toenails should not be overlooked.
- Patients with short duration of symptoms can be treated with one or two applications of antiscabietic agents if applied properly to all sites. Treatment failure may occur if patient has chronic scabies or has not applied the medicine properly. In some patients, reapplication of antiscabietic agent or continuous application of a non-irritating drug like permethrin for seven days may be recommended. It may take 4-8 weeks for complete remission of symptoms in scabies.
- Eczematization in children should be taken care of properly and to be treated by giving 5-10 mg of prednisolone or 4-8 mg of methylprednisolone or 6 to 12 mg of deflazacort daily along with an antibiotic like azithromycin from the beginning of the therapy for 7-15 days (in younger children it can be used as per body weight). It will cause rapid drying of the lesions and allow the application of antiscabietic agent over eczematized areas. After a week, the remaining lesions are treated with local corticosteroids, while systemic corticosteroids are withdrawn.
- In cases of secondary infection, antibiotics like azithromycin should be given.
- Treat all close contacts and household members if they have minimal clinical evidence of scabies.
- Symptoms may persist upto 3 weeks after eradication of mites, local emollients combined with topical. corticosteroids may be applied.
- Nodular lesions are quite persistent and itchy. Persistent nodules after proper antiscabietic treatment should be treated with local application of corticosteroids and tacrolimus 0.1%. Patient may require oral steroid in the dose of 4-8 mg methylprednisolone or 6 to 12 mg of deflazacort per day for a period of 4-6 weeks. Intralesional steroids and cryotherapy may also be used for recalcitrant lesions.
- In children, scalp and face should be treated, taking care to avoid perioral and periorbital skin. Gloves are necessary for hands of thumb sucking infants and toddlers to avoid oral absorption of drug.
- Antihistamine agents should be given throughout the treatment for symptomatic relief from pruritus.
- European Guidelines for Management of Crusted Scabies.
- A topical scabicide (permethrin 5% cream or benzyl benzoate lotion 25%) repeated daily for 7 days then twice weekly until cure.
- Oral ivermectin 200 micrograms/kg on days 1, 2 and 8 should be added. For severe cases, based on persistent live mites on skin scrapings at follow-up visit, additional ivermectin treatment might be required on days 9 and most 15 or on days 9, 15, 22 and 29.

TICKS

Etiopathogenesis

Ticks are mainly classified into three groups: Hard ticks (Ixodidae), Soft ticks (Argasidae) and Nuttalliellidae.

They are important vectors of diseases like relapsing fever, rickettsial infections (Rocky Mountain spotted fever, Mediterranean spotted fever, Q fever and ehrlichiosis), Lyme disease, Colorado tick fever, babesiosis and tularemia.

Ticks penetrate the human epidermis with distal mouth parts, feed on blood and deposit various anticoagulant and anti-inflammatory substances, which result in acute and chronic dermatoses.

Clinical Features

- Acute manifestations are erythema, papules, nodules, bullae, ulceration and necrosis.
- Granulomas, alopecia, and secondary bacterial infection may be seen in chronic cases. Localized foreign body type reactions have been reported due to retained mouth parts or improper tick removal.
- Non dermatologic findings include anaphylaxis, fever, headache, flu like symptoms, abdominal pain, vomiting, tick paralysis (reversible disorder ascending motor weakness and flaccid paralysis due to salivary neurotoxin). Death may occur due to involvement of respiratory musculature.
- Cutaneous manifestations of Lyme's disease include erythema migrans, lymphocytoma, acrodermatitis chronica atrophicans, morphoea and other sclerotic skin disorders.

Treatment

Tick removal is the mainstay of treatment, which causes rapid resolution of the signs and symptoms.

Prevention

It is advised to wear light-colored, long-sleeved clothes and footwear, tucking pants into socks and taping the exposed edges. Insect repellents containing N, N-diethyl-3-methylbenzamide (DEET) or picaridin are applied to exposed areas of skin and permethrin can be applied to clothing. Presence of ticks should be examined frequently and all ticks must be removed, either manually or by commercial kits.

Antimicrobial prophylaxis with doxycycline may be sometimes used for prevention of diseases such as lyme disease.

Lyme's Disease/Borreliosis

It is caused by Borrelia burgdorferi, which is transmitted by ticks. Incubation period for Lyme's disease is 1-2 weeks.

Clinical features: It has three clinical stages:

- **Stage 1:** Erythema Chronicum Migrans (ECM): Initially patient develops asymptomatic erythematous papules over the site of bite, which gradually spread (2-3 cm/day) forming annular erythematous pattern also known as bull's eye appearance. The center of lesion may become indurated, with vesiculation and necrosis. Subsequently patient develops multiple smaller annular lesions. These rashes are accompanied by constitutional symptoms like fever, malaise and arthralgia.
- **Stage 2:** In few months, patient develops multiple systemic symptoms like arthralgia, lymphadenitis, carditis, meningitis, neuritis, panniculitis and ocular involvement which characterise this stage..
- **Stage 3 :** Over a period of one to ten years, patient develops acrodermatitis chronica atrophicans, juxtra-articular nodules, arthritis and progressive encephalomyelitis. Acrodermatitis chronica atrophicans presents with thin atrophic or cigarette paper like skin over distil extremities with visible cutaneous blood vessels. Juxtra-articular nodules represent fibrous proliferation over elbow and knee.

Diagnosis: Detection of antibody in serum by ELISA and western blot.

Treatment: Treatment should be done according to stage of disease.

- **Stage 1:** Doxycycline 100 mg bd for 2-3 weeks.
- **Stage 2:** Doxycycline 100 mg bd for 2-3 weeks or injection ceftriaxone 2 gm for 2 weeks.
- **Stage 3:** Injection ceftriaxone 2 gm for 2 weeks.

SPIDERS

The clinical syndrome following the bite of spider is called **"Arachnidism"**.

BLACK WIDOW SPIDER

Black widow spider and the brown recluse spider are the most common causes in reported cases of serious spider bite. While the former has a milder outcome, bite of the latter has severe implications.

Etiopathogenesis

The black widow spider, or *Latrodectus mactans,* is a potentially dangerous spider found mainly in southern Canada, the United States, Cuba and Mexico. It is coal-black in color and has globular body (1 cm in diameter) with a red-orange hourglass marking on ventral abdomen. It spins its web and lives in cool, dark places.

Clinical Features

α-Latrotoxin, is the potent black widow neurotoxin, which is responsible for its effects. It leaves two red, punctate marks and local swelling, burning, stinging and intense pain at the site of bite. This is followed by severe cramping abdominal pain and spasmodic muscular contractions, which peak in about 3 hours. Irritability, sweating, anxiety, agitation, priapism and hypertension have been noted. Although most of the children recover in 2-3 days, rarely it can be fatal.

Treatment

Treatment includes analgesics, benzodiazepines (diazepam), calcium gluconate, and specific antivenin. Intravenous opioids can be used for symptomatic relief.

BROWN RECLUSE SPIDER ("Violin" Or Fiddle Back Spider)

Etiopathogenesis

The brown recluse spider (Loxosceles reclusa), is one of the most dangerous spiders.

It has an oval, tan to dark brown body with a dark brown violin-shaped marking extending dorsally from the eyes to the distal cephalothorax. It lives in human altered environments. Its venom contains numerous enzymes, mainly SMD 2 (Sphingomyelinase D2), as well as alkaline phosphatase, esterase, adenosine triphosphatase (ATPase) and hyaluronidase.

Clinical Features

Within 6 hours of bite, pruritus, pain, and/or erythema develop at the site. In 24 hours, perilesional red ring, blue purple discoloration, followed by occasional hemorrhagic blisters and increased pain can develop. Ultimately, gangrenous ulceration with necrosis and eschar formation occurs (Figure 6.7). Targetoid lesion (Red, white and blue sign/marble plaque sign) has also been demonstrated. The affected area is often anaesthetic. Acute generalized exanthematous pustulosis has been seen in some cases which can be confused with drug eruptions.

Systemic findings may include chills, fever, nausea and joint pain. Rarely, severe hemolysis, renal failure, pulmonary edema, lymphangitis, erysipelas, cellulitis and necrotizing fasciitis have also been reported.

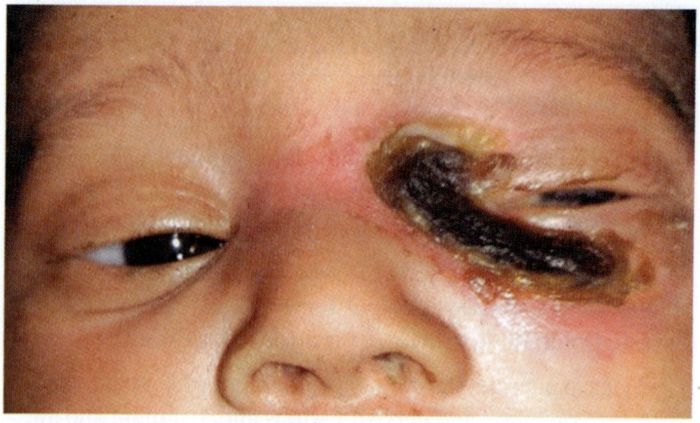

Figure 6.7: Spider bite

Treatment

Conservative treatment measures for these patients include rest, ice compression, and elevation of the affected area. Antibiotics should be given if secondary bacterial infection is suspected. Aspirin, antihistamines, dapsone and tetanus vaccination may be considered.

SCORPIONS

Etiopathogenesis

- Scorpions are photophobic arachnids that hide in the day and hunt in night. They are found worldwide, particularly in the tropics.
- In India, Buthidae family are the most toxic scorpions found.
- Children younger than 10 years are at greater risk of developing severe scorpion envenomation. Hence stings in children should be watched carefully, especially during the first 4 hours.
- Its venom is in curved stinger at the tip of the tail, through which it releases two agents: a localized hemolytic toxin and a dangerous neurotoxic venom. Their venom also contains histamines, kinins and 5-hydroxy tryptamine.

Clinical Features

Painful burning sensation, redness with swelling, discoloration, necrosis, lymphangitis, and occassionally, disseminated intravascular coagulation or renal failure can occur due to hemolytic toxin. The neurotoxic venom may produce local numbness and a severe reaction consisting of sweating, salivation, tightness in the throat, abdominal cramps, cyanosis, muscle jerking, tongue fasciculations, convulsions, respiratory paralysis and death, particularly in small children. Tachycardia, hypertension, pulmonary edema, and shock may also develop.

Treatment

Tourniquet above the area of the sting should be applied immediately. Application of ice or cold water should be done. Serotherapy, which is the administration of scorpion antivenin, is a controversial therapy.

CLASS: INSECTA

This class includes thousands of species present throughout the world, out of which common pathogenic infestations will be discussed here:

- **Pediculosis.**
- **Fleas.**
- **Blister beetle.**
- **Bed bugs.**

PEDICULOSIS

Pediculosis or lice infestation is caused by blood sucking insects with six legs. They lay their eggs on hair shafts or clothing seams. Three species of lice of the order Anoplura affect humans: *Pediculus humanus capitis* (head louse), *Pediculus humanus corporis* (body louse) and *Phthirus pubis* (pubic louse). While pediculosis capitis is typically restricted to the scalp, patients with pediculosis corporis present with widespread symptoms, frequently involving the truncal areas.

Head louse or pediculosis capitis is the predominant infestation during childhood with a prevalence of 10-40% in school children. *Pediculus humanus corporis* (body louse) serves as a vector for diseases such as epidemic typhus, trench fever, and relapsing fever. Bartonella quintana transmission via louse infestation has also been linked to endocarditis.

Epidemiology

- It is distributed worldwide.
- Females are affected more than males.
- Overcrowding, poor hygiene and low socioeconomic status are predisposing factors but pediculosis affects children with high socioeconomic status also.
- Upto 50% of persons might have suffered from pediculosis some time in their life.

Etiopathogenesis

- Lice are wingless, dorsoventrally flattened, crawling insects.
- It is an obligate ectoparasites and complete their life cycle on human host.
- They feed by directly inserting their mouth parts into host blood vessel.
- Louse has three pairs of legs with claws adapted to cling to hair or body clothes.
- Head louse and body louse are similar in structure. They are greyish white insects 3-4 mm long, male is slightly smaller.
- The pubic or crab louse is different in appearance from the head or body louse. Its body is broader and less elongated. The second and third pair of legs have heavy claws for grasping hairs.
- Female louse firmly cements its newly laid eggs to the proximal hair shaft close to the scalp or skin for warmth.
- The eggs or nits are oval with an operculum or lid.
- After 6-8 days the emerging louse nymph comes out from the operculated end, ready for its first meal.
- After the ovum has hatched, the empty egg case or nit remains firmly cemented to the hair shaft.
- Life span of an adult louse is 17-28 days, female louse lays an average of 3-5 eggs per day.

Clinical Features

Pediculosis Capitis

- Transmission is by head to head contact, role of fomites like combs or hats is controversial.
- Main symptom is pruritus, due to sensitization to the saliva and faecal material of the louse, pruritus may be absent in initial weeks of infestation.
- Scratching injures the insects and limits the degree of infestation.
- Occipital region is the most commonly affected site. Secondary bacterial infections with posterior cervical and occipital lymphadenopathy may occur.
- Examination reveals nits, firmly cemented to hair shaft (Figure 6.8), live insects are often missed.
- In children with long hair, bite reactions may be seen on the back and sides of neck.
- Secondary infection causes recurrent pyodermas, matting of hair or foul smelling discharge. Children with recurrent pyodermas, especially in the occipital region, should be examined for pediculosis.

Differential Diagnosis

Nits should be distinguished from hair casts, white Piedra, black Piedra and Seborrheic capitis (true nits of pediculosis

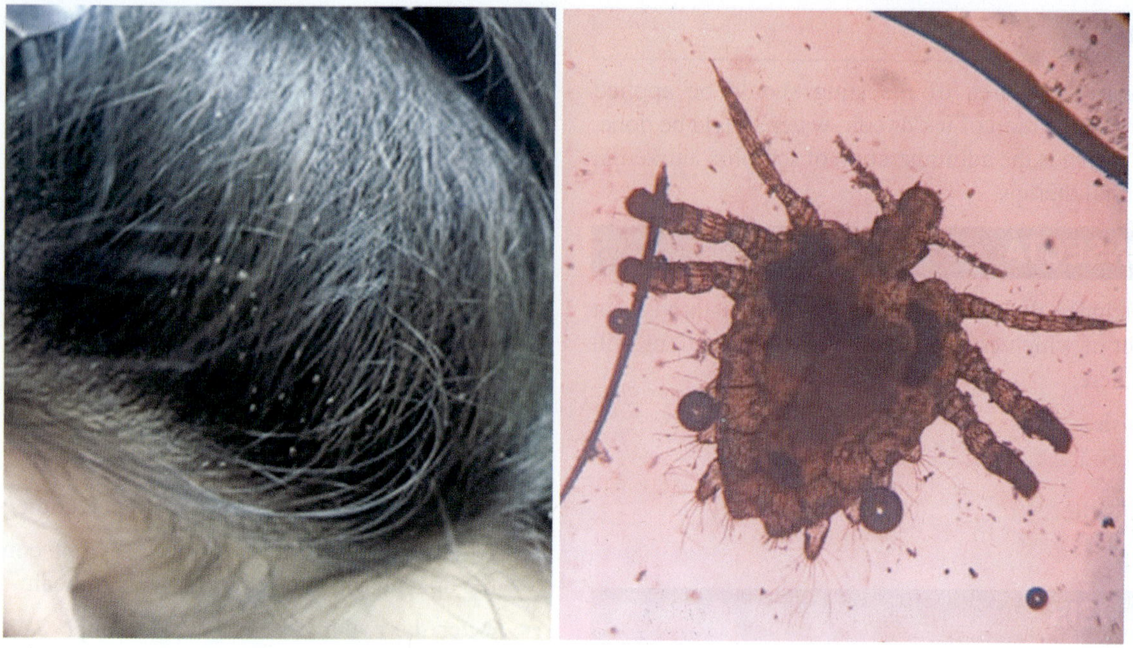

Figure 6.8: Pediculosis capitis showing nits

are firmly attached to hair, while scales of seborrheic capitis come off easily).

Pediculosis Corporis (Figure 6.9)

- Body louse is similar in morphology to head louse.
- It is rarely seen in children.
- Transmission is via infested clothing or bedding.

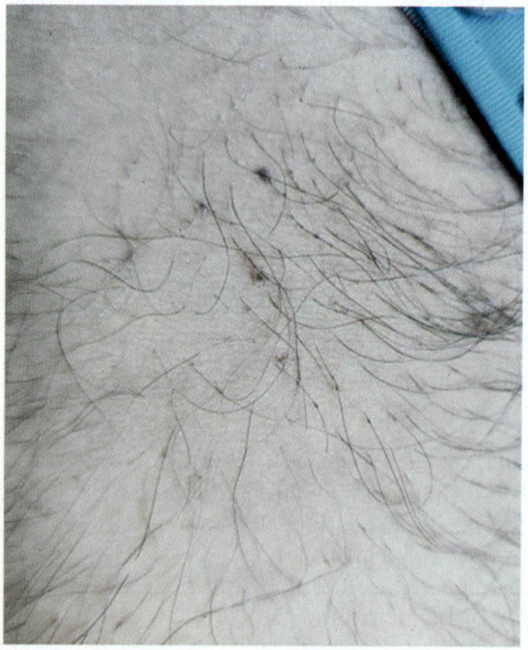

Figure 6.9: Pediculosis Corporis

- Body louse infestation is also known as vagabond disease, which may present with itching over the back. Bite reactions are seen as erythematous papules, weal's in areas of skin clothing. Signs may be limited to linear excoriations on the trunk and neck along with post inflammatory hyperpigmentation. Self-negligence may lead to eczematization, secondary infection, lichenification or lymphadenopathy. Skin changes tend to be concentrated around the waist and in the axillary folds, areas where clothing seams contact the integument.
- Lice and eggs are found in seams of clothing next to skin.
- Disease is eradicated by change of clothing and bedding.
- Atopic or contact dermatitis, pruritus secondary to systemic disease, and neurodermatitis may present with similar symptoms, and should be considered in the differential diagnosis.

Pediculosis Pubis

- Caused by *Phthirus pubis* (crab or pubic lice) which is broader (Figure 6.10) and smaller (1.5-2 mm) than head louse.
- It is less common in children.
- Transmitted by sexual or close body contact, infests pubic hair of adults.
- Patient presents with itching and scratching in pubic area, upper thighs or in axilla.

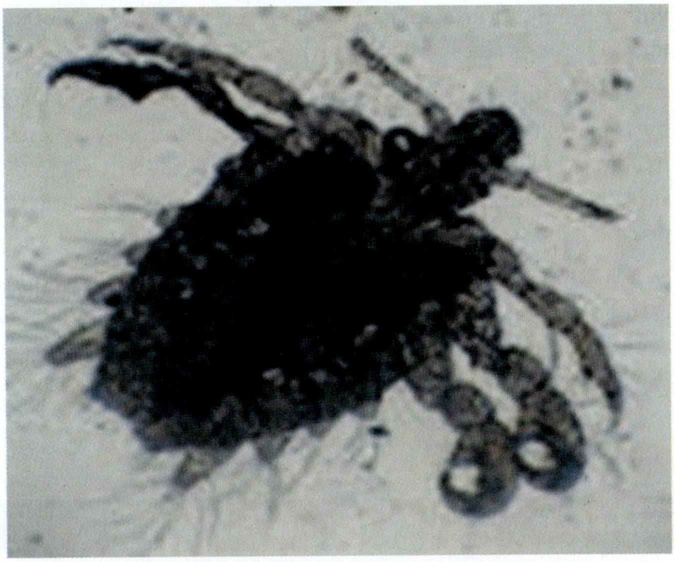

Figure 6.10: Pubic louse

- Louse is well-camouflaged, can be easily overlooked or mistaken for freckles or scabs which are close to pubic hair as brownish specks.
- It can affect hair of eyelashes in children, with symptoms of blepharoconjunctivitis (also known as pediculosis ciliaris and phthiriasis palpebrum).
- Bluish brown hemosiderin laden-macules known as 'maculae cerulae' are seen at site of bites.

Management

General Considerations

- Lotion formulations should be thoroughly applied near the root of hair and left for 12 hours.
- Treatment should be repeated after 7-10 days to kill newly born lice.
- Lotions are preferred over shampoos as the later expose the insects to relatively short period, at low concentration, which may allow the development of resistance.
- For removing nits and to kill ova, the hair should be combed with a fine toothed comb dipped in pediculocides.
- All pediculocides are similar in their ability to kill adult lice, but vary in their ovicidal activity.
- Gamma benzene hexachloride (lindane) is less commonly used nowadays, since resistance has been reported.

Pediculocidal Drugs

Permethrin (1%)

- It is both ovicidal and pediculocidal.
- Single application is adequate, can be repeated after one week if live lice are observed.
- *Side effect:* Mild irritation.

Malathion (0.5%)

- Both ovicidal and pediculocidal.
- Single application is sufficient.
- Safe, but has unpleasant odour.

Lindane (1%)

- Only pediculocidal, hence repeat application is recommended to kill the larvae, which hatch out of ova.
- Neurotoxic, if absorbed through impaired skin barrier, but no adverse effects reported after use of shampoo locally.

Treatment of Pediculosis Capitis

- Pediculocides are formulated as shampoo (lindane), cream rinse (permethrin 1%), lotion (malathion 0.5%, lindane 1%, permethrin 1%).
- Shampoos and cream rinses have shorter application times and higher failure rates.
- Lotions are applied for long hours and have greater efficacy.
- Secondary infection should be treated with systemic antibiotics, analgesics, antipyretics. If hairs are badly matted, they should be shortened.

Treatment of Pubic Lice

- Repeat application of pediculocide after one week is required.
- Treatment of spouse or partner may be done.
- Other hair bearing areas of scalp and body should be examined and treated adequately.

Treatment of Eyelash Infestation

- Treatment with pediculocides is not recommended because of potential ocular irritation and toxicity.
- Application of plain petroleum jelly twice daily for a week or removal of lice and nits manually with fine forceps or application of freshly prepared 20% fluorescein eye drops to the lid margin is quite effective.

Treatment of Pediculosis Corporis

- Laundering of clothes in hot water to kill lice and eggs, use of hot iron, particularly to seams of clothing and change of bedding are effective measures.

FLEAS

Etiopathogenesis

Fleas (Siphonaptera) are uniquitously present among animals and humans.

Most common species, which attack humans, are the human flea (Pulex irritans), the cat flea (Ctenocephalides felis), and the dog flea (Ctenocephalides canis). Fleas play a role in the transmission of several infectious diseases as a component of epidemiologic cycles that also include animals and humans. Examples include plague (*Yersinia pestis*), bartonellosis and murine typhus.

Clinical Features

- The most common clinical finding seen in case of flea bite in a sensitized individual, is an urticarial wheal or papule with a centrally located hemorrhagic punctum (papular urticaria).
- Young children are highly susceptible and wheals may progress and develop into tense bullae in them. Flea bites can be clinically diagnosed with specific features like multiple and grouped bites in linear or irregular clusters on the arms, forearms, or legs.
- Bites in a linear configuration (the "breakfast, lunch, and dinner" sign); are common and is because of their tendency to jump and crawl but not fly.

Treatment

Local skin reactions can be treated with systemic non sedating antihistamines, mild topical steroid and antibiotic preparations and astringent. Suspected animal carriers should be treated. Cleaning/spraying of carpets, floors, crevices, and other potentially infested areas should be considered. They are present in large numbers in and around any infected individual. Animal flea sprays and powders must be repeated every 2 weeks during the summer months to be effective.

CUTANEOUS MYIASIS

It is an infestation of larva or maggots of fly, order Diptera and presents in three different forms:

- Furuncular form
- Migratory form
- Wound form

Furuncular myiasis: It is most commonly caused by Dermatobia hominis and Cordyloabi anthropophaga. Boil like nodule with central pore occur, through which serosanguinous or purulent fluid is discharged. In few days, a cavity is formed with pain and pruritus. Patient can feel sensation of moving larva. Lesions resolve with scarring.

Migratory myiasis or creeping myiasis: It is caused by Gastrophilus intestinalis, which presents initially as small papule, which progresses to form linear, raised burrows in the skin, producing the migratory pattern. Patient complains of pricking and pain sensation.

Wound myiasis: Infestation of maggot into open wounds results in wound myiasis, which presents with extensive tissue destruction and necrosis resulting in bleeding and pain. It is caused by Cochliomyia and Chrysomya.

Treatment includes oral or topical ivermectin, turpentine mineral oil and manual removal of larva.

BLISTER BEETLES (Figure 6.11)

Blister beetles (Meloidae and Oedemeridae family beetle) contain cantharidin in their genitalia, which is a vesicant. It causes acute irritant contact dermatitis, commonly seen in Asia and tropical areas. The symptoms appear within few hours of contact with beetle. Vesicant toxin comes from saliva of beetle, which produces painful blisters at the site of salivation.

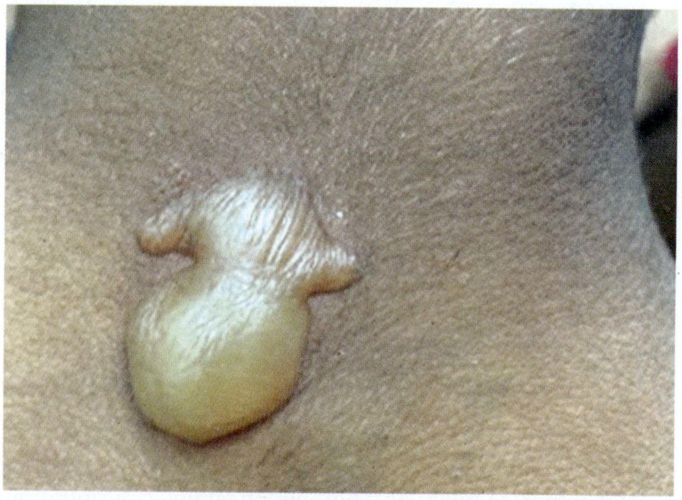

Figure 6.11: Blister beetle dermatitis

Treatment

Treatment depends on the extent and site of lesions. Simple aseptic drainage of large bullae and cool compresses alleviate the symptoms. If vesicles are not ruptured, they usually resolve in 3 to 4 days with desquamation and healing. Topical steroid can be used for symptomatic relief.

PAEDERUS DERMATITIS (Figure 6.12)

It is caused by Nairobi fly, order coleoptera (rove beetle). These beetles are usually found in decaying vegetables and animal material in rainy season. Patient presents with linear streak of erythema which appears within 1-2 days after exposure to beetle, followed by vesiculation and pustulation. The lesions heals in a week. Other features include kissing lesions, which occur over two adjacent flexural surfaces, periocular dermatitis or conjunctivitis (Nairobi eye), and balanitis. Diagnosis is made by clinical examination. Treatment includes cleaning of the affected area with soap and water to remove toxin followed by topical steroid application.

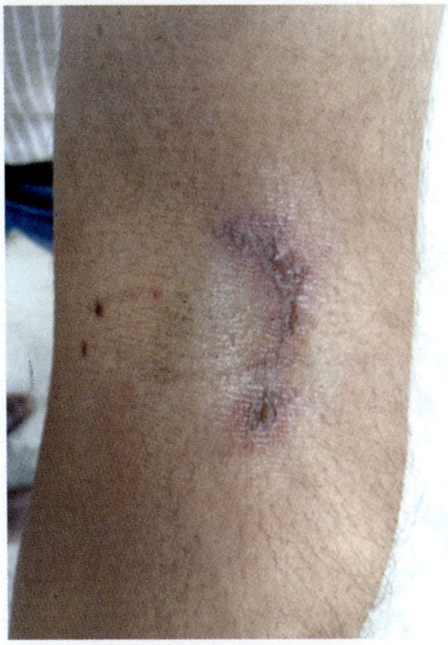

Figure 6.12: Paederus dermatitis (kissing lesion)

BED BUG

- Bedbugs are true bugs of the order Hemiptera and family Cimicidae.
- Bedbugs are obligate, blood feeding insects that inhabit human dwellings and may cause skin reactions in humans.
- Bedbugs are present worldwide. Spread of infestation can occur through transportation of items, harboring bedbugs, as may occur with travel or acquisition of used furniture, or through direct movement of bedbugs in multifamily buildings or institutions.
- Bedbugs do not live on humans. Rather, they tend to inhabit cracks and crevices of mattresses, cushions, bed frames, or other structures. Bedbugs are attracted to the host by warmth and carbon dioxide and generally feed at night while the victim sleeps.
- Skin reactions to bedbugs vary, ranging from no reaction to pruritic papules or wheals, purpuric macules, or bullae. Reactions are typically noticed upon awakening or within a few days after the bites. A linear series of bites is a potential but not consistent finding.
- Confirmation of the diagnosis of bedbug bites requires detection of bedbugs in the victim's environment. Inspection of the victim's residence by a professional pest control service is the preferred method for detection.
- Management of bedbug infestation consists of eradication of the infestation through employment of a professional pest control service. The primary methods include application of insecticides and heat treatment. When such interventions are not feasible, physical removal of detected bedbugs may reduce the severity of infestation but is unlikely to eradicate the infestation.
- Bedbug bites resolve spontaneously. Topical corticosteroids and oral antihistamines may reduce associated pruritus. Psychologic support services can be beneficial for some victims.

RICKETTSIAL DISEASES

Rickettsia are obligate intracellular, gram-negative coccobacilli. These are transmitted by blood sucking arthropod vectors like lice, fleas, ticks and mites. Classification of rickettsial diseases is given in Table 6.4.

Table 6.4: Classification of Rickettsial diseases

Disease	*Organism*	*Vector*	*Mammalian host*
Typhus group			
Epidemic typhus (Louse borne typhus)	R. prowazekii	Louse	Human
Endemic/murine typhus (Flea borne typhus)	R. typhi	Flea	Rodents
Scrub typhus (Mite borne typhus)	O. tsutsugamushi	Mite	Rodents
Spotted fever group			
Rocky mountain spotted fever	R. rickettsiae	Tick	Rodents
Indian tick typhus	R. conorii	Tick	Rodents
Rickettsial pox	R. akari	Mite	Mice
Others			
Q fever	C. brunetti	Nil	Cattles
Trench fever	R. quintana	Louse	Human

The patients present with undifferentiated acute febrile illness, headache, malaise and skin rashes.

Rocky Mountain Spotted Fever

Rashes appear over wrist and ankles in 2-3 days of tick bite, which later become more widespread.

Rickettsial Pox

Patient presents with erythematous indurated patch over mite bite site which later forms eschar. Cutaneous rash develops over face, trunk and extremities. These rashes closely resemble varicella infection.

Epidemic Typhus Or Louse Borne Typhus/ Brill-Zinsser Disease

It is presents with abrupt onset of fever, severe headache and rashes. Rashes are blotchy, initially occur over trunk and then spread to extremities.

Endemic/Murine Typhus/Flea Borne Typhus

It is a less severe form of typhus.

Scrub Typhus

It presents with fever headache and rashes. Patient initially develops erythema and induration over site of mite bite which later forms dry scab like lesion (eschar). Other features include rashes over trunk and generalized lymphadenopathy.

Diagnosis of Rickettsial Disease

Serology is the mainstay for diagnosis. Indirect immuno-fluorescent test is the most superior test to detect rickettsial antigen. Other tests include Weil-Felix test, complement fixation test and latex agglutination test.

Treatment of Rickettsial Disease

Most of the Rickettsial disease are self-limiting Treatment includes oral antibiotics doxycycline (drug of choice), macrolides or chloramphenicol and supportive treatment.

INSECT BITE REACTION

It is a common skin reaction to arthropod bite, sting or contact with body part of arthropods. First exposure doesn't produce reaction. Subsequent exposure results in hypersensitivity reaction against the exposed products of arthropods. Most common identified causes are human flea (pulex irritans) and mites. Other arthodpods are also implicated like bed bugs (cimex lectularius and cimex hemipterus), mosquitoes and beetles.

It is commonly seen in childhood and presents with chronic and recurrent relapsing papular urticaria (misnomer as it is not urticaria). It presents with pruritic papules and vesicles with excoriations.

Treatment: Symptomatic treatment using topical corticosteroids and antihistamines.

PARASITIC DISEASES

Protozoan and helminths are endoparasite (living in body of host) causing various diseases in human. Classification of important cutaneous diseases caused by protozoan and helminths are described in Table 6.5.

Table 6.5: Classification of important cutaneous diseases caused by protozoal and helminthic infections (Parasites)

Protozoal diseases		
• Leishmaniasis • Amoebiasis • Toxoplasmosis		
Diseases caused by helminths		
Nematodes	***Trematodes (Flukes)***	***Cestodes (Tape worms)***
• Onchocerciasis • Anchylostomiasis • Strongyloidiasis • Filariasis • Cutaneous larva migrans • Enterobiosis vermicularis	• Schistosomiasis • Cercarial dermatitis	• Cysticercosis

INFECTIONS WITH PROTOZOA

Pathogenic protozoan species which cause diseases in humans are:

- **Leishmania.**
- **Amoeba.**
- **Toxoplasma.**

CUTANEOUS LEISHMANIASIS

Leishmaniasis is caused by several species of intracellular protozoa of the genus *Leishmania. Leishmania* causes a spectrum of cutaneous disease. The range of clinical manifestations may be attributed to variability in parasite virulence and variability in the host immune response. At one end of the spectrum, mucosal leishmaniasis (ML) and leishmaniasis recidivans (LR) are caused by oligoparasitic disease associated with a marked cellular immune response. The center of the spectrum consists of localized cutaneous leishmaniasis (LCL), which is the most common clinical presentation. At the opposite end of the spectrum, diffuse cutaneous leishmaniasis (DCL) is caused by polyparasitic disease with a predominance of parasitized macrophages and no granulomatous inflammation.

Four major diseases that affect the skin, mucosal tissues and some viscera are:

- Cutaneous leishmaniasis.
- Mucosal leishmaniasis.
- Diffuse (anergic) Cutaneous leishmaniasis.
- Visceral leishmanias – kala azar, post kala azar dermal leishmaniasis.

In India, cutaneous leishmaniasis is endemic in northern parts of Rajasthan whereas visceral leishmaniasis is seen in eastern India, mainly in Bihar, West Bengal and Assam. Amongst the cases of cutaneous leishmaniasis, 15% occur in children under 14 years of age.

Etiopathogenesis

- Caused by protozoa belonging to family Trypanosomatidae and genus Leishmania.
- It is transmitted to the vertebrate host by the bite of the sand-fly of genera *Phlebotomus* or *Psychodopygus* (Old world) and Lutzomyia (New world).
- It is a dimorphic parasite living in the host macrophages as amastigotes which are round-oval forms, 2-3 µm in diameter.
- In cultures and in gut of the sand flies they adopt a promastigote form, which is elongated, 15-25 µm ×3 µm in size, with a long anterior flagellum.
- Sandflies contain abundant promastigotes in their proboscis, which are injected into the host, about 10-200 per bite.
- The promastigotes are phagocytosed by macrophages and transformed into amastigotes. Amastigotes are obligate intracellular parasites.
- The disease presentation depends on the immune response by the host, a good immune response results in localized Cutaneous form of leishmaniasis, with poor immunity diffuse nodular form is seen.

Histopathology

- Initial papular lesions show dermal infiltrate of lymphocytes and plasma cells with vacuolated sub-epidermal macrophages containing abundant amastigotes (LD bodies). Leishman Donovan bodies are seen in 70% of the cases. By Giemsa stain, the parasite is stained metachromatically and the kinetoplast bright red.
- Older, ulcerated lesions show epidermal hyperplasia. Dermis shows disorganized granulomas formed by epithelioid cells, vacuolated macrophages, lymphocytes and plasma cells. Giant cells as well as fibrinoid or caseation necrosis may be seen resembling tuberculosis. Amastigotes are difficult to demonstrate in older lesions.

Clinical Features

Localized Cutaneous Leishmaniasis

- Commonly seen in India.
- *L. donovani, L. tropica* and *L. major* are the causative organisms.
- It is most frequent clinical form in both children and adults.
- It commonly affects the exposed parts of the body, like face and extremities.
- Mostly presents as a single lesion, but multiple lesions and extensive ulcers may also occur.
- Incubation period ranges from 2 weeks to 12 months.
- At the site of inoculation, erythema with a papule, nodule (Figure 6.13) or plaque (Figure 6.14) forms which gradually increases in size and eventually ulcerates.

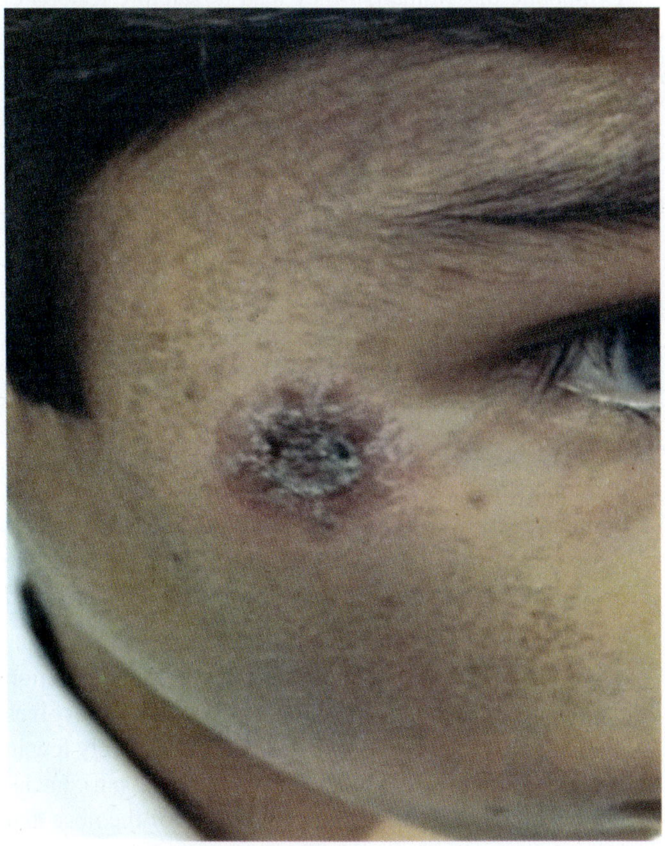

Figure 6.13: Cutaneous leishmaniasis (nodule)

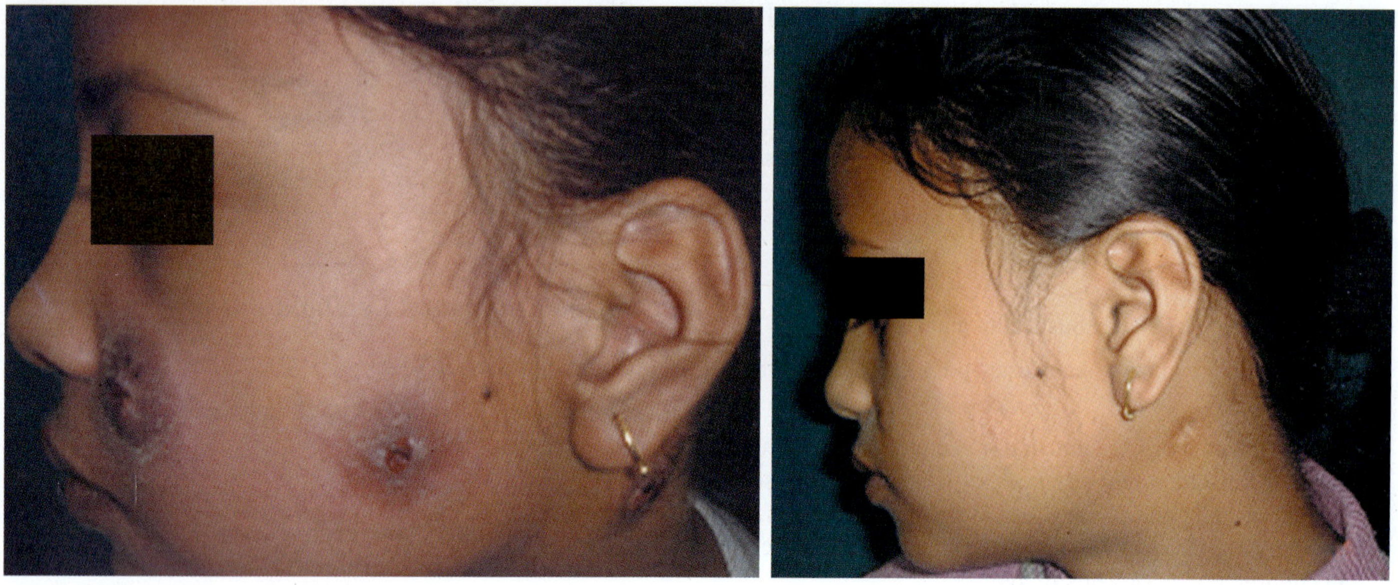

Figure 6.14: Cutaneous leishmaniasis (plaque) before treatment (A) and after treatment with ketoconazole, rifampicin and dapsone (B)

- The ulcer is painless, with well-defined, thick, raised, erythematous borders and a hard indurated base. It may be covered with a thick crust or may have a verrucous appearance.
- Lymphatic dissemination may lead to satellite lesions or regional lymphadenopathy.
- Lesions are usually self resolving, within 6-12 months, leaving behind an atrophic or pigmented scar. Following resolution of the initial lesion(s), it is possible that reactivation of the initial lesion(s) may occur during the subsequent year.
- According to the morphology two major types are seen: the wet (moist/rural) form shows ulceration and is caused by *L. major*, while the dry (urban) form shows less ulceration, is covered by a thick crust and is caused by *L. tropica*.
- *L. major* infection typically has a short incubation period, and ulcers may expand in one to two months to ≥ 6 cm in diameter. Multiple lesions are common. Frequently, ulcers are covered with a thick crust, and nodular, plaque-like lesions are common. Epithelialization of the ulcer bed usually occurs within six months.
- *L. tropica* infection is typically a more chronic infection than cutaneous leishmaniasis due to *L. major*; it evolves over months to years. The skin lesions are relatively few in number and sometimes relatively small (1 to 2 cm). Facial lesions may be larger, and a predilection for the nose and forehead may be observed. They are very dry and appear crusted. Spontaneous resolution is slow, usually over one to two years or longer. *L. tropica* can be associated with the complication of LR (leishmaniasis recidivans).
- **Leishmaniasis recidivans (LR):** Leishmaniasis recidivans (LR) refers to a relatively uncommon syndrome caused by *L. tropica* infection. Following healing of the primary lesion, persistent organisms can cause new papules to form around the margin of the scar. Skin biopsy demonstrates few parasites but a robust granulomatous, cell-mediated immune response. LR can occur following trauma in the area of a prior lesion many years after initial healing. Ulcerated lesions give a crateriform appearance often referred to as "volcano sign".

Mucocutaneous Leishmaniasis

- It is rare in children and is uncommon in India.
- May occur a month to years after the initial cutaneous lesion occurs, which may not be noticed.
- Invasion of mucosa from a contiguous cutaneous lesion occurs, usually over the nose or upper lip. Concomitant cutaneous and mucosal lesions are found is less than 30% of the patients.
- Mucosal leishmaniasis (ML), also known as espundia, occurs in the New World and is caused by the *Viannia* subgenus, especially *L.V. braziliensis*, *L.V. guyanensis*, and *L.V. panamensis*.
- Nasal, buccopharyngeal, conjunctival or penile mucosa may be involved.
- Nasal mucosa involvement may lead to nasal blockage, rhinorrhoea, epistaxis, nodular infiltration, ulceration or perforation.

- Oral lesions may cause halitosis, dysphagia and secondary bacterial infections.

Diffuse Cutaneous Leishmaniasis

- Uncommon in India.
- Diffuse cutaneous leishmaniasis (DCL) is a rare syndrome that occurs mainly in the setting of *L.L aethiopica*, *L.L mexicana* and *L.L. amazonensis* infection. It begins as a localized lesion that does not ulcerate; rather, amastigotes disseminate via macrophages in other areas of the skin.
- It is characterized by soft nodules or plaques on the face and extensor limb surfaces, which disseminate slowly affecting most of the body surface.
- The evolution of the lesions is chronic, possibly lifelong and the lesions have large amounts of amastigotes.
- Patients with DCL usually have a defect in the cell-mediated immune response and are anergic to *Leishmania* antigen.
- Successful treatment of DCL is difficult.

Visceral Leishmaniasis

- Endemic in Bihar, West Bengal and Assam.
- It is also known as 'Kala azar', occurs mainly in India and Pakistan and refers to the brownish-black pigmentation of skin, which is commonly seen.
- The disease disseminates from the cutaneous lesion to macrophages of spleen, bone marrow, liver and lymph nodes.
- The patient presents with prolonged fever, fatigue, weight loss with hepatosplenomegaly and lymphadenopathy.
- Bone marrow and spleen involvement may cause anemia, thrombocytopenia and leucopenia.

Post Kala Azar Dermal Leishmaniasis

- It occurs in 20% of patients suffering from visceral leishmaniasis and usually occurs weeks or months after treatment.
- The clinical manifestations of PKDL are variable. Hypopigmented macules to infiltrated papules, plaques and nodules can be seen (Figure 6.15). Children predominantly have the hypopigmented form with little or no papular lesions. Black pigmentation of skin may be seen.

Complications

- Atrophic scars causing cosmetic problem is associated with cutaneous leishmaniasis.
- Secondary bacterial infections, dysphagia, dysphonia, fistulas can occur in mucocutaneous leishmaniasis.

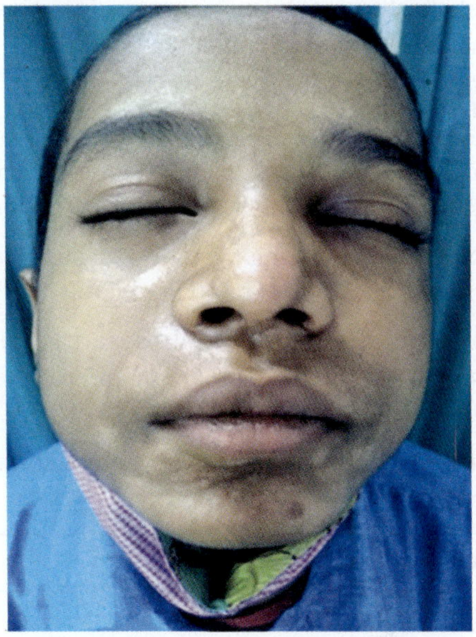

Figure 6.15: PKDL with infiltrated hypopigmented papules and plaques over face

Diagnosis

- Clinical appearance of lesion, geographical location of patient is important.
- Slit skin smear from the edge of lesion, stained with Giemsa stain shows amastigotes in 80-90% cases. Slit skin smear shows amastigotes more frequently than biopsy.
- Culture in NNN (Novy, MacNeal, Nicolle) media.
- Skin biopsy would also reveal amastigotes.
- Direct and indirect immunofluorescence.
- Leishmanin (Montenegro) test indicates active disease if present with appropriate clinical findings.
- Polymerase chain reaction is one of the most sensitive diagnostic tests for CL.
- Serology – rk39 rapid antigen dipstick test based on recombinant k39 protein is also done.

Differential Diagnosis

- Bacterial ulcers.
- Pyoderma gangrenosum.
- Scrofuloderma, lupus vulgaris.
- Fungal infections like sporotrichosis, chromomycosis, paracoccidioidomycosis.

- Nasal lesions resemble rhinosporidiosis, nasal scleroma or lepromatous leprosy.
- Visceral leishmaniasis may be confused with histoplasmosis, leukemia or lymphoma.

Treatment

- Sodium stibogluconate is given 20 mg/kg once daily IM for14-21days, patient should be followed up for 2 years.
- Amphotericin B-0.5-1mg/kg daily as slow intravenous infusion upto a total dose of 20 mg/kg.
- Ketoconazole, rifampicin and dapsone can be used in a combination (Figures 6.14). Care should be taken to avoid hepatotoxicity.
- Local therapy in the form of electrocauterization, curettage and cryotherapy.

Prevention

Vector control methods include:

- Fully covered clothing of children to avoid bite of sand-fly at exposed sites.
- Use of mosquito nets, pesticides, insect repellents and house painting with pesticide are other measures.

Treatment of post kala azar dermal leishmaniasis:

Post kala azar dermal leishmanisis can be treated by miltefosine, amphotericin B and liposomal Amphotericin B. Duration and dose regimen given in Table 6.6.

Table 6.6: Treatment of PKDL

Drugs	*Duration*	*Dose*
Miltefosine	4 weeks	Adult > 12 years-50 mg bd Children 2-12 years-2.5 mg /kg once daily
Amphotericin B (Non liposomal)	4 months (20 days on and 20 days off therapy)	1 mg/kg/day infusion 60 -8- doses over 4 months
Liposomal Amphotericin B	3 weeks	5 mg/kg /day infusion two times/week

AMOEBIASIS

Etiopathogenesis

Amoebiasis is caused by Entamoeba histolytica, which usually affects intestines but may metastasize to the liver, lungs, brain and skin. Amoebic ulcers on skin may be necrotic with verrucous borders having some associated subcutaneous swelling.

Clinical Features

Intensely painful serpiginous ulcers with undermined edges and erythematous rim about 2 cm wide is seen. Haemopurulent exudate, necrotic slough affecting anal region, spreading as sloughing coalescing ulcers may also be seen. Regional lymph nodes are usually enlarged.

Poor prognosis is seen in neglected cases of infant age group, but with early diagnosis, treatment response is good. History of dysentery is not essential for diagnosis of amoebiasis with skin involvement.

Management

Microscopic examination of cutaneous lesional edge, serological tests are helpful. Motile trophozoites containing red blood cells is diagnostic. The goal of therapy is to eliminate the invading trophozoites and to suspend carriage of the organism. Local cleaning of ulcers may be required.

First line:

- Metronidazole, followed by a luminal agent such as paromycin, diiodohydroxyquin or diloxanide furoate.

Second Line:

- Tinidazole 2000 mg orally once a day for 3-5 days.
- Nitazoxanide 500 mg orally twice a day for 3 days.

TOXOPLASMOSIS

Etiopathogenesis

Toxoplasmosis is caused by an intracellular protozoan Toxoplasma gondii. Cats are definitive hosts and rodents and birds are the intermediate hosts. Humans are infected incidentally, by eating raw infected meat or by ingesting oocysts in contaminated food or water.

Clinical Features

Toxoplasmosis causes four types of disease in humans:

1. **An acute febrile lymphadenopathy.**
2. **Fetal infection, causing brain damage.**
3. **Ocular disease, usually due to reactivation of fetal infection.**
4. **Disseminated disease in immunocompromised patients, causing fulminating encephalitis.**

In the congenital disease, macular and haemorrhagic eruptions are predominantly present. Abnormal hair growth and exfoliative dermatitis have been reported. In the acquired disease, macular, maculopapular, papular and haemorrhagic eruptions, followed by scarlatiniform desquamation are seen. Various other lesions like vesicles and bullae, nodules, livedo reticularis, urticaria and an eruption like pityriasis lichenoides have been described.

Diagnosis

- Demonstration of the organism in biopsy.
- Serological tests, The Sabin Feldman dye test, which measures mainly IgG antibodies.
- Direct agglutination of formalinized parasites, useful for screening, detects IgM and IgG antibodies.
- Indirect fluorescence, can distinguish IgM from IgG antibodies, as can an IgM ELISA.

Management

- The sulphonamides and pyrimethamine (Daraprim) with folinic acid are used for treatment. Trimethoprim plus sulfamethoxazole is the treatment of choice for central nervous system toxoplasmosis in immunocompromised patients.

NEMATODE INFECTIONS

It includes six commonly seen diseases:

- Onchocerciasis.
- Ancylostomiasis.
- Strongyloidiasis.
- Filariasis.
- Cutaneous larva migrans.
- Enterobiosis vermicularis.

ONCHOCERCIASIS

Onchocerciasis is also known as 'river blindness'. It is caused by the filarial nematode, Onchocerca volvulus, the blackfly vector which breeds near fast flowing rivers and streams. It is the second most common infectious cause of blindness after trachoma.

Clinical Features

- The most common symptoms and signs are pruritus, dermatitis, nodules and, in areas of high endemicity, blindness.
- In children, in early cases in endemic areas, the skin has an infiltrated appearance and obliteration of surface markings. This is confined to one body area and is often present with small itching papules or pustules.
- In Europeans, localized oedema, blotchy erythema and urticated papules are common early signs on exposed areas.
- Acute swelling on the face and cheeks with erythema and itching, known as erisipela de la costa, is also a manifestation of acute phase. The lesions may heal with scarring.
- Lichenified onchodermatitis may represent an extreme form of the clinical pattern. It is a lichenified itchy rash confined to one limb or contiguous area, which is characteristically hyperpigmentation and is known in Arabic areas as Sowda. It is accompanied by gross enlargement of the regional lymph nodes. These findings are seen in young population of Africa. Atrophy and depigmentation are other long-term sequelae of onchocerciasis.
- **Leopard skin:** Patches of hypopigmentation, with islands of normal appearing skin, but large coalescent sheets of depigmentation is seen in late stage disease. It is an indicator of the prevalence of onchocerciasis in the population.
- The major complication of onchocerciasis is severe visual impairment and blindness.
- Regional lymphadenopathy may cause hanging groin/ genital elephantiasis.
- **Onchocercomata:** Asymptomatic, 0.5-1 cm nodular lesions.

Investigations

Microscopic examination of corneoscleral punch, histopathology and filarial immunofluorescence test or enzyme linked immunosorbent assay (ELISA).

Management

First Line:

- Doxycycline, 100 mg daily for 6 weeks.

Second Line:

- Ivermectin 100-200 μg/kg as single dose to be retried every 6-12 months until asymptomatic.

Third Line:

- Suramin, nodulectomy.

ANCYLOSTOMIASIS ('GROUND ITCH', 'UNCINARIAL DERMATITIS', 'DEW ITCH')

Etiopathogenesis

Ancylostomiasis is caused by Ancylostoma duodenale, Necatoramericanus, Strongyloides stercoralis (round worm) which are widely distributed in the tropics and subtropics.

Adult worms live in the jejunum passing eggs in the faeces. Eggs under favorable conditions hatch into motile rhabditiform larvae, further moulting into the infective filariform larvae, which is capable of penetrating intact human skin. After penetrating the skin, larvae migrate via the bloodstream to the lungs, pass up the bronchial tree, are swallowed and pass down the oesophagus, reaching the duodenum and jejunum.

Clinical Features

Ground itch arises as larvae penetrates the skin, papular or papulovesicular rash mostly occurs on the feet accompanied by generalized urticaria. Adult worms in the gut cause abdominal pain, diarrhoea and occasionally, melena. Later, features of iron deficiency anaemia, hypoproteinaemia and retarded development can be seen.

Clinical Variant: Loeffler Syndrome: Eosinophils accumulate in the lung in response to a parasitic load. Patients complain of a dry unproductive cough, which usually resolves after 2-3 days, but may last up to 3 weeks.

Management

Ground itch is diagnosed clinically. Eosinophilia and patchy pneumonitis are characteristic of Loeffler syndrome. Eggs of parasite can also be demonstrated in the faeces.

Ground itch is treated symptomatically with an anti-pruritic cream. Pulmonary symptoms, if severe, respond to corticosteroids.

- Albendazole 400 mg single dose.
- Mebendazole 100 mg twice daily for 3 days.
- Pyrantel pamoate 11 mg/kg/day for 3 days.

STRONGYLOIDIASIS

Etiopathogenesis

Strongyloidiasis is caused by roundworm. Strongyloides stercoralis, which is prevalent in warm damp climates. Adult male and female worms release eggs, which hatch to form rhabditiform larvae in faeces, which further moult into infective filariform larvae. Penetration of the skin by filariform larvae may cause dermatitis. Adult worms give rise to duodenitis and jejunitis, which result in diarrhoea and malabsorption. Autoinfection may lead to hyper infection which presents with severe symptoms.

Clinical Features

Initial infection is similar to that seen in hookworm infection. Urticaria and raised IgE levels are often observed. In larva currens, the urticarial weal and flare of migrating subcutaneous larvae may be seen, especially around the anus and buttocks. Intestinal infection causes abdominal pain, diarrhoea and, if severe, weight loss or stunting of growth in children. They move at a rate of several centimetres an hour and can traverse the abdomen in a single day, which can disappear the next day.

Complications

In hyperinfection or disseminated strongyloidiasis, which occurs in immunosuppressed patients, severe diarrhoea, fluid and electrolyte loss; fever, abdominal distension, cough, dyspnoea, mental changes and shock may develop.

Investigations

Worms and ova can be demonstrated in the faeces by direct examination. Strongyloides antibody tests, invasive methods such as examining samples of jejunal juice (obtained by a 'string test' or entero test capsule), jejunal biopsy or video capsule endoscopy are other methods.

Management

Ivermectin in a single oral dose of 200 μg/kg body weight, to be repeated on day 2 or day 14, is the treatment of choice. Faecal and jejunal samples can be examined for larvae after 3 and 6 months.

FILARIASIS

Lymphatic filariasis is caused by the worms Wuchereria bancrofti, Brugia malayi or B. timori of which W. bancrofti is the most common. The adult worms lie in the lymphatics and the resulting inflammatory response is the cause of the main pathological feature, i.e., lymphatic obstruction. Leakage of lymph may contribute to tissue damage. The disease is transmitted by many species of anthropophilic mosquitoes of the genera Culex, Aedes, Mansonia and Anopheles.

Clinical Features

Swelling, tenderness and erythema on the arms, legs or scrotum are the initial signs. Swelling may be firm, and fixed nodules and urticaria have also been described. Cellulitis is common, may be mild or severe and is recurrent. In the severest form, it presents with fever, sweating and tender enlargement of lymph nodes, particularly the inguinal lymph nodes. Lymphangitis may occur. Other complications include orchitis, hydrocele, scrotal oedema, and recurrent epididymitis. Abscesses may form in limb muscles, deep or superficial.

Management

First Line:

- Diethylcarbamazine 200 mg orally every 12 hours for 12 days, to be repeated after 10 days.

Second Line:

- Ivermectin 0.15-0.2 mg/kg orally single dose (treatment of choice for patients with concurrent onchocerciasis).

CUTANEOUS LARVA MIGRANS

Cutaneous larva migrans is a disease characterized by the penetration of the human skin by the larvae from hookworms.

Etiopathogenesis

- Cutaneous larva migrans is seen mainly in tropical countries.
- Cutaneous larva migrans is caused by non-human species of hookworms like *Ancylostoma braziliense, Ancylostoma caninum, Uncinaria stenocephala* and *Bubostomum phlebotomum.* Rarely, it is caused by *Necator americanus* and *Strongyloides stercoralis.*
- Cats and dogs are the definitive hosts of *A. braziliense.* The adult worms live in the intestines of their hosts and eliminate their eggs in the faeces that are deposited in the soil. Under appropriate conditions of humidity temperature and oxygenation, the eggs hatch in 7 days to produce larvae.
- Larvae remain viable in the soil for several weeks.
- Humans are accidentally infected by direct contact with the infected larvae through hair follicles or fissured or intact skin.

Clinical Features

- At the site of penetration of the larvae, a reddish, edematous papular lesion is observed.
- As the larva migrates, an erythematous, linear or serpiginous track (Figure 6.16) is formed that advances 1-2 cm per day.
- Sometimes vesicobullous lesions are observed over or around the track.

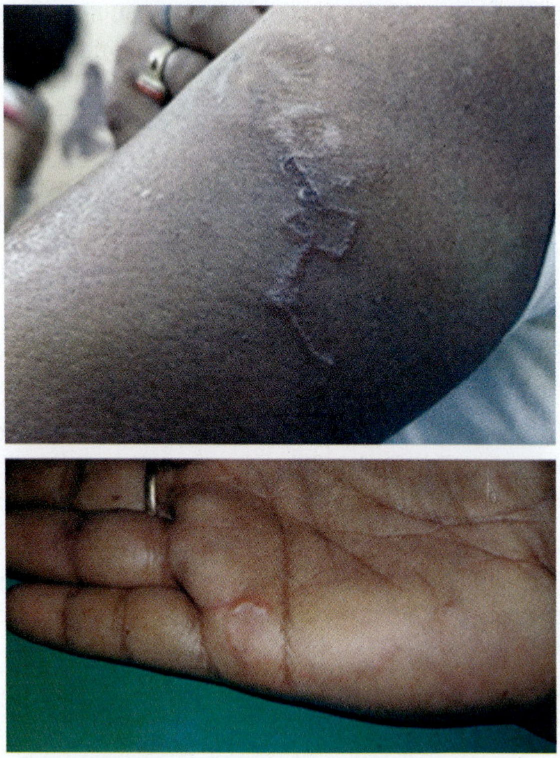

Figure 6.16: Cutaneous larva migrans

- Pruritus is usually associated which may lead to secondary bacterial infection.
- Most common sites of infection are dorsal and plantar aspect of the feet.
- Cutaneous tracks that arise from follicular lesions may present with folliculitis, with buttocks being the most common sites.
- Loeffler's syndrome is a rare association with larva migrans, characterized by pulmonary infiltrates and peripheral eosinophilia.

Diagnosis

- Clinical diagnosis is based on typical serpiginous cutaneous tracks associated with severe pruritus and history of exposure to contaminated area.
- Eosinophilia and a rise in total serum IgE is suggestive but not diagnostic of cutaneous larva migrans.

Differential Diagnosis

- Larva currens, caused by *Strongyloides stercoralis,* can be distinguished from cutaneous larva migrans by its greater speed, about 10 cm/hour, which is usually seen on buttocks and trunk.

- Differential diagnosis with disease shaving serpiginous skin lesions like granuloma annulare, erythema annulare centrifugum etc.

Treatment

- Oral albendazole, single dose of 400 mg or 10-15 mg/kg.
- Oral thiabendazole, 25 mg/kg every 12 hours for 3-4 days. Thiabendazole 10-15% solution or ointment can also be applied at the end of the track on skin.
- Single dose ivermectin 200 μg/kg can be safely used in children above 5 years.
- If secondary bacterial infection is present, a systemic or topical antibiotic should be given.

Prevention

- Cat and dog owners should be advised about proper disposal of animal faeces to avoid contamination of the soil.
- Wearing appropriate footwear to avoid infection by contaminated soil.

ENTEROBIUS VERMICULARIS (PINWORM)

- It is one of the most common nematode infections worldwide. Enterobiasis occurs in both temperate and tropical climates.
- The life cycle of *Enterobius* begins with egg deposition by gravid adult female worms in the perianal folds. Autoinfection occurs by scratching the perianal area and transferring infective eggs to the mouth with contaminated hands. Person to person transmission can occur by eating food touched by contaminated hands or by handling contaminated clothes or bed linens.
- Most *Enterobius* infections are asymptomatic. The most common symptom of enterobiasis is perianal itching, which occurs predominantly at night. Occasionally, the worm burden is so high that abdominal pain, nausea and vomiting develop.
- Enterobiasis can be diagnosed via examination of cellophane tape for eggs after pressing to the perianal skin. The utility of stool examination is limited since worms and eggs are not generally passed in stool.
- For patients with enterobiasis, treatment with albendazole, mebendazole, or pyrantel pamoate is recommended. Simultaneous treatment of the entire household is warranted, given high transmission rates among families.

TREMATODE INFECTIONS

Schistosomiasis

Schistosomiasis or bilharziasis is a systemic disease, which is caused by different species of human schistosomes or blood flukes. A second group of non-human schistosomes causes cutaneous symptoms only. This occurs when cercariae penetrate into the skin, but further development of flukes is arrested and there are no sequelae ('swimmer's itch' or cercarial dermatitis).

Clinical Features

It may present as:

- Schistosomal dermatitis.
- Urticarial reactions.
- Paragenital granulomas and fistulous tracts.
- Ectopic cutaneous schistosomiasis.

Management

The treatment of choice for all schistosome species is praziquantel (20 mg/kg twice in 1 day).

CESTODE INFECTIONS

Cysticercosis

Etiopathogenesis

Taenia solium (pork tapeworm) causes human intestinal infection (taeniasis), and the lodging of larval stage (Cysticercus cellulosae) in various organs, especially the subcutaneous tissue, muscle and brain results in cysticercosis.

The growing cyst in these organs provokes a non-specific inflammatory reaction, which gives rise to fibrosis and calcification.

Human infections with Cysticercus cellulosae are due to: ingestion of eggs in contaminated food or drink; eggs from an individual's own intestinal infection being introduced into the mouth on dirty hands; or internal autoinfection as a result of vomiting.

Clinical Features

The cysticerci form nodules in the subcutaneous tissue of the muscles, eye, eyelid, lungs and brain and other organs, interfering with their functioning.

Cysticercosis cellulosae cutis is the term coined for disease in the skin where subcutaneous nodules 1-2 cm in diameter are formed. They are rubbery, firm, rounded and painless.

Investigations

Examination of gravid proglottids for exact identification, histology of an excised cyst, Serology, X-ray examination showing calcification in the muscle, CT scan for typical appearances in the brain and muscles showing cysts as round non-enhancing hypodense lesions are methods of diagnosis.

Management

Surgical removal of individual subcutaneous cysts can be done. Cerebral disease is treated with praziquantel 50 mg/kg daily for 10 days, under steroid cover.

CERCARIAL DERMATITIS

Cercarial dermatitis is a group of dermatoses caused by penetration of the skin by free-living cercarial stages of non-human schistosomes.

Clinical Features

Tingling sensation after contact with water is the first sign of an infection. This lasts for about 1 hour with fine macular erythema. After few hours, a second phase of multiple itchy papules with surrounding erythema occurs which may form vesicles or oedematous lesions. It resolves within a week.

Clinical Variants

- Fresh water avian cercarial dermatitis.
- Sea water avian cercarial dermatitis.
- Fresh water mammalian cercarial dermatitis.

Management

Symptomatic treatment with antihistamines or topical hydrocortisone is advised. Preventative measures like control of vegetation in endemic areas or of the snail population are advised.

7 CHAPTER Cutaneous Tuberculosis

Contents

Tuberculosis of the skin is mainly caused by *Mycobacterium tuberculosis* (*M. tuberculosis*) but sometimes *M. bovis* and rarely *Bacillus Calmette-Guerin (BCG)* can also be responsible. The disease has a wide clinical spectrum from a localized tubercular chancre to a widespread miliary tuberculosis depending upon the route of infection, immune status of the patient and previous sensitization with tuberculosis.

Epidemiology

The incidence of cutaneous tuberculosis appears to be low as compared to pulmonary tuberculosis. In India where tuberculosis prevalence is high, cutaneous manifestations of tuberculosis (including overt infection or tuberculids) are found in less than 0.1% of patients seen in dermatology clinics.

- *Sex:* Male: female ratio is 1.3:1.
- *Age:* Most patients show clinical infection within the first 3 decades of life.
- Scrofuloderma and lichen scrofulosorum are common in children whereas lupus vulgaris is common in adults.

Classification

There are different ways of classifying cutaneous tuberculosis depending upon route of infection, immunity of the host and bacillary load.

According to route and host immunity:		
1.	***Exogenous Route***	
	Host Immune status	
	Naïve:	• Primary inoculation tuberculosis • Tuberculosis verrucosa cutis (TVC) • Lupus vulgaris (occasionally)
2.	***Endogenous Route***	
	Host immunity Status	
	High:	• Lupus vulgaris • Scrofuloderma
	Low:	• Metastatic tubercular abscess • Miliary tuberculosis • Orificial tuberculosis
3.	***TB due to BCG***	
		• Normal primary complex-like reaction • Perforating regional adenitis • Post vaccination lupus vulgaris
4.	***Tuberculids***	
		• Lichen Scrofulosorum • Papulonecrotic tuberculid • Facultative tuberculids • Nodular vasculitis • Erythema nodosum (EN)

According to bacillary load:
Paucibacillary TB
• Tuberculosis verrucosa cutis
• Lupus vulgaris
• Tuberculids
Multibacillary TB
• Scrofuloderma
• Orificial TB
• Acute miliary TB
• Tubercular gumma
• Tubercular chancre

Pathogenesis

- Primary inoculation tuberculosis results from direct inoculation of mycobacteria into the skin or mucosa of an individual who was not previously infected with tuberculosis or was not immunized with the BCG vaccine. Since mycobacteria do not penetrate intact skin, initiation of infection almost always follows an injury, usually in children. Common sites include the face and other exposed parts of skin.
- After mycobacteria gain entry into the skin, they multiply in tissue macrophages and spread to regional lymph nodes. An inflammatory papule develops in 2-4 weeks at the inoculation site that breaks down into a firm, non-healing, shallow, nontender, undermined ulcer with a granulomatous base. Painless regional lymphadenopathy is evident at 3-8 weeks. Numerous bacilli are present at the inoculation site and in regional lymph nodes. This ulcero-glandular complex is the skin analog to the primary complex in lungs.
- As with all tubercular infections, the clinical course depends upon the host-immune response. If host response is good, epithelioid granulomas are evident in the skin and lymph nodes. Number of tubercle bacilli progressively decreases. The primary lesion heals with scarring after 1-3 months. With a less effective host immune response, bacterial load remains high and healing is delayed for upto 12 months. Regional nodes may suppurate, erode and perforate the surface of overlying skin (scrofuloderma). Latent foci of infection can remain at the site and progress to lupus vulgaris or tuberculosis verrucosa cutis. Hematogenous dissemination of mycobacteria from skin can rarely result in tuberculosis at other sites (particularly bones and joints) or progress catastrophically to acute miliary disease with a fatal outcome.

Clinical Features

Following clinical presentations are seen in patients of cutaneous tuberculosis. Lupus vulgaris, scrofuloderma and TVC are common presentations while other presentations are uncommon and are only seen occasionally.

PRIMARY INOCULATION TUBERCULOSIS

- This type of cutaneous tuberculosis is commonly seen in children having no natural or artificial immunity against *M. tuberculosis*.
- A tubercular chancre develops at the site of inoculation.
- The bacillus enters skin through abrasions or minor injuries. After 2 to 4 weeks a papule develops on the inoculation site which ulcerates and forms a painless tubercular chancre with undermined edges and shallow granular hemorrhagic base.
- Ulcer becomes indurated and forms thick crust.
- Lesions are seen on face, hands and lower extremities.

TUBERCULOSIS VERRUCOSA CUTIS (TVC)

- TVC occurs after direct inoculation of tubercular bacilli into the skin of individuals previously infected with *M. tuberculosis*.
- Individuals, especially children from lower socio-economic groups, can contract this infection after contact with tubercular sputum. In India, walking barefoot and the habit of spitting are associated with the spread of infection.
- Lesions most commonly occur on the hands, and in children, the lower extremities.
- Infection starts as an asymptomatic, warty papule often mistaken for verrucsa vulgaris. Slow growth and irregular peripheral extension occur. The lesion may show central involution with an atrophic scar (Figure 7.1). It is usually solitary, and regional nodes are not affected unless secondary bacterial infection occurs.
- Lesions may evolve and persist for years. Spontaneous resolution with scarring can occur.
- Histology shows pseudoepitheliomatous hyperplasia with marked hyperkeratosis and a dense inflammatory infiltrate of neutrophils and lymphocytes. Abscesses form in the superficial dermis. Epithelioid cells and Langhans giant cells are seen, but typical tubercles and acid-fast bacilli are rarely seen.

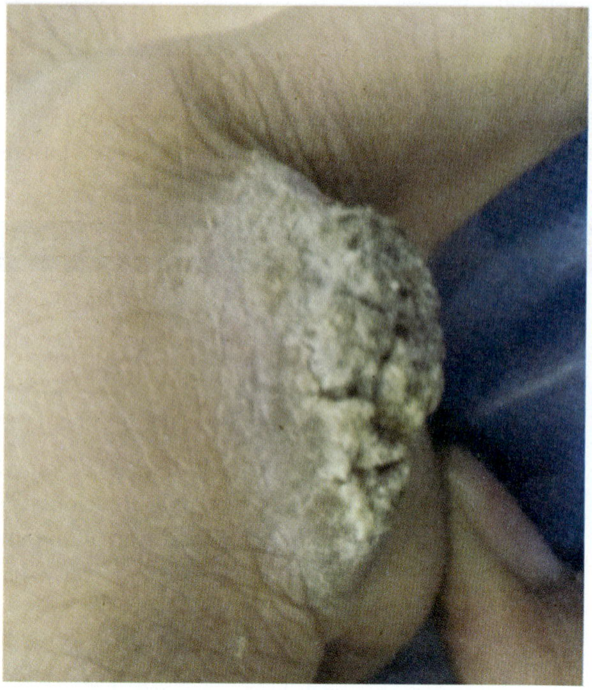

Figure 7.1: Tuberculosis verrucosa cutis

Differential Diagnosis

- Warts (verruca vulgaris).
- Deep fungal infections, e.g., blastomycosis, chromomycosis etc.
- Lesions due to other mycobacteria particularly *M. marinum* infections.
- Hypertrophic lichen planus.

LUPUS VULGARIS

- Lupus vulgaris is a chronic and progressive form of cutaneous tuberculosis that occurs in tuberculin sensitive patients.
- It is the most common form of cutaneous tuberculosis.
- Lesions appear in normal skin as a result of direct extension of underlying tubercular foci, lymphatic or hematogenous spread, after primary inoculation, BCG vaccination, or in scars of old scrofuloderma.
- Lesions usually are solitary, and more than 90% involve the head and neck in western countries. In India, buttocks and lower limbs are the most common sites (sites of trauma in children).
- Small, sharply marginated, red-brown papules of gelatinous consistency (apple-jelly nodules) slowly evolve by peripheral extension and central atrophy into large plaques.
- Chronic asymptomatic lesions with atrophy, scarring and active border should arouse suspicion of cutaneous tuberculosis.
- Cartilage (nose, ears) within the affected area is progressively destroyed, leading to deformity; bone is usually spared. Buccal, nasal and conjunctival mucosae may be involved primarily or by extension.
- Clinical variants are seen in the following forms:
    - *Plaque form:* Disease extension occurs with little central atrophy. Scaling can occur, especially on the lower legs where it may resemble psoriasis. Irregular scarring is common and the active edge may be thickened and hyperkeratotic (Figure 7.2 and Figure 7.3).

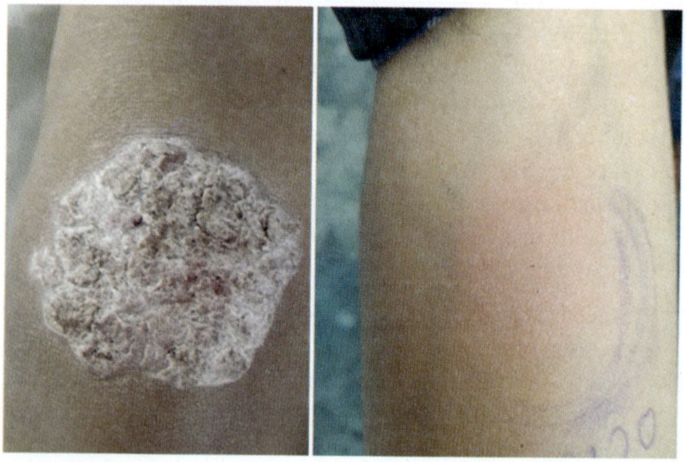

Figure 7.2: Lupus vulgaris with positive tuberculin test

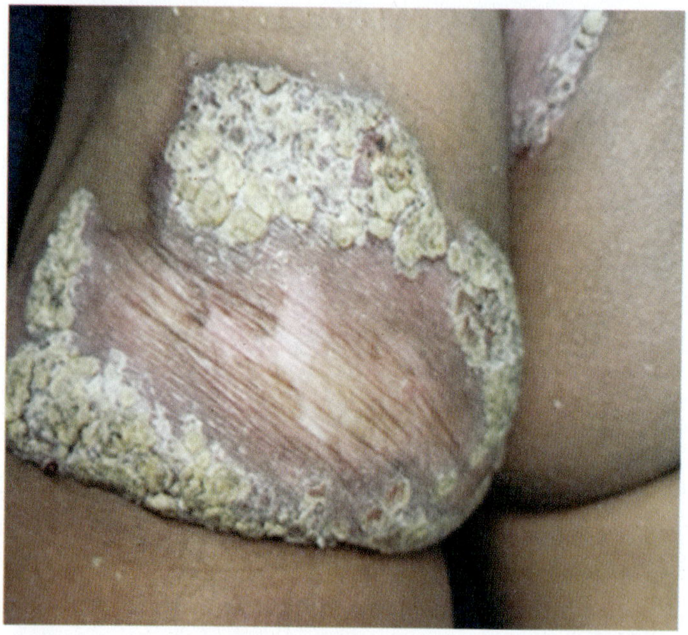

Figure 7.3 : Lupus vulgaris showing central atrophy and scarring

- *Ulcerating form:* Scarring and ulceration predominate. Crusts form over areas of necrosis. Deep tissues and cartilage are invaded by eventual scarring that produces contractures and deformity.
- *Vegetative form:* This form is characterized by necrosis, ulceration and proliferative and papillomatous granulation tissue.
- *Nodular form:* This form is characterized by a relative absence of ulceration and scarring. Large soft tumors occur, especially on ear lobes.

- Histologically, the most prominent feature is a typical granulomatous tubercle with epithelioid cells, Langhans giant cells, and a mononuclear infiltrate. Caseation necrosis is minimal, and acid-fast bacilli are rare. Tissue histology varies with secondary changes of abscess formation, ulceration, atrophy and scarring.
- Lesions often persist for years before diagnosis and can be disfiguring. In long-standing lupus vulgaris, squamous cell carcinoma can occur and can be confused with the disease itself.

Differential Diagnosis

- Sarcoidosis.
- Discoid lupus erythematosus (DLE).
- Leprosy.
- Deep fungal infections, e.g., blastomycosis.
- Lupoid leishmaniasis.

SCROFULODERMA

- Scrofuloderma results from breakdown of skin overlying a tubercular focus, usually a lymph node but also at the skin over infected bones or joints.
- Lesions present as firm, painless, subcutaneous nodules (Figure 7.4) that gradually enlarge and suppurate and then form ulcers and sinuses in overlying skin. Ulcers have undermined edges and a floor of granulation tissue. After healing, atrophic scars are seen.
- Tubercle bacilli usually can be isolated from the purulent discharge.
- Tuberculin sensitivity is usually marked.
- Spontaneous healing can occur but often takes years and is accompanied by the formation of hypertrophic scars. Lupus vulgaris may develop in the vicinity of healing scrofuloderma.

Differential Diagnosis

- Lymphadenitis due to *Mycobacterium avium intracellulare.*

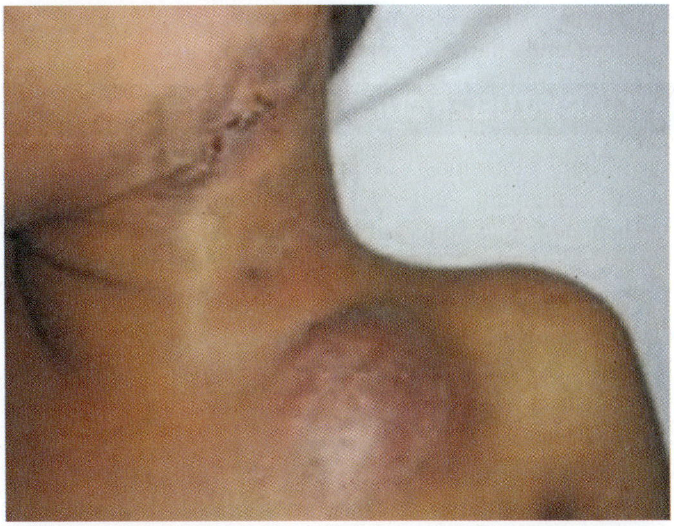

Figure 7.4: Scrofuloderma showing sinuses at the angle of mandible and cold abscess at upper part of chest

- Other mycobacterial infections, e.g., *M. scrofulaceum.*
- Sporotrichosis.
- Actinomycosis.
- Hidradenitis suppurativa.

METASTATIC TUBERCULAR ABSCESS (Tubercular Gumma)

- It is a variant of scrofuloderma that occurs following hematogenous spread of mycobacteria to the skin in tuberculin sensitive individuals.
- Painless, fluctuant, subcutaneous abscesses form singly or at multiple sites, then break down into fistulas and ulcers resembling scrofuloderma (Figure 7.5).

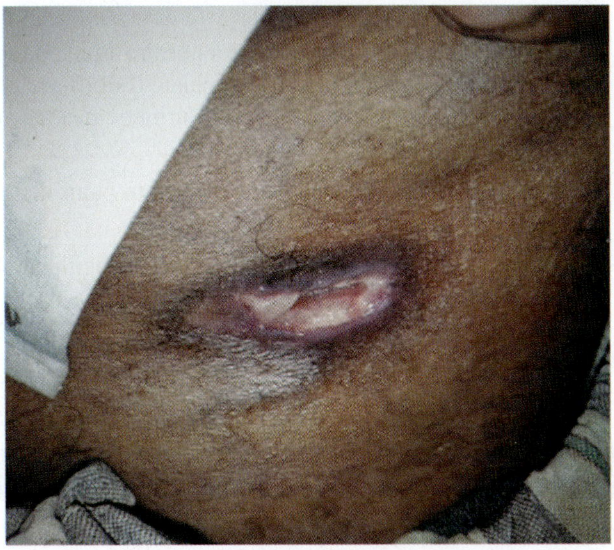

Figure 7.5: Metastatic tuberculoar absecess with sinus formation

- Typically, these lesions occur in malnourished children or in severely immunosuppressed patients.

MILIARY TUBERCULOSIS OF THE SKIN

- Miliary tuberculosis of the skin is a rare manifestation of fulminant miliary tuberculosis, resulting from hematogenous spread of mycobacteria to multiple organs, including skin. The initial site of infection usually is pulmonary or meningeal.
- Disseminated lesions occur on all parts of the body, especially the trunk. Lesions erupt as small (millet-sized) red macules or papules. Purpura, vesicles and central necrosis are common.
- Disease occurs predominantly in children and may be coincidental with other infections such as measles. The bacillary load is high, which is consistent with an overwhelming infection. Miliary tuberculosis of the skin is also seen in immunosuppressed individuals infected with HIV. Affected patients are gravely ill, and the prognosis is poor.

Orificial Tuberculosis

- Uncommon in children.
- Orificial tuberculosis results from autoinoculation of mycobacteria into the periorificial skin and mucous membranes in patients with advanced tuberculosis.
- Underlying disease can be pulmonary, intestinal, or genitourinary tuberculosis. Infectious mycobacteria shed from these foci are inoculated into surrounding mucous membranes and skin.
- Patients typically are older men. Tuberculin sensitivity is strong. The site of the periorificial lesion is often determined by trauma.
- The tip and lateral margins of the tongue are affected most frequently; however, hard and soft palate lesions are also common. Perianal skin, the vulva, the urinary meatus, and the glans penis also are described sites.
- Lesions start as red papules that evolve into painful, soft, punched out, shallow ulcers.
- Histopathologically, tubercles with acid-fast bacilli can be found in the deep dermis and ulcer walls.

Differential Diagnosis

- Aphthous ulcers.

TUBERCULIDS

Tuberculids are symmetrical generalized skin lesions in tubercular patients due to hypersensitivity reaction to tubercle bacillus or its products. The basic features of tuberculids are:

- Strongly positive tuberculin test.
- Evidence of manifest or past tuberculosis.
- Good response to antitubercular therapy.
- Skin biopsy and culture are negative for tubercular bacilli, however PCR can detect mycobacterial DNA in some forms of tuberculids.

Depending on the type of main lesions tuberculids can be classified as follows:

- **Micropapular:** Lichen scrofulosorum.
- **Papular:** Papulonecrotic tuberculid.
- **Nodular:** Erythema induratum of bazin; nodular tuberculid.

Lichen Scrofulosorum

- Lichen scrofulosorum is an eruption of asymptomatic, closely grouped, 0.5-3 mm, perifollicular, lichenoid papules affecting children and young adults with underlying tuberculosis.
- Papules may be skin colored, yellowish or reddish brown.
- They are present on abdomen, chest, back and proximal limbs.
- The eruption becomes more extensive in few weeks and then slowly regresses for months without scarring.
- Recurrences are possible. The response to anti-tubercular drugs is not as remarkable as that seen in other tuberculids.
- Tuberculin test is strongly positive.

Differential Diagnosis

It should be differentiated from other conditions having grouped papular lesions:

- Lichen nitidus.
- Lichen spinulosus.
- Lichen planus.
- Micropapular forms of sarcoidosis.
- Phrynoderma.

Papulonecrotic Tuberculid

- It occurs as a chronic and recurrent symmetric eruption of necrotizing papules appearing in clusters and healing with varioliform scars.
- Lesions appear on the extensor aspects of extremities (knees, elbows, buttocks, lower trunk) in a symmetric distribution, often in clusters. Individual lesions are asymptomatic, small, dusky-red papules with a central

punctum or crust. Involution is common after 6-8 weeks and leaves pitted scars (Figure 7.6).

- New crops of lesions may continue for months or years.
- In children it may be associated with phlyctenular conjunctivitis.

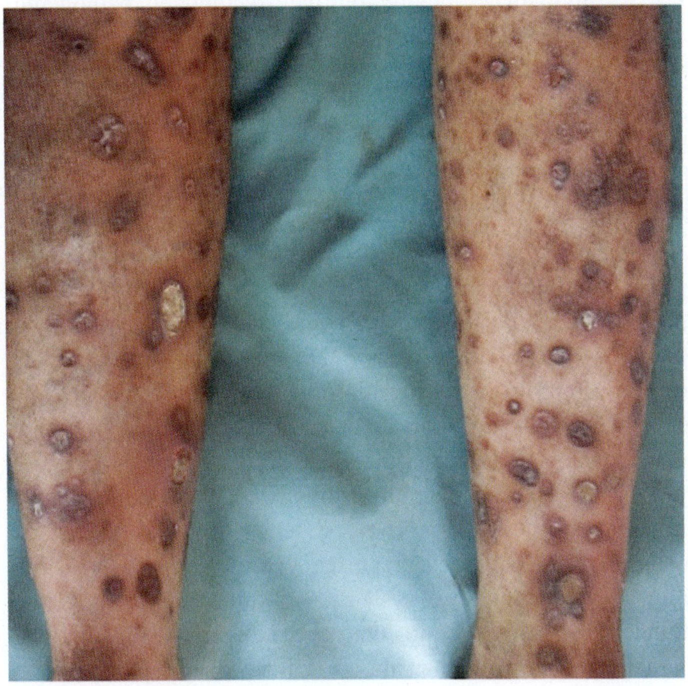

Figure 7.6: Papulonecrotic tuberculosis with varioliform scar

- Histologically, these lesions show a wedge-shaped necrosis of the upper dermis extending to and involving the epidermis. Epithelioid cells and, infrequently, Langhans giant cells are seen. An obliterative granulomatous vasculitis with fibrin present in vessel walls and lumen is typical.

Differential Diagnosis

- Pityriasis lichenoides et varioliformis acuta.
- Prurigo.
- Leucocytoclastic necrotizing vasculitis.

Erythema Induratum (Bazin Disease)

- Erythema induratum is a persistent or recurring condition associated with past or active tuberculosis.
- Lesions arise in small numbers as tender indurated plaques and nodules that may progress to ulceration and scarring. It occurs on the posterior aspect of legs, mostly in women (< 10% of affected patients are men) in temperate countries. In India nodular vasculitis is seen as one of the presentation of tuberculosis (Figure 7.7). It should be differentiated from nodular vasculitis due to other causes.
- Pre-existing erythrocyanotic circulatory disease may predispose patients to lesions and an increased prevalence is seen during cold weather.

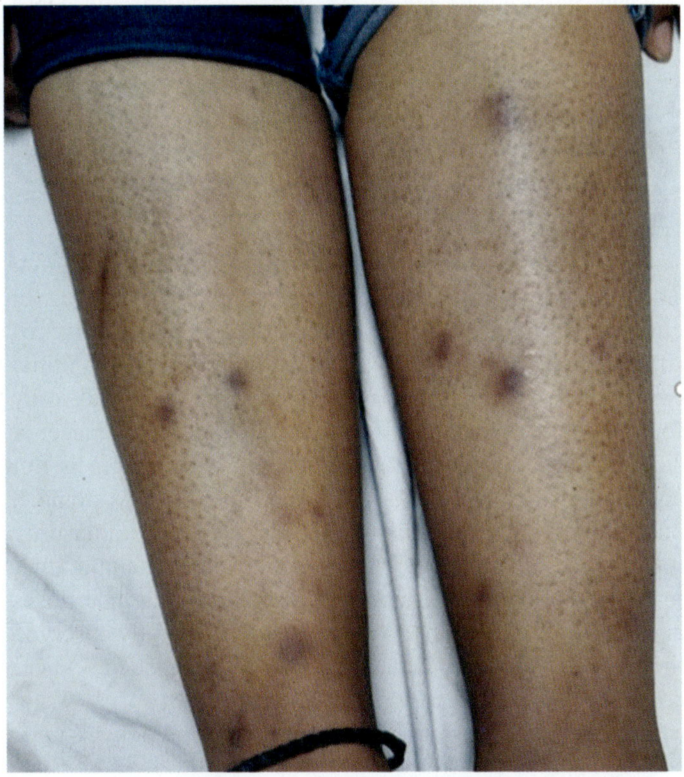

Figure 7.7: Nodular vasculitis

Diagnosis

The absolute criteria for diagnosis of cutaneous tuberculosis are the positive culture for *M. tuberculosis* from the lesion or PCR identification of mycobacterial DNA. The other diagnostic criteria include:

- History and clinical examination of the lesion.
- Mantoux test.
- X-ray chest.
- Skin biopsy with AFB staining and/or culture.
- Ziehl-Neelsen acid fast stain, while highly specific for mycobacteria, requires at least 10,000 bacilli per ml; a more sensitive auramine-rhodamine fluorescent stain (Auramine O) is used nowadays.
- Routine culture uses a non-selective egg medium (Lowenstein-Jensen) and often requires more than 3-4 weeks to yield the bacilli because of the 22-hour doubling

time of *M. tuberculosis*. Radiometric broth culture (BACTEC radiometric system) of clinical specimens significantly reduces time (2-6 days) for mycobacterial recovery.

- Polymerase chain reaction (PCR) amplification techniques can be used to detect *M. tuberculosis*-specific DNA sequences and detects small numbers of mycobacteria in clinical specimens.
- Another screening test is the QuantiFERON TB Gold test, which quantifies the release of interferon-γ in whole blood upon stimulation with *M. tuberculosis* antigens.

Treatment

The multi-drug 6-month regimen is highly effective for cutaneous tuberculosis. Three drugs consisting of rifampicin, isoniazid and pyrazinamide are given for initial two months followed by rifampicin and isoniazid only for remaining 4 months. If patient develops intolerance or side effects, ethambutol may be used. Streptomycin is not commonly used. All drugs are taken on an empty stomach once daily. Tuberculous meningitis is treated with a four-drug regimen for 2 months followed by isoniazid and rifampin for 7 to 10 more months. The antitubercular drugs with their doses and main side effects are given in Table 7.1. Directly observed therapy or DOTs is a good alternative for those patients where compliance is poor. It is given on alternate days.

Table 7.1: Antitubercular drugs

Drugs	*Daily dose in mg/kg*	*Main side effects*
Rifampicin	10	Hepatitis, Thrombocytopenia
Isoniazid	5-10	Peripheral neuropathy, Hepatitis
Pyrazinamide	35	Hepatitis, Hyperuricemia
Ethambutol	15-25	Optic neuritis
Streptomycin	20-40	Deafness

NON-TUBERCULOUS MYCOBACTERIA (NTM)

The non tuberculous mycobacteria (NTM) or atypical mycobacteria usually do not cause disease in humans. In case of human infections they tend to occur in immunocompromised individuals. In healthy immunocompetent children, cervical lymphadenitis has been observed to result from NTM infection.

Ernest Runyon put these human disease associated bacteria into four groups (Runyon classification):

- **Photochromogens** (Develop pigments in or after being exposed to light): *M. kansasii*, *M. simiae* and *M. marinum*.
- **Scotochromogens** (become pigmented in darkness.): *M. scrofulaceum* and *M. szulgai*.
- **Non chromogens:** *M. avium complex* (MAC), *M. ulcerans*, *M. xenopi*, *M. malmoense*, *M. terrae*, *M. haemophilum* and *M. genavense*.
- **Rapid growers** include four well-recognized, pathogenic, rapidly growing, nonchromogenic species: *M. chelonae*, *M. abscessus*, *M. fortuitum* and *M. peregrinum*. Other examples which cause disease rarely, *M. smegmatis* and *M. flavescens*.

M. Marinum

M. marinum causes a skin infection termed as swimming pool granuloma or fish-tank granuloma. After an incubation period of 2 to 3 weeks or in some cases upto 9 months, it begins with a nodule or pustule that eventually forms an ulcer or abscess. Extremities are the most common sites. Multiple secondary lesions in a linear, sporotrichoid distribution may develop. If untreated, the skin lesion resolves in 1 to 3 years with scarring. Complications like severe disseminated infection in immunocompromised, tenosynovitis, arthritis and osteomyelitis, have been reported. Besides surgical excision and warm compresses, systemic antimicrobial therapy like tetracycline, minocycline, doxycycline, clarithromycin, sulfamethoxazole-trimethoprim, linezolid and rifampin, alone or in combination with ethambutol have been tried but with less satisfactory results.

M. Ulcerans

M. ulcerans is the causative organism of an ulcerative skin disease called Buruli ulcer, which is common in Africa, Central and South America and Asia. It usually begins after trauma by grass or a thorn and a painless nodule develops at that site which progresses to form abscess and later, a shallow ulcer. It most commonly occurs on lower extremities. The ulcer may remain for months to years and heals spontaneously with scarring and lymphedema. Surgical and systemic antibiotic therapies have been tried with variable results.

Rapid Growers

M. fortuitum, M. chelonae and *M. abscessus* are referred to as rapid growers. They may cause abscess formation after trauma or surgery and in postsurgical scars. In paediatric age group, *M. fortuitum* is the most common rapid grower to cause disease. *M. abscessus* infection has been implicated in causation of inflammatory skin lesions like papules, pustules and nodules over palms and soles in children. Some authors describe it as "M. abscessus hand-and-foot disease". Systemic antibiotic like clarithromycin is recommended after diagnosis is confirmed.

8 CHAPTER Leprosy

Contents

Leprosy is one of the oldest diseases known to mankind. It has been described in Vedas, written as early as 1400 BC in India. In India, where it is known as "Kushtha". Leprosy is a chronic granulomatous disease caused by *Mycobacterium leprae (M. leprae)*. It mainly affects the skin and peripheral nervous system. The skin lesions and deformities were historically responsible for the stigma attached to the disease.

Gerhard Armauer Hansen discovered *M.leprae* in Norway in 1873. It was the first bacillus to be associated with human disease but could not be cultivated in artificial culture media so far. Leprosy is also known as 'Hansen's disease' after the name of Armauer Hansen.

EPIDEMIOLOGY

The global prevalence of leprosy is reported to be 0.25 case per 10,000 population. As per WHO report of 2017 there were 2,10,671 registered new cases of leprosy from 150 countries of world. Most of the cases come from tropics and sub tropics. Sixty percent of the world's leprosy cases are in India. India has achieved the elimination target of less than 1 case per 10,000 (0.66/10,000) but 6 states including Bihar, Chhattisgarh, Jharkhand, West Bengal, Odisha, Uttar Pradesh, Delhi and Dadar and Nagar Haveli are yet to achieve it. The prevalence rate in India steadily continued to be 0.67/10000 in 2018. The percentage of childhood leprosy cases among the newly detected leprosy cases in India ranged from 8.7 to 10.14% between 2005 and 2017. The worldwide prevalence of leprosy has decreased drastically since the introduction of multidrug therapy (MDT) in 1982.

High leprosy child rate is an index of prevalence of leprosy in the general population, high transmission in the community, efficiency of control programs and higher likelihood of leprosy afflicted familial contacts. The peak age of onset is between 10 and 20 years. It is rare in infants. It affects more males than females. Male to female ratio in adults is around 2:1. In adults, the lepromatous type of leprosy is more common in men than in women, with a male to female ratio of 2:1. In children, the tuberculoid form predominates with no sex preference. Leprosy occurs in persons of all races. Leprosy is endemic in Asia. It is more a rural than urban disease. The incubation period is 6 months to 40 years or longer. The mean incubation period is 4 years for tuberculoid leprosy (TT) and is 10 years for lepromatous leprosy (LL).

EPIDEMIOLOGICAL INDICATORS OF LEPROSY

Epidemiological indicators are helpful to identify burden of disease and endemicity of leprosy.

Prevalence of leprosy: Denotes number of cases on MDT /10,000 population at a given point of time.

Elimination of leprosy: The term is used when prevalence of leprosy is below 1/10000 population.

Annual New Case Detection Rate (ANCDR): Total number of new cases /10,000 population in a given year.

Grade 2 disability rate: Number of patients who have grade 2 disability in a given year/10,000 population.

Cure rate: Number of patients cured with MDT in a given year/10,000 population.

ETIOPATHOGENESIS

M. leprae is an obligate intracellular, acid-fast, straight or slightly curved, rod like acid fast bacillus. It is 3-8 microns in length. It lies in cigar shaped bundles called globi. It is less acid and alcohol fast as compared to *M. tuberculosis. M. leprae* is a slow growing bacterium with mean generation time ranging from 18 to 42 days, whereas *M. tuberculosis* takes only 20 hours to grow. It has an affinity for macrophages and Schwann cells. Their slow replication within the Schwann cells eventually stimulates a cell-mediated immune response, which creates a chronic inflammatory reaction. As a result, swelling occurs in the perineurium, leading to ischemia, fibrosis and axonal death. This is seen in the tuberculoid pole of the disease.

In the lepromatous pole, the patient has specific absence of this cell mediated immune response (CMI) leading to widespread dissemination of lepra bacilli and a macrophage type of cell response.

Humans are the primary reservoir of *M. leprae.* Animal reservoirs of leprosy have been found in nine-banded armadillos, chimpanzees and monkeys.

The area's most commonly affected, are the superficial peripheral nerves, skin, mucous membranes of the upper respiratory tract, anterior chamber of the eyes and the testes. These areas tend to be the cooler parts of the body. Tissue damage depends on the degree to which cell-mediated immunity is expressed, the type and extent of bacillary spread and multiplication, the appearance of tissue-damaging immunologic complications (lepra reactions), and the development of nerve damage and its sequel.

The strength of the host's immune system influences the clinical spectrum of the disease.

Strong cell-mediated immunity (leading to formation of IFN-γ, IL-2) and a weak humoral response results in mild forms of disease, with a few well-defined skin lesions, asymmetrical nerves involvement and lower bacterial load (tuberculoid pole).

A strong humoral response (leading to formation of IL-4, IL-10) but relatively absent cell-mediated immunity against *M. leprae,* results in lepromatous leprosy (LL), with widespread lesions, extensive skin and nerve involvement and high bacterial load.

TRANSMISSION OF LEPROSY

The transmission of leprosy is occurred by droplets from the nose and mouth. Prolonged close contact with untreated leprosy patients is needed for transmission. Casual contact with an infected individual, such as handshakes, hugs, meal sharing, or sitting close to each other, does not transmit the disease. Furthermore, as soon as the patient starts treatment, they stop spreading the illness.

CLASSIFICATION

There are several classifications of leprosy but the Ridley-Jopling classification has been widely accepted. It is based on clinical, histological, bacteriological and immunological parameters. As per this classification, leprosy is a spectral disease with 5 subgroups: Tuberculoid (TT), borderline tuberculoid (BT), mid borderline (BB), borderline lepromatous (BL) and lepromatous (LL). **Salient features of different spectrum of leprosy are described in Table 8.1.** The cell-mediated immunity declines from TT to LL and the bacterial load goes inversely as lowest at TT to highest at LL. Subsequently subpolar forms of TT and LL were proposed as TTp and TTs for tuberculoid pole and LLp and LLs for lepromatous pole. This classification does not include 'indeterminate' and 'pure neuritic' forms of leprosy.

For treatment purpose WHO has classified leprosy in two groups:

Paucibacillary Leprosy (PB): It includes tuberculoid, indeterminate and borderline tuberculoid forms of leprosy. Slit smear examination is negative and number of lesions is less than 5 in these cases with or without one nerve involvement.

Multibacillary Leprosy (MB): It includes lepromatous, borderline lepromatous and mid borderline forms. Slit smear is positive and number of lesions is more than 5 in these cases. One or more nerves may be involved.

Table 8.1: Salient features of different types of leprosy

	TT	*BT*	*BB*	*BL*	*LL*
Number of lesions skin lesions	Single lesion or 1-3	Few lesions (3-10)	Multiple countable lesions (11-30)	Multiple uncountable lesions	Innumerable lesions
Shape of lesion	Variable	Large lesions	Variable	Small	Small
Sensation on lesion	Anesthetic	Hypoesthetic	Hypoesthetic	Hypoesthetic or normoesthetic	Usually normoesthetic
Symmetry of lesions	Asymmetrical	Asymmetrical	Asymmetrical	Almost symmetrical	Symmetrical
Morphology of lesion	Well defined patches or plaques	Patches or plaques with satellite lesions	Punched out lesions with slopping edges (saucer shaped or swiss cheese), annular, dimorphic lesions	Macules, patches, plaques or nodules	Macules, patches, plaques, nodules with diffuse infiltration of skin with leonine facies
Nerve involvement	Single nerve	Few, asymmetric involvement	Multiple, asymmetric involvement	Multiple nerves with almost symmetrical pattern	Multiple nerve in symmetrical pattern
Histology					
Granuloma	Compact, well defined epithelioid granuloma invading/abutting the basal layer of epidermis	Epithelioid cell granuloma with plenty of lymphocytes	Ill-defined macrophage granuloma which is poor in lymphocytes	Ill-defined granuloma with many lymphocytes, perineural fibroblast proliferation resulting in onion peel or onion skin appearance	No granuloma, diffuse foamy macrophages or foamy histiocytes (Virchow cells)
Granz zone	Absent	May Present	Well defined grenz zone	Well defined grenz zone	Prominent grenz zone
AFB	Negative	Negative or few bacilli may be seen	+ to ++	++ to +++	++++ to ++++++
Lepromin test	Strongly Positive	Positive	Positive/ negative	Negative	Negative
Immunological response to AFB (cell mediated)	Excellent immunity	Good immunity	Fair immune response	Poor immune response	Very poor immune response

Clinical Features

The onset of leprosy is usually gradual and insidious. Mostly the first signs of leprosy are seen on skin but if the neural component predominates first sign may be numbness, tingling or pain in the extremity. Early skin sign is usually the lesion of indeterminate leprosy and single patch lesions are most commonly detected in exposed areas but a complete examination is important to screen for lesions in hidden sites. Multibacillary cases have also been commonly recorded in Indian childhood leprosy cases.

Indeterminate Leprosy

It is an early phase of leprosy when the immunological response has not yet developed. Clinically, it is seen as one to three ill-defined hypopigmented macules. Sensations are doubtful and nerves around the lesion may be thickened.

Lesions are generally present over face, extensor surface of limbs, buttocks and trunk.

M. leprae is negative in skin lesion but may be positive in nerve.

Lepromin reaction may be positive or negative to doubtful.

Most of the lesions may heal spontaneously but some cases may go to determinate forms of leprosy like tuberculoid, borderline or lepromatous type.

Tuberculoid Leprosy (TL)

- Lesions may be macules or plaques. Plaques are usually single, but may be 1 to 3 in number, well defined, thickened, erythematous or skin colored with raised edges and flattened hypopigmented center.
- The surface of the lesions is well-defined, hypopigmented, dry, may be scaly and hairless (Figure 8.1).

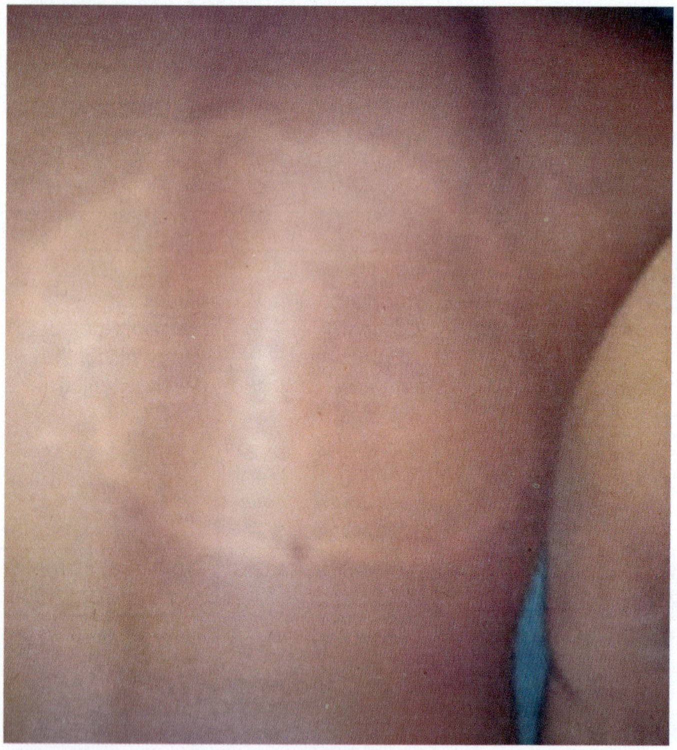

Figure 8.1: Tuberculoid leprosy

- Lesions are hypo-aesthetic or anaesthetic and a nearby sensory nerve may be thickened.
- Since the immunity is strong, there may be spontaneous cure.
- Skin smear is negative for *M. leprae*.
- Lepromin test is strongly positive.

Borderline Tuberculoid Leprosy (BT)

- BT lesions are hypopigmented or erythematous plaques or macules with well-defined irregular margins. They tend to break on the border and form characteristic satellite lesions (Figures 8.2 and 8.3).

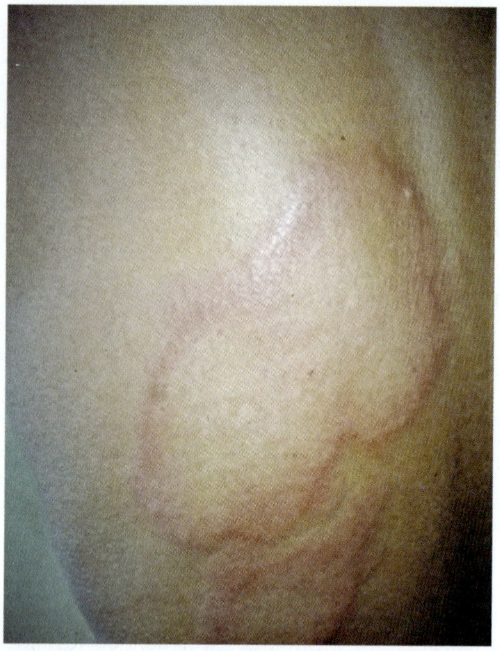

Figure 8.2: Borderline tuberculosis with satellite lesion over lower left back

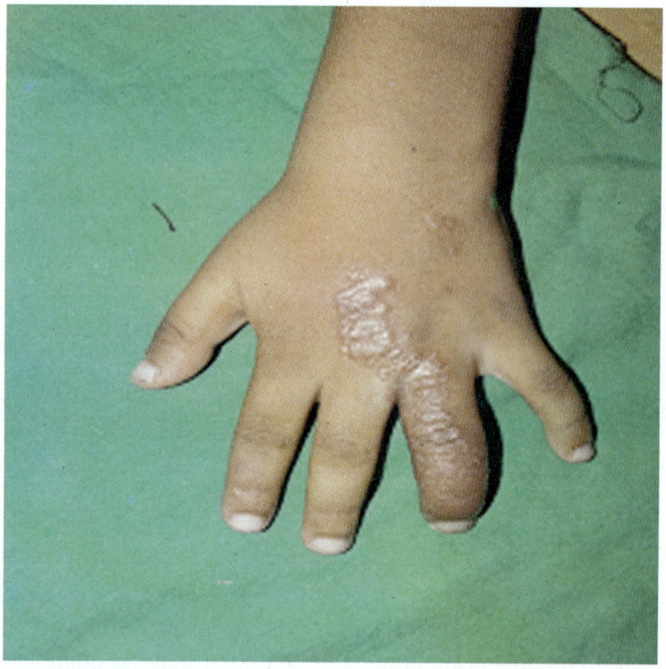

Figure 8.3: Borderline tuberculoid leprosy with satellite lesions (Dorsum of hand)

- Lesions may be 3 to 10 in number and are present on a localized region or one half of the body.

- They are dry, hairless and show variable degree of anesthesia.
- Nerves near the plaque may be thickened and sensory changes may be seen along the distribution of the nerve.
- Skin smear for AFB is negative.
- Lepromin test is weakly positive.

Midborderline or Borderline Borderline Leprosy (BB)

- It is the most unstable part of spectrum when patients either upgrade or downgrade to a stable form.
- BB lesions are mixture of BT and BL lesions.
- Lesions are bilateral but asymmetrical infiltrated plaques with sloping edges and punched out center (saucer shaped). They are of variable size and shape, and can be upto 30 in number but may be even more.
- The sensory loss over the lesions is variable, some show complete loss while others show partial loss.
- They are seen mostly on trunk, face and extremities.
- Nerves are thickened bilaterally but asymmetrically and may be tender.
- Skin smear is positive, BI (bacteriological index) is 2+ or 3+.
- Lepromin test is weakly positive or negative.

Borderline Lepromatous Leprosy (BL)

- Lesions of BL are mixture of BB and lepromatous leprosy. They are more widespread than BB but not symmetrical as in lepromatous leprosy.
- BL lesions may be macular, annular plaques (Figure 8.4) or even nodules.
- They are shiny, copper colored and more infiltrated in the center than at the periphery.
- Macules are multiple, poorly defined and are of variable shape and size. They are not as symmetrical as in LL.
- Sensations are intact in macules but in long standing lesions, temperature and pain may be impaired.
- Multiple nerves are thickened asymmetrically.
- Lepromin test is usually negative.
- Slit-skin smear is positive, BI is 3+ or 4+.

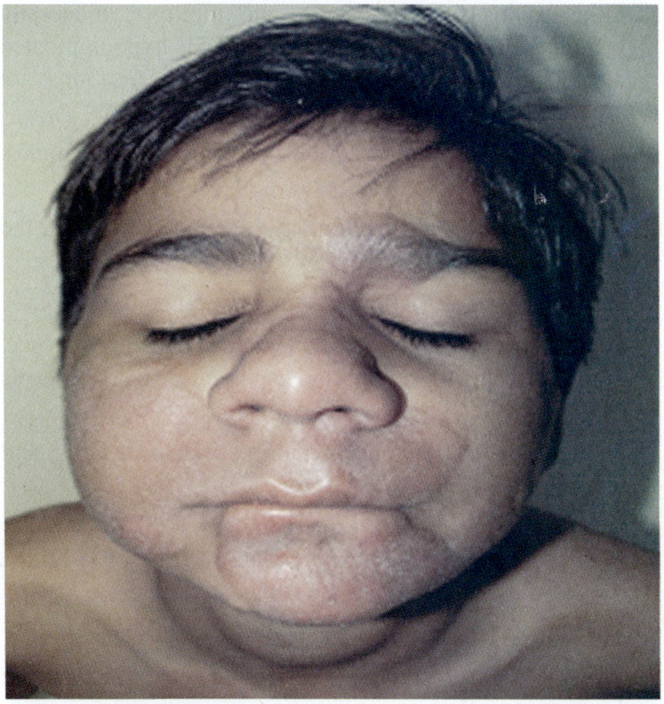

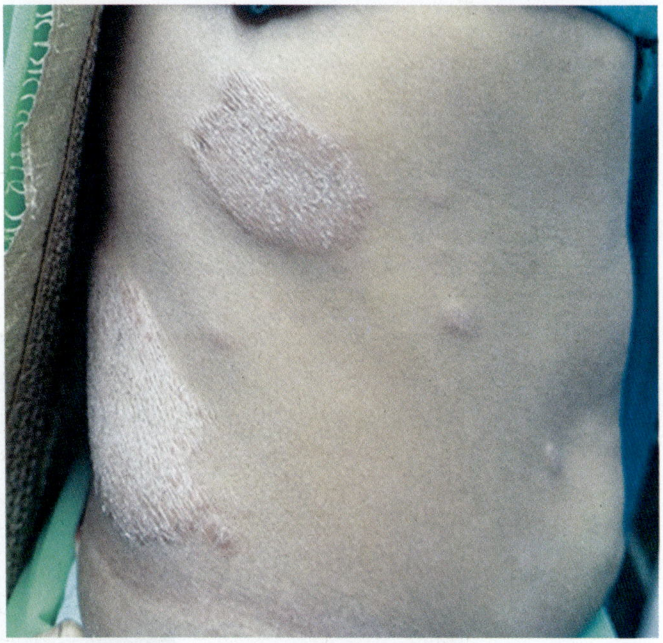

Figure 8.4: Borderline lepromatous leprosy

LEPROMATOUS LEPROSY (LL)

- Lepromatous leprosy is a multisystem disease involving skin, mucosa, nerves, reticuloendothelial system, upper respiratory tract, eyes, testes, adrenals and other viscera but sparing the central nervous system.
- It is infectious form of disease and large number of lepra bacilli are discharged from upper respiratory tract.

- Skin lesions in early stages are multiple, bilaterally symmetrical, smooth, shiny, ill defined, hypopigmented or coppery colored macules. Hair and sensations are preserved over the lesions.
- In later stages skin gets infiltrated and forms papules, nodules (Figure 8.5) and plaques.
- Gradually skin may develop waxy in appearance with the loss of skin creases.
- Pain and touch sensations are unimpaired on the lesions.
- Lesions are distributed characteristically mainly on face, dorsal aspects of forearms and hands and extensor aspects of lower legs.
- Axillae, eyelids, palms, scalp, perineum, groins and midline of the back are spared.
- Infiltration, furrowing and nodulation of skin over eyebrows, nose and lips and collapse of the nose bridge results in the characteristic 'leonine facies'.
- The skin of legs becomes ichthyotic and thickened.
- Variable degree of loss of eyebrows and eyelashes may be present.
- In later stages sensory loss starts initially on dorsum of hands, the forearms, feet and the lower legs which extends proximally to finally result in 'glove and stocking' type of sensory deficit.
- Multiple nerves are thickened bilaterally, the commonly involved are: greater auricular, supraclavicular, ulnar, cutaneous nerves of the forearm, superficial branch of the radial and median nerve at wrist, lateral popliteal, sural and posterior tibial nerves.
- Nerve involvement may result into various deformities like facial palsy, claw hand, ape hand, wrist drop, foot drop and trophic ulcers.
- Testicular atrophy may result in sterility, impotence and gynecomastia.
- Lepromin test is negative.
- Slit-skin smear is highly positive with BI upto 6+ with or without globi.

HISTOID LEPROSY

Histoid leprosy is a rare variant of lepromatous leprosy with characteristic clinicopathological manifestations and bacterial morphology. It was first described by wade in 1963. The prevalence of histoid is 2.79% to 3.6%. It occurs in two forms:

1. Relapse after dapsone monotherapy in presence of Dapsone resistance.
2. De-novo histoid hansen

Clinical Features

Clinically it presents with dermal and subdermal, firm, oval or dome-shaped, red or skin coloured nodules and plaques over an apparently normal skin (Figure 8.6). These lesions have regular pattern and the overlying skin is shiny and stretched. Lesions are usually located on the posterior and lateral aspects of arms, buttocks, thighs, dorsum of hands and on the lower part of the back and over the bony prominences, especially over the elbows and knees.

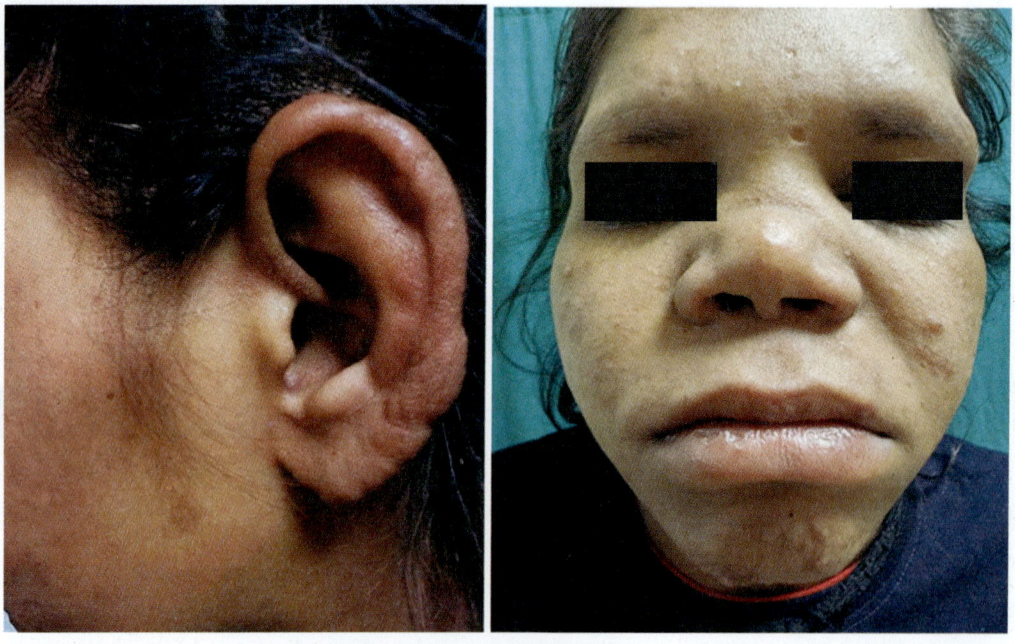

Figure 8.5: Lepromatous leprosy

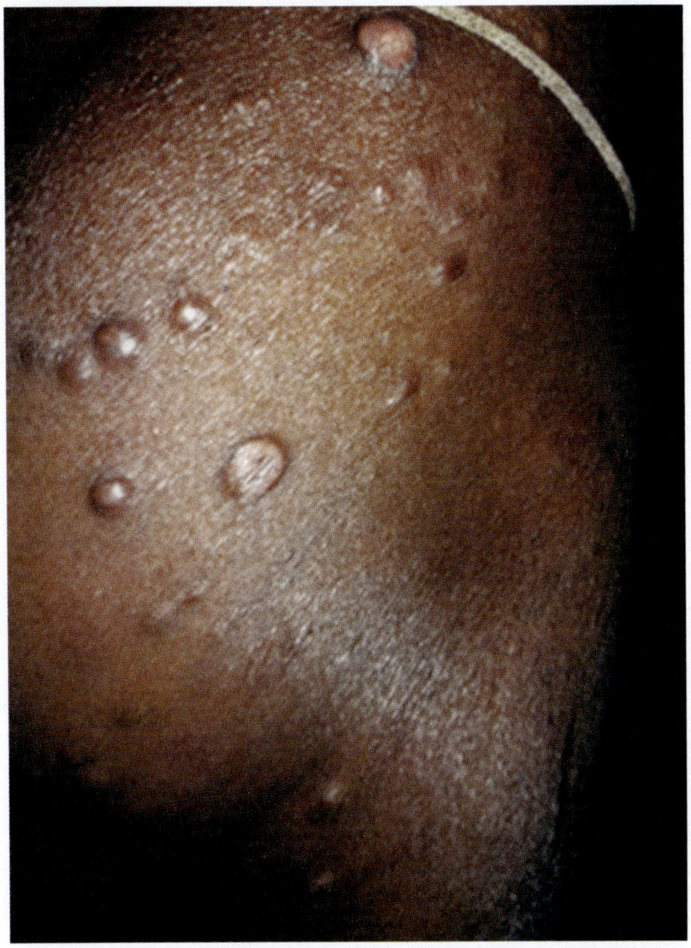

Figure 8.6: Histoid Hansen

On acid fast stain bacilli appears long with tapering ends, as compared to ordinary lepra bacilli with hight bacteriological index may be 5+ to 6+ and morphological index. Histology shows, epidermal atrophy due to dermal expansion of leproma and an acellular band (Unna band or Grenz zone) located immediately below the epidermis. Leproma consists of fusiform (spindle shape) histiocytes arranged in a whorled, criss-cross or storiform pattern and it cover with pseudo capsule. Three different variant has been described based on histopathology:

1. Pure fusocellular
2. Fusocellular with epitheloid component
3. Fusocellular with vacuolated cells-MC

Differential Diagnosis

- Dermatofibromas
- Neurofibromas
- Fibro histiocytoma

Difference between histoid and lepromatous leprosy Table 8.2.

Table 8.2: Showing difference between histoid leprosy and lepromatous leprosy

Histoid leprosy	*Lepromatous leprosy*
Enhanced immune response against *M. leprae* in these patients compared with lepromatous leprosy with respect to both cell mediated immunity and humoral immunity	Less immune response against *M. leprae* compared to histoid
Despite adequate number of macrophages, they lack the functional property to kill bacilli	In lepromatous macrophages have good killing properties
Spindle shape histiocytes are the characteristic cells	Foamy macrophages are the characteristic cells
Bacilli are longer in size and vary high in number as compared to lepromatous leprosy	Bacilli are normal in size and less in number as compared to histoid leprosy

PURE NEURITIC LEPROSY

Pure neuritic leprosy presents with signs and symptoms of nerve damage without involvement of skin. It constitutes 5 to 10% of leprosy cases in India. Patients may present with sensory or motor changes in the distribution of the involved nerves. Single or multiple nerves may be involved which may be thickened and tender. The commonly affected nerves are ulnar, median, radial, lateral popliteal, posterior tibial and facial.

It should be differentiated from hereditary sensory and motor neuropathy. Its diagnosis is questionable when there is only motor deficit and no sensory deficit. Nerve biopsy is the gold standard. FNAC and USG of peripheral nerves are also valuable tools for diagnosis.

MACULOANAESTHETIC LEPROSY

It is a variant of BT leprosy. Typical lesions are well defined, anaesthetic macules with dry surface, bacilli are scanty or absent. Some authors call it 'low resistant tuberculoid leprosy'.

LUCIO LEPROSY

It is diffuse, non-nodular, slow progressive form of leprosy commonly seen in Mexico. The skin looks waxy, and shiny with diffuse infiltration of involved skin leads to loss of hair, thickened upper eyelid looks sleepy. If these cases left untreated results in Lucio phenomenon. Lucio phenomenon presents as well defined angulated bizarre shape ulcerations mainly on extremities.

Histopathologically there is necrosis of epidermis with dermal histiocyte and neutrophilic infiltrate around nerve fibres, blood vessels and adnexa.

SYSTEMIC MANIFESTATIONS IN LEPROSY

Leprosy may affect multiple organ systems, most common with multibacillary leprosy. Systemic manifestation includes, renal amyloidosis, hepatic amyloidosis, laryngeal involvement, orchitis, ocular leprosy, arrhythmias, ventricular hypertrophy and coronary artery disease etc. The gastrointestinal tract and female reproductive system, central nerve system are almost always spared.

Laryngeal Leprosy

Laryngeal involvement is the Late feature in leprosy. Two different type of laryngeal involvement seen in leprosy:

1. **Fibrotic:** Fibrosis leads to vocal cords immobile and which causes hoarseness of voice.
2. **Ulcerative type:** Thickening, nodulation and ulceration leads to pain and gradually narrowing of glottis resulting stridor.

Ocular Leprosy

Ocular manifestations occurs due to involvement of fifth and seventh cranial nerves, direct infiltration of *M. leprae* and lepra reaction. Clinical features of eye involvement are madarosis, lagophthalmos, reduce corneal sensation, corneal ulceration, scleritis, iridocyclitis, cataract, glaucoma etc.

Lagophthalmos

It occurs due to involvement facial nerve, which supplies orbicularis oculi muscle which is responsible for closing the eyes. Lagophthalmos results in exposure keratitis, corneal ulceration. Treatment includes lateral tarsorrhaphy, canthoplasty and temporalis muscle transfer.

Iridocyclitis

It is an inflammation of iris and ciliary body, commonly seen in multibacillary leprosy with type 2 lepra reaction. Treatment of iridocyclitis includes steroid eye drops and oral steroids.

Bone Changes in Leprosy

Polyarthralgia, joint pain, periostitis, osteitis, osteoporosis, osteomyelitis, resorption of bones over hands and feet are the common features of bone seen in leprosy. Resorption is usually start from meta-tarsals bone, most pronounced changes take place at the distal end and bone can become thin and pointed an appearance known sucked candy bone. Later tarsal bones may become disintegrated.

LEPRA REACTIONS

During the course of untreated or treated leprosy, the immune system may produce inflammatory reactions which are of two types:

Type 1 Reaction

Upgrading or reversal reaction occurs in patients with borderline leprosy because of their immunological instability and results from sudden increase in cell-mediated immunity. It generally occurs in first 6 months after starting therapy. This reaction can cause fever and inflammation of the pre-existing skin and peripheral nerve lesions, resulting in skin edema, erythema, and tenderness and worsening nerve function. This reaction, particularly if not treated early, contribute significantly to nerve damage. Because the immune response is increased, these reactions are termed reversal reactions, despite the apparent clinical worsening. On the other hand, if reaction is associated with reduction in immunity, which is a natural tendency of borderline leprosy to downgrade towards lepromatous pole, it is called **'downgrading reaction'.**

Type 2 Reaction (Erythema Nodosum Leprosum or ENL)

Erythema nodosum leprosum is systemic inflammatory reaction that appears to be a vasculitis or panniculitis and probably involves circulating immune complex deposition in blood vessels and has increased T-helper cell function. Patients may develop erythematous and painful papules or nodules that may pustulate and ulcerate. They appear in crops and heal spontaneously in 2-3 weeks. Fever, neuritis, lymphadenitis, orchitis, arthritis (particularly in large joints, usually knees), and glomerulonephritis may also be seen. Hemolysis or bone marrow suppression may cause anemia, and hepatic involvement may cause mild abnormalities in liver function tests.

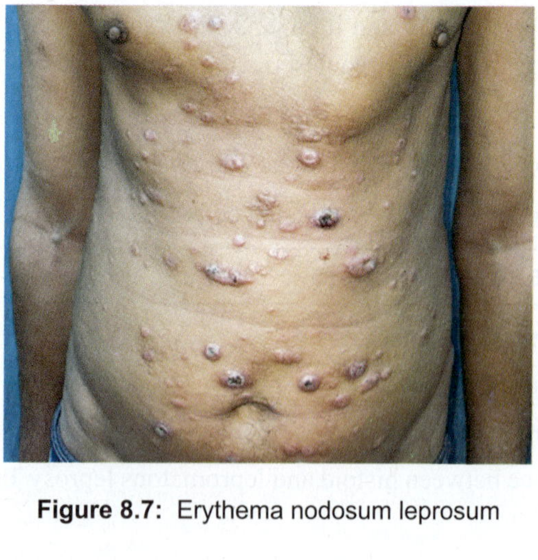

Figure 8.7: Erythema nodosum leprosum

Treatment of lepra reactions includes continuing MDT, systemic corticosteroids for immunosuppression and symptomatic medication. Clofazimine is also helpful because of its anti-inflammatory properties. Its dose can be increased upto 4-6 mg/kg/day during ENL reaction. Thalidomide is also helpful to control acute and chronic ENL with dose ranging from 3 to 9.5 mg/kg/day.

DEFORMITY, DISABILITY AND TROPHIC ULCERS IN LEPROSY

Deformity

Deformities are visible consequences of impairment due to leprosy. These deformities may result in rehabilitation and destitution. They are classified into three types:

- **Specific deformity:** These deformities are due to direct infiltration or direct result of disease process resulting in tissue damage e.g. leonine facies, nasal septal perforation, madarosis, sagging of earlobe (buddha ear), rat bitten helix appearance, palatal perforation, reaction hand, frozen hands, intrinsic plus deformity, twisted toe, testicular atrophy, gynecothelia etc.
- **Paralytic deformity:** These deformities are due to motor nerve damage e.g. lagophthalmos, claw hand, ape thumb deformity, 'Z' thumb deformity, claw toes and foot drop.
- **Anesthetic deformities:** These deformities are the consequences of sensory nerve damage e.g. anosmia, corneal damage, digital resorption, trophic ulcers, tarsal disintegration, callosities etc.

Disability

Disability is defined as inability or difficulty to perform a task. WHO grading (1998) for disability in leprosy is defined as:

Disability grading for hand and feet:

- **Grade 0:** No anaesthesia, no visible deformity or damage.
- **Grade 1:** Anaesthesia present, but no visible deformity or damage.
- **Grade 2:** Visible deformity or damage.

Disability grading in eyes:

- **Grade 0:** No eye problem due to leprosy, no evidence of vision loss.
- **Grade 1:** Eye involvement due to leprosy present but vision not severely affected (vision 6/60 or better; can count finger at 6 meter distance).
- **Grade 2:** Severe visual impairment (vision worse than 6/60; inability to count finger at 6 meter distance), also includes lagophthalmos, iridocyclitis and corneal opacity).

Trophic Ulcers

Trophic ulcers in leprosy are due to sensory, motor and autonomic nerve impairment. Motor deformity, continuous high pressure, infection, lack of proper care and malnutrition contributes in formation of recurrent trophic ulcers. Common sites are ball of great toe, tip of toe and dorsum of proximal interphalangeal joints.

Various stages of trophic ulcer in leprosy is given in Table 8.3.

Table 8.3: Stages of trophic ulcer in leprosy

Stage	*Clinical findings*	*Treatment*
Threatened ulceration	• Burning sensation, • Deep plantar tenderness, oedema, puffiness • Splaying of toe	• Rest and leg elevation for 3- 7 days with splint
Concealed ulceration	• Blister formation	• Cover the blister with bulky layer of sterile gauze with bandage. • Rest for 3-7 days. • Patient may need below knee plaster cast with provision of walking for 3 weeks.
Open ulceration		
Acute ulceration	• Pain, redness, oedema, swelling, pus discharge with lymphadenopathy	• Bed rest with elevation of limb, hydrocolloid dressings, oral antibiotics
Chronic simple ulceration	• Raised hyperkeratotic edges, indurated hard base with unhealthy granulation tissue and mild discharge	• Debridement with dressing and below knee walking plaster cast for 6 weeks • Skin graft if ulcer size is > 2 cm
Chronic complicated ulcer	• Recurrent ulceration • Ulcer extending up to bones and joints with associated deformity • Deep sinus formation with pseudo-epitheliomatous hyperplasia • Malignant transformation can occur	• Wound debridement with oral antibiotics • Offloading measures • Treat osteomyelitis if present • Reconstructive surgeries

Management of trophic ulcer: Trophic ulcers require proper wound care which includes debridement of the wound and dressing by using silver base cream like silver sulphadiazine, hydrogel with silver ion. When there is excessive exudation, hydrocolloid dressings can be used.

Platelet derived growth factors (Becaplermin), platelet rich fibrin, topical phenytoin, topical insulin and hyperbaric oxygen therapy may also be used. Offloading methods include bed rest, air cushion, water bed, plantar boots, removable cast, specialized microcellular rubber footwear etc.

Differential Diagnosis

Leprosy has to be differentiated from other diseases presenting with hypopigmented or erythematous patches or plaques or with annular or nodular lesions, e.g., tinea versicolor, vitiligo, psoriasis, granuloma annulare, syphilis, leishmaniasis, neurofibromatosis and xanthomas. Uncommon presentation with ENL may be misdiagnosed as vasculitis or pyoderma. Sensory loss over the lesions and presence of thickened and tender nerves are cardinal signs to diagnose leprosy. In one Ethiopian study, following criteria had a sensitivity of 97% with a positive predictive value of 98% in diagnosing leprosy. Diagnosis was based on 1 or more of 3 cardinal features:

Hypopigmented or reddish patches with definite loss of sensation.

Thickened and tender peripheral nerves.

Acid fast bacilli on skin smears examination or biopsy.

The doubtful cases should be confirmed by examination of tissue smears for AFB staining and histopathology.

Investigations

Tissue Smear Testing/Slit-Skin Smears

After making the skin bloodless by pinching it between thumb and fingers, an incision is made by number 15 BP scalpel blade and fluid and pulp is obtained by scraping with it. Material is usually taken from pinna of ear, eyebrows, nasal mucosa or from lesions. The fluid and pulp are placed on a glass slide and stained by using Ziehl Neelsen method to look for organisms. They are seen as pink rod shaped bacilli (Figure 8.8) either scattered or in clumps. The bacteriologic index is then determined as the number of organisms per 100 × with oil immersion. BI ranges from 0 to 6. It helps in monitoring the response of treatment. The slit smear positivity varies from 10.9% to 46%.

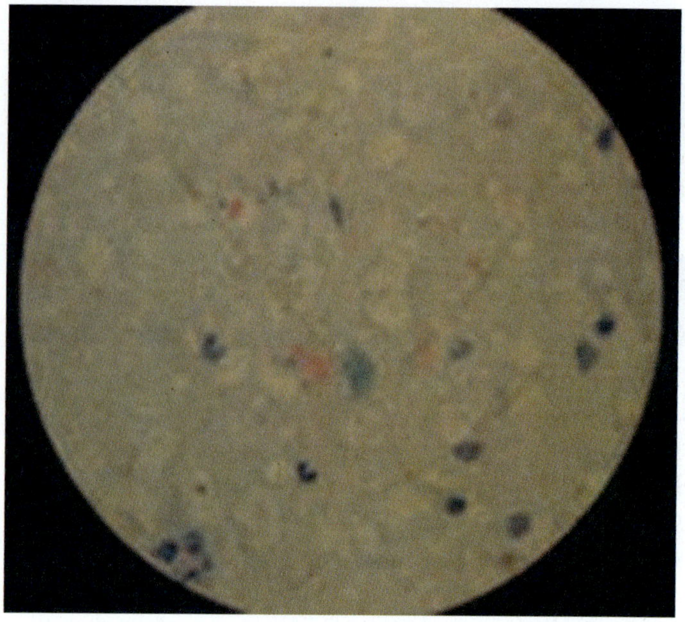

Figure 8.8: AFB stain

Skin Biopsy

Skin biopsy is helpful in confirmation of diagnosis in doubtful cases as in indeterminate leprosy or other granulomatous disorders. It is also helpful in correct classification of the disease. The histopathology correlation may be evident in 52% to 70% patients. Histology of the different types of leprosy is as follows:

Indeterminate leprosy: Histological findings are non-specific. Histiocytes and lymphocytes are scattered, with some concentration around dermal appendages and nerves. At times, an acid-fast bacillus may be observed in a nerve bundle. The number of dermal mast cells may be increased.

Tuberculoid: Well-developed epithelioid cell granulomas are observed in the papillary dermis, often around neurovascular structures. The granulomas are surrounded by lymphocytes, which extend into the epidermis. Langhans giant cells are common. Dermal nerves are destroyed or swollen because of the granulomas. Acid-fast bacilli are not observed.

Borderline Tuberculoid: Well-developed epithelioid cell granulomas are apparent and diffuse, but few or no Langhans giant cells are observed. Fewer lymphocytes are present in this form as compared to TT. Bacilli are absent or rare, but they can be found in dermal nerves and in the arrector pilorum. Nerves are moderately swollen.

Borderline or mid borderline: There is diffuse epithelioid cell granuloma with scanty lymphocytes and no giant cells. The papillary zone of the dermis is clear and nerves are swollen by cellular infiltrate. AFB are present in moderate number.

Borderline Lepromatous: Smaller granulomas with some foamy macrophages and numerous lymphocytes are observed. Nerves often have an onion skin appearance as a result of invasion of the perineurium. A few epithelioid cells may be observed.

Lepromatous leprosy: A diffuse infiltrate of foamy macrophages is present in the dermis below a subepidermal grenz zone. An enormous number of acid-fast bacilli are present within the foamy macrophages, singly or in clumps, called globi. Lymphocytes are scanty and giant cells are typically absent. Numerous bacilli invade the nerves, but these are fairly well preserved with little infiltrate.

Histoid leprosy: There are spindle shaped clusters of histiocytes in a whorled or parallel pattern. In paucibacillary histoid leprosy, these clusters are in the papillary and mid dermis. Multibacillary histoid leprosy has a grenz zone with the histiocytes located in the mid and deep dermis.

LEPROMIN TEST

This test indicates host resistance to *M. leprae.* Its results do not confirm the diagnosis, but they are useful in determining the type of leprosy.

A positive finding indicates good cell-mediated immunity against *M. leprae,* which is observed in tuberculoid pole of leprosy. A negative finding suggests a lack of resistance to disease and is observed in lepromatous pole of leprosy. A negative result also indicates a poor prognosis.

To perform this test, lepromin antigen is injected into the forearm. An assessment of the reaction at 48 hours is called Fernandez reaction, and a positive result indicates hypersensitivity to antigens of *M. leprae* or mycobacteria that cross react with *M. leprae*. When the reaction is read at 3-4 weeks, it is called the Mitsuda reaction, and a positive result indicates that the immune system is capable of mounting an efficient cell mediated response.

Serology against *M. leprae* and polymerase chain reaction (PCR) testing are also used to study leprosy but not routinely done. Antigen used for serodiagnosis are phenolic glycolipid-1 (most common), lipoarabinomannan, MMP-I, MMP-II, Early secretory antigen target 6 kDa (ESAT-6), Culture filtrate protein -10 (CFP-10), Leprosy IDRI diagnostic -1(LID -1), Protein advances diagnostic of leprosy (PADL) and 35 kDa protein. ELISA, lateral flow assay, dipstick, haemagglutination are the various method used for serodiagnosis in leprosy. Gene sequence which used in leprosy are RLEP, Rpo-T, Sod-A, 16s rRNA, 4-alpha gluconotransferase, 18kDa antigen, 36 kDa antigen and Hsp 65 kDa groEL. Plain radiographs of hands and feet may be useful to detect and monitor leprosy-related changes.

Treatment

The early institution of multi-drug therapy is the best for prevention of deformities and disabilities that could have a huge impairment of quality of life in children.

Dapsone has remained the sheet anchor in the treatment of leprosy since 1940. This was used as a single drug which led to the development of resistance. W.H.O. introduced multi drug therapy (MDT) for leprosy in 1982 consisting of three drugs namely rifampicin, dapsone and clofazimine for a fixed period of twelve months.

Rifampicin is given once a month. No toxic effects have been reported in the case of monthly administration. The urine may be colored slightly reddish for a few hours after its intake, this should be explained to the patient while starting MDT. Few patients develop flu like syndrome after taking monthly rifampicin which last for 2-3 days.

Clofazimine is most active when administered daily. The drug is well tolerated and virtually non-toxic in the dosage used for MDT. The drug causes brownish black discoloration and dryness of skin. However, this disappears within few months after stopping treatment. This should be explained to patients when starting MDT regimen for multibacillary leprosy.

Dapsone is very safe in the dosage used in MDT and side effects are rare. The main side effect is allergic reaction, causing itchy skin rashes and exfoliative dermatitis. Patients known to be allergic to any of the sulpha drugs should be given dapsone with caution after challenge dose. Hepatitis, peripheral neuritis, psychosis, haemolytic anemia, DDS syndrome, etc. are uncommon side effects.

Multi drug regimens for different types of leprosy are as follows: (Tables 8.4 and 8.5)

Table 8.4: Multi-drug therapy for children 10-14 years of age

Type of leprosy	*Monthly supervised*	*Daily self administered*	*Duration of therapy*
Paucibacillary	Rifampicin 450 mg	Dapsone 50 mg	6 months
Multibacillary	Rifampicin 450 mg Clofazimine 150 mg	Clofazimine 50 mg alternate day Dapsone 50 mg	12 months

Table 8.5: WHO multi-drug therapy regimen for more than 14 years of age

Type of leprosy	*Monthly supervised*	*Daily self administered*	*Duration of therapy*
Paucibacillary	Rifampicin 600 mg	Dapsone 100 mg	6 months
Multibacillary	Rifampicin 600 mg Clofazimine 300 mg	Clofazimine 50 mg Dapsone 100 mg	12 months

For children less than 10 years of age:

Multibacillary (MB-child) Rifampicin – 10 mg/kg monthly, Clofazimine – 6 mg/kg monthly and 1 mg/kg daily, Dapsone – 2 mg/kg daily.

Duration – 12 months.

Paucibacillary (PB-child) Rifampicin – 10 mg/kg monthly, Dapsone – 2 mg/kg daily.

Duration – 6 months.

RELAPSES AFTER MDT

WHO 1988 definition for relapse: As per WHO, relapse is defined as, a patient who has successfully completed an adequate course of MDT but subsequently develops signs and symptoms of disease either during the surveillance period (2 years for PB and 5 years for MB) or thereafter.

There are different aspects of relapse:

1. **Microbiological relapse:** When a patient becomes acid fact bacilli positive after becoming negative or persistent high bacillary index or increase in bacillary index by 2+. Other methods to assess microbiological relapse are line morphological index, fluorescent diacetate ethidium bromide (FDA-EB) staining, laser microprobe mass analysis (LAMMA) and molecular testing.
2. **Immunological relapse:** In lepromatous leprosy phenolic glycolipids (PGL)- immunoglobulin M (IgM) and natural disaccharide ND-O-Bovine serum antigen are increased during relapse. Th1 and Th2 immune type of interleukin profile may also be useful to identify relapse.
3. **Histological relapse:** Reappearance of granuloma in PB and new spindle cell macrophage with foamy cytoplasm in MB are indicators of relapse.

Becx-Bleumink criteria for relapse:

1. New skin lesions.
2. New activity in previous existing lesions.
3. Bacteriological index 2+ or more.
4. New nerve function impairment.
5. Histopathological evidence of relapse in skin and nerve
6. Lepromatous activity in eye

Predisposing factor for relapse:

There are various factors involved in relapse of disease:

- Persisters in dermal nerves, smooth muscles, lymph nodes, iris, bone marrow and liver.
- Inadequate and irregular treatment.
- Monotherapy.
- High initial bacillary index.
- Lepromin test negativity.

Difference between relapse and resistance are given in Table 8.6.

Table 8.6: Difference between relapse and reversal reaction

	Relapse	*Reversal reaction*
Time course	Seen 1 year after release from treatment	Usually seen within 6 months of release from treatment
Spectrum	In any spectrum	BT, BB, BL
Skin lesions	Increase in number and size of lesions No ulceration of lesions Oedema is rare	Increased erythema, pain, swelling and tenderness in lesions Few new lesions Ulceration can occur in severe form of reaction Oedema of hands and feet
Nerve	New nerve involved with gradual progression in sensory and motor function	Acute painful neuritis, nerve abscess, sudden onset of motor and sensory deficit
Skin smear	AFB smear positivity may occur in previously negative patients	Decreased bacteriological index with granular and fragmentation of bacilli
Systemic steroids	No response	Significant improvement in 2-3 weeks

DRUG RESISTANT LEPROSY

Drug resistance has been reported for dapsone since 1964, for rifampin since 1976 and for ofloxacin since 1996. Mouse foot pad assay to determine *M. leprae's* susceptibility to anti-leprosy drugs has been the gold standard for drug susceptibility testing, but it is laborious and expensive, hence molecular methods were developed for the detection of mutations associated with dapsone, rifampicin and fluoroquinolone resistance. Recent studies have identified point mutations in the ***folP1*** **gene,** which encodes dihydropteroate synthase (DHPS) in dapsone-resistant *M. leprae.* Rifampicin resistance is associated with mutations in the ***rpoB*** **gene** that encodes the β subunit of RNA polymerase. Resistance to ofloxacin is known to be associated with mutation in ***gyrA*** **gene** encoding the A subunit of DNA gyrase in *M. leprae.* No molecular target has been defined for clofazimine.

The Guidelines Development Group (GDG) of WHO in 2018 recommended (Table 8.7) that for leprosy patients with rifampicin resistance, at least two of the following second-line drugs should be given: clarithromycin, minocycline, or a quinolone (ofloxacin, levofloxacin or moxifloxacin), plus clofazimine daily for 6 months, followed by clofazimine plus one of the second-line drugs daily for an additional 18 months. In case of rifampicin plus ofloxacin resistance, a quinolone should not be chosen; therefore, the recommended regimen is clarithromycin, minocycline and clofazimine for 6 months followed by clarithromycin or minocycline plus clofazimine for an additional 18 months.

Table 8.7: WHO guidelines for treatment of drug resistant leprosy

Resistance type	*Treatment*	
	First 6 months (daily)	Next 18 months (daily)
Rifampicin resistance	Ofloxacin 400 mg + minocycline 100 mg + clofazimine 50 mg	Ofloxacin 400 mg OR minocycline 100 mg + clofazimine 50 mg
	Ofloxacin 400 mg + clarithromycin 500 mg + clofazimine 50 mg	Ofloxacin 400 mg + clofazimine 50 mg
Rifampicin and ofloxacin resistance	Clarithromycin 500 mg + minocycline 100 mg + clofazimine 50 mg	Clarithromycin 500 mg OR minocycline 100 mg + clofazimine 50 mg
Ofloxacin can be replaced by levofloxacin 500 mg or moxifloxacin 400 mg		

VACCINES IN LEPROSY

These are biological agents that have both immunoprophylactic and immunotherapeutic properties, which work by boosting the immune system against foreign antigens. Various mycobacteria have been observed to share common antigens with *M. leprae.* They show cross reactivity and have the potential to generate immune response against *M. leprae.*

Impact of immune-prophylaxis: Immunotherapy improves protective cell-mediated immunity against leprosy in both patients and their contacts. By shortening the length of treatment, lowering the relapse rate and reducing medication resistance, it lowers mortality and morbidity. Additionally, it leads to the effective elimination of persisters and viable bacilli, which improves the skin lesions.

It is still debatable whether vaccine is needed in high endemic areas of leprosy. It is due to the low prevalence, low transmission rate, changing profile of the disease, effective and widely available MDT, so, vaccines may not be efficacious. However, in high risk groups, areas of high endemicity and close family contacts, it might be useful. The vaccines mentioned in the immunotherapy section can also be used for immuneprophylaxis.

First generation vaccines:

Non cultivable vaccine

- Killed *M. leprae*
- Killed *M. leprae* + BCG (Convit vaccine)
- Acetoacetylated *M. leprae*

Cultivable

- BCG (Attenuated *M. bovis*)
- BCG + *M. vaccae*
- Killed *M. welchii* (*M. indicus pranii*)
- Killed ICRC (*M. avium intracellulare* complex)
- *M. habana*
- *M. vaccae*

Second generation vaccines: In second generation vaccines, only immunological subunit is used for vaccine. These are prepared by recombinant technology, which enhance immunity.

- HMW PP 1 glycoprotein (Sonicated fraction of ICRC bacilli or *Mycobacterium avium intracellulare* complex).
- *M. leprae* 35 kDa protein.

Following are commonly tried preparations as immunotherapy in *M. leprae* infection:

- **Bacillus Calmette Guerin:** Bacillus Calmette Guerin (BCG), is a live vaccine containing *M. bovis* which produces specific as well as nonspecific immunomodulatory effect in leprosy.
- **Bacillus Calmette Guerin + Killed *M. leprae*:** Combination of BCG with killed *M. leprae* was shown to enhance the bacterial clearance in patients of LL undergoing treatment and also resulted in histological upgrading.
- **Mycobacterium Indicus Pranii (MIP):** MIP is a rapid growing, nonpathogenic and cultivable mycobacteria classified under Group IV Runyon classification of mycobacteria. It is a killed vaccine and due to common antigens with *M. leprae* it has immunomodulatory effect in leprosy patients.

- **Indian Cancer Research Centre (ICRC):** Its organism belongs to *Mycobacterium avium intercellulare* complex and is cultivable mycobacteria, which was isolated from leprosy patients and showed cross-reactive antigens to *M. leprae.*
- **Mycobacterium Vaccae:** It is a rapid growing and nonpathogenic mycobacteria which also shares few common antigens with *M. leprae* and *M. tuberculosis,* hence, induces *in vitro* and *in vivo* immunomodulatory effect in leprosy patients. It is administered intradermally as a killed vaccine in the dose of 108 organisms/ml.

LEPVAX

A mixture of three prioritized antigens (ML2055, ML2380 and ML2028) with the T helper 1 (Th1) biased adjuvant formulation Glucopyranosyl Lipid Adjuvant in stable emulsion (GLA-SE), when injected into mice, has shown to reduce *M. leprae* infection levels. A single chimeric fusion protein comprising the above-mentioned antigens, LEP-F1, was found to be efficacious. Experimental studies in armadillos have shown that *M. leprae* infection induces neuropathy that mimics the pre-clinical silent neuropathic situation that develops in leprosy patients. Hence administration of LepVax after *M. leprae* infection (post-exposure immunoprophylaxis) was performed in armadillos and it has shown to be safe and efficacious, especially in reducing sensory nerve damage. It also delayed/ alleviated motor nerve damage in some experimental animals infected with high doses of *M. leprae.*

CHEMOPROPHYLAXIS

Chemoprophylaxis is defined as administration of drugs which are capable of preventing an infection or keep illness in falling trend. Contact in leprosy is defined as someone who had regular or interrupted contact with index case during last one year. Guideline development group recommends single dose rifampicin for chemoprophylaxis in leprosy contacts after excluding leprosy and tuberculosis. Single dose rifampicin dose regimen according to age is given in Table 8.8.

Table 8.8: Chemoprophylaxis (Single dose rifampicin) in leprosy contacts dose regimen

Age/weight	*Dose of SDR*
15 years or above	600 mg
10-14 years	450 mg
6-9 years (weight 20 kg or above	300 mg
Less than 20 kg (2 years or above)	10-15 mg/kg

Dapsone 100 mg once or twice weekly for 2 years, ROM (Rifampicin 600 mg + Ofloxacin 400 mg + Minocycline 100 mg) single dose have also been tried.

NATIONAL LEPROSY ERADICATION PROGRAMME (NLEP)

The National Leprosy Eradication Programme was launched in 1983. Subsequently, in 1991, at the 44th World Health Assembly, WHO and its member states committed to eliminate leprosy as a public health problem by the year 2000 and they defined elimination as prevalence below one case per 10,000 population. To enhance this process of elimination, the first World Bank supported project on NLEP was started in the year 1993-94. In India, the global target of leprosy elimination by end of the year 2000 was not attained. The prevalence rate in March 2001 remained at 3.7/10,000 population. Afterwards, the Second World Bank supported National Leprosy Elimination Project was started from 2001-02 for a period of 3 years. This project formulated the following strategy towards leprosy elimination in India:

- **Decentralization of NLEP to states and districts.**
- **Integration of leprosy services with General Health Care (GHC) system.**
- **Leprosy training of GHS functionaries.**
- **Surveillance for early diagnosis and prompt MDT, through routine and special efforts.**
- **Intensified information, education and communication (IEC) activities using local and mass media approaches.**
- **Prevention of disability (POD) and care.**
- **Monitoring and evaluation on regular (monthly/ quarterly/ annually) basis as well as with special efforts such as independent evaluation, leprosy elimination monitoring, annual survey(s) and validation of progress towards leprosy elimination, etc.**

The 2nd National Leprosy Elimination Project successfully ended on December 31, 2004 and at the end of the second project as on March 31, 2005, the prevalence rate was 1.34/10,000.

Finally after a well planned decades long programme, India achieved the goal of elimination of leprosy as a public health problem (less than 1 case per 10,000 population) in December, 2005. As on December 31, 2005, prevalence rate recorded in the country was 0.95 per 10,000 population. Prevalence rate in year 2021-22 was 0.45 per 10,000 population.

Recent programme milestone and implementation (form directorate general of health services):

Year	Milestones	Implementation
2016-17	Newer initiatives in the programme- Three Pronged strategy including chemoprophylaxis	Leprosy Case Detection Campaign (LCDC) – 14 day active case detection campaign in high endemic districts Focused Leprosy Campaign (FLC) – non-endemic districts, Special plan for hard to reach areas Single Dose Rifampicin (SDR) implementation to eligible contacts of new cases Immunotherapy - MIP Vaccine as pilot phase
2017	Sparsh leprosy awareness campaign (SLAC)	Increasing awareness, addressing high level of stigma and discrimination – special Gram Sabha meeting
2017-18	Introduction of "NIKUSTH" ASHA based Surveillance for Leprosy Suspects (ABSULS)	Real time monitoring of leprosy patients across the country and facilitating better monitoring and evaluation of NLEP ABSULS - Active surveillance of leprosy suspects with prioritizing leprosy case detection by ASHA & treatment follow up
2018-2019	Sparsh Leprosy Elimination Campaign (SLEC) 150th Birth anniversary of Mahatma Gandhi Ji	Enhancement of recently launched initiatives – LCDC, SLAC Grade 2 Disability target to reduce <1case/Million & reduce backlog of Reconstructive surgery cases Grade II disability investigation
2018-19	WHO Guidelines for Diagnosis, treatment and prevention of Leprosy	Evidence based recommendations in accordance with procedures established by the WHO Guidelines Review Committee Independent Evaluation of NLEP by WHO (2019)
2019	Convergence of leprosy screening under major programme of national health mission	1. Comprehensive primary health care of Ayushman bharat - Community Based Assessment Checklist (CBAC) to screen 30 + population at HWCs 2. Rashtriya Bal Swasthya Karayakaram to screen children
2020	Active Case Detection and Regular Surveillance (ACD & RS) Convergence under Rashtriya Kishore Swasthya Karyakaram (RKSK)	ACD & RS guidelines rolled out – active case finding to be continuous and regular Flexibility for states to plan and implement Frontline workers (FLWs) RKSK – screening and counselling of adolescent children District Award Scheme for achievements in NLEP

Achievements during 2020 (form directorate general of health services):

- Percentage of Grade II Disability (G2D)/visible deformity among new cases decreased from 3.05% in 2018-19 to 2.39% (2019-20).
- The G2D amongst new cases/ million population decreased from 2.65/million population as on 31st March, 2019 to 1.94/ million population as on 31st March 2020.
- Child cases percentage has reduced from 7.67% as on 31st March 2019 to 6.86 % as on 31st March 2020.

9 CHAPTER Eczemas

Contents

Eczema can be defined as an inflammatory reaction pattern of skin, clinically characterized by itching, erythema, edema, formation of papulovesicular lesions, blistering, oozing and crusting in acute stage and scaling and lichenification in chronic stage. Eczema is a common condition in adults as well as in children. **Lichenification** is defined as thickening of skin, hyperpigmentation and prominent skin creases and occurs due to constant itching and rubbing of the lesion.

Eczemas can be classified according to their cause, site of involvement or morphology (Table 9.1).

Table 9.1: Classification of eczema

Etiological classification	*Topological classification*	*Morphological classification*
Endogenous eczema		
Atopic dermatitis	Perioral dermatitis	Discoid or nummular eczema
Seborrheic dermatitis	Facial dermatitis	Pompholyx
Nummular dermatitis	Hand eczema	Hyperkeratotic eczema
Pompholyx	Foot eczema	Vesiculopustular eczema
Pityriasis alba	Diaper dermatitis	Nodular prurigo
Stasis dermatitis		Papular urticaria
Perioral dermatitis		
Lichen simplex chronicus		
Juvenile plantar dermatosis		

Contd.

Exogenous eczema		
Allergic contact dermatitis		
Irritant contact dermatitis		
Infective dermatitis		
Photodermatitis		
Phytophotodermatitis		
Dermatophytid		
Post traumatic eczema		

The common types of eczemas are discussed below:

IRRITANT CONTACT DERMATITIS (ICD)

Irritant contact dermatitis is a non-specific response of the skin to direct chemical damage. It results from repeated exposure to irritants like soap, cleansers and solvents. It is mostly an occupational disease in adults and is relatively uncommon in children.

Epidemiology

Occupation

It plays a major role in irritant contact dermatitis, especially of hands. Workplace exposure is commonly seen in hair dressers, cooks, construction workers, etc.

Age

Irritant contact dermatitis may occur at any age. It results from direct contact with diaper and excessive moisture which in combination of occlusive effect and presence of fecal and urinary waste results in maceration of the skin and disruption of stratum corneum. Infants and children have a drier and thinner skin that does not tolerate soaps and solvents as efficiently as older individuals.

Sex

ICD is more common in females as compared to males in adults, but no sex predilection is seen in children.

Etiopathogenesis

Irritant contact dermatitis is the clinical result of inflammation arising from the release of proinflammatory cytokines from keratinocytes, usually in response to chemical stimuli. The main pathophysiological changes are skin barrier disruption, epidermal cellular changes and cytokine release.

A wide range of chemicals with sufficient concentration or duration of exposure are capable of acting as cutaneous irritants. Common cutaneous irritants include detergent and water. Most cases of home workers eczema are irritant contact dermatitis resulting from repeated exposure to low grade cutaneous irritants, particularly soap, water and detergents. Solvents are another cause of cutaneous irritation because they remove essential fatty acids and oils from the skin, which increases the transepidermal water loss and renders the skin susceptible to the increased direct toxic effects of other previously well-tolerated cutaneous exposures.

Clinical Features

Following clinical features are usually seen:

- History of sufficient exposure to a cutaneous irritant is noted and onset of symptoms occurs within minutes to hours of exposure in simple acute irritant contact dermatitis.
- The onset of signs and symptoms may be delayed by weeks in cumulative irritant contact dermatitis. Cumulative irritant contact dermatitis is a consequence of multiple incidents of subthreshold damage to the skin, with the time between exposures being too short for damaging skin barrier function. Patients with sensitive skin (i.e., atopic individuals) have a decreased irritant threshold or a prolonged restoration time, making them more vulnerable to clinical irritant contact dermatitis. Cumulative irritant contact dermatitis is not dependent on exposure to a potent irritant, but exposure to weak irritants, which initiate the reaction. Often, the exposure (i.e., by water) is not only at work but also at home.
- Pain, burning, stinging or discomfort, exceeding pruritus early in the clinical course may occur. These patients report both itching and pain caused by fissuring of the hyperkeratotic skin.
- Individuals with history of atopic dermatitis are more susceptible to irritant contact dermatitis, particularly of the hands.
- Other causes of contact dermatitis (particularly allergic contact dermatitis) must be excluded by history and/or by patch testing to the relevant allergens (Table 9.1). Patch testing should be negative for all possible allergens.

- Macular erythema, hyperkeratosis and fissuring are seen in cumulative irritant contact dermatitis. Erythema and vesiculation is seen more in acute irritant dermatitis (Figure 9.1).
- Healing process begins promptly on withdrawal of exposure to the offending agent.

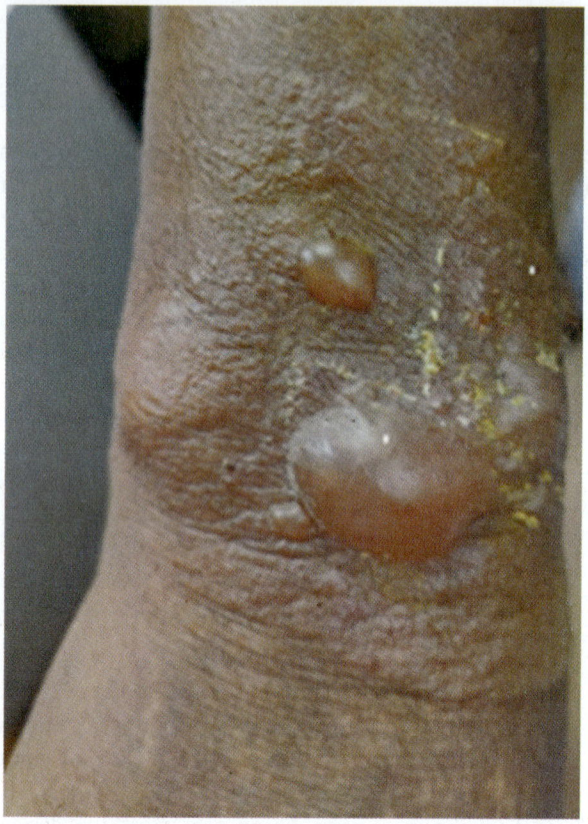

Figure 9.1: Irritant contact dermatitis showing sharply marginated erythematous plaque with vesiculation

Differential Diagnosis

- Atopic dermatitis.
- Allergic contact dermatitis.
- Tinea corporis, tinea manuum.
- Asteatotic dermatitis.
- Seborrheic dermatitis.

Investigations

- A bacterial culture can be obtained in cases complicated by secondary bacterial infection.
- A KOH examination may be performed and samples for mycological examination may be obtained to exclude superficial tinea infections or candidal infections, depending on site and morphology of lesions.
- Findings of significantly elevated serum immunoglobulin E levels are occasionally useful to substantiate an atopic diathesis in the absence of a personal or family history of atopy.
- Patch testing can be performed to diagnose contact allergies, but no patch test exists that proves that a cutaneous irritant is responsible for a particular case of irritant contact dermatitis. Diagnosis rests on exclusion of allergic contact dermatitis and history of sufficient exposure to a cutaneous irritant.
- Skin biopsy can help to exclude other disorders, such as tinea or psoriasis. All clinical cases of dermatitis are similar histologically. Skin biopsy of lesions of the palms and soles has several differences from skin of other sites. The stratum corneum and epidermis are particularly thick on the palms and soles. This makes the histologic differentiation from psoriasis more difficult.

Treatment

- Acute irritant contact dermatitis reactions to potent irritants (e.g., acids, alkaline solutions) are comparable to a chemical burn and can be graded like thermal burns (i.e., first, second or third degree burns). With appropriate symptomatic management, the prognosis for this type of irritant contact dermatitis is usually good unless the dermis is damaged, no permanent scarring occurs.
- Topical corticosteroids play a limited role in treatment of irritant contact dermatitis. They do not address the disease process directly, but may be helpful for super-imposed eczematous features.
- Creams containing dimethicone and zinc may be particularly helpful in restoring the epidermal barrier in persons with irritant contact dermatitis and atopic dermatitis.
- Most soaps and detergents are alkaline and induce an increase in cutaneous pH, which affects the physiologic protective acid mantle of the skin by decreasing the fat content. Disruption of stratum corneum and changes in pH are key elements in the induction of irritant contact dermatitis and pruritus by soaps. These conditions are exacerbated in the winter months in patients with dry, sensitive skin. Application of emollients may help in decreasing these effects.
- Thus, use of bland emollients, avoidance of irritants and use of bland barrier creams such as those containing dimethicone are the mainstays of treatment for irritant contact dermatitis. A number of agents commonly used in therapeutic products for skin (e.g., propylene glycol, lactic acid, urea, salicylic acid) may produce further skin inflammation and should be avoided.

ALLERGIC CONTACT DERMATITIS (ACD)

Allergic contact dermatitis is inflammation of the skin manifested by varying degrees of erythema, edema and vesiculation. It is a delayed type of hypersensitivity resulting from cutaneous contact with a specific allergen to which the patient has developed sensitivity.

Mechanism

The basic cellular sequence of events in allergic contact dermatitis is manifested by type IV cell-mediated hypersensitivity reaction. It is convenient to divide the process into (i) The induction of the state of specific hypersensitivity and (ii) The elicitation of a reaction in a previously sensitized individual.

1. **Induction:** An allergen penetrating the skin, combines with class II molecules present on Langerhans cells. Langerhans cells carrying an allergen drain via the lymphatics to the paracortical areas of the regional lymph nodes. Here, because of the dendritic morphology of the Langerhans cells, there are multiple contacts with T cells. Interleukin 1 (IL-l) is released by the Langerhans cells and IL-2 by T cells, causing proliferation of specific T cells. These effector cells are released into the circulation while some return to the skin. Thus, the person gets sensitized to this specific allergen.
2. **Elicitation:** On challenging a sensitized individual with an allergen, allergen-carrying cells and specific T cells interact in the skin and release cytokines. These cytokines cause more T cells to be attracted to the area and cause inflammatory effects, resulting in the development of an eczematous reaction which is seen as contact dermatitis.

At present there is no way of determining an individual's susceptibility of being sensitized to a particular allergen but it also depends on the sensitizing capacity of the substance and duration of exposure to it.

Epidemiology

Allergic contact dermatitis has been said to be uncommon in children but recent studies have shown that ACD may be more common than the aforementioned belief. Consideration of allergic contact factors is important in the evaluation of eczematous skin conditions in the young patients also.

Among 158 Danish children aged upto 14 years, 77 were allergic to one or more allergens, the most common of these was nickel, followed by chromate and then rubber chemicals. In a Spanish study, allergic contact factors were observed in 378 children out of 1023, upto the age of 14 years, who were patch tested. The most common allergen in this series was nickel, followed by mercurial compounds and then cobalt and chromate. Allergic reactions were more common in children aged over 8 years. Nickel, followed by cobalt, chromate and then fragrance substances, were most common allergens in 60 out of 125 children under the age of 12 years in a Scottish study. Similar sequences of reactions have been reported from other countries including Italy, Portugal and Germany.

In reports of the incidence of contact allergy in children with atopic dermatitis, there has been a spectrum of results in comparisons with non-atopic groups. The reported incidences have been, higher, equal or lower.

Clinical Features

The clinical features of allergic contact dermatitis in a child are similar to those well recognized in an adult.

- Most commonly an allergic contact dermatitis is obvious with an eczematous reaction occurring at the site of skin contact, e.g., shoe material (Figure 9.2), dyes (Figure 9.3), clothing (Figure 9.4), artificial jewellery and metallic articles, etc.

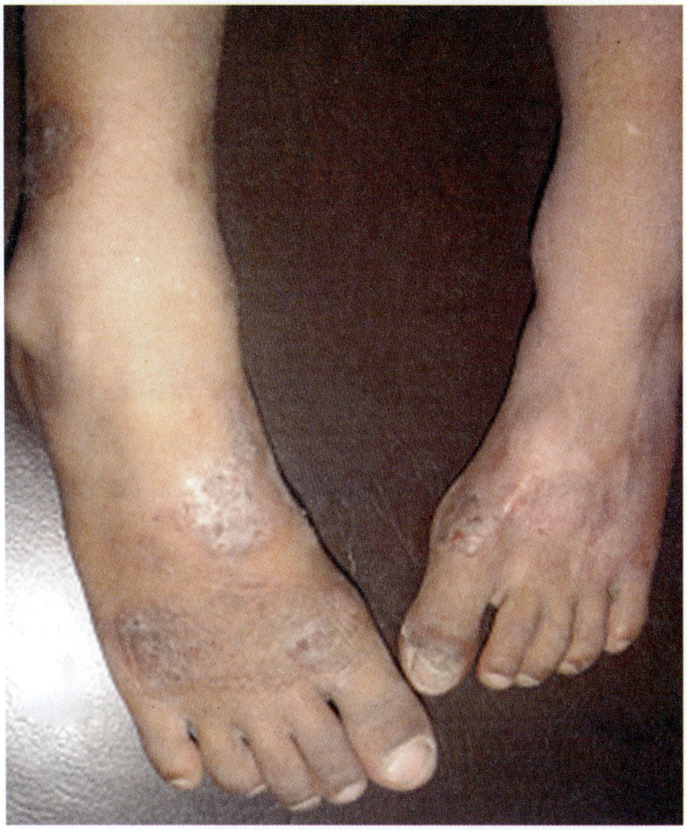

Figure 9.2: Allergic contact dermatitis due to shoe material

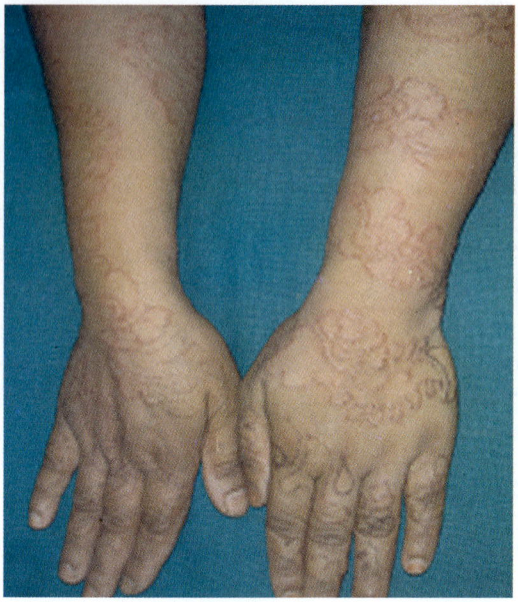

Figure 9.3: Allergic contact dermatitis due to henna with dye

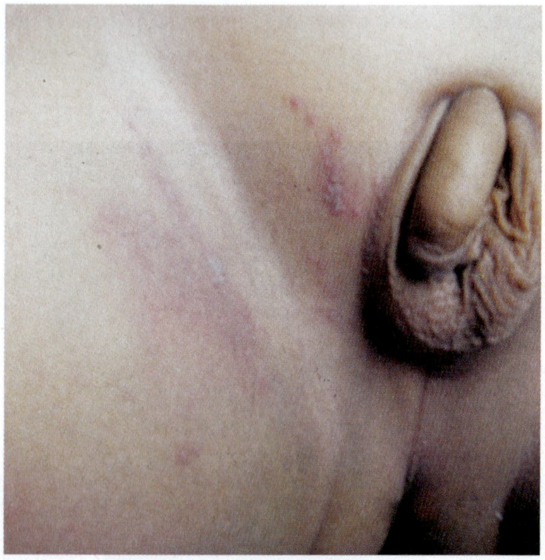

Figure 9.4: Allergic contact dermatitis due to clothing

- A streaky dermatitis usually suggests a plant (such reactions are more of phototoxic than of contact allergic type).
- A facial dermatitis, particularly with marked eyelid involvement, can be seen with airborne allergens or due to application of cosmetics.
- There may be diffuse skin involvement or failure of an existing eczema to improve with topical treatment, raising the suspicion of a superimposed contact dermatitis with topical medicaments.
- Flare of contact dermatitis may occur due to ingestion of an allergen to which hypersensitivity has been induced previously through the skin.
- Because of the great variability in the features of allergic contact dermatitis, it is always worth considering the presence of allergic contact factors when assessing eczema of any clinical type.
- Differences between irritant contact dermatitis and allergic contact dermatitis are described in Table 9.2 given below. Table 9.2 enumerates the differences between irritant and allergic contact dermatitis.

Table 9.2: Differences between ICD and ACD

	Irritant contact dermatitis	***Allergic contact dermatitis***
Definition	Nonspecific response to an irritant or caustic chemical or a series of contactants	Delayed type hypersensitivity reaction resulting from cutaneous contact with a specific allergen
Onset	Within minutes to hours of exposure	Within a few days of exposure
Clinical spectrum	Ranges from a mild irritant reaction with transient erythema to a much more florid dermatitis with oedema, inflammation, pain and vesiculation	Ranges from pruritic papules and vesicles on an erythematous base to lichenified pruritic plaques. Occasionally, erythroderma, exfoliative dermatitis may occur
Lesions	Well defined borders, confined to site of exposure	Not well defined borders, may get generalized
Patch test	Negative	Positive (to which the person is allergic) but not always
Diagnosis	Distinguishable by exclusion of allergic contact dermatitis and history of sufficient exposure to a cutaneous irritant	Distinguishable by a careful history and patch testing
Histopathology	Less pronounced	More pronounced
Spongiosis **Other findings**	In chronic irritant contact dermatitis hyperkeratosis, parakeratosis, acanthosis and elongation of the rete ridges may be seen	In chronic allergic contact dermatitis hyperkeratosis, acanthosis and parakeratosis may be seen along with dermal inflammatory infiltrate

Important Allergens

The following is a review of those substances that are more likely to be observed as allergens. Table 9.3 shows the sources of these allergens in daily life.

Table 9.3: List of antigens used in Indian standard series along with substances of daily use

S. No.	Antigen	Substance
1.	Vaseline	Emollients
2.	Balsam of Peru	Perfumes, flavouring agents in foods, soaps, aromatherapy oils
3.	Formaldehyde	Cosmetic preservative, soaps, shampoos, tanning agent for leather
4.	Mercaptoparaben/ meraptobenzothiazole	Antioxidant in rubber
5.	Potassium bichromate	Cement, paints, printing materials, soaps, detergents, wood preservatives, metal alloys, dental prosthesis
6.	Nickel sulphate	Artificial jewellery, coins, water taps, buttons, zips, utensils, soaps and detergents, eye shadow, mascaras, pigments in glass, pottery, enamel
7.	Cobalt sulphate	Cement, paints, varnishes, blue enamel, colored crayons, soaps, detergents
8.	Colophony	Pine trees, paper, adhesive dressings, printing ink, cosmetics
9.	Epoxy resins	Paints, varnishes, flooring, glues, stabilizers in plastic, aircraft materials
10.	Paraben mix	Preservatives in topical medicaments, bandages, cosmetics
11.	Paraphenylenediamine	Hair dyes, tattoos, photocopier, printing ink, photography developing material
12.	Parthenium	Weed-*Gazar Ghas*
13.	Neomycin sulphate	Topical medicament
14.	Benzocaine	Anaesthetic agents
15.	Wool alcohol	Medicaments, emollients, cosmetics, waxes, polishes, bath additives
16.	Chlorocresol	Preservatives in topical creams, hand cleansers, cosmetics, metal working fluids
17.	Fragrance mix	Perfumes, cosmetics, moisturizers, deodorants, aftershaves, soaps, toiletries
18.	Thiuram mix	Rubber gloves, shoes, car tyres, masks, cables, hoses, kneeling mats, mattresses
19.	Nitrofurozone/ nitrofurazone	Topical medicaments
20.	Black rubber mix	Rubber gloves, shoes, car tyres, masks, cables, hoses, kneeling mats, mattresses

Nickel

Nickel has been reported as the most common allergen. It is more common in girls than boys and ear piercing is the most important predisposing factor. In females, nickel sensitivity may increase the risk of developing hand eczema. Imitation jewellery and other items such as zips, buckles and studs release nickel onto the skin. Dietary avoidance of nickel is not usually advocated. Reactions to cobalt generally occur in association with nickel. Isolated and significant cobalt sensitivity is rare.

Chromate

The most likely relevance of chromate sensitivity is its presence in leather, and especially shoes, where chromium salts are used in the tanning process.

Chromate sensitivity can be associated with hand or foot eczema, which has 'endogenous' characteristics and persists after chromate avoidance.

Mercurials

The organic mercurial thimerosal (thiomersal) is preservative that is widely used in vaccines. Although many individuals, patch tested to it, will react, these reactions are rarely of clinical significance and, as a rule, individuals allergic to thimerosal can still receive vaccinations containing it.

Aluminium

It is known that children may develop cutaneous granulomas in relation to immunizing substances containing aluminium hydroxide. The prognosis in these patients is good with spontaneous resolution. These children have a positive patch test to metallic aluminium or aluminium salts. Presumably, the aluminium sensitivity is lost with time as the sensitivity is exceedingly rare in adults.

Rubber Chemicals

The thiuram mix, carba mix, mercaptobenzothiazole, mercapto mix are generally used in rubber. The thiurams and carbamates are accelerators needed in the process of vulcanization and may be present in the rubber used for items such as gloves, grips and balloons etc. The same or similar substances are also used as fungicides. Mercaptobenzothiazole and the mercapto mix chemicals are more likely to be encountered in rubber that is used for making shoes.

Polyurethane is a synthetic elastomer (rubber) that 'rubber-sensitive' individuals can use. The soles of shoes and the elastic of garments are usually made up of polyurethane.

Perfume

Fragrances are ubiquitous and a child has as much exposure to perfume substances as an adult. Generally, the advice given to a fragrance-sensitive individual is to use fragrance free products of which there are many readily available. Balsam of Peru is a marker of fragrance sensitivity in addition to the standard fragrance mix. It is used in some medicaments also.

Colophony

Colophony (resin) is obtained after distillation of volatile fractions from the oleoresin obtained from certain trees of the Pinaceae family. It has a variable composition. Allergic reactions to it are not rare and its presence in some adhesive plasters is well-known. Individuals may also be exposed to it in preparations used for treating verrucae, certain soaps and in the gripping powder used by gymnasts.

Medicaments

Many topical medicaments are potential contact allergens. Because of differences in availability and popularity there are wide variations in the importance of these worldwide. Among antibiotics, the most common sensitizer is neomycin. Topical antihistamines and anaesthetics, including promethazine and benzocaine, are important potential allergens in some countries.

There is a growing appreciation of the potential of topical corticosteroids themselves to cause contact allergy. Tixocortol pivalate (used as a marker for hydrocortisone sensitivity), hydrocortisone-17-butyrate, budesonide and clobetasol propionate are among the most important of these allergens. If a reaction to a topical steroid is observed, it is important to patch test with a range of other steroids to determine the spectrum of sensitivity. Betamethasone esters, appropriately diluted, are useful in steroid-sensitive individuals as allergy to betamethasone is rare.

Preservatives

Preservatives are added to water-containing cosmetics, medicaments and other products to reduce the growth of bacteria and fungi.

Parabens have a falsely bad reputation; genuine allergic reactions to them are rare in children. Minor irritant reactions can be seen on testing to the parabens mix, which can be proven by negative reactions on testing with the individual components. Individuals allergic to parabens can often tolerate the use of products containing them.

Other examples of preservatives that occasionally cause problems are benzyl alcohol and chloroxylenol, glutaraldehyde is present in some wart preparations.

Vehicle Ingredients

Lanolin (wool alcohols), cetearyl alcohol or cetyl stearyl alcohol and propylene glycol are used as vehicles in creams and ointments and sometimes cause allergic contact reactions.

Rhus

Poison ivy, poison oak and poison sumac contain a potent allergen which is present in the oleoresin. The acute dermatitis develops after direct contact with the plant but may occur from indirect exposure such as from fumes of burning plant material. The eruption is characteristically papular/vesiculobullous with a streaky distribution. Cross-reactions may occur with the oleoresins of other plants including mango, cashew and Japanese lacquer tree.

INVESTIGATIONS IN ALLERGIC CONTACT DERMATITIS

Patch Testing

Patch testing remains the objective way of screening for the presence of contact sensitivity. Therefore, it can be used in the evaluation of eczema of any clinical type. Although patch testing has been well established in the investigation of the adult patients, it has been relatively little used in the children. It has been suggested that the concentration of allergens used on children should be less than those for adults, but there are observations that children tolerate adult concentrations well and it is now generally accepted that the dilutions of allergens used when patch testing the children should be the same as those for adults.

For patch testing, suspected allergens are applied on upper back and occluded with micropore tape for 2-3 days. If patient is allergic to an allergen, a reaction in form of erythema, vesicle or eczema develops (Figure 9.5) which is read as:

Clinical findings	*Grading*
Normal skin	0
Minimal erythema	+
Erythema	++
Erythema and edema	+++
Erythema and vesicular/bullous lesions	++++

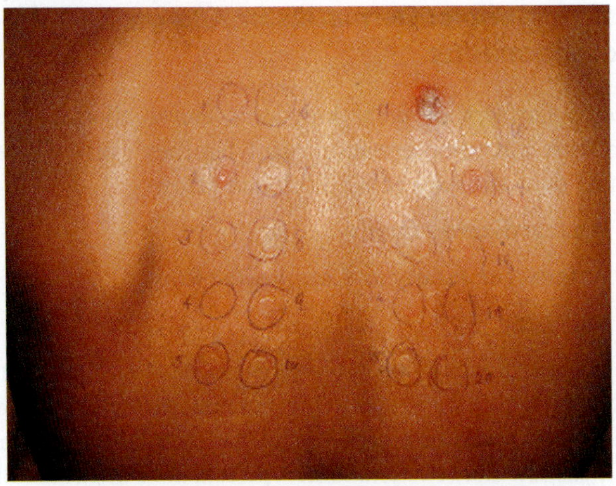

Figure 9.5: Patch test showing positive reaction

Several types of chambers are available for the application of allergens to the skin. The most widely used and often taken as the 'standard', is the Finn chamber. This is an 8 mm aluminium chamber. Allergens diluted in petroleum can be introduced directly into the chamber; solutions of allergens need to be absorbed onto filter paper discs placed within the chamber. Finn chambers have the advantage that a large number of allergens can be applied if necessary, the only limitation is the skin area available for application and which will be less in infants.

Patches should be applied to the upper quadrants of the back unless there is a particular reason why this should not be done. Such a reason may be the presence of active eczema on the back. In such cases allergens may be applied to the front of the trunk, upper arms or thighs; these are not, however, 'standard' sites and anatomical variations in skin thickness and the degree of occlusion will alter allergen penetration and elicitation of response.

In infants and small children there is a tendency for the patch test micropore tapes to become loose. This tendency may be reduced by covering the patches with fabric adhesive plaster.

Under ideal circumstances, allergens are applied for 2 days and the site of application is kept dry. Readings should be made at two days after application with, a second reading at four days. A single reading is unsatisfactory as it may not be possible to distinguish an irritant (false positive) reaction from an allergic one.

In the older child an established 'standard' series of allergen as used on adults should be applied. In India we use Indian standard series which contains around 20 common antigens.

Aimed testing with a particular allergen or components of a product, may be required when a child presents with dermatitis on a particular site. Otitis externa will require testing with medicaments, foot eczema with components of shoes and facial eczema with skin-care products and airborne allergens. It may be appropriate to test for allergy to topical corticosteroids, topical antimicrobials and components of vehicle bases in patients who do not show expected response to these medicaments or disease gets exacerbated after their use. Such 'aimed' testing should be considered in each case.

In the infant or young child, it may be required to test with a few selected allergens because of practical considerations. In the event of an atopic dermatitis being evaluated it is important that potential medicament allergens are included in test battery. Photo contact allergy is exceedingly rare in children.

Dubious reactions may be further evaluated by repeated open application test. This requires the application of an agent or product several times daily for two to three days to the skin of the upper arm or other suitable site. A response, often papular, indicates a positive reaction.

Allergic reactions are interpreted as being of current, old or of unknown significance. A decision regarding its relevance requires information on potential environmental exposure and knowledge of the formulation of products such as medicaments and toiletries.

Thin Layer Rapid Use Epicutaneous Test (TRUE Test)

This is a ready to use patch test with incorporation of allergens into hydrophilic gels coated on a water impermeable sheet of polyester and dried as a thin film. In TRUE test two strips of 12 antigens each are applied on the back. It is well standardized, accurate, and easy to performed test.

Photo patch test:

Photo-patch test is indicated in photoallergic contact dermatitis in which UV radiation exposure is required to induce reaction.

Atopic patch test:

Atopic patch test is indicated in protein contact dermatitis or atopic children with food allergy. In photo patch test intact protein allergen is used in test chamber and reading is taken after 24 to 72 hours. In atopic patch test, prick test kit is used, as there is no separate standard kit available for atopic patch test.

Repeated Open Application Test (ROAT):

ROAT is indicated when patch test is doubtful. Allergen is applied twice daily for 28 days over upper arm or flexor aspect of forearm and findings are noted.

Spot test:

Inexpensive and rapid test to detect specific allergen for example Dimethylglyoxime (DMG) test for nickel, acetyl acetone for formaldehyde, Nitroso-R for cobalt, Diphenyl carbazide for chromate.

Invitro test:

Invitro test can be accurate and sensitive over patch test to detect contact allergen e.g. allergy specific lymphocyte transformation test (LTT), Lymphocyte migration inhibition test (LMIT), lymphocyte procoagulant activity test, etc.

Treatment

Treatment primarily involves removing the allergen from the individuals's environment. Oral antihistamines are prescribed to relieve the pruritus. Topical or oral corticosteroids may be used in the acute phase of the condition, but definitive treatment is avoidance of the responsible allergen.

PLANT DERMATITIS

Contact with plant products or extract, results in development of adverse reaction in different forms and includes, irritant contact dermatitis, allergic contact dermatitis, photoallergic contact dermatitis, phytophotodermatitis, pseudo-phyto-dermatitis, contact urticaria etc.

Irritant Contact Dermatitis

This is the most common plant dermatitis. Commonly seen in farmers, grocers and florists due to direct contact with plant irritants. In acute forms it presents with erythema, oedema, papules and vesicles. In chronic form it presents with hyperkeratosis and fissuring. It presents in different forms:

1. **Mechanical ICD:** It is due to physical injury by plant trichrome, thorns or spine and presents with erythematous papules and nodules e.g. prickly pear cactus dermatitis.
2. **Chemical irritant dermatitis:** It occurs due to deposition of plant chemical products in skin epidermis e.g. calcium oxalate (in Dieffenbachia raphide and Daffodils mucus), isothiocyanates (in mustard, papaya, cabbage), bromelain (in pineapple), capsaicin (in Solanaceae family plant).

Management includes avoidance of irritants, protective gloves, barrier cream, topical corticosteroids and topical calcineurin inhibitors.

Contact Urticaria

It is an urticarial inflammatory cutaneous eruption which occurs due to contact with plant products. Some patients may develop anaphylactoid reactions to chemicals e.g. celery plant, urtica plant.

Allergic Contact Dermatitis or Allergic Photodermatitis

Several families of plant kingdoms cause allergic contact dermatitis but some common plant families causing allergic contact dermatitis are being discussed below:

- **Anacardiaceae family**
- **Asteraceae family or Compositae family**
- **Alliaceae**

Anacardiaceae family: This is the most common family of plants which causes allergic contact dermatitis. Poison ivy, poison oak, poison sumac, Mangifera indica (mango tree), cashew nut (cauterization type reaction, brownish black thickened sheets of skin) belongs to genus Toxicodendron which contain strongly allergenic oleoresin called urushiol.

Alliaceae family: Onion, garlic, chives etc. belong to this family and contain diallyl disulfide, allyl propyl disulfide and allicin. They cause contact dermatitis in homemakers and caterers, mostly over finger tips.

Asteraceae family or compositae family (daisy family, sunflower family or chrysanthemum family): This is the second largest family of flowering plants which contain sesquiterpene lactone as allergen. Parthenium, Chrysanthemum, Dahlia, Helianthus annus, Xanthium strumarium, magnolia stellate are few examples which cause allergic contact dermatitis.

Parthenium (Congress Grass, Fever Few, Bitterweed) Dermatitis

Parthenium dermatitis is a common cause of plant dermatitis in India which is caused by Parthenium hysterophorus (hybrid species of Parthenium confertum and Parthenium bipinnatifidum). Most common allergens in parthenium are sesquiterpene lactones, which are lipophilic in nature. These allergens are present in highest concentration in trichrome of the plant which is seen on the undersurface of the leaves. Parthenin is the most common sesquiterpene lactones, others being coronopilin, tetraneurin A, hymenin, hysterin, ambrosin, dihydro-iso-parthenin etc.

Clinical Patterns of Parthenium Dermatitis

- Classical air borne contact dermatitis
- Chronic actinic dermatitis
- Mixed pattern
- Exfoliative dermatitis or erythroderma
- Prurigo nodularis like lesions

- Vesicular hand eczema or pompholyx type
- Perianal dermatitis
- Photosensitive lichenoid eruption
- Hand and feet dermatitis
- Lichen nitidus like

Common patterns of parthenium dermatitis are described below:

Air borne contact dermatitis (ABCD):

This is the most common type of contact dermatitis produced by Parthenium. It involves eyelids, neck, V area of the neck, and retroauricular area, cubital fossa and popliteal fossa. Clinically it presents as chronic dermatitis and lichenification.

Chronic actinic dermatitis (CAD):

It manifests as lichenified papules and plaques on sun exposed skin, including forehead, rim of the ears, cheeks, V area of the neck, nape of the neck, extensor aspect of the forearms and hands, while sparing eyelids, retroauricular areas, under surface of the chin and depth of the skin folds.

Mixed pattern:

It represents a transition phase from classic ABCD to CAD pattern in natural history of Parthenium dermatitis.

HAIR DYE DERMATITIS

It is a common cause of allergic contact dermatitis due to cosmetics. About 70-80% of hair dyes available in market contain Para-Phenylene-Diamine (PPD), which is the major allergen causing hair dye dermatitis (discovered by Hoffman 1863).

Types of hair dyes:

- Vegetable hair dyes: Henna, fenugreek and walnut are commonly used natural hair dyes.
- Metallic hair dyes: Silver and lead salts are commonly available metallic dyes.
- Synthetic hair dyes.
  - Direct hair dyes.
    - Temporary hair dyes.
    - Semi-permanent hair dyes.
  - Oxidative or permanent hair dyes.

Permanent hair dyes are the most popular hair dye products. They are composed of three main components:

1. Primary intermediate (PPD) and coupler
2. Oxidants (hydrogen peroxide)
3. Alkali (ammonia)

When PPD or primary intermediate is mixed with oxidizer, it produces oxidized products which further react with coupler to form hair color. Hydrogen peroxide diffuses natural hair melanin causing lightening of natural hair color while ammonia causes cuticle swelling and separation. Both ammonia and hydrogen peroxide thus act as developer.

PPD is a colorless, low molecular weight arylamine derivative with high protein binding capacity. Oxidative intermediate of hair dye, benzoquinone or brandowski based trimer are responsible for allergic reaction. Source of PPD other than hair dyes include, dark color cosmetics, photographic developer, black henna tattoos, photocopy ink, printing ink, X-ray film fluid etc.

Clinical Features

Hair dye dermatitis is most commonly seen in people using hair dye to colour the hair, hairdressers, textile workers etc. Clinical presentation includes, irritant contact dermatitis, allergic contact dermatitis, contact urticaria, contact leukoderma, contact anaphylaxis. Common site for contact dermatitis is scalp margin, beard and hands (in hairdressers). It may also cause lichenoid reaction, erythema multiforme like eruption and lichen planus pigmentosus like lesions. Prolonged exposure to PPD may lead to renal problems, lenticular changes and malignancy (bladder carcinoma, myelodysplastic syndrome, leukemia and lymphomas).

CEMENT DERMATITIS

It is the most common occupation dermatitis in construction industry. In purified form, cement is non allergenic, accidental contamination with chromate, nickel, and cobalt leads to allergic reaction. Hexavalent form of chromate causes significant allergic response as compared to trivalent. Allergy to cement may cause irritant contact dermatitis (due to caustic and hygroscopic action), chrome ulcers (protein denaturation due to hexavalent chromium) and allergic contact dermatitis (chromium, nickel, cobalt).

Diagnosis

Diagnosis is usually done by clinical presentation and performing patch test with potassium dichromate 0.5%, nickel sulphate 5% and cobalt sulphate 1%.

Management

Management includes prevention of sensitization by adding ferrous sulphate, personal protective measures (butyl or nitrile gloves and waterproof boots) and barrier cream (tartaric, silicone, glycine etc.). Anti-chrome solution, sodium dithionate may be used to clean cement from the exposed skin. Treatment includes, topical steroids, oral steroids, cyclosporine and azathioprine.

Cement Burn

It is a type of alkali burn due to cement, occurs due to reaction between cement and sweat, which produces alkaline hydroxide ions (OH^-, pH >12). Hydroxide ions result in protein denaturation and liquefactive necrosis of saponified fat. It is commonly seen with kneeling or standing in cement and limited to lower limb with deep second or third degree burn.

Treatment includes saline irrigation till neutral pH is achieved, antibiotics and grafting.

NUMMULAR OR DISCOID DERMATITIS

The Latin word 'nummulus', meaning little coin, signifies the disc-shaped configuration of the well demarcated eczematous patches seen in nummular dermatitis. The condition is defined by its clinical appearance.

Etiology

Although the specific cause is not known, several factors have been incriminated as possible etiological agents. It has been suggested that bacteria may play a role either directly or through the mechanism of hypersensitivity. Antistreptolysin O titre is more often elevated in patients with nummular dermatitis than in control subjects.

Other etiological agents mentioned in the literature are asteatosis, external irritants, infected wounds, nutritional deficiency and emotional conflict. There are few studies that reveal the relevance of contact allergy in nummular dermatitis. Nummular dermatitis in children is frequently associated with dry skin and therefore is most often seen in winter months. The disorder is exacerbated by soaps, wool and other materials that are mechanically irritating. There is no high incidence of atopy in these patients.

Clinical Features

Nummular dermatitis is defined by its typical morphological appearance. It is characterized by an acute eruption of well-demarcated, coin shaped lesions (Figures 9.6A and B), 1-5 cm in diameter. These lesions are edematous, bright red, oozing and crusted. Initially, they consist of patches or papules or vesicles on an erythematous base which by peripheral extension and confluence, become coin shaped. Over 1-2 weeks, they progress towards a chronic phase, in which less vesicular, red, scaly discs are seen. Central clearing may result in ring-shaped lesions. Severe pruritus occurs in the lesional sites and excoriation enhances secondary infections. Although the extent of involvement may be limited to few lesions, the presence of numerous lesions is the rule. Lesions may coalesce to form large patches.

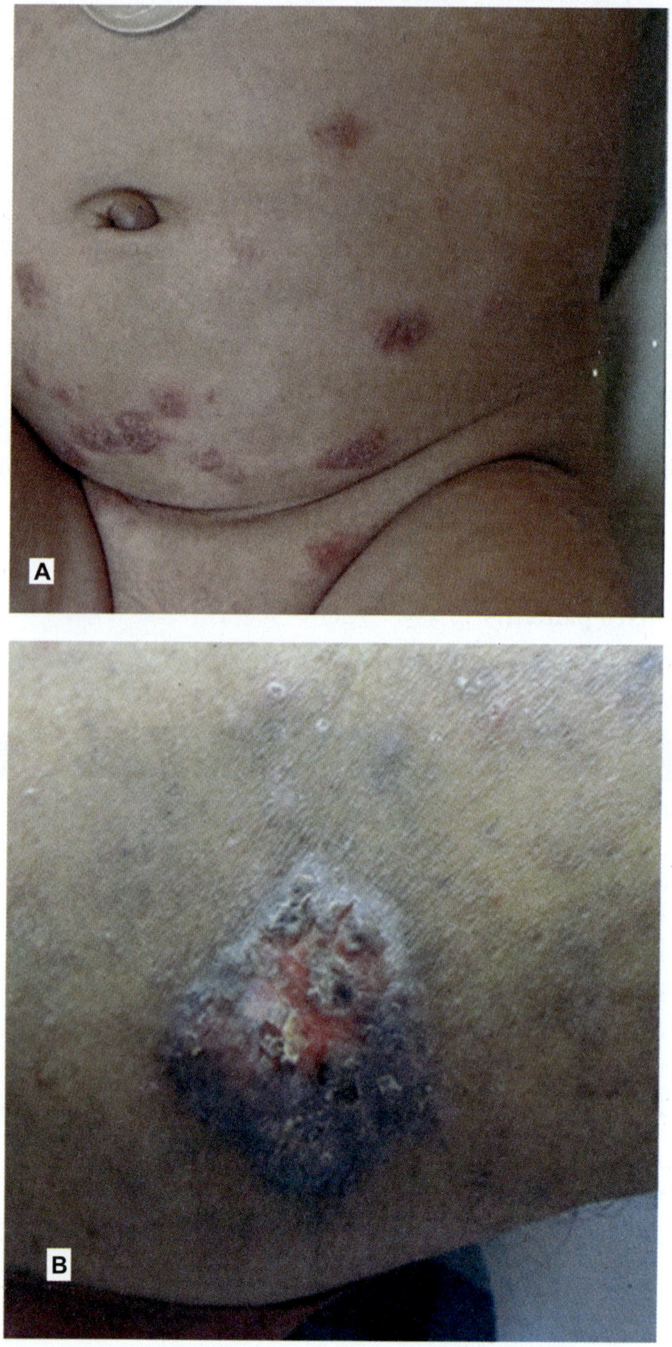

Figures 9.6A and B: Discoid or nummular eczema

At onset, patches are predominantly located on the extensor surfaces of the lower extremities and subsequently spread to the upper extremities, in particular the dorsal aspect of the hands and the trunk. Involvement of the face is unusual. The eruption runs a remitting and relapsing course and is worse during the winter months. The exacerbations that occur in winter have been associated with increased dryness of the skin.

Differential Diagnosis

- Impetigo.
- Tinea corporis.
- Contact dermatitis.
- Pityriasis rosea.
- Seborrheic dermatitis.

Prognosis

In most patients, the condition persists for many months. Parents should be counselled that the disease may be expected to improve only slowly.

Treatment

As extremes of heat and humidity aggravate the condition, sudden changes in environment, should be minimized. Irritating clothing such as woolen garments and synthetic materials should be avoided. Bathing should be recommended regularly and immediately after bathing an emollient must be applied.

For oozing lesions, the use of wet compresses is helpful. Dry lesions may benefit from the application of a topical steroid cream. In the more chronic stages, daily application of a steroid ointment is an acceptable treatment.

As bacterial infections appear to play a pathogenic role in some cases, appropriate systemic antibiotic therapy may be instituted. Antihistamines may relieve pruritus when the nummular dermatitis is severe. For widespread lesions short course of oral steroids, preferably deflazacort in tapering doses is helpful in bringing out rapid control of disease.

HAND ECZEMA

Hand eczema is defined as dermatitis largely confined to hands with only minor involvement of other parts.

Morphological Classification of Hand Eczema

- Hyperkeratotic hand eczema
- Pompholyx
- Fingertip eczema
- Nummular or discoid dermatitis
- Recurrent focal palmar peeling
- Ring eczema
- Apron eczema
- Wear and tear dermatitis or dry palmar dermatitis

Important hand eczemas are described below:

POMPHOLYX

Pompholyx or vesicular eczema of palms and soles is a recurrent acute eczematous eruption, composed of discrete, well visible vesicles situated mostly on the palms and soles, and along the sides of fingers and toes. When pompholyx occurs on the palmar surfaces or along the sides of fingers, it may be called cheiropompholyx, and when on the soles or along the sides of toes, podopompholyx.

Epidemiology

Pompholyx in childhood is an infrequent condition, but in adults, pompholyx is believed to account for about 5-20% of all cases of hand eczema.

Etiopathogenesis

The cause of pompholyx is unknown. Pompholyx is often worse in warm weather. As the synonym dyshidrotic eczema denotes, it was thought to result from excessive sweating, but it is now recognized that the term 'dyshidrotic eczema' is a misnomer. Pompholyx has also been attributed to stress and emotional liability.

Literature suggests that pompholyx is a manifestation of the atopic diathesis. In different studies, 40-50% of patients affected by pompholyx had a personal or family history of atopy.

A number of recent investigators have come to believe that pompholyx is an expression of allergy to nickel. Pompholyx can be induced in nickel-sensitive subjects by oral administration of high doses of nickel. Other primary irritants, such as soluble oils used by metal workers and direct contact allergens (paraphenylenediamine, benzisothiazolinone, dichromate's, perfumes, fragrances and balsams) can also cause pompholyx, but almost always in adults. However, glue components, chrome salts, dyes and rubber present in shoes can cause contact allergy and also provoke pompholyx in children and adolescents. In some children, pompholyx may occur as a reaction to dermatophyte or Candida infection on the feet or hands. Bacterial infection can also provoke similar reactions. Finally, pompholyx can be induced by medications, e.g., antiseptics, antimycotics, neomycin, aspirin, methotrexate and mycophenolate mofetil.

Pathology

The evolving lesions of pompholyx show eczematous changes, i.e., foci of spongiosis and vesicles in the epidermis, edema of the papillary dermis and a superficial perivascular predominantly lymphocyte infiltrates; eosinophils can be observed occasionally. Histological features of lichen simplex chronicus may be the hallmark of chronic lesions. In impetiginized lesions, histology shows intraepidermal vesicular-pustules together with bacteria.

Clinical Features

Pompholyx is classically characterized by the sudden onset of crops of tense, clear vesicles, which have been described to be 'sago-like' (Figure 9.7). It may occur at any age but is rare under the age of 10 years. The eruption, generally bilateral, can affect the sides of fingers and toes, palms and soles. Erythema may be present. Subjective symptoms are generally present during or before the attack in the form of pruritus or prickling. Pruritus may sometimes be severe. Vesicles, usually discrete at the beginning, may become confluent and form large multiloculated bullae, especially on the feet. Generally, the blisters are distributed symmetrically.

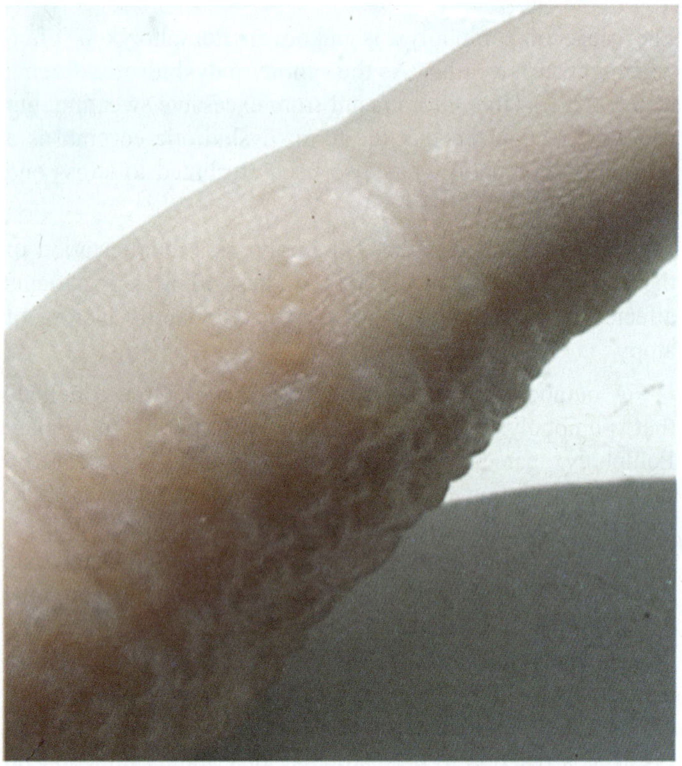

Figure 9.7: Pompholyx showing vesiculation

Recurrences are common, that last for a few days to a few weeks and subside spontaneously in 2-3 weeks with desquamation. When secondary infection of primary blisters occurs, pustular lesions may develop. Erosions and ulceration may also complicate the clinical appearance. Secondary lymphoedema can occur but constitutional symptoms, such as fever etc. are rare.

Differential Diagnosis

- Infantile acropustulosis.
- Hand, foot and mouth disease.
- Blistering distal dactylitis.
- Localized bullous pemphigoid.
- Recurrent palmoplantar pustulosis.

Treatment

Treatment of pompholyx should be based around avoiding the offending cause. This includes avoidance of any contact with nickel-containing metals, low-nickel diet, eradication of the fungus and local hygiene.

Treatment of pompholyx associated with atopy, the common form in children, involves symptomatic treatment, including topical corticosteroids of medium or high potency, zinc oxide ointments and oral antihistamines. Topical steroids are widely used for management of the condition. Zinc oxide can be used in the acute phase for their mild anti-inflammatory and protective properties. Oral antihistamines are useful to alleviate the itching. A short course of oral steroids is sometimes indicated, but it may be justified for severe cases only.

In acute phase, management of pompholyx also includes soaks or wet dressings to cleanse the affected area and to relieve discomfort by potassium permanganate solution (dilution 1: 10,000). Large bullae can cause discomfort or even pain and may be punctured. Systemic antibiotics should not be used unless impetiginization supervenes. Secondary bacterial infection is most likely due to staphylococci, thus an appropriate antibiotic should be prescribed. Harsh detergents should be avoided. As the acute phase subsides, the wet dressing or soaks should be discontinued and replaced with protective topical treatments. Tar preparations are indicated for cases of chronic pompholyx which have entered into hyperkeratotic phase.

FINGER TIP ECZEMA

Fingertip eczema is a type of hand dermatitis in which eczematous changes effect the fingertip. The patient usually presents with dryness, chapping, scaling and fissuring. Secondary bacterial infection cause redness, oozing, crusting and pain. Nail dystrophy or onycholysis can be a complication of eczema (Figure 9.8).

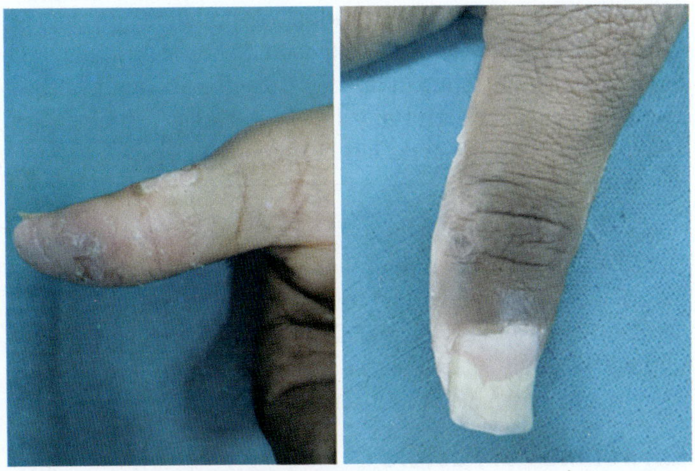

Figure 9.8: Hand eczema with onycholysis

LICHEN SIMPLEX CHRONICUS

Lichen simplex chronicus (LSCh) describes the localized eczematous skin changes that occur as a result of long-term rubbing and scratching.

Etiology

The etiology of LSCh is unknown. It may be the result of repeated rubbing and scratching, which is motivated by localized and intense pruritus. The area's most commonly affected are those within easy reach of the patient. Itching and scratching are most intense during periods of stress.

The initial event that precipitates the lesions may be a transient irritation such as an insect bite or a pre-existing skin disorder (e.g., atopic dermatitis, seborrheic dermatitis or contact dermatitis), or LSCh may appear on apparently normal skin. The cause of the intense pruritus responsible for the lesions of LSCh must be carefully investigated in each individual patient.

Some believe that patients with LSCh are more readily prone to scratching in response to a minimal to moderate stimulus than normal control subjects.

Clinical Features

Although LSCh may appear at any age, it is a relatively uncommon skin disorder in childhood, it most often begins in adolescence or young adulthood. LSCh is more common in women than in men. Patients with atopic dermatitis may develop lichenification of their lesions accompanying or preceding LSCh.

Lichenification is defined by the accentuation of normal skin markings with hyperkeratosis and pigmentation. The plaques appear as areas of diffuse, thickened, erythematous, hyperpigmented skin (Figure 9.9), with slight scaling and frequently with multiple excoriations. The most common location is on the nape of the neck. Other regions frequently affected are the dorsum of feet, legs, wrists and ankles, but almost any area of body may be affected.

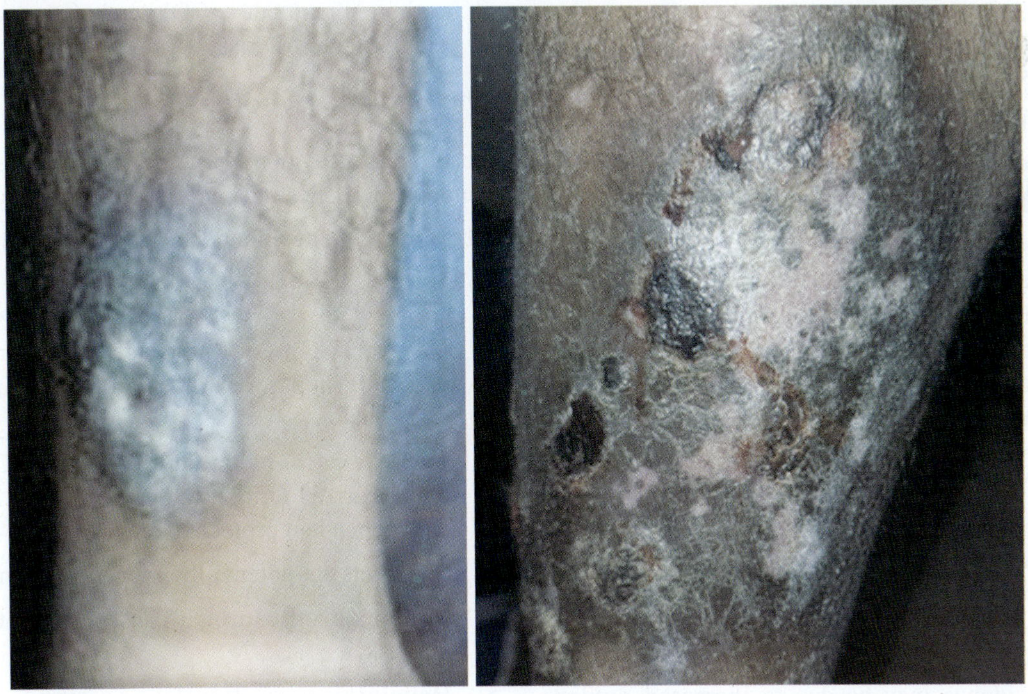

Figure 9.9: Lichen simplex chronicus

Prognosis

The course of LSCh is chronic, with multiple exacerbations and partial remissions. These clinical fluctuations are the result of changes in the intensity of pruritus, and thereby the amount of scratching and rubbing.

Differential Diagnosis

- Atopic dermatitis.
- Lichen planus.
- Psoriasis.
- Tinea corporis.

Treatment

Therapy is focused on the cause of pruritus and towards breaking the itch-scratch cycle. The lesions do not resolve if rubbing and scratching persists. Topical applications of medium potency corticosteroid preparations like mometasone furoate 0.1% cream are used to control pruritus and decrease inflammation. In recalcitrant cases, a potent topical corticosteroid preparation like clobetasol, betamethasone or halobetasol is recommended for a short period.

Tacrolimus and pimecrolimus are effective treatments for atopic dermatitis and provide a therapeutic alternative to topical corticosteroids.

In the case of superimposed bacterial infection, topical or systemic antibiotics are indicated. Administration of oral antihistamines may help to relieve the pruritus.

In the presence of underlying psychopathology, which may include attention deficit or hyperactivity disorder, consultation with a child psychologist or psychiatrist may be necessary.

ATOPIC DERMATITIS

Atopic dermatitis (AD) is an eczema characterized by intense itching and a relapsing course in infants and children with a personal or family history of atopic disorders. In 1923, Coca and Cooke used the term "Atopy" for the first time to describe a diathesis presenting as triad of asthma, allergic rhinitis and eczema. It is a common skin disorder, affecting upto 10% of infants. It coexists with asthma or rhinitis in upto 80% of cases. Nearly 70% of patients have a family history of atopy. Though much of the dermatitis resolves during childhood, the inflammatory susceptibility remains. The disorder as seen in India is relatively mild in its manifestation but incidence and basic susceptibility are the same. Recent studies suggest an increase in the incidence of atopic dermatitis. The cause of this increased incidence may be due to increased outdoor pollution, increased concentration of pollutants in highly insulated buildings, increased exposure to house dust mite and food additives, a decline in the breastfeeding and an increased awareness of parents and physicians. A higher prevalence in urban areas than rural areas has been reported.

Etiopathogenesis

Genetic factors, maternal/intrauterine factors and environmental factors play important role in etiopathogenesis of atopic dermatitis and environmental factors have been extensively studied to establish their role in causation of the disease process and they have been briefly described here:

Environmental Factors

- **Climate:** Symptoms increase with latitude. UV radiation facilitates conversion of trans-urocanic acid into immunosuppressive cis-urocanic acid isoform. Lower outdoor temperatures lead to disease worsening.
- **Urban versus rural living:** Higher eczema burden is seen in cities as compared to countryside.
- **Diet:** Fresh fruits have protective effect whereas fast food triggers it.
- **Breastfeeding and delayed weaning:** Exclusive breastfeeding for 6 months helps in allergy prevention.
- **Obesity and physical exercise:** Obesity has positive association with AD.
- **Pollution and tobacco smoke:** Nitrogen oxides (NO_2), carbon monoxide (CO) and fine particle pollution contribute to AD risk.

The Hygiene Hypothesis

According to 'hygiene hypothesis' atopic dermatitis is more common in smaller and higher socio-economic status families.

- **Basic hygiene:** Frequency of washing and use of household cleaners and wet wipes is associated with increased risk of AD between 2.5 and 3.5 years age group.
- **Day care homes:** Associated with increased microbial exposure (in particular respiratory tract infections) and is a risk factor.
- **Farm environment and animals:** Consumption of unpasteurized farm milk during the first 2 years of life is an independent protective factor.
- **Pets:** Pets are potentially protective against AD.
- **Endotoxin exposure:** It causes up to 50% reduction in AD risk.
- **Helminthic parasites:** Have a protective effect in AD.

- **Childhood infections and vaccinations:** Chickenpox, mumps, whooping cough and measles vaccination have either positive or no associations.
- **Microbiome of the gut and skin:** Presence of more Staphylococcus aureus and coliforms as early gut microflora results in higher risk of development of AD.
- **Antibiotics:** Increase the risk of developing AD.

Immunopathogenesis: T cells infiltrate early in the disease process. CD4+:CD8+ cells ratio is about 7:1. CLA+ (skin homing receptor) and predominantly CD45RO+ cells are present. Eosinophils may also be present. Allergen specific Th2 cells are critical in AD pathogenesis. They induce IL-4, IL-5 and IL-13 cytokines which down regulate filaggrin expression in keratinocytes thereby inducing further epidermal barrier disruption. In chronic cases IL-5, granulocyte-macrophage colony-stimulating factor (GM-CSF), IL-12 and IFN-γ predominate. IL-31 directly signals to neurons mediating pruritus in AD.

'**Atopic march**' is the progression within an individual from AD to other atopic diseases like allergic rhinitis, food allergy and asthma.

Role of IgE: Th2 cells induce B cell to switch IgE antibody production. Antibodies produced by plasma cells in lung and skin bind to high affinity receptor (Fc epsilon RI) on mast cells, basophils, Langerhans cells and eosinophils, which after internalization and cellular activation, immediately releases preformed or newly synthetized inflammatory mediators. Histamine causes vasodilation (classical wheal and flare) and itch.

Clinical Features

Atopic dermatitis is an itchy, chronic, fluctuating disease that is slightly more common in boys than in girls. The age of onset is between 2 and 6 months in 75% of cases and 90% of cases are seen before 5 years of age, but AD may start at any age, even before the age of 2 months in some cases.

Clinically, patients have itching, macular erythema, papules or papulovesicles, eczematous areas with crusting, lichenification and excoriation, dryness of the skin and secondary infection.

There are three phases of AD:

1. **Infantile phase** **(0-2 years)**
2. **Childhood phase** **(2-12 years)**
3. **Adolescent phase** **(12-18 years)**

Infantile Phase

The disease often starts on face as erythematous patches with itchy oedematous papules (Figure 9.10). The disease gradually involves other parts of body, extensor surface of limbs being most commonly involved areas. Continuous itching and rubbing may cause further eczematization, secondary infection and lymphadenopathy.

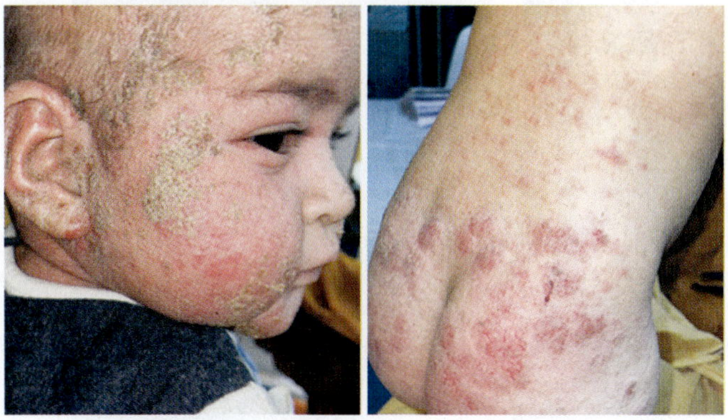

Figure 9.10: Atopic dermatitis on face and back

Childhood Phase

The disease changes its pattern and most commonly involved sites are flexural areas of elbows and knees (Figure 9.11), sides of neck, wrists and ankles. Sides of neck may have reticulate pigmentation known as 'atopic dirty neck'. Lichenification may occur gradually and hand eczema may occur.

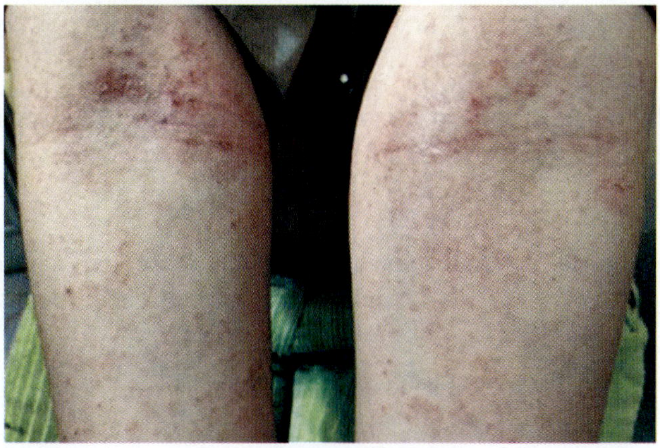

Figure 9.11: Atopic dermatitis showing lesions over flexure aspect of elbow

Adult Phase (Adolescent Phase)

Flexural involvement (Figure 9.12) is common. Hand dermatitis may be the only manifestation. Dermatitis of the upper eyelid is another frequent finding. Atopic dermatitis can be diffuse or patchy on the body. Localized patches are seen over nipples of adolescent and young women. Associated features are dry skin, ichthyosis and keratosis pilaris.

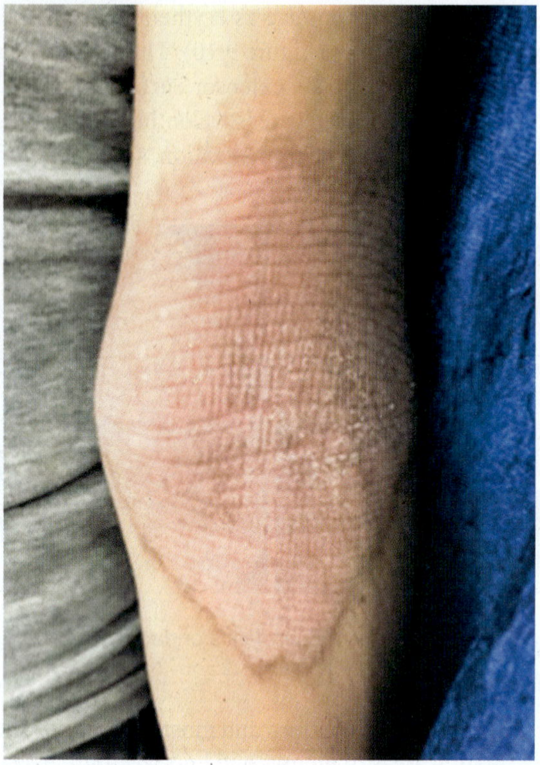

Figure 9.12: Atopic dermatitis showing flexural lichenification

Ocular abnormalities: Dennie-Morgan fold on lower eyelid, non-specific conjunctival irritation, keratoconjunctivitis, keratoconus, cataract (atopic cataract) which is almost always bilateral and symmetrical.

Major Clinical Features for Diagnosis of Atopic Dermatitis

- Pruritus.
- Typical morphology and distribution, facial and extensor involvement in infants and children and flexural lichenification or linearity in adults.
- Chronic or chronically relapsing dermatitis.
- Personal or family history of atopy (asthma, allergic rhinitis, atopic dermatitis).

Minor Clinical Features for Diagnosis of Atopic Dermatitis

1. Early age at onset.
2. Xerosis.
3. Ichthyosis/palmar hyperlinarity/keratosis pilaris.
4. Tendency towards nonspecific hand or foot dermatitis.
5. Nipple eczema.
6. Cheilitis.
7. Itch when sweating.
8. Perifollicular accentuation.
9. Immediate (type 1) skin test reactivity.
10. Elevated serum IgE mediated immunity.
11. Recurrent conjunctivitis.
12. Dennie-Morgan infraorbital folds.
13. Keratoconus.
14. Anterior subcapsular cataracts.
15. Orbital darkening.
16. Facial pallor/facial erythema.
17. Pityriasis alba.
18. Anterior neck folds.
19. Intolerance to wool or lipid solvents.
21. Food intolerance.
22. Environmental/emotional influence.
23. White dermographism.

Associated Disorders

Other manifestations of atopy are allergic rhinitis (Hay fever), asthma. Onset is later than eczema.

Other patterns of eczema are also commonly seen in patients of AD, e.g., infantile dermatitis, allergic contact dermatitis, lip-lick cheilitis (perioral eczema). These patients also have increased incidence of drug sensitivity (anaphylactoid drug reactions), reactions to insect stings and bites, food allergy (abdominal symptoms), alopecia areata and urticaria.

Complications

- Impact on quality of life:
  - *Psychological aspects:* Disturbed sleep pattern, behavioral difficulties.
  - Growth delay.
- Secondary bacterial infection by staphylococci and streptococci.
- *Viral infections:* Herpes infection.
- Cartilaginous pseudocyst of external auricle.
- Sudden death.

Diagnosis

According to the UK refinement of Hanifin and Rajka's diagnostic criteria of atopic dermatitis (eczema), for diagnosis of atopic dermatitis, a child must have an itchy skin condition (or parental report of scratching or rubbing in a child) plus three or more of the following:

1. Onset <2 years of age (not used if child is under 4 years).
2. History of skin crease involvement (including cheeks in children < 10 years).
3. History of a generally dry skin.
4. Personal history of other atopic disease (or history of any atopic disease in first degree relative in children under 4 years).
5. Visible flexural dermatitis (or dermatitis of cheeks/ forehead and outer limbs in children under 4 years).

Differential Diagnosis

- Scabies.
- Infantile seborrheic dermatitis.
- Contact dermatitis.
- Dermatophytosis.
- Keratosis pilaris.
- Lichen simplex chronicus.
- Nummular dermatitis.
- Juvenile palmoplantar dermatosis.
- Impetigo.
- Drug eruptions.
- Perioral dermatitis.
- Pityriasis alba.
- Photodermatitis.

AD like conditions with immunocompromised state:

- Agammaglobulinemia.
- Anhidrotic ectodermal dysplasia.
- Ataxia-telangiectasia.
- Coeliac disease.
- Cystic fibrosis (heterozygote).
- Histidine depletion.
- Hurler's syndrome.
- Hyper IgE syndrome.
- Hyper-eosinophilic syndrome.
- Jung's disease.
- Nephrotic syndrome.
- Netherton's syndrome.
- Phenylketonuria.
- Wiskott-Aldrich syndrome.

Less common diseases to be considered are metabolic and nutritional deficiency disorders, e.g., phenylketonuria, multiple carboxylase deficiency and zinc deficiency, etc. Other differential diagnoses for AD are number of less common disorders, e.g., severe combined immunodeficiency disorder, DiGeorge syndrome, hypogammaglobulinemia, Wiskott-Aldrich syndrome, ataxia telangiectasia, hyper-immunoglobulin IgE syndrome, Omenn syndrome, Netherton syndrome and Langerhans cell histiocytosis, etc.

Prognosis

There is generally a tendency towards spontaneous improvement with increasing age and upto 50% to 70% of cases show remission by the age of 13 years. Prognosis is worse if both parents are atopic.

Investigation

There is no confirmatory test for diagnosis of AD. Elevated serum IgE levels occur in 80-90% of patients. There may be eosinophilia. Routine allergy testing, dietary testing and environmental or dietary manipulation are often not productive.

Treatment

The mainstay of treatment is to control inflammation. Topical corticosteroids of appropriate strength for the patient's age and affected area are applied twice daily to inflamed skin for 10-21 days. Topical immunomodulators, e.g., tacrolimus ointment 0.03% for children aged 2-15 years and 0.03% and 0.1% for adults, or pimecrolimus cream 1% daily initially and less frequently later may also be used as an effective topical immunomodulator. Their use can avoid the adverse effects associated with chronic topical steroid application. They are especially helpful for atopic dermatitis of the face, eyelids, or in patients with limited areas of involvement.

Appropriate antihistamines should be used to control itching, preferably non-sedating in school-going children.

Oral antibiotics such a dicloxacillin, azithromycin and cephalexin are administered to control secondary infection. Topical mupirocin cream twice daily for 5 days may be helpful, if infection is mild.

For acute lesions and severe flares, wet dressings with Burrow's solution is applied for 20 minutes two or three times a day, followed by the application of a topical steroid.

Topical corticosteroids, e.g., Mometasone cream or Desonide cream is applied twice daily on affected areas initially to control the disease. Once lesions subside, steroids should be applied less frequently either once a day or on alternate day. They can also be diluted with a combination of Vitamin E and aloe vera cream. For larger body areas steroid lotions, e.g., betamethasone lotion diluted in equal amount of oil or aloe-vera + vitamin E lotion may be used to reduce side effects of topical corticosteroids. Appropriate antihistamines should be used to control itching.

For extensive disease and oozing lesions wet compresses with normal saline may be done twice daily. The disease should be controlled with short course of oral steroids and systemic antibiotic should be given to control infection. Once lesions get dried, topical steroids should be applied.

Systemic Treatment Options are in Severe Cases of Atopic Dermatitis

- Immunosuppressants
  - Oral corticosteroids
  - Cyclosporine
  - Azathioprine
  - Methotrexate
  - Mycophenolate mofetil
- Immune response modifiers
  - Gamma interferon.
  - Leukotriene inhibitors.
  - Anti-IgE antibodies (Omalizumab).
  - High dose intravenous immunoglobulins.

General Measures

Atopic individuals, generally have dry skin so they should be promoted to use oil and emollient creams liberally. Aggravating environmental factors such as excessive sweating, extremes of cold and heat, stress, offending foods, etc. should be avoided. They should be advised to wear light colored cotton clothing. Woolen clothing should be worn after wearing cotton clothes underneath. Excessive use of soaps and detergents should be avoided. Evening primrose oil and traditional Chinese herbs

Table 9.4: Indications for the use of different preparations of topical corticosteroids (TCS)

Potency (Class)	*Type of dermatoses*	*Extent of dermatoses*	*Duration of use*	*Location of dermatoses*	*Usage in infants and children*	*State of the epidermis*
Super-potent (0)	To be used in dermatoses resistant to high or intermediate potency TCS	Extensive application should be avoided (>50 g weekly)	Should be used for short term only (2-3 weeks at a time)	Should not be used on face, axilla, submammary areas or groins	Should be avoided in infants and children <12 years	Best suitable for thick, cornified or hypertrophic epidermis
High (II and III)	Severe	Extensive application should be avoided (>50 g weekly)	Should be used for short term only, if applying to atrophy prone areas or groins	Should not be used over face, axilla, submammary areas or groins	Should be avoided in infants and children <12 years	Suitable for thick, cornified/ or hypertrophic epidermis
Intermediate (IV and V) moderately potent	Mild to moderate	Suitable for short term treatment of extensive AD	Extended use (>1-2 weeks) should be avoided in infants and children	Trunk and extremities	Avoid extended use (1-2 weeks) in infants and children	Suitable for short-term use on thin skin; less effective on thicker skin
Low potent (VI and VII)	Mild	Suitable for treatment of large areas	For long term treatment	Best choice for face, axilla, groin and other moist, occluded areas	Safe in infants and children	Best suitable for thin skin; not effective on thick skin

are also being used, Tables 9.4, 9.5 and 9.6 illustrate the corticosteroids used in AD.

Table 9.5: Some commonly used corticosteroid preparations according to their potency

Class I (Ultra high potent)
1. Clobetasol propionate cream 0.05% 2. Halobetasol propionate cream 0.05%
Class II (High)
1. Betamethasone dipropionate ointment 0.05% 2. Mometasone furoate ointment 0.1% 3. Fluocinonide ointment or cream 0.05% 4. Halcinonide ointment or cream 0.1%
Class III
1. Fluticasone propionate ointment 0.005% 2. Betamethasone valerate ointment 0.01% 3. Triamcinolone acetonide ointment 0.1% 4. Betamethasone dipropionate cream 0.05%
Class IV (Moderate)
1. Fluocinolone acetonide ointment 0.025% 2. Mometasone furoate cream 0.1% 3. Triamcinolone acetonide cream 0.1% 4. Hydrocortisone valerate ointment 0.2%
Class V
1. Betamethasone dipropionate lotion 0.02% 2. Betamethasone valerate cream 0.1% 3. Fluocinolone acetonide cream 0.025% 4. Triamcinolone acetonide lotion 0.1% 5. Hydrocortisone valerate cream 0.2% 6. Hydrocortisone butyrate cream 0.1%
Class VI (Low)
1. Betamethasone valerate lotion 0.05% 2. Desonide cream 0.05% 3. Clobetasone butyrate cream 0.05%
Class VII
1. Hydrocortisone acetate 0.5% to 2.5%

Table 9.6: Amount of topical corticosteroid required according to site and age

Anatomic area	***Finger Tip Unit (FTU) required***			
	Age: 3-6 months	***Age: 1-2 years***	***Age: 3-5 years***	***Age: 6-10 years***
Face and neck	1	1.5	1.5	2
Arm and hand	1	1.5	2	2.5
Leg and foot	1.5	2	3	4.5
Anterior trunk	1	2	3	3.5
Posterior trunk and buttocks	1.5	3	3.5	5

FTU–A finger-tip unit (FTU) is the amount of ointment expressed from a tube with a 5 mm diameter nozzle, applied from the distal skin crease to the tip of the index finger.

PITYRIASIS ALBA

Definition

Pityriasis alba (PA) is a common low grade eczematous dermatosis, characterized by ill-defined erythematous or hypopigmented patches with fine scales which subside to leave areas of hypopigmentation. It is regarded as a minor form of atopic dermatitis by some authors.

Epidemiology

Epidemiological data are highly variable. In India estimated incidence in children is around 8.4%. Its prevalence in general population is estimated to be around 1%, but in atopic individuals it may be upto 32%.

Etiopathogenesis

Exact cause of pityriasis alba is not known. As this condition is quite common in children. Various factors like infection, nutritional factors, atopy, dryness of skin, obesity, over-eating especially at night and sleeping immediately after the night meal, excessive use of cosmetics and topical preparations, etc. have been implicated. Role of UV light may be important in large number of patients and they should be advised to avoid exposure to sunlight. Worm infestations have been falsely implicated to cause pityriasis alba.

Clinical Features

Pityriasis alba occurs predominantly in children between 3 and 16 years of age. Both sexes are equally susceptible.

The individual lesion is a rounded or oval patch, 0.5 cm to 2.0 cm in diameter, red, pink or skin colored and has fine scaling. Common sites involved are face, especially cheeks (Figure 9.13), chin and around lips. Neck, shoulder and arms are involved in around 20% of children. Trunk and limbs may be involved sometimes. Initially, the erythema may be conspicuous and there may be minimal serous crusting. Later, the erythema subsides completely, and shows only persistent fine scaling and hypopigmentation.

Course: The course of pityriasis alba is extremely variable. Most cases persist for some months, and some may show hypopigmentation for a year or more after scaling subsides.

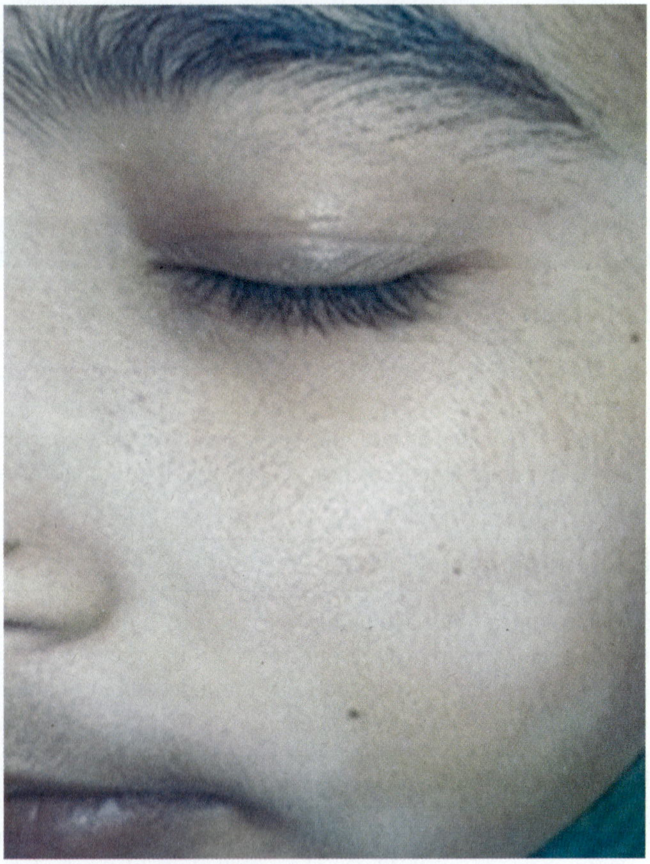

Figure 9.13: Pityriasis alba on face

The average duration of the common facial form in children is a year or more. There may be recurrence after some interval.

Differential Diagnosis

- Vitiligo.
- Indeterminate leprosy.
- Psoriasis.
- Discoid eczema.
- Tinea faciei.
- Tinea versicolor.

Diagnosis

Pityriasis alba is mostly diagnosed clinically. Age, fine scaling and distribution of the lesions usually suggest diagnosis.

Treatment

There is no definite treatment for pityriasis alba as course of disease is variable. In the morning, patient is advised to use an emollient cream like a combination of Vitamin E and aloe vera. In the evening, mild diluted local corticosteroid cream (e.g., mometasone cream diluted with Vitamin E and aloe vera cream) is advised. Tacrolimus ointment (0.03%) may also be used in these cases. Sunscreens with sun protection factor 15 (SPF-15) or more should be used in daytime. Response is generally good.

Persistent hypopigmentation causes worry and concern to the patients/parents and induces them to seek medical advice. Patient may be assured that hypopigmentation will persist for some time but will not be permanent. In case of persistent hypopigmentation, local psoralen in form of 10 drops of methoxsalen lotion mixed in 5 grams of emollient cream may be applied during night. Most of the patients will regain adequate pigmentation in 15-20 days.

PERIORAL DERMATITIS

Perioral dermatitis is characterized by inflammatory papules clustered around the mouth and occasionally at other sites, particularly the periocular and perinasal areas.

Etiopathogenesis

Perioral dermatitis is probably an allergic response to a variety of exogenous factors. The most common of these is the use of topical corticosteroids on the face. Reactions to substances such as toothpaste, creams or antiseptic solution have been implicated in some cases.

Perioral dermatitis is considered by some to be a variant of rosacea, but most patients lack the flushing and telangiectasia that are characteristic of rosacea. Steroid rosacea in prepubertal children is well documented and has features that are identical to perioral dermatitis. The granulomatous variant of perioral dermatitis occurs commonly in racially pigmented children, but the reasons for this are not known.

Clinical Features

Perioral dermatitis includes perinasal and periocular lesions in some of the cases. The vermilion border of the lip is usually spared. Involvement of the lips and corners of the mouth is more likely to be due to a specific contact allergen. In most cases, small erythematous papules are present superimposed on a background of erythema and scaling. In severe cases, pinpoint vesiculopustular lesions may be evident. In the granulomatous form of perioral dermatitis, lesions are often discrete, small, firm, dome shaped, flesh-coloured papules without erythema or scale (Figure 9.14). Some cases show overlapping clinical features of these two disease variants.

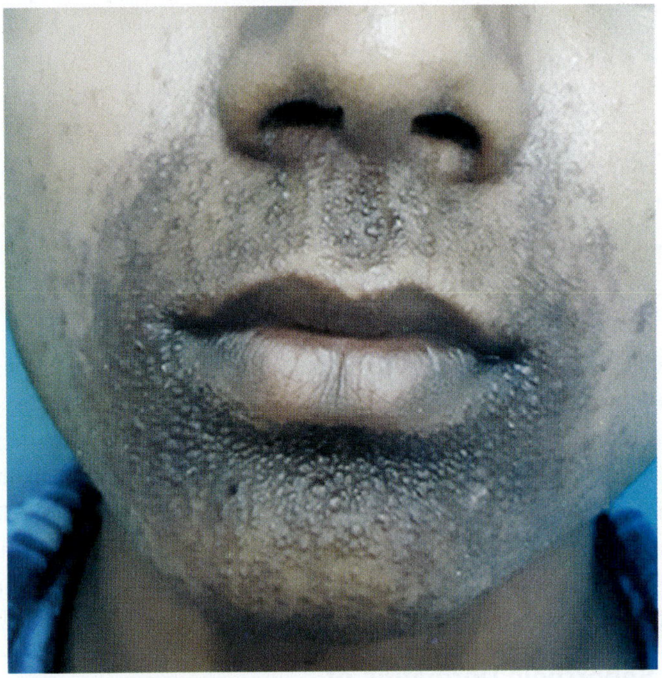

Figure 9.14: Perioral dermatitis

Differential Diagnosis

- Contact dermatitis.
- Atopic dermatitis.
- Acne rosacea.
- Lip licking dermatitis.
- Folliculitis, impetigo.
- Acrodermatitis enteropathica.
- Sarcoidosis.

Prognosis

The condition generally has a good prognosis, but pinpoint scarring has been reported in a few cases. The condition, if left untreated, can wax and wane for months to years, but with treatment generally resolves within a few months. Recurrences may develop after cessation of treatment.

Treatment

In severe, long standing disease, the response to therapy is slow, with occasional relapses over many months, whereas mild disease normally clears within a few weeks. Removal of the inciting factor such as topical corticosteroids or toothpaste must be done. Offending topical steroid should be replaced with an emollient cream. Low-or medium-potency topical corticosteroids like mometasone furoate 0.1% desonide 0.05%/ hydrocortisone 1% cream may be helpful which may be diluted with emollient cream and may be used initially, but care must be taken not to use mid- or high-potency steroids, which can exacerbate the disease. In less severe cases, topical therapy with metronidazole gel or cream applied twice daily may be curative. Tacrolimus ointment has also been reported as an effective treatment for steroid induced cases.

Oral tetracycline 250 mg twice daily is very effective in treating more recalcitrant cases but should not be given to children of less than 9 years of age because of the risk of causing irreversible dental staining. Oral azithromycin 10 mg/kg once a day for 3 days may be effective in cases with secondary infection. Isotretinoin, given orally, has been reported to be effective for granulomatous perioral dermatitis unresponsive to other therapies.

SEBORRHEIC DERMATITIS

Seborrheic dermatitis is a papulosquamous disorder occurring areas rich of sebaceous glands and characterized by erythematous, sharply marginated plaques with greasy looking scales. The lesions may be pruritic and may cause irritation on affected area.

Etiology

Etiology is unknown, there is no evidence for an increased sebum production associated with this eruption in children. Sebum secretion was found to be normal. In few cases *Pityrosporum ovale* is isolated and considered as a causative agent.

At birth, sebaceous glands are active due to stimulatory effect of maternal androgens, when the androgens level declines the glands become inactive upto the onset of puberty. At the age of 13 years, the usual age of onset of puberty, the indigenous androgen secretion again stimulates activity of sebaceous glands. In first few months, if seborrheic dermatitis develops it is called infantile seborrheic dermatitis whilst that occurring after the onset of puberty is called seborrheic dermatitis of adolescence.

Thus, based on age incidence in pediatric population, seborrheic dermatitis is of two types:

- Infantile seborrheic dermatitis.
- Seborrheic dermatitis of adolescence.

Infantile Seborrheic Dermatitis (ISD)

Infantile seborrheic dermatitis is an asymptomatic papulo-squamous skin disease of early infancy. The Braze and Rook diagnostic criteria for ISD include early onset, scalp and flexural involvement, erythematosquamous lesion and absence of pruritus.

ISD is usually localized on areas of increased sebaceous gland concentration. It is a superficial inflammatory process, the eruption lacks sharp margination. It generally disappears within a few months even without treatment.

Clinical Features

The disease usually begins in the first month of life and clears by the fourth month.

Usually, ISD begins in the napkin area or on the scalp (known as cradle cap) as non-itchy erythematous or grey papulosquamous eruption (Figure 9.15) which may spread to affect the face, forehead, eyebrows and retroauricular areas. The lesion does not have sharp borders and most of the body folds, e.g., axilla, inguinal, intergluteal fold and creases of neck may be involved. Sometimes other parts of the body, e.g., chest and back may be affected. Itching is not seen and if itching is an important feature other disease like atopic dermatitis should be excluded.

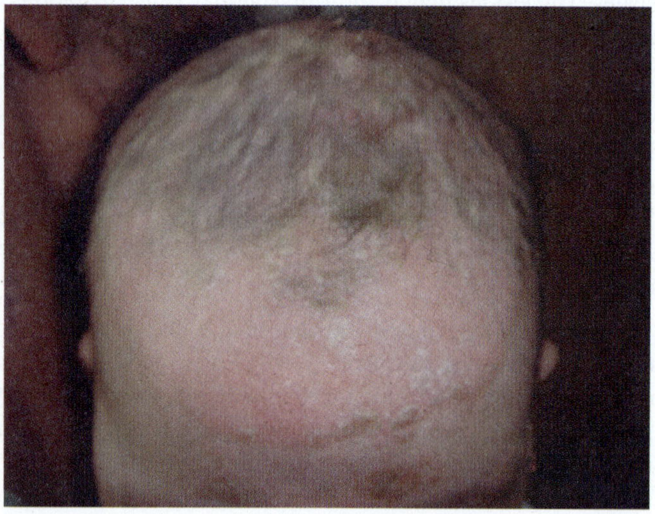

Figure 9.15: Cradle cap

Prognosis

The prognosis in ISD is much better than in atopic dermatitis. The disease usually clears in a few weeks and does not recur.

Differential Diagnosis

The diagnosis of ISD is based on clinical criteria. Differential diagnosis includes:

- Neonatal erythroderma.
- Atopic dermatitis.
- Psoriasis.
- Contact dermatitis.
- Langerhans cell histiocytosis.
- Immunodeficiency disorders.

Treatment

Usually no treatment is required. Reassurance should be given to the parents. Topical emollients may be prescribed. If disease is widespread, mild corticosteroid lotion may be applied, initially twice a day and later only once a day. Oral fluconazole is also effective and accelerates the response. It is available as 50 mg dispersible tablets and may be used in 2-3 mg/kg as single oral dose for 7-10 days. Ketoconazole shampoo should be avoided in infants because irritant reaction may occur.

Seborrheic Dermatitis of Adolescence

Clinical Features

- The scalp appearance of seborrheic dermatitis varies from mild, patchy scaling (dandruff) to widespread, thick, adherent crusts (Figure 9.16). From the scalp, seborrheic dermatitis can spread onto the forehead, eyebrows nasolabial folds, retroauricular groove and upper part of trunk. Blepharitis may also be evident (Figure 9.17).
- Skin lesions manifest as branny or greasy scaling over red, inflamed skin. Behind the ears there may be redness and greasy scaling and a crusted fissure (Figure 9.18). Often develops in retroauricular groove. This feature differentiates it from tinea capitis in which lesions are seen either on the helix or on the pinna or on the posterior surface of the ear (ear sign). Presternal or interscapular involvement is quite common.

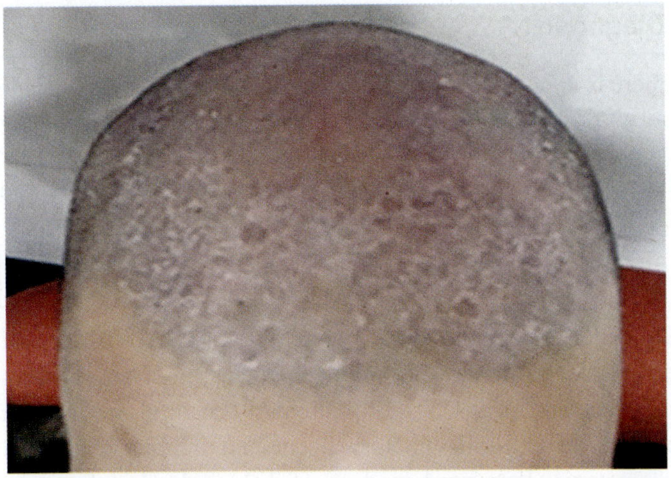

Figure 9.16: Seborrheic capitis

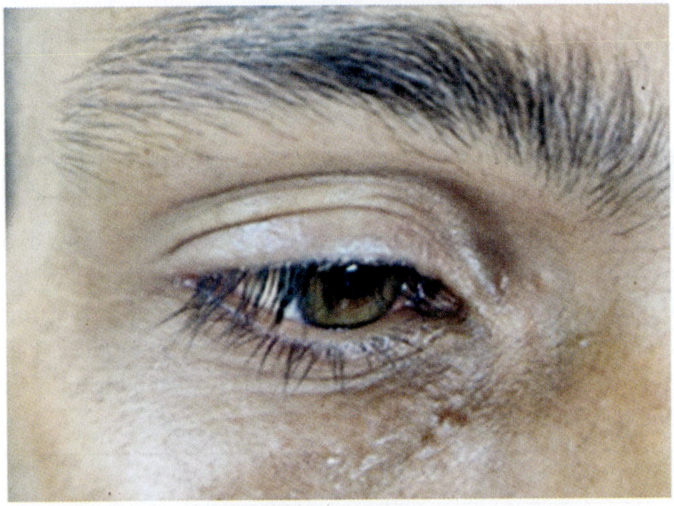

Figure 9.17: Blepharitis

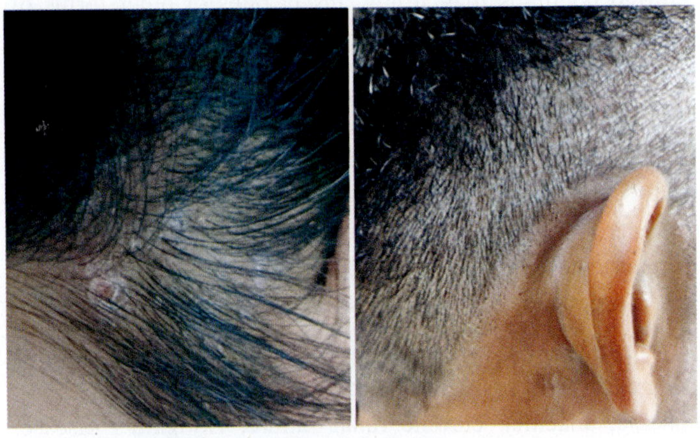

Figure 9.18: Seborrheic dermatitis involving scalp and retro-auricular fold

- Distinct truncal pattern of seborrheic dermatitis may occur as annular or geographic petaloid scaling. Pityriasiform variety which can be seen on the trunk and the neck and is characterized by a generalized erythematosquamous eruption, somewhat similar to, but more extensive than pityriasis rosea.
- Seborrheic dermatitis is particularly severe in HIV infected patients and may progress to erythroderma.
- Seborrheic dermatitis is common in winter and early spring and is usually precipitated by stress and poor hygiene.

Differential Diagnosis

- Psoriasis.
- Atopic dermatitis.
- Pityriasis rosea.
- Seborrheic type of tinea capitis.
- Drug eruptions, e.g., chlorpromazine or cimetidine.
- Pemphigus foliaceus.
- Darier's disease.
- Histiocytosis X.

Treatment

Seborrheic dermatitis of scalp should be treated with ketoconazole 2% shampoo, once or twice a week. For severe scaling steroid lotion diluted with emollient such as coconut oil applied at night and shampooing at morning is quite effective. Seborrheic dermatitis of face should be treated with low potency diluted steroid cream. For unresponsive disease oral fluconazole 2-3 mg/kg daily or alternate day or oral ketoconazole 3-5 mg/kg/day for 7 to 10 days is quite effective and bring longer remission. Washing with soap and water removes lipid layer over skin and decreases the growth of *Malassezia*. Antihistamines should be used for symptomatic relief from pruritus. Later the remission may be maintained with ketoconazole 2% shampoo once or twice in a week.

PAPULAR URTICARIA

Definition

Papular urticaria is a common skin disorder of children characterized by recurrent itchy papular eruptions. The papules may be surrounded by a variable degree of erythema. It is an immunologically mediated disorder and is most often caused by the feeding bites of blood-sucking insects such as mosquitoes or other arthropods. There may be history of similar lesions in siblings.

Etiology

Papular urticaria is a specific acquired hypersensitivity reaction to contents of injection of foreign proteins of biting insects into skin of sensitized children. Insects like mosquitoes, bedbugs, fleas, ticks, mites and dipterous insects other than mosquitoes may also cause papular urticaria. There is usually seasonal variation depending upon habit of offending insects.

Pathogenesis

Biting of insect may induce immediate IgE mediated reaction resulting into a wheal formation which may have a central punctum. This reaction is followed by delayed type of hypersensitivity reaction resulting into intensely itchy indurated papules which lasts for weeks to months.

Clinical Features

Papular urticaria is commonly seen in children between 2-10 years of age. The disease is most commonly seen in summer months. Repeated reaction in a particular season may lead to hyposensitization and ultimately cure of disease.

Most patients have widespread wheals and indurated papules which have central haemorrhagic punctum (a classic bed bug bite reaction is 2-5 mm erythematous papule or wheal with central haemorrhagic punctum) (Figure 9.19). The lesions heal in 10-14 days but recurrent cropping leads to continuation of the disease. In severe reaction, vesicles and bullae may also be seen. The lesions are distributed chiefly over exposed parts but in case of insects like tick, it may be seen over covered parts also. Lesions are grouped in clusters. Secondary infection and modification of lesion by trauma, eczematization may be seen.

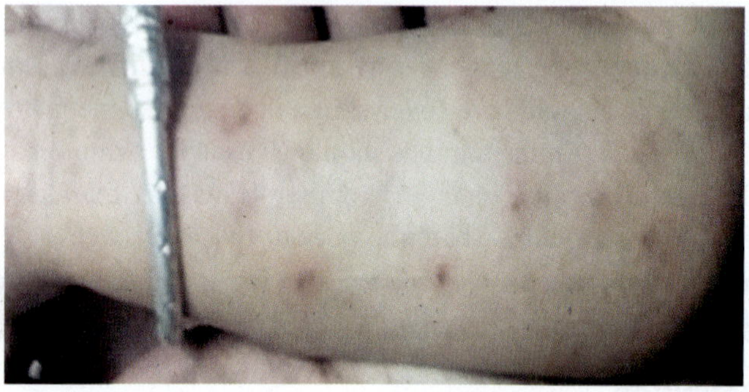

Figure 9.19: Papular urticaria showing excoriated papules and haemorrhagic punctum

Differential Diagnosis

- Scabies.
- Eczematous dermatitis.
- Folliculitis.
- Pyoderma.

Diagnosis

There is no confirmatory test and diagnosis of disease is made on clinical grounds. Age of the patient, characteristic itchy papular lesions, pattern of distribution, history of similar lesions in siblings, response to preventive measures are features suggestive of papular urticaria.

Treatment

Education of parents about preventive measures like use of protective clothing, mosquito repellents, and insecticides is necessary. Dapsone is particularly helpful because it acts as an anti-inflammatory agent and inhibits neutrophil chemotaxis. It is used in dose of 1-2 mg/kg/day. Dapsone may cause haemolytic anaemia in individuals who have G-6-PD deficiency so its estimation before starting dapsone is advisable. Topical steroids and antihistamines are helpful. In severe cases short course of oral steroids may also be used. Topical and oral antibiotics are used for secondary infections.

PRURIGO NODULARIS

It represents a nodular reaction pattern to intense pruritus due to focal scratching. It is a chronic dermatitis, characterized by intensely pruritic nodules that are difficult to treat, occurring mainly on the extensor aspect of the lower extremities. The disease is more common in adults but may affect both children and adolescents.

Etiology

In many patients the cause of the initial lesion is unclear. Prurigo nodularis may follow insect bites or other forms of localized inflammation. The lesion itself is intensely pruritic, which sets up a vicious cycle of scratching, mechanical trauma, reactive hyperplasia, infection, scarring and attempted healing.

The atopic diathesis has been implicated as a contributing factor in the development of prurigo nodularis. In some patients a history of local trauma or insect or arthropod bites is reported. The chronic scratching may be a manifestation of stress or more severe psychological disturbances.

Prurigo nodularis may occasionally result from the pruritus of underlying systemic disorders like obstructive biliary disease, anaemia, chronic renal failure, Hodgkin's disease, leukemia, polycythemia rubra vera, hypo and hyperthyroidism, diabetes mellitus, parasitic infections, drug reactions, gluten enteropathy and other forms of malabsorption. Of all systemic disorders associated with prurigo nodularis, the most common in children is Hodgkin's lymphoma.

Clinical Features

The lesions of prurigo nodularis are most often irregular nodules of 0.5-3 cm in diameter. The surface of these nodules may be keratotic or depressed. The early lesion is erythematous and may appear urticarial. However, all lesions tend to become pigmented with time. Crusting and scaling may cover recently excoriated lesions. Irregular rings of hyperpigmentation are sometimes seen around the nodules. There may also be areas of hypopigmentation or active keloid formation. As a result of repeated excoriation, the nodules may become infected.

The lesions are most prevalent on the extensor aspect of the thighs and legs and, occasionally, the upper extremities (Figure 9.20). They are usually grouped and numerous, but may vary in number from 2 to 200. New lesions develop intermittently, but old ones tend to persist and remain pruritic. Lesions leave scarring and pigmentary changes. The surrounding skin is usually normal apart from signs of previous lesions.

Prognosis

Prurigo nodularis is a chronic condition that can be very frustrating to the child and the family. When there is an underlying condition, improvement may be achieved by treating the associated disorder.

Differential Diagnosis

Hypertrophic lichen planus may easily be confused with prurigo nodularis. Most patients with this form of lichen planus will have typical lesions of lichen planus in other locations.

Treatment

The goal of therapy is symptomatic relief of pruritus. Oral antihistamines are an important aspect of treatment. They are especially useful at bedtime, when relief from the distractions of daytime activity often leads to an increase in pruritus. Because xerosis is often a contributing factor, emollients are of significant value. Topical corticosteroids are important part of therapy. Intralesional corticosteroids may be of value in the treatment of chronic lesions. Topical capsaicin may be helpful. Ultraviolet radiation for severe and generalized cases of prurigo nodularis has also been used.

NON- ECZEMATOUS CONTACT DERMATITIS

Non-eczematous contact dermatitis is more common than eczematous contact dermatitis where classical signs of eczematous dermatitis (acute, subacute and chronic) are absent. Many clinical forms of non-eczematous dermatitis are reported in literature e.g.

- Erythema multiforme like contact dermatitis
- Pigmented purpuric contact dermatitis
- Pigmented contact dermatitis
- Pustular contact dermatitis
- Granulomatous contact dermatitis
- Lymphomatoid contact dermatitis

Erythema multiforme is the most common type of non-eczematous contact dermatitis. Diagnosis can be done by performing patch test.

ASTEATOTIC ECZEMA (ECZEMA CRAQUELE/ WINTER ECZEMA)

This type of eczema is commonly seen in individuals having excessive dry skin. It commonly affects legs, arms, forearms, hands and back. Clinical features include dry, scaly itchy skin with 'crazy paving pattern' specifically over legs. Flare is seen during winters. Dry and cracked skin over finger pulp produces depression and distorted finger pulp which is known

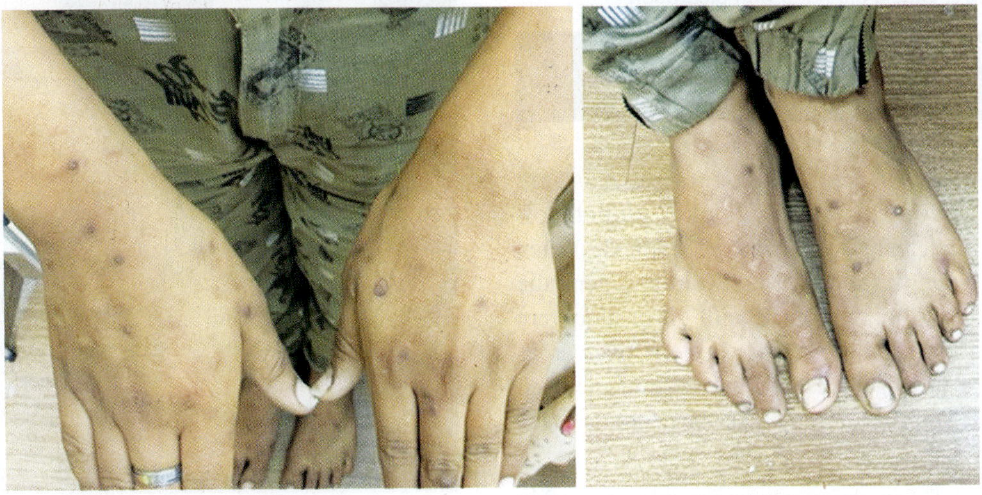

Figure 9.20: Prurigo nodularis lesions over dorsal aspect of bilateral hand and feet

as parchment pulps. Treatment includes, avoidance of sudden change in temperature, emollients, oil bath and mild topical steroids.

STASIS DERMATITIS (Figure 9.21)

It is an acute, subacute and chronic dermatitis due to venous hypertension occurs on lower extremities. It is an early sign of venous hypertension. It presents with pruritis, reddish brown discoloration, and oedema at ankle region. Late stage of venous stasis may result in ulceration, atrophic scar and lipodermatosclerosis. Diagnosis is based on clinical examination. Venous doppler may help to identify abnormal lower leg vein and their venous blood flow. Management include topical steroids, calcineurin inhibitor, pentoxifylline and compression therapy,

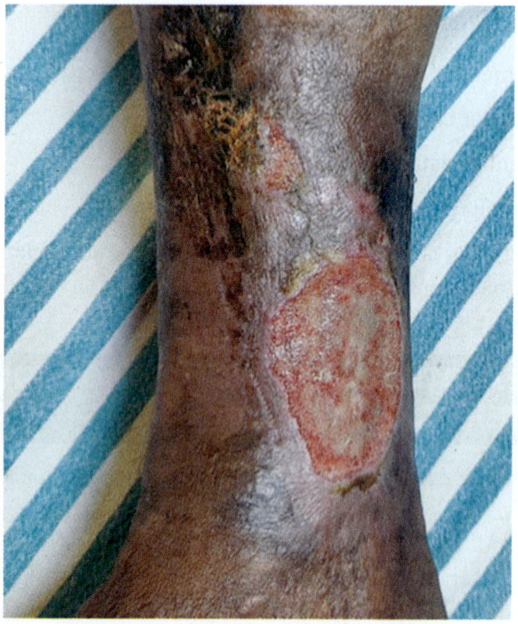

Figure 9.21: Stasis changes with ulceration

PRACTICAL TIPS OF USING LOCAL STEROIDS

- When smaller areas are involved or lesions are hypertrophied, topical steroids like clobetasol/ betamethasone in cream form may be applied. When large areas of body, flexural creases, scalp and genitalia are involved, steroid lotion diluted with oil or aloe vera + Vitamin-E lotion should be used. Lesions over areas of thin skin like face, genitals and in children medium potency topical steroids like mometasone furoate 0.1% are indicated.
- The use of the FTU in dermatology provides a readily understandable measure for both patients and doctor. It should be given according to the age of the patient and site of dermatoses (Table 9.6). A finger-tip unit (FTU) is the amount of ointment expressed from a tube with a 5 mm diameter nozzle, applied from the distal skin crease to the tip of the index finger.
- In case of thick, hyperkeratotic dry lesions over palms and soles, corticosteroid cream may be mixed with salicylic acid ointment to improve penetration.

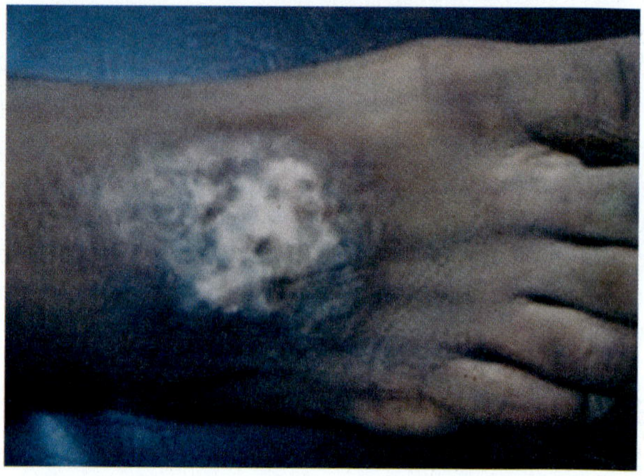

Figure 9.22: Hypertrophic eczema

- Intralesional triamcinolone acetonide injections may be given fortnightly in thick hypertrophic lesions (Figure 9.22). In case of oozing lesions, a short course of oral prednisolone may prove beneficial. Steroids may be tapered after symptomatic relief.
- Chronic hyperkeratotic lesions over legs, palms and soles are difficult to treat. Oral psoralen plus ultraviolet A therapy (PUVA therapy) may give additional benefit in such patients. Topical tar along with steroids is also given (Figure 9.23).

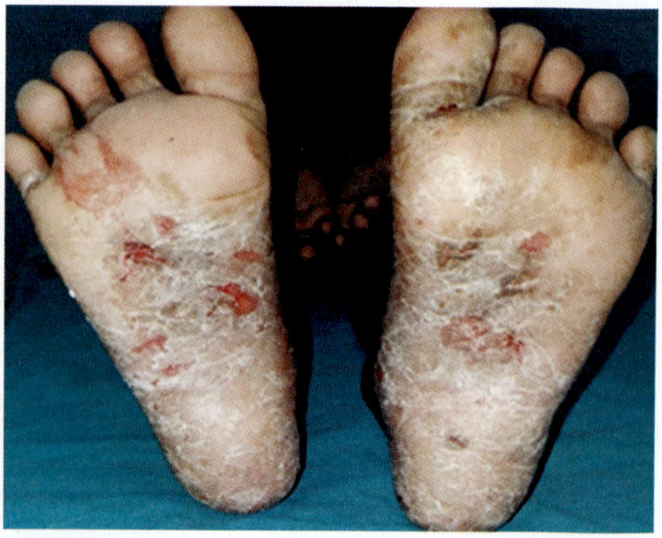

Figure 9.23: Hyperkeratotic planter eczema with fissure

10 CHAPTER Photobiology and Photodermatosis

Contents

PHOTOBIOLOGY

The science of photobiology focuses on role of Ultraviolet (UV) and visible light on human skin. The light coming from sun (solar spectrum) has a wide range of electromagnetic radiations. It ranges from very short wavelength, below 200 nm (cosmic rays, X-rays, γ-rays), ultraviolet rays (200-400 nm), visible light (400 nm -700 nm), infrared rays to very long wavelength radio and television waves. UV radiation has been explored for a long time for damaging and beneficial effects on human skin. Many dermatological disorders are caused or exacerbated by UV rays while on the other hand, they are useful in dermatology for detection of the diseases (wood's lamp) and in management of many dermatosis (phototherapy). Depth of penetration of UV radiation in skin depends on wave length, more the wavelength, deeper the penetration.

UV radiations are categorised into three subtypes (Figure 10.1):

UV C (200-280 nm): This is filtered by ozone layer of atmosphere and does not reach the earth's surface.

UV B (280 - 320 nm): UV B reaches earth's surface and it penetrates the superficial layer of skin up to the epidermis and causes sunburn, delayed tanning, epidermal hyperplasia, photoageing and carcinogenesis. It is filtered by ordinary window glass. It is further subdivided in two types:

- Broad band UV B (280-320 nm)
- Narrow band UV B (monochromatic, 311-313 nm)

UV A (320-400 nm): It penetrates into deep dermis and causes both immediate and delayed tanning, photoageing and photo carcinogenesis. It passes through ordinary window glasses. It is subclassified into two types:

- UV-A2 (320-340 nm)
- UV- A1 (340-400 nm)

Visible light (400-700 nm): Visible light is the part of electromagnetic spectrum that is visible to human eyes.

Infrared red radiation (700 nm-1 mm): This spectrum is also known as thermal spectrum and is categorized into three types:

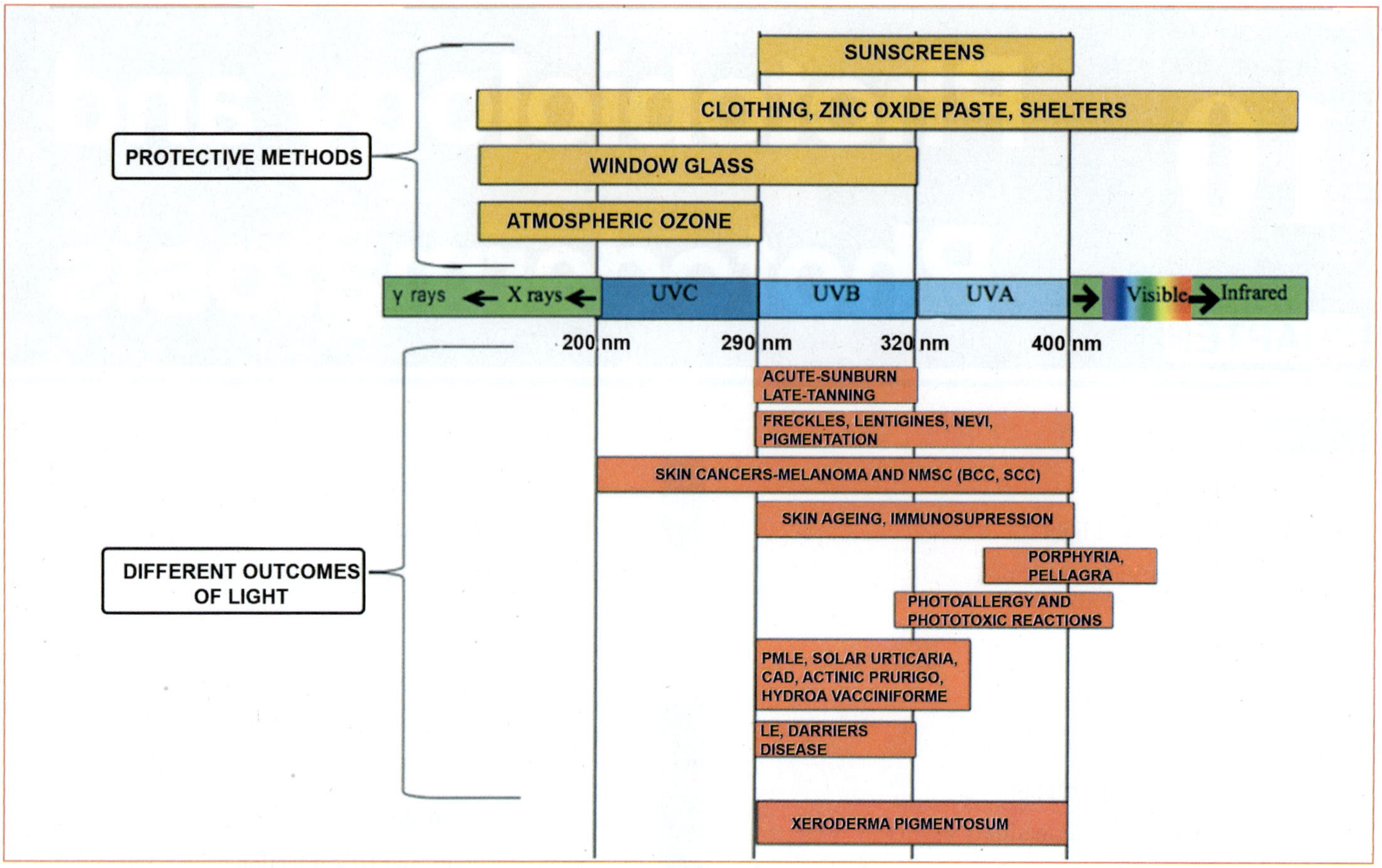

Figure 10.1: Spectrum of light, outcome on skin and protective measures

- IR-A /Near infrared (700 μm-1.4 μm)
- IR-B /Mid infrared (1.4 μm-3 μm)
- IR-C /Far infrared (3 μm-1mm)

ARTIFICIAL SOURCES OF LIGHT

There are many artificial sources of light, e.g., incandescent lamps (emit visible and infrared light), fluorescent lamps (emit visible light and UV A), and light emission diodes (LED, emit visible light). They are used in humans for recreational tanning, occupational and therapeutic purposes (phototherapy).

SKIN AND ULTRA VIOLET RADIATION

When UV radiations reach on a surface, they are either reflected, transmitted, absorbed or scattered. In the skin they are absorbed by structural molecules known as chromophores e.g. DNA, transurocanic acid (t UCA), melanin, porphyrin, aromatic amino acid containing protein. After absorption two types of responses occur:

1. **Direct response:** Chromophores undergo structural changes when they absorb UV radiation e.g. dipyrimidine formed in DNA molecule. After structural changes these molecules initiate biological responses.
2. **Indirect response:** In indirect response, chromophore is not the molecule that causes the biological response but it transfers the energy to another molecule e.g. after transfer of energy to oxygen, reactive oxygen species (ROS) are formed, which damage cellular components such as DNA and membranes.

Normal effects of UVR on skin: Normal effects of UV radiation at molecular and cellular levels on skin are:

- Photo damage and repair of skin
- Formation of reactive oxygen species (ROS) that damage DNA & cell membranes
- Melanogenesis
- Vit D synthesis
- Keratinocyte apoptosis or sunburn cells
- Langerhans cell depletion
- Epidermal hyperplasia, dermal inflammatory infiltrate
- Change in gene expression

Clinical effects of UV radiation on skin (Table 10.1):

Table 10.1: Clinical effects of UV radiations on skin

Acute	*Chronic*
Erythema	Skin cancer
Tanning Immediate and persistent pigment darkening Delayed tanning	Photoageing

Acute Effects

Acute effects occur within seconds to weeks after exposure to UVR.

1. **Erythema:**

   Erythema is the most common inflammatory response due to UVB exposure which occurs within 6 hours and reaches its peak at about 24 hours. Clinically it presents with erythema associated with pain, tenderness, burning sensation.

   Minimum Erythema Dose (MED): Amount of UVR that will produce minimal erythema of skin (sunburn or redness) within few hours.

2. **Tanning:**

   Three different types of tanning occur in response to UVR:

   - Immediate pigment darkening (IPD)
   - Persistent pigment darkening (PPD)
   - Delayed tanning or melanogenesis (DT)

   Immediate pigment darkening (IPD): Upon exposure to UV A and visible light, the already existing colourless melanin precursors undergo an immediate photooxidation that results in a temporary grey coloration which disappears in fifteen minutes. In people with fair complexion, it is nearly unnoticeable, but in those with darker skin, it is clearly noticeable.

   Persistent pigment darkening (PPD): This reaction occurs due to higher UVA doses causing a brown hue, which peaks two hours after post irradiation and lasts for one to five days. PPD results from a more prolonged oxidation of melanin precursors rather than from fresh melanin synthesis.

   Delayed tanning (Neomelanogenesis/DT): Delayed tanning, occurs when basal epidermal melanocytes stimulate the production of additional melanin, which is subsequently transported by dendrites to nearby keratinocytes and redistributed towards the skin's surface. Usually, it becomes noticeable three days after radiation. When stratum corneum sheds over a few weeks, tanning fades away.

Chronic Effects

1. **Skin cancers:**

   UV radiation exposure is associated with various cutaneous premalignant (actinic keratosis) and malignant skin cancers (basal cell carcinoma, malignant melanoma, squamous cell carcinoma). Risk of UV induce skin cancer depends on skin type.

2. **Photoageing:**

   Photoageing presents with fine and course skin wrinkling, telangiectasia, yellowish discoloration and irregular patchy pigmentation. Histological changes include, flattened dermo-epidermal junction, skin thickening and atrophy, elastin and collagen tissue degeneration.

UV Protection

Natural protective unit in skin is melanin and cornified layer of epidermis. UV protective measures include, appropriate clothing, avoid outing in afternoon light (10 am-3 pm) and sunscreen application.

SUNSCREEN

These are photoprotective topical preparations, which reflect or absorb sunlight and protect the skin from the short term and long-term effects of ultraviolet radiation. The common indications for the use of sunscreens in dermatology are:

- Sunburn
- Freckling
- Photoaging
- Skin cancer
- Photoallergic reactions
- Photosensitivity diseases (Polymorphous light eruption, Solar urticaria, Chronic actinic dermatitis, Persistent light reaction, Lupus erythematosus, Xeroderma pigmentosum, Albinism)
- Photoaggravated dermatoses

Ideal Sunscreen Properties

- Combined physical and chemical protection
- Broad spectrum
- Cosmetically elegant
- Non irritant
- Non allergic or inert

- Non comedogenic
- Photostable
- Economical

Classification of Sunscreen

Inorganic sunscreens

Inorganic agents function by reflecting, scattering or absorbing UV radiation. Their opaque nature and "whitening effect" can be minimized by the use of micronized or ultra micronized particles. e.g. zinc oxide, titanium dioxide, iron oxide, kaolin, calamine, ichthammol, talc etc.

Organic Sunscreens

Organic sunscreens are active ingredients that absorb UV radiation within a particular range of wavelengths, depending on their chemical structure. Organic sunscreens are further divided into UVB and UVA filters:

1. **UVB filters:**
   - PABA derivatives – Padimate O
   - Cinnamates – Octinoxate, Cinoxate
   - Salicylates – Octisalate
   - Octocrylene
   - Ensulizole
2. **UVA filters:**
   - Benzophenones (UVB and UVA2 absorbers) – Oxybenzone, Sulisobenzone, Dioxybenzone
   - Avobenzone or Parsol 1789 (UVA1 absorber)
   - Meradimate (UVA2 absorber)

   The sunscreen molecules with the strongest UVA filter is avobenzone; however, it has the drawback of being photo unstable.
3. **Newer generation broad spectrum (UVA + UVB) filters:**
   - Ecamsule (Mexoryl SX),
   - Silatriazole (Mexoryl XL),
   - Bemotrizinol (Tinosorb S),
   - Bisoctrizole (Tinosorb M)

Tinosorb M combines the advantage of both organic and inorganic UV conventional filters.

Systemic Sunscreens

Many compounds exhibit a systemic photoprotective impact. Examples of such substances include beta-carotene, corticosteroids, ascorbic acid, beta-tocopherols (a combination of vitamins A, C, and E), retinol, selenium, green tea, antihistamines, aspirin and indomethacin.

Sun Protection Factor (SPF)

It is a ratio between minimum erythema dose of photoprotected skin to minimum erythema dose of non photoprotected skin.

Grading system for SPF

- **Low SPF:** 2-15
- **Medium SPF:** 16-30
- **High SPF:** 31-50
- **Highest SPF:** > 50

Critical Wavelength

The wavelength below which 90% of the sunscreen's UV absorbency occurs.

Broad Spectrum Sunscreen

Critical wavelength > 370 nm and UVA protection factor > 4.

Water-resistant Sunscreen

Maintains the label SPF value after two sequential immersions in water for 20 minutes (total 40 minutes).

Recommendation for Sunscreen Applications

Whenever going into the sun, sunscreen should be adequately applied to all sun exposed regions (at a concentration of 2 mg/cm^2). It should also be allowed to dry completely and reapplied after swimming, strenuous activity, considerable perspiration, or towelling.

Teaspoon Rule

- 3 ml (slightly more than half tea spoon)
  - For each arm
  - For face and neck
- 6 ml (slightly more than a tea spoon)
  - For each leg
  - For the chest
  - For the back

Note: It is not recommended to use sunscreen on infants under six months old. Of all the sunscreen ingredients, oxybenzone is the most common cause of contact dermatitis (photoallergy).

PHOTODERMATOSIS

Photodermatoses are heterogeneous group of disorders characterized by an abnormal sensitivity of skin to sunlight which is responsible for local or generalized eruptions. Uncommon in children, the most frequent of them such as sunburn and phototoxicity are fortunately benign, brief and spontaneously resolving. Some of them disappear spontaneously after few years like polymorphic light eruptions, which are rather observed in children older than 10 years of age. In case of persistence, rare diseases should be considered and investigated with specific tests (photo tests, blood examination, genetic investigations), as some metabolic or genetic disorders may be revealed by photosensitivity, especially before the age of 3 years.

Photosensitivity Disorders

Idiopathic

- Polymorphic light eruptions (PLE).
- Actinic prurigo.
- Hydroa vacciniforme.
- Chronic actinic dermatitis.
- Solar urticaria.
- Juvenile spring eruptions.

Nutritional

- Pellagra.

Metabolic

- Porphyrias.
- Hartnup disease.

Genetic

- Xeroderma pigmentosum.
- Cockayne's syndrome.
- Bloom's syndrome.
- Kindler syndrome.
- Rothmund-Thomson syndrome.

Autoimmune

- Lupus erythematosus.
- Dermatomyositis.

Drug Induced Photosensitivity

- Antibiotics (Tetracyclines, Sulfonamides, Fluoroquinolones).
- Antifungals (Griseofulvin, Voriconazole).
- Non-steroidal anti-inflammatory drugs (NSAIDs).
- Retinoids.
- Amiodarone etc.

Chemical Induced Photosensitivity

- Psoralens
- Sunscreen
- Chemical dyes

Clinical Features

- The majority of patients complain of pruritus, burning or tingling sensation over sun exposed parts of body.
- The duration of exposure required to induce these symptoms depend upon the underlying disease and environmental conditions.
- Erythema and swelling on exposed parts of the body (face, upper back, upper chest, extensor aspect of forearm) are common features in patients suffering from photosensitive disorder.
- In an acute episode apart from erythema, patients can develop blisters.
- With repeated exposure, patient may develop butterfly erythema on face, persistent plaques, telangiectasia and poikilodermatous changes.
- Specific clinical diagnosis in a particular case can be made by combination of signs and symptoms suggestive of a particular photosensitive disease.

Clinical Findings in Photosensitive Patients

- **Butterfly rash:** SLE, Pellagra, Cockayne's syndrome, Bloom's syndrome, Rothmund-Thomson syndrome.
- **Blisters:** Kindler syndrome, Bloom's syndrome, Rothmund-Thomson syndrome.
- **Dermatitis:** Pellagra, SLE, polymorphic light eruption.
- **Telangiectasia:** Rothmund-Thomson syndrome, Xeroderma pigmentosum, Cockayne's syndrome, Bloom's syndrome.
- **Poikiloderma:** Kindler syndrome, juvenile dermatomyositis, Rothmund-Thomson syndrome.
- **Hypertrichosis:** Congenital erythropoietic porphyria, juvenile dermatomyositis.

Investigations

- Photo testing with ultraviolet and sometimes with visible light, patch tests and the combination (photo patch test) are occasionally helpful when there is diagnostic difficulty. In photo patch testing, suspected photoallergens are applied in two sets. One set is removed after 24 hours and ultraviolet irradiation is given and again covered. Both test sites are then compared after 72-96 hours.

- Serological tests may help to exclude connective tissue diseases.
- Testing to exclude metabolic causes may be helpful, e.g., plasma porphyrin levels, ANA, etc.

POLYMORPHIC LIGHT ERUPTION (PLE)

PLE is the most common photodermatosis. Females are affected twice as frequently as males. About 15% of adolescents and young adults will suffer to some degree at some time. The disease starts in summer with gradual improvement in autumn but pattern may vary in different patients. Different patients show different patterns, so the disease has been given the name of polymorphic light eruption. The lesions develop on sun exposed parts of body, e.g., dorsum of hands, extensor aspects of forearm, upper back and 'V' area of chest, chin, bridge of nose, helix and pinna of ear, sometimes on dorsa of feet after few minutes to 24 hours of sun exposure. Clinically, most commonly three types of skin lesions are encountered in children viz.:

- Erythematous patches with scaling and papules present over face and forearms (Figure 10.2).
- Hypopigmented patches with scaling are present over face (Figure 10.3) and forearms in a symmetrical distribution. It should be differentiated from pityriasis alba, which is also a commonly encountered entity in children. Generally, patients of pityriasis alba have hypopigmented patches which may be asymmetrical, in contrast to photosensitivity where they are bilaterally symmetrical. In some patients the border of hypopigmented plaques may be raised (Figure 10.4).

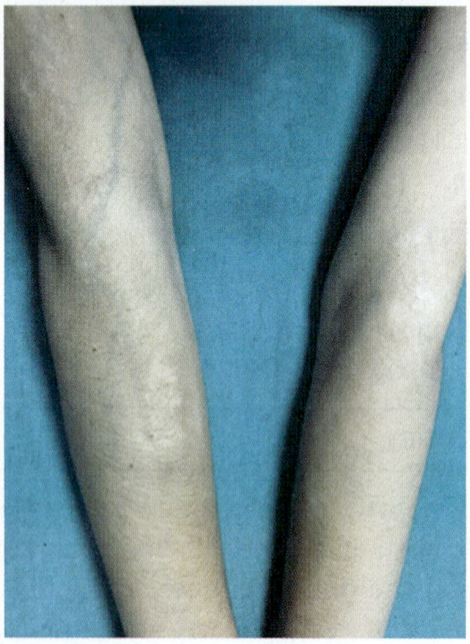

Figure 10.2: Polymorphic light eruption (PLE)

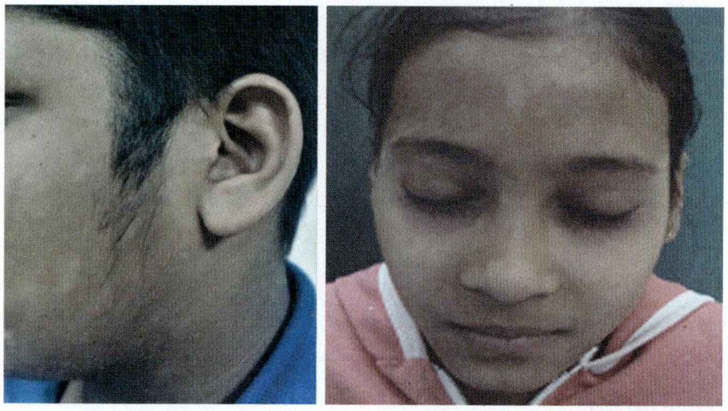

Figure 10.3: PLE showing lesions mimicking pityriasis alba

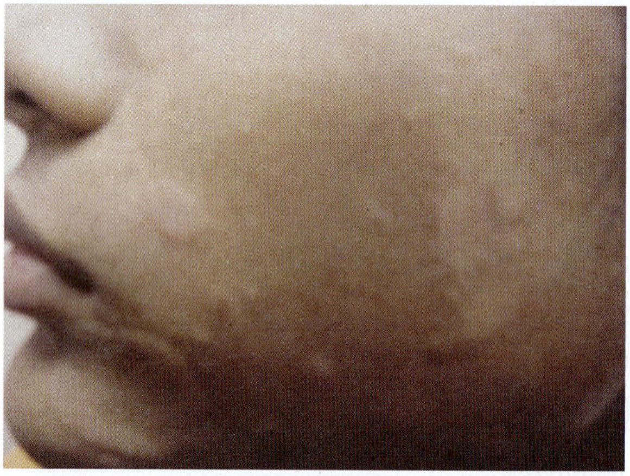

Figure 10.4: PLE showing hypopigmented plaques with raised borders

- Plaques with central hyperpigmentation and peripheral hypopigmentation. Few papular lesions may be present around the plaque (Figure 10.5).
- Sometimes eczematous plaques (Figures 10.6, 10.7 and 10.8), vesicles and urticarial lesions may occur in severe cases.

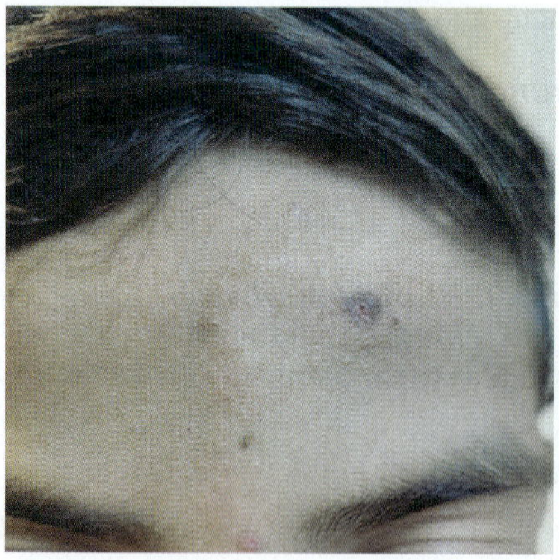

Figure 10.5: Hyperpigmented plaque with surrounding papules over forehead in PLE

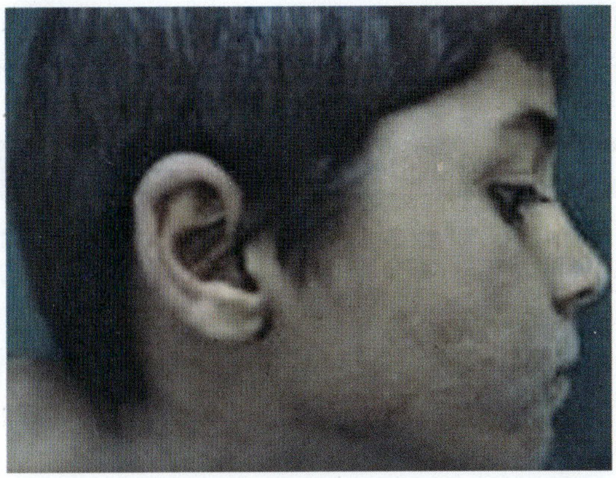

Figure 10.6: Severe PLE showing eczematous lesions on ear and face change

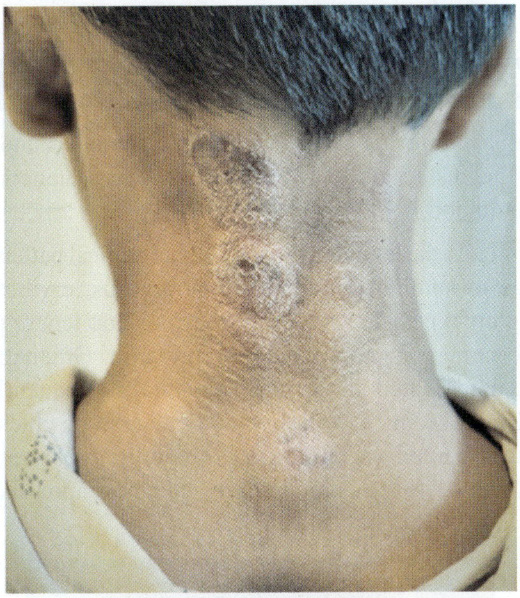

Figure 10.7: Severe PLE showing eczematous plaque on neck

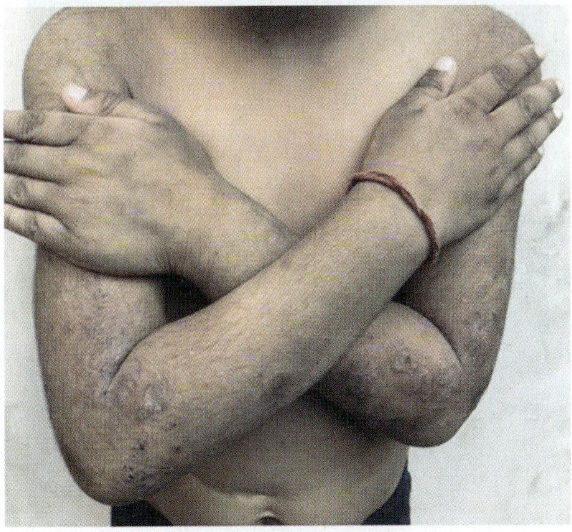

Figure 10.8: Severe PLE showing eczematous lesions on arms and forearms

Treatment

- In general, topical steroids like 1% hydrocortisone, mometasone and fluticasone can be used over the lesions on the face, whereas betamethasone and more potent steroids like clobetasol may be used at extra facial sites.
- An acute eruption can be treated with emollients and mild to moderate potency topical steroids. Oral steroids are sometimes needed. Antihistamines may be used to control pruritus. Severe cases may benefit from short courses of PUVA (Psoralen and UVA treatment) in the spring to artificially 'harden' the skin.
- Prophylactically, few measures like wearing broad brimmed hat, protective clothing, avoidance of sunlight and application of sunscreen should be done. Densely weaved and loose fitting clothing screen UVB more effectively. Sunscreens are compounds which provide protection from UV radiation when applied to skin, the efficacy of sunscreen in blocking UVB radiation is expressed as sun protection factor (SPF).
- There are two types of sunscreens viz. UV absorbing chemicals, i.e., chemical sunscreens and UV scattering or blocking agents, i.e. physical sunscreens. For Indian skin types, a sunscreen with SPF–15 to 25 is sufficient. It should be applied at least 20 minutes before going in the sun. Repeat applications may be required after 4 hours for two more times in the afternoon. Sunscreens may be water resistant (maintaining their SPF after 40 min. of water immersion) or waterproof (maintaining their SPF after 80 min. of water immersion).

JUVENILE SPRING ERUPTION

Juvenile spring eruption may be a variant of PLE, but is clinically distinct. The lesions consist of tiny blisters on the ear, 1-2 hours after exposure to intense sunlight. They cause itching and pain. The lesions are transient, usually lasting for 2 weeks. This is typically a disorder of early spring, but may occur throughout the summer and may recur on annual basis throughout childhood. Photo tests are normal and provocation tests are negative.

Treatment

Topical corticosteroids may be used. The important aspect is to use a broad spectrum sunscreen to prevent the eruption, but benefit is variable. Physical barriers are most effective.

CHRONIC ACTINIC DERMATITIS

Chronic actinic dermatitis is a rare condition affecting mainly middle-aged and elderly men. Rarely it is also seen in children, which often follows years of chronic dermatitis.

Clinically lichenified plaques on light exposed skin are present. Initially it is worse in the summer but can become perennial. In long standing cases, it may become disseminated and may involve non sun exposed areas also.

There is usually little doubt about the diagnosis, but possibility of a drug induced photodermatosis or airborne contact dermatitis should also be considered.

Leonine facies is seen in long-standing cases (Figure 10.9).

Treatment

Light avoidance, sunscreens and topical steroids.

Chronic cases may require systemic steroids and/or other immunosuppressants (azathioprine).

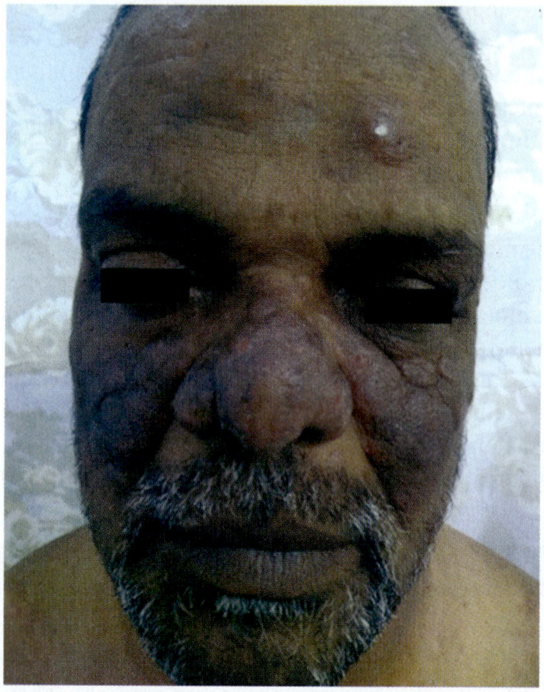

Figure 10.9: Chronic actinic dermatitis

SOLAR URTICARIA

Solar urticaria is a rare disorder in which wheals appear minutes after exposure to sunlight and is associated with pruritus, stinging and erythema. Usually sun exposed skin is affected but unexposed areas may also be involved if thin clothing is worn. There may be mucosal involvement with tongue and lip swelling. Rash disappears after sun exposure ceases and this is key to diagnosis.

Treatment

Sun avoidance, sunscreens and antihistamines are useful. PUVA can be helpful as well as phototherapy with UVA or UVB. Desensitization treatments may be carried out in spring but effects may be short-lived and maintenance treatment may be needed.

ACTINIC PRURIGO

Actinic prurigo is a rare condition, which tends to be familial although etiology is unclear. It rarely occurs in Europe and Asia but is seen more commonly in Central and South America.

It often occurs in childhood with papules and excoriation on sun-exposed skin. Conjunctiva and lips can be affected sometimes.

Treatment

Sunscreens, topical steroids, systemic steroids and PUVA are useful. Antimalarials and thalidomide may also be used.

HYDROA VACCINIFORME

Hydroa vacciniforme (HV) is a chronic photodermatosis that usually begins in childhood and resolves spontaneously by early adulthood.

Clinically the lesions follow a distinct clinical pattern. After exposure to sunlight, child develops pruritus, erythema and swelling on exposed parts. Later, they develop tender papules which become vesicular (hydroa) and tense. Gradually, they become umbilicated and hemorrhagic and subsequently form crust (which seems to follow clinical course of chickenpox, hence it is named vacciniforme). The crust separates out in about a week leaving behind depressed chickenpox-like scars (Figure 10.10).

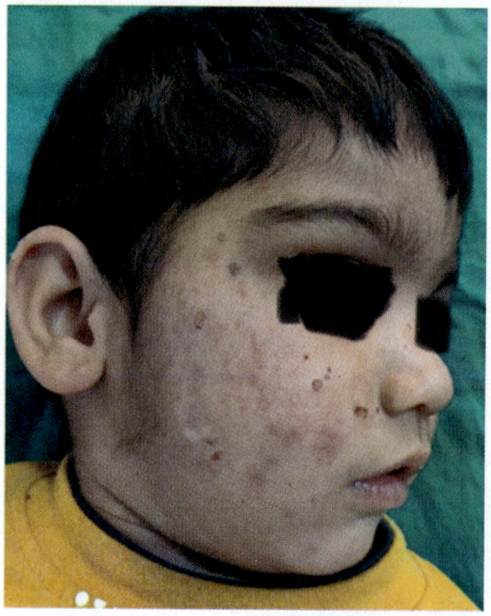

Figure 10.10: Hydroa vacciniforme

Treatment

Sunscreens, topical steroids, systemic steroids and PUVA therapy should be used. Antimalarials may also be used.

NUTRITIONAL DEFICIENCY PHOTODERMATOSES

Pellagra (Figure 10.11) is due to inadequate dietary intake of niacin or its precursor (tryptophan). It is usually seen in children with malabsorption syndromes and in adolescents with anorexia nervosa. Apart from systemic symptoms, child may develop dermatitis plaques confined to sun exposed sites, e.g., face, neck, dorsal surface of hands and feet. The plaques are well defined, which subside and leave dusky brown-red discoloration. On the neck, the plaque appears as broad collarette of erythematous pigmented rash known as *Casal's necklace*. Measurement of the urinary excretion of N1- methyl nicotinamide and/or pyridine is helpful in suspected cases. Treatment of pellagra consists of administration of high-protein diet and nicotinic acid or nicotinamide. If good diet is maintained, complete recovery is the rule.

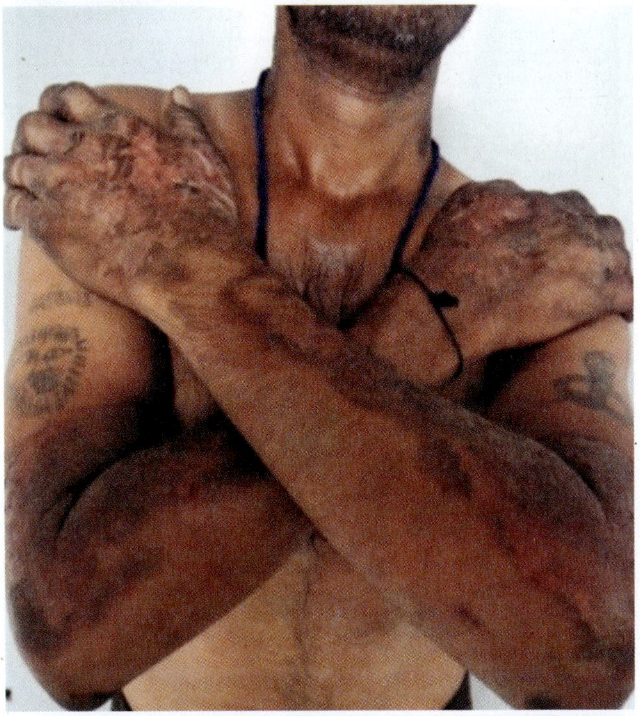

Figure 10.11: Pellagra

METABOLIC PHOTODERMATOSES

Congenital erythropoietic porphyria (CEP) or Gunther's disease manifests during infancy. It is a rare autosomal recessive disease characterized by cutaneous fragility, photosensitivity and tendency for scarring and mutilation. Children develop photosensitivity (redness and burning) on exposed parts of the body followed by blisters, which heal by scarring. Hypertrichosis, hemolytic anemia, progressive splenomegaly, photophobia, excessive tearing, keratoconjunctivitis, loss of eyelashes and ectropion may occur. The urine is dark and deciduous teeth are red in color (erythrodontia). The disease is slowly progressive in nature and has mutilating tendency.

Erythropoietic protoporphyria (EPP) is an autosomal dominant disorder characterized by photosensitivity, which is variable and unpredictable. Often the parents are unaware of their child's photosensitivity. The age of onset is between 3-5 years. The child develops pain immediately after exposure to sunlight. The skin gradually becomes yellowish, thickened and waxed over dorsa of hands and feet.

Hartnup disease is a rare inborn error of metabolism with autosomal recessive inheritance. It is characterized by pellagra like cutaneous eruptions, neurologic abnormalities and a specific aminoaciduria. Cerebellar ataxia is a prominent feature which manifests as unsteady, wide-based gait.

GENETIC PHOTODERMATOSES

These disorders are differentiated from each other on the basis of their clinical features and age of presentation.

Xeroderma pigmentosum (XP) is characterized by photosensitivity, photodamage and cutaneous malignancies. The cells of patient with XP have defect in DNA repair. Generalized progressive freckling and photophobia are common presenting features.

Children with **Cockayne's syndrome** look cachectic and dwarf. Weight is more affected than height, hence it is termed "cachectic dwarfism". Freckling and cutaneous malignancies are not features of Cockayne's syndrome as compared to XP.

Bloom's syndrome is characterized by growth retardation, immunodeficiency, photosensitivity, telangiectasia and pigmentation.

Kindler syndrome is characterized by acral blister formation in infancy and childhood, photosensitivity, generalized progressive poikiloderma. Characteristically, the photosensitivity and blister formation improves with age.

Children suffering from **Rothmund-Thomson syndrome** may have transient photosensitivity, short stature, sparse hair, hypoplastic nails, cataract, hypogonadism and mid face hypoplasia.

AUTOIMMUNE PHOTOSENSITIVE DISORDERS

The connective tissue diseases, which manifest in childhood with photosensitivity are lupus erythematosus and juvenile dermatomyositis (Chapter 15).

EXOGENOUS PHOTODERMATOSES

Drug-induced Photosensitivity

Photosensitivity reactions can occur as adverse effects of some commonly prescribed topical or systemic medications. Reactions can be phototoxic (where the damage to the tissues is direct), or photoallergic (where the damage is immunologically mediated).

Lichenoid reactions, subacute cutaneous lupus erythematosus or pseudoporphyria can also occur. Commonly implicated medications include:

- **Antibiotics:** Tetracyclines, fluoroquinolones, sulfonamides.
- Non-steroidal anti-inflammatory drugs.
- **Diuretics:** Furosemide, bumetanide.
- **Antidiabetics:** Sulfonylureas.
- **Neuroleptics:** Phenothiazines.
- **Antifungals:** Terbinafine, griseofulvin, itraconazole, voriconazole.
- **Other drugs:** Amiodarone, enalapril, oral contraceptives, diltiazem.

Phototoxic reactions tend to be more common and resemble severe sunburn. Their onset can be rapid.

Photoallergic reactions tend to resemble allergic contact dermatitis and they can have delayed onset (24-72 hours).

Lichenoid reactions appear as erythematous, violaceous papules and plaques. Hydroxychloroquine and captopril are common culprit drugs.

Lupus-like reactions resembling subacute cutaneous lupus erythematosus can occur with some drugs, e.g., hydrochlorothiazide, calcium channel blockers, ACE inhibitors and some antifungal agents.

Treatment

- Topical corticosteroids, systemic, if severe.
- Sunscreens (if they are not the cause of the photosensitivity).
- Avoidance of causative agent.

Complications of repeated phototoxic injury include premature skin ageing and increased risk of skin cancer.

PHYTOPHOTODERMATITIS

This is a photosensitivity reaction caused by exposure to certain plants (either due to ingestion or contact with skin) followed by exposure to sunlight. Common plants causing phytophotodermatitis are:

- Celery.
- Giant hogweed.
- Parsley.
- Parsnip.
- Angelica.
- Mustard.
- Chrysanthemums.
- Lime, lemon, fig.
- Fennel, dill, anise, etc.

Burning erythema and blistering occur about 24 hours after exposure. Pruritus is not usual. The patients show diffuse erythema, vesiculation and sometimes edema over exposed parts of the body (Figure 10.12). Desquamation and hyperpigmentation may follow. The disease shows seasonal variation and is usually self-limiting.

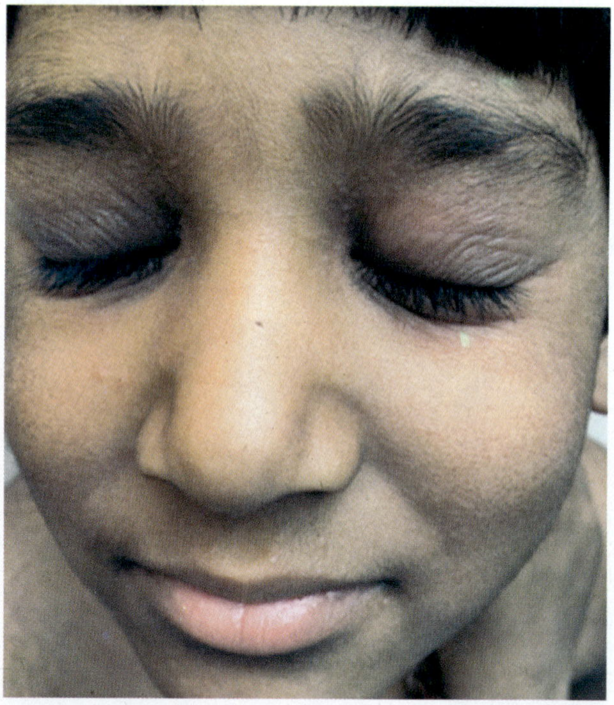

Figure 10.12: Phyto photodermatitis change

Treatment

Avoidance of plants and sunlight.

Topical steroids and sunscreens are useful, systemic steroids and azathioprine may be required for severe and persistent cases.

PHOTOSENSITIVITY AND HIV INFECTION

Photosensitivity is seen when CD4 + T cells count is less than 200 and more commonly when CD4 + T cells count is less than 50.

Photosensitivity may be associated with ingestion of photosensitizing medication especially NSAIDs, trimethoprim- sulfamethoxazole but the skin eruption often does not improve even when the medication is discontinued.

CHAPTER 11 Urticaria and Reactive Erythemas

Contents

Urticaria is defined as transient, evanescent, erythematous or oedematous swellings of the dermis usually associated with itching. It is not a disease entity but is a common reaction pattern to various kinds of stimuli.

Epidemiology

Urticaria and angioedema are common disorders (1 to 2% of the patients in general dermatological practice). The incidence of the problem is about 15-20% in general population. Although persons of any age may experience urticaria or angioedema, the lesions occur most frequently after adolescence with the highest incidence in young adults. Recurrent episodes are more prevalent in females.

Pathogenesis

Urticaria is due to local increase in permeability and vasodilatation of vessels, i.e., capillaries and venules.

Histamine is the major mediator of urticaria, which mainly acts by binding to H1 receptors. It is released from mast cells, which get activated by allergic or non-allergic pathway.

Histamine and other mediators act upon H1 and other receptors present in the skin and induce erythema, flare and weal response. H2 receptors may also contribute. Other inflammatory cells attracted by chemoattractant mast cell derivatives may amplify and prolong the weals.

Non-allergic activation occurs by neuropeptides such as substance P, some foods, e.g., strawberries, drugs like morphine, codeine and vancomycin etc.

Allergic mast cell activation occurs by a variety of agents which could be responsible for majority of cases of acute and chronic urticaria. IgE receptors on mast cells play an important role in causing immediate hypersensitivity response resulting in urticaria.

Besides histamine, other mast cell secreted substances like PGD2, LTC4, IL-4, TNF-alpha may also contribute in the evolution of urticaria.

Etiological Factors

1. **Genetic:** Mutations in histamine related genes, such as FcεRI and HNMT (Histamine N methyl transferase), have been proposed to play a role in histamine metabolism and mast cell activation. Leukotriene overproduction has been proposed as a pathogenic mechanism and several genetic variants of leukotriene related genes, including ALOX5, LTC4S and the PGE2 receptor gene, prostaglandin E receptor 4 (PTGER 4) gene, have been linked to it.

   Autosomal dominant trait: Angioedema caused by C1 esterase deficiency.

   Autosomal dominant trait: Cold urticaria and physical urticaria.

   Association of HLA-DR4 has been found in chronic idiopathic urticarias.
2. **Allergic and immunological.**
3. **Insect bite: Papular urticaria.**
4. **Physical agents**
   - Pressure
   - Vibration
   - Heat
   - Cold
   - Sunlight
   - Exercise.
5. **Emotional stress:** Stress and depression may aggravate or induce urticaria.
6. **Medications:** Any drug may cause urticaria. However, common drugs include penicillin, nonsteroidal anti-inflammatory drugs (aspirin, indomethacin), sulfonamides, thiazide diuretics, oral contraceptives, angiotensin converting enzyme inhibitors, codeine, morphine, curare and its derivatives, radiocontrast substances.
7. **Infections and infestations:** Sinusitis, tonsillitis, sore throat, dental abscesses, urinary tract infection, hepatitis, infectious mononucleosis, and parasites (Ankylostoma, strongyloides, echinococcus) may cause urticaria.
8. **Food:** Nuts, eggs, fish, seafood, chocolate, meat, cow's milk, fruits (strawberries, bananas, apples, plums, pineapples, and citrus fruits), vegetables (carrots, peas, beans, and garlic), mushrooms, fermented foods, spices, and spirits. Important causal factors include preservatives such food colours, azo dyes, salicylates, and derivatives of benzoic acid.
9. **Inhalants:** Grass, pollens, mould, spores, animal danders and house dust etc.
10. **Implants:** Dental prosthesis and metal pins.
11. **Systemic diseases:** Thyroid diseases and connective tissue diseases such as systemic lupus erythematosus, Sjogren syndrome, rheumatoid arthritis, lymphoma, leukaemia, etc.
12. **Latex and latex products:** Cause contact urticaria.
13. **Idiopathic:** Urticaria due to unknown cause.

Clinical Manifestations

In general, urticaria is characterized by circumscribed, raised, erythematous to pale pink edematous swellings. Edema involves the superficial portion of the dermis only. Weal is a transient, well demarcated superficial pink or pale swelling of dermis due to reversible exudation of plasma in skin that fades within hours without leaving a mark.

When the edematous process extends into the deep dermis and/or subcutaneous and submucosal layers, it is known as *angioedema.*

Anaphylaxis is a sudden, severe, life-threatening, systemic reaction often involving the skin due to mast cell mediator release, which may be allergic or non-allergic.

Pruritus is intense, with a desire to rub the lesions rather than to itch.

The individual lesions of urticaria arise suddenly which usually do not persist longer than 24 to 48 hours. Urticaria may continue to recur for indefinite period.

Systemic symptoms: Headache, dizziness, sensation of a lump in the throat, hoarseness, wheezing, shortness of breath, nausea, vomiting, abdominal pain, diarrhea, arthralgia may occur.

ASSOCIATIONS OF URTICARIA

Urticaria may associated with other autoimmune diseases like:

- Thyroid disease
- Celiac disease
- Diabetes mellitus
- Connective tissue diseases (Systemic lupus erythematosus, Rheumatoid arthritis, Sjogren syndrome, dermatomyositis)
- Vitiligo

Classification of Urticaria

Ordinary urticaria

- Acute
- Intermediate/episodic
- Chronic

Immune complex urticaria

- Serum sickness
- Urticarial vasculitis
- Papular urticaria
- Physical and cholinergic urticaria
- Contact urticaria
- Angioedema

ORDINARY URTICARIA

Acute Urticaria

Episodes of lesions of less than 6 to 8 weeks duration are considered *acute* whereas those with longer duration are termed *chronic.*

Acute idiopathic urticaria (Figure 11.1): In more than 50% of patients with acute urticaria, no well-defined cause is identified.

Acute allergic urticaria (Immunologic IgE and IgE receptor-dependent urticaria): It is IgE mediated hypersensitivity reaction in individuals with a personal or family history of asthma, rhinitis or eczema. This can be provoked by antigens such as foods, shellfish, nuts and chocolate, drugs and therapeutic agents, notably penicillin, aeroallergens, and Hymenoptera venom. Urticaria in patients with helminthic infestations has also been attributed to IgE-dependent processes.

Acute non-allergic urticaria: This is a non-IgE dependent urticaria. The histamine release is non-immunological, and is due to intolerance to certain substances, therefore can occur after first time exposure to substance.

Urticaria in patients receiving radiographic contrast media, opiate analgesics, polymyxin B, curare and *d*-tubocurarine, angiotensin-converting enzyme (ACE) inhibitors, hepatitis B virus infection, streptococcal throat infections in children and Epstein-Barr virus infection are due to non-allergic release of histamine.

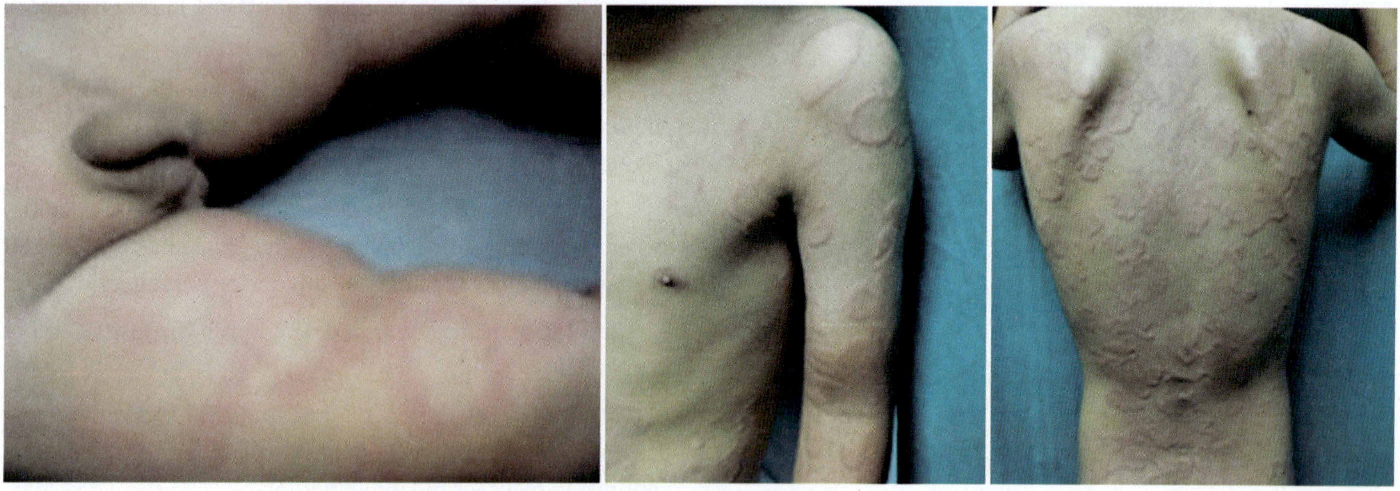

Figure 11.1: Acute urticaria

Episodes of urticaria last upto one week and may be associated with fever and arthralgia.

Chronic Urticaria

Wheals (Figure 11.2) are present on most days for longer than 6 weeks. Most of chronic urticarias are idiopathic or have some autoimmune basis.

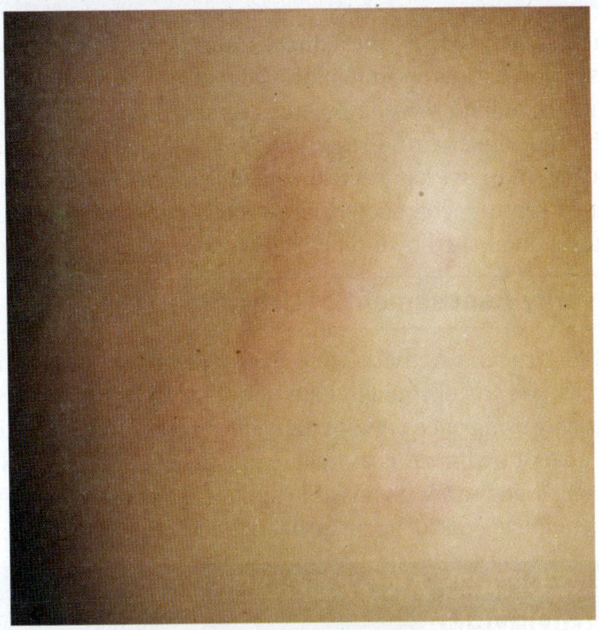

Figure 11.2: Chronic urticaria

IMMUNE COMPLEX MEDIATED URTICARIA

Serum Sickness

It is a type III hypersensitivity reaction, resulting from the administration of heterologous serum to humans. Serum sickness occurs 7 to 21 days after the administration of the offending agents like vaccination, antivenom, rituximab etc. It is manifested by fever, urticaria, lymphadenopathy, myalgia, arthralgia and arthritis. Symptoms are usually self-limiting and last for 4 to 5 days.

Urticarial Vasculitis

In urticarial vasculitis cutaneous lesions resemble with that of the urticaria with histological evidence of leukocytoclastic vasculitis. It is type III hypersensitivity reaction, which is generally idiopathic but in few cases it is associated with hepatitis B, hepatitis C, EBV and collagen vascular diseases. The lesions last for more than 48 hours, while in urticaria lesions resolve within 48 hours. It is rare in children (peak incidence is in fourth decade). Urticaria and urticarial vasculitis difference given in below Table 11.1.

Table 11.1: Differences between urticaria and urticarial vasculitis

	Urticarial vasculitis	*Urticaria*
Pain and burning sensation	Present	Absent
Duration of wheal	>24 hours	<24 hours
Residual changes	Residual bruise like changes or pigmentation usually present	No residual changes seen
Systemic symptoms	Usually present like abdominal pain, arthritis	Absent
Laboratory findings	Increased acute phase reactant e.g. CRP	Acute phase reactant are normal
Histology	Findings of vasculitis present	No vasculitis features

- **Papular urticaria (Immediate IgE mediated reaction):** Papular urticaria consists of wheals due to injection of foreign protein by insect bite in sensitive subjects. This reaction may sometimes evolve into a delayed hypersensitivity reaction resulting into multiple erythematous papules commonly seen on the legs and on exposed parts of children.

PHYSICAL URTICARIA

1. **Dermographism:** It is the most common form of physical urticaria. It appears as a linear weal with a flare at sites at which the skin is briskly stroked with a firm object (Figure 11.3). A transient weal appears rapidly and usually fades within 30 minutes.

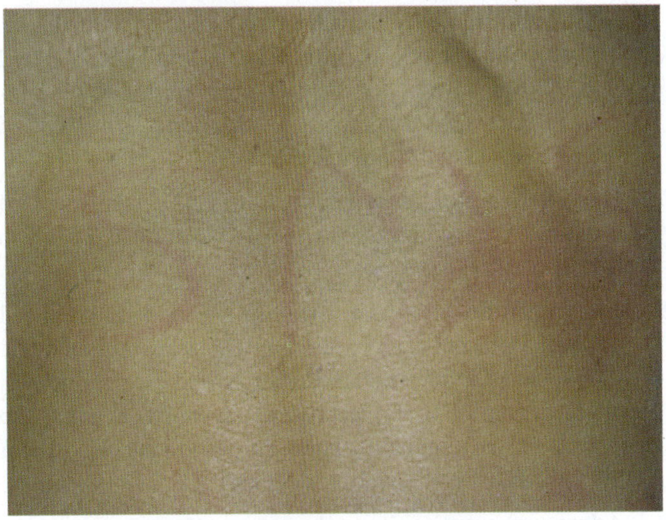

Figure 11.3: Dermographism

Types of Dermographism

- **Delayed dermographism:** Develops 3 to 6 hours after stimulation, either with or without an immediate reaction, and lasts for 24 to 48 hours. The clinical eruption is composed of linear red nodules.
- **Symptomatic/factitious urticaria.**
- **Cholinergic dermographism:** A rare form that develops as punctate wheals.

2. **Pressure urticaria:** Pressure urticaria appears as erythematous, deep local swellings, often painful. It arises after 30 minutes to 6 hours, if constant pressure has been applied to the skin and may be associated with fever, chills and arthralgia as well as with an elevated ESR.
3. **Vibratory angioedema:** It occurs as an acquired idiopathic disorder in association with cholinergic urticaria, or after several years of occupational exposure to vibration.
4. **Cold-induced urticaria:** Out of acquired and inherited forms of cold-induced urticaria/angioedema, acquired forms are more common. Attacks occur within minutes after the appropriate exposures that include cold foods or liquids, application of ice and changes in ambient temperature. The elicitation of a wheal after the application of ice is called *cold contact test.*
5. **Solar urticaria:** It develops within minutes after exposure to the sun or artificial light sources. Symptoms of pruritus, erythema, wheals, are occasionally accompanied by angioedema with bronchospasm and syncope.
6. **Cholinergic urticaria:** Cholinergic urticaria is also known as *generalized heat urticaria.* It develops after an increase in core body temperature, such as during a warm bath or shower, exercise, or episodes of pyrexia, etc. The eruption appears as distinctive, pruritic, small, 1 to 2 mm wheals, surrounded by erythema. Systemic features may include dizziness, headache, wheezing, shortness of breath, nausea, vomiting and diarrhea.
7. **Heat urticaria:** Local heat urticaria is a rare form of urticaria. Wheals develop within minutes of exposure to locally applied heat.
8. **Exercise-induced anaphylaxis:** Exercise induced urticaria presents as pruritus, urticaria, angioedema (cutaneous, laryngeal and intestinal), and syncope that is distinct from cholinergic urticaria. In most patients, the wheals are not punctate but are larger in size. There is a high prevalence of an atopic diathesis.
9. **Adrenergic urticaria:** Adrenergic urticaria occurs as wheals surrounded by a white halo and develops during emotional stress. The lesions can be elicited by the intracutaneous injection of noradrenaline.
10. **Aquagenic urticaria and aquagenic pruritus:** Contact of the skin with water of any temperature results in pruritus alone or rarely, urticaria. The eruption consists of small wheals reminiscent of cholinergic urticaria.

CONTACT URTICARIA

Urticaria may occur after direct contact with a variety of substances, e.g., latex proteins, powder in gloves, food and food additives, animal secretions, drugs, grass, pollen, caterpillars, fungi and algae. Cross-reactivity to fruits such as bananas, avocado and kiwi has been found. Associated manifestations include rhinitis, conjunctivitis, dyspnea and shock. The risk group is dominated by biomedical workers.

Severity Assessment of Urticaria

UAS7 (Urticaria Activity score over 7 days) assesses the itch severity and wheal count in chronic spontaneous urticaria over a week by using once or twice daily diary based documentation. The goal of treatment is to treat the disease until it is cured, as efficiently and safely as possible aiming at a continuous UAS7 = 0, complete control and a normalization of quality of life.

HEREDITARY AND ACQUIRED ANGIOEDEMA

It is a dominantly inherited disorder which is characterized by recurrent attacks of angioedema involving skin (Figure 11.4), mucous membranes, respiratory and gastrointestinal tracts. Urticaria is not a manifestation. There is a functional deficiency of the inhibitor of the activated first component (C_1) of the complement system.

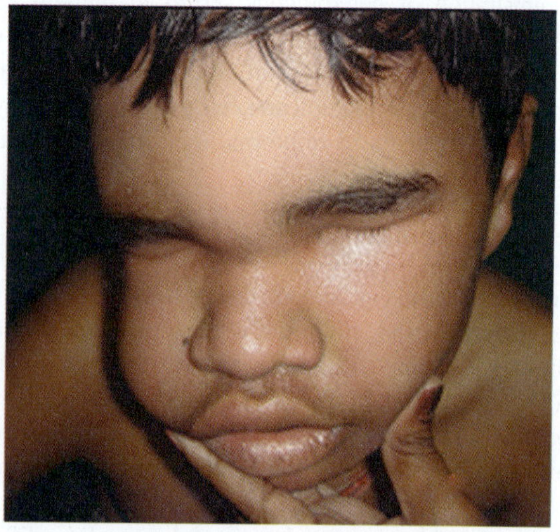

Figure 11.4: Angioedema

Angioedema without Wheal

It is characterized by recurrent deep localized swelling of subcutaneous tissue or submucosal tissue (lips, eyelids, genitalia, respiratory tract and gastrointestinal tract). It is of two types:

- **Acquired angioedema**
- **Hereditary angioedema**

Acquired Angioedema: It is classified into three different types:

1. **Idiopathic:** No cause can be identified. These patients have normal C1INH and there is no familial history of angioedema. It is of two types:

   A. ***Idiopathic Histamine responsive – Acquired Angioedema (IH-AAE):*** These patients respond to antihistamines.

   B. ***Idiopathic Histamine non responsive – Acquired Angioedema (I non H-AAE):*** No Response to antihistamines.

2. **Drug induced:**

   A. ***ACE (Angiotensin Converting Enzyme) inhibitor induced AAE:***

   ACE inhibitors may cause angioedema by inhibiting ACE which results in reduced bradykinin metabolism. Most cases develop within 3 weeks of commencing treatment but can occur at any time even after more than 10 years. It is rare with angiotensin receptor blockers.

   B. ***NSAIDs induced AAE:***

   NSAIDs specific IgE antibodies binds to high affinity IgE receptor on surface of mast cells, thereby triggering massive production of inflammatory mediators causing angioedema.

3. **Acquired C1 inhibitor deficiency:**

   This is most commonly seen in patients older than 40 years. They have no family history of angioedema. It can occur either due to continuous complementary system activation (e. g lymphoproliferative disease) or due to C1 inhibitor autoantibodies (systemic lupus erythematosus, Sjogren syndrome etc).

Hereditary Angioedema

This rare disorder presents with recurrent swelling of the skin and mucous membranes throughout life, often associated with nausea, vomiting, colic and urinary symptoms. These attacks may occurs regularly within every few days or weeks. Abdominal symptoms may occur in the absence of skin changes and cause great diagnostic difficulty. A positive family history is usually present. Oestrogen contraception and hormone replacement therapy usually exacerbates it. It is classified into three types:

Type 1: Genetic C1 esterase inhibitor deficiency or low concentration (C1 INH-HAE).

TYPE II: Normal C1 esterase INH with low activity.

Type III: Normal concentration and activity of C1 esterase INH but it is inhibited by autoantibodies. Clinically patients present with recurrent episodes of angioedema. Family history of angioedema is present in more than one generation.

Clinical Variants

Clarkson syndrome (Systemic capillary leak syndrome)

This uncommon condition is characterised by recurrent episodes of fluid leakage into many organs, including the skin. There have been reports of angioedema. There is an increased possibility of developing a severe shock-like state and death rates are high. Immunoglobulin G (IgG) paraproteinaemia is present.

Gleich syndrome (Episodic angioedema with eosinophilia)

There have been reports of recurrent bouts of angioedema linked to pyrexia, blood eosinophilia, and eosinophil infiltration of the dermis. It is a known consequence in hypereosinophilic syndrome, however there is no indication of systemic involvement or progression to cardiomyopathy. Treatment with prednisolone ends each episode.

Investigations

Investigations are usually normal in majority of the patients of urticaria. Routinely they should be avoided in acute urticaria but in cases of chronic urticaria following guidelines may be used:

In all patients:

- Detailed history and physical examination.
- Provocative tests for physical urticaria.

In selected patients as per findings of history and physical examination:

- Complete blood count with differential count.
- Erythrocyte sedimentation rate.
- Liver function tests, hepatitis viral markers.
- Antinuclear factor and other tests for collagen vascular disorders.
- Thyroid function tests.

- Serum antibodies against different environmental antigens, e.g., food, plants, drugs etc. (RAST) is not of much help.
- Urinalysis with culture and sensitivity.
- Stool examination for ova and parasites.

Table 11.2: Important history points in urticaria patients

History point to be elicited in urticaria patients	*Associated diseases with chronic urticaria*
• Duration of urticaria • Frequency of wheal • Diurnal variations • Seasonal variations • Duration of individual lesions • History of exposure to contact allergens • Symptoms of pain, burning • Residual changes • History of angioedema • Familial of personal history of atopy and urticaria • Physical stimuli • History of constitutional symptoms	• Thyroid disease • Celiac disease • Diabetes mellitus • Connective tissue diseases (Systemic lupus erythematosus, Rheumatoid arthritis, Sjogren syndrome, dermatomyositis) • Vitiligo

Differential Diagnosis

- Erythema multiforme.
- Bullous pemphigoid.
- Urticaria pigmentosa.
- Cellulitis and thrombophlebitis.
- Other causes for edematous conditions resembling angioedema, i.e., congestive heart failure, renal insufficiency, myxedema, etc.

Treatment

An approach to the management of chronic urticaria/ angioedema includes:

- Identification and removal of precipitating cause whenever possible.
- Administration of H1 and H2 antihistamines.
- Systemic glucocorticoids for moderate to severe unresponsive episodes.
- Avoidance of epinephrine except in instances of respiratory tract compromise or cardiovascular collapse.

First Line Therapy

Treatment of acute urticaria: With meticulous history of the patient the cause of urticaria may be elicited in majority of patients with acute urticaria. Therefore, it is worth removal of all suspected triggers (e.g., infections, drugs, food, drinks and inhalants, etc.).

Antihistaminic drugs: Non-sedating antihistamines should be given as first line of treatment. They may be combined with sedating type of antihistamines when required. Non sedating newer generation anti-histamines can be given in day time and sedating one at night time.

Oral steroids can be administered periodically in cases not controlled by antihistamines. Few resistant cases may require other immunosuppressant, e.g., cyclophosphamide in addition to oral corticosteroids.

Treatment of chronic urticaria: Non-sedative anti-histaminics alone or with combination of sedating and non-sedating drugs along with H2 blockers are to be given as per need of patients.

The role of steroids in chronic urticaria is controversial but still it can be worth tried in severe or refractory cases.

Antibiotic, antifungal and anthelmintic therapy may help in eliminating infections as a cause of chronic cases.

These may be prescribed even empirically in cases of chronic urticaria.

Treatment of physical urticaria: In the treatment of the physical urticarias, awareness and avoidance of the inciting stimulus are important. Antihistamines used prophylactically are helpful in some forms of physical urticaria.

In hereditary angioedema, therapy is directed towards treatment of the acute attack, to preoperative, prophylaxis, e.g., dental surgery, and to chronic prophylactic suppression of attacks.

Second Line Therapy (Targeted Therapy)

Mast cell inhibitors like ketotifen and cromolyn sodium may be tried. Oral steroids are prescribed in resistant cases. Leukotriene receptor antagonists have been shown to benefit in aspirin sensitive urticaria and may be of value in delayed pressure urticaria and autoimmune urticaria when added to antihistamines. Doxepin, a tricyclic antidepressant with H1 and H2 antihistaminic activity, has been used at night in a starting dose of 10-30 mg.

Third Line Therapy (Immunomodulatory)

Intravenous immunoglobulin (IVIG) infusions, at 0.4 g/kg/day for 5 days (total 2 g), cyclosporin, tacrolimus, mycophenolate mofetil, methotrexate and cyclophosphamide are indicated in chronic resistant urticaria.

Fourth Line Therapy

Many large phase III trials of omalizumab (anti-IgE) have shown very good results in H1 antihistamine unresponsive chronic spontaneous urticaria.

Newer Therapy for Urticaria

Dupilumab (block IL-4R alpha subunit of IL-4 and IL-13), Mepolizumab (IL-5 antagonist) and Benralizumab (act on IL-5 receptors on basophils and eosinophils) are off label drugs which are recently being used in treatment of chronic spontaneous urticaria.

Management of Angioedema

The management of mast cell mediator induced angioedema is essentially the same as for chronic spontaneous urticaria patients with wheals.

Hereditary angioedema with normal C1INH is an emergency. The following can be tried:

- Icatibant (bradykinin receptor 2 antagonist).
- Plasma derived C1INH.
- Recombinant C1INH.
- Ecallantide (kallikrein inhibitor).
- Plasma derived C1INH.
- Tranexamic acid.
- Anabolic steroids (danazol, stanozolol).

Acquired C1INH deficiency is also an emergency and can be treated with:

- Plasma derived C1INH.
- Bradykinin receptor 2 antagonist–Icatibant.

Management of Anaphylaxis

Injection of epinephrine via the intramuscular/subcutaneous route is the treatment of choice in anaphylaxis. Diluted epinephrine (1:1000) should be given IM into the anterolateral thigh at a dose of 0.01 mg/kg, and can be repeated every 5 min to 15 min.

Children with systemic allergic reactions should carry epinephrine autoinjectors at all times. Children and their families need to be educated about the proper usage of the emergency devices.

Initial management of the pediatric patient with anaphylaxis should include a thorough, rapid assessment of the airway, breathing and circulation, with immediate administration of IM epinephrine.

PLAN FOR MANAGEMENT OF URTICARIA IN CHILDREN

- Children have acute urticaria more commonly than chronic urticaria. They should be given one course of deworming agents (albendazole) and antibiotics to eliminate the possibility of infection (Streptococcal sore throat) and infestations, which may be an important cause in this age group.
- Sedative antihistamines, e.g., hydroxyzine, chlorpheniramine, dexchlorpheniramine may be used in preschool children. These antihistamines act well and sedation is not a major concern in children of this age group. These antihistamines should also be the first choice for infants in syrup form.
- School going children require attention in school and during studies, so newer non-sedating antihistamines, e.g., cetirizine or levocetirizine should be the first choice.

They can be prescribed once a day or twice a day as per the patient's need. They can be given in syrup form in infants also:

- In patients who respond poorly to one group of antihistamines, can be managed by combining two different group of antihistamines. Combination of conventional antihistamines, e.g., cetirizine with 5-HT antagonist, cyproheptadine works well in many cases. Cyproheptadine has disadvantage of causing sedation.
- Third generation antihistamines, e.g., fexofenadine which are very less sedative, can also be used. They are costlier, which may be a disadvantage in patients who require long-term therapy in chronic urticaria. They can be combined with conventional antihistamines and cyproheptadine in refractory cases of urticaria.
- Steroids have not much role in the management of urticaria. They can be given as short course in severe refractory cases.
- Role of food and food additives is not clear in children. Different prick and serological tests are not much useful. Patients can be advised to avoid colouring agents, chocolates, cold drinks, processed foods etc. especially in patients with chronic urticaria.

REACTIVE INFLAMMATORY ERYTHEMAS

Multiple skin conditions can present with arcuate, annular, circinate, figurate, gyrate, polycyclic, reticular and serpiginous pattern due to reactive changes occurring in skin. They tend to spread peripherally while complete or partial clearing occurs centrally. Various diseases included under this term are:

- Erythema multiforme.
- Annular erythema of infancy.
- Erythema annulare centrifugum.
- Erythema gyratum repens.
- Erythema marginatum.
- Necrolytic migratory erythema.

Annular Erythema of Infancy

It is similar to erythema annulare centrifugum which occurs in young individuals, may start in infancy which has a self-limiting course without systemic symptoms. Clinically it presents as polycyclic annular erythematous plaques, expanding upto 2-3 mm/days with central clearing. Lesions are localized to the face, trunk and proximal limbs, individual lesion lasts from two to several days. New lesions may appear in cyclic pattern, every 5-6 weeks. Heavy intestinal colonization of candida albicans, Malassezia infection and Epstein Barr virus infection etc have been considered to be triggering factors. Histologically dermal perivascular and interstitial lymphocytic infiltrates is seen. Treatment includes topical corticosteroids and calcineurin inhibitors.

Erythema Annulare Centrifugum

Clinically it presents as annular polycyclic erythematous plaques of variable size with scaling over advancing edge (Figure 11.5). Lesions first appears as erythematous indurated papules that slowly enlarge to form a ring or arciform lesion, as the central area flattens and fades. The lesions may be static a varied rate of expansion (usually 2-3 mm /day) may be seen to reach maximum size of 6-8 cm. Common sites are buttocks, thighs and arms, lesions may last for few months. EAC is a reactive process which may be precipitated by drugs, infections or malignancy.

EAC is classified into two types:

- **Superficial:** Presents with pruritis and scaling, histology usually shows parakeratosis, spongiosis, epidermal hyperplasia and papillary dermal oedema.
- **Deep:** Presents with non-scaly, non-pruritic lesions, histology shows sleeve like infiltrates, melanophages and necrotic keratinocytes.

Treatment includes topical corticosteroids, topical calcineurin inhibitor and topical vit. D analogues.

Erythema Gyratum Repens

Erythema gyratum repens is a rare disorder due to fibroblast induced ground substance alterations. In around 80% of cases it may be associated with underlying malignancy (bronchial and oesophageal) and is commonly seen in males. Clinically it presents as creeping, mobile (1cm/day), concentric, palpable, erythematous plaques showing wave like bands, trailing scales which gives a wood grain appearance. Ichthyosis and bulla within erythema can also be seen. Severe pruritus is commonly seen on torso. It spares the face, hands and feet. Histology shows hyperkeratosis, parakeratosis, acanthosis and tightly

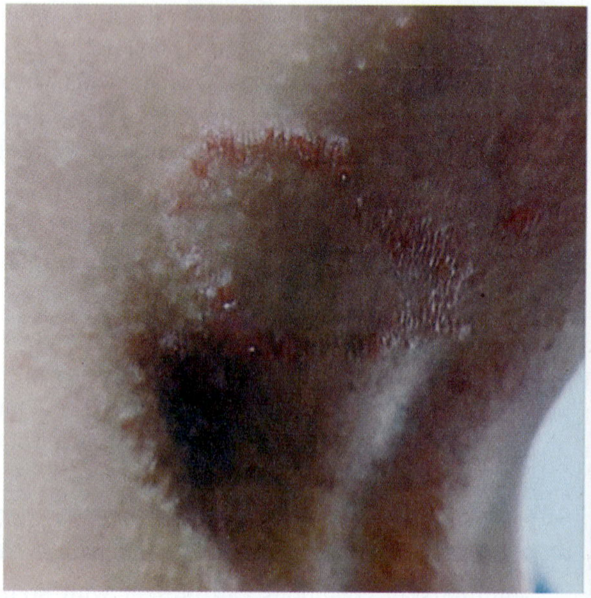

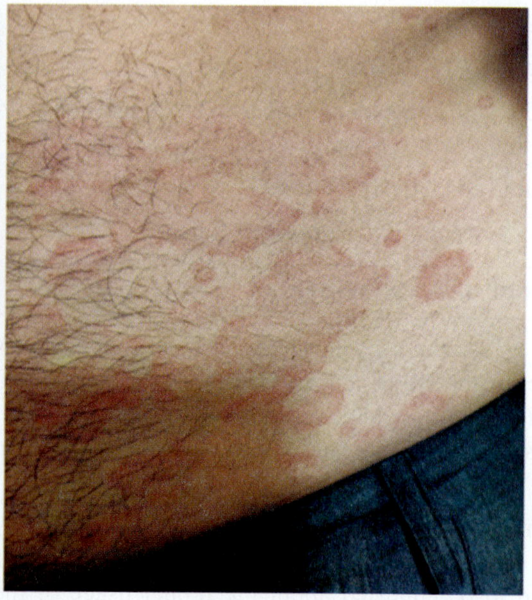

Figure 11.5: Erythema annulare centrifugum

cuffed superficial perivascular infiltrate of lymphocytes with endothelial swelling. Treatment is to identify the underlying cause and treat accordingly.

Necrolytic Migratory Erythema (NME)

- Necrolytic migratory erythema (NME) is due to glucagonomas (glucagon secretory tumours) and reduced levels of histidine and tryptophan amino acid.
- Clinically it presents as annular or arciform erythematous macules and papules associated with pruritus and burning sensation. The lesions enlarge gradually and develop blisters in the central area which erodes and necrotise, leaving behind hyperpigmented areas over groin, lower extremities, trunk and face (perioral and peri anal areas). Other clinical features include cheilitis, beefy erythematous glossitis and dystrophic nails.
- **Glucagonoma syndrome:** Presents with weight loss, sore mouth, diarrhoea, weakness, mental status changes and diabetes mellitus.
- **Pseudo-glucagonoma syndrome:** NME can also be associated with various non glucagonoma secretory conditions e.g. cirrhosis of liver, pancreatitis, celiac disease, inflammatory bowel disease etc.
- Treatment includes somatostatin injections.

Erythema Marginatum

Erythema marginatum, is most frequently seen in patients with acute rheumatic fever. Even though it is an uncommon cutaneous manifestation, acute rheumatic fever and other uncommon illnesses can be accurately diagnosed with it. It is characterised as a nonpruritic, evanescent, blanchable macular rash, that typically affects the trunk and extremities. It is also seen in psittacosis and hereditary angioedema and is a self-limiting condition.

CHAPTER 12 Acne

Contents

INTRODUCTION

Acne vulgaris is an inflammatory disease of adolescence and young adults involving **pilosebaceous** glands, characterized by comedones, papules, pustules, nodules or pseudocysts and later on scars as sequel. It is a disorder of pediatrician's concern also as it is seen commonly in adolescents.

Epidemiology

Acne vulgaris commences around 12-13 years of age, but most of the cases are seen during middle or late teenage. It is often considered as early manifestation of puberty and in females it may precede menarche by about 1 year. The problem may continue into twenties and sometimes in older age groups (some may have the disorder upto thirties). Acne in males is more common in adolescence while females are affected more commonly in adulthood. Acne is prevalent worldwide.

Etiology

Acne is a multifactorial disease although, the basic cause is unknown. There are various factors suggested in the pathogenesis:

Follicular plugging: Overgrowth of epithelium on the follicular opening, due to genetic and environmental factors, results in retention of sebum and increased concentration of bacteria and free fatty acids.

Bacterial colonization: *Propionibacterium acnes,* now known as *Cutibacterium acnes,* colonizes the pilosebaceous ducts and breaks down the triglycerides. The free fatty acid so formed, causes inflammatory changes by type IV immune reaction.

Sebum secretion: The sebum secretion is controlled by the testosterone hormone. The sebaceous glands are unusually more sensitive to androgens, resulting in increased sebum secretion.

Inflammation: Pro-inflammatory cytokines like IL-1 induce follicular epidermal hyperproliferation and comedone formation.

Hormonal: Androgens (to a major extent) and thyroid and growth hormones (to a minor extent) are the main stimulants for excess sebum secretion.

Genetics: The condition is familial in 50% cases with acne.

Clinical Features

Acne is a largely asymptomatic, polymorphic disease but patients may complain of pain and tenderness in the lesions.

The lesions of acne vary from small papules, pustules, comedones, to larger nodules and scars. They can be divided into two types:

Non-inflammatory Lesions

The lesions are comedones, which may be either open or closed comedones.

- ***Open comedones (black heads):*** They appear as flat or slightly raised lesions with central dark colored follicular impaction of keratin and lipid.
- ***Closed comedones (white heads):*** They are pale, slightly elevated small papules and do not have clinically visible orifice.

Other Type of Comedones

- **Submarine comedones:** These are large comedonal structures with a diameter of more than 0.5 cm which are found deeper within recurring inflammatory nodular lesions and are connected to the skin.
- **Sandpaper comedones:** They are several tiny, white heads which are often dispersed across the forehead and have a rough texture.
- **Macrocomedones:** These are large whiteheads with a diameter of more than one millimeter.

Inflammatory Lesions

They vary from small papules to pustules to large tender fluctuant nodules (previously they were called cysts or nodulocystic, but as they are not true cyst, so the term nodules or severe nodular acne is used). Nodules are more common in males. Some patients have multiple nodules, some being quite deep. Sinus formation between nodules may occur. Extensive and disfiguring scars may form on the face and back. Such disease has been named as 'acne conglobata'.

Scars

Scars are sequel of acne, ranging from mild hyperpigmented to extensively depressed and/or hypertrophic (keloidal) scars.

Depressed Scars

Depressed scars occur as a result of loss or damage to tissue.

- **Ice pick scars** are sharp, narrow (<2 mm), deep, depressed scars, wider at the surface and narrow at the base. They extend vertically to deep dermis or subcutaneous tissue. Wider superficial, atrophic scars,1 mm to 4 mm in diameter with irregular edges may also develop.
- **Box scars:** Box scars are wide, spherical to oval depressions with vertical edges which are well defined.
- **Rolling scars:** These are wider scars which may reach up to 5 mm in diameter. Scars look undulating and with superficial shadowing due to fibrous anchorman of the dermis to subcutis.

Elevated Scars

Usually occur as a result of increased tissue formation.

- **Hypertrophic:** Elevated, fibrotic scars, more common in males and frequently seen in the mandibular area of the face and back. They do not extend beyond the original inflammation.
- **Keloidal:** These are keloids developing in acne lesions which extend beyond the extent of original inflammation, are more common in males, on the chest, back and shoulders.
- **Papular:** Raised, papular and fibrotic scars, most commonly seen on the chin and nose.
- **Bridging scars and sinus tracts:** Multiple linear scars, joined together by epithelial tracts containing foul-smelling products of sebum.

Grading of Acne Vulgaris

Lesions of acne can be classified as:

- **Grade I (Mild):** Comedones, occasional papules (Figure 12.1).

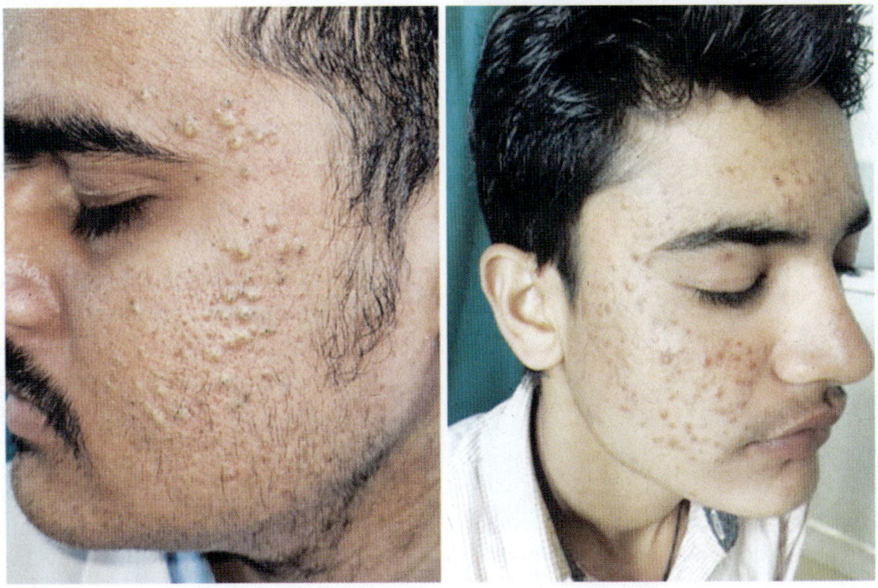

Figure 12.1: Mild grade acne with comedones

- **Grade II (Moderate):** Comedones, papules and few pustules (Figure 12.2).
- **Grade III (Severe):** Pustules, nodules, abscess and cysts (Figure 12.3) with or without widespread scarring (Figure 12.4).

Sites

The predominant site of acne is face and to lesser extent on the shoulders, back, upper chest and upper arm. On the face,

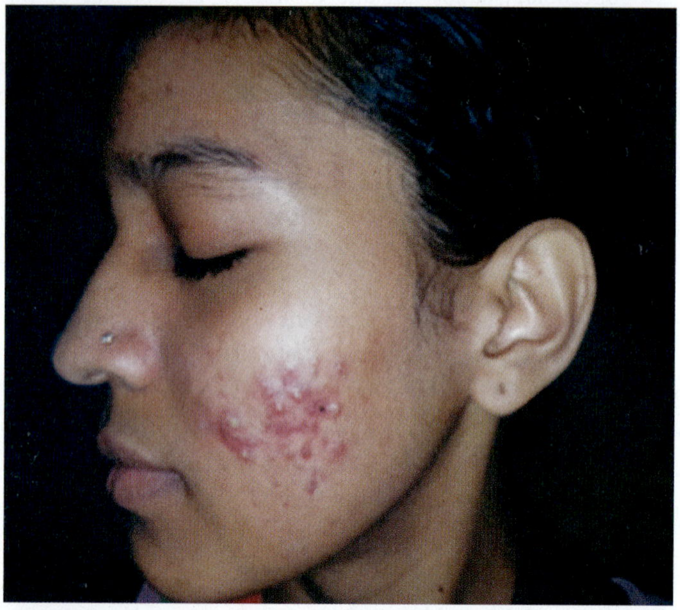

Figure 12.2: Moderate grade acne with papules and pustules

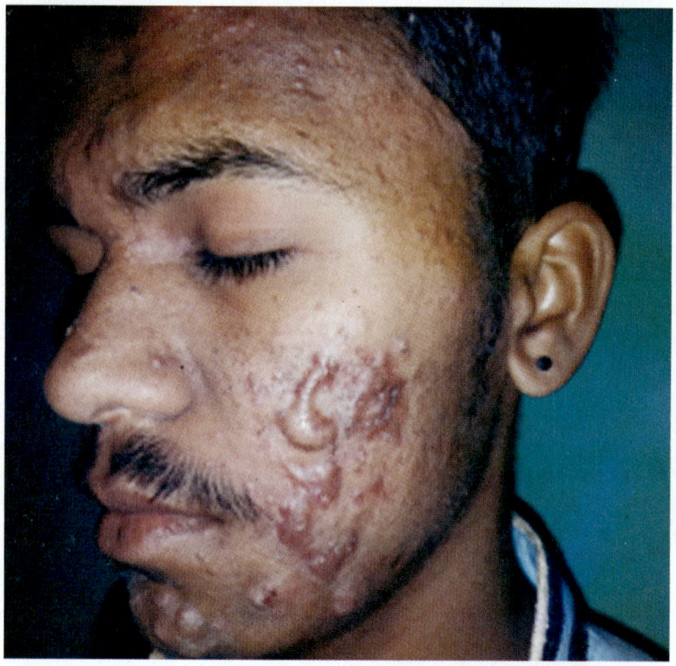

Figure 12.3: Severe grade acne with nodule and cyst formation

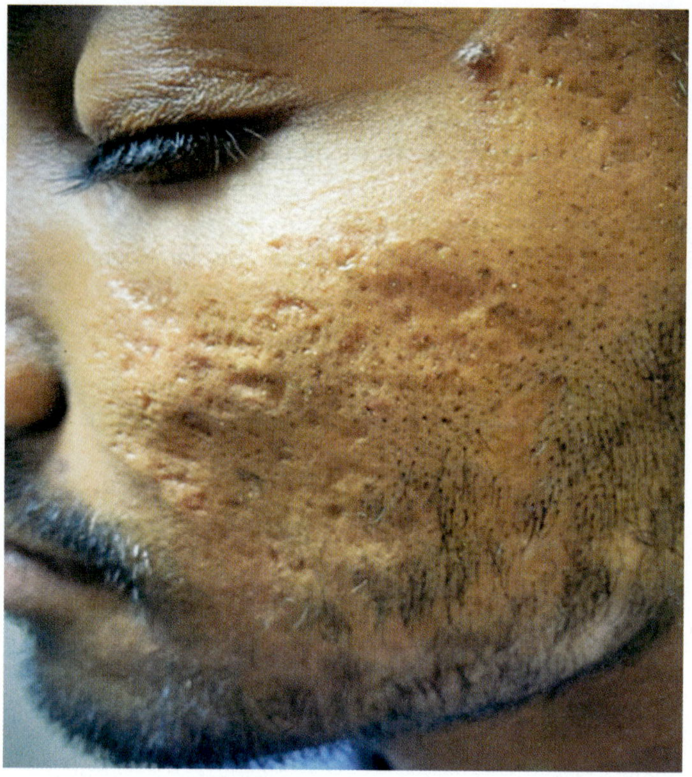

Figure 12.4: Acne scars

cheeks, center of forehead and chin are most commonly affected. If lesions of acne are present on unusual sites then possibility of acneiform eruptions due to drugs should be considered.

VARIANTS OF ACNE

Neonatal acne: It has been renamed as neonatal cephalic pustulosis (NCP). It presents in the first few weeks of life due to influence of maternal hormones, as papules and pustules on the cheeks, chin, eyelids and forehead. Comedones are absent. NCP represents follicular or poral colonization with *Malassezia sympodialis* and *M. globosa*. It is usually self-limiting.

Infantile acne: It is less common than NCP and starts between 3-6 months of age. It is seen more frequently in boys (5:1), due to high testosterone level and may last up to 3 years. It clinically presents with comedones, inflammatory lesions including nodules and cysts, and in some cases, even scars. Treatment includes oral erythromycin and topical clindamycin. Oral isotretinoin is indicated for nodular/scarring infantile acne.

Mid-childhood acne: It occurs between 1-7 years of age and is very rare. Clinically it is similar to infantile acne, but denotes hyperandrogenism.

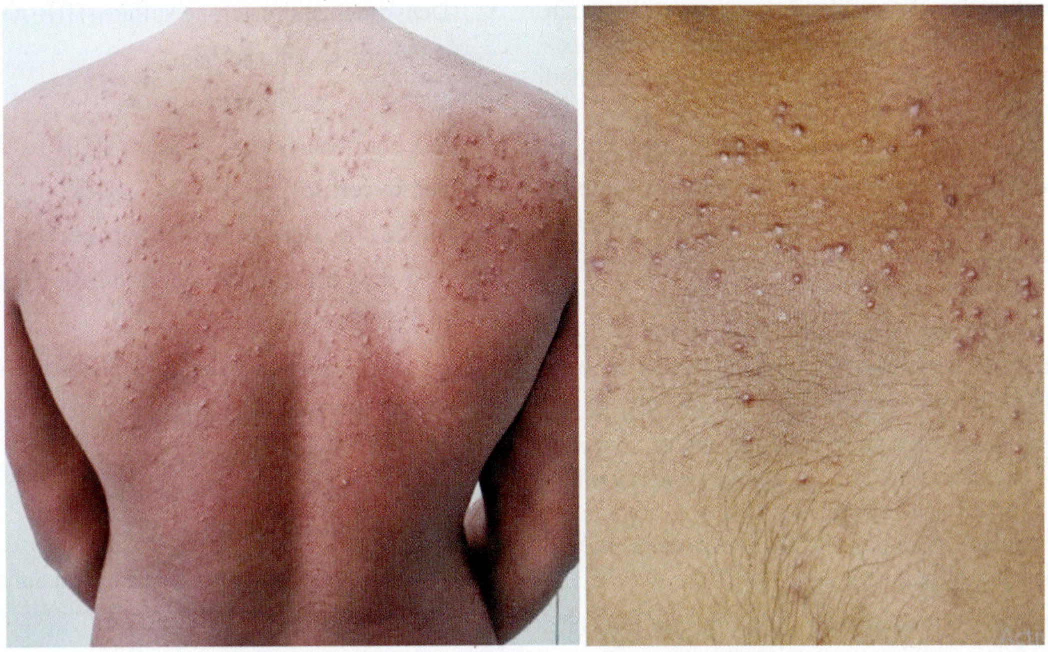

Figure 12.5: Monomorphic lesions in drug induced acne

Prepubertal acne: It represents early adrenarche and may appear as early as at 8 years of age. It is more common in girls. Which is predominantly comedonal. It begins at central part of forehead. Raised levels of DHEAS and free testosterone are found. Macrolides are the treatment of choice. Tetracyclines may be given above the age of 8 years. Cephalexin is an option in less than 8 years age group.

Drug induced acne: Papulopustular, monomorphic type of lesions rather than comedones (Figure 12.5), appear suddenly in a non-teenager and coincides with the drug ingestion. Drugs such as corticosteroids, androgens, anabolic steroids, antipsychotics, anti tubercular, halogens, vitamin B and oral contraceptives are mainly implicated.

Acne excoriee: It is a variant of neurotic excoriation where patients either have only facial or predominant facial involvement. Few patients develop lesions after picking acne lesions while majority did not have acne at any time. The lesions are polymorphic, new lesions are crusted, excoriated erosions, predominantly on the sides of the neck, chin, upper chest, shoulders and upper arms. After healing, the lesions become white with central atrophy and hyperpigmentation at the periphery. They leave pink or red scars, some of which may be hypertrophic. It is more common in females with a mean age of 30 years.

Psychiatric comorbidities include body dysmorphic disorder (BDD), depression, anxiety, obsessive compulsive disorder (OCD), delusional disorder, personality disorder and social phobias.

Acne conglobata: Severe form of acne characterized by cysts, intercommunicating sinuses and abscess formation with multi-porous comedones (Figure 12.6).

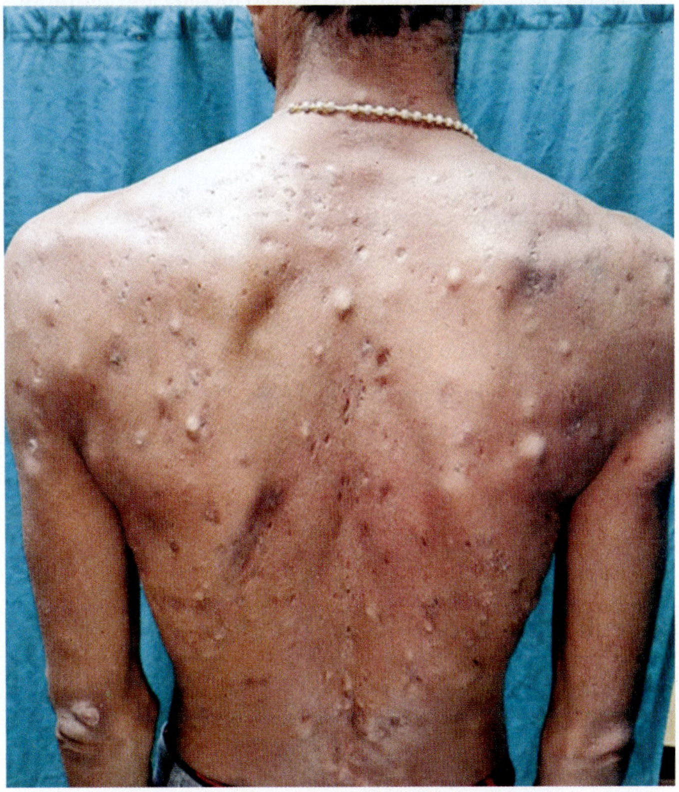

Figure 12.6: Showing acne conglobata

Acne fulminans: Crusted and ulcerated lesion of acne along with fever, myalgia and arthralgia.

Occupational acne: Acne like lesions may occur in previously non acne prone patients after exposure to occupational agent. Chloracne is caused by certain polyhalogenated organic compounds.

Cosmetic acne: It is a contact acneiform eruption caused by or aggravated by cosmetic products. Clinically it presents with multiple grouped comedones with scattered bumps on the site of cosmetic application. Treatment includes non comedogenic moisturizers.

Acne mallorca/Acne aestivalis: Polymorphic light eruption induced by ultra violet A radiation (sudden acneiform eruptions after sun exposure are observed).

Adult acne: If acne occurs beyond the age of 25 years and it commonly occurs in females. The common site for adult acne is on lower third of face and jaw line. It may be associated with hormonal acne and premenstrual flare in females . They are relatively resistant to treatment.

Persistent acne: Continuation of acne from adolescence to adult life or middle age is known persistent acne.

Hormonal acne: Occurs due to increase production of androgen and related hormones. When to suspect hormonal acne:

- Severe acne resistant to oral retinoid therapy and antibiotics
- > 25 years of age onset acne
- Hirsutism
- Irregular menstrual periods
- Cushingoid features
- Increased libido or virilisation
- Presence of acanthosis nigricans
- Androgenetic alopecia
- Pre pubertal acne
- Lesions along the jaw line and chin
- New onset adult acne
- Pre menstrual acne
- Cystic acne or vary severe acne
- Rapid relapse

Investigations for Hormonal Acne

Following investigation should be done in suspected cases of hormonal acne:

- FSH/LH ratio
- Prolactin
- Testosterone free and total
- Androstenidione
- Dehydroepiandrosterone sulfate (DHEAS)
- 5-Dihydroxytestosterone
- 17- alpha hydroxyprogesterone
- Sex hormone binding protein (SHBP)
- Serum cortisol
- Single dose dexamethasone suppression test
- Low dose dexamethasone suppression test
- S. ACTH level
- High dose dexamethasone suppression test
- Corticotropic releasing hormone RH IV then measure S. cortisol and ACTH
- Fasting and postprandial insulin
- Fasting blood sugar /HbA1c
- Ultrasound abdomen for ovarian and adrenal assessment

Associations of Acne

Acne may be associated with several disorders which have underlying metabolic abnormalities including resistance to insulin, androgenic hormone imbalance, as well as due to increased growth factor receptor 2 (FGFR2) signaling. A few conditions which are linked to acne are briefly described below:

- **Polycystic Ovary Syndrome (PCOS):** Women with PCOS are predisposed to developing acne due to elevated androgen and insulin resistance, among other factors.
- According to the Rotterdam criteria, PCOS is diagnosed when:

Rotterdam diagnostic criteria for PCOS	
1.	Oligo or anovulation
2.	Clinical and biochemical signs of hyperandrogenism **Clinical:** Acne, hirsutism, acanthosis nigricans **Biochemical:** Serum total testosterone > 70 ng/dl, Dehydroepiandrosterone (DHEA) >248 ug/dl, FSH/LH ratio >1.
3.	Polycystic ovaries: >12 ovarian follicle, each measuring 2 - 9 mm thick wall or enlarged ovary > 10cc Two out of three criteria are required for diagnosis of PCOS. **Exclusion:** Hyperthyroidism, congenital adrenal hyperplasia, androgen secreting tumors and Cushing syndrome

- **Late onset congenital adrenal hyperplasia**: It is also known as non-classical congenital adrenal hyperplasia which occurs due to 21 hydroxylase deficiency leading to raised serum 17 alpha hydroxyprogesterone. Severe, refractory to treatment and atypical forms of acne are seen. Treatment includes low dose oral prednisolone or dexamethasone.

- **Cushing disease:** Cushing's disease is due to overproduction of ACTH by pituitary gland and resulting hypercorticism. In adolescents before puberty, it can result in acne.
- **Acromegaly:** Excessive production of growth hormone and insulin like growth factor 1 (IGF-1), stimulates sebaceous gland differentiation leading to acne.
- **SAPHO Syndrome** (Synovitis, Acne, Pustulosis, Hyperostosis, Osteitis syndrome): It presents with sudden onset hemorrhagic and ulcerative acne on face and trunk.
- **SAHA Syndrome (Seborrhea, Acne, Hirsutism and Androgenetic alopecia):** It presents in female with acne, hirsutism, androgenetic alopecia and acne.
- **PAPA Syndrome (Pyogenic arthritis, Pyoderma gangrenosum, and Acne):** It is an autosomal dominant autoinflammatory disease present with recurrent sterile erosive arthritis in childhood, recurrent pyoderma gangrenosum and nodulocystic acne.
- **PAPASH syndrome:** Pyogenic arthritis, Pyoderma gangrenosum, Acne and Hidradenitis suppurativa.
- **PASH syndrome:** Hereditary autoinflammatory disease characterised by a combination of Pyoderma gangrenosum, acne and hidradenitis suppurativa.
- **Apert Syndrome:** It is a rare autosomal dominant disorder caused by mutations in fibroblast growth factor receptor (FGFR-2). Incidence is about 1 in 65,000 individuals.

It is also known as acrocephalosyndactyly, and is characterized by craniosynostosis, premature fusion of the cranial sutures and early epiphyseal closure resulting in various deformities of the skull, hands and feet.

The development of widespread, severe, pustular acne around puberty is a characteristic feature in these patients.

Differential Diagnosis

Rosacea: It affects older individuals, and begins as a rash and telangiectasia on erythematous background. Later on papules and pustules are formed, but comedones, nodules and scars are characteristically absent. This disease is confined to face in majority of the patients.

Pseudofolliculitis barbae: This is caused by ingrowth of hair, occurs in men with curly hair on the neck and beard area.

Hidradenitis suppurativa: It is a chronic relapsing inflammatory disease of apocrine gland follicles, characterized by induration, scarring, destruction of skin appendages and sinus formation usually on axillae, perineal region and perianal areas.

Milia: They are small, pinhead sized, white colored lesions in infraorbital region, which may be confused with white heads.

Other diseases: Gram negative folliculitis, kerion and pityrosporum folliculitis are uncommon diseases sometimes mimicking acne.

Investigations

In female patients having features of hyperandrogenism, e.g., hirsutism, obesity, menstrual abnormalities; possibility of polycystic ovarian syndrome should be considered and investigated. In routine, patients do not require investigations except when isotretinoin therapy is planned.

Treatment

There are four major principles in treating acne vulgaris:

- Decreasing sebum secretion.
- Correction of altered pattern of follicular keratinization.
- Decreasing the population and activity of *P. acnes*.
- Control of inflammation.

General advice: Patient should be explained about the nature of the disease as acne is an age-related problem which may persist for 4-6 years. Adequate therapy will keep the disease under control and prevent scarring. This will help in boosting the patient's confidence and faith in treatment.

In India, the habit of oiling with mustard oil and amla oil may be comedogenic and patients should be advised to stop it. If they are fond of applying oil, small amounts of coconut oil may be allowed on head.

Diet: There is little evidence that diet containing spices, chocolates, alcohol and dairy products (except for iodine containing foods), causes acne. In general, dietary restrictions are not of much help.

Approach for Therapy

Adolescent patients at the age of 10-14 years usually have mild, non-inflammatory lesions like comedones and few papules or pustules. These patients should be given counselling about the nature of disease and not to fiddle with lesions which will help in reducing development of scarring. They should be prescribed topical anti-comedogenic agent, tretinoin 0.025% at night, along with local antibiotic cream, e.g., clindamycin 1-2% cream in the morning. Tretinoin is irritant if improperly applied, so it should be applied only on lesions and if irritation occurs it should be applied on alternate days. It is also a good drug for acne on the back and chest.

Local Therapy

Topical acne therapies are designed to be used as "field therapy," meaning the entire face needs to be treated. The "spot-treatment" of individual acne lesions is neither advised nor effective. Patients should be instructed to use a "pea-sized" amount of topical medication for the entire face. To combat irritation, all patients should be encouraged to utilize skin moisturizers and sun protection while on therapy. Moisturizers should, specifically, be "non-comedogenic" and sunscreens should be at least with a SPF of 30.

Delivery system:

- Cream based advised for dry skin.
- Gel based for oily skin.
- Lotions are preferred for larger areas.
- Soaps and face washes can be used as adjectives.

Special precautions

- Infants and neonates and patients with sensitive skin are treated with lower concentrations of required drug.
- Retinoids are avoided in pregnancy.

1. **Local antibiotic preparations** (Clindamycin 1-2%, erythromycin 2-4%, clarithromycin 1-2%): They are available as creams or lotions. These agents suppress the activity of P. acnes, so are used in mild to moderate forms of acne with inflammation.
2. **Benzoyl peroxide (2.5 or 5%):** It acts as antimicrobial agent. It also has anti-inflammatory activity by decreasing hydrolysis of triglycerides, so it can be used in both inflammatory and non-inflammatory acne.
3. **Azelaic acid (10-20%) cream:** It is effective in reducing follicular keratinization and also acts as an antimicrobial agent.
4. **Retinoids Tretinoin (0.025-0.05%) gel or cream:** It increases epidermal cell turnover and decreases cohesiveness of stratum corneum. It is mainly effective for comedones, but it is also useful in inflammatory acne. As dryness is quite common with this agent, it can cause irritation and photosensitivity. It should be started with lowest concentration with only night-time application. Adapalene (0.1% gel) is a newer form of topical retinoid with less irritation, so it can be used at daytime.

Systemic Therapy

When the child develops pustules, nodules or other inflammatory lesions, systemic drugs should be given.

Oral antibiotics

Oral antibiotics are the mainstay of treatment in moderate to severe acne. These agents inhibit the growth of P. acnes. The antibiotics also inhibit various enzyme activities and modulate chemotaxis, lymphocyte function and proinflammatory cytokines, thus their benefit may be obtained through mechanisms other than a direct effect on bacteria. Flowing antibiotics are commonly used for the treatment of acne:

- **Tetracycline:** It is given 1 gm daily in divided doses. It should not be given to children below 8 years of age, as it may cause pigmentation of teeth.
- **Doxycycline:** 100 mg once or twice a day.
- **Minocycline:** 50-100 mg once or twice a day. It may cause blue-black pigmentation in a dose-dependent manner.
- **Azithromycin:** 500 mg once a day for 3 days in a week.
- Cotrimoxazole and ciprofloxacin can also be used with similar results.
- Oral antibiotics are used initially (usually for 6-8 weeks) to control the inflammatory lesions. Once it is achieved, they must be stopped.

Oral Isotretinoin

It is a retinoid with remarkable action in severe to very severe acne, and now is the drug of choice for the same. It inhibits sebum secretion, reduces inflammation, and also reduces the load of bacteria.

Side Effects of Isotretinoin

- Common mucocutaneous side effects like cheilitis, facial dermatitis, dry skin, blepharoconjunctivitis, nasal dryness and soreness can be countered by the use of lubricants.
- Other uncommon side effects like arthralgia, myalgia, headache, achilles tendonitis, depression, mood changes, urticaria, vasculitis and night blindness, are not seen with lower doses but should be kept in mind.
- Isotretinoin is teratogenic and before prescribing isotretinoin, it should be ensured that the female patient is not pregnant. She should be advised not to get pregnant until 1 month after stopping the isotretinoin.
- Raised serum lipids and abnormal liver function test.

Oral isotretinoin is a good choice. For severe nodulocystic acne the recommended dose of isotretinoin is 0.5-1 mg/kg/day for 20-24 weeks, which results in long-term remission. At this dose, the patients develop many mucocutaneous or other side effects. For moderate grade acne, isotretinoin at lower doses (20 mg alternate days) acts well with minimal side effects. Once remission is achieved, usually in 4-6 months, the patients can be maintained on topical therapy alone. Baseline blood counts, fasting lipid profile and liver function tests are done and repeated at 4 and 8 weeks and if they are normal or unchanged and dose of isotretinoin is not increased, no further tests are needed to be done.

Hormonal Therapy

Indications

1. Failed standard antibiotic/combination regimens.
2. Menstrual control and/or contraception required along with acne therapy.
3. When oral isotretinoin is inappropriate or not available. With the introduction of isotretinoin, which is more effective, hormone therapy is less preferred in those females where isotretinoin is not contraindicated.

Treatment of hormonal acne:

Drugs used in the treatment of hormonal acne fall into four categories:

Androgen receptor blockers:

- Spironolactone
- Flutamide
- Cyproterone acetate

Oral contraceptives and GnRH analogues

Commonly used oral contraceptives are:

- Crisanta (EE 0.03 mg + Drospirenone 3 mg)
- Femilon (EE 0.02 mg + Desogestrel 0.15 mg)
- Yasmin (EE 0.03 mg + Drospirenone 3 mg)

GnRH analogues can be used in combination with other topical and oral therapies for acne for better results:

- Nasal sprays (to be given 2-3 times a day): Nafarelin and Buserelin
- Subcutaneous injections (once daily): Buserelin and Leuprolide
- Intramuscular depot injection (to be given monthly): Triptroelin
- Subcutaneous implant (to be given monthly): Leuprolide, Goserelin

Glucocorticoids:

- Low-dose prednisolone (2.5-5 mg)
- Dexamethasone 0.25-0.75 mg

Enzyme inhibitors (5a-reductase inhibitors):

- Finasteride - type 2 5 α-Reductase inhibitor
- Dutasteride -inhibits both the isoenzymes
- Turosteride - is a potent inhibitor of type 2 isoenzyme

Antiandrogens

Cyproterone acetate (2 mg) combined with 35 µg of ethinyl estradiol once daily for 21days followed by 7 days interval with placebo pills can be used in female patients who are resistant to other treatments.

Once acne is controlled, conventional triphasic pills such as Trinordiol (ethinylestradiol 35 µg, levonorgestrol 50 µg) can be prescribed which suppresses sebum production.

Physical Therapies

Incision and Drainage of Cysts

Intralesional triamcinolone (2.5-10 mg/ml): 0.1-0.2 ml may be injected intralesionally for nodules and cystic type of acne lesions. It can be repeated after every 2-3 weeks.

Dermabrasion: It is used to remove or lessen scars and post acne pigmentation.

Photodynamic therapy: Recently, visible light (phototherapy or deep penetrating light therapy) has been successfully employed to treat mild to moderate acne. Intense violet/blue light (405-420 nm) is generated by purpose-built fluorescent lighting, dichromic bulbs, LEDs or lasers. It decreases the number of inflammatory acne lesion by 60-70% in four weeks of therapy, particularly when the *P. acnes* is pretreated with δ-aminolevulinic acid (ALA), which increases the production of porphyrins.

Laser Treatment

Laser surgery has been used to reduce the scars left behind by acne. Since lasers and intense pulsed light sources cause thermal damage to the skin, they may cause hyperpigmented macule (spots) formation or may cause long-term dryness of the skin.

Specific Points

- Never prescribe short courses of different antibiotics, as it may lead development of drug resistance.
- Tetracylines should not be prescribed to children below 8 years of age and to pregnant females.
- Make sure that female is not pregnant before, during and upto 1 month after stopping isotretinoin therapy.

Course and Prognosis

Acne vulgaris clears by the age of 24-25 years in most of cases, but few patients may continue to develop acne till thirties or forties.

MANAGEMENT OF ACNE SCARS

- **Surgical techniques:** Punch excision of ice pick scars is easy and gives good early result. Punch autograft is used when treating deep ice pick scars. The donor site is usually postauricular skin. Subcision involves subcutaneous sectioning of dermal adhesions with a sharp needle (18 G). It is often associated with neocollagenesis.
- **Resurfacing techniques:** The aim is to restore skin contour by inducing neocollagenesis. These include TCA peeling, phenol peeling, microdermabrasion, laser abrasion, selective thermolysis with Fraxel laser, and resurfacing by radiofrequency and electrosurgery. Resurfacing is indicated in U and W scars. The side effects are erythema and pigmentation. Spot TCA peeling is a good technique for V and deep U scars.
- **Microdermabrasion:** This involves planning of the skin by mechanized means utilizing the projection of micromarbles consisting of aluminum oxide on scars. Chemabrasion is term used when microdermabrasion is combined with a peeling agent.
- **Lasers:** Intense Pulse Light (IPL) acts by heating the dermis and stimulating neocollagenesis. It has weak activity and may be helpful in red, hypertrophic scars. Light-Emitting Diode (LED) acts by photobiomodulation and is used for superficial U scars, erythema (acne macules) and pigmentation. It is a safe and painless procedure but the efficacy is low. Ablative laser resurfacing, although effective, is associated with excessive tissue reaction as erythema and edema, and with complications such as pigmentation and scarring. It is less suited for skin types V and VI. Fractional photothermolysis, a new concept, using 1,550-nm erbium-doped fiber laser, creates microscopic thermal wounds to achieve skin rejuvenation without significant side effects. Clinical improvement averaged 51-75% in nearly 90% of patients. Side effects are transient erythema and edema without dyspigmentation, ulceration, or scarring.
- **Fillers:** The aim is to lift the depression caused by scars, by injecting a filler underneath. Resorbable filler such as hyaluronic acid is a good option as it lasts for 6-12 months and is indicated for scars with gentle slopes without sclerosis. Non resorbable fillers carry the risk of granuloma formation. Autologous fat transfer can also be done.
- **Dermabrasion:** It is a higher risk procedure with prolonged down-time and considerable risk of pigmentary disturbances.

ROSACEA

It is a chronic disease characterized by erythema, telangiectasia and edema with recurrent episodes of papules and pustules, particularly in the central area of the face. It occurs most frequently in middle aged women. Although the exact cause of rosacea is unknown, the following factors have been considered e.g. vascular abnormalities, Demodex folliculorum, gram negative bacteria, *Helicobacter pylori* and fluorinated topical steroids. Other suggested contributing factors are ultraviolet radiation, increased toll like receptor 2 (TLR2) activity, proteases activity and cathelicidin production. Familial history seen in 25 % of patients. Rosacea is classified into four subtypes:

1. **Erythematotelangiectatic:**

   It presents with frequent episodes of flushing, erythema and telangiectasia, which is aggravated by sun exposure, diet (hot, spicy food, alcohol) etc. It is most common subtype of rosacea.

2. **Papulopustular type:**

   This type of rosacea presents with inflammatory papules, pustules with surrounding erythema and telangiectasia over centro facial area. In severe cases lesions coalesce to form plaques with edema of face.

3. **Phymatous type:**

   In this subtype, rhinophyma is most common, which presents as thickening of skin on distal part of nose with prominent follicular opening. In advanced stage nose may acquire bulbous appearance. There is no pain and erythema. Other types of phyamtous rosacea are otophyma (ear) and metaphysis (forehead skin).

4. **Ocular rosacea:**

   Ocular rosacea presents with stinging and burning sensation, blepharitis, pain, redness and photophobia in both eyes.

Management

General measures include, broad spectrum sunscreen, washing face with lukewarm water, moisturizers and avoiding spicy food and beverages. For erythematotelangiectatic rosacea, topical alpha receptor agonists (brimonidine, oxymetazoline), vascular lasers, low dose beta-blocker's, botulinum toxin may be used. For papulopustular rosacea, topical metronidazole, azelaic acid, topical sulphur, alpha receptor antagonists, oral antibiotics (tetracyclines, erythromycin), low dose isotretinoin and topical acaricides (ivermectin, crotamiton, permethrin) have been tried.

For phymatous type, skin peeling agents, electrocautery, low dose isotretinoin, ablative CO_2 laser are recommended.

CHAPTER 13

Papulosquamous Disorders

Contents

Papulosquamous disorders are a group of diseases which are predominantly associated with scaly papules and/or plaques. Though there are many conditions which come under this group, but the following diseases which are of practical value will be discussed here:

- **Psoriasis**
- **Lichen planus**
- **Lichen nitidus**
- **Pityriasis rubra pilaris**
- **Pityriasis rosea**
- **Pityriasis lichenoides chronica**
- **Reiter's disease**

PSORIASIS

Psoriasis is a chronic inflammatory, genetically influenced disease of the skin and joints. It is characterized clinically by the presence of well-defined erythematous, scaly plaques mainly over extensor surfaces of the body and scalp.

Epidemiology

- Psoriasis is a common disease prevalent throughout the world with variable prevalence of 0.1% to 3% in different populations.
- There is a wide ethnic variation with increased prevalence in Caucasians than in brown or black populations.
- The age of onset in psoriasis is bimodal. Type I psoriasis which accounts for more than 75% of cases occurs in the age group of 15 to 40 years. Type II psoriasis begins after 40 years of age.
- There is no sex predisposition, although women develop the disease earlier than men.

Etiopathogenesis

Exact etiology of psoriasis is unknown but the following factors play a major role in the development of the disease:

- **Genetic predisposition:** Genetic basis of psoriasis is now well established. Around 30% of psoriasis patients have an affected first degree relative. Concordance of psoriasis is seen in 65% of identical twins. Psoriasis patients have increased frequency of HLA-B13, HLA-B17 and HLA-Cw6. 75% of juvenile psoriasis patients are positive for HLA-Cw6. Nine psoriasis susceptibility loci on different chromosomes have been identified and have been named as PSORS 1-9. PSORS 1 which is situated on chromosome 6 has been found to be associated with psoriasis in 35% to 50% cases. PSORS 2 is located on chromosome 17 which is responsible for CARD 14 gain of function mutation. It results in constitutive activation of NF-kB pathway, leading to plaque psoriasis, pustular psoriasis and pityriasis rubra pilaris. Based on the association of HLA, psoriasis has recently been classified into two types. Type I has strong association with HLA-Cw6, B-13 and Bw57 and starts before 40 years of age. About two thirds of patients have type I psoriasis. Family association is present and the disease is more severe in this type. Type II has much weaker association with HLA, there is no family tendency and nail changes and arthritis are more common.
- **Environmental factors:** Many environmental factors have been implicated in the etiology of psoriasis which play an important role in genetically predisposed individuals in causation and exacerbation of disease. The important factors are:

1. ***Trauma:*** Psoriatic lesions show Koebner's phenomenon, i.e., develop more at the site of physical, chemical and surgical trauma.
2. ***Infection:*** Infections have been seen to provoke psoriasis in about 40% cases. Streptococcal infection is associated with guttate and plaque psoriasis. Other infections include hepatitis C, HIV, herpes simplex and cytomegalovirus infections.
3. ***Drugs:*** Certain drugs like lithium salts, antimalarials, beta blockers, NSAIDs and ACE inhibitors may provoke or exacerbate the disease.
4. ***Other factors:*** Sunlight, alcohol intake, smoking, stress and hypocalcemia are the other provocative factors.

Immunopathogenesis

There is now enough evidence to suggest that psoriasis is a T cell mediated chronic inflammatory disease of skin and joints. Specific antigens involved in psoriasis have not yet been identified but there could be several including bacterial, viral or autoantigens and superantigens that interact with the antigen presenting cells (APCs) like Langerhans cells in the epidermis. These cells migrate to the lymph nodes where they activate the CD4 resting memory cells. Activated T cells enter the circulation, and reach dermis and epidermis where they help to activate APCs. Plasmacytoid dendritic cells are first activated which in turn stimulate myeloid dendritic cells. These activated myeloid dendritic cells produce TNF-α, IL-12, and IL-23 cytokines leading to activation of Th1, Th17 and Th 22 cells, which in turn secrete inflammatory cytokines TNF-α, IL-17, and IL-22 respectively. These cytokines, particularly IL17, subsequently stimulates keratinocytes, which then generate chemokines (CXCL1, CXCL8, CCR5), cytokines (IL-1, IL6, IL8), and antimicrobial peptides (LL37 or cathelicidin, β-defensins, and S100 proteins), all of them contribute to the propagation of inflammation and epidermal proliferation. Psoriasis is primarily driven by the IL-23/IL-17 pathogenic axis. The nuclear factor-kappa B (NF-κB), MAP Kinase, phosphodiesterase 4 pathway and signal transducer and activator of transcription (STAT), are the main cell signalling pathways, which are impaired in psoriasis. It is also now well recognised that JAK (Janus kinase)/STAT signalling pathways are also primarily involved in the pathogenesis of psoriasis. Psoriasis development is highly dependent on STAT 3 in keratinocytes.

- **Epidermal hyperplasia:** Before the current evidence of immunological pathogenesis, psoriasis used to be considered as a disease of keratinocyte proliferation and abnormal differentiation. In psoriatic lesions, the keratinocyte cell cycle time is reduced to about 8 times from 311 hours to 36 hours and the number of dividing cells is doubled resulting in hyperkeratosis.

Comorbidities in Psoriasis

Psoriasis is associated with a number of comorbid conditions. Immune dysregulation and chronic inflammation play an important role in the development and progression of psoriasis. As psoriasis progresses, persistent inflammatory dysfunction by causing increase in Th1 cytokines (TNF alfa, IL-2, IL-6, IFN gamma), may drive the development of comorbid conditions such as cardiovascular diseases. Metabolic syndrome is the most common comorbidity associated with psoriasis. For metabolic syndrome to be diagnosed, at least three of the following should be present:

- Central obesity (waist circumference >90 cm in men and >80 cm in women).

  Plus, two of the following four factors:
  - Triglycerides >150 mg/dl.
  - HDL cholesterol <40 mg/dl in men and <50 mg/dl in women.
  - Fasting glucose >100 mg/dl.
  - Blood pressure > 130/85 mm Hg.

Obesity is a relevant risk factor for psoriasis, and increased BMI is known to be associated with an increased risk of psoriatic arthritis. Emerging data suggest that the association of psoriasis with metabolic syndrome occurs early in course of the disease as psoriasis is associated with obesity and elevated lipids even in childhood.

There is also a significant statistical association of psoriasis with Crohn's disease (x7 fold higher risk) and ulcerative colitis (x3 fold higher risk). This could be because Crohn's disease, ulcerative colitis and psoriasis share the same susceptibility loci (6P21), IL-23 receptor and IL-12B genes and are driven by Th-1 cytokines such as TNF-alpha.

Patients with severe psoriasis and psoriatic arthritis have increased impact on the quality of life of patients.

Classification of psoriasis: Classification of psoriasis described in Table 13.1.

Table 13.1: Classification of psoriasis
Based on morphology of lesions
Chronic plaque psoriasis
Guttate psoriasis
Pustular psoriasis
Unstable psoriasis
Erythrodermic psoriasis
Rupioid psoriasis
Elephantine psoriasis
Ostraceous psoriasis
Based on site on involvement
Scalp psoriasis
Palmoplantar psoriasis
Nail psoriasis
Genital psoriasis
Flexural psoriasis
Follicular psoriasis
Ocular – Blepharitis, keratitis, conjunctivitis, uveitis etc.
Mucosal – Geographical tongue, erythema of mucosa, annular plaques on mucosa etc.
Other atypical forms of psoriasis
Seborrheic psoriasis
Annular psoriasis
Circinate psoriasis
Nummular psoriasis
Photosensitive psoriasis
Linear psoriasis

Clinical Features

Psoriasis is a chronic inflammatory disease with classical presentation of itchy/non-itchy, well defined, symmetrical, erythematous plaques covered with silvery white scales with extensor distribution. Psoriasis may be classified (Table 13.1) according to clinical appearance, morphology and localization. Their various clinical presentations of psoriasis include:

Chronic Plaque Psoriasis (Psoriasis Vulgaris)

- It is the most common form of psoriasis. The lesions are well defined erythematous or "salmon pink" colored plaques of variable size covered with silvery white scales (Figure 13.1 A, B).
- Lesions are distributed bilaterally symmetrically on extensor surfaces of the body particularly on elbows and knees.
- Itching is variable in intensity and may be even absent.
- Plaques are oval or irregular in shape, raised and may vary from one to several centimeters in size. Plaques may coalesce together and form large plaques commonly on legs and sacral region. Sometimes lesions may become annular by central clearing of the plaque.
- Lesions may also appear as follicular, nummular, linear, circinate, gyrate and serpiginous.
- Koebner phenomenon is positive in about 20% of cases.
- When psoriatic scales are removed successively with a glass slide, bleeding points appear on a smooth, glossy red membrane (Bulkeley's membrane). This phenomenon is known as "Auspitz's sign".

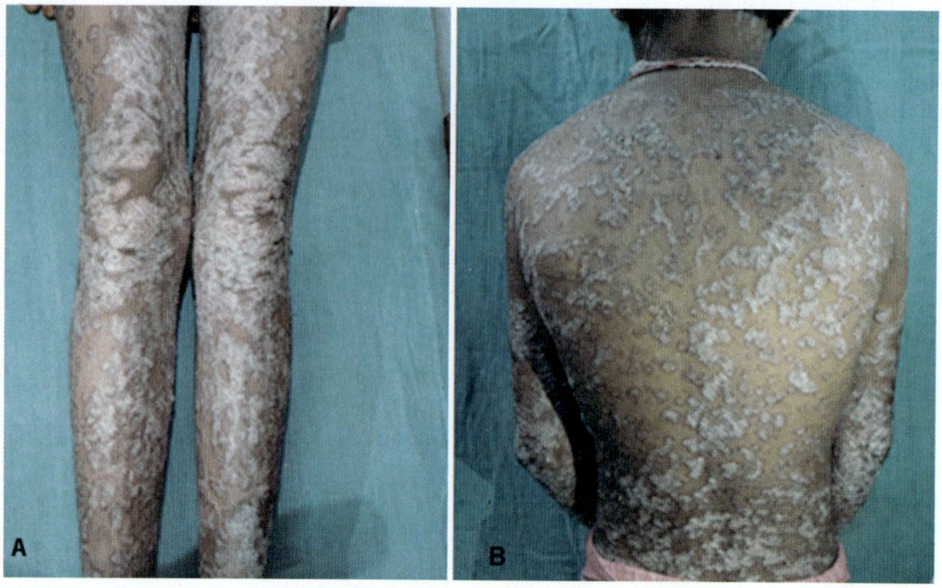

Figure 13.1: Plaque type psoriasis (A and B)

- **Candle grease sign:** On scratching a psoriatic plaque with glass slide, scales fall off and reveal a shiny candle like surface.
- In resolving lesions, a peripheral halo may be seen around lesions, known as Woronoff ring.
- Resolved lesions may show post-inflammatory hypomelanosis.
- **Psoriatic march:** This provides a framework to explain how psoriatic inflammation causes cardiovascular comorbidities via atherosclerosis, independently from the presence of additional cardiovascular risk factors. According to this concept psoriasis is a chronic systemic inflammatory disorder as evidenced by elevated biomarkers for systemic inflammation. These is also increase in leptin and resistin which results in insulin resistance and may drive atherosclerosis through immunomodulation.

Severity of psoriasis can be assesses by using BSA (Body Surface Area) and PASI score (Psoriasis Area and Severity Index).

PASI (Psoriasis Area and Severity Index)

The PASI is a widely used instrument in psoriasis trials to assess and grade the severity of psoriasis and the patient's response to treatment. It produces a score ranging from 0 to 72. A 75% reduction in the PASI score (PASI 75) is the current benchmark for most clinical trials. PASI is calculated by dividing the body into four regions: Head (H), Upper extremities (U), Trunk (T) and Lower extremities (L). The extent of psoriatic involvement is graded (Area, A) as follows:

- 0 = no involvement;
- 1 = 1% to 9%;
- 2 = 10% to 29%;
- 3 = 30% to 49%;
- 4 = 50% to 69%;
- 5 = 70% to 89%;
- 6 = 90% to 100%.

Each of these areas are assessed separately for erythema (E), induration (I) and scaling (S), which are rated on a scale of 0 (none) to 4 (very severe).

The following formula is used to calculate the PASI score:

PASI : 0.1 x (EH + IH + SH) x AH + 0.2x (EU + IU + SU) x AU + 0.3x (ET +IT + ST)x AT + 0.4 x (EL +IL +SL) x AL.

- **Mild disease** – PASI < 5
- **Moderate disease** – PASI between 5-10
- **Severe disease** – PASI more than 10

GUTTATE PSORIASIS

It is the most common form of psoriasis found in children, seen in upto 44% of pediatric population. Lesions are drop-like (guttate), round or oval, measure from 2-6 mm in diameter and generally occur in a symmetrical distribution over the trunk and proximal aspects of the extremities (Figure 13.2) and occasionally the face, scalp, ears and distal aspects of the extremities. Guttate psoriasis is often, but not necessarily, triggered by group A streptococcal infection of the upper respiratory tract in about two thirds of patients. The latency period between streptococcal infection and the appearance of skin lesions is typically 1 to 3 weeks. Although guttate psoriasis may clear spontaneously, 40% of affected children progress to the chronic plaque type.

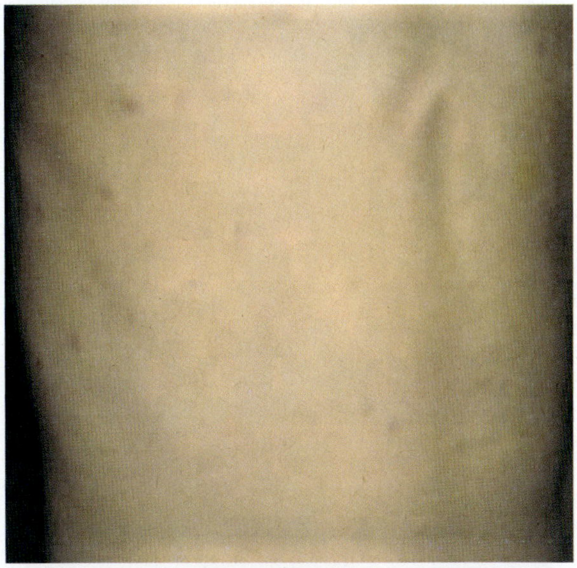

Figure 13.2: Guttate psoriasis

SCALP PSORIASIS

Scalp is involved in psoriasis in about 50% cases. It may be involved alone or as a part of generalized involvement of body. Whole scalp can be involved diffusely or there may be discrete, well defined, erythematous plaques with silvery white scales on scalp particularly on frontoparietal (Figure 13.3) or occipital region.

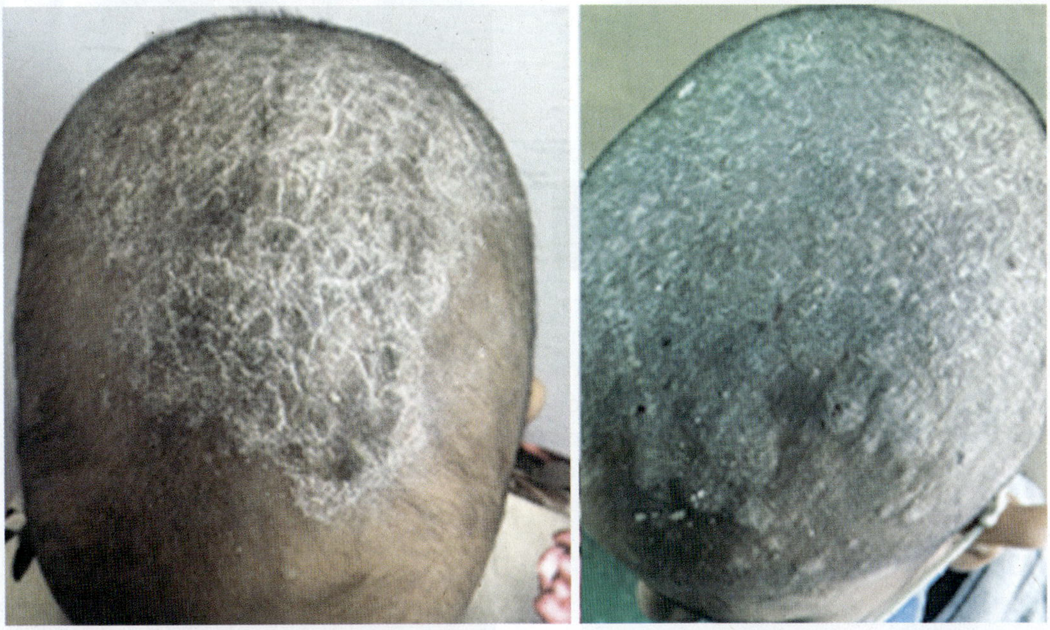

Figure 13.3: Scalp psoriasis

NAIL PSORIASIS (Figure 13.4 A, B)

Nail involvement in psoriasis is seen in 10-55% cases in adults and upto 80% cases in psoriatic arthritis patients, it is uncommon in children. Nail psoriasis may be seen without involvement of skin. Psoriatic nail changes include irregular pitting on nail plate, oil spots (yellowish nail bed discoloration surrounded by an erythematous halo), thickening and brittleness, onycholysis, subungual hyperkeratosis, paronychia and splinter hemorrhages. The nail becomes discolored and dystrophic.

NAPSI (Nail psoriasis severity index): The NAPSI was intended to both quantify the severity of psoriatic nail disease as well as assess the efficacy of drug therapy by looking at the nail involvement. The nail divided into four quadrants with each quadrant being assessed for nail matrix disease (pitting, lunular red spots, crumbling, and leukonychia) and nail bed disease (onycholysis, splinter haemorrhages, subungual hyperkeratosis and salmon-patch dyschromia). Each nail is given a score of 0 to 8 for a total score of 0 to 80 for the fingernails and 0 to 160 if the toenails are also included in the analysis.

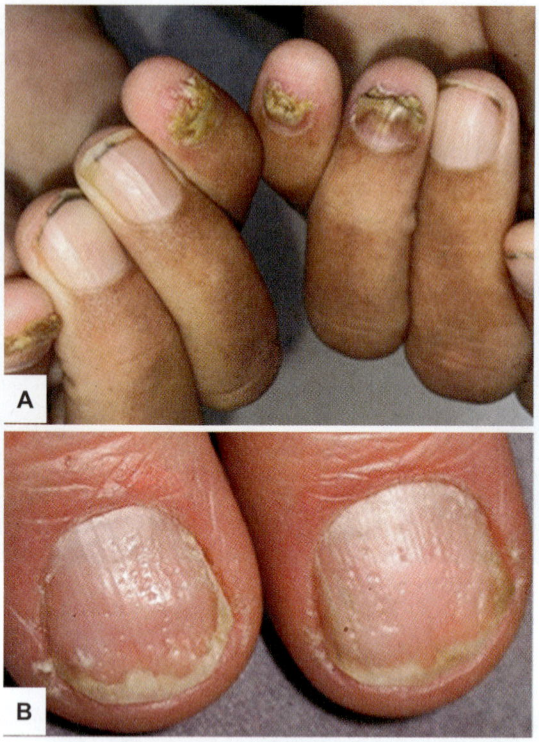

Figure 13.4: Nail psoriasis (A and B)

FLEXURAL (INVERSE) PSORIASIS (Figure 13.5)

About 2-6% of patients develop psoriasis in flexural distribution involving major skin folds such as groins, axillae, submammary region, gluteal cleft, perianal region and retroauricular region. Flexural psoriasis is uncommon in children. Lesions are extremely erythematous and lack typical scaling. Scales are fine and moist. In the absence of other typical lesions, it may be difficult to differentiate flexural psoriasis from intertrigo, seborrheic dermatitis, erythrasma and candidiasis.

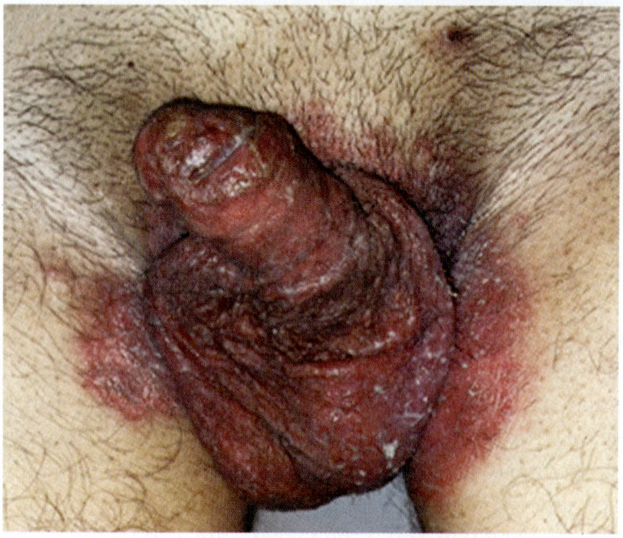

Figure 13.5: Flexural psoriasis with genital lesion

PALMOPLANTAR PSORIASIS (Figures 13.6 and 13.7)

Well-circumscribed red scaly plaque or generalized thickening and scaling of entire palms and soles are the most common clinical presentation of palmoplantar psoriasis. Palmoplantar psoriasis tends to be a chronic persistent condition and more commonly associated with nail dystrophy as compared to chronic plaque psoriasis. Hyperkeratotic eczema is the close differential diagnosis for palmoplantar psoriasis.

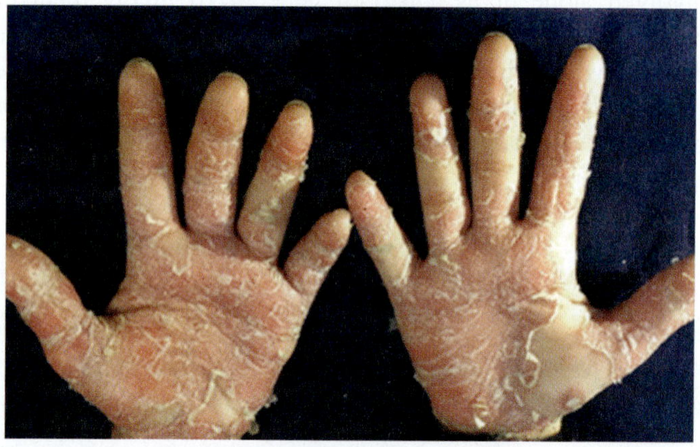

Figure 13.6: Palmar psoriasis

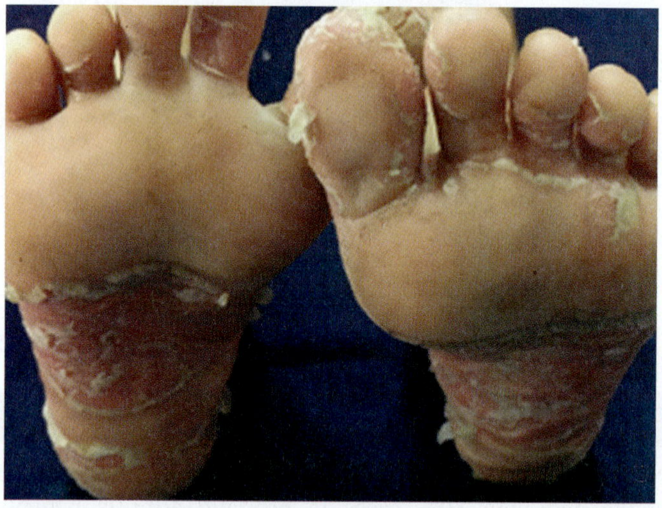

Figure 13.7: Plantar psoriasis

LINEAR PSORIASIS

Linear psoriasis is characterized by a linear distribution of well-defined erythematous scaly papules and plaque along the Blaschko's lines (Figure 13.8).

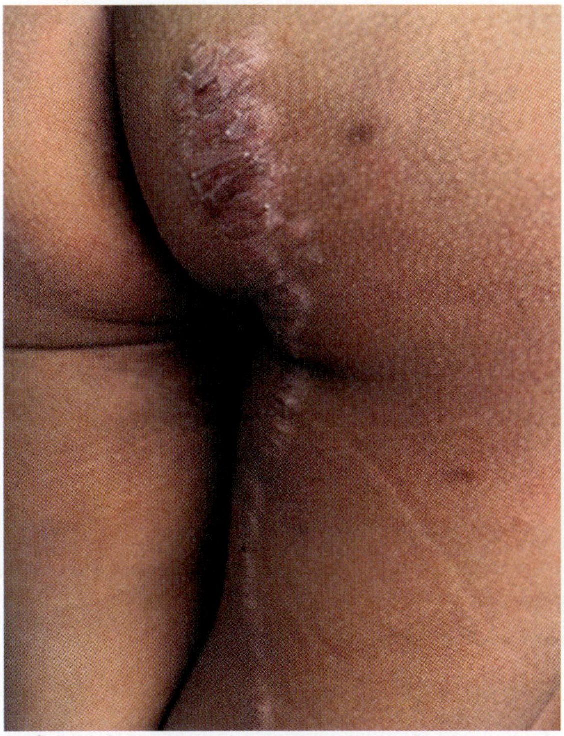

Figure 13.8: Linear psoriasis

ERYTHRODERMIC PSORIASIS

Erythroderma is characterized by generalized erythema and fine scaling involving more than 90% of body surface area. Psoriasis is an important cause of erythroderma accounting for about 30% of cases. It can evolve from pre-existing plaque psoriasis gradually or can occur suddenly. The most common causes that can lead to development of erythroderma include, reaction to certain drugs like lithium, beta-blockers, antimalarials, steroid withdrawal, vigorous tar or dithranol therapy, infection and emotional stress. Clinically there is generalized itching, intense erythema, superficial, fine, white scaling all over the body (Figure 13.9 A, B). In addition edema, fissures, exudation and nail dystrophy may be present. Persistent skin inflammation and exfoliation may lead to protein loss, hypo or hyperthermia, dehydration, electrolyte imbalance, renal failure and cardiac failure. Other complications include, staphylococcal septicemia and pneumonia.

PUSTULAR PSORIASIS

Pustular psoriasis may be localized or generalized. It is characterized by presence of erythema and sterile pustules (Figure 13.6). It may be triggered by pregnancy, sudden withdrawal of steroids, hypocalcemia and infection. Pustular psoriasis can be classified into localized and generalized type.

A. **Generalized pustular psoriasis**

   Clinical variants (based on morphology and natural history):

   (i) Acute generalized pustular psoriasis (von Zumbusch).

   (ii) Subacute annular and circinate pustular psoriasis (Figure 13.10).

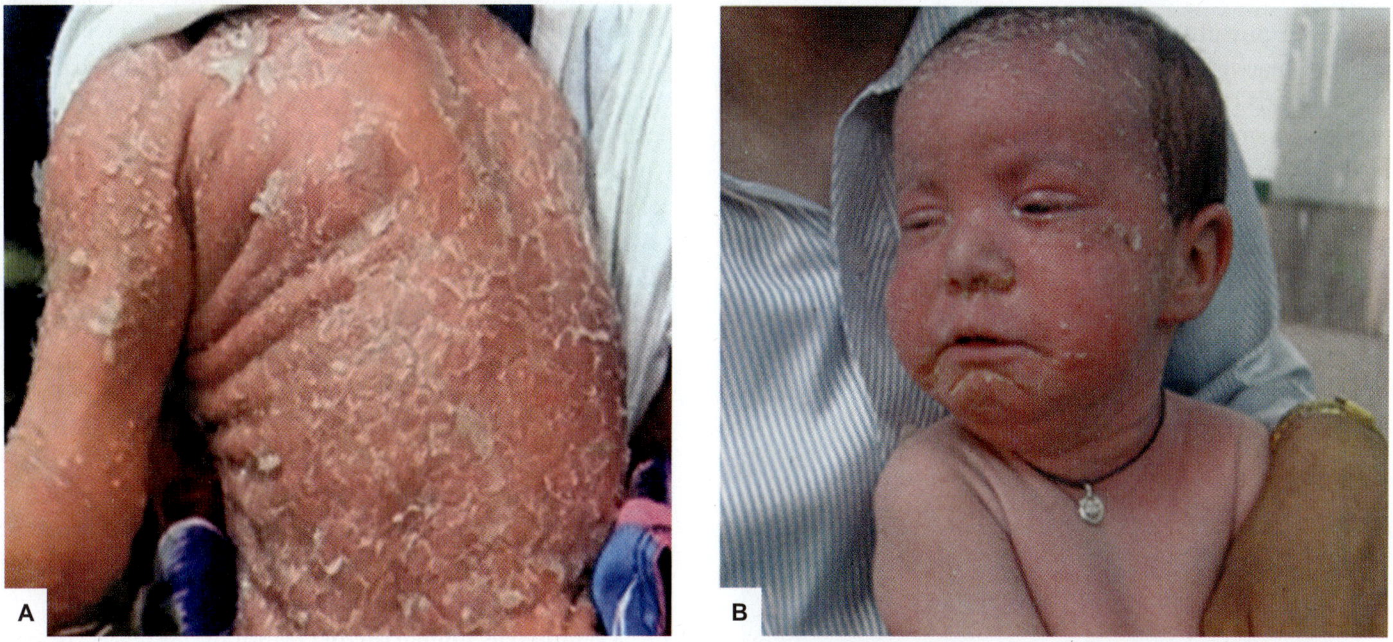

Figure 13.9: Erythrodermic psoriasis (A and B)

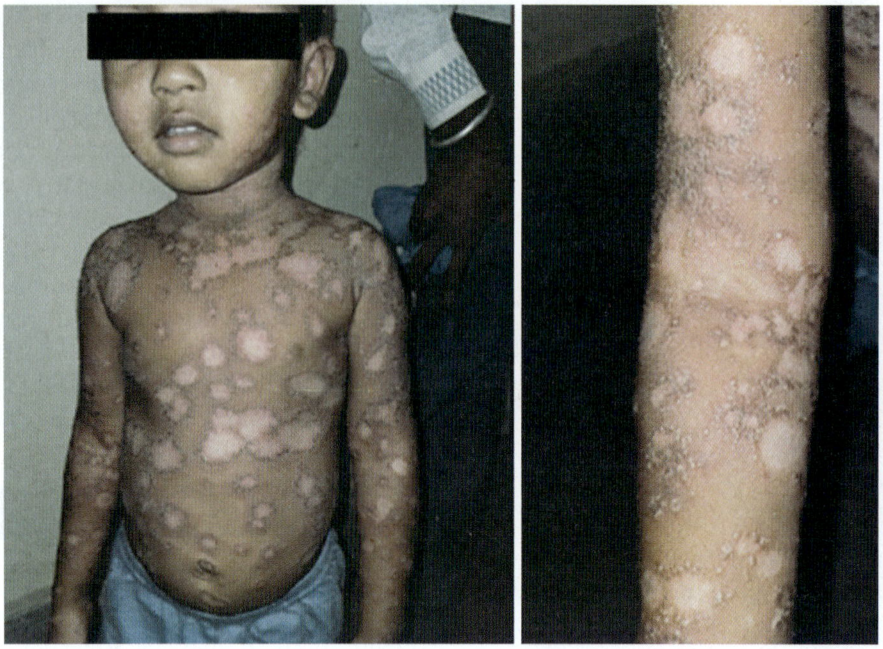

Figure 13.10: Subacute or circinate pustular psoriasis

Other specified forms (based on age or precipitants):

(i) Acute generalized pustular psoriasis of pregnancy (impetigo herpetiformis).

(ii) Infantile and juvenile generalized pustular psoriasis.

B. Localized pustular psoriasis

(i) Palmoplantar pustulosis (Figure 13.11).

(ii) Acrodermatitis continua of Hallopeau.

Localized pustular psoriasis: It may be seen in two forms: palmoplantar pustulosis and acropustulosis. Palmoplantar pustulosis is more common in females and presents as numerous, small, sterile pustules on erythematous plaques, bilaterally symmetrical on palms and soles. Acropustulosis type of localized pustular psoriasis is a chronic and persistent variant where fingertips show pustular lesions over glazed erythema and scaling. Nails may be destroyed and there could be osteolysis of distal phalanx.

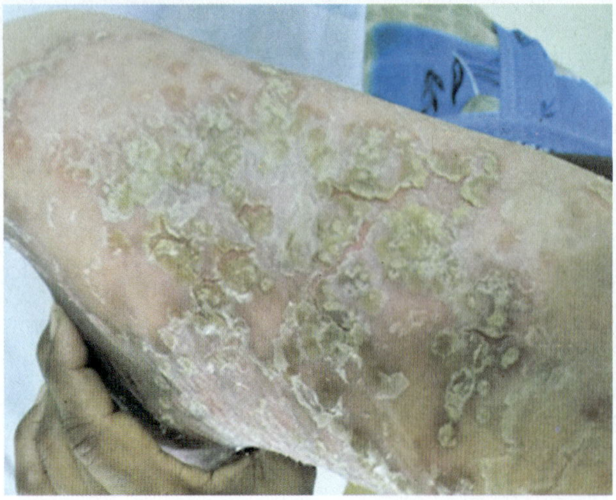

Figure 13.11: Localized pustular psoriasis: Plantar surface

Generalized pustular psoriasis: It is a severe form of pustular psoriasis characterized by multiple erythematous plaques studded with tiny, sterile pustules that may coalesce to form lake of pus (Figure 13.12A). Uninvolved skin also shows erythema and pustules. It may be associated with fever, arthralgia and malaise. Pustules dry up and form scales or crusts. It is followed by development of new crop. Generalized pustular psoriasis may also be of exanthematic type, annular type and localized type. Oral psoriasis is an extremely rare condition. Benign migratory glossitis or geographical tongue is well documented oral lesion-in psoriasis (Figure 13.12 B).

PSORIATIC ARTHRITIS

Psoriatic arthritis is a seronegative inflammatory arthritis associated with psoriasis of skin. In 70% of cases arthritis develops years after skin changes of psoriasis but in 10% to 15% cases arthritis precedes the skin lesions. In psoriatic arthritis HLA-B7 and HLA-B27 are more commonly found. Psoriatic arthritis involves both peripheral joints and axial skeleton causing pain, stiffness and swelling. Rheumatoid factor is negative. Clinically five different patterns are seen.

1. **Asymmetric oligoarthritis:** Most of the cases belong to this group. Less than five joints are involved asymmetrically. Interphalangeal and metacarpophalangeal

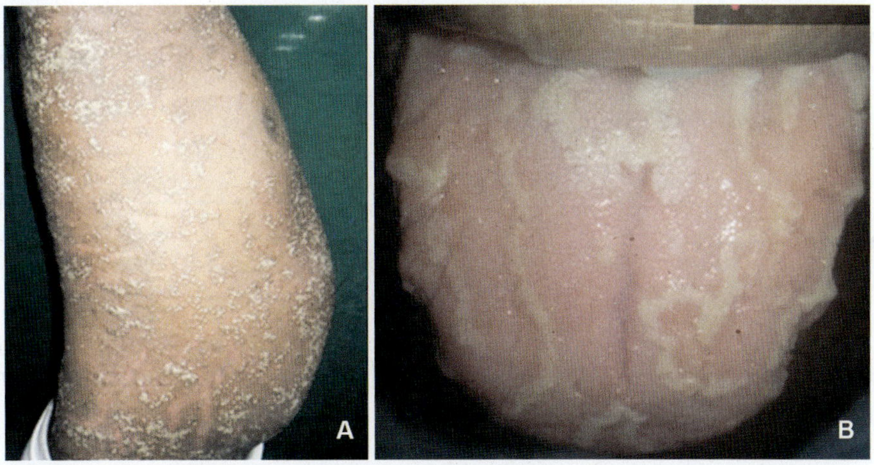

Figure 13.12: Generalized pustular psoriasis with geographical tongue (A and B)

joints are usually involved but hip and knee joints may also be affected. Dactylitis is a common feature of psoriatic arthritis which is due to inflammation of joints and tendons of the fingers leading to swelling and tenderness of the whole digit, also known as "sausage digit".

2. **Symmetric polyarthritis:** It resembles rheumatoid arthritis. Five or more joints are involved symmetrically.
3. **Distal interphalangeal joint arthritis:** It occurs only in 5% cases of psoriatic arthritis. Distal interphalangeal joints are mainly involved.
4. **Arthritis mutilans:** It is a severe form of arthritis causing destruction of bones and ankylosis of joints. There may be complete dissolution of phalanges.
5. **Spondyloarthritis:** It affects the sacroiliac joints and the apophyseal joints of the spine.

Diagnosis of psoriatic arthritis is based on clinical picture, history of psoriasis, negative rheumatoid factor and radiological changes. Radiological changes include mainly, erosion and new bone formation. There is loss of joint space, periostitis and lysis of the terminal phalanges. There is the pencil-in-cup appearance of the phalanges resulting from the reduced middle phalanx with bony proliferation at the base of distal phalanx. Classification of psoriatic arthritis (CASPER) criteria (Table 13.2) use for inflammatory arthritis.

Table 13.2: Classification of psoriatic arthritis (CASPER) criteria

Criteria	*Description*	*Points*
Psoriasis	Current psoriasis	2
	Personal history of psoriasis	1
	Psoriasis in a first- or second-degree relatives	1
Typical psoriatic nail involvement	–	1
Negative rheumatoid factors	–	1
Dactylitis	Current dactylitis	1
	History of dactylitis	1
Radiological evidence of psoriatic arthritis (Juxta articular new bone formation)	–	1
3 or more point out of 5 categories required for diagnosis of psoriatic arthritis		

Contd.

Diagnosis

Diagnosis of psoriasis is mostly done on clinical basis. It can be confirmed by histopathological examination (Figure 13.13) which is characterized by:

- Hyperkeratosis and parakeratosis.
- Absence of granular cell layer.
- Regular elongation, branching and clubbing of rete ridges.
- Collection of neutrophils in stratum corneum (Munro's micro abscess) and Malpighian layer (spongiform pustule of Kogoj).
- Supra-papillary thinning.
- Regular elongation of dermal papillae with clubbing of their upper ends. Marked edema and perivascular infiltrate of lymphocytes, histiocytes and neutrophils is seen in papillary dermis.

Differential Diagnosis

The psoriatic lesions are to be differentiated from:

1. **Seborrheic dermatitis:** Seborrheic distribution, greasy yellowish scales.

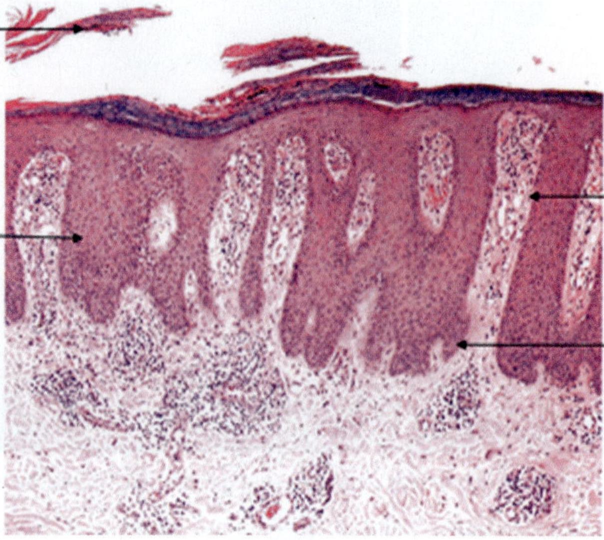

Figure 13.13: Showing histology of psoriasis

2. **Lichen simplex chronicus:** Thickened skin, hyperpigmentation and exaggeration of skin markings.
3. **Candidiasis:** To be differentiated from flexural psoriasis. Collarette scaling and satellite pustular lesions, candida positive.
4. **Pityriasis rosea:** To be differentiated from annular psoriasis. Lesions are distributed in inverted Christmas tree pattern and presence of herald patch.
5. **Tuberculoid leprosy:** Sensory loss, dry, hairless lesions and thickened nerve.
6. **Discoid lupus erythematosus:** Lesions are depigmented, atrophic, scarred and show 'carpet tack' sign.
7. **Tinea corporis:** Scaly well-defined lesions with central clearing. Fungus positive in KOH preparation.
8. **Syphilis:** Secondary syphilis lesions may mimic psoriasis lesions. Serology positive for syphilis.

Course and Prognosis

Psoriasis is a lifelong disease with variable period of remissions and exacerbations, however, the course and prognosis varies with the type of psoriasis. Guttate psoriasis is usually self-limiting and resolves within 12-16 weeks. Psoriatic erythroderma, pustular psoriasis and psoriatic arthritis are severe and persistent conditions.

Treatment

Though, there is no cure for psoriasis, but various topical and systemic therapeutic regimens can keep the disease in remission for long time. There are three main components of psoriasis therapy: topical therapy, phototherapy and systemic therapy.

- **Topical therapy:** Many patients of psoriasis can be treated with topical therapy alone. The important drugs used in topical therapy include:
  - ***Emollients:*** Liquid paraffin and white soft paraffin are used once or twice daily to remove dryness, relieve itching and reduce scaling. They can be combined with keratolytic agents like salicylic acid.
  - ***Salicylic acid:*** It is used as 2% to 6% ointment twice daily over thick lesions as keratolytic agent. It is commonly used with emollients, anthralin, tar and corticosteroids.
  - ***Coal tar:*** Coal tar has traditionally been used in psoriasis in **Goeckerman's regimen**. It consists of daily application of 1 to 5 percent crude coal tar, leaving it on body for 24 hours. The excess tar is removed by vegetable oil and then skin is exposed to ultraviolet light followed by bath. Tar acts by inhibition of DNA synthesis and sensitizing the skin to UVA.
  - ***Anthralin (Dithranol):*** It is used in plaque psoriasis as 0.05 to 0.1%, incorporated in petrolatum or zinc paste. 1-2% salicylic acid can also be added to it. Anthralin concentration is gradually increased upto 5% on weekly basis. It can also be used as short contact therapy where 2-4% anthralin in water soluble vehicle is applied for 5 to 30 minutes and then washed off. **Ingram regime consists of 0.1-0.5% anthralin ointment application and selective UVB phototherapy.** Anthralin acts as antiproliferative and

anti-inflammatory agent. Irritation and staining are the main side effects.

- *Corticosteroids:* Topical corticosteroids are highly effective in plaque and scalp psoriasis involving limited areas. Potent steroids like clobetasol propionate 0.05% or betamethasone dipropionate 0.05% are used as ointment for thick lesions and as cream for skin folds and flexural areas. In scalp psoriasis, they are used in solution or foam forms. They can be used alone or in combination with anthralin, coal tar and salicylic acid. Prolonged and inappropriate use may cause side effects like atrophy, striae, telangiectasia, folliculitis, milia and infection. Extensive use over large area may induce systemic side effects including HPA axis suppression and Cushing's syndrome.
- *Tazarotene:* Tazarotene is new generation retinoid which is beneficial in psoriasis by its anti-proliferative and anti-inflammatory action. It is used as 0.1% or 0.05% gel once daily at bed time. Mild to moderate skin irritation can be seen as side effect. It can be combined with corticosteroid for better results.
- *Calcipotriol:* It is a synthetic Vitamin D_3 derivative. It reduces epidermal cell proliferation and enhances keratinocyte differentiation. It is used as 50 µg/gm ointment, cream or lotion for plaque psoriasis, as monotherapy or in combination with phototherapy. Calcipotriol when combined with betamethasone dipropionate is highly effective in treating plaque psoriasis. The most common side effects are irritation, itching and redness.

- **Phototherapy:** Phototherapy in psoriasis has been in use for nearly a century. Broad-band UVB, narrow-band UVB, PUVA and excimer laser are used to treat psoriasis effectively.
  - *Broad-band UVB:* Ultraviolet radiation of the wave length 290 to 320 nm (UVB) is very useful in treating mild to moderate eruptive plaque psoriasis. Psoriatic lesions are rubbed with petrolatum before UVB exposure to enhance the UVB effect. Therapy is given thrice a week for three months. Remission for 3-6 months may be achieved. It may be combined with tar or anthralin.
  - *Narrow-band UVB:* Narrow-band (311-313nm) phototherapy is more effective than broad-band UVB in treating psoriasis. Stable or guttate psoriasis cases with more than 20% body area involvement can be treated with narrow-band UVB. Therapy is given two to four times a week in sub-erythemogenic doses. In 80% of cases this results in clearing of 90% of lesions in 20-30 sittings. Narrow-band therapy is most effective therapy with fewer side effects. It can be combined with topical steroids, calcipotriol or anthralin.
  - *PUVA therapy:* PUVA therapy consists of oral administration of psoralens followed by exposure to ultraviolet A(UVA). 8-methoxypsoralen (8-MOP) 0.6 mg/kg body weight is given on alternate days followed by exposure to UVA. PUVA chambers are used for UVA exposure after two hours for 10-15 minutes. Sunlight can be used alternatively in cases of non-availability of PUVA chamber (PUVASOL). Remission up to one year has been seen after 30 sittings. Short-term side effects include redness, swelling, blisters, nausea, vomiting, photo onycholysis and photo keratitis. Long-term side effects result due to high cumulative UVA doses. They are seen as PUVA lentigines, hypertrichosis, wrinkles, loss of elasticity and actinic keratosis. Risk of skin cancer and premature cataract formation are the other serious side effects. PUVA is contraindicated in children below 12 years. UVA-opaque glasses are to be used for eye protection.
  - *Bath PUVA:* Psoralen can be applied topically followed by UVA exposure to avoid the side effects of ingested psoralens. 8-MOP in the concentration of 0.5-4.5 mg/L followed by UVA given 2 to 4 times a week results in clearance of lesions in 60-90% patients.
  - *Excimer laser:* 308 nm excimer laser treatment and monochromatic excimer light have been found to be very safe and effective in treating psoriasis.
- **Systemic therapy:** Systemic drugs commonly used for psoriasis include retinoids, methotrexate, cyclosporin A and biologicals.
  - *Retinoids:* Retinoids are derived from Vitamin A. Etretinate was used in the treatment of psoriasis but it was discontinued due to its long-term storage in fat leading to serious side effects. Acitretin, an active metabolite of etretinate, is now used for treatment of severe psoriasis. It is more effective in pustular psoriasis than in other types of psoriasis. The exact mode of action of retinoids in psoriasis in not known but it interferes with various cytokines, thus reducing the inflammation. It also modulates the differentiation of epidermis. Acitretin is started in low doses of 10 to 25 mg/day and gradually increased to 50 mg/day. It can also be used in combination of phototherapy in plaque psoriasis. It is contraindicated in pregnancy due to its teratogenicity. The main side effects of acitretin include cheilitis, dryness of nasal mucosa and lips, hair loss, hyperlipidemia and disseminated idiopathic skeletal hyperostosis. Major limitation of oral retinoids (acitretin) in children is the risk of growth retardation due to premature closure of epiphyses on long-term use. Therefore, bone and spine radiology

together with regular growth parameter assessment should be applied in children on long-term retinoid therapy.

- ***Methotrexate:*** Methotrexate, a dihydro folate reductase (DHFR) antagonist, is now widely used in the treatment of moderate to severe psoriasis not responding to topical and other systemic therapies. Generalized pustular psoriasis, erythrodermic psoriasis and psoriatic arthritis are the other important indications. It is immunosuppressive, antiproliferative and anti-inflammatory drug. Two dosage schedules are commonly used: single weekly oral, intravenous or intramuscular dose of 10-25 mg once a week or 7.5 mg to 22.5 mg in three equal weekly oral doses at 12-hourly intervals once a week. Before starting therapy complete blood count, renal and hepatic function tests are done. Side effects include malaise, bone marrow suppression, nausea, vomiting, stomatitis and hepatotoxicity. It is contraindicated in pregnancy. Folic acid 5 mg/day if given with methotrexate can reduce the side effects such as nausea and megaloblastic anemia. In children, advantages of MTX include the efficacy and weekly oral dose (0.2–0.7 mg/kg/week). Dose escalations of 1.25–5 mg/week until the achievement of clinical benefits, followed by a slow tapering to a maintenance dosage, is advised. Generally, MTX-associated side effects are less frequent and less severe in children, probably due to the low frequency of concomitant medications and comorbidities at the pediatric age.
- ***Cyclosporin:*** It is an immunosuppressive drug obtained from a fungus. It selectively inhibits the release of interleukin-1 and interleukin-2 which plays a major role in activation of T lymphocytes. Most of the reports indicate a favorable response with CYA in childhood psoriasis.
  - *Indications:* Erythrodermic psoriasis, generalized and localized pustular psoriasis and psoriatic arthritis.
  - *Dosage:* Starting dose is 2.5-5 mg/kg body weight per day; it can be increased by 0.5 to 1mg/kg body weight per day.
  - *Side effects:* Hypertension, nephrotoxicity, hyperlipidemia, increased risk of infections, arthralgia, nausea, vomiting and increased risk of malignancy.
- ***Other drugs:*** Fumaric acid esters, hydroxyurea and mycophenolate mofetil are the other drugs which have been found useful in treatment of psoriasis.
- ***Biological therapies:*** Recent realization that psoriasis is an immune system dysfunction has led to the development of new therapies which target the immune system. These drugs are called "biological therapies" as they are different engineered proteins produced in living organisms. They interfere with the specific components of the immune response.

BIOLOGICALS IN PSORIASIS

1. **TNF alfa inhibitors – Etanercept, Infliximab, Adalimumab**

   Etanercept: It is available as 25 mg dose per vial as a sterile, white, preservative free lyophilized powder for parenteral administration, after reconstitution with 1 ml of the supplied sterile bacteriostatic water for injection. The adult dose is 50 mg/week, given subcutaneously for 3 months.

   Infliximab: It is given IV in doses of 5 or 10 mg/kg, over a period of 2 hours at weeks 0, 2, 6 and may be followed by repeat single infusions at 8-12 weeks intervals.

   Adalimumab: It is given as 40 mg S/C every other week.

   Certolizumab and Golimumab are other TNF antagonists are in various stages of clinical development.
2. **Secukinumab** is a fully recombinant human IgG1 that selectively binds to and neutralizes the pro-inflammatory cytokine IL-17A. It is given as an induction dose of 300 mg every week for 5 weeks and thereafter as a maintenance regimen of 300 mg once a month administered subcutaneously.
3. **Itolizumab:** It is a humanized recombinant anti-CD6 monoclonal antibody. It is available as a preservative-free, single-use 25 mg/5 ml vial and is administered intravenously at a dose of 1.6 mg/kg once every 2 weeks for the first 3 months and then once a month for the next 3 months (total infusion is 250 ml) over an infusion period of not less than 3 hours. Alefacept is a bivalent recombinant fusion protein composed of the first extracellular domain lymphocyte function antigen 3 (LFA-3), fused to the hinge CH2 domain and CH3 domain of human IgG1. It is given by intramuscular or intravenous route with a dose of 10-15 mg IM weekly or 7.5 mg IV weekly and a 12-week course is recommended.
4. **Alefacept:** It is a bivalent recombinant fusion protein composed of the first extracellular domain lymphocyte function antigen 3 (LFA-3), fused to the hinge CH2 domain and CH3 domain of human IgG1. It is given by intramuscular or intravenous route with a dose of 10-15 mg IM weekly or 7.5 mg IV weekly and a 12-week course is recommended.
5. **Efalizumab** is a recombinant humanized monoclonal IgG1 antibody that binds to CD11a, a subunit of leukocyte

function-associated antigen 1 (LFA-1) in a dose of 1 mg/kg weekly as a subcutaneous, self-administered injection for 12 weeks, following a first conditioning dose of 0.7 mg/kg.

6. **Ustekinumab:** It is a fully human monoclonal antibody targeting IL-12 and IL-23, given as 45 mg or 90 mg subcutaneously at weeks 0 and 4 and then every 12 weeks.
7. **Apremilast:** It is an oral phosphodiesterase 4 inhibitor, approved by the FDA in the management of psoriatic arthropathy (PsA). The recommended maintenance dose is 30 mg twice daily. A two-week titration pack containing 10 mg, 20 mg and 30 mg tablets is available to facilitate the initiation of therapy. Patients with severe renal impairment (Creatinine Clearance of less than 30 ml/min) require a modified dosing schedule with a maintenance dose of 30 mg once daily. The most common adverse effects are diarrhea, nausea and headache. Other side effects include upper respiratory tract infection, vomiting, nasopharyngitis, upper abdominal pain, hypersensitivity, dyspnea, cough and skin rash.
8. **Biosimilars:** They are regarded as the biological equivalent of a chemical generic drug. They are similar, but not exactly identical, to the original innovator biological agent. The first biosimilars of the mAb infliximab were approved in 2013 by EMA under the brand names of Remsima and Inflectra. Amgevita, Cyltezo and Imraldi are biosimilars of Adalimumab whereas Benepali and Erelzi are of Etanercept.

CHILDHOOD PSORIASIS

Psoriasis in children differs from that of adults in the following aspects:

- Prevalence of childhood psoriasis is 0.1% to 3% of pediatric population.
- It is more common in females than in males.
- In studies from India, most patients developed psoriasis at the age of 6 to 10 years.
- Familial prevalence is greater in childhood psoriasis than in adult onset psoriasis.
- Bacterial and viral infections especially streptococcal infection causing upper respiratory tract infection and perianal dermatitis, physical and psychological trauma are common triggering factors in childhood psoriasis.
- As compared to adults the lesions of childhood psoriasis are more pruritic, thinner, softer and less scaly (Figure 13.14 A, B).
- In infants under the age of 2 years, the most frequent presentation is "diaper rash".
- Childhood psoriatic lesions are more common on face than in adults. The other sites involved are axillae, groin, palms soles, genital and perianal area, knees, elbows, nails and scalp.
- Psoriatic erythroderma, arthropathy and pustular psoriasis are rare in children.
- Guttate psoriasis is the classical pattern of childhood psoriasis but not uncommon in India, plaque type psoriasis is more common in children.
- Mucosal involvement is common in childhood psoriasis but it is rare in India.

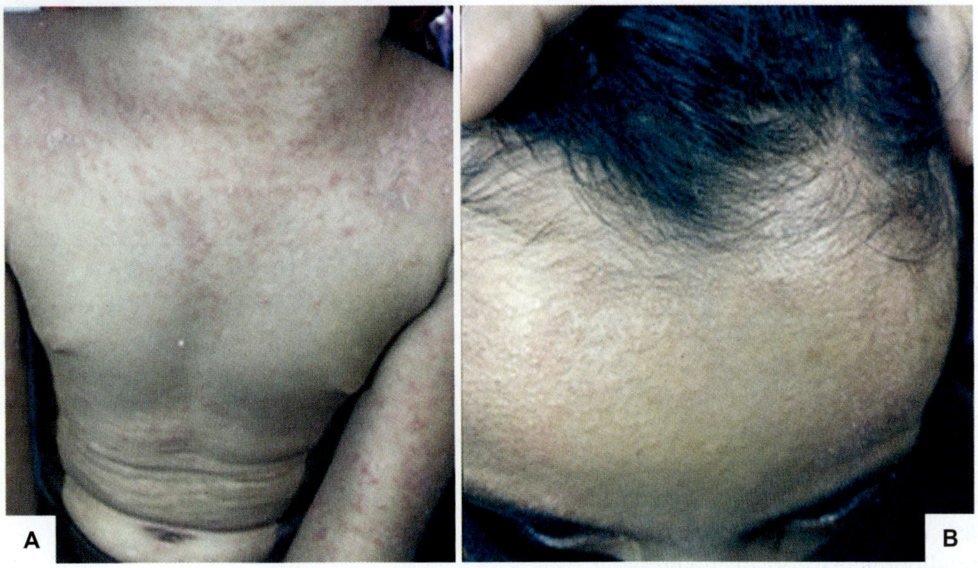

Figure 13.14: Childhood psoriasis (A and B)

- Low potency topical steroids are used in children. Calcipotriol is effective and safe in children.
- Systemic therapies are not indicated in children but in most severe cases retinoids, methotrexate, phototherapy and PUVA may be considered in older children.

LICHEN PLANUS (LP)

Lichen planus is an inflammatory, papulosquamous disorder of skin, mucous membrane, hair and nail, of unknown etiology, characterized by formation of shiny, flat topped, polygonal, violaceous, papular lesions.

Epidemiology

Worldwide prevalence of lichen planus is less than 1%. In India incidence of 0.38% has been reported in one study. Females are affected more than males. It is considered to be rare in children but it is not uncommon in Indian subcontinent. It is extremely uncommon in infants. The average age of onset is fourth decade in males and sixth decade in females. In children the average age of onset of 7.1 to 8.4 years has been reported in some studies.

Etiopathogenesis

The exact etiology of lichen planus is unknown but immunological mechanism is thought to be operative. Apoptosis of keratinocytes is the main event brought about by activation of cell mediated immunity. Infectious agents (HIV, HCV, HHV-7, *Helicobacter pylori,* etc.), drugs (antihypertensive like- beta blockers, ACE inhibitors, penicillamine, gold salts, etc.), vaccination (influenza, DPT, etc.), chemical and occupational exposures like those in furniture industries, photograph developers, dentists, etc., are involved in the pathogenesis. Genetic predisposition has also been recorded with familial incidence and association of HLA-3, HLA-5, HLA-B7 and HLA-B18 with lichen planus.

Pathogenesis includes three stages:

1. Lichen planus specific antigen recognition
2. Cytotoxic lymphocyte activation
3. Keratinocyte apoptosis

Following antigen recognition (autoantigen or exogenous), CD8+ T-cells are activated to upregulate cytokines associated with a Th1 immune response, like IFN gamma , TNF alfa, IL-2, IL-6 and IL-8. There is increased expression of vascular endothelial adhesion molecules (intercellular adhesion molecule-1 [ICAM-1] and vascular cell adhesion molecule [VCAM]) and mast cell degranulation is also observed. MMP-9 (matrix metalloproteinase-9) overexpression causes disruption of the basement membrane resulting in the transit of T-cells into the epidermis.

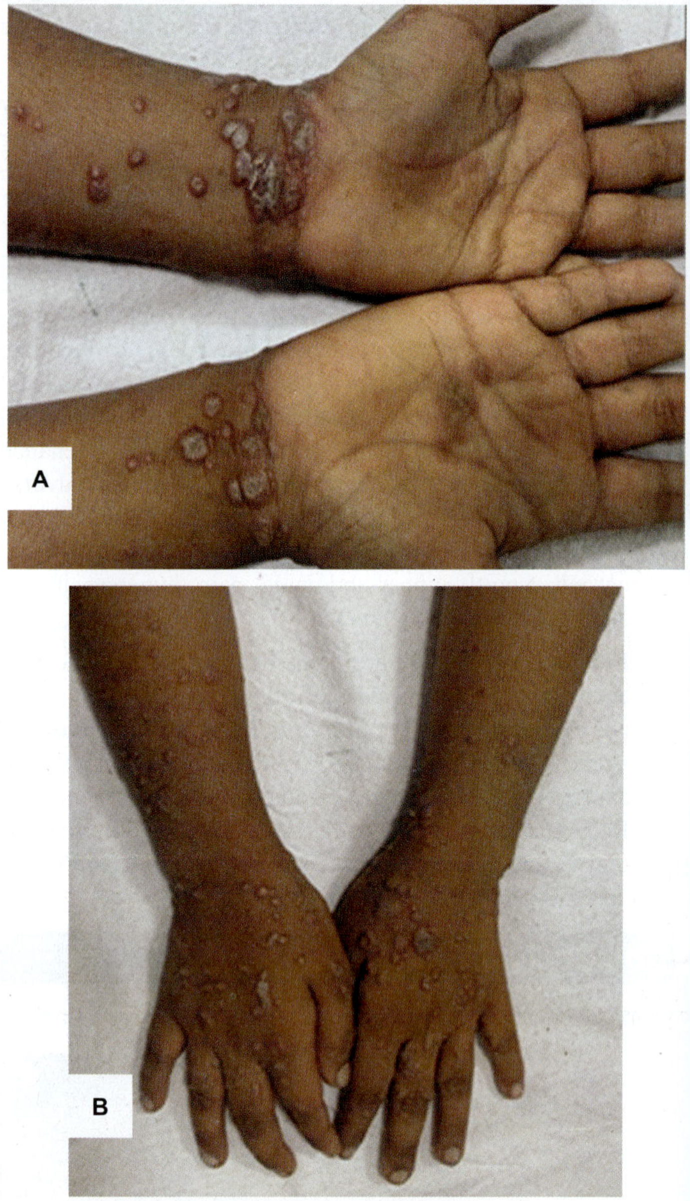

Figure 13.15: Classical lesions of lichen planus (A and B)

Clinical Features

- Lesions of lichen planus are intensely pruritic, shiny, violaceous, flat-topped papules (Figure 13.15 A, B), variable in size from pinpoint to a centimeter or more in diameter.
- Surface of the papules shows fine white reticulate lines known as Wickham's striae.
- New lesions may develop over site of injury or scratch mark or on scars (Koebner phenomenon) (Figure 13.16).

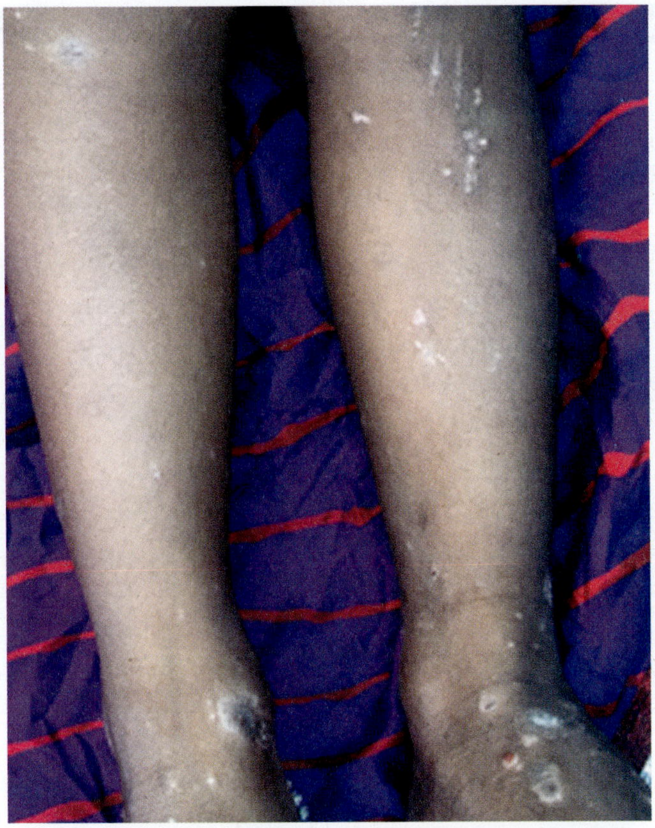

Figure 13.16: Lichen planus with Koebner phenomenon

- Papules may remain discrete or may be arranged in groups, in lines (Figure 13.17) or in circles.
- Lesions are generally seen on front of wrist, lumbar region and around ankles. Other body areas may also be involved.
- After few months papules flatten and leave behind hyperpigmentation persisting for months and years.
- Some papules may thicken and persist for a longer period forming lichen planus hypertrophicus.
- Mucosa is involved in 30-70% cases and sometimes may be involved even without involvement of skin. The buccal mucosa and tongue are most commonly involved, but lesions can be seen around anus, on the genitalia and in the larynx. White streaks forming a lacework on the buccal mucosa are characteristic lesions of lichen planus. They may be present on inner surface of cheeks, gums and lips.
- Acute lichen planus lesions may resolve in 6 to 18 months while chronic lesions persist for a long time.
- Lichen planus may be associated with diabetes, candidiasis, ulcerative colitis, alopecia areata, vitiligo, dermatomyositis, systemic lupus erythematosus and pemphigus.

Lichen planus and lichenoid drug eruption differences are given in Table 13.3:

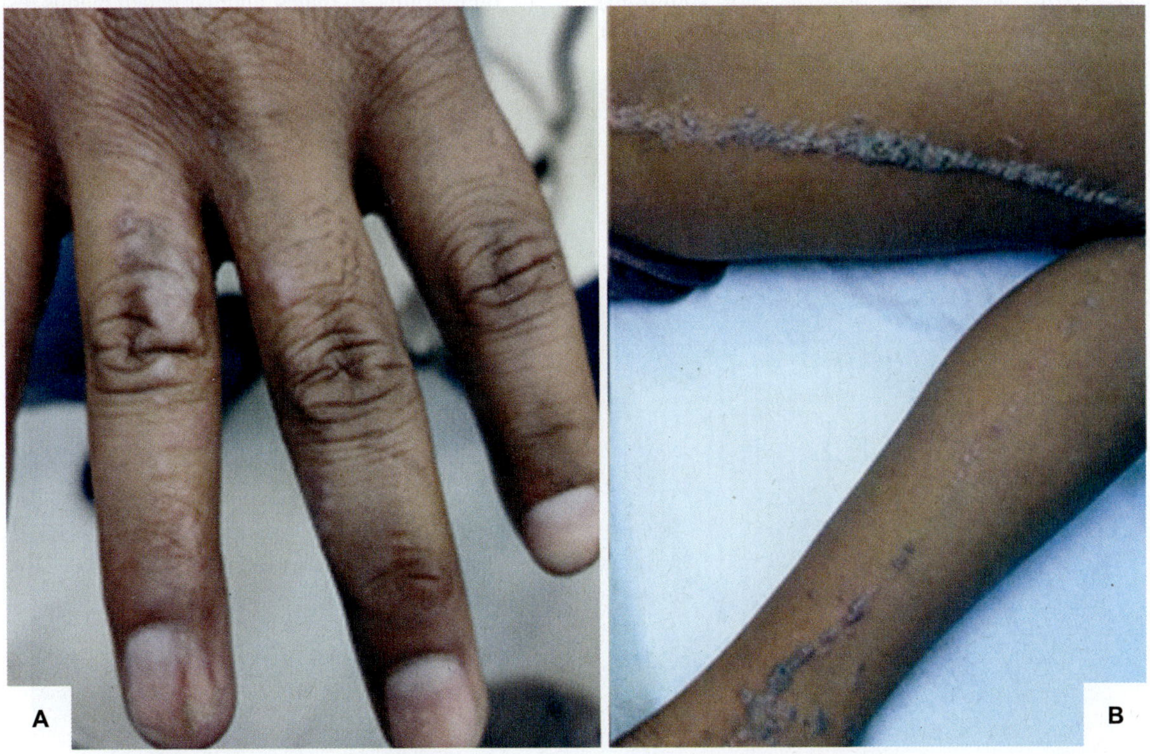

Figure 13.17: Linear lichen planus with nail involvement (A and B)

Table 13.3: Showing difference between lichen planus and lichenoid drug eruption		
	Lichen planus	***Lichenoid drug eruption***
Aetiology	Autoimmune	Drug induced
Trigger	Unknown, possible triggers are trauma, infections, medications and dental implant	Drugs like beta blockers, antimalarials, Terbinafine ACE inhibitors, NSAIDS, Thiazide diuretics, penicillamine, mepacrine, isoniazid, Methyldopa etc.
Latent period	Unknown	Few weeks to months
Morphology of lesions	Polygonal, flat topped, violaceous papules	Scaly or eczematous papules and plaques
Wickham's striae	Present	Absent
Distribution of lesions	Flexural (wrists, forearms, lower legs)	Generalized or photo distributed
Mucosal lesions	Usually, present	Absent
Nail involvement	Usually, present	Absent
Scalp involvement	Common	uncommon
Isomorphic phenomena	Common	Uncommon
Colloid bodies	Occasional	Multiple
Parakeratosis	Absent	Present
Focal spongiosis and eosinophils	Absent	Present
Course and prognosis	Self limiting	Take longer time to resolve

Variants of Lichen Planus

- **Mucosal lichen planus:** Lesions involving only mucous membranes without skin involvement is seen in about 15% cases. Oral and genital mucosae are commonly involved. Oral lesions may be reticular (Figure 13.18), erosive, atrophic, bullous or plaque. Erosive type oral lichen planus may rarely develop into squamous cell carcinoma. Genital lichen planus may occur alone or in combination with oral lesions or as a part of generalized lesions. In females, lesions are painful, white, lacy erosions on introitus. In males, annular lichen planus lesions are seen on shaft, glans penis, prepuce and scrotum.

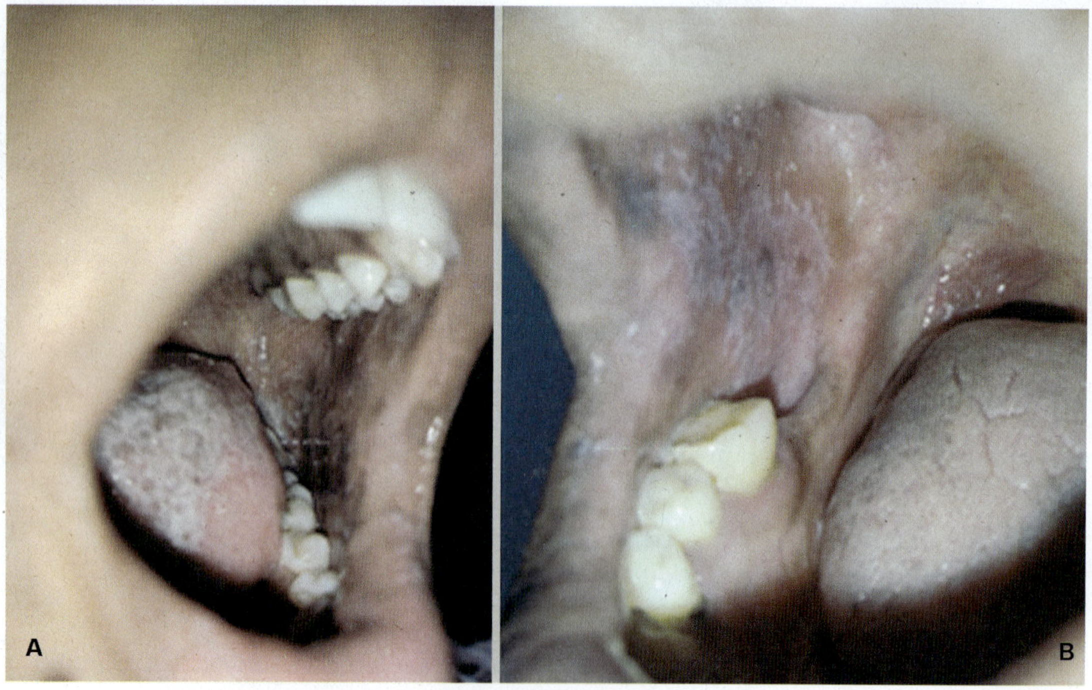

Figure 13.18: Mucosal lichen planus (A and B)

- **Lichen planus hypertrophicus:** Lesions are thick, hypertrophied, hyperpigmented generally seen over shins and ankles (Figure 13.19). Some lesions may show central depigmentation and peripheral ring of hyperpigmentation. There is severe itching and lesions heal with scarring.

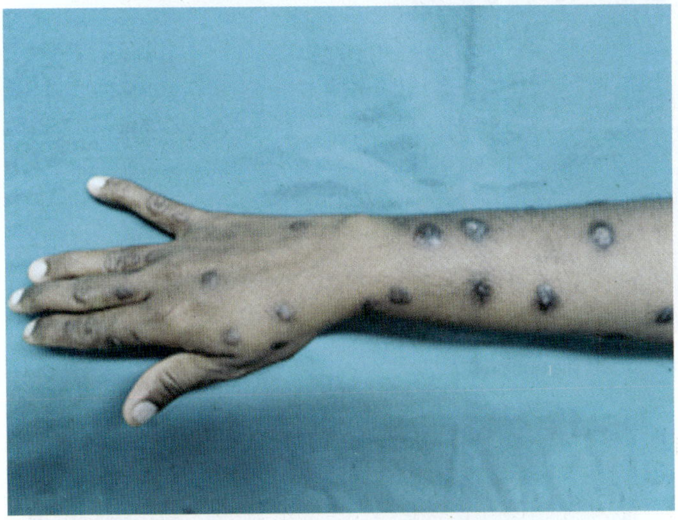

Figure 13.19: Hypertrophic lichen planus

- **Lichen planus atrophicus:** Papule or plaque lesions become atrophic in the center. They are seen on trunk and lower limbs.
- **Guttate or eruptive lichen planus:** Multiple small, discrete, erythematous, pinhead to 1cm size papular lesions appear in crops, distributed widely over trunk (Figure 13.20).

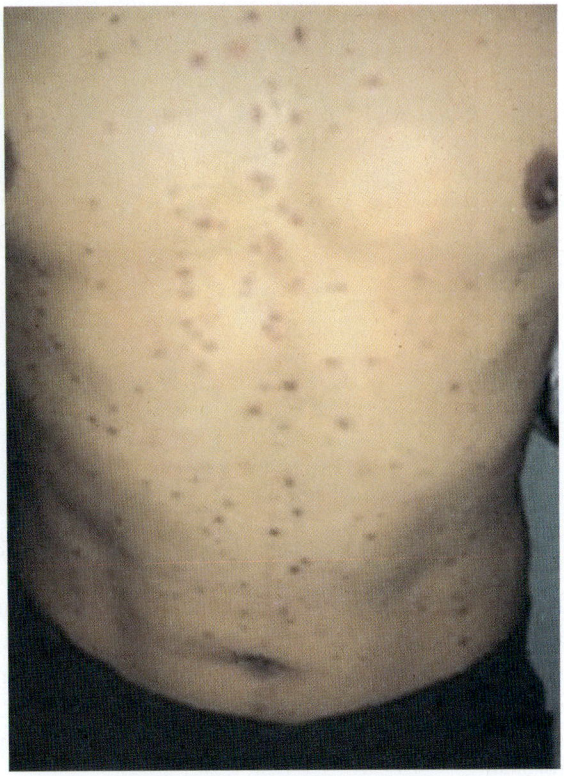

Figure 13.20: Guttate lichen planus

- **Follicular lichen planus (Lichen planopilaris):** Lesions are violaceous or hyperpigmented, follicular, hyperkeratotic papules present over trunk, medial aspects of proximal extremities and scalp (Figure 13.21). On scalp, lesions are followed by cicatricial alopecia.

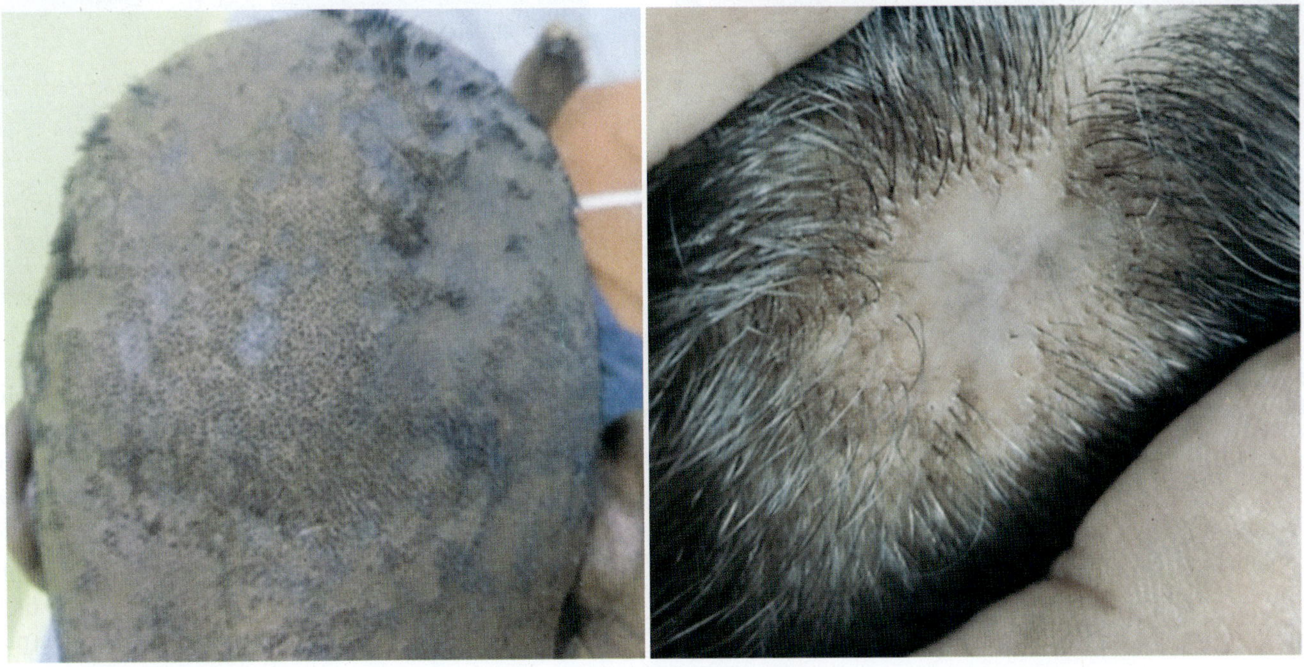

Figure 13.21: Lichen planopilaris

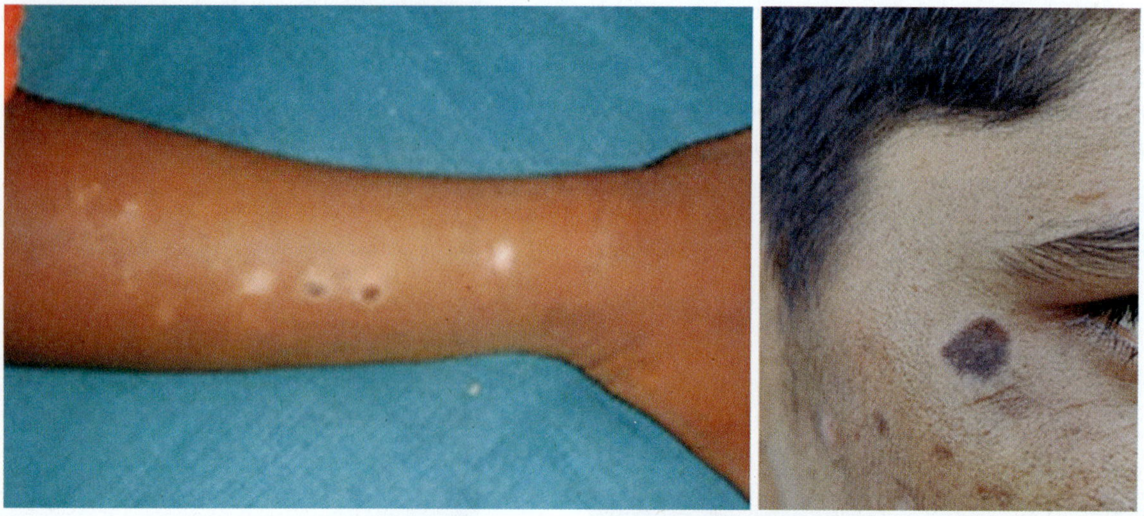

Figure 13.22: Actinic lichen planus

- **Actinic lichen planus:** It is generally seen in children and young adults in tropical countries during spring and summer. Sunlight is the predisposing factor. Lesions are seen on face, outer area of forearms (Figure 13.22), dorsa of hands and neck. Sometimes melasma like lesions can be seen.
- **Lichen planus pigmentosus:** Slate grey to brownish black macular pigmentation is seen on face (Figure 13.23), neck and upper limbs. Typical lichen planus lesions may or may not be seen.

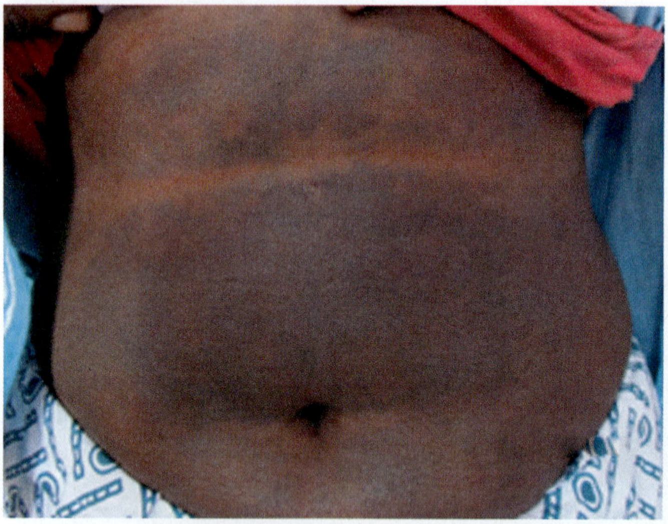

Figure 13.23: Lichen planus pigmentosus

- **Annular lichen planus:** Multiple small and few large annular lesions with central atrophy surrounded by narrow rim of erythema are commonly seen on shaft and glans penis (Figure 13.24).

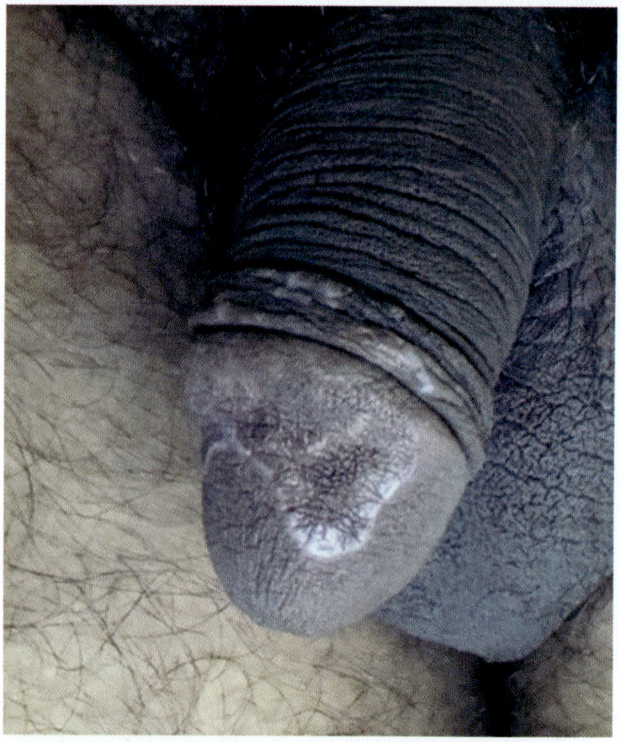

Figure 13.24: Showing annular genital lichen planus

- **Bullous lichen planus:** In Bullous lichen planus, blisters arise on or near the lesion of lichen planus due to severe liquefactive degeneration of basal cell layer. Histology shows typical lichenoid changes with subepidermal bulla. Direct and indirect immunofluorescence are negative.
- **Lichen planus pemphigoides:** Lichen planus pemphigoides presents with sudden appearance of large bulla both on involved and uninvolved sites of lichen planus.

Such type of lesions can also be seen in paraneoplastic pemphigus. Histology shows subepidermal bulla without typical lichenoid changes. Direct immunofluorescence shows linear deposition of IgG and C3 in perilesional skin and on indirect immunofluorescence circulating antibody against C- terminal of NC16A domain of bullous pemphigoid antigen is seen.

- **Nekam's disease (Keratosis Lichenoides Chronica):** It presents with linear or reticulately arranged violaceous papules and nodules on buttocks and extremities with seborrheic dermatitis like eruption on face. Individual papules and nodules have verrucous surface with keratotic plugs. On removal of plugs, surface reveals irregular indentations. Recurrent oral aphthae can also be seen. Histology shows chronic dermatitis with lichenoid changes.
- **Nail involvement:** It occurs in about 10% cases. Finger nails are more frequently involved than toe nails. Nail changes include focal or diffuse thinning, exaggerated longitudinal lines, distal splitting, pterygium formation, melanonychia, erythronychia, leukonychia, proximal onycholysis and pup tent nails (Figure 13.25).

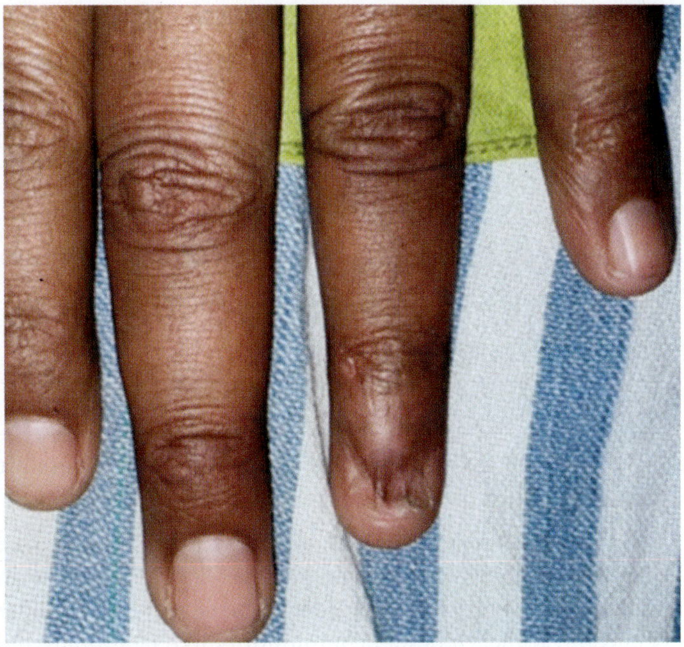

Figure 13.25: Nail lichen planus showing pterygium of ring finger

Diagnosis

Diagnosis of lichen planus is made on clinical grounds; it may be confirmed by characteristic histopathology which shows the following features: (Figure 13.26)

1. Compact hyperkeratosis.
2. Wedge shaped hypergranulosis.
3. Elongated rete ridges which may appear flattened known as "saw-tooth" appearance.
4. Liquefaction degeneration of the basal cell layer.
5. Multiple apoptotic basal cells called colloid body may be present singly or in groups at dermoepidermal junction and in papillary dermis.
6. A band like, dense, lymphocytic infiltration is seen at papillary dermis.
7. Incontinence of melanin.
8. Small separation between dermis and epidermis may be present (Max-Joseph spaces).

Differential Diagnosis

Lichen planus is to be differentiated from:

1. Lichenoid eruption caused by drugs or color developers.

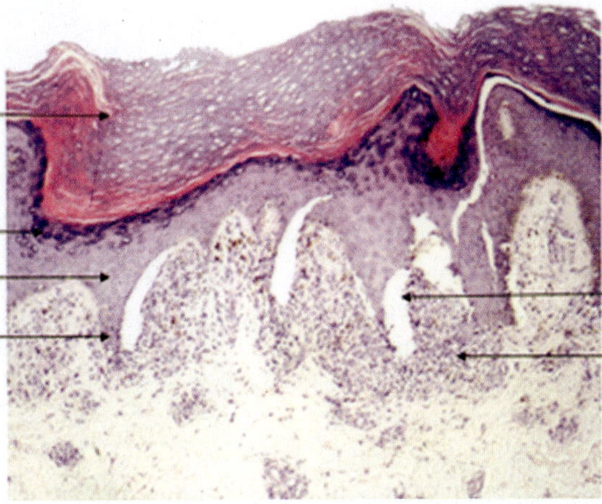

Figure 13.26: Showing lichen planus histology

2. Plane warts, pityriasis rosea, lichen amyloidosis.
3. Hypertrophic LP from nodular prurigo, lichen simplex chronicus.
4. Atrophic LP from morphea, lichen sclerosus et atrophicus.
5. Annular LP from granuloma annulare.
6. Guttate LP from guttate psoriasis.
7. Oral LP from leukoplakia, oral pemphigus.
8. LP nails from onychomycosis, nail psoriasis.

Treatment

Lichen planus may resolve spontaneously after a variable period. Treatment involves topical and systemic therapies.

Topical therapy: Potent topical corticosteroids like clobetasol propionate 0.05% are the mainstay of treatment in lichen planus. For LP hypertrophicus they can be given under occlusion. Topical calcineurin inhibitors like tacrolimus and pimecrolimus are also useful.

Systemic therapy: In widespread eruptive lichen planus, erosive oral LP and progressive nail LP, systemic corticosteroids, e.g., prednisolone 1-2 mg/kg/day is given for one or two weeks then tapered. Acitretin and cyclosporine may be used in those cases who do not respond to corticosteroids. Other systemic agents like griseofulvin, dapsone, hydroxychloroquine, metronidazole, methotrexate, cyclophosphamide and azathioprine have also been used in cutaneous, oral and nail LP. Antihistamines are used to alleviate the itching.

LICHEN NITIDUS (LN)

Lichen nitidus is a lichenoid dermatosis of unknown etiology characterized by minute, skin colored, numerous, grouped asymptomatic papules of size 1-2 mm. Children and young adults are commonly involved.

Etiology

Exact etiology is not known but it is thought to be a variant of lichen planus.

Clinical Features

Lesions are asymptomatic tiny pinpoint to pinhead sized, flat or dome-shaped, shiny papular lesions. They are discrete lesions but are arranged in groups (Figure 13.27A). They are seen on forearms, wrists, penis, abdomen, chest, buttocks and knees. Palms and soles may also be involved. Lichen nitidus lesions can coexist with lichen planus lesions. Oral lesions in lichen nitidus are rare. Involvement of palms, soles and nails are rare. Other variants of LN are—confluent, hemorrhagic, linear, perforating, vesicular, spinous follicular, generalized and actinic.

Diagnosis

Diagnosis of lichen nitidus is mainly clinical but in doubtful cases it can be confirmed by histopathology which is quite characteristic.

The salient features of histopathology of lichen nitidus are:

- There is a well-defined infiltrate of lymphocytes, histiocytes and few langhans giant cells immediately below epidermis.
- The epidermis is flattened and sometimes there is liquefaction degeneration of basal cells.
- The rete ridges at the margin of the infiltrate are elongated and encircle the infiltrate giving a claw like pattern (ball in clutch appearance) (Figure 13.27B).

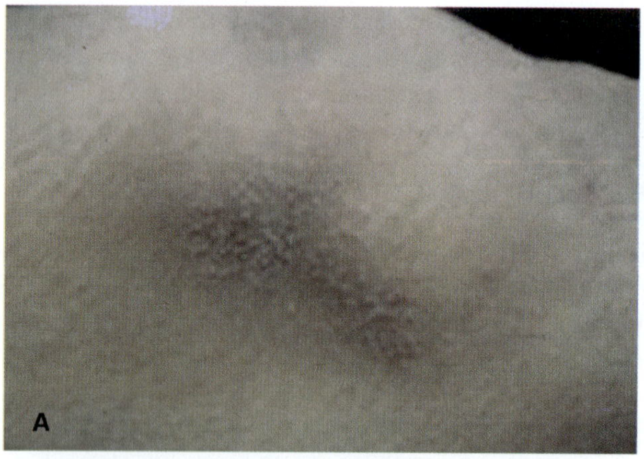

Figure 13.27 A: Lichen nitidus over knee

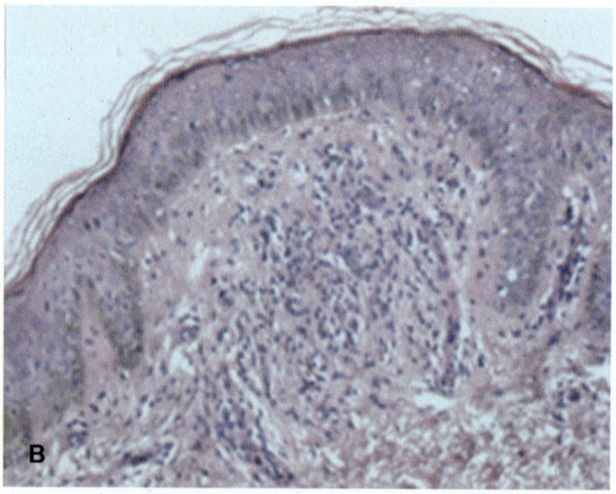

Figure 13.27B: Claw like acanthotic rete ridge encircling lymphohistiocytic granuloma

Differential Diagnosis

Lichen nitidus is to be differentiated from:

- Lichen scrofulosorum.
- Phrynoderma.

Treatment

- As the disease is asymptomatic and self-limiting, no treatment is required in most of the cases.
- In those cases where treatment is required, topical corticosteroids are prescribed.
- Generalized lichen nitidus can be treated with systemic corticosteroids, PUVA or narrow band UVB phototherapy.

PITYRIASIS RUBRA PILARIS (PRP)

Pityriasis rubra pilaris is an uncommon chronic papulosquamous disorder characterized by reddish orange scaly plaques, acuminate follicular papules and palmoplantar keratoderma.

Etiology

The etiology is unknown. Family history is positive in some cases with autosomal dominant pattern. Disorder of Vitamin A metabolism has also been implicated in the etiology. Immunological abnormality, bacterial and viral infections have also been blamed as etiological factors.

Clinical Features

The disease occurs in three age groups viz early childhood (upto 10 years), late childhood (11-19 years) and adulthood in fifth decade. The average incidence is 1 in 5000 of population. In adults both sexes are affected equally but in children males are affected more than females.

- The characteristic lesions of PRP are widespread, small, acuminate follicular papules with pinkish yellow scales (mica like) that coalesce to form plaques with islands of normal skin (island of sparing) (Figure 13.28). These plaques are present symmetrically on the trunk and limbs. Keratosis pilaris is also seen.
- Keratosis pilaris. Scalp shows diffuse erythema and scaling simulating seborrheic dermatitis.
- PRP begins at scalp and then descends down to whole trunk resulting into erythroderma with islands of normal skin within the affected area.
- Dorsal aspect of proximal phalanges show follicular hyperkeratosis, which is surrounded by an erythematous perifollicular halo. Palpation of these lesions give a sensation of 'nutmeg grater'. This sign is considered pathognomonic of PRP.
- The scaling is fine and branny and is most marked on face.
- There is yellowish orange hyperkeratosis of palms and soles with painful fissures (Figure 13.28). It is often termed as 'PRP sandal'.
- The nails are thickened, brittle with longitudinal ridging and splinter hemorrhage.
- Oral mucosa may rarely be involved showing diffuse, lacy white plaques resembling lichen planus.

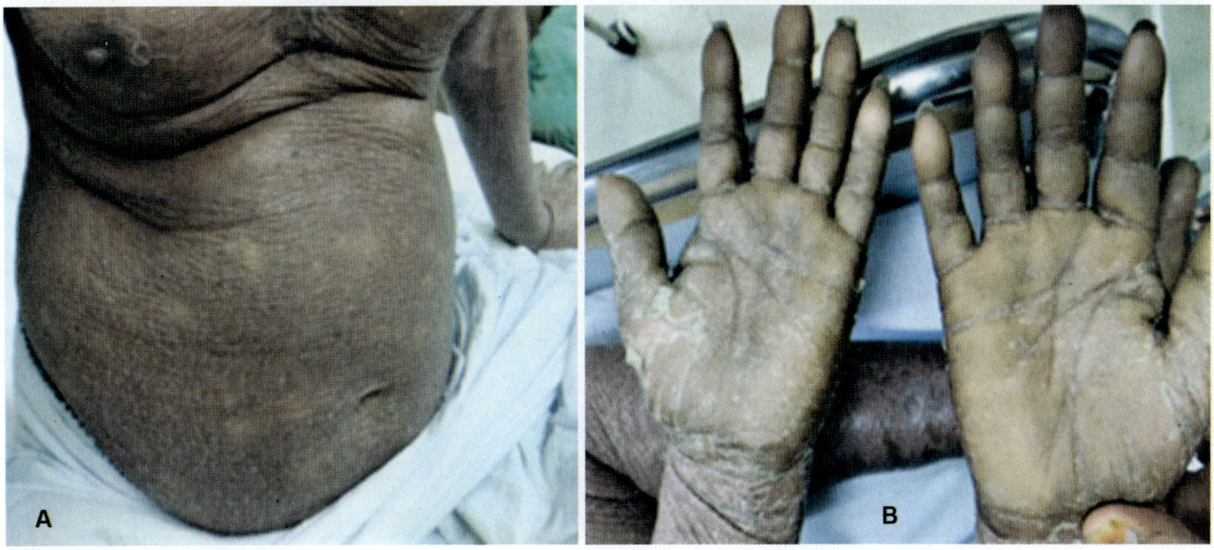

Figure 13.28: Classical adult type PRP showing island of sparing with yellowish hyperkeratosis of palms (A and B)

Classification

PRP has been classified into five types on the basis of age of onset, clinical features and prognosis.

1. **Type I (Classical adult type):** This is the most common type of PRP seen in more than 50% cases. It affects the adults and has acute onset. Progression of the disease is cephalocaudal. It carries a good prognosis with spontaneous resolution in 80% cases within 1 to 3years.
2. **Type II (Atypical adult type):** It accounts for about 5% cases. Clinical features are atypical with lamellar ichthyosiform scaling and eczematous changes. Scalp hair is sparse. Disease persists for a long time.
3. **Type III (Classical juvenile type):** It is similar to classical adult type except that it starts in first two years of life. It is seen in about 10% cases. Spontaneous resolution is seen in 1 to 2 years.
4. **Type IV (Circumscribed juvenile type):** Circumscribed plaques of erythematous follicular papular hyperkeratosis are seen on elbows and knees resembling psoriasis (Figure 13.29). It affects the pre-pubertal children and accounts for about 25% cases. The prognosis is uncertain.
5. **Type V (Atypical juvenile type):** It begins at birth or in the first year of life and overlap with icthyosis and erythrokeratoderma. Erythematous follicular hyperkeratosis and scleroderma like changes are seen in hands and feet. Most cases of familial PRP belong to this group and run a chronic course. This accounts for about 5% of cases.
6. **PRP associated with HIV:** A variant of PRP associated with HIV shows acne conglobata and filiform pattern of keratosis. Elongated follicular plugs or lichen spinulosus like lesions are seen. PRP type VI has been proposed for this type of PRP.

Diagnosis

The diagnosis of PRP is mainly clinical. It can be supplemented by histopathological findings which are as follows:

1. Diffuse hyperkeratosis.
2. Follicular keratin plug surrounded by perifollicular parakeratosis.
3. Focal or confluent hypergranulosis.
4. Thick suprapapillary plates, broad rete ridges, narrow dermal papillae.
5. Sparse perivascular infiltrate, mostly of lymphocytes, in the superficial dermis.

Differential Diagnosis

PRP is to be differentiated from:

1. Psoriasis.
2. Phrynoderma.
3. Erythrokeratoderma.
4. Follicular eczema.
5. Keratosis pilaris.
6. Lichen scrofulosorum.

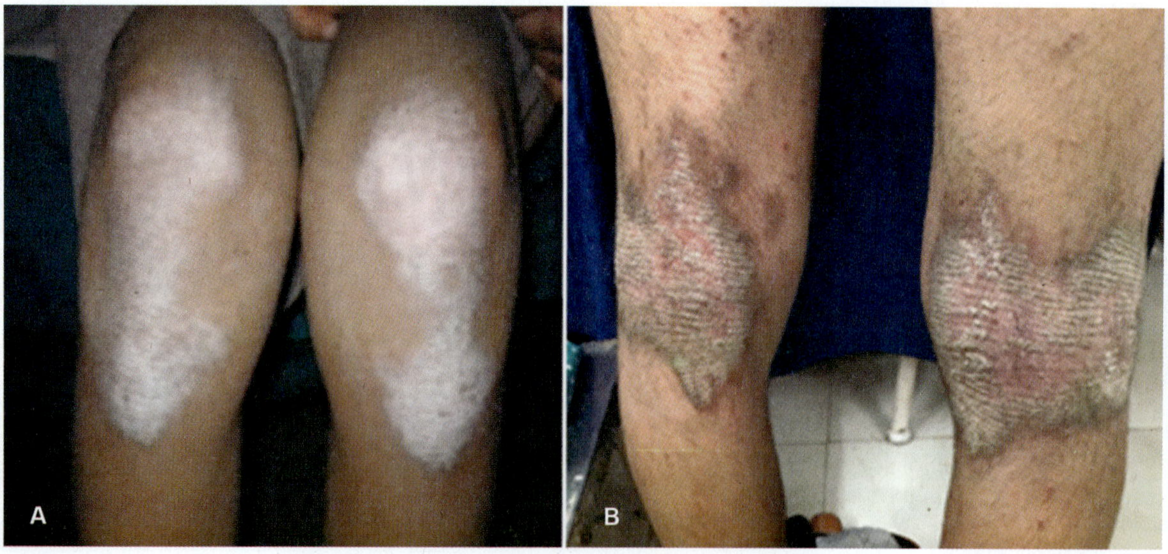

Figure 13.29: Circumscribed juvenile type PRP (A and B)

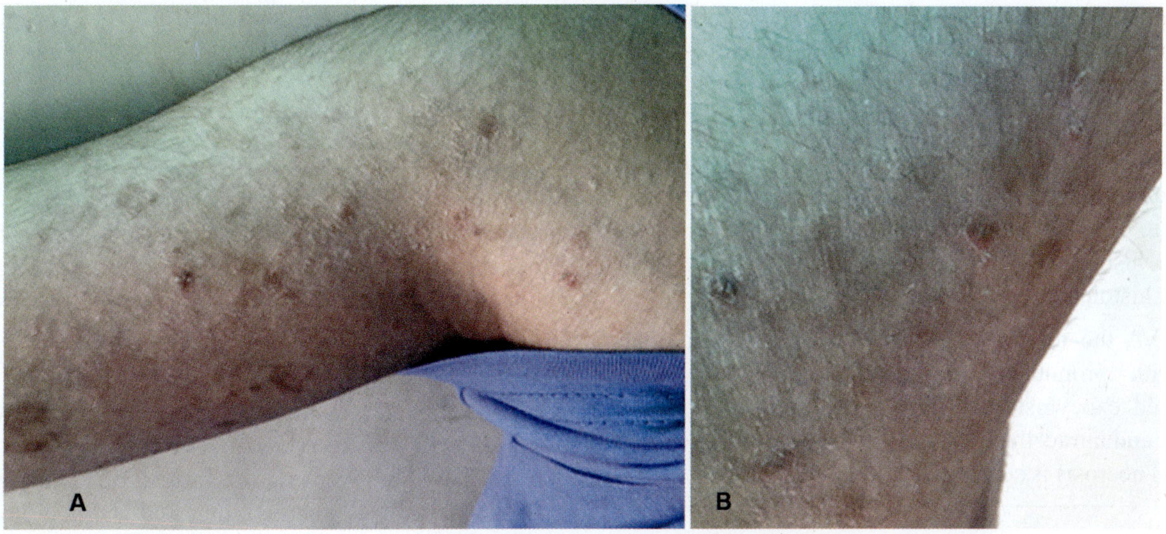

Figure 13.30: Pityriasis lichenoides chronica (A and B)

Treatment

Topical therapy: Topical emollients with mild keratolytics like 3% salicylic acid ointment is used to reduce itching and scaling. Topical corticosteroids, pimecrolimus and calcipotriol may be used for limited area.

Systemic therapy: Oral Vitamin A 50,000 IU three times daily with Vitamin E, isotretinoin 1mg/kg/day and acitretin 0.5-0.75 mg/kg/day are the drugs used in systemic therapy. Clinical improvement with retinoids takes 4 to 6 weeks' time. Systemic corticosteroids have no role in PRP. Narrowband phototherapy is useful. Cyclosporin, methotrexate, azathioprine, infliximab and efalizumab have been found to be effective in PRP in different studies.

PITYRIASIS LICHENOIDES (PL)

PL an uncommon dermatitis, previously included in the parapsoriasis group.

The pathogenic mechanism is unclear although infectious or drug related hypersensitivity reactions versus premycotic lymphoproliferative disorder are the main theories.

Variants: Pityriasis lichenoides et varioliformis acuta (PLEVA), pityriasis lichenoides chronica (PLC), and febrile ulceronecrotic Mucha-Habermann disease (FUMHD) are clinical variants of this group of disorders.

PLC has a gradual manifestation of very small red to brown flat maculopapular with mica-like scales (Figure 13.30); it also follows a relapsing course but with long periods of remission.

PLEVA (Figure 13.31) generally presents as an acute-to-subacute skin eruption of multiple, small, red papules that develops into polymorphic lesions and vacillates with periods of varying remissions as well as possible sequelae of hyper/hypopigmentation and varicella-like scars.

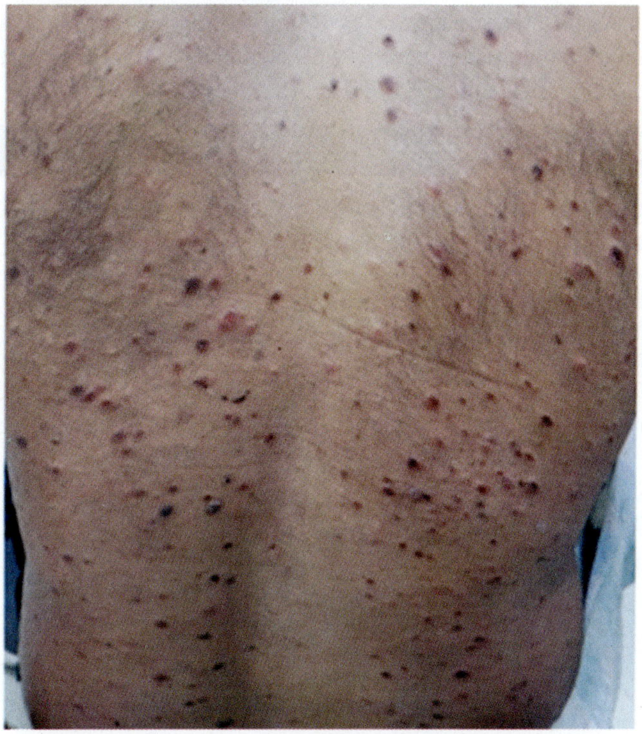

Figure 13.31: Pityriasis lichenoides et varioliformis acuta (PLEVA)

FUMHD is an acute and severe generalized eruption of purpuric and ulceronecrotic plaques with associated systemic involvement and a mortality rate of up to 25%; hence, it should be approached as a dermatologic emergency.

Differential diagnosis for PLEVA includes lymphomatoid papulosis, arthropod bite reactions, varicella, Gianotti-Crosti syndrome, erythema multiforme, pityriasis rosea, guttate psoriasis, vasculitis and secondary syphilis.

Histopathological findings include dermal, wedge-shaped, lymphocytic infiltrate, epidermal spongiosis, parakeratosis, and variable necrosis of keratinocytes. PLC demonstrates more subtle histology whereas, FUMHD exhibits the most exaggerated histological features.

In PLEVA the infiltrate obscures the dermal epidermal junction with pronounced vacuolar alteration of basal layer. Marked exocytosis of lymphocytes and erythrocytes, intercellular and intracellular edema leading to variable degree of epidermal necrosis is seen.

Treatment

For PLEVA and PLC– phototherapy, topical corticosteroids, tetracycline, erythromycin, methotrexate, calciferol, chinoline and acridine derivates, cyclosporine, intravenous gamma globulin and retinoids.

Aggressive treatment with immunosuppressant and/or immunomodulating agents as well as intensive supportive care are recommended for FUMHD.

REITER'S DISEASE

It is also known as reactive arthritis, which is characterized by triad of conjunctivitis, urethritis, and non-gonococcal arthritis.

Etiology

Reiter's disease is triggered by genitourinary infection (Chlamydia trachomatis, Mycoplasma hominis, and Ureaplasma urealyticum) or gastrointestinal tract infection (Salmonella enteritidis, Shigella flexneri, Yersinia enterocolitica and Campylobacter jejuni). It may be associated with HLA-B27 and HLA-B51 positivity .

Clinical Features

Symptoms of disease appears after few days to weeks of genitourinary infection or gastrointestinal tract infections. Patients present with acute onset of asymmetric oligoarthritis, mainly involving weight bearing joints, the lower extremities, sacroiliac joint and the lumbar spine. Tendinitis and enthesitis are the prominent features of Reiter's disease.

Extra-articular manifestations include eye involvement (conjunctivitis, anterior uveitis episcleritis and keratitis), genitourinary involvement (urethritis, cervicitis, prostatitis, cystitis or circinate balanitis), mucosal and skin involvement (mucosal ulcers, psoriasiform hyperkeratotic lesions, keratoderma blennorrhagica and erythema nodosum), cardiac involvement (carditis, aortitis, conduction and valvular abnormalities) and nail changes (onycholysis, subungual keratosis and pitting of nails).

Treatment

The goal of treatment is to provide symptomatic relief and prevent chronic articular complications. Non-steroidal anti-inflammatory drugs (NSAIDS) are the initial treatment of choice in the acute phase. Systemic use of glucocorticoids is limited to patients with severe polyarthritis, cardiac and ocular manifestations.

Disease modifying antirheumatic drugs (DMARDs), mainly sulfasalazine are effective in both acute and chronic arthritis. Methotrexate and azathioprine can be used in chronic arthritis.. Biologicals like infliximab and etanercept can also be used for refractory cases.

14 CHAPTER Vesiculobullous Disorders

Contents

Vesiculobullous disorders are broadly classified into inherited disorders and acquired disorders. Vesiculobullous lesions vary considerably in etiology, age of occurrence and the pattern of the lesions. The morphology of the blister often provides a visual clue to the location of the lesion within the skin. Blisters localized to the epidermal layers are thin walled and relatively flaccid and tend to rupture easily. Subepidermal blisters are thick walled, and tense. In addition to a complete history and examination, bacterial culture and histologic assessment of biopsies, laboratory investigations involving immunofluorescence and electron microscopy may be required to establish the final diagnosis. In the newborns, presence of vesicular or pustular lesions evokes justifiable concern to clinicians, because life-threatening bacterial and viral infections may present in this manner.

Primary vesiculobullous lesions include vesicles, bullae or pustules. These may secondarily lead to erosions or ulcers.

- **Vesicle:** Fluid filled blister <0.5 cm in diameter.
- **Bulla:** Fluid filled blister >0.5 cm in diameter.
- **Pustule:** Vesicle or bulla filled with pus.
- **Erosion:** Lesion due to partial loss of epidermis.
- **Ulcer:** Lesion due to complete loss of epidermis.

This chapter presents an overview of approach to vesiculobullous disorders. Classification of vesiculobullous disorder is described in Table 14.1 and vesiculobullous disorders at birth/neonates is given in table 14.2 and as per level of cleavage is given in Table 14.3.

<table>
<tr><th colspan="2">Table 14.1: Classification of Vesiculobullous disorders</th></tr>
<tr><td>Inherited disorders</td><td>Epidermolysis bullosa
Bullous Congenital Ichthyosiform Erythroderma
Incontinentia pigmenti
Darier's disease
Hailey-Hailey disease
Grover disease</td></tr>
<tr><td>Inflammatory dermatosis</td><td>Miliaria
Erythema Toxicum Neonatorum (ETN)
Transient Neonatal Pustular Melanosis (TNPM)
Suckling blisters
Eosinophilic pustular dermatosis
Urticaria pigmentosa
Stevenson Johnson syndrome (SJS) / Toxic Epidermolysis Necrosis (TEN)
Pustular psoriasis</td></tr>
<tr><td>Infection</td><td>Bullous Impetigo
Staphylococcal Skin Scalded Syndrome (SSSS)
Pemphigus syphiliticus /vesiculobullous type of congenital syphilis
Herpes simplex
Varicella zoster infection (varicella/ herpes zoster)
Cytomegalovirus (CMV)
Epstein-Barr virus (EBV)
Candidiasis
Hand foot mouth disease</td></tr>
<tr><td>Metabolic</td><td>Acrodermatitis enteropathica
Porphyria</td></tr>
<tr><td>Immunobullous</td><td>Intraepidermal:
• IgA pemphigus
    o Intra epidermal neutrophilic type
    o Subcorneal Pustular dermatosis
• Pemphigus foliaceous and its variants
    o Pemphigus erythematosus (Senear-Usher syndrome)
    o Endemic pemphigus
    o Pemphigus herpetiformis
• Pemphigus vulgaris and its variants
    o Pemphigus vegetans
• Drug induce pemphigus
• Paraneoplastic pemphigus
Subepidermal:
• Bullous pemphigoid
• Cicatricial pemphigoid
• Pemphigoid gestationis
• Linear IgA bullous Dermatosis
• Dermatitis herpetiformis
• Epidermolysis bullosa acquisita
• Bullous systemic lupus erythematosus
• Lichen planus pemphigoids</td></tr>
</table>

Table 14.2: Vesiculobullous disorders at birth/in neonates

	Common causes	*Uncommon causes*
Inherited disorders	–	Incontinentia pigmenti Bullous congenital ichthyosiform erythroderma Epidermolysis bullosa (Junctional and dystrophic type)
Inflammatory dermatoses	Miliaria Erythema toxicum neonatorum	Urticaria pigmentosa Generalized mastocytosis Transient pustular melanosis Sucking blisters Eosinophilic pustular dermatosis Drugs causing Stevens-Johnson Syndrome (SJS) Toxic Epidermal Necrolysis (TEN)
Infections	Impetigo neonatorum	SSSS (Staphylococcal scalded skin syndrome) Congenital syphilis Herpes simplex (Intrauterine and neonatal) Herpes zoster, Cytomegalovirus (CMV), Epstein-Barr virus (EBV), varicella (neonatal and fetal infection) Candidiasis
Autoimmune disorders	–	Pemphigus vulgaris Pemphigus foliaceous Herpes gestationis Chronic bullous dermatosis of childhood (CBCD)
Metabolic disorders	–	Acrodermatitis enteropathica

Table 14.3: Vesiculobullous disorders according to the level of cleavage of the bulla

Sub corneal	Bullous impetigo Staphylococcal scalded skin syndrome (SSSS) Candidiasis Bullous congenital ichthyosiform erythroderma (BCIE) Pemphigus foliaceous, pemphigus erythematosus Acropustulosis of infancy Subcorneal pustular dermatosis Pustular psoriasis
Spinous	Insect bites Dermatitis Hailey-Hailey disease Incontinentia pigmenti Viral infections – H. simplex, H. zoster
Supra basal	Pemphigus vulgaris
Subepidermal	Epidermolysis bullosa simplex, SJS, TEN, FDE
Subepidermal (BMZ damage)	Junctional and dystrophic Epidermolysis bullosa, EB acquisita CBCD Bullous pemphigoid Dermatitis herpetiformis Porphyria cutanea tarda

Mechanism Responsible for The Split Epidermis or Different Mechanism of Blister Formation

Acantholysis

Loss of coherence between keratinocytes due to breakdown of intercellular connections results in formation of acantholytic cells. Acantholytic cells are rounded keratinocytes with peripherally condensed cytoplasm and perinuclear halo. Nuclei are large which display prominent nucleoli and peripheral condensation of chromatin. It occurs due to abnormalities of the tonofilament desmosome complexes, e.g. pemphigus.

Cytolysis

Disruption of keratinocytes caused by a large amount of mechanical forces like friction and heat overwhelming the desmosomal plaques and structural matrix e.g. friction blister, burn.

Reticular Degeneration

It is a subset of cytolysis, occurs due to intracellular oedema or ballooning degeneration after viral infections, which leads to rupture of keratinocyte membrane and their death. The remaining desmosomal components and ruptured keratinocyte membranes appear as an irregular meshwork giving a reticulated appearance e.g. herpes infection.

Spongiosis

It is an intense intercellular oedema resulting in stellate appearance of keratinocytes and disruption of desmosomes resulting in vesicle formation e.g. eczema.

Basement Membrane Zone Disruption

It occurs due to primary structural deficiencies as well as from immunologically mediated damage to the dermo epidermal junction e.g. epidermolysis bullosa, bullous pemphigoid.

EPIDERMOLYSIS BULLOSA (EB)

Epidermolysis bullosa is a rare group of inherited disorders which manifests as blistering or erosion of the skin, in response to little or no apparent trauma.

Epidemiology

- The exact prevalence of epidermolysis bullosa is unknown. Milder variants have an incidence of 1 per 50,000 births. The more severe varieties are believed to occur in 1 per 500,000 births.
- The incidence is equal in both sexes.
- Some forms of EB are more prevalent in certain races, e.g., EB simplex, ogna variant is seen more often in the Norwegians.

Classification of Epidermolysis Bullosa

Based on the level of cleavage of the skin blister, EB can be divided into 3 types:

1. **Epidermolysis bullosa simplex (EBS):** Intraepidermal cleavage, at level of basal keratinocytes, above the basement membrane.
   - Localized subtype (Weber-Cockayne EBS).
   - Generalized subtype (Koebner EBS and Dowling–Meara EBS).
   - EBS with muscular dystrophy.
   - Autosomal recessive lethal EBS.
   - EBS with mottled pigmentation.
2. **Junctional epidermolysis bullosa (JEB):** Blisters form within the basement membrane.
   - Herlitz JEB.
   - Non-Herlitz JEB.
   - JEB with pyloric atresia.
   - Progressive JEB.
3. **Dystrophic epidermolysis bullosa (DEB): Blisters form beneath the basement membrane.**
   - Dominant dystrophic EB.
   - *Recessive dystrophic EB:* Hallopeau-Siemens EB and non-Hallopeau-Siemens EB.

Etiopathogenesis

- Cytolysis causes blisters in the epidermis or basement membrane zone of the skin.
- In epidermolysis bullosa simplex, cytolysis causes blisters in the basal or spinous layers of the epidermis and keratinocytes often have abnormal density and organization of keratin filaments.
- In junctional epidermolysis bullosa, the epidermis separates from the basal lamina, forming a blister cavity in the plane of the lamina lucida. Hemidesmosomal structure and density of basal cells are frequently diminished.
- In dystrophic epidermolysis bullosa, the basal lamina remains attached to the epidermis, but the blister cavity forms beneath the lamina densa of dermoepidermal junction, and anchoring fibrils may appear abnormal, reduced in number, or altogether absent.

Clinical Features

- Clinical features are summarized in Table 14.4. EB as such is not a common skin disease, the common incidence shown in the table, means it is commoner out of all the varieties of EB.
- **History:** Important findings in epidermolysis bullosa (EB) include the age of onset, the size, frequency and location of blisters and the possible inciting factors (e.g. heat, trauma etc.).

Table 14.4: Summary of clinical features of epidermolysis bullosa (Figures 14.1 to 14.5)

Type	*Time of presentation*	*Inheritance*	*Clinical features*	*Mucous membranes/ Nail/Teeth*	*Associated features*	*Prognosis*
Epidermolysis bullosa simplex (EBS)						
Weber-Cockayne EBS (more common)	Childhood	AD	Localized to palms, soles, waist or neck, no scarring, more in summers	Normal	Hyperhidrosis of palms, soles exacerbates the bullae	Good
Koebner EBS (rare)	At birth or infancy	AD	On occiput, back or legs in infancy, hands and feet in childhood, no scarring	Normal	Aggravated by warm weather, hyperhidrosis of palms and soles	May improve after puberty
Dowling-Meara EBS (rare)	At birth or infancy	AD	Herpetiform blisters on trunk, limbs, neck No scarring	Mucous membranes (MM), nails involved	Milia, hyperpigmentation seen	Severe in infancy, better with age
EBS with muscular dystrophy (rare)	At birth or early infancy	AD	Blisters on hands and feet, then generalized	Nail deformities, MM involvement, scarring, alopecia	Muscle weakness early or late onset, milia present	Poor
Autosomal recessive lethal EBS (rare)	At birth	AR	Generalized, more on distal limbs	Normal, oral mucosa mildly affected	No scarring or milia seen	Poor
EBS with mottled pigmentation (rare)	At birth or infancy	AD	Reticulate pattern of macular pigmentation over trunk, limbs	Hair, teeth normal Nails involved MM-normal	Punctate keratoses on palms and soles	Improves with age
Junctional epidermolysis bullosa (JEB)						
Herlitz JEB (common)	At birth or soon after birth	AR	Severe generalized blistering, skin fragility, difficult to handle child, erosions slow to heal	MM, nails, teeth involved, Larynx may be involved	Sepsis or multiorgan failure may occur	Poor, child may die in early infancy due to infection
Non-Herlitz JEB (rare)	At birth	AR	Generalised blisters, Scalp involvement causes alopecia	MM, nails, teeth involved	Pigmentation and nevi seen	Improves with age
JEB with pyloric atresia (rare)	At birth	AR	Generalized skin and mucosal blisters	Nails, teeth involved	Non-bilious vomiting in newborn	Very poor
Progressive JEB (rare)	5-8 years	AR	Hands, feet, knees, elbows (sites of friction)	Nails, teeth involved	Finger contractures, deafness	Good
Dystrophic epidermolysis bullosa (DEB)						
Dominant dystrophic EB (rare)	At birth or early infancy	AD	Hands, feet, elbows, knees (sites of friction)	Nail dystrophy, MM, teeth– Normal	White papules on trunk Pasini variant	Good
Hallopeau-Siemens EB (rare)	At birth or early infancy	AR	Large, flaccid bullae at sites of friction, Healing slow, scarring present	Dystrophic nails, scarring alopecia, carious teeth, MM involved	Flexural contractures, esophageal strictures, inability to protrude tongue	Poor-death by 3-4 decade
Non-Hallopeau-siemens EB (rare)	At birth	AR	Skin and mucosae are fragile	Changes are localized	Few complications	Good

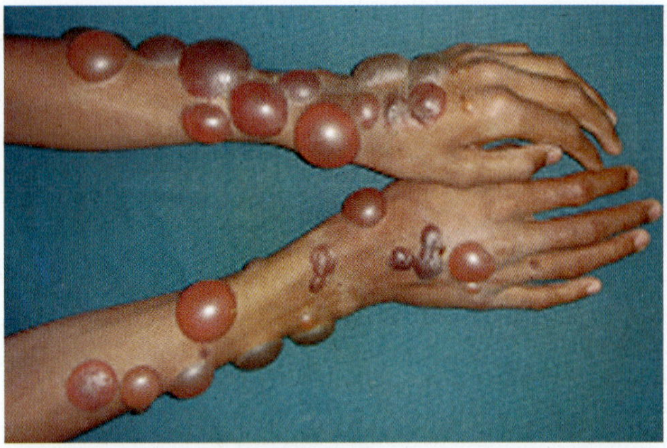

Figure 14.1: Dystrophic epidermolysis bullosa

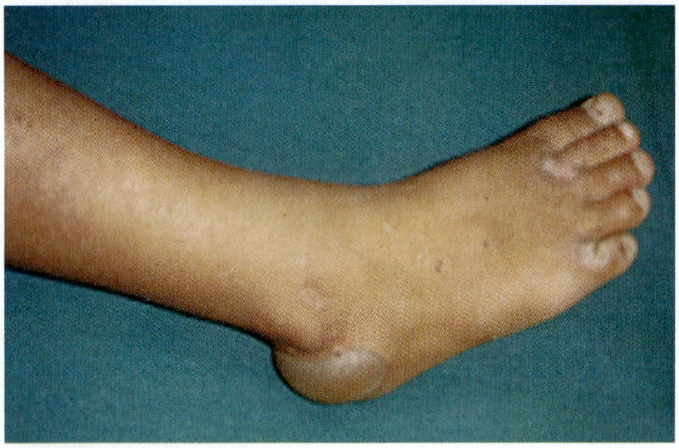

Figure14.2: Epidermolysis bullosa simplex showing bulla

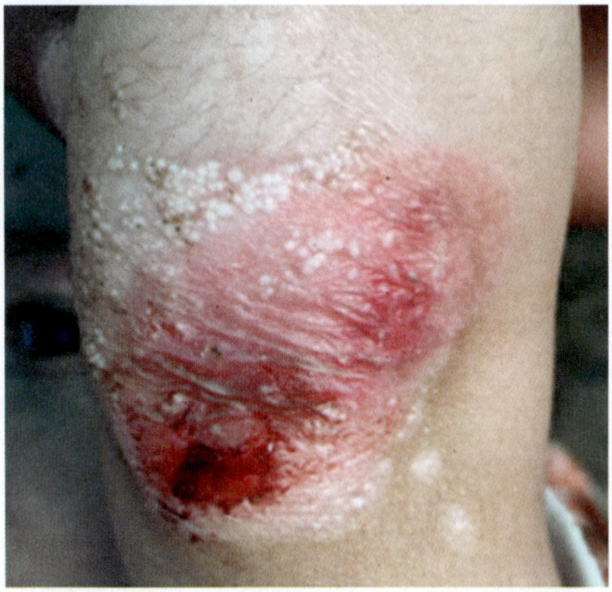

Figure 14.3: Dystrophic epidermolysis bullosa showing milia and scars

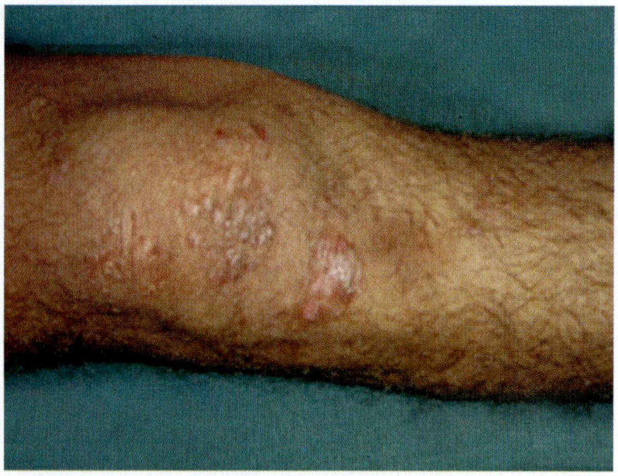

Figure 14.4: Epidermolysis bullosa showing scarring and lichenoid eruption

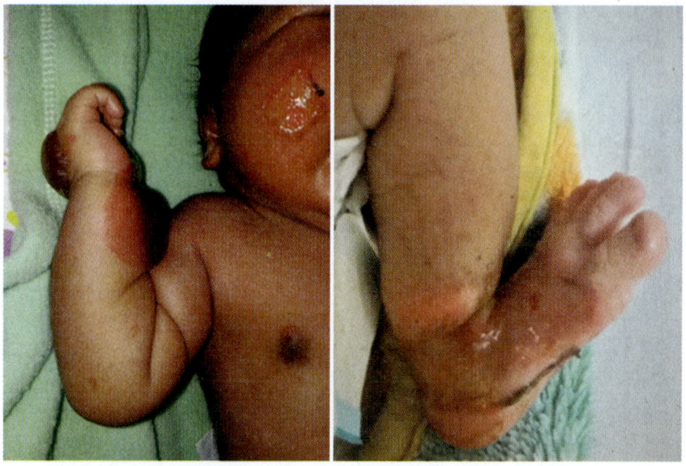

Figure 14.5: Epidermolysis bullosa showing hemorrhagic bulla and superficial erosion over cheek and feet

- Family history of blistering disease should be elicited. Isolated cases can be due to spontaneous mutation or incomplete penetrance of an autosomal dominant trait.
- Mucosal involvement should be searched including oral, nasopharyngeal, ocular, genitourinary, gastrointestinal and respiratory symptoms.
- A complete physical examination should be performed with emphasis on inspecting all skin areas and mucosal surfaces. Evaluate the size, location and character of the blisters.
- Examine the patient for involvement of the nails, hair or teeth.
- Areas prone to pressure, trauma, or excessive heating have more blistering, e.g. fingers, hands, elbows, feet, legs and diaper area (in infants).

Differential Diagnosis

- Burns.
- Staphylococcal scalded skin syndrome (SSSS).
- Toxic epidermal necrolysis.
- Congenital syphilis.
- Benign familial pemphigus.
- Porphyria cutanea tarda.
- Ectodermal dysplasia.

Diagnosis

Diagnosis of EB cannot be satisfactorily done using clinical or histopathological parameters. Use of immunohistochemistry is the mainstay of diagnosis. Nevertheless, clinical diagnosis and histopathology are useful in narrowing the range of possible diagnosis and predicting prognosis.

- **Skin biopsy:** It is primarily used to determine the level of cleavage of the bulla. The sample of biopsy should be taken carefully. Old and secondarily infected bullae should be avoided. It should be taken from small bullae. Bullae can be induced by rubbing the normal skin with a finger or India rubber for a minute and then biopsied.
- Electron microscopy determines the level of skin cleavage in epidermolysis bullosa (EB) and permits visualization and semi quantitative assessment of specific structures.
- **Immunofluorescence mapping (IFM):** IFM, when coupled with the use of specific monoclonal antibodies, can provide considerable insight into not only the major type of epidermolysis bullosa but also into the structural protein most likely mutated.
- **Mutation analysis:** It is the ultimate means of determining them mode of inheritance and the precise site and type of molecular mutation. It is the recommended technique for prenatal and pre implantation diagnosis. It is very labor intensive and expensive to perform.

Treatment

- **General care of infants and neonates:** Prevention of secondary infection by appropriate antibiotics, correction of nutrition and anemia is required in most of the patients.
- Prevention of trauma is the most important preventive measure, soft clothes and shoes should be used.
- Application of emollients is helpful.
- Care of eyes, teeth, oral mucosa, esophagus, nails is necessary in case they are involved.
- Prevention of deformity by appropriate movement and change of postures.
- The treatment of epidermolysis bullosa (EB) is primarily preventive and supportive. Once blistering has occurred, the blister should be punctured with a sterile needle or a blade. This may prevent the accumulation of fluid and pressure and may thus prevent the blister from extending.
- Open wounds should be covered with nonadherent dressings such as petrolatum impregnated gauze. Tape and any significant pressure to the skin must be avoided.
- Application of mupirocin or fusidic acid topical ointments to treat open or partially healed wounds may be useful to decrease the overgrowth of *Pseudomonas* and staphylococcal organisms.
- Surgical procedures can correct the deformities of epidermolysis bullosa caused by repeated episodes of blistering and scarring of the hand.
- Skin grafting may be done in patients with epidermolysis bullosa who have chronic, nonhealing ulcers especially in generalized recessive dystrophic EB.
- Drug therapy is not currently a component in the treatment for epidermolysis bullosa (EB). Systemic corticosteroids may be used in short, intermittent courses when disease is progressive, but their long-term use is not recommended because of the risk of complications. Other systemic drugs like phenytoin, tetracycline, minocycline, cyclosporine, retinoic acid, have been used with variable results. Vitamin E can be used because of its healing properties and no risk of side effects. Botulinum toxin has been tried in cases of EB with beneficial effect.
- Genetic counselling should be done for the parents to explain the risk of having the disorder in other children. Gene therapy, by addition of a normal gene or deletion of a particular mutation may open new doors for treatment.

SUBEPIDERMAL BLISTERING DISORDERS

Chronic Bullous Dermatosis of Childhood (CBDC, Linear IGA Disease)

It is an acquired blistering disease of skin and mucous membranes, characterized by blisters and erosions. CBDC is now known as linear IgA dermatosis as IgA gets deposited in linear fashion at the basement membrane zone.

Epidemiology

- Incidence of adult linear IgA dermatosis is estimated to be 0.1-1 in every 250,000 population per year.
- Estimates have not been reported for linear IgA dermatosis in children.
- There is a slight female preponderance; with the female to male ratio being 1.6:1.
- Linear IgA dermatosis has a bimodal age of onset. Disease in children occurs from 6 months to 10 years, with a mean of 5 years (pre-school age), while the disease in adults occurs from 14-80 years of age.
- Drug induced disease is more likely to occur in the older population because this group often receives treatment for multiple medical conditions.

Etiology

HLA: There is a strong association between linear IgA disease and HLA-B8, Cw7 and DR3.

Drugs

- **Antibiotics:** Vancomycin, ampicillin, cefamandole, penicillin, sulfamethoxazole-trimethoprim, moxifloxacin, amoxicillin-clavulanic acid.
- **Anticonvulsants:** Phenytoin, vigabatrin.
- **Others:** Diclofenac, glibenclamide, iodine contrast agent, lithium carbonate.
- **Preceding illnesses:** Such as typhoid, brucella, tuberculosis, varicella, herpes zoster and upper respiratory infections have all been reported in association with linear IgA dermatosis.

Malignancy

- Reported in as many as 5% of cases.
- Lymphoproliferative malignancies, specifically Hodgkin's disease, non-Hodgkin lymphoma and chronic lymphocytic leukemia have been described. Also reported with solid tumors, such as bladder carcinoma.

Association with Autoimmune Disorders

Systemic lupus erythematosus, dermatomyositis, rheumatoid arthritis, polymyalgia rheumatica, hypothyroidism, chronic hepatitis, Crohn's disease, ulcerative colitis, multiple sclerosis, acquired hemophilia and IgA nephropathy have been described with CBDC.

Pathogenesis

- Linear IgA dermatosis is an autoimmune disease which is histopathologically characterized by the linear deposition of IgA at the basement membrane zone (BMZ).
- Antibody deposition leads to complement activation and neutrophil chemotaxis, which eventuates in loss of adhesion at the dermo-epidermal junction and in blister formation in subepidermal zone.
- The mechanism of loss of self-tolerance to target antigens is unknown.

Clinical Features

- Prolonged period of prodromal itching or transient pruritus or burning may occur before lesions appear.
- The classic lesions of linear IgA dermatosis are clear and/or hemorrhagic, round or oval vesicles or bullae on normal (Figure 14.6), erythematous, or urticarial skin. Cutaneous manifestations may also include erythematous plaques, blanching macules and papules, or targetoid erythema multiforme like lesions.
- Bullae may be discrete or arranged in a herpetiform pattern, often described as cluster of jewels sign. Alternatively, vesicles and bullae may be seen at the edge of annular or polycyclic lesions, the appearance of which has been described as the **string of beads or cluster of jewels** sign (Figure 14.7).
- The distribution of linear IgA dermatosis differs between adults and children. Lesions in children are typically localized to the lower abdomen and anogenital areas with frequent involvement of the perineum (Figure 14.8). Other sites of involvement include the feet, hands and face, particularly the perioral area.
- In adults, the trunk and the limbs are most commonly affected. Involvement of the perineum and the perioral area is less frequent than in children.
- Crusts, excoriations, erosions or ulcers may be present.
- Oral manifestations are common in children and adults with linear IgA dermatosis. Oral lesions include vesicles, ulcerations, erythematous patches, erosions, desquamative gingivitis or erosive cheilitis and they may precede skin lesions.
- Ocular symptoms, such as grittiness, burning, or discharge may be present.
- Review of medication taken in past few days may be helpful.

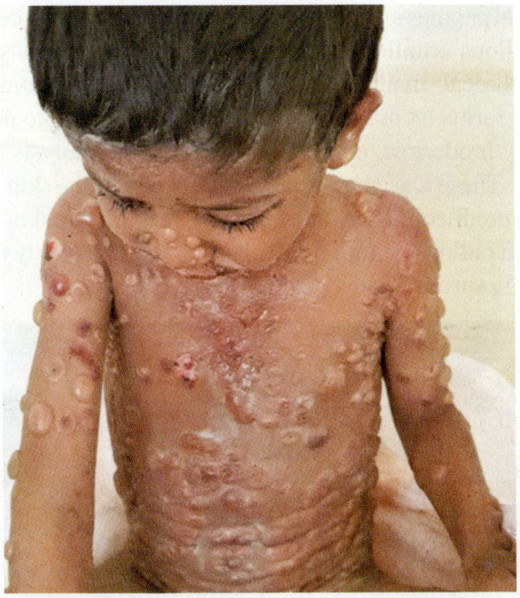

Figure 14.6: Chronic bullous disease of childhood

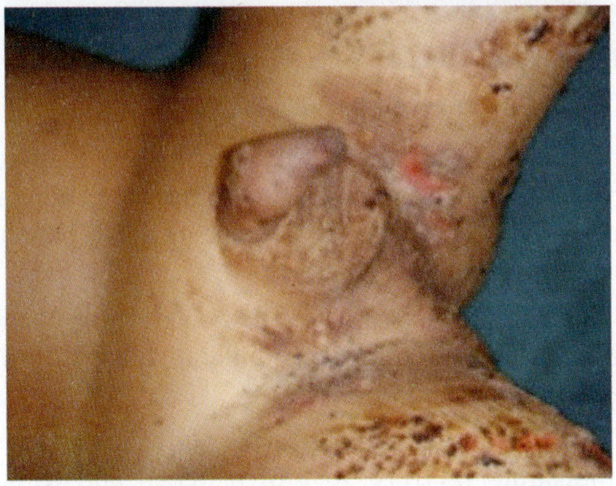

Figure 14.7: Chronic bullous disease of childhood showing involvement of perineum

Differential Diagnosis

- Bullous impetigo.
- Epidermolysis bullosa acquisita.
- Childhood bullous pemphigoid.

Prognosis

Spontaneous remission occurs in most cases in 3-6 years, only few cases persist after puberty.

Treatment

- Bullae do not need special care, as long they remain intact.
- Ruptured lesions and erosions should be covered with sterile dressings.
- Infected lesions may be treated with topical mupirocin and sterile dressing changes twice daily.
- Drug induced disease may be treated merely by withdrawal of the offending agent.
- Most patients respond to dapsone (2 mg/kg/day) or sulfapyridine.
- Oral corticosteroids, like prednisolone, 0.5-2 mg/kg per day, may be used along with dapsone to control the acute phase. Corticosteroids are gradually tapered in few weeks and the child may be maintained on oral dapsone only. If recurrence occurs with dapsone alone, oral corticosteroids may be given for longer period and newer oral steroids, e.g., methylprednisolone or deflazacort may be used to reduce the systemic side effects. Recently, rituximab has also been tried in refractory cases, with good results.
- Anti-inflammatory agents and antibiotics may be given if necessary.

BULLOUS PEMPHIGOID

Bullous pemphigoid (BP) is a chronic, autoimmune, subepidermal, blistering skin disease that rarely involves mucous membranes.

BP is characterized by the presence of immunoglobulin G (IgG) autoantibodies specific for the hemidesmosomal BP

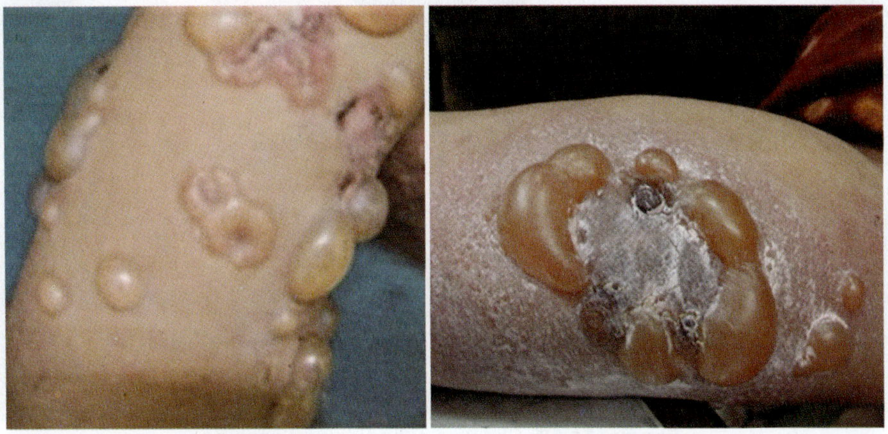

Figure 14.8: Chronic bullous disease of childhood showing cluster of jewels sign

antigens BP 230 (BPAg1) and BP180 (BPAg2). Usually affects older age groups (50-70 years), but uncommonly, BP can be seen in infants and children.

Immunopathogenesis of Bullous Pemphigoid

Initially, loss of immune tolerance leads to formation of antibodies against BP180 and BP230 antigen, NC16A domain of BP 180 being dominant antigen in bullous pemphigoid. This area of BP180 is the main target of the autoreactive B and T cell responses in BP. A significant number of eosinophils and to a lesser extent, neutrophils migrate to the dermis which degranulate as a result of BP autoantibodies, triggering an inflammatory response. Numerous cytokines (IL-4, IL-5, IL-13, TNF alpha), chemokines (CXCL-9, CXCL-10, CCL-17, CCL-22), hydrolytic degradation enzymes (neutrophil elastase, matrix metalloprotease 9) and reactive oxygen species are released leading to development of subepidermal blister and tissue injury.

Associations of BP

Bullous pemphigoid may be associated with various malignancies, most commonly with gastrointestinal tract malignancy. Neurological and psychiatric disorders have been associated with bullous pemphigoid which includes parkinsonism, dementia, multiple sclerosis, bipolar disorder and stroke.

Drug induce Bullous Pemphigoid

Common drugs which can cause bullous pemphigoid are PD1-inhibitor (pembrolizumab, nivolumab), dipeptidyl peptidase-4 inhibitors or gliptins (sitagliptin, saxagliptin, vildagliptin), penicillamine, potassium iodide, penicillin, gold, frusemide, captopril etc.

Clinical Features

Bullous pemphigoid patients initially present with pruritic urticarial papules and plaques which are subsequently converted into bullous eruptions. Occasionally urticarial lesions are the main clinical manifestation of bullous pemphigoid. Other clinical forms includes vesicular, vegetative, prurigo nodularis like, erythrodermic, eczematous, toxic epidermolysis necrosis like etc. These tense bullae arise on any part of the skin surface, with a predilection on the flexural areas of the skin (Figure 14.9). In bullous pemphigoid, nikolsky sign is usually negative and bulla spread sign is positive.

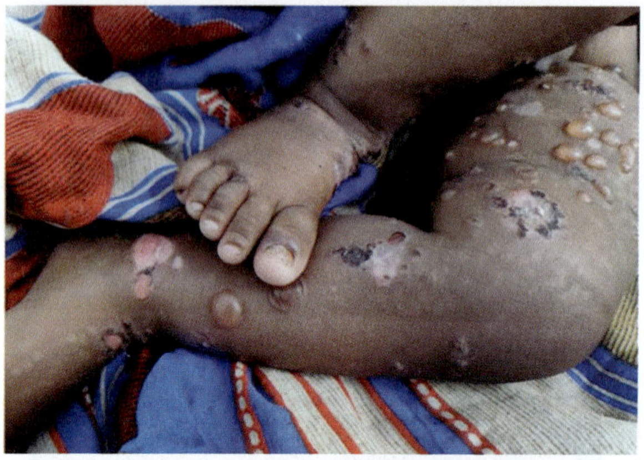

Figure 14.9: Bullous pemphigoid

- In infants affected with BP, the blisters tend to occur frequently on the palms, soles and face; genital areas are rarely affected. Sixty percent of these patients have generalized blisters.
- Histopathologic examination demonstrates a subepidermal blister having polymorphous inflammatory infiltrate, with an eosinophil predominance.
- DIF studies on normal appearing perilesional skin usually demonstrate IgG (70-90% of patients) and complement C3 deposition (90-100% of patients) in a linear fashion at dermoepidermal junction.
- DIF pattern analysis shows 'n' serration pattern. Salt split technique depicts roof pattern of immune deposits.

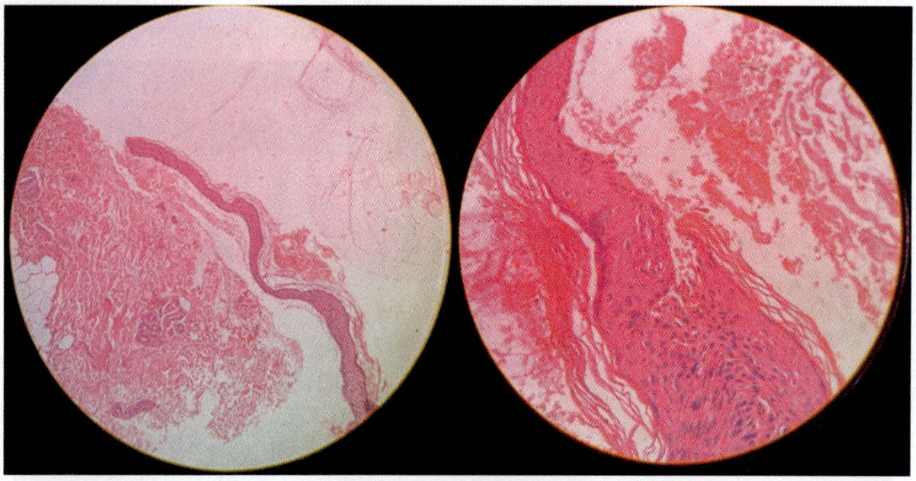

Figure 14.10: Showing subepidermal splitting

Treatment

Topical: Potent topical steroids are usually preferred when disease limited to < 10 % of body surface area.

Systemic: Systemic therapy is required in moderate to severe cases, which includes, oral prednisolone at the dose of 0.5-1 mg/kg/day, oral doxycycline 100 mg twice daily, and oral dapsone 1-1.5 mg/kg/day. Nicotinamide, azathioprine, mycophenolate mofetil, methotrexate, IVIG, Rituximab, omalizumab are other systemic drugs which may be used in the management of BP.

MUCOUS MEMBRANE PEMPHIGOID/ CICATRICIAL PEMPHIGOID (MMP/CP)

It is a chronic progressive subepidermal blistering disorder characterized by predominant involvement of mucous membranes and occasionally the skin. The oral and ocular mucosa are the most commonly affected sites while nasopharynx, oesophagus, larynx and anogenital region may also be involved. It is clinically characterised by blistering, ulceration, severe scarring and milia formation. Most common oral lesion is desquamating gingivitis. MMP can be triggered by medications such as methyldopa, clonidine and D-penicillamine.

Autoantigens involved in MMP are bullous pemphigoid antigen 2 (BPAg 2), bullous pemphigoid antigen 1 (BPAg1), integrin subunits α6/β4, laminin-332 (also called epiligrin and laminin-5). Antibody against β4 subunit of integrin is associated with predominant ocular involvement, laminin -332 is associated with solid organ tumors. There are several ocular grading systems for the severity of MMP, including Foster, Mondino and Tauber.

Histology of vesicle shows subepidermal cleft formation with mixed inflammatory infiltrate. Immunofluorescence shows linear IgG and C3 deposition along basement membrane.

Treatment: For mild to moderate disease, topical steroid and tetracycline mouthwash is sufficient. Systemic steroids are indicated in severe oral, ocular, laryngeal and oesophageal involvement. Other treatment options include dapsone, cyclophosphamide, azathioprine, minocycline and IVIG.

ANTI-P200 PEMPHIGOID (ANTI-LAMININ GAMMA-1 PEMPHIGOID)

Anti-p200 pemphigoid is a rare subepidermal autoimmune bullous disease caused by antibody formation against 200-kDa protein localized within the lower zone of basement membrane. Clinically it presents with polymorphic lesions which may mimic bullous pemphigoid, mucous membrane pemphigoid or inflammatory epidermolysis bullosa.

Histology shows subepidermal split with mixed cellular infiltrate. Salt split shows immunofluorescence on dermal side of split.

Treatment

Topical steroids, oral prednisolone (0.5 mg /kg/day), dapsone (1-1.5 mg /kg/day), tetracycline azathioprine are indicated in management of p200 bullous pemphigoid.

DERMATITIS HERPETIFORMIS

Dermatitis herpetiformis (DH) is an autoimmune blistering disorder associated with gluten sensitive enteropathy.

It is commonly found in adults 20-40 years of age; rare in children.

HLA-DQ2 and HLA-DQ8 are associated with the susceptibility of DH. About 90% of individuals with celiac disease have HLA-DQ2, while other patients have a relatively modest percentage of lower risk heterodimers (such as HLA-DQ8). Ten to fifteen percent of DH patients may have first degree relatives who are affected.

Although most patients are asymptomatic, more than 90% have an associated gluten sensitive enteropathy. Around 15-25% patients with celiac disease develop dermatitis herpetiformis.

Dermatitis herpetiformis is characterized by grouped erythematous papules with vesicles, which may form plaques.

It is exquisitely pruritic, and the vesicles are often excoriated to erosions by the time of physical examination (Figure 14.11).

The lesions of dermatitis herpetiformis are located mainly on the extensor surfaces of the elbows, knees, buttocks and back. Lesions usually resolve with post inflammatory hypopigmentation and hyperpigmentation.

Histopathological examination shows subepidermal cleft with microabscesses containing neutrophils and eosinophils at the tip of dermal papilla.

To confirmation of diagnosis requires direct immunofluorescence of a skin biopsy specimen which shows deposition of immunoglobulin A (IgA) in a granular pattern in the upper papillary dermis.

Anti TTG, anti ETG, anti endomysial, antigliadin and anti-reticulin antibody detected in serum of DH patients.

Treatment

Dapsone and gluten free diet are the mainstay of treatment. Gluten is present in many cereals like wheat, barley, rye and oats. Other treatment option includes sulfasalazine, azathioprine, cyclosporin, colchicine, nicotinamide etc.

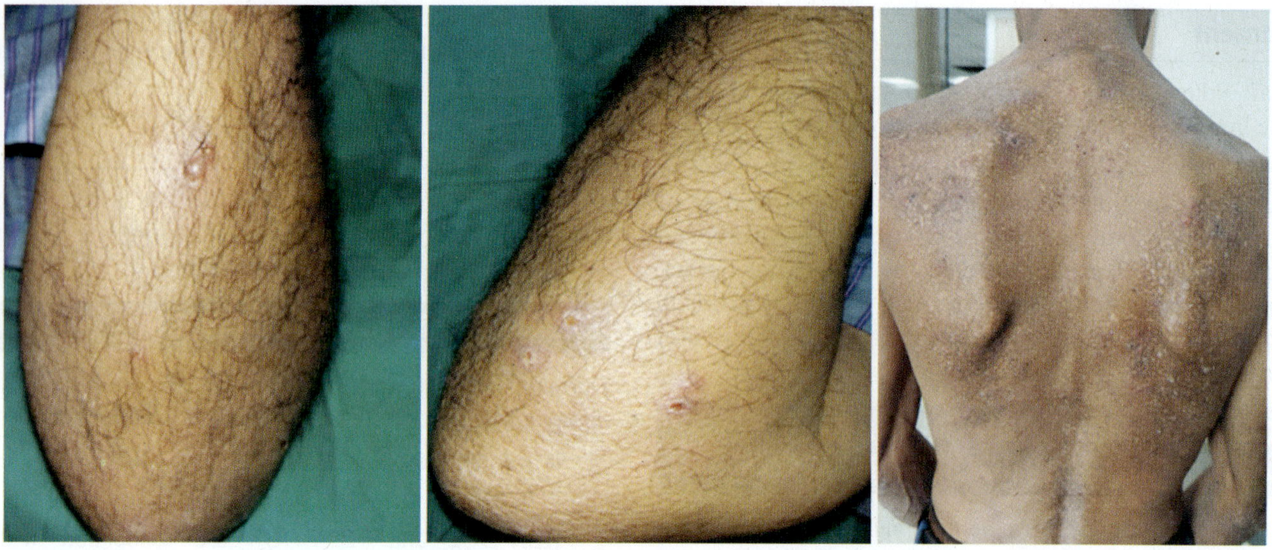

Figure 14.11: Dermatitis herpetiformis

PEMPHIGOID GESTATIONIS/ HERPES GESTATIONIS (PG/HG)

It is a rare specific dermatosis of pregnancy with similar pathophysiology as of bullous pemphigoid. Target autoantigen is BPAG2 (BP 230) and collagen XVII (BP 180).

Herpes gestationis usually occurs in third trimester. In subsequent pregnancies it recurs before third trimester with more serious course. It usually resolves within 2 months after delivery. Low birth weight, prematurity may occur but there is no increased risk of stillbirth and abortion.

Clinically it is characterised by polymorphic lesions including erythematous urticarial papules and plaques which evolve into subepidermal vesicles and bullae. Eczematous or erythema multiforme like lesions can also be seen. Initially, the lesions begin in the periumbilical region and then spread to the abdominal area, as well as to the limbs. Face and mucous membranes are rarely affected.

When validating a diagnosis, direct immunofluorescence staining (DIF) is the most specific and sensitive test. Along the dermoepidermal junction, it displays positive linear C3 deposition in 100% of the cases and IgG in 30% of the cases.

Treatment

Topical corticosteroids, oral prednisolone (0.3–0.5 mg/kg), and in certain situations, the inclusion of immunosuppressant medications like azathioprine or cyclosporine for disease control are all part of the treatment.

EPIDERMOLYSIS BULLOSA ACQUISITA

It is an acquired, trauma induced blistering disease, with autoantibodies against type VII collagen and is usually seen in 40-60 years of age, occasionally reported in children. Few cases have been reported in association with thyroid carcinoma, multiple myeloma, uterine and cervical carcinoma etc. Clinically it is subdivided into inflammatory and noninflammatory phenotypes. In non-inflammatory variant (classical EBA), flaccid blisters are seen at trauma prone areas like elbows, knees, hands and feet. Mucosal lesions, milia and scarring may be seen. Inflammatory form of EBA mimics other chronic blistering dermatosis like bullous pemphigoid, mucous membrane pemphigoid, linear IgA bullous dermatosis. It presents with widespread blistering, not localized to trauma prone sites. No specific treatment is required; avoidance of trauma should be done.

BULLOUS SYSTEMIC LUPUS ERYTHEMATOSUS

Bullous SLE presents with tense vesicles, bullae and erosions on normal or erythematous skin, predominantly on sun exposed areas. Mucosal surfaces can also be involved. Lesions heal without milia and scarring. Bullous systemic lupus erythematosus is associated with worsening of lupus nephritis.

Histopathological findings include subepidermal split, neutrophilic infiltrate and papillary micro-abscesses in upper dermis with mucin deposition. Direct immunofluorescence study shows linear or granular IgG, IgM, IgA and C3 deposition at dermo-epidermal junction.

Diagnostic criteria for bullous systemic lupus erythematous:

1. Diagnosis of systemic lupus erythematosus based on ACR criteria.
2. **Clinical features:** Vesiculobullous eruption.
3. Histology examination: Subepidermal cleft with neutrophilic predominant infiltrates.
4. Direct immunofluorescence: Linear or granular IgG, IgM and IgA deposition.
5. Positive circulating antibodies against collagen VII.

Treatment

Dapsone is the treatment of choice. Other treatment option includes oral steroids, azathioprine and rituximab.

KINDLER'S SYNDROME

It is a rare autosomal recessive subtype of epidermolysis bullosa which presents with skin fragility, acral blistering, photosensitivity, poikilodermatous lesions, skin atrophy, pseudo-syndactyly, along with mucosal involvement. Palmoplantar hyperkeratosis and nail dystrophy can also be seen. It occurs due to loss of functional mutations in FERMT1 gene resulting in defective kindlin-1 protein.

Treatment includes standard skin care, blister care, use of moisturizers, avoidance of trauma, photoprotection, lubricant eye drops, optimal oral hygiene and management of gastrointestinal and urethral complications. Screening for premalignant keratoses should be done at regular intervals.

INTRAEPIDERMAL BLISTERING DISORDERS

Pemphigus Vulgaris (PV)

It is an autoimmune blistering disease of the skin and mucous membranes characterized histologically by intraepidermal blister and immunopathologically by circulating IgG antibody directed against the cell surface of keratinocytes (desmoglein 3 and desmoglein 1). These antigens are part of desmosomes of epidermal cells. Antibodies against these antigens lead to lysis of cell junctions and formation of acantholytic cells.

The disease is less common in children than adults, it may occur in neonates due to transplacental transfer of maternal antibodies. In western countries it occurs in younger age.

Etiopathogenesis

Genetic predisposition may play a role. Pemphigus may be seen in association with other autoimmune diseases like thymoma, lymphoproliferative disorders (paraneoplastic pemphigus), bullous pemphigoid, SLE (pemphigus erythematosus) etc.

Theories of Pemphigus Vulgaris Pathogenesis

The exact pathogenesis behind the formation of blisters is not clearly understood, however several theories have been proposed which include:

1. **Stearic hindrance by autoantibodies:**

   This long-standing theory states that the binding of autoantibodies to the extracellular domain of desmogleins causes loss of intercellular adhesion and acantholysis.

2. **Desmoglein compensation hypothesis:**

   The different distribution patterns of DSG1 and DSG3 in the skin and oral mucosa support this theory. It describes that if both DSG1 and DSG3 are present and only one is inactivated by autoantibodies then the other will compensate and provide adhesion, but if only one DSG is present and is attacked by the autoantibodies, then the acantholysis will occur. However, accumulating data suggest that this theory is unable to justify the disease presentation of PV. Blistering in patients with autoantibodies against both DSG1 and DSG3 should not only be restricted to suprabasal level but rather should appear across the entire epidermis. Nonetheless, this does not seem to happen.

Newer theories

1. **Antibody induce apoptosis/Outside-in-signalling theory:**

   Binding of various desmoglein and non desmoglein antibodies to the keratinocytes results in activation of various signalling pathways like EGFR, p38 signalling, MAP kinase and JAK STAT kinase, resulting in increased levels of caspases 8 and 9 which cause extrinsic and intrinsic apoptosis of the keratinocytes respectively.

2. **Basal cell shrinkage and apoptolysis hypothesis:**

   When the pathogenic autoantibodies bind to the desmosomes, a series of various signal-transduction pathways trigger the rupture of the cytoskeleton, resulting in the collapse and shrinkage of the basal keratinocytes.

3. **Oxidative stress mediated YAP (Yes-Associated Protein) dysregulation:**

   Reduction of antioxidants, increased oxidative stress and dysregulated YAP expression leads to disruption of cell-to-cell adhesion.

4. **Multiple hit hypothesis:**

   According to this hypothesis multiple antibodies are involved in the pathogenesis of pemphigus which include anti-desmoglein, anti-desmocollin, anti-desmoplakin antibodies along with non-desmosomal antibodies like anti-acetylcholine receptor, anti-mitochondrial, anti-pamphaxin, anti-thyro-peroxidase and anti-annexins antibodies.

5. **T-cell dysregulation:**

T cells are critically involved in both the effector and regulatory immune responses and have been demonstrated to have a variety of defects that contribute to PV immunopathogenesis.

Drug induced PV: Drugs reported most commonly in association with PV include penicillamine, captopril, rifampin and other thiol-containing compounds.

Clinical Features

- PV presents with oral lesions in 50-70% of patients. Mucosal lesions may develop before skin lesions develop or they may be the sole manifestation of the disease. Intact bullae are rare in the mouth. Most patients have ill-defined, irregularly shaped, gingival, buccal or palatal erosions, which are painful and slow to heal. The erosions extend peripherally with shedding of the epithelium. Patient is often unable to eat or drink because of the painful lesions. Lack of oral hygiene may cause oral candidiasis.
- The primary cutaneous lesion of PV is a flaccid blister, which usually arises on normal appearing skin but may be found on erythematous skin. Affected skin often is painful but rarely pruritic. Rupture of blisters produces painful erosions which is the most common skin presentation (Figure 14.12). Erosions often are large because of their tendency to extend peripherally with the shedding of the epithelium.
- **Nikolsky's sign:** In patients with active blistering, firm sliding pressure with thumb especially over bony prominences, separates normal appearing epidermis, producing erosion. This sign is not specific for PV and is found in other active blistering diseases also.
- Lesions are seen on face, trunk, axillae, groins and scalp.
- Pemphigus vegetans (Figure 14.13) is a localized form of pemphigus vulgaris having vegetative plaques in

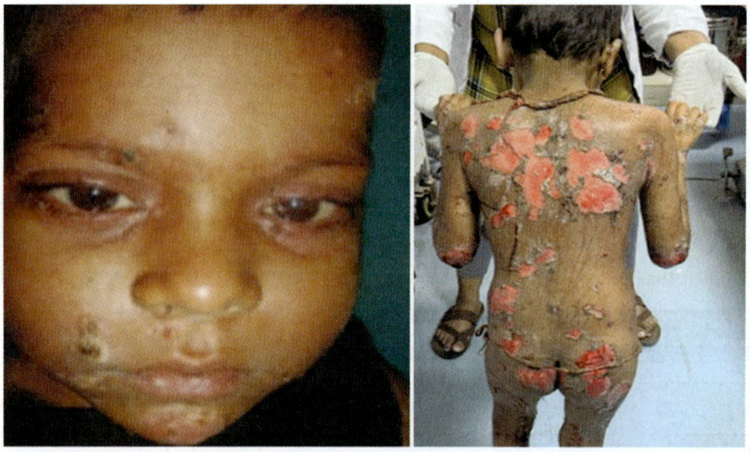

Figure 14.12: Pemphigus vulgaris

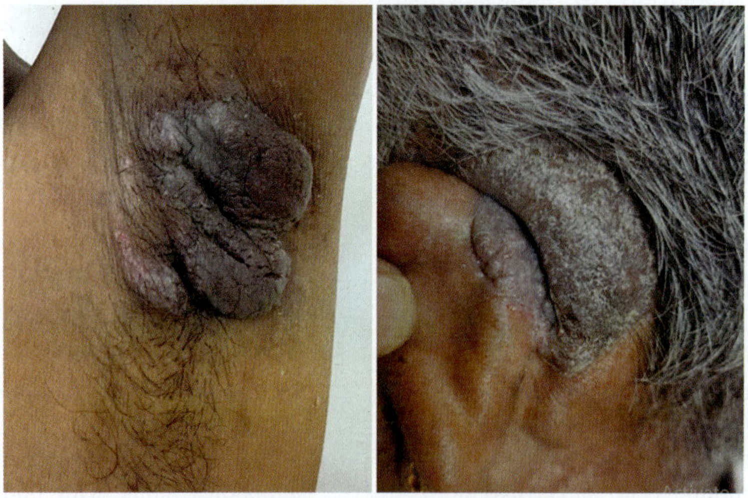

Figure 14.13: Pemphigus vegetans

intertriginous areas due to papillomatous response. It is divided in two types: Neumann and Hallopeau.

- The Neumann type is more severe, refractory to treatment and oral mucosa is usually involved while Hallopeau has an indolent course and oral mucosa is not usually involved.
- To measure the distribution, severity and extent of disease is assessed by using Autoimmune Bullous Skin Intensity and Severity score (ABSIS) or Pemphigus Disease and Area Index (PDAI).

PEMPHIGUS FOLIACEOUS

It is an autoimmune skin disorder characterized by the loss of intercellular adhesion of keratinocytes in the upper parts of the epidermis (acantholysis), resulting in the formation of superficial blisters. IgG antibodies are present mostly against desmoglein 1. Oral mucosal involvement is uncommon.

Clinical Features

- The primary cutaneous lesions are small, superficial blisters; however, these flaccid bullae are difficult to find because they are transient, easily rupture and transform into erosions.
- Scaly, crusted erosions (Figure 14.14) on an erythematous base confined mainly to so called seborrheic areas (e.g., face, scalp, upper part of the trunk) are commonly seen.
- The erosions can become numerous, showing a tendency to generalize. Occasionally, erythroderma develops.
- The erosions may be accompanied by a burning sensation and local pain.
- In contrast to PV, in pemphigus foliaceous, little or no involvement of the mucous membranes occurs.
- Variants of pemphigus foliaceous are pemphigus herpetiformis, pemphigus erythematosus and endemic pemphigus.
- Pemphigus herpetiformis presents with papulovesicular lesions on erythematous base over extensor surfaces.
- Pemphigus erythematosus or Senear-Usher syndrome presents with features of both lupus erythematosus and pemphigus foliaceous. DIF study shows deposition of IgG and C3 at basement membrane zone and in intraepidermal area. It shows ANA positivity.
- Endemic pemphigus or fogo selvagem (wildfire) or Brazilian pemphigus is caused by autoimmune response to black fly (*Simulium Nigrimanum)* saliva.

PEMPHIGUS NEONATORUM

- Disease occurs due to transplacental transfer of autoantibodies against intercellular substances.
- In neonates, desmoglein 3 is present throughout the epidermis, desmoglein1 has lesser expression. Hence, pemphigus foliaceous is rare in neonates.
- Neonates present with vesicles, bullae and erosion of skin with mucous membrane involvement.
- No active treatment is required, spontaneous recovery occurs within 3 weeks, as the levels of antibodies subside.

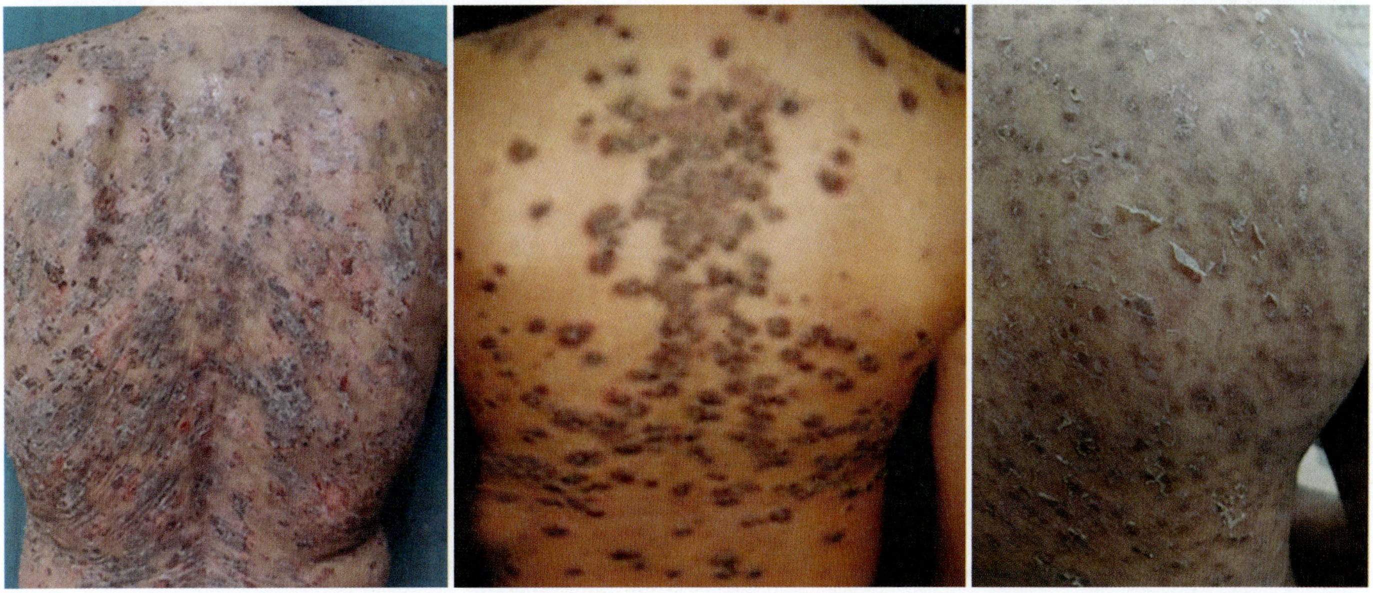

Figure 14.14: Pemphigus foliaceous

Differential Diagnosis of Pemphigus

- Pemphigus herpetiformis.
- Bullous pemphigoid.

Investigations

1. Tzanck preparation from the base of a blister or oral erosion shows acantholytic cells.
2. In pemphigus vulgaris histopathology (Figure 14.15) from early vesicle or from the edge of the lesion demonstrates an intraepidermal blister. The earliest changes consist of intercellular edema with loss of intercellular attachments in the basal layer. Suprabasal epidermal cells separate from the basal cells to form clefts and blisters. Basal cells are separated from one another and stand like a row of tombstones on the floor of the blister, but they remain attached to the basement membrane. Blisters contain some acantholytic cells. Histopathology can help in differentiating PV from pemphigus foliaceous, which demonstrates a more superficial epidermal cleavage. Blistering is preceded by eosinophilic spongiosis in some patients. The superficial dermis has a mild, superficial, mixed inflammatory infiltrate, which includes few eosinophils.

   Histopathology can help in differentiating pemphigus vulgaris from pemphigus foliaceous. In pemphigus foliaceous bulla are seen in upper epidermis.
3. DIF on normal appearing perilesional skin usually shows IgG deposited on the surface of the keratinocytes in and around lesions (Fish net appearance). IgG1 and IgG4 are the most common subclasses. Antibodies are deposited throughout the epidermis. The best site for taking specimen for DIF is normal perilesional skin. When DIF is performed on lesional skin, false-positive results can be observed.
4. IIF by using patient's serum, demonstrates the presence of circulating IgG autoantibodies that bind to epidermis. Circulating intercellular antibodies are detected by IDIF in 80-90% of patients with PV. The titer of circulating antibodies correlates with disease course..
5. Other investigations include ELISA to detect circulating anti desmoglein antibodies.

Treatment

Pemphigus vulgaris is an autoimmune disease; hence immunosuppressant drugs like systemic corticosteroids are the mainstay of treatment. These patients have multiple ulcers and raw skin surface which requires management like burns in some cases, which includes barrier nursing, IV fluids, appropriate systemic antibiotics, care of mouth, eyes and prevention of bed sores. Septicemia is major cause of death in severe cases.

Introduction of steroids has greatly reduced mortality in pemphigus patients. Prednisolone (1-2 mg/kg/day) should be given initially. In mild to moderate cases it should be given orally, while in severe cases IM or IV route should be used. Once the disease is under control which takes around 2-4 weeks, steroids should be gradually tapered and most of the patients can be maintained on 5-10 mg/day of prednisolone, which may take years before steroids can be completely stopped.

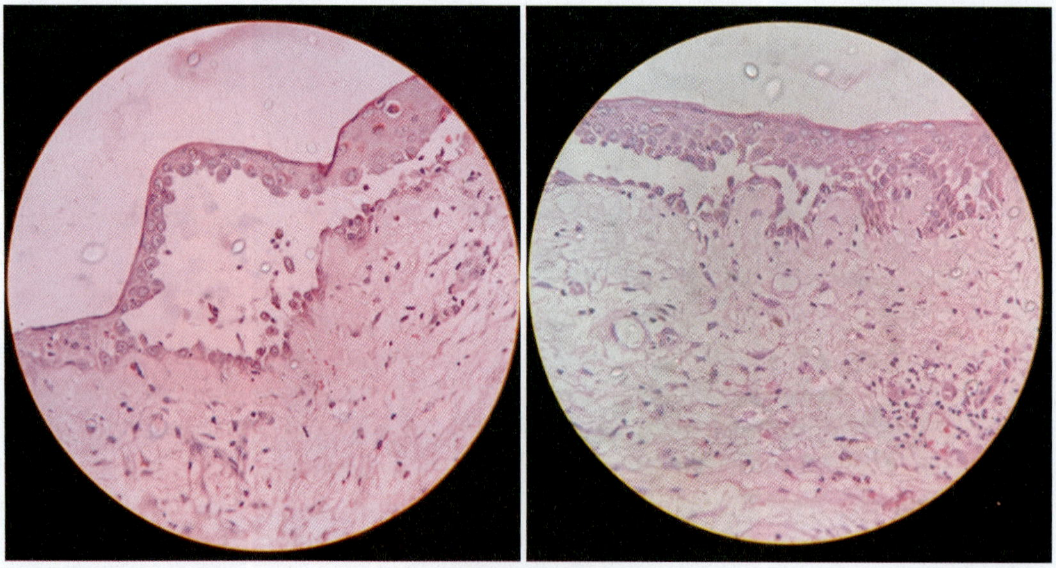

Figure 14.15: Sub-corneal splitting with row of tomb appearance with acantholytic cells

The patients who respond poorly to oral steroids or who require high maintenance dose need some steroid sparing agent. They also have adjuvant effect. Immunosuppressants like azathioprine (1-3 mg/kg/day), cyclophosphamide (1-2 mg/kg), cyclosporin (3-5 mg/kg/ day) can be used, but with caution in children. Azathioprine has side effects like bone marrow suppression and possibly increased incidence of myeloproliferative disorders. Cyclophosphamide can lead to hemorrhagic cystitis, increased risk of bladder and other cancers. Because of the gonadal side effects like azoospermia, amenorrhea and sterility, cyclophosphamide is less popular in children. For these reasons, azathioprine is a better choice in children. Patients with oral lesions may have superimposed candidiasis which should be taken care of. Use of high dose dexamethasone pulse (2 mg/kg) for 3 consecutive days, pulse therapy is helpful to bring remission in complicated cases and refractory cases requiring higher doses of corticosteroids. Dexamethasone pulse should be repeated after 28 days for total of 12–14 cycles.

Pemphigus foliaceous is easier to control than pemphigus vulgaris and its prognosis is better. Dapsone (1-2 mg/kg/day) can be used for steroid sparing effect.

Other treatment options in pemphigus include mycophenolate mofetil, methotrexate, cyclosporin, monoclonal antibodies like rituximab, plasmapheresis, photopheresis, gold etc.

- **Rituximab:** It is a chimeric monoclonal antibody against CD20 B cell receptors. It acts by depleting B cells through three mechanism: Antibody dependent cellular cytotoxicity, Complement mediated cytolysis and inhibition of signaling and apoptosis. FDA approved non dermatologic indications are Non-Hodgkin B-cell lymphoma, CD20+ Chronic lymphocytic leukemia, Rheumatoid arthritis. Other uses, not approved by FDA, are Pemphigus vulgaris and foliaceous, Paraneoplastic pemphigus, Dermatomyositis, Cutaneous lupus erythematosus etc.
- Rituximab is administered by two regimens. In lymphoma protocol it is given in the dose of 375 mg per square meter of body surface area which is repeated every weekly for four weeks. In Rheumatoid arthritis protocol rituximab is given as two 1000 mg intravenous infusions separated by 2 weeks.
- Common contraindications are pregnancy, breast-feeding, hypersensitivity to murine protein, severe heart insufficiency, uncontrolled infection, active tuberculosis, active HBsAg and HCV infection, Late onset cytopenias have also been reported in rituximab treated patients.
- The adverse effects are not common which includes hypertension, nausea, upper respiratory infections, arthralgia, pyrexia and pruritis. Infusion reaction can occur 30-120 minutes after starting of infusion which is characterized by fever, chills, flushing, pruritis, urticaria, shortness of breath, wheezing, hypotension and anaphylaxis.
- Prior to administration, patients should be premedicated with paracetamol 1000 mg and chlorpheniramine 10 mg I.V. bolus dose, hydrocortisone 100 mg I.V. bolus dose, ondansetron 8 mg to prevent or attenuate possible infusion related reaction. Premedication must be given at least 30 min prior to infusion. Antihypertensive should be stopped 12 hours prior to infusion. Vitals should be measured every 15 minutes for first hour of infusion thereafter every 30 or 60 minutes.
- Increased incidence of infections such as bacterial, viral and fungal may be seen during and upto 12 months after rituximab therapy. Reactivation of tuberculosis may occur, so it is important to exclude tuberculosis by performing chest X-ray, tuberculin test, CBNAAT and QuantiFERON-TB Gold. Hepatitis B, C and HIV infections should be excluded by serological tests before starting of therapy. It can also reactivate JC virus which may lead to progressive multifocal leukoencephalopathy.
- Complete blood counts (CBC) should be performed every 2 weekly during rituximab treatment and every 1-3 months thereafter.

Patient's attendants should be briefed about the nature of the disease and requirement of long-term management.

PARANEOPLASTIC PEMPHIGUS

- It is an autoimmune blistering disorder, involving skin and mucous membranes and is associated with neoplasms. Antibodies are formed against desmoplakins, envoplakin, periplakin, BP-180, BP-230, plectin, plakophilin, desmocollins, and desmoglein. Plakin are the major antigen target in paraneoplastic pemphigus.
- Revised criteria for diagnosis of PNP (Camisa and Helm criteria):

Major criteria:

- Polymorphic mucocutaneous eruptions (papules, vesicles, bullae, erosions, plaques, lichenoid).
- Concurrent neoplasia.
- Specific immunoprecipitation pattern.

Minor criteria:

- **Histology:** Acantholysis.
- **DIF:** Intercellular and basement membrane deposition of IgG and C3.

- **IIF:** Anti-desmoplakin antibody on rat bladder urothelium.
- Three major criteria or two major and two minor criteria are required for diagnosis of PNP.

Underlying malignancy should be searched for and treated. Treatment of malignancy usually leads to resolution of skin lesions. Other treatment modalities similar to those given in pemphigus have been tried.

Lymphoproliferative neoplasms are the most commonly associated malignancies e.g. Non-Hodgkin's lymphoma followed by chronic lymphocytic leukemia and Castleman disease. Others include sarcomas such as follicular dendritic cell sarcomas, thymomas, squamous cell carcinoma of skin and vagina, and carcinomas of the lung, stomach and colon.

IgA PEMPHIGUS

IgA pemphigus is a rare autoimmune vesiculopustular eruption, seen mainly in adults, characterized by IgA autoantibodies against desmocollin 1 or desmoglein 1 or 3. Flaccid pustules and bullae are seen on an erythematous base with itching. Axilla and groin are common sites. Two types have been recognized: Intraepidermal neutrophilic type and subcorneal pustular dermatosis type. It has a chronic benign course. Dapsone is the drug of choice, PUVA therapy, colchicine and mycophenolate mofetil have also been tried.

SUBCORNEAL PUSTULAR DERMATOSIS(SCPD)/ SNEDDON - WILKINSON DISEASE

It is a rare vesiculopustular disorder with subcorneal bullae and abundant neutrophils, predominantly affecting flexural areas. Very small pustules arise in crops over erythematous skin, which rupture to form dry, peeling skin and crusts. Treatment consists of dapsone, retinoids and steroids to suppress the flares.

Drugs and Pemphigus

Drug induced pemphigus: Drug induced pemphigus regresses without treatment after withdrawal of the offending drug. Clinically, it resembles pemphigus foliaceus or pemphigus herpetiformis. Histologically, it is different from PV because of uneven and partial supra basal acantholysis. In drug induced pemphigus, keratinocyte cohesiveness is disrupted due to biochemical acantholysis. Cysteine-cysteine bonds which are present between normal keratinocytes are replaced by drug-cysteine bonds, known as non-antibody medicated acantholysis.

Drug triggered pemphigus: In drug triggered pemphigus, drugs appear to be primarily a trigger or facilitator of the dysimmune process. The disease self-perpetuates with all the features of spontaneous pemphigus, including mucocutaneous involvement and suprabasal antibody mediated acantholysis. The disease continues even after the precipitating drug has been eliminated.

Medications suspected of triggering PV are classified in three groups:

1. Thiol drugs
2. Phenol drugs
3. Non-thiol non-phenol drugs

Thiol group: These medications cause immunological acantholysis by antigenically conforming membrane desmogleins, which in turn produces antibody mediated pemphigus vulgaris. For example, piroxicam, gold sodium thiomalate, penicillamine, captopril, penicillin and its derivatives (mostly aminopenicillins), and thiamazole.

Phenol group: Phenol exposed genetically predisposed keratinocytes release IL-1α and TNF-α resulting in increased protease activity (plasminogen activator) leading to acantholysis. e.g. cephalosporins rifampicin, levodopa, heroin and aspirin.

Non-thiol and non-phenol drugs: These medications promote immune acantholysis through a number of mechanisms, such as increased target antigen expression on keratinocyte membranes, excessive immune system activation through increased antibody production, heightened local immune response and keratinocyte release of plasminogen activators. For example, ACE inhibitors, nifedipine, NSAIDs, and enalapril.

INHERITED ACANTHOLYTIC DISORDERS

Hailey-Hailey Disease

It is also known as familial benign chronic pemphigus. It is a rare hereditary disorder characterized by vesicular eruption localized to intertriginous areas like axilla, groins, neck and perianal region. Disease exacerbates in summer.

Treatment includes avoidance of excessive exposure to hot and humid environment to reduce sweating, vitamin A, retinoids, topical and systemic corticosteroids.

Darier's Disease

It is a rare congenital acantholytic disorder, transmitted as autosomal dominant trait. The disease is characterized by multiple, warty, papular lesions over seborrheic areas of body (Figure 14.16A and B). Acrokeratosis verruciformis of hopf, plane wart like lesions are seen on dorsa of hands (Figure 14.17C). Palmoplantar keratoderma and pitting are common

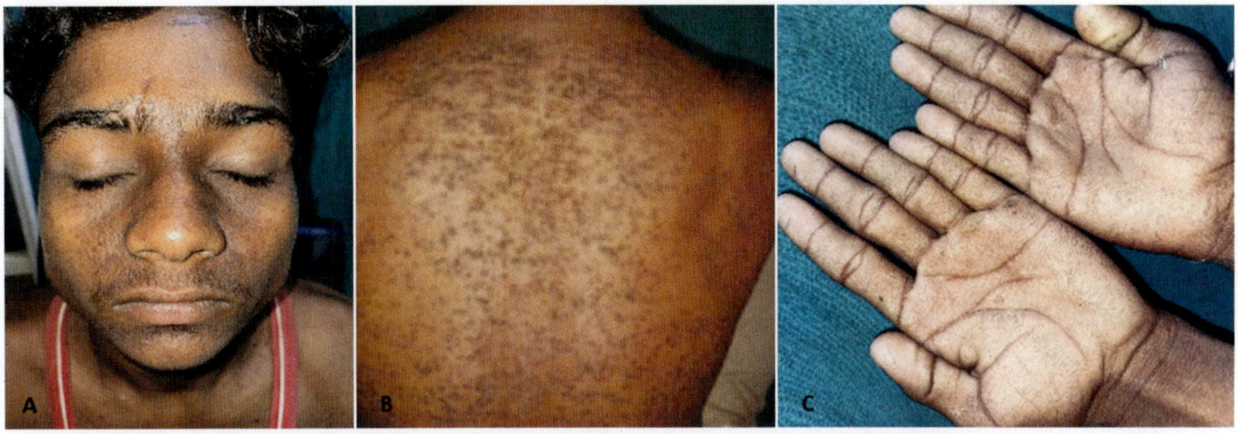

Figure 14.16: Darier's disease showing warty greasy papules over seborrheic distribution (A and B) and palmer pitting (C)

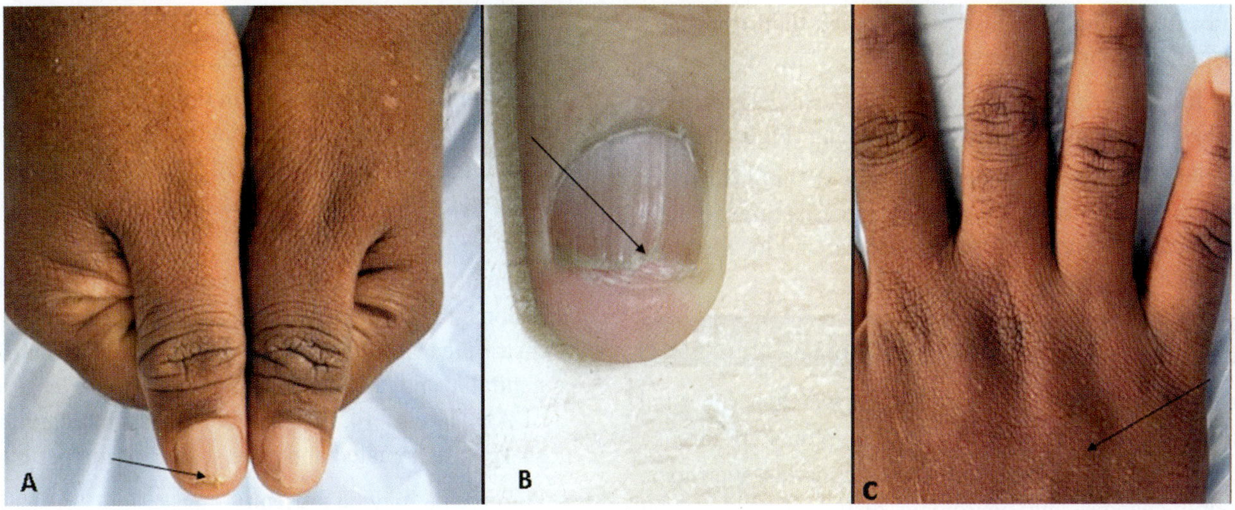

Figure 14.17: Darier disease showing 'V' shape nicking with longitudinal streaking of nail (A) & (B) Acrokeratosis verruciform lesion on dorsal surface of hand (C)

finding (Figure 14.16C) with occasional hemorrhagic macules. Mucosal involvement presents with cobblestone papules. Nail fragility, white and red longitudinal bands terminating in V-shaped nicks are typical for Darier disease (Figure 14.17A and B). Dyskeratosis or premature keratinization of corneocytes with **corps ronds and grains** is seen on histopathology. Oral Vitamin A, topical and oral retinoids are the mainstay of treatment.

GROVER DISEASE (TRANSIENT ACANTHOLYTIC DERMATOSIS)

It presents with intense pruritic small erythematous crusted papules and vesicles on chest , back and arms. Drugs associated with this condition are BRAF inhibitors like dabrafenib, vemurafenib. Histological examination shows acantholysis with or without dyskeratosis. Treatment includes moisturizer, topical steroids, vit D3 analogue, oral retinoids and oral corticosteroids.

MISCELLANEOUS BLISTERING DISORDERS

BLISTER BEETLE DERMATITIS

- It is an irritant dermatitis produced by the insects known as 'Blister Beetles'. Common beetles causing the disease are *Lytta vesicatoria, Mylabris* and *Paederus* (Rove beetle) species.
- The insect has small sacs at the joints of legs. These sacs have cantharidin (pederin in case of *Paederus* species) containing fluid inside. During sleep, the insect may get crushed in between the skin surfaces or between the skin

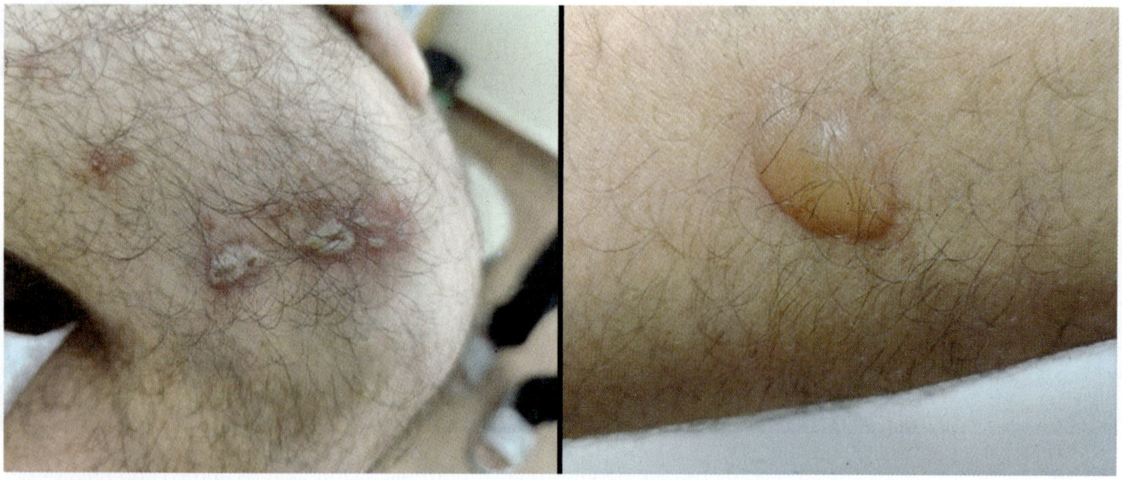

Figure 14.18: Blister beetle dermatitis

and bed resulting in release of vesicating fluid from sacs, causing severe irritant dermatitis locally.

- The lesions are grouped vesiculobullous lesions with localized erythema and crusting or oozing (Figure 14.18).
- Treatment consists of administration of antihistamines orally and prevention of secondary bacterial infections. In severe cases, a short course of systemic and local steroid therapy will be beneficial.

ACRODERMATITIS ENTEROPATHICA (AE)

It is an inborn error of zinc metabolism which is inherited as an autosomal recessive disorder. Symptoms in infancy typically include periorificial and acral dermatitis, diarrhoea, behavioural changes and neurologic disturbances. In older children, failure to thrive, anorexia, alopecia, nail dystrophy, and repeated infections are most common.

Etiology

- Defective gene SLC39A4 encodes for a zinc transporter due to which there is less absorption of zinc from the gut.
- Breast milk has a protein, which helps in absorption of zinc, hence the deficiency does not manifest until breast milk is discontinued. Zinc deficiency may also be seen due to:
  - Inadequate intake.
  - Malabsorption.
  - Excessive loss.
  - Prolonged parenteral nutrition without zinc supplemen-tation.
  - Low birth weight, preterm babies.

Clinical Features

- Symptoms typically appear in the first few months of life, when an infant is weaned from breastfeeding. AE can also develop in full term breastfed infants as a result of zinc deficiency in breast milk and decreased maternal plasma zinc levels.
- **Dermatitis:** Erythematous, vesiculobullous, or pustular lesions that lead to dry, scaly, or eczematoid lesions, distributed around periorificial areas, e.g., mouth, anus, genitalia and acral areas of the body are characteristic of AE (Figure 14.19). The borders of affected areas are sharply demarcated and have scaling at the periphery.
- Paronychia may be present.
- **Alopecia:** Partial or total hair loss may be evident.
- Diarrhea.
- Growth retardation, bacterial and fungal infections and behavioural changes may also be seen.
- Patients are miserable and depressed. Infants are inconsolable and may withdraw from social contact.

Differential Diagnosis

- Atopic dermatitis.
- Biotin deficiency.
- Candidiasis.
- Epidermolysis bullosa.

Investigations

- In most patients with AE, plasma zinc concentrations is low (<50 µg/dl) but it is not diagnostic.

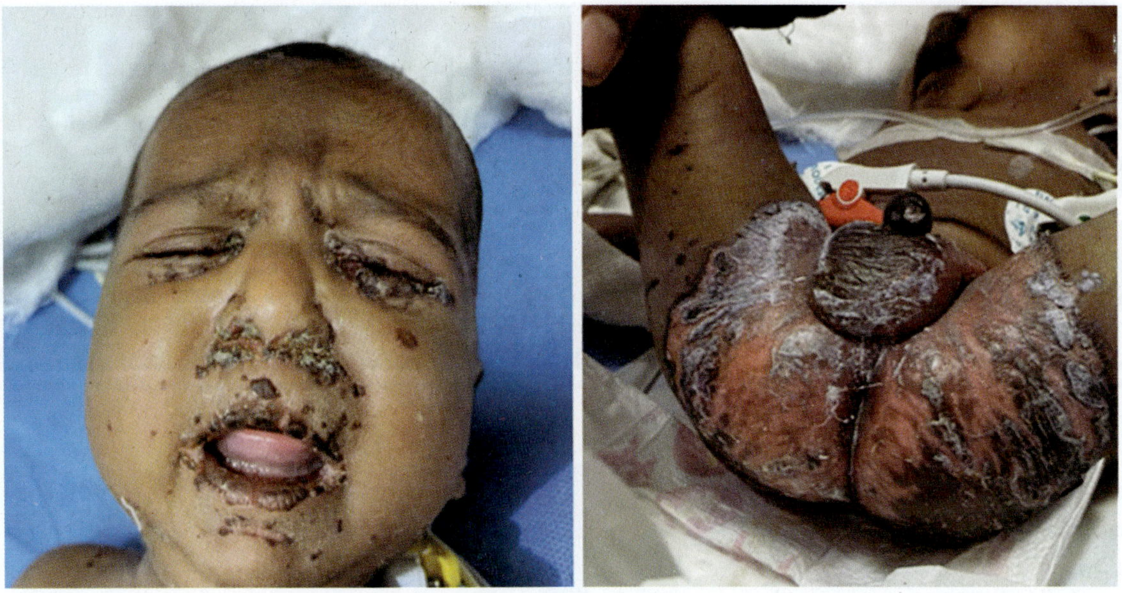

Figure 14.19: Showing acrodermatitis enteropathica- erythematous erosive rashes around perioral, perinasal and perianal area

- Production of serum alkaline phosphatase depends on zinc; therefore, a low level of alkaline phosphatase may support a diagnosis of AE.

Treatment

- In patients with AE, zinc gluconate or sulfate is administered orally at a dosage of 1-3 mg/kg/day. Although the intravenous dosage have not clearly been estimated, amounts of 300-1000 µg/kg/day may be sufficient for rapid reversal of symptoms.
- Clinical response is observed within 5-10 days. Zinc therapy has to be maintained throughout the patient's life span, though periods of remission are reported. Exacerbation during pregnancy or the stress, may require an increase in dose. In acquired zinc deficiency, treatment can be stopped after the precipitating cause.
- Warm compresses and Vaseline applied three times a day to areas of weeping or crusting is helpful.

15 CHAPTER Connective Tissue Diseases

Contents

Connective tissue diseases are heterogeneous group of chronic multisystem inflammatory disorders including systemic lupus erythematosus, progressive systemic sclerosis, dermatomyositis and polymyositis, mixed connective tissue disease and Sjögren's syndrome, etc. Patients can present with similar clinical features, particularly the initial presentation, which frequently makes the diagnosis of a specific disease difficult. The incidence of connective tissue diseases is much lower in children than in adults and the clinical picture is more variable. Clinical signs, such as fatigue, fever, or weight loss, may precede any systemic organ involvement and in children, mucocutaneous manifestations develop more frequently during the varying disease course. This chapter summarizes recent information on epidemiology, clinical manifestations, diagnostic procedures and treatment strategies of the different connective tissue diseases, concentrating on specific problems in childhood.

CLASSIFICATION OF CONNECTIVE TISSUE DISEASES

1. **Lupus erythematosus**
   - Acute cutaneous lupus erythematosus (ACLE)
   - Subacute cutaneous lupus erythematosus (SCLE)
   - Chronic cutaneous lupus erythematosus (CCLE)
   - Systemic lupus erythematosus (SLE)
   - Neonatal lupus erythematosus (NLE)
   - Drug induced lupus erythematosus
2. **Antiphospholipid syndrome (APLA)**
3. **Polymyositis and Dermatomyositis (PM/DM)**
4. **Localized scleroderma**
   - Morphea
   - Eosinophilic fasciitis
5. **Systemic sclerosis (SSc)**
6. **Sjogren syndrome**
7. **Raynaud syndrome**
8. **Mixed connective tissue disease (MCTD)**
9. **Relapsing Polychondritis (RP)**

ANTINUCLEAR ANTIBODY (ANA)

Antinuclear antibodies are class of antibodies, which bind to components of the nucleus. Presence of these antibodies is a defining feature of connective tissue diseases. ANA can be detected by indirect immunofluorescence technique where mouse kidney or rat kidney are used as substrate. Now-a-days Hep 2 cell lines are most commonly used. ANA can also be detected by radioimmune assay, ELISA and immunoblot technique. ANA titres of more than 1:160 is considered diagnostic for connective tissue disorders. The ANA titres can fluctuate according to disease severity. Other than CTD it can be found positive in pregnancy, neoplasms and chronic infection. The prevalence of ANA positivity and different patterns of ANA are discussed below in Table 15.1 and 15.2.

Table 15.1: Prevalence of ANA positivity

Disease	Prevalence
SLE , Drug induced LE	95-100%
SCLE	60-80%
Discoid lupus erythematosus (DLE)	5-60%
Mixed connective tissue disease (MCTD)	95-100%
Systemic sclerosis	90-95%
Sjogren syndrome	75%
Rheumatoid arthritis	50-75%
Dermatomyositis	30%

Table 15.2: Patterns of ANA

Pattern		Associations
• Homogenous	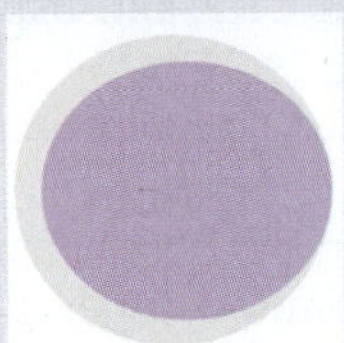	Anti-histone antibody – drug induced LE Anti-ds DNA- Correlates with development of lupus nephritis and disease activity
• Peripheral rim	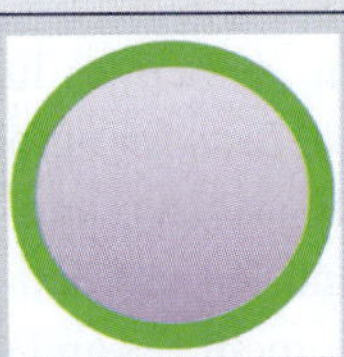	Nuclear laminas – SLE, linear morphea Nuclear pore – polymyositis
• Speckled particulate	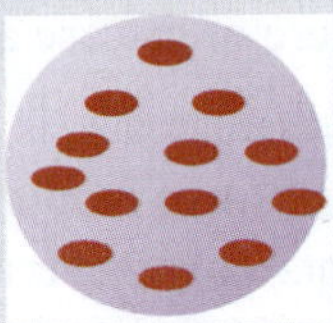	Fine speckled- anti-Ro, anti-La, anti-ribonucleoprotein, anti-Ki, anti-Mi-2 Coarse speckled – U1 RNP, Anti Smith
• Anticentromere	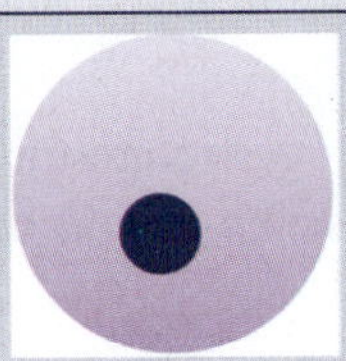	CREST syndrome
• Nucleolar	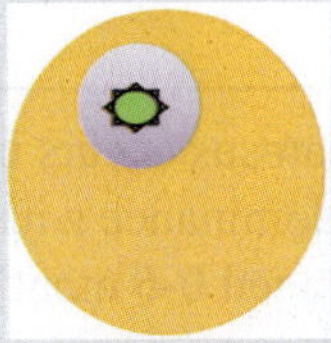	Anti-Scl 70/ anti-DNA topoisomerase I- Specific for PSS Anti-RNA polymerase III – Renal risk Anti-fibrillarin – Specific for U3RNP, risk of pulmonary artery hypertension Anti-PM-Scl – Overlap syndrome

Term Used for Different Overlap Connective Tissue Diseases

Undifferentiated connective tissue disease: Signs and symptoms of connective tissue disease are present but does not meet full criteria to diagnose a specific collagen connective tissue disease.

Overlap syndrome: In overlap syndrome, patient satisfies two or more systemic connective tissue disease criteria.

Mixed connective tissue disease: It is a separate connective tissue disease with specific diagnostic criteria and anti U1RNP positivity.

SYSTEMIC LUPUS ERYTHEMATOSUS (SLE)

Lupus erythematosus (LE) occurs less frequently in children. Most cases take the form of systemic lupus erythematosus (SLE). Two patterns of LE are seen in children:

1. Neonatal LE.
2. Childhood LE (tends to have more severe disease as compared to adults).
3. Adult LE

Neonatal Lupus Erythematosus (Figure 15.1)

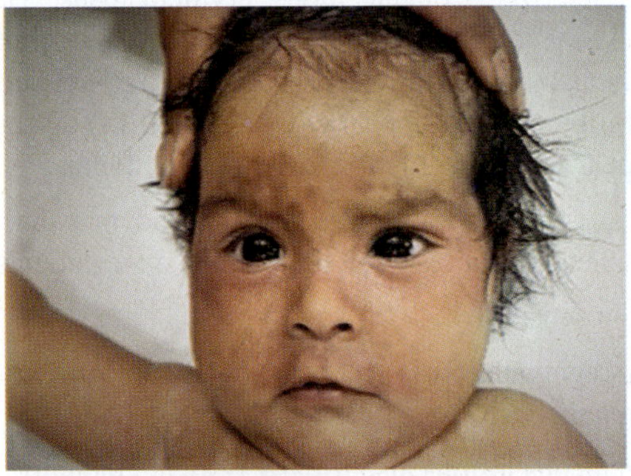

Figure 15.1: Neonatal lupus erythematosus

Epidemiology

Neonatal lupus erythematosus occurs in 1 in every 20,000 live births. It has female predominance with female to male ratio of 3:1 and affects children aged 0-6 months.

Neonatal lupus erythematosus results from maternal transfer of autoantibodies (LE factor and antinuclear antibodies); however, most infants exposed to these antibodies *in utero* do not develop disease. It is a rare syndrome and occurs in 1 in 200 patients with anti-Ro antibodies. The antibodies associated with heart block and with cutaneous disease are different, anti-Ro (SS-A) antibody against the 52/60-kd protein is associated with congenital heart block, while anti-La (SS-B) antibody against the 50-kd protein is associated with cutaneous disease.

Only small percentages of neonates exposed to these antibodies develop disease; therefore, other factors, which trigger the disease, may also be involved. These are genetic predisposition, viral infections, hormones and other unknown environmental factors. The risk of neonatal lupus erythematosus or congenital heart block developing in a woman who tests positive for anti-Ro antibody who has never had a child with neonatal lupus erythematosus or congenital heart block, is less than 1%, whereas the risk for a mother who has had an affected infant, it is approximately 25%.

Clinical Features (Table 15.3)

Neonatal lupus erythematosus that affects the heart is usually discovered on physical examination at birth but may be recognized with ultrasonography *in utero*. Mothers may be asymptomatic or have symptoms of lupus erythematosus or Sjögren's syndrome. When carefully questioned, they may report dry eyes, arthralgia, myalgia or arthritis.

Cutaneous Manifestations

- Annular erythematous plaques with slight scaling characterize neonatal lupus erythematosus. Head and neck are the most commonly affected areas, but lesions may also appear on the arms and trunk. They are present at birth or always appear within 2 months of age and rarely appear when the infant is older than 6 months.
- Telangiectasia is often prominent and may be the sole cutaneous manifestation reported in some patients.
- Photosensitivity.
- Dyspigmentation is frequent, but, with time, it resolves spontaneously.
- Cutaneous lesions also usually resolve gradually.

Cardiac manifestations

- Complete congenital heart block (CHB) is the usual finding, but incomplete heart block and prolongation of the QT interval are also found. Heart blocks present as bradycardia *in utero* or at birth.
- Heart failure is a well-recognized complication during the neonatal period.

Other manifestations

- Hepatosplenomegaly is an occasional transient finding. Transaminase elevation is often present.
- Pneumonitis may manifest as tachypnea or tachycardia.
- Thrombocytopenia may cause petechiae.

Table 15.3: Summary of clinical findings in neonatal lupus erythematosus

Skin manifestations	*Systemic manifestation*
Photosensitivity	Congenital heart block
Annular erythematous plaques with light scale	Hepatosplenomegaly
Telangiectasia	Pneumonitis
Dyspigmentation	Thrombocytopenia

Clinical lesions that indicate systemic activity in lupus erythematosus include photosensitivity, lupus hair, periungual telangiectasia, cutaneous vasculitis including nail fold infarcts, elevated ESR or CRP, anti-dsDNA antibody titers and decreased complements.

Investigations

- Neutropenia, thrombocytopenia and elevated liver enzymes and deranged renal functions may be found.
- Children in whom systemic lupus erythematosus is suspected serological tests for autoimmune disorders, e.g., antinuclear antibody (ANA), anti-double stranded DNA, anti-Sm, anti-RNP, anti-Ro, and anti-La antibodies should be done. Serum complement C3 and C4 levels are decreased and provide a measure of disease activity.
- Neonatal lupus erythematosus is related to the anti-Ro Antibody, which is positive in more than 90% of patients. Occasionally, patients only have anti-La or anti-U1RNP antibodies. Rheumatoid factor and VDRL test may also be positive.
- Respiratory, renal, gastrointestinal, cardiovascular and central nervous systems should be evaluated to rule out complications.

- Electrocardiography reveals heart block in a patient in whom neonatal lupus erythematosus is suspected.
- Skin biopsy is also useful.

Treatment

- Neonatal lupus erythematosus that affects the skin, blood, spleen, or liver is usually self-limiting and resolves without intervention within 2-6 months.
- In severe cases, when heart block occurs, cardiac failure and death may occur. A pacemaker is often required.

Follow-up

- Patients with neonatal lupus erythematosus may be more prone to develop lupus erythematosus later because of their genetic predisposition. Their non-affected siblings are also at higher risk for development of systemic lupus erythematosus.
- Patients with cardiac involvement require regular monitoring to assess cardiac function and the need for a pacemaker.

Prognosis

- Generally, skin disease is self-limiting.
- Hepatosplenomegaly is self-limiting, although death due to hepatitis may occur.
- Thrombocytopenia is self-limiting; however, if severe thrombocytopenia is present, bleeding can affect the prognosis.
- Cardiac involvement is associated with a poor outcome in many patients, including some who receive pacemakers.

Childhood Lupus Erythematosus (Juvenile SLE)

Children have more severe disease, though clinical picture, course and treatment are same as in adults with SLE. CNS involvement occurs in 30-40% of cases and high involvement of renal system (87%) is seen in childhood LE. Enlargement of liver, spleen and lymph nodes are more common in children. Disease causing mutations or risk alleles (complement genes, TREX 1) may be enough to cause disease in pediatric age group, while in adults, environmental factors accumulate over time to cause disease expression. Thus, genetic factors play a major role in juvenile disease.

Epidemiology

Lupus erythematosus of childhood occurs in 6/100,0000 children annually. It affects prepubertal and post-pubertal children. Female predominance varies from 4:1 before puberty to 8:1 afterwards. Peak age of onset is between 12 and 14 years. Onset before the age of 5 is extremely uncommon and is referred to as early onset SLE. Approximately 10-20% of patients with SLE develop disease before the age of 16 years. Acute LE in 20% cases is diagnosed before the age of 20.

Clinical Features

Juvenile onset of SLE manifests acutely, aggressively with severe clinical presentations.

- Lesions of discoid lupus erythematosus or subacute cutaneous LE, malar rash (Figure 15.2), photosensitivity, arthralgia, arthritis and fever may be the presenting symptoms. The patient may give history of rash, which is slightly scaly eruption on the face and periorbital skin (Raccoon eye sign/Owl eye/Eye mask).

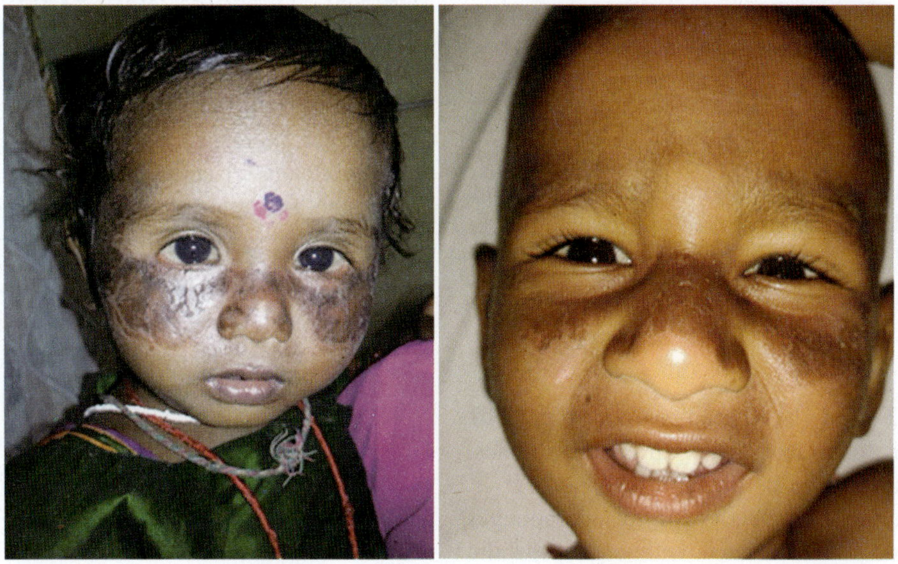

Figure 15.2: Malar rash in a child with lupus erythematosus

- Adults with discoid lupus erythematosus have a low risk of systemic disease. However, risk of systemic disease appears to be greater in children. Inflammatory multiorgan involvement and tissue damage is more common in juvenile SLE. Fever, hematological and lymphadenopathy are more common.
- Malar rash, mucocutaneous involvement, hematological abnormalities, seizures, renal involvement, urinary cellular casts and proteinuria, lymphadenopathy and fever are far more common in juvenile SLE.

Adult Lupus Erythematosus

Systemic lupus erythematosus (SLE) is a systemic chronic autoimmune disease with a relapsing and remitting course. Its prevalence is higher in reproductive age group women, with a female to male ratio of 9:1.

Pathogenesis

The pathogenesis of SLE involves a complex interaction of genetic predisposition, environmental precipitants, immunological and hormonal factors.

1. **Genetic susceptibility**
   - A genome wide association study (GWAS) has mapped > 90 SLE susceptibility loci.
   - A large number of genes are important which include Interferon regulatory factor 5 (IRF5), signal transducer and activator of transcription 4 (STAT4), B-lymphoid tyrosine kinase (BLK) and integrin alpha M (ITGAM).
2. **Environmental factors**
   - Exposure to oral contraceptives, ultraviolet B (UVB), certain drugs, Epstein-Barr virus (EBV) infection, silica and cigarette smoking may act as precipitating factors.
   - Important drugs implicated in inducing SLE are hydralazine, procainamide, isoniazid, minocycline and TNF-α inhibitors. Procainamide and hydralazine are associated with the highest risk of inducing SLE, with 30% and 5% to 10%, respectively.
3. **Abnormal innate and adaptive immune responses**

Role of T Cells

Imbalance of Th1/Th2 cells: Th cells can be divided into Th1 and Th2 cells according to the secretion of different cytokines. Th1 cells secrete tumor necrosis factor-α (TNF-α), IL-2, IFN-γ, which are involved in the activation of macrophages and CD8+ T cells and are associated with organ specific autoimmune diseases. Th2 cells secrete IL-4, IL-6, and IL-10, which can promote the activation of B lymphocytes and induce the production of IgG1. Normally, the two types of cells regulate and inhibit each other through cytokines to maintain the immune balance. In SLE, the balance is broken, active SLE is characterized by decreased function of Th1 and hyperfunction of Th2, which leads to excessive activation of B cells, generation of autoantibodies and tissue injury.

T follicular helper (Tfh) cells are subset of CD4 positive T cells, which are essential for germinal center induction, proliferation, isotype switching and somatic hypermutation. Pathological expansion of Tfh cells in SLE is directed by the interaction of the Tfh cells with the OX40 ligand expressed on myeloid antigen presenting cells. The expression of the OX40 ligand is induced by TLR7 activation from circulating RNA-containing immune complexes. This pathologic expansion of the Tfh cell subset contributes to enhanced antibody production and loss of tolerance in SLE patients.

Regulatory T (Treg) cells are a unique T cell subset population that suppresses the immune response and maintains self-tolerance, suppressing autoreactive lymphocytes in healthy individuals. The development of Treg cells is dependent on IL2 activity. In SLE, an imbalanced T cell cytokine profile characterized by decreased IL2 leads to impaired Treg cell development and function.

Role of B cells

B cells contribute to the pathogenesis through their response to antigens and autoantibody production. The pathways involved in the aberrant activation of B cells include the toll like receptor (TLR) pathway, stimulation via beta cell activating factor (BAAF) and B cell receptor (BCR) mediated activation.

Role of the complement system

Complement dysfunction (C1q, C3, C4) is proposed to accelerate several steps in the pathogenic pathways of SLE, such as impaired clearance of apoptotic debris and immune complexes, increased autoreactive CD+8 T cell activity and tissue damage by activation of the inflammatory cascade in organs with immune complex deposition.

Clinical Features (Table 15.6)

SLE exhibits a broad spectrum of presentation, ranging from mild mucocutaneous disease to severe, life threatening disease with multiorgan involvement.

1. **Constitutional symptoms**
   - Seen in more than 90% of patients.
   - Fatigue, malaise, fever, anorexia and weight loss are common.

- SLE may be an infrequent cause of fever of unknown origin.

2. **Mucocutaneous manifestations**
    - More than 80% of patients with SLE suffer from mucocutaneous involvement.
    - Lupus specific lesions include:
        1. Acute cutaneous lupus erythematosus (ACLE) includes localized malar and generalized rash,
        2. Subacute cutaneous lupus erythematosus (SCLE) includes annular and papulosquamous rash and
        3. Chronic cutaneous lupus erythematosus (CCLE)
    - Oral and nasal ulcers are common in SLE and are often painless. They may occur anywhere in the oral cavity but are commonly seen over hard palate, the buccal mucosa and the vermilion border of lips as gradually occurring erythema, macules, petechiae, erosions, or ulcers.
    - Photosensitivity is seen in more than 90% of cases.
    - Gilliam classification of skin lesions associated with Lupus Erythematosus is given in Table 15.4.

Table 15.4: Gilliam classification of skin lesions associated with Lupus Erythematosus

Lupus erythematosus specific lesions	*Lupus erythematosus non-specific lesions*
• **Acute cutaneous lupus erythematosus** o Localized: malar rashes, butterfly rash o Generalized: maculopapular rash, photosensitive rash • **Subacute cutaneous lupus erythematosus** o Annular-Lupus marginatus, autoimmune annular erythema o Papulosquamous-Psoriasiform, pityriasiform. • **Chronic cutaneous lupus erythematosus** o Classical discoid lupus erythematosus o Hypertrophic DLE o Verrucous DLE o Lupus profundus or lupus panniculitis o Lupus tumidus o Chilblain lupus o Mucosal DLE - oral/conjunctival o Lichenoid DLE (Lichen planus overlap)	• **Cutaneous vascular disease** o ***Vasculitis:*** ◊ Leukocytoclastic vasculitis ◊ Urticarial vasculitis ◊ Polyarteritis nodosa like vasculitis o ***Vasculopathy:*** ◊ Degos disease like lesions ◊ Secondary atrophie (livedoid vasculitis) o Periungual telangiectasia o Livedo reticularis o Thrombophlebitis o Raynaud's phenomena o Erythromelalgia • **Non scaring alopecia** o Lupus hair o Telogen effluvium o Alopecia areata • Sclerodactyly • Rheumatoid nodules • Calcinosis cutis • Urticaria • Cutis laxa • Anetoderma • Acanthosis nigricans • Leg ulcers • Non-specific bullous lesions • Erythema multiforme (Rowell syndrome)

3. **Musculoskeletal manifestations**
   - Approximately 80 to 90% of patients with SLE have musculoskeletal involvement at some point during their disease course.
   - Symptoms range from mild arthralgias to deforming arthritis.
4. **Neuropsychiatric manifestations**
   - Both central (CNS) and peripheral (PNS) nervous systems can be involved.
   - Most common CNS manifestation is intractable headaches, reported in more than 50% of cases. Other CNS manifestations include focal or generalized seizures, aseptic meningitis, demyelinating syndrome including optic neuritis and myelitis, disorders of movement such as chorea and cognitive dysfunction, and high risk for ischemic strokes.
   - Cranial and peripheral neuropathies, mononeuritis multiplex, autonomic neuropathies and syndromes mimicking Guillain Barré syndrome and Myasthenia gravis are manifestations of peripheral nervous system involvement.
   - Psychiatric manifestations may range from depression and anxiety to psychosis.
5. **Renal manifestations**
   - Lupus nephritis is a well-known and common complication of SLE.
   - Hypertension, hematuria, proteinuria, lower extremity edema and elevation in creatinine shall raise suspicion for lupus nephritis.
   - Thrombotic microangiopathy, interstitial nephritis, lupus vasculopathy, vasculitis and arteriolosclerosis are other complications that can occur.

   Wire loop appearance is typical for lupus nephritis, which is characterized by thickening and hyalinization of the glomerular tuft's capillary basement membrane on biopsy. **International society of nephrology classification of lupus nephritis (Table 15.5).**
6. **Pulmonary manifestations**
   - Pleuritis is the most common pulmonary manifestation.
   - Other manifestations include exudative pleural effusions, acute lupus pneumonitis, interstitial lung disease which may be nonspecific interstitial pneumonia (NSIP) or usual interstitial pneumonia (UIP), diffuse alveolar hemorrhage associated with capillaritis, pulmonary arterial hypertension, pulmonary embolism (with or without antiphospholipid antibody syndrome) and shrinking lung syndrome.

Table 15.5: International society of nephrology classification of lupus nephritis

Class	*Description*
I (Minimum mesangial LN)	Normal glomeruli with mesangial immune deposition on electron microscopy
II (Mesangial proliferative LN)	Mesangial hypercellularity without subendothelial immune deposition
III (Focal LN)	Segmental glomerulonephritis involving less than 50 % of all glomeruli
IV (Diffuse LN)	Glomerulonephritis involving more than 50 % of glomeruli
V (Membranous LN)	Global or segmental subendothelial immune deposition
VI (Sclerosing LN)	More than 90% glomeruli sclerosed

7. **Gastrointestinal manifestations**
   - Any part of the gastrointestinal tract may be involved in SLE.
   - Manifestations include esophageal dysmotility, mesenteric vasculitis, lupus enteritis, peritonitis and ascites, protein losing enteropathy, pancreatitis and lupoid hepatitis.
8. **Hematologic and reticuloendothelial manifestations**
   - Anemia is present in more than 50% of patients, most commonly due to chronic disease. Other causes of anemia in SLE include iron deficiency anemia, coomb's positive autoimmune hemolytic anemia, red blood cell aplasia and microangiopathic hemolytic anemia, which may be associated with antiphospholipid antibody syndrome.
   - Leukopenia secondary to neutropenia or lymphopenia is also frequent and severe.
   - Thrombocytopenia can be mild or severe due to autoantibodies against platelets, glycoprotein IIb/IIIa, or thrombopoietin receptor. May be associated with antiphospholipid antibody syndrome also.
   - Pancytopenia can also be seen and may be associated with myelofibrosis.
   - Soft non tender lymphadenopathy is common in SLE, however rare cases of Kikuchi-Fujimoto disease have also been reported.
   - Splenomegaly is also common in SLE.
9. **Eye involvement**
   - Keratoconjunctivitis sicca is frequently seen in SLE in the presence or absence of secondary Sjogren syndrome.

- Other ocular manifestations are retinal vasculitis, optic neuritis, uveitis, scleritis, peripheral ulcerative keratitis and episcleritis.
- Drug induced ocular damage, including steroid induced glaucoma or cataract and hydroxychloroquine induced retinal maculopathy may be seen.

10. Ear involvement

- May lead to sudden sensorineural hearing loss.

11. Pregnancy complications

- SLE patients with positive antiphospholipid antibodies are at high risk of spontaneous abortions, fetal loss and pre-eclampsia. Increased incidence of spontaneous thrombosis may be seen.
- Anti-Ro (SSA) and Anti-La (SSB) antibodies can cross the placenta leading to fetal heart block and neonatal lupus. Risk is 2% with the first pregnancy but increases to 20% if there is a history of neonatal lupus in a past pregnancy.
- SLE flares may be seen in pregnancy, especially if the disease was uncontrolled in the six months preceding pregnancy.

Table 15.6: Summary of clinical findings in systemic lupus erythematosus

Skin manifestations	*Systemic manifestations*
• Photosensitivity • Malar rash • Maculopapular rash • Chilblain • Discoid rash • Bullous lesions • Toxic epidermal necrolysis like lesions • Hypertrophic (verrucous) lupus • Subacute LE like annular and polycyclic lesions • Oral ulceration • Diffuse thinning of hair	• *Musculoskeletal manifestations:* Arthritis, arthralgia, tendonitis and myositis. • *Gastrointestinal manifestations:* Hepatosplenomegaly, chronic abdominal pain, hepatitis, ascites, mesenteric thrombosis. • *Cardiac manifestations:* Pericarditis, endocarditis, valvular insufficiency, conduction defect, ischemia and cardiac failure. • *Pulmonary:* Acute pneumonitis, pleurisy, infective pneumonia, pulmonary hemorrhage, pneumothorax, impaired pulmonary diffusion. • *Neurologic manifestations:* Seizures, headache, chorea, pseudotumor cerebri, cerebral venous thrombosis, aseptic meningitis, chorea, global cognitive deficits, transverse myelitis, peripheral neuropathy, mood disorders and psychosis. • *Renal manifestations:* Hypertension, edema of the lower extremities, electrolyte abnormalities, and acute renal failure, nephritis, nephrotic syndrome. • *Eye:* Uveitis, scleritis, episcleritis, conjunctivitis, retinal hemorrhage. • *Hematological:* Uveitis, scleritis, episcleritis, conjunctivitis, retinal hemorrhage • Lymphadenopathy • Hepatosplenomegaly

Investigations

- Hematological: Hemoglobin, total leukocyte count, differential leukocyte count, platelets and reticulocyte count, ESR.
- Serum electrolytes, liver function test and kidney function test.
- Urinary status (protein/creatinine ratio, 24-hour urine protein and microscopic examination of urinary sediments).
- Infrared thermography for Raynaud's phenomenon can be done.
- Immunological: Antinuclear antibody (in children ANA may not be specific, background positivity may be triggered by infections in up to 25% cases), anti-double stranded DNA antibody, anti-Smith (Sm) antibody, lupus anticoagulant, antiphospholipid antibody, anti-Ro (Ro/SSA), anti-La (La/SSB) antibodies associated with Sjögren syndrome and anti-ribonucleoprotein (anti-RNP) antibodies, complement C3 and C4, C-Reactive Protein (CRP), Rheumatoid factor (RF), VDRL. The incidence of ANA negative SLE has been estimated to be 1–5%.

Different antibody profile in systemic lupus erythematosus given in Table 15.7.

Table 15.7: Antibody profile in systemic lupus erythematosus

Antinuclear antibody	ANA is used for screening, diagnosis, and as a prognostic biomarker of SLE It is highly sensitive with sensitivity ranging from 95% to 97% but has low specificity of 20%. Positive ANA does not confirm the diagnosis of SLE.

Contd.

Anti-dsDNA	Anti-dsDNA antibodies are highly specific (96%) for SLE. It correlates with disease activity and predicts the development of lupus nephritis. It's levels can be undetectable during treatment and increase during a flare, especially in active nephritis.
Anti-Smith Antibody	Anti-Sm antibodies are highly specific for SLE (99%). Anti-Sm antibodies correlate with SLE disease activity and have relatively static expression in serum unlike anti-dsDNA antibodies, which show fluctuations with disease activity.
Anti Ro/SSA and Anti La /SSB antibody	Anti-Ro antibodies are seen in up to 50% of cases of SLE and anti-La antibodies in up to 20%. These are associated with subacute cutaneous lupus (SCLE), photosensitivity and neonatal lupus. These antibodies are highly associated with Sjögren syndrome with 90% specificity and can be used to assess secondary Sjögren syndrome in patients with SLE.
Antiphospholipid antibodies	Antiphospholipid antibodies are found in 30-40% of patients with SLE. They are of three types- Lupus anticoagulant antibody (LAC), beta-2 glycoprotein, anticardiolipin antibody.
Anti-Ribosomal P (Anti-P)	It is present in 10-20% of SLE patients and correlates with neuropsychiatric lupus, lupus hepatitis and lupus nephritis
Anti-histone antibody	It is positive in drug induced lupus (67-100%).
Anti U1 RNP	Positive in approximately in 25% of SLE patients. Highest levels are seen in mixed connective tissue disease.

- Radiological: X-ray of chest and involved joints should be done. Other imaging studies should be guided by clinical manifestations and may include the following:
  - MRI of the brain.
  - Renal ultrasonography, DMSA (Dimercapto-succinic acid) and DTPA (Diethylenetriamine pentaacetic acid) scan for assessing renal functions.
  - High resolution CT scan to diagnose and evaluate pulmonary fibrosis.
  - Dual energy X-ray absorptiometry (DEXA) to evaluate bone density.
  - Histopathological: Skin biopsy is a useful diagnostic tool.
  - Other Tests: Pulmonary function tests, including diffusing capacity of the lung for carbon monoxide (DLCO), screening for comorbidities and assessment of vaccination status.

Diagnosis is based on clinical, laboratory and immunological findings. ARA criteria was in use for long time for diagnosis of SLE (Table 15. 8). SLICC (Table 15.9) criteria has also been validated for diagnosis of SLE. Newer ACR/ EULAR criteria may also be used (Table 15.10).

Table 15.8: American college of rheumatology 1998 revised criteria for classification of systemic lupus erythematosus

	Criteria	*Definition*
1.	Malar rash	Fixed erythema, over malar area tending to spare nasolabial fold
2.	Discoid rash	Erythematous plaques with adherent keratotic scaling and follicular plugging, atrophic scaring
3.	Photosensitivity	Skin rashes as a result of unusual reaction to sunlight
4.	Oral ulcers	Painless oral or nasopharyngeal ulceration
5.	Arthritis	Two or more peripheral joint involvement, non-erosive arthritis, associated with tenderness, swelling or effusion
6.	Serositis	Pleuritis - History of pleuritis pain, pleural rub, evidence of plural effusion Pericarditis - Documented by ECG, pericardial rub, evidence of pericardial effusion
7.	Renal manifestation	Persistent proteinuria - > 500 mg / day or > 3+ of quantitation not done
8.	Haematological manifestation	Haemolytic anaemia with Reticulocytosis Leukopenia - < 4000/mm^3 on two or more occasions Lymphopenia - < 1000/mm^3 on two or more occasions Thrombocytopenia - <100000/mm^3 in absence of offending drugs
9.	Neurological manifestation	Seizures - In the absence of offending drugs and metabolic derangement Psychosis- In the absence of offending drugs and metabolic derangement

Contd.

10.	Immunological features	Anti-dsDNA Antibody or Anti-Sm antibody or Positive finding of APLA
11.	Antinuclear antibody	Abnormal high titre by immunofluorescence or any equivalent test in absence of drugs known to associated with drug induce lupus syndrome
≥ 4 out of 11 criteria should be present, serially or simultaneously, during any interval of observation to classify as systemic lupus erythematosus		

Table 15.9: Systemic Lupus International Collaborating Clinics (SLICC) classification criteria for systemic lupus erythematosus (SLE), 2012

	Clinical criteria	
1.	Acute cutaneous lupus	Lupus malar rash (does not include malar discoid), bullous lupus, toxic epidermal necrolysis variant of SLE, maculopapular rash, photosensitive lupus rash in the absence of dermatomyositis; or sub-acute cutaneous lupus.
2.	Chronic cutaneous lupus	Classic discoid rash, hypertrophic (verrucous) lupus, lupus panniculitis (profundus), mucosal lupus, lupus erythematosus tumidus, chilblain lupus, discoid lupus/lichen planus overlap.
3.	Oral ulcers	Palate, buccal, tongue or nasal ulcers in the absence of other causes
4.	Non-scarring alopecia	Diffuse thinning or hair fragility with broken hairs in the absence of other causes
5.	Synovitis	Involving two or more joints characterized by effusion or swelling or tenderness in two or more joints and at least 30 min of morning stiffness
6.	Serositis: pleurisy or pericarditis	More that 1-day duration of pleural/pericardial effusions or pleural/pericardial rub
7.	Renal disorder	Persistent proteinuria (>0.5 g/day) or cellular casts
8.	Neurological disorder	Seizures, psychosis, mononeuritis multiplex, myelitis or acute confusional state in the absence of other causes
9.	Haemolytic anaemia	
10.	Leukopenia	< 4000/mm^3 at least once or lymphopenia <1000/mm^3
11.	Thrombocytopenia	<100 000/mm^3 at least once
Immunological criteria		
1.	ANA above reference laboratory range	
2.	Anti-dsDNA antibody above reference laboratory range (or more than two fold	
3.	Anti-Sm antibody: presence of antibody to Sm nuclear antigen	
4.	Antiphospholipid antibody positivity	
5.	Low complement (low C3, C4 or CH50)	
6.	Direct Coomb's test in the absence of haemolytic anaemia	
	Criteria required for diagnosis of SLE: 1. Four criteria, with at least one clinical criteria and one immunological criteria Or 2. Lupus nephritis + ANA OR anti-dsDNA antibody positivity	

Contd.

Table 15.10: New 2019 ACR/EULAR criteria for SLE

Antinuclear antibody (ANA) titer of 1:80 on HEp-2 cell or equivalent test positive	
If absent – does not classify as SLE If present, apply supportive criteria	
Supportive criteria Occurrence of criterion on at least one occasion is sufficient and criteria need not occur simultaneously and within each score, only highest weighted criterion is counted toward the total score	
Clinical Criteria	***Score***
Constitutional	
• Fever	2
Hematologic	
• Leukopenia	3
• Thrombocytopenia	4
• Autoimmune haemolysis	4
Mucocutaneous	
• Non-scarring alopecia	2
• Oral ulcers	2
• Subacute cutaneous or discoid lupus	4
• Acute cutaneous lupus	6
Neurological	
• Delirium	2
• Psychosis	3
• Seizures	5
Serosal	
• Pleural or pericardial effusion	5
• Acute pericarditis	6

Contd.

Musculoskeletal involvement	
• Joint involvement	6
Renal	
• Proteinuria > 500 mg/day	4
• Renal biopsy histological class II or V lupus nephritis	8
• Renal biopsy histological class III or IV lupus nephritis	10
Immunological Criteria	***Score***
Antiphospholipid antibodies	
• Anticardiolipin antibodies or anti β2GP1 antibodies or lupus	2
• Anticoagulant antibodies	
Complement proteins	
• Low C3 or Low C4 level	3
• Low C3 and Low C4 level	4
SLE specific antibodies	
• Anti-dsDNA antibody or anti-Smith antibody	6
Total score	-
To classify as systemic lupus erythematosus score should be 10 or more if entry criteria fulfilled	

Treatment of SLE

Goals of treatment

Goal of treatment is to induce remission or low disease activity. When complete remission occurs clinical activity is absent without use of systemic steroids or immunosuppressant's which is infrequent. Low disease activity is achieved by maintenance of disease with by lowest dose of systemic steroids with or without immunosuppressant (while preventing flare ups). Systemic lupus erythematosus disease activity index (SLEDAI) score ≤3 on antimalarials or SLEDAI ≤4, PGA≤1 with glucocorticoids ≤7.5 mg of prednisone and well tolerated immunosuppressant is considered low disease activity. Depending on the degree of organ involvement, flares in SLE can be treated either by increasing the dosage of ongoing treatment (glucocorticoids, immunomodulating drugs) or moving to new drugs or combining existing therapies.

Hydroxychloroquine (HCQ)

Unless contraindicated, HCQ is advised for all SLE patients at a dose of not more than 5 mg/kg/real body weight. When there are no risk factors for retinal toxicity, ophthalmological screening (using spectral domain-optical coherence tomography or visual fields testing) should be carried out at baseline, five years later and annually after that.

Glucocorticoids

Glucocorticoids are the mainstay of treatment. Juvenile SLE require higher doses of corticosteroid and other immunosuppressants. Prednisolone 1-2 mg/kg/day is used initially to control disease activity, which is gradually tapered when remission occurs. For long-term maintenance therapy, glucocorticoids should be reduced to less than 7.5 mg/day of prednisolone or of prednisone equivalent and if feasible, stopped. Methylprednisolone pulse offers an instant therapeutic benefit. The tapering or withdrawal of glucocorticoids can be accelerated by the prompt beginning of immunomodulatory drugs.

Immunosuppressive therapies: It is advisable to think about adding immunosuppressive or immunomodulating medications such as mycophenolate, azathioprine, or methotrexate. Immunosuppressants are advised when patients are unable to lower their steroid dosages below what is considered safe for long term usage or as initial therapy in cases of organ threatening illness or when they are not responding to HCQ (alone or in combination with steroids). Mycophenolate mofetil has lesser side effects, cyclophosphamide is preferred for severe manifestations, particularly CNS disease and lupus nephritis. When other immunosuppressive treatments are not working for a patient with severe organ-threatening or life threatening SLE, cyclophosphamide might be given as "rescue" therapy. Intravenous pulse therapy is preferred because of less side effects compared to oral therapy. Azathioprine is useful for maintenance in lupus nephritis, while methotrexate may be used mainly in cases associated with lupus nephritis. Chlorambucil, isotretinoin, IV immunoglobulins may be added as steroid sparing agents.

Biologics

If patients do not respond well to standard therapy (HCQ and steroids in combination with or without immunosuppressive drugs), which is characterised by persistent disease activity that prevents steroid tapering and/or frequent relapses, biologicals like belimumab, anifrolumab, sifalimumab, tabalumab, telitacicept, should be added. Rituximab may be used in cases of organ threatening disease, which does not respond to traditional immunosuppressive medications, or in patients who are intolerant or have contraindication for them.

Treatment for Specific Manifestations

Cutaneous Disease

Sunscreen, topical steroids, topical calcineurin inhibitors, antimalarial medications, and/or systemic steroids are the first line treatments for skin disease in patients with systemic lupus erythematosus. Dapsone, mycophenolate, retinoids, methotrexate, or other medications can be added in non-responsive cases which require high dose steroids.

Neuropsychiatric Disease

Glucocorticoids and immunosuppressive medications are used to treat neuropsychiatric disorder associated with SLE when the symptoms are thought to be indicative of an inflammatory condition; antiplatelets and anticoagulants are used to treat atherothrombotic and antiphospholipid antibody syndrome (APLA) related symptoms.

Haematological Disease

For the acute management of lupus thrombocytopenia, high dose oral or pulse steroids and intravenous immunoglobulin is used. Immunosuppressive/steroid sparing medications like cyclosporine, azathioprine, or mycophenolate can be used to maintain response. Treatment options for refractory instances include cyclophosphamide or rituximab.

Renal Disease

As the most effective and least toxic first line treatment, mycophenolate or low dose intravenous cyclophosphamide are advised. Analogous regimens may be explored for individuals at high risk for renal failure (lowered glomerular filtration rate, histological fibrous crescents or fibrinoid necrosis, or tubular atrophy/interstitial fibrosis), high dose intravenous cyclophosphamide may also be employed. Mycophenolate or azathioprine need to be utilised for maintenance treatment. When treating severe nephrotic syndrome or incomplete renal response, mycophenolate and a modest dose of calcineurin inhibitors may be used.

Follow-up

- Every 3 to 6 months depending on course of treatment. In case of lupus nephritis, initially every 2 to 4 weeks for first 2 to 4 months then every 3 to 6 months.
- Ocular examination of patients taking hydroxychloroquine should be done every 6 months.

Prognosis

- Survival rate is around 85% at 10 years and 77% at 15 years after onset of disease.
- With recent update in options of management, many juvenile SLE patients in later life have conceived and delivered healthy infants successfully which is perhaps a reflection of better control of disease.

DISCOID LUPUS ERYTHEMATOSUS (DLE)

DLE is uncommon in children and less than 3% of patients with DLE develop disease before the age of 10 years. Lupus can occur in all age groups, but DLE occurs more frequently in women in their fourth and fifth decades of life. Twenty-five percent of patients with SLE may develop typical discoid lesions at some point during their illness, and 1% to 5% of patients with discoid lupus may develop SLE.

The clinical features of childhood DLE are similar to those of adult DLE in presentation and chronicity. Clinically the lesions are discoid plaques, which are characterized by well-circumscribed, elevated, indurated red to purplish plaques with adherent scale and fine telangiectasia. They are exacerbated by exposure to UV light (photosensitivity). If they are not well treated, then hyper or hypopigmentation with scarring and atrophy develops (Figure 15.3).

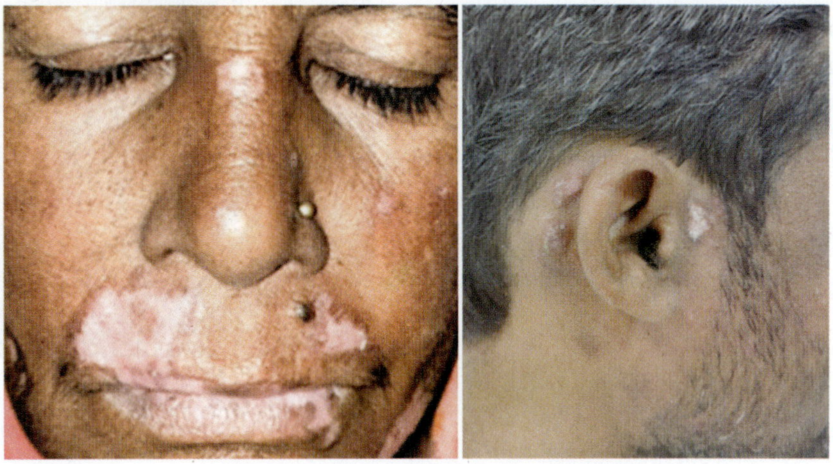

Figure 15.3: Discoid lupus erythematousus

Follicular plugging with adherent scales are characteristic of DLE. A thick scale when lifted, the under surface shows follicular projections **(tin tack sign)**. Scarring of the concha due to lesions of DLE is called as Shuster's sign and it can be present in 30% of the cases.

Cutaneous lesions are usually localized in sun exposed areas like face and scalp and is known as limited DLE whereas, in disseminated form other sites below neck are also involved like arms, legs, hands, fingers, back, chest, abdomen. 25% of cases rarely DLE follows lines of Blaschko. A very slow progression of DLE to SLE is seen in 0 to 28% of patients, in months to decades.

Clinical Variants of DLE

1. **Chilblain lupus:** It is predominantly seen in females, presents with red to dusky purplish scaly papules and plaques, which are exacerbated by cold exposure, commonly seen over toe and finger tips. It can be associated with Raynaud's phenomena, cold agglutinins and cryofibrinogenaemia. These patients are usually positive for anti Ro antibody. In chronic stage, fingers and toes may become atrophic with dystrophic nails and resorption of digits.
2. **Lupus panniculitis or Lupus erythematosus profundus:** This is an unusual clinical variant of LE, which presents as well-defined erythematous nodules with areas of atrophy. It shows lobular subcutaneous infiltration.
3. **Tumid lupus:** Tumid lupus presents with swollen, indurated, brawny, warm, tense plaques over cheeks or proximal limbs.
4. **Lupus erythematous telangiectoides:** It is a disseminated type of discoid lupus erythematosus, which presents with reticulate telangiectasia, usually over arms, legs.
5. **Lupus erythematous gyratum repens:** This is a migratory gyrate annular erythema with histology similar to discoid lupus erythematosus.
6. **Verrucous DLE:** It presents with hyperkeratotic plaque over hands and feet.

Histopathology: Following are prominent histopathological features of chronic cutaneous lupus erythematosus:

- Epidermal atrophy
- Follicular plugging
- Basal cell vacuolar degeneration
- Interface dermatitis (small lymphocytic infiltrate at dermo-epidermal junction)
- Basement membrane thickening (appreciated on Periodic acid Schaff staining)
- Perivascular and peri-adnexal lymphocytic infiltrate.
- Variable degree of mucin in dermis

Treatment

First line therapy is strict photoprotection, sunscreen, topical steroids or intralesional steroids and topical calcineurin inhibitors. If lesions are non-responsive or patients have a widespread disease, need systemic therapy. Antimalarials (hydroxychloroquine) consider fist line systemic drugs for chronic LE. Other systemic drugs include methotrexate, mycophenolate mofetil, steroids, azathioprine, thalidomide, systemic retinoids and clofazimine.

SUBACUTE CUTANEOUS LUPUS ERYTHEMATOSUS (SCLE)

SCLE is extremely rare in childhood. The mean age of onset of SCLE ranges from 50 to 52 years. Patients with SCLE present with erythematous, non-scarring papulosquamous or annular polycyclic lesion (Figure 15.4) in a photosensitive distribution with scaling, pigmentary changes, and telangiectasia (Figure 15.5) associated with mild systemic symptoms, musculoskeletal complaints being the most prominent. Anti-nuclear and anti-Ro antibodies are frequently present. Although the classic presentation is in the form of annular or papulosquamous lesions, poikilodermatous, erythrodermic, and bullous SCLE have also been reported.

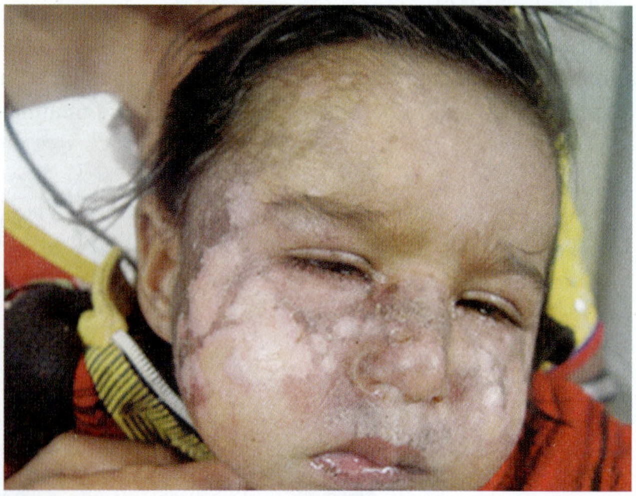

Figure 15.4: Child with SCLE showing annular scaly plaque with erythema of skin

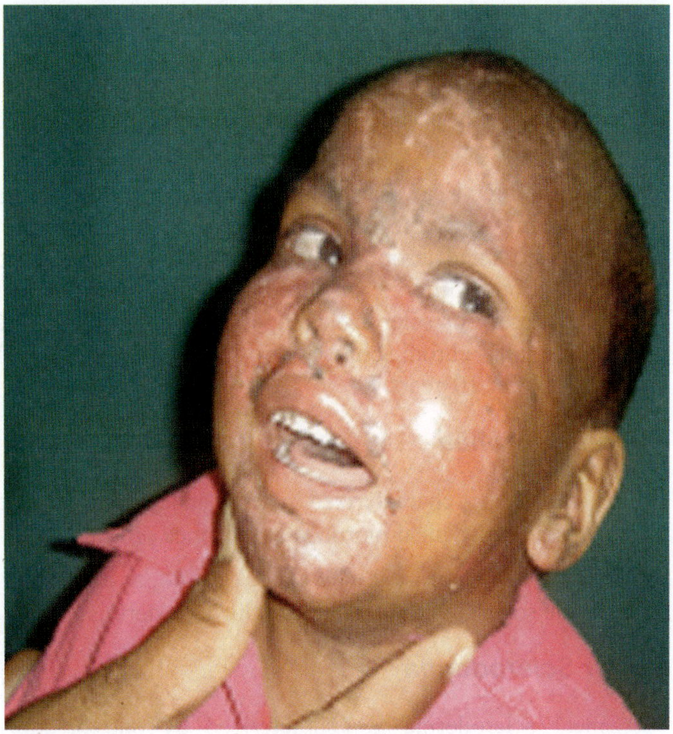

Figure 15.5: Child with SCLE showing erythema, scaling, telangiectasia and photosensitivity

SCLERODERMA

Scleroderma is a spectrum of disorders characterized by fibrosis affecting dermis, subcutaneous tissue, lungs, kidneys, gastrointestinal tract etc. If scleroderma occurs without systemic involvement, it is known as morphea, which can be localized, or generalized. If it is associated with systemic involvement, it is known as systemic sclerosis.

Pseudo-Scleroderma

A group of illnesses marked by skin induration or atrophy resembling to that seen in progressive systemic sclerosis (PSS) or localised scleroderma are together referred to as pseudo-scleroderma. Scleroderma mimics are given in Table 15.11.

Table 15.11: Pseudo-scleroderma or scleroderma mimic

Congenital

- Stiff skin syndrome
- Premature ageing syndromes
  - Acrogeria (Werner's syndrome)
  - Progeria

Inflammatory dermatosis or autoimmune dermatosis

- Eosinophilic fasciitis
- Graft vs Host disease (GVHD)
- Scleredema (Page no. 509)
- Scleromyxodema
- Amyloidosis
- Carcinoid syndrome
- Phenylketonuria
- Porphyria cutanea tarda (PCT)
- Nephrogenic systemic fibrosis (NSP)
- Lichen sclerosis et atrophicans (LSA)

Endocrinological disorders

- Thyroid disease
- Diabetic cheiroarthropathy

Chemical induced

- Toxic oil syndrome (aniline contaminated rapeseed oil)
- Eosinophilia myalgia syndrome (L-tryptophan)

Drug induces

- Bleomycin, carbidopa, pentazocine

Occupational

- Polyvinylchloride
- Silicosis
- Epoxy resins

Miscellaneous

- Paraneoplastic

MORPHEA

Epidemiology

The frequency of morphea ranges between 3 and 4 cases per million of population. Morphea has female predominance with a female to male ratio of 3:1 to 4:1. Children are more likely to develop localized forms of scleroderma than adults. Localized scleroderma can result in major facial or limb asymmetry, flexion contractures and disability. Linear scleroderma tends to affect children and adolescents more frequently. Morphea en plaque is more common in adults.

Classification

Morphea can be classified as following categories:

Localized morphea

- **Plaque morphea**
  - **Morphea en plaque**
  - **Guttate morphea**
  - **Keloid morphea**
  - **Atrophoderma of Pasini and Pierini**

- **Bullous morphea**
- **Linear scleroderma**
- **Deep morphea**

Generalized morphea

Localized Morphea

Plaque Morphea

Plaque morphea is often confined to the dermis only.

- **Morphea en plaque:** Morphea en plaque is the most prevalent form of this group. It usually involves the trunk most commonly (Figure 15.6). The disease is characterized by one or more circular areas of induration, usually larger than 1 cm in diameter, with varying degree of pigmentary changes. An erythematous or violaceous halo (lilac ring) around the lesion, which is often evident during early disease, corresponds with inflammatory state. As the disease progresses, the skin becomes sclerotic. Once inflammation subsides, the center of the lesion becomes whitish. After months to years, the skin softens and becomes atrophic, and a residual area of hypopigmentation or hyperpigmentation might occur. Distinctive borders usually separate the plaques from the normal surrounding skin.
- **Guttate morphea:** Guttate morphea is an uncommon condition usually occurring on the upper trunk. Typically, it presents as multiple oval lesions between 2 and 10 mm in diameter. The lesions often manifest as faint erythema, followed by mild induration and hypopigmentation or hyperpigmentation.
- **Keloid morphea:** Keloid morphea is a rare condition, which presents as nodules that resemble keloids in the presence of typical morphea.
- **Atrophoderma of Pasini and Pierini:** Atrophoderma of Pasini and Pierini presents as asymptomatic, hyperpigmented atrophic patches with well demarcated "cliff drop borders" on the trunk. No pronounced inflammatory or sclerotic changes are present. This rare condition has chronic course, with spontaneous resolution usually after 10 years.

Bullous Morphea

Bullous morphea is characterized by tense subepidermal bullae in the presence of typical morphea or morphea profunda.

The lesions can occur on the face, neck, trunk, or extremities and may be superficial or extend into the deep dermis.

Linear Scleroderma

- Linear scleroderma is characterized by one or more linear streaks with induration that can involve dermis, subcutaneous tissue, muscle and bone. It occurs on the extremities, face, or scalp of children and adolescents. It is subdivided into linear morphea, en coup de sabre and progressive hemifacial atrophy (Parry-Romberg syndrome).
- **Linear morphea:** Linear morphea is the most common form of morphea in children and it is characterized by

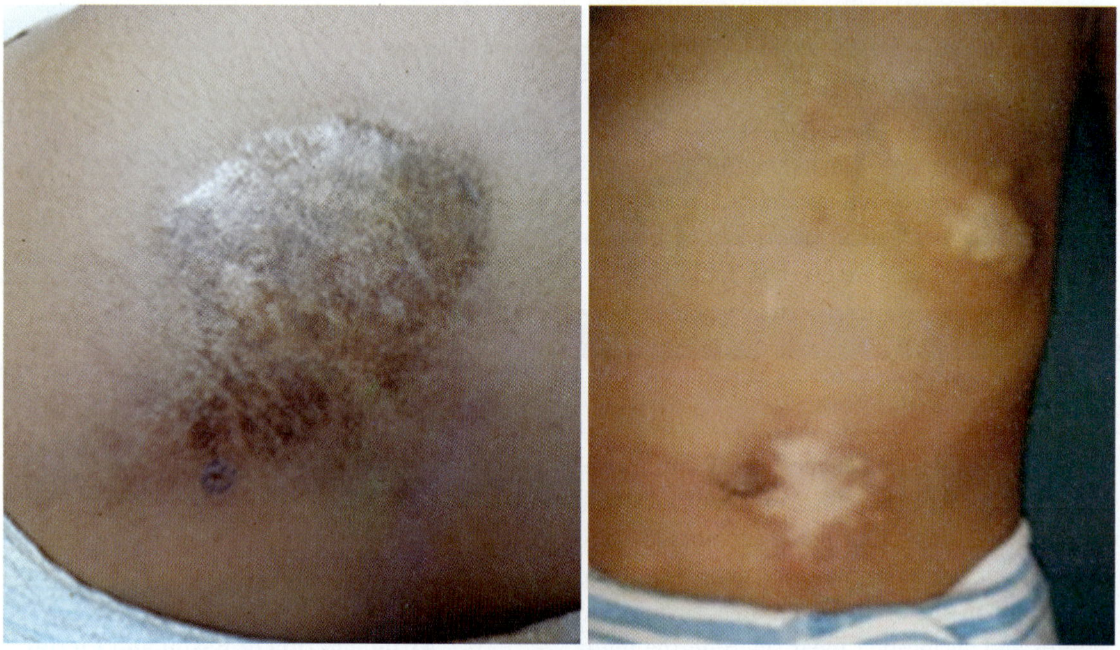

Figure 15.6: Plaque morphea

discrete linear induration that primarily affects the extremities (Figure 15.7). In more than 90% of patients, the involvement is unilateral. Linear morphea is complicated by deformities, joint contractures, and severe limb atrophy. The process can affect the growth of bony structures.

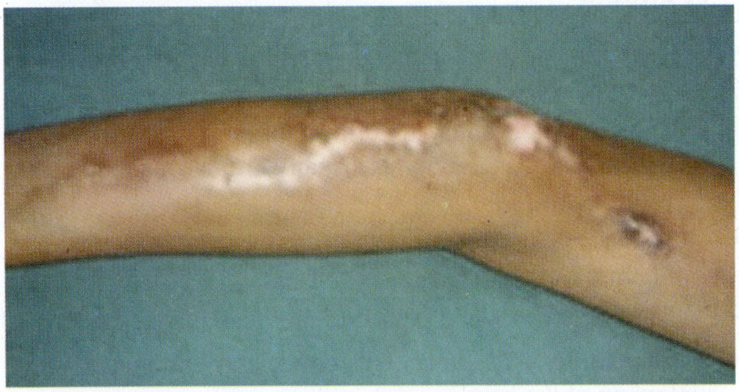

Figure 15.7: Linear morphea

- **En coup de sabre:** If the face or scalp is affected with linear scleroderma, the involvement is often compared to a stroke of sabre. Typical lesion starts with contractions and firmness of the skin over the affected area. Commonly lesion starts from nose and extends to forehead and scalp in a linear fashion (Figure 15.8). Eventually, an ivory, irregular, sclerotic plaque with hyperpigmentation at the edge develops. Seizures along with eye and teeth abnormalities need to be ruled out.

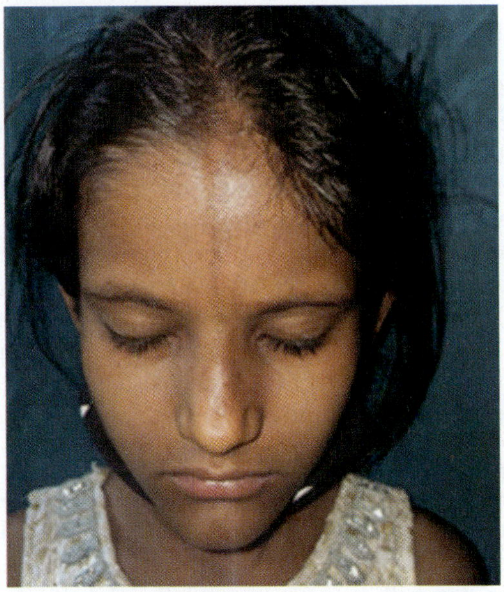

Figure 15.8: En coup de sabre

- **Progressive hemifacial atrophy (Parry-Romberg syndrome):** In progressive hemifacial atrophy, primary lesions occur in the subcutaneous tissue, muscle and bone. The disease usually begins in the first two decades of life (Figure 15.9).

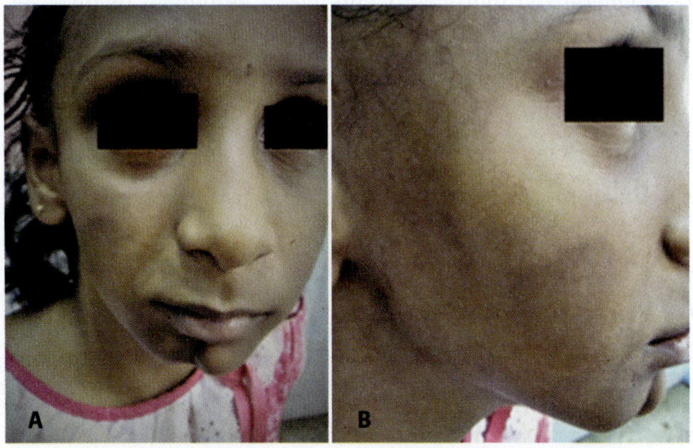

Figure 15.9A and B: Progressive hemifacial atrophy

Deep Morphea

Deep morphea is a rare condition primarily involving the deep dermis, subcutaneous tissue, fascia, or superficial muscle. The lesions are more diffuse than in linear scleroderma and do not demonstrate a linear pattern. Subtypes include subcutaneous morphea, morphea profunda, disabling pansclerotic morphea of childhood and eosinophilic fasciitis.

- **Subcutaneous morphea:** Subcutaneous morphea primarily involves the panniculus or subcutaneous tissue. The onset of sclerosis is usually rapid, occurring within a period of few months.
- **Morphea profunda:** In morphea profunda, the entire skin is thickened, bound down and taut. Patients develop sclerosis of the deeper skin. Onset usually occurs before age 14 years. The extensor aspect of the extremities and trunk develops sclerotic plaques that extend deep into the subcutaneous tissue, fascia, muscle and bone. The lilac ring is usually absent.
- **Disabling pansclerotic morphea of childhood:** Disabling pansclerotic morphea of childhood is an aggressive and mutilating variant of morphea. It is characterized by generalized, full thickness involvement of the trunk, extremities, face and scalp. The fingertips and toes are usually spared.
- **Eosinophilic fasciitis:** Eosinophilic fasciitis is characterized by a painful peaud' orange appearance involving the extremities, proximal to the hands and feet. The fascia is the predominant level of involvement. The natural course of disease is not well defined, but disease seems to spontaneously regress or remains unchanged for years.

Generalized Morphea

- Generalized morphea occurs when individual plaques of morphea become confluent lesions.
- It can affect more than two anatomical sites, including the upper trunk, breasts, abdomen and upper thighs.
- Arms, legs, face, neck and scalp may also be involved.
- Bullae may develop in localized areas, particularly around the abdomen.
- Keratoses and calcinosis may occur.
- Contractures may occur in limbs and mobility may be restricted.

Investigations

- Anti-nuclear antibodies can be detected in 46-80% of patients with morphea. The most common pattern is homogeneous, but this is non-specific.
- ESR may be increased in eosinophilic fasciitis, in some forms of linear and localized morphea.
- A polyclonal gammopathy may occur in patients with morphea or eosinophilic fasciitis.
- Skin biopsy–All subtypes of morphea shows similar findings with early active inflammatory infiltrate and as lesions evolve, collagen bundles are thickened. Skin sclerosis occur in late fibrotic phase.

Treatment

- Most patients with plaque morphea experience spontaneous remission and require no specific treatment. Treatment depends entirely on the severity of the disease.
- Intralesional injections of corticosteroids might be helpful in early stages.
- Vitamin E locally as well as orally may be given.
- In linear scleroderma and deep morphea, aggressive treatment, including systemic corticosteroids, may be necessary. Topical corticosteroids may also be useful.
- If the lesions spread (as in generalized morphea), anti-inflammatory or immunosuppressive medications may be required.
- Occasionally, other disease modifying agents, including d-penicillamine, azathioprine, sulfasalazine, methotrexate and cyclophosphamide, are necessary to control severe inflammatory process.
- Daily antimalarial agents may be beneficial, especially when lesions are highly inflammatory.
- Plasmapheresis may be useful in some patients.
- Severe localized scleroderma can be treated successfully with psoralen plus ultraviolet A (PUVA) bath photo-chemotherapy.
- Occlusive treatment with tacrolimus ointment can be useful in localized scleroderma.

Prognosis

- In general, localized and regional fibrosing disorders carry a good prognosis.
- Plaques like lesions tend to improve with time. The duration of the activity is usually 3-5 years, but some lesions persist longer.
- Residual pigmentation may persist for long time in about one third of the patients.
- Linear lesions tend to persist longer than plaque lesions.
- Contractures may limit joint movements and may lead to clawing of the hands.
- Facial hemi-atrophy persists.
- Individuals with the severe inflammatory subtypes, En coup de sabre, linear scleroderma, and Parry-Romberg disease can have severe functional limitations.

SYSTEMIC SCLEROSIS

Systemic sclerosis is a connective tissue disease of unknown etiology. Characteristic features include fibrosis of the skin, subcutaneous tissues and of internal organs as well as abnormalities of the vascular and immune system.

Etiopathogenesis

One of the earliest processes thought to occur in juvenile systemic sclerosis is vascular injury. This results in upregulation of endothelial cell adhesion molecules, which facilitates local platelet aggregation and infiltration of inflammatory cells. This endothelial injury is manifested clinically as Raynaud's phenomenon, pulmonary hypertension and renovascular hypertension. Fibrosis in systemic sclerosis is caused by increased production of collagen by fibroblast, which are liberated by infiltrating cells. Autoimmunity and genetic factors may also play some role in etiology of systemic sclerosis.

Epidemiology

The overall prevalence of SSc ranges between 38 and 341 cases per million persons, while the incidence rates vary from 8-56 new cases per million persons annually globally. Systemic sclerosis is rare. Female to male ratio is 15:1 in adults. A child must be younger than 18 years at the time of disease onset to meet the criteria for juvenile systemic sclerosis. The youngest patient documented with juvenile systemic sclerosis was only a few months old at disease onset.

Systemic sclerosis classified into two types (Table 15.12):

1. Limited systemic sclerosis
2. Diffuse systemic sclerosis

Difference between two are described in Table 15.12.

Table 15.12: Difference between limited and diffuse systemic sclerosis

Diffuse systemic sclerosis	*Limited systemic sclerosis*
Onset and progression of skin changes are rapid	Onset and progression of skin changes are slow
Sclerosis of skin extend to proximal limb (above elbow and knee), trunk and face	Sclerosis is limited to extremities and face
Short or concomitant Raynaud's phenomena with skin changes	Long history of Raynaud's phenomena before onset of skin changes
Modified Rodnan Skin Score (MRSS) > 14	Modified Rodnan Skin Score (MRSS) <14
Skin disease may plateau and improve in 2 to 3 years	No plateau stage
Lung fibrosis more common	Less common
Gastrointestinal disease is universal	Less common
Low risk of cardiac and scleroderma renal crisis	High risk
Digital ulceration and calcinosis are common	Uncommon findings
High risk of organ related complications	Less common
Anti RNA polymerase III positivity in 25 % of patients, anti-topoisomerase positive in 30% of cases.	Anticentromere antibodies present in 50% of patients
Poor prognosis due to multisystem involvement	Better prognosis

Clinical Features

- Raynaud phenomenon is the most common finding at the time of diagnosis and is present in approximately 75% of patients. Cold exposure or stress may induce vasoconstriction of fingers with the episodic pallor and cyanosis, followed by erythema. Other skin changes such as induration and sclerodactyly are the next most common symptoms.
- Swelling and puffiness of the hands and fingers, polyarthralgia, or polyarthritis of the hands, fingers, feet and toes are also early symptoms. Systemic sclerosis is characterized by visceral involvement in addition to skin changes. This involvement may manifest as dysphagia, gastroesophageal reflux, dyspnea, palpitations, arthritis, muscle weakness and neuropathies. Children have less incidence of interstitial lung disease (ILD), pulmonary artery hypertension (PAH) and gastric reflux when compared to adults. Mortality is lower as compared to adults.

Cutaneous Manifestations

- Diffuse puffiness of the hands and feet, which may be followed by development of tautness of the skin.
- Barnett's sign (scleroderma neck sign): It is ridging and tightening of the skin of the neck on extending the head with a visible and palpable tight band over platysma in the hyperextended neck.
- Prayer sign is the inability to extend the fingers which can occur either due to intrinsic pathology of hands or tendons of forearms. In scleroderma, fibrosis of skin leads to limitation of movements.
- Hyperpigmentation or hypopigmentation: Commonly misdiagnosed as vitiligo (Figure 15.10A). Several other

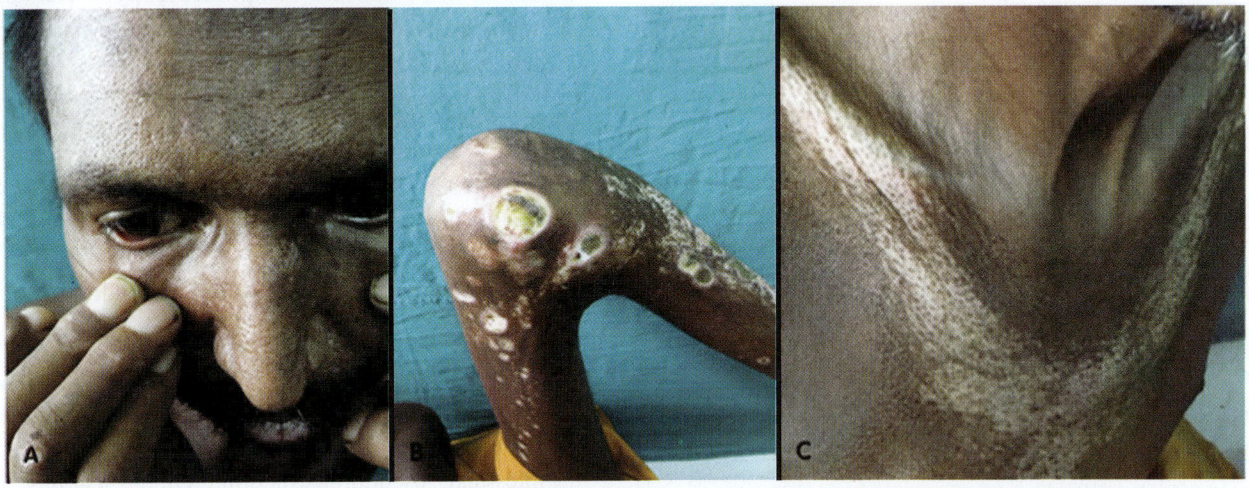

Figure 15.10: (A) Inability to retract lower eyelids, (B) Calcinosis cutis with cutaneous ulceration and (C) Dyspigmentation in systemic sclerosis

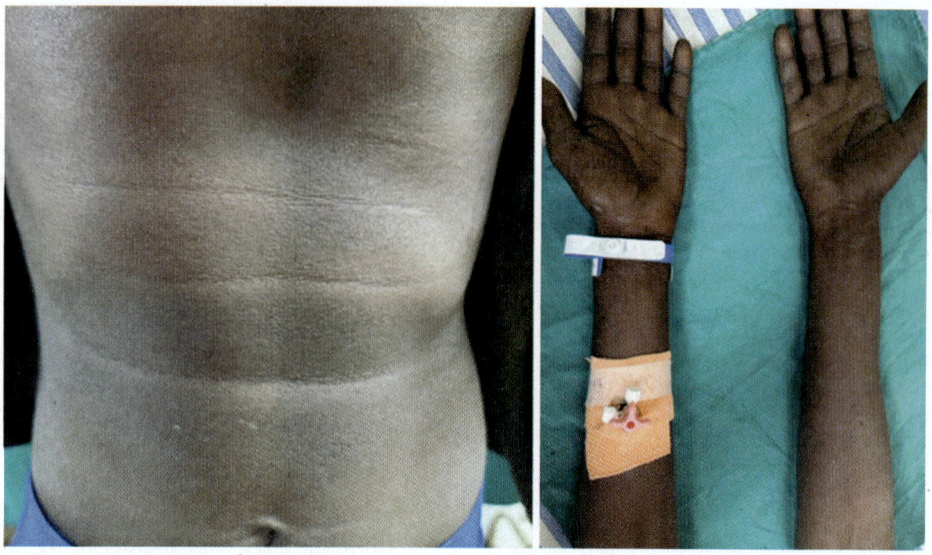

Figure 15.11: Diffuse hyperpigmentation in systemic sclerosis

patterns of pigmentation include diffuse generalized hyperpigmentation (Figure 15.11) or Addisonian like pigmentation, reticulate hyperpigmentation, and streak like hyperpigmentation along vein.

- Telangiectasias.
- Calcinosis cutis (Figure 15.10B).
- **Face:** There is pursed lips, flattened and lost facial folds and features, difficulty in opening the mouth and chewing. Inability to retract lower eyelids is known as Ingram sign (Figure 15.10C). Stafne's sign is widening of the periodontal ligament space secondary to increase in the collagen synthesis and increase in the bulk of the ligament.

The extent of skin sclerosis can be measured by Modified Rodnan skin score (MRSS) (Table 15.13). Other methods for assessing skin thickening include durometry, 20 MHz ultrasound and optic coherence tomography.

Table 15.13: Modified Rodnan Skin Score (MRSS) to measure skin sclerosis

Site	*Score*	
Face	0-3	
Anterior chest	0-3	
Abdomen	0-3	
	Right	*Left*
Upper arm	0-3	0-3
Forearm	0-3	0-3
Hand	0-3	0-3
Fingers	0-3	0-3
Thigh	0-3	0-3
Leg	0-3	0-3
Feet	0-3	0-3

Contd.

Maximum score: 51
Thickening and tethering grading
0 – normal
1 – possible thickening
2 – unable to pinch skin
3 – unable to move the skin (skin fixed to deeper tissue)
Note: This scoring system omits back and neck area

Peripheral Vascular Manifestations

- **Raynaud's phenomenon:** Pallor, cyanosis, suffusion and tingling of the fingers, which occurs abruptly and episodically usually after exposure to cold. Mizutani's sign (round finger pad sign) is disappearance of peaked contour on finger pads, especially on ring finger.
- **Abnormal nailfold capillaroscopy:** Hemorrhages, abnormal or dilated loops, mega-capillaries, arborization and avascular areas may be seen.

Gastrointestinal Manifestations

- **Esophageal dysmotility:** Detected by newer diagnostic techniques in 90% of patients (Symptomatic dysphagia is seen in only 24% of patients).
- **Esophageal reflux:** Seen in 30% of children.
- Patient may develop significant weight loss and diarrhea, possibly due to malabsorption.
- Involvement of small bowel results in bacterial over growth, atonic dilation of small bowel, which results in intestinal pseudo-obstruction. Other features include gastric antral vascular ectasia, mucosal atrophy, constipation, diverticulitis etc.

Pulmonary Manifestations

- Interstitial pulmonary fibrosis, inflammatory alveolitis and pulmonary hypertension either alone or in combination.

Cardiac Manifestations

- **Heart failure:** Most common cause of death in juvenile systemic sclerosis, although often complicated by concomitant pulmonary hypertension.
- Arrhythmias, pericarditis, myocardial fibrosis and contraction band necrosis of coronary vessels may be seen.

Musculoskeletal Manifestations

- Sclerodactyly (i.e., tightening of the skin over the fingers), often with a tapered appearance of the fingertips and flexion contractures.
- **Digital tuft resorption:** Observed on radiographs, known as acro-osteolysis.
- **Chronic myopathy:** Mild weakness and minimal muscle enzyme elevations.
- **Myositis:** Not uncommon in systemic sclerosis, must be distinguished from other connective tissue diseases.
- Long bone growth arrest and fibrotic bands that involve the joint capsule in long-standing cases.
- Contractures of the fingers and toes.
- **Subcutaneous calcinosis:** Seen in 19% of patients diagnosed with juvenile systemic sclerosis, usually involving extensor surfaces of both upper and lower extremities.
- **Arthritis and arthralgia:** Inflammatory arthritis with true synovitis may occur, often resembling the pattern observed in rheumatoid arthritis, affecting joints such as the metacarpophalangeal, proximal interphalangeal, wrist, and ankle joints. Although erosions are uncommon, they may occur, particularly in association with periarticular calcinosis.

Renal Manifestations

- Kidney involvement may be subtle which may manifest as slow rise in creatinine levels.
- Scleroderma renal crisis occurs in approximately 10% of systemic sclerosis patients, predominantly in those with diffuse cutaneous systemic sclerosis, and typically manifests within three years of diagnosis. Risk factors for the development of scleroderma renal crisis include African-American race, pericardial effusion, tendon friction rubs, new-onset anemia, diffuse cutaneous systemic sclerosis, anti-RNA polymerase III antibody, and high-dose (or chronic low-dose) corticosteroids. Indicators of poor outcomes in scleroderma renal crisis encompass male gender, advanced age at onset, and serum creatinine levels exceeding 3 mg/dL.
- Scleroderma renal crisis (SRC) is an important renal complication. Features of SRC include microangiopathic hemolytic anemia, azotemia, microscopic hematuria, elevated plasma renin levels and hypertension. Fall in 24-hour creatinine clearance of 20 ml/min from the previous value or a creatinine clearance of <60 ml/min and new persistent proteinuria of >500 mg/day indicate impending renal crisis.
- Renal changes have been reported in only 13% of cases of juvenile systemic sclerosis, but patients who develop proteinuria or hypertension are at increased risk of death.
- The renal lesion is a slowly progressive vasculitis characterized by intimal proliferation, medial thinning and adventitial fibrosis. Decreased blood flow and glomerular function also occur.

Neurological Manifestations

- Although seizures are rare in systemic sclerosis, 3% of patients may develop seizures at some time during their disease.
- Peripheral neuropathy, such as carpal tunnel syndrome, is a rare manifestation and is caused by fibrotic impingement of a nerve.
- Trigeminal neuropathy can also be seen in patients with facial skin involvement.

Classification criteria for diagnosis of systemic sclerosis is given in Table 15.14.

Table 15.14: ACR/EULAR Classification criteria for systemic sclerosis

Item	*Sub item*	*Score*
Skin thickening of the finger of both hands Extending proximal to MCP joints		9
Skin thickening of fingers (only count highest score)	Puffy fingers Whole finger, distil to MCP	2 4
Fingers tip lesions (only count the highest score)	Digital tip ulcer Pitting scars	2 3
Telangiectasia		2

Contd.

Abnormal nailfold capillaries		2
Pulmonary artery hypertension or interstitial lung disease		2
Raynaud phenomena		3
Scleroderma-related antibodies (any of anticentromere, anti-topoisomerase 1 or anti-RNA polymerase III)		3
Patients having a total score of 9 or more are classified as having definite systemic Sclerosis		

Investigations

- Systemic sclerosis may be associated with anemia, thrombocytosis and sometimes with eosinophilia.
- Hematuria, proteinuria and cellular casts are ominous signs in patients with systemic sclerosis and may represent impending renal insufficiency.
- MRI of proximal muscles may show edema. Electromyography abnormalities and creatine phosphokinase elevation are seen in patients with myositis.
- Muscle biopsy may show perifascicular or interfascicular inflammation. Necrosis and phagocytosis of muscle fiber is visible as micro infarcts. Intramuscular vessels show endothelial hyperplasia and thus results into obliteration.
- Baseline evaluation of cardiac status by ECG should be done.
- Rheumatoid factor (RF) is present in 17% of patients with juvenile systemic sclerosis, slightly less than in those with adult-onset disease (25%).
- Immunologic tests are often helpful in diagnosis of juvenile systemic sclerosis. Patients often have a positive ANA finding as nucleolar staining. Following autoantibodies may be found:
  - ***Anti-SCL 70 antibodies:*** Specific for topoisomerase I is found in 28-34% of cases.
  - ***Anti-centromere antibodies:*** Only found in 7-8% of juvenile systemic sclerosis cases compared with 21-23% of adult systemic sclerosis cases.
  - Anti-fibrillin, anti-PM-Scl, anti-RNA polymerase I or II, anti-U1RNP, anti-ku, anti-Sm, anticardiolipin antibodies may be found.

Autoantibody profile and associated clinical features in systemic sclerosis are described in Table 15.15.

Table 15.15: Autoantibodies in systemic sclerosis

Antibody	***Disease association***
Anti-Scl-70 or anti-topoisomerase1	Diffuse cutaneous disease Interstitial lung disease and lung fibrosis Association with high mortality
Anticentromere antibody	Limited systemic sclerosis Telangiectasia Pulmonary artery hypertension
Anti-ribonucleoprotein polymerase	Rapidly progressive diffuse systemic sclerosis Hypertensive renal crisis Associated with malignancy Risk of isolated pulmonary artery hypertension
Anti-fibrillarin (Anti U3 RNP)	Diffuse systemic sclerosis Cardiac involvement Poor prognosis
PM-Scl U1 -RNP Anti-Ku	Associated with overlap syndrome

Imaging Studies

- Although once commonly performed in patients with systemic sclerosis, barium swallow with small bowel follow through has been replaced by esophageal manometer and endoscopy. Scintigraphy procedures are new non-invasive and quantitative procedure.
- High resolution CT (HRCT) scan of the lungs has been helpful in diagnosis and in assessing the progress of diffuse interstitial pneumonitis and pulmonary fibrosis.
- Although HRCT remains the imaging study of choice when monitoring patients with juvenile systemic sclerosis for early evidence of interstitial pneumonitis and pulmonary fibrosis, the diffusing capacity of the lung for carbon monoxide (DLCO) test is the most sensitive for detecting early evidence of pulmonary fibrosis.
- Right heart catheterization may be needed in case of PAH.

Histopathology

- It is useful in early inflammatory disease, which shows mild inflammatory infiltrate of lymphocyte, plasma cells, and histiocytes around dermal vessels, eccrine ducts with thickening of collagen bundle within papillary and reticular dermis. In later stages, there is thickening and hyalinization of blood vessels along with narrowing of lumen. There may be thinning of epidermis with disappearance of rete ridges. Atrophic sebaceous and sweat glands due to surrounding fibrosis may be seen.

Treatment

- **Systemic steroids:** Mainly prednisone, 1-2 mg/kg/day, which is gradually tapered.
- **Collagen modulators:** D-penicillamine, relaxins and interferons.
- **Vasoactive agents:** Captopril, nifedipine and pentoxifylline.
- **Immunosuppressants:** Azathioprine, cyclophosphamide, cyclosporine and methotrexate.
- ACE inhibitors and angiotensin receptor blockers (ARBs) for long-term management of hypertension, renal insufficiency and renal crisis.
- For treatment of gastrointestinal manifestations proton pump inhibitors can be given.
- For treatment of pulmonary artery hypertension bosentan, sitaxentan and sildenafil are useful.
- The arthritis in systemic sclerosis may respond to NSAIDs.

Complications

- Complications include subcutaneous calcinosis, esophageal dysfunction to the point of malnutrition and wasting.
- Hypertension is an indicator of advanced renal disease, and hypertensive crises occasionally occur.

Prognosis

- Although it is a severely debilitating disease with significant morbidity and mortality, the prognosis of children with systemic sclerosis appears to be better than in adult patients with systemic sclerosis.
- Over the past 30 years, the prognosis of systemic sclerosis has improved, with 5-year survival rates reaching up to 80%. However, patients with advanced PAH have a less than 50% 2-year survival rate. Additionally, patients with systemic sclerosis-related PAH have a poorer prognosis compared to those with idiopathic PAH.
- The survival of juvenile systemic sclerosis at 5 years, 10 years, 15 years and 20 years after diagnosis is 89%, 80-87.4%, 74-87.4% and 69-82.5%, respectively. These survival rates are significantly higher than those reported in patients with adult onset systemic sclerosis.
- The most common causes of death are secondary to complications of cardiac, renal or pulmonary involvement.

Systemic sclerosis management guideline Table 15.16.

Table 15.16: Management of systemic sclerosis

Symptoms	*Investigations*	*First line therapy*	*Second line therapy*
Systemic sclerosis-Raynaud's phenomenon	Raynaud's provocative test Nail fold capillaroscopy	• Dihydropyridine type calcium channel antagonists (Nifedipine) • PDE-5 inhibitors (Sildenafil and Tadalafil) • Selective serotonin reuptake inhibitor (SSRI-Fluoxetine)	• Endothelin receptor antagonist (Bosentan) • Intravenous iloprost • Antiplatelets agents
Skin	MRSS Durometer	• Azathioprine • Methotrexate	• PUVA therapy
Pulmonary artery hypertension	Pulmonary function test Right heart catheterization	• Endothelin receptor antagonist (Bosentan) • PDE-5 inhibitors (Sildenafil and Tadalafil)	• Intravenous Epoprostenol • Intravenous iloprost
Interstitial lung disease	Pulmonary function test Bronchoalveolar lavage High resolution computed tomography Six minute walk test	• Cyclophosphamide	• Mycophenolate mofetil • Azathioprine
Hypertensive renal disease	Blood pressure monitoring Urine routine and microscopy Renal function test Glomerular filtration rate (GFR)	ACE inhibitors (Enalapril, captopril) Angiotensin receptor blockers (ARB) (Telmisartan, losartan) Avoid high dose steroid	Calcium channel blockers (Nifedipine) Prostacyclin

Contd.

Gastrointestinal	Barium swallow Esophageal scintigraphy Upper GI endoscopy Hydrogen breath test Colonoscopy (for lower GI)	Proton pump inhibitor H2 blockers Prokinetics	-
Cardiac	Electrocardiography (ECG) Echocardiography (2D-ECHO) Cardiac MRI	Diastolic dysfunction – diuretics and if systolic dysfunction – ACE inhibitors Cyclophosphamide Mycophenolate mofetil	-

RAYNAUD'S PHENOMENON

Raynaud's phenomenon is characterized by transient reversible attacks of color changes due to vascular ischemia, triggered by cold exposure. It is classified into two types (Table 15.17):

1. Primary Raynaud's phenomenon (Raynaud's disease)
2. Secondary Raynaud's phenomenon (Raynaud's syndrome)

Table 15.17: Showing differences between primary and secondary Raynaud's phenomenon

Primary Raynaud's phenomenon	***Secondary Raynaud's phenomenon***
It is an exaggerated physiological response to cold exposure and stress.	Exaggerated pathological response to cold exposure and stress
More common and symmetrical changes	Less common and asymmetric changes
Usually occurs in second or third decade	More common in fourth and above decade
Symptoms are mild (ulceration, pitted scars and gangrene is not seen)	Symptoms are severe (may be associated with digital ulceration, pitted scars, gangrene formation in critical ischemic condition)
Normal capillaries on nail fold capillaroscopy (NFC)	Abnormal nail fold capillaries
Idiopathic	Associated with other diseases like autoimmune collagen vascular disease, drugs (ergot derivates, bromocriptine, cocaine, amphetamine, estrogen, ephedrine), hypothyroidism, pheochromocytoma
Increased frequency of migraine and prinzmetal angina	Not increased
Family history usually present	No family history
Negative autoimmune profile	Usually, positive autoimmune profile as it is frequently associated with connective tissue disease
Requires symptomatic treatment	Requires aggressive treatment

Management of Raynaud's Phenomenon

General measures and life style changes: Lifestyle measures such as avoiding aggravating factors (cold exposure), wearing gloves, keeping trunk warm, cessation of smoking and avoidance of vibration exposure is key to management. Occupational therapy may be provided.

Medical management: Calcium channel blockers are first line of treatment for Raynaud's phenomenon. In this class, sustained release dihydropyridine class calcium channel blockers like nifedipine, amlodipine, felodipine are preferred as monotherapy. They should be started at low dose and adjusted to maximum effective dose with minimum side effects. If inadequate response or unacceptable side effects develop with calcium channel blockers, phosphodiesterase inhibitor (tadalafil, sildenafil) or angiotensin receptor blockers (telmisartan, losartan) may be added. Other first line treatments include, selective serotonin receptor inhibitors (fluoxetine, sertraline, paroxetine, and escitalopram etc.), topical nitroglycerine ointment, pentoxyphylline, alpha receptor antagonist (prazosin) etc. For recurrent or severe ischemia, prostaglandin analogue (Epoprostenol, Iloprost), endothelin -1 receptor inhibitors (bosentan), botulinum toxin and aspirin are indicated. When gangrene occurs, amputation of affected digit with selective sympathectomy can be done.

ACQUIRED INFLAMMATORY MYOPATHIES

Acquired inflammatory myositis are classified into different subtypes:

1. **Polymyositis**
2. **Dermatomyositis**
3. **Inclusion body myositis**
4. **Granulomatous myositis**
5. **Infective myositis**

DERMATOMYOSITIS

Dermatomyositis (DM) is a systemic, autoimmune inflammatory muscle disorder and vasculopathy that commonly affects persons between the ages of 40 and 50. DM primarily affects the skin and the skeletal muscles. Juvenile DM manifests similar to adult onset dermatomyositis but, less likely to develop pulmonary disease, cardiac disease and malignancy. However, more likely to develop calcinosis, vasculitis (cutaneous and systemic) and metabolic abnormalities. Bohan and peter criteria is used to diagnose DM (Table 15.18).

Table 15.18: Diagnosis of JDM has been based on five criteria (Bohan and Peter classification)
These include:
1. Characteristic skin rash
2. Proximal muscle weakness
3. Elevated muscle enzymes
4. Myopathic changes on electromyography
5. Abnormal muscle biopsy findings
Definitive diagnosis: Typical skin findings in combination with 3 other criteria are necessary to make the diagnosis
Probable diagnosis: Patients with the characteristic rash who fulfill only two criteria
Possible diagnosis: Patients with characteristic rash and one any other finding

- The new proposed criteria have been expanded to include typical MRI and ultrasonography findings, nail fold capillaroscopy, presence of calcinosis and dysphonia.
- Amyopathic dermatomyositis refers to characteristic skin changes without muscle weakness or elevated muscle enzymes for longer than 6 months. One quarter of patients may progress to clinically significant myositis.
- Unlike adults, juvenile polymyositis is less common than JDM, and inclusion body myositis is rare in children. Cancer associated myositis and interstitial lung disease is uncommon in children.

Epidemiology

Dermatomyositis commonly affects persons between the ages of 40 and 50 years. The condition is more common in women than in men, with incidence rates being 3.98 and 4.68 per 1,000,000, respectively. The median age of onset of JDM is 6.8 years in girls and 7.3 years in boys.

Clinical Features

- Constitutional, respiratory and gastrointestinal symptoms may occur within 3 months of onset of dermatomyositis.
- Eruption of skin is associated with pruritus in 38% of individuals. Occasionally the dermatosis of DM occurs in isolation, when it is known as amyopathic DM (DM sine myositis).
- Photosensitive rashes may occur.
- Muscle involvement can be insidious with demonstration of functional limitations such as difficulty in getting out of bed or tiring easily by sports activities.
- Other common symptoms include fever, dysphagia, dysphonia or hoarseness, myalgia, arthralgia, abdominal pain and malena from gastrointestinal involvement as a consequence of vasculopathy.

Cutaneous Features (Table 15.19)

- The eyelids and face may be swollen with a heliotrope rash, which is seen as purple or dusky mauve color in the periorbital region with overlying scales (Figure 15.12A). Periorbital edema is sometimes present. **Confluent**

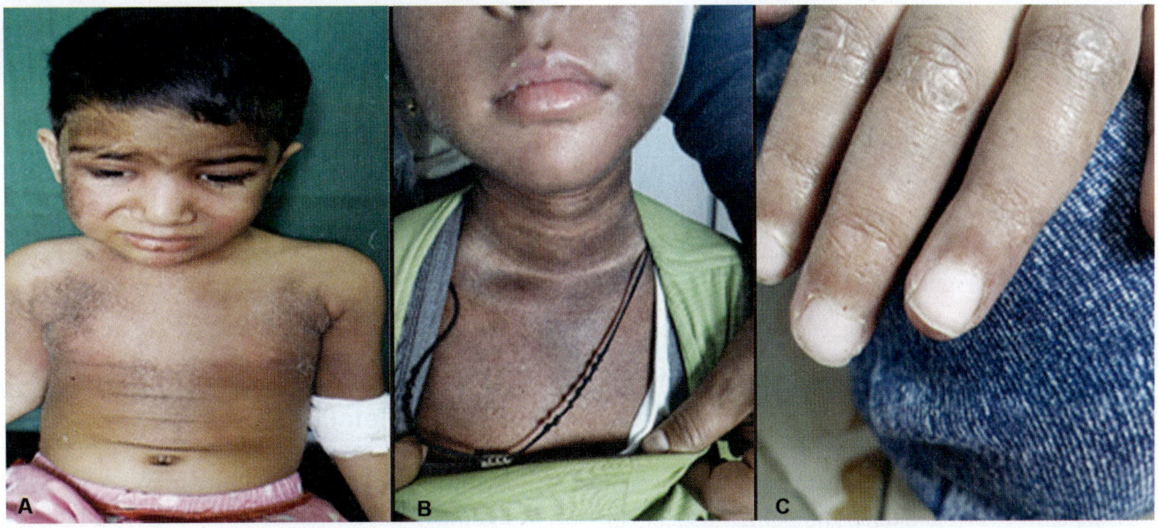

Figure 15.12: (A) Confluent rashes over face and trunk with periorbital erythema, (B) Confluent fixed macular erythema over chest and neck or V sign, (C) Periungual telangiectasia with ragged cuticle or Samitz sign

Table 15.19: Cutaneous manifestations of dermatomyositis		
1.	Pathognomic	Gottron's sign, Gottron's papules
2.	Characteristic	Heliotrope rash, mechanic's hand, periungual telengiectasia, V-sign, Shawl sign
3.	Compatible	Calcinosis cutis, poikiloderma
4.	Less common	Erythroderma, facial edema, cutaneous vasculitis, panniculitis, lipodystrophy
5.	Rare	Acanthosis nigricans, hypertrichosis, PRP like rash, urticaria, urticarial vasculitis, flagellate erythema, malignant atrophic papulosis, popular mucinosis, follicular hyperkeratosis

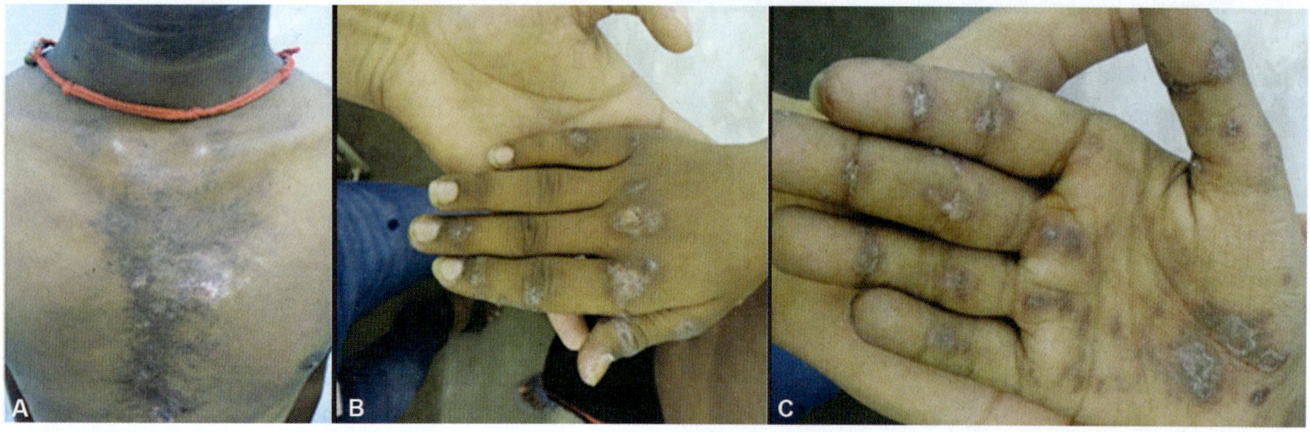

Figure 15.13: (A) A case of dermatomyositis showing Poikiloderma like rash with (B) Gottron sign and (C) Inverse Gottron sign

macular violaceous erythema on the anterior neck and chest in patients of dermatomyositis is called "V" sign (Figure 15.12B).

- Fixed macular erythema across the shoulders ('shawl sign') (Figure 15.14) and over lateral thighs and hips (holster sign) may be seen.
- Malar rash in photosensitive distribution with sparing of the nasolabial folds may occur, making it difficult to distinguish from systemic lupus erythematosus.
- Gottron's papules are shiny, elevated, violaceous papules and plaques present over the bony prominences such as metacarpophalangeal joints, proximal interphalangeal joints, distal interphalangeal joints, elbows, knees and ankles.
- **Gottron's sign:** Scaly erythematous eruption seen on the dorsa of hands, metacarpophalangeal joints, and proximal interphalangeal joints (Figure 15.13B).
- **Inverse Gottron's sign:** Scaly papules over palmer aspect of hands (Figure 15.13C).
- Hypertrophic, ragged cuticles (Samitz's sign) may accompany periungual erythema (Figure 15.12C).
- Mechanic's hands may occur, with hyperkeratosis and peeling of the skin over the lateral and palmar aspects of the fingers.

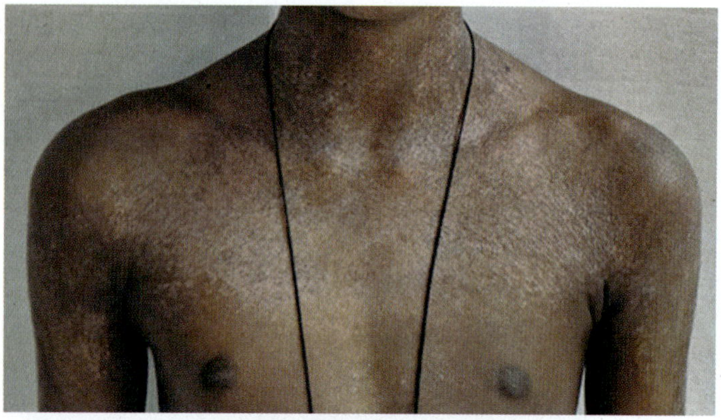

Figure 15.14: Fixed macular erythema across the shoulders (shawl sign)

- Hypertrichosis and lipoatrophy not seen in adults may also be seen in children.
- Poikilodermatous skin lesion (Figure 15.13A).
- Less common findings related to complement deposition and associated with a more severe disease course include cutaneous and mucosal ulcerations.

Musculoskeletal Features

- Symmetrical proximal muscle weakness involving the deltoid muscles, quadriceps muscles, or both is a prominent clinical finding in DM. The patients may demonstrate

Gower's sign. This sign is seen in severe myopathies, occurs when the patient attempts to stand up from the floor, patient first sits up, then assumes a quadriplegic position, and climbs up his own legs by using arms to pushup.

- Although calcinosis is rare in adults with dermatomyositis, it occurs in 20-40% of individuals with JDM. The deposits are firm, white or flesh colored nodules over bony prominences. The most commonly affected sites include the elbows, knees, and extremities, and onset is within 3 years of diagnosis but may occur as long as 20 years after diagnosis.

Other Features

- Diffuse vasculopathy may be associated with vasomotor instability, such as Raynaud's phenomenon, livedo-reticularis, or vascular infarctions on the medial canthus of the eyelids.
- Rarely, pneumatosis intestinalis or colonic perforation may occur.

Juvenile dermatomyositis differs from adult diseases in presentation with higher calcinosis cutis, vasculitis, insulin resistance, lipoatrophy and a lower association with malignancy.

Investigations (Table 15.20)

- Erythrocyte sedimentation rate (ESR) is commonly elevated.
- Levels of muscle enzymes such as aspartate amino-transferase, lactate dehydrogenase, creatine kinase, and aldolase may be elevated early in the disease course. Creatine kinase levels may initially be within the reference range in approximately 10-40% of patients and may return to normal within a few months of disease onset.
- Elevated antinuclear antibody level may be seen in approximately half of patients with DM. Generally, the extractable nuclear antigens (SS-A, SS-B, Sm, RNP) are negative.
- Electromyography (EMG) reveals a reduction of the motor unit action potentials in the proximal muscles and fibrillation potentials suggestive of fiber splitting, necrosis and vacuolization. However, the EMG findings may be normal in approximately 19% of children.
- Muscle biopsy is the most accurate test to confirm the diagnosis of dermatomyositis and to exclude other causes of muscle weakness or skin rash. Muscle biopsy should be obtained on weak muscles as identified by physical examination or contralateral to the abnormal muscles, as identified by electromyography.
- Unlike adult myositis, a muscle biopsy is not usually performed to confirm the diagnosis of JDM; however, it is needed in the workup of juvenile polymyositis.
- Skin biopsy may be helpful and histopathological findings are similar to that seen in subacute LE.

Table 15.20: Summary of laboratory findings in juvenile dermatomyositis

Investigation	*Finding*
Hemogram and ESR	ESR may be raised
Liver function tests	SGOT may be raised
Renal function tests	No specific finding
Urine and stool examination	No specific finding
24 hours urine protein and creatine excretion	24 hours urinary creatine raised (Best index of disease activity)
ECG	May show conduction abnormalities
Chest X-ray, pulmonary function test and HRCT scan of chest	May show features of interstitial lung disease
Barium swallow ± Esophageal manometry	May show abnormal esophageal motility
Muscle enzymes	Raised aspartate aminotransferase, lactate dehydrogenase, creatine kinase and aldolase
Antinuclear antibody	Positive in 50% of patients.

Dermatomyositis specific antibodies and myositis associated antibodies (Table 15.21):

Myositis specific antibodies are usually not associated with other connective tissue diseases. They are helpful in identifying specific phenotype and prognosis.

Table 15.21: Dermatomyositis specific antibodies and myositis associated antibodies	
Dermatomyositis specific antibodies and their related features	
TIF-1 gamma/ $p^{155/140}$ (Transcriptional Intermediary Factor -1 gamma)	In juvenile DM - Severe cutaneous disease, lipodystrophy In adult DM - Malignancy
NXP-2 (Anti-nuclear matrix protein 2)/P140	In juvenile DM- Calcinosis In adults - Malignancy
MDA 5/CADM -140 (Melanoma differentiation associated gene 5)	Rapidly progressive interstitial lung disease, Clinically amyopathic dermatomyositis High mortality rate Arthritis
Anti Mi-2 antibody	Classical cutaneous dermatomyositis Excellent prognosis
Anti t- RNA synthetase antibody (anti-Jo1 most common type)	Anti-synthetase syndrome which is characterised by fever, myositis, interstitial lung disease, arthritis, mechanical hands, Raynaud's phenomenon
Anti SRP (Signal Recognition Particle) & Anti-3-Hydroxy 3- Methyl Glutaryl Coenzyme A Reductase (HMGCR)	Severe necrotizing autoimmune myopathies Poor prognosis
Myositis associated antibodies and their associated features	
Pm/Scl	Overlap syndrome
U1 RNP	Overlap syndrome
Anti Ro	Overlap syndrome

Treatment

- Avoidance of sun exposure, judicious use of sunscreens that protect against ultraviolet A and B rays, and the use of topical corticosteroids are approaches used to treat skin manifestations of DM.
- Hydroxychloroquine at a dose no greater than 5-7 mg/kg/day may be beneficial.
- Topical tacrolimus (0.1%) has been used to treat cutaneous disease.
- Medical therapy for calcinosis in DM has been controversial due to inconsistent responses. Diltiazem at doses of 240-480 mg (3-6 mg/kg/day) have been used with varying success rates. Other agents used with little success include bisphosphonates, aluminium hydroxide, probenecid, and local corticosteroid injections. Calcinosis cutis may regress overtime.
- For active muscle disease, oral corticosteroids are the mainstay of treatment. High doses (Prednisolone 1-2 mg/kg/day) are initially used until improvement or 4-6 weeks with a slow taper to avoid relapse. Weaning of steroids often occurs over 1-2 years. For refractory or severe disease, pulse therapy with intravenous methylprednisolone is used at a dose of 30 mg/kg, with maximum dose of 1 gm daily for 3 days each month.
- Second line agents are routinely added for steroid sparing effects and for recalcitrant or refractory disease. Methotrexate, cyclosporin, cyclophosphamide, azathioprine, mycophenolate mofetil and hydroxychloroquine are the commonly used second line agents.
- Pulmonary disease can be arrested using anti-inflammatory and immunosuppressive agents.
- Intravenous immunoglobulin (IVIG) may also be used in patients with DM who are steroid-resistant or steroid dependent at a dose of 1 gm/kg/day on 2 consecutive days, or 2 gm/kg/day on day one, then every month thereafter, generally for 6 months.
- Rituximab can be considered (1 gm 2 weeks apart).
- Biologic agents such as the anti-TNF agents have had mixed results.
- Although not usually recommended, areas of calcinosis that cause significant disfigurement, pain, or compromised physical function may be resected. Sometimes, resected areas may be complicated by draining sinuses, infection and ulceration, and calcinosis may recur. For calcinosis cutis diltiazem (2-4 mg/kg), colchicine (0.5 mg/kg), minocycline (50-100 mg/kg) can be tried.

Complications

Calcinosis cutis is a common complication. If skin break down occurs, then secondary bacterial infection may occur. Joint contractures with long-term immobility, calcinosis, or both may occur.

Prognosis

The average disease duration has widely varied from 1.5 years to throughout the lifespan. More extent of damage at presentation leads to poor prognosis. Calcinosis cutis is single poor prognostic factor suggesting chronic disease. Presence of nail fold capillaries and gottron papules early in the course are poor marker. In general, children with JDM are able to lead normal lives with full recovery, compared with adults. Delayed or inadequate treatment with corticosteroids is a predictor of poor outcome and a prolonged disease course.

MIXED CONNECTIVE TISSUE DISORDERS

Mixed connective tissue disease remains a controversial diagnosis. Some rheumatologists view mixed connective tissue disease as a separate disease; others classify the disorder as an undifferentiated connective tissue disease or overlap syndrome, which may have features of lupus erythematosus, progressive systemic sclerosis, rheumatoid arthritis and myositis. Mixed connective tissue disease (MCTD) was first recognized by Sharp and colleagues in 1972. People with MCTD are diagnosed as SLE. As the disease progresses other signs and symptoms become apparent MCTD is diagnosed. M:F ratio is 1:16 and the onset of MCTD can occur at any age but typically occurs in people aged 15-25 years.

Diagnostic criteria for MCTD (Table 15.22):

- Anti-RNP antibody is frequently positive.
- Direct immunofluorescence study of apparently normal skin reveals particulate ('speckled') epidermal nuclear staining.

LICHEN SCLEROSUS ET ATROPHICUS

This subset of morphea has a predilection for the anogenital area. Lichen sclerosus typically occurs in the fifth or sixth decades of life, but 10% to 15% of all cases occur in prepubertal children, with girls out numbering boys with a ratio of 10: 1. Adolescents also can have lichen sclerosus with female predominance. It is a benign but chronic condition of the skin characterized by ivory or white shiny macules (Figure 15.15) and papules that form hypopigmented plaques. Comedones like plugs may be seen on surface, which disappear as lesion ages leaving behind smooth porcelain white plaque. (Figure 15.16). A figure of eight pattern often is present encircling the vulva and anus. The skin becomes thin and fragile and may fissure, bruise, excoriate and bleed easily. Purpura may be present. Typical symptoms of anogenital lichen sclerosus include itching, bleeding, and hemorrhagic blisters; hence can be confused with sexual abuse. Lichen sclerosus can be associated with considerable dysuria and/or pain during defecation, which can result in holding of urine and bowels leading to nocturnal enuresis and sleep disturbances. An increased association with autoimmune-related diseases (e.g., vitiligo, alopecia areata) may be seen.

Table 15.22: Different diagnostic criteria for MCTD

SHARP criteria for MCTD		*Requirements for diagnosis of MCTD*
Major criteria	***Minor criteria***	
1. Myositis 2. Pulmonary involvement – PAH / Proliferative change on biopsy / Diffusion capacity < 70 of normal on Pulmonary function test 3. Raynaud's phenomena or oesophageal hypomotility on manometry 4. Swollen hands 5. Anti-ENA (extractable nuclear antigen) titer > 1: 10000 U1-Rnp Positive and Anti-Sm Negative	1. Alopecia 2. Malar rash 3. Anemia 4. Leucopenia 5. Thrombocytopenia 6. Pleuritis 7. Pericarditis 8. Arthritis 9. History of swollen hands 10. Mild myositis 11. Trigeminal neuralgia	• At least four major criteria plus essential criteria – anti-U1-RNP titer of at least 1:4000 and exclusion criteria: positivity for anti-Sm antibody. OR • Any of the two major criteria out of 1, 2 and 3 plus 2 minor criteria + anti-U1-RNP titer of at least 1:1000.

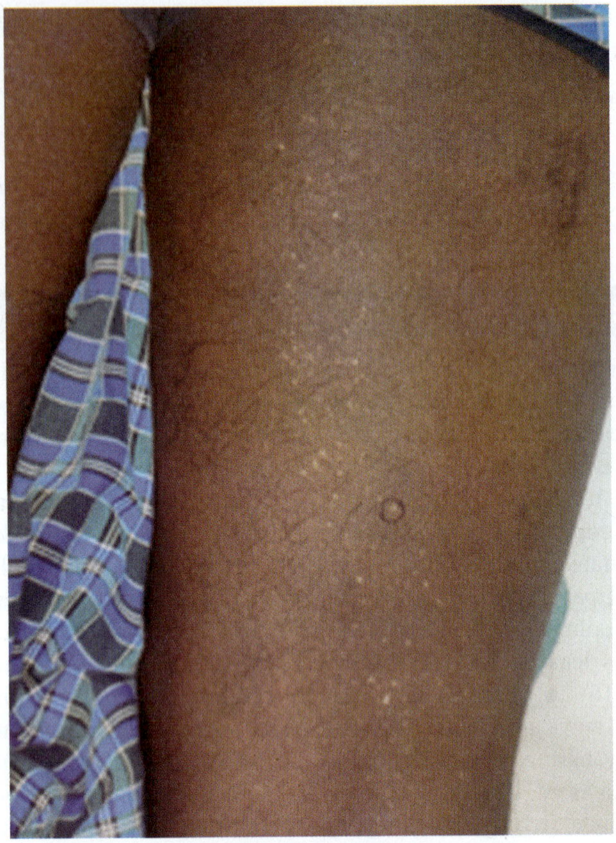

Figure 15.15: Extragenital lichen sclerosis atrophicus

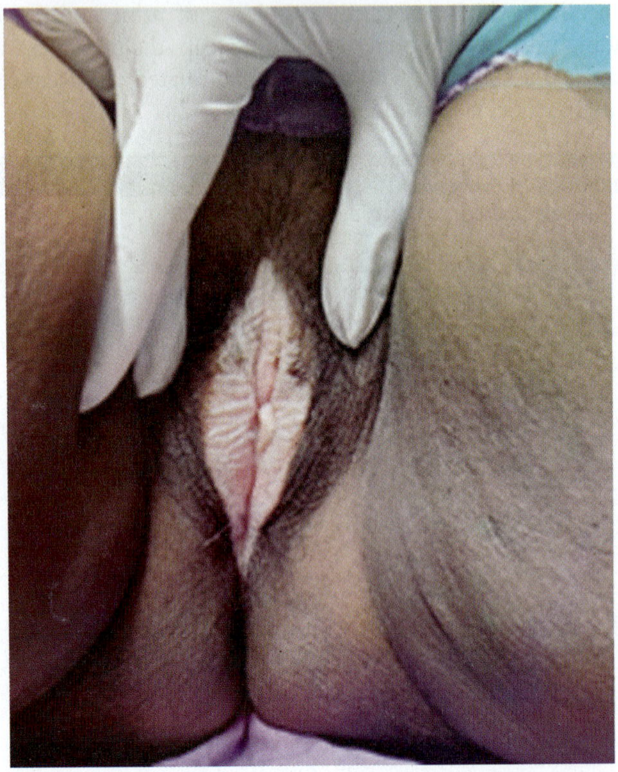

Figure 15.16: Genital lichen sclerosis et atrophicus

Treatment

Asymptomatic extragenital lichen sclerosus usually requires no treatment. Genital lichen sclerosus may respond to potent topical corticosteroids. The calcineurin inhibitors (i.e., tacrolimus, pimecrolimus) have been found to help some patients. Circumcision may benefit in phimosis accompanied by lichen sclerosus of male genitalia. Non-ablative lasers such as the pulsed dye and Er: YAG lasers, have been reported to benefit persons with lichen sclerosus. Cryotherapy of affected genital lesions is also reported to reduce the area involved. Narrow-band UVB, psoralens plus ultraviolet A (PUVA), and photodynamic therapy using a photosensitizer with laser light activation are also reported to be anecdotally beneficial.

Prognosis

Prognosis is good for acute genital cases, especially in pediatric age group that may resolve spontaneously. Prognosis is poor for extragenital cases and for chronic atrophic genital disease.

RELAPSING POLYCHONDRITIS (RP)

- It is an inflammatory disorder, episodic in nature, characterized by recurrent inflammation of cartilaginous tissues and eventual destruction of affected tissues.
- The disorder mainly affects the eyes, respiratory tract, nose and ears.
- **Diagnostic criteria:** By McAdams and colleagues - Any three or more of the following clinical features should be present:
    1. Bilateral auricular chondritis.
    2. Nasal chondritis.
    3. Respiratory tract chondritis.
    4. Non-erosive seronegative inflammatory polyarthritis.
    5. Ocular inflammation.
    6. Cochlear and/or vestibular dysfunction.
    7. Compatible histological features in a cartilage biopsy specimen.

RHEUMATOID ARTHRITIS (RA)

RA is symmetrical, progressive and long lasting autoimmune arthritis. It manifests as joint stiffness, erythema, effusion, discomfort, and swelling. These characteristic symptoms are more noticeable or worse in the morning or following extended periods of inactivity or sleep. Proximal interphalangeal, metacarpophalangeal and metatarsophalangeal joints of the hands and feet are most commonly affected; the distal interphalangeal and interphalangeal joints of thumb are spared. Wrist and ankle joints may also be affected. Although the lumbar spine is spared, cervical spine may be affected. This distinguishes the condition from other inflammatory arthropathies. The ulnar deviation, swan neck, boutonniere and Z-thumb deformities are specific hand malformations and these deformities can be repaired.

Within the extra-articular symptoms of RA, cutaneous involvement has been well described. These are classified into two types **(Table 15.23)** :

- Specific cutaneous features
- Non-specific features

Table 15.23: Showing specific and non-specific cutaneous manifestation of rheumatoid arthritis

Specific cutaneous features	*Non-specific features*

• Rheumatoid nodules
• Accelerated nodulosis
• Rheumatoid vasculitis
• Felty syndrome
• Neutrophilic dermatosis:
  o Sweet's syndrome
  o Pyoderma gangrenosum
• Granulomatous dermatitis:
  o Interstitial granulomatous dermatitis with arthritis
  o Palisaded neutrophilic and granulomatous dermatitis
	• Raynaud's phenomenon
	• Palmar erythema
	• Urticaria
	• Cutaneous atrophy
	• Skin xerosis or ichthyotic changes
	• Nail changes

Specific Cutaneous Features in Rheumatoid Arthritis

Rheumatoid nodules

It is the most common extra-articular manifestation of RA, observed in about 20-25% of patients. They manifest as asymptomatic, solitary or many skin coloured deep subcutaneous nodules which are typically located on traumatic sites such as on occiput, olecranon process, extensor surface of forearms, fingers and feet. Rheumatoid nodules may occurs in sclera and leads to scleromalacia. These nodules are indicative of severe form of RA. Three separate zones have been identified histologically: an innermost zone of central necrosis surrounded by perivascular infiltrate of chronic inflammatory cells and an outermost zone of palisading granulomas.

Accelerated rheumatoid nodulosis

There have been reports of accelerated rheumatoid nodulosis in patients receiving methotrexate for an extended period of time. The lesions are most commonly found on hands, especially on the proximal interphalangeal and metacarpophalangeal joints. It has been observed that they may or may not shrink after stoppage of methotrexate. Etanercept has also been associated with accelerated rheumatoid nodulosis.

Rheumatoid vasculitis

Less than 1% of patients have rheumatoid vasculitis (RV), a notable but uncommon symptom of RA. Individuals with rheumatoid nodules, joint erosions, and/or long-term seropositivity are more likely to develop it. Petechiae, visible purpura, ulceration, digital infarcts, peripheral gangrene are some of the common presenting symptoms. Leg ulcers at the pretibial or lateral malleolus may be acute, painful and punched out. Bywaters was the first to describe the transient, painless purpuric or pigmented lesions in the folds, edges and pulps of the nails, which are thought to be benign lesions with little possibility of progression.

Felty syndrome

Felty syndrome presents with triad of splenomegaly, leukopenia and arthritis. Leg ulcers, rheumatoid nodules and darkening around the shins and ankles are seen.

Granulomatous dermatitis

- **Palisaded neutrophilic and granulomatous dermatitis:** It is seen in patients with RA and other connective tissue diseases, which presents as symmetrical, erythematous to violaceous plaques, papules and nodules on multiple body sites.
- **Interstitial granulomatous dermatitis with arthritis:** This rare syndrome occurs in middle aged women who have positive rheumatoid factor and severe RA. Clinically, the lesions appear as erythematous to violaceous papules, nodules, and plaques which are symmetrical, may be painful. A burning sensation in the axilla, trunk and inner parts of the thighs may be felt. Rope sign is characteristic indurated, erythematous to violaceous linear cord which extends from axilla to iliac crest. Interstitial histiocytic granulomas are pathognomic.

Neutrophilic dermatosis

Pyoderma gangrenosum, Sweet's syndrome, palisaded neutrophilic granulomatous dermatitis and rheumatoid neutrophilic dermatosis are among the neutrophilic dermatoses associated with RA. Rheumatoid neutrophilic dermatosis (RND) presents as asymptomatic papules, nodules or plaques on the extensor surfaces of limbs, especially over the hands, forearms, neck and trunk. In the absence of vasculitis, a substantial neutrophilic infiltration is observed histologically.

When RA improves, the lesions disappear without specific treatment.

Non-specific Features

RA can lead to atrophic skin, resulting in increased fragility and susceptibility to bruises. Pale or even translucent skin may appear on the dorsal surface of the hands due to atrophy of the skin over interphalangeal joints. Nail changes include longitudinal ridging, clubbing, brittle nail, onycholysis, red lunula and periungual erythema with telangiectasia etc. Other feature are Raynaud's phenomenon , chronic urticaria and palmar erythema.

JUVENILE IDIOPATHIC ARTHRITIS

It is the most common chronic rheumatic disease of unknown aetiology in childhood and predominantly presents with peripheral arthritis.

Type of JIA

- Systemic juvenile idiopathic arthritis–most common subtypes, characterized by recurrent fever and rash.
- Oligoarticular juvenile idiopathic arthritis–seen in young female patients, is usually accompanied by anti-nuclear antibody positivity and anterior uveitis.
- Seropositive polyarticular juvenile idiopathic arthritis–an analogue of adult rheumatoid arthritis, is seen in less than 10% of paediatric patients.
- Seronegative polyarticular juvenile idiopathic arthritis–an entity more specific for childhood, appears with widespread large and small joint involvement.
- Enthesitis related arthritis–characterized by enthesitis and asymmetric lower-extremity arthritis. This disease subtype represents the childhood form of adult spondyloarthropathies, with human leukocyte antigen-B27 positivity and uveitis but commonly without axial skeleton involvement.
- Juvenile psoriatic arthritis–characterized by a psoriatic rash, accompanied by arthritis, nail pitting and dactylitis.

Disease complications include growth retardation, osteoporosis, life-threatening macrophage activation syndrome with multi-organ insufficiency.

The first-line treatment includes disease-modifying anti-rheumatic drugs (methotrexate, sulphasalazine, leflunomide) in combination with corticosteroids. Intra-articular application of steroids seems to be an effective treatment modality, especially in monoarthritis. Biological agents like etanercept, infliximab, adalimumab, anakinra, canakinumab should be added in the treatment of unresponsive patients.

SJÖGREN SYNDROME (SS)

It is an autoimmune disorder characterised by lymphocytic infiltration of exocrine glands, resulting in glandular dysfunction with a female to male ratio of 9:1.

It can be classified into two types:

1. **Primary Sjögren's syndrome (pSS)** occurs in the absence of other autoimmune diseases and is characterised by keratoconjunctivitis sicca (dry eyes) and xerostomia (dry mouth), collectively called the sicca syndrome.
2. **Secondary Sjögren's syndrome** presents along with other autoimmune diseases such as rheumatoid arthritis (RA) and systemic lupus erythematosus.

Epithelial cells of the glands, cytokines, T lymphocytes and BAFF have all been demonstrated to contribute to the pathogenesis of this condition.

Skin Manifestations

Xeroderma, pruritus and scaling; Subacute cutaneous lupus erythematosus like skin rashes and annular erythema, including Sweet disease like lesions; Raynaud syndrome; Hyperglobulinaemic purpura and inflammatory vasculitis including polyarteritis nodosa like lesions; Vitiligo; Abnormalities of sweating; Amyloidosis; Alopecia.

Non cutaneous features of Sjögren syndrome: Joint symptoms: arthralgia and arthritis; Myalgia and myositis; sinusitis and deafness; Tracheal and oesophageal reflux; Interstitial pneumonitis, pulmonary fibrosis and pulmonary hypertension; Interstitial nephritis; primary biliary cirrhosis; Fatigue; Neurological abnormalities: migraine, neuropathies and cerebral vasculitis.

Revised classification criteria for Sjogren's syndrome:

1. **Ocular symptoms** – at least one of:
   a. Dry eyes for more than 3 months.
   b. Sensation of sand or gravel in the eyes.
   c. Need for tear substitutes more than 3 times a day.
2. **Oral symptoms** – at least one of:
   a. Dry mouth for more than 3 months.
   b. Recurrently or persistently swollen salivary glands.
   c. Need liquids to swallow dry food.
3. **Ocular signs** – at least one of the following two tests to be positive:
   a. Schirmer test, performed without anaesthesia ($\leq$ 5 mm in 5 min).
   b. Rose bengal score or other ocular dye score.

4. **Histopathology** – in minor salivary glands, focal lymphocytic sialoadenitis (focus score ≥ 1)
5. **Salivary gland involvement** – a positive result for at least one of the following diagnostic tests:
    a. Unstimulated whole salivary flow (≤ 1.5 ml in 15 min).
    b. Parotid sialography showing the presence of diffuse sialectasias (punctate, cavitary or destructive pattern), without evidence of obstruction in the major ducts.
    c. Salivary scintigraphy showing delayed uptake, reduced concentration and/or delayed excretion of tracer.
6. **Autoantibodies** – presence in the serum of antibodies to Ro (SSA) or La (SSB) antigens, or both.

For primary Sjögren syndrome: The presence of any four of the six criterion mentioned above, so long as either criteria 4 (histopathology) or 6 (serology) is positive.

For secondary Sjögren syndrome: The presence of serial number 1 or 2 criterion plus any two out of 3, 4 and 5 criterion.

Treatment

Symptomatic treatment for the dryness of the eyes is by lubricating agents, such as 0.5% methylcellulose eye drops. Artificial saliva can be prescribed and steam inhalations or an air humidifier may help dryness of the respiratory tract. Systemic corticosteroids are effective in reducing parotid swelling. Chloroquine or hydroxychloroquine sulphate and Ciclosporin may reduce histopathological progression.

The main challenge in treatment of CTD are drugs being untested and not approved for use in paediatric age group. These drugs can interfere with growth and sexual maturation, hence, should be judiciously used.

16

CHAPTER

Disorders of Oral Cavity

Contents

A large number of diseases involves the oral mucosa. These may be limited to the oral cavity or involve other systems. A thorough knowledge of these diseases is essential to make an accurate diagnosis, particularly when oral involvement is the presenting feature.

A complete oral examination is an essential part of any dermatologic examination. Often the oral cavity is examined in a fleeting manner. Diseases of the oral cavity may be congenital or acquired later in life. They may be localized to the buccal mucosa or the tongue, or may be part of generalized diseases (See Table 16.1).

Morphologically, they may present as:

- Papules and nodules.
- Stomatitis and mucosal ulcers.
- White lesions or plaques.
- Pigmented lesions.

Important oral cavity lesions in children are discussed below.

CONGENITAL DISEASES OF ORAL MUCOSA

Cysts of Oral Mucosa

Epstein's pearls, Bohn's nodules, and dental lamina cysts are all variations of a cystic lesion seen on the alveolar or palatal mucosa of neonates. Clinically, all of these cysts appear

Table 16.1: Disorders of buccal mucosa

Congenital		*Acquired*	
Common	***Uncommon***	***Common***	***Uncommon***
Sucking pads	Cysts	Aphthous stomatitis	Epulis
Fordyce's spots	Natal teeth	Candidiasis	Squamous papilloma
	Congenital epulis	Trauma	Leukoplakia
	Congenital fistulae	Mucocele	Malignancy
	Congenital ranula	Abscess	

similarly as small, white papules or translucent cysts. There may be one or multiple lesions. No treatment is indicated because they resolve spontaneously.

Epstein's pearls occur at the junction of the hard and soft palates. They most likely represent remnants of epithelial tissue entrapped during palatal fusion.

Bohn's nodules develop from heterotopic salivary glands and are found on the facial and lingual surfaces of the alveolar ridges and on the palate, away from the midline.

Lesions on the crest of the alveolar ridge are known as dental lamina cysts, alveolar cysts, or gingival cysts of the newborn. They are derived from dental lamina, the ectodermal portion of the tooth bud.

Fordyce's Spots

Fordyce's spots are collections of normal sebaceous glands within the oral cavity. Although present at birth, they often do not become clinically apparent until puberty. They present as 1-3 mm, white to yellow papules most commonly on the mucosa of the lips but can occur on any mucosal surface (Figure 16.1). They are of no medical significance and require no intervention.

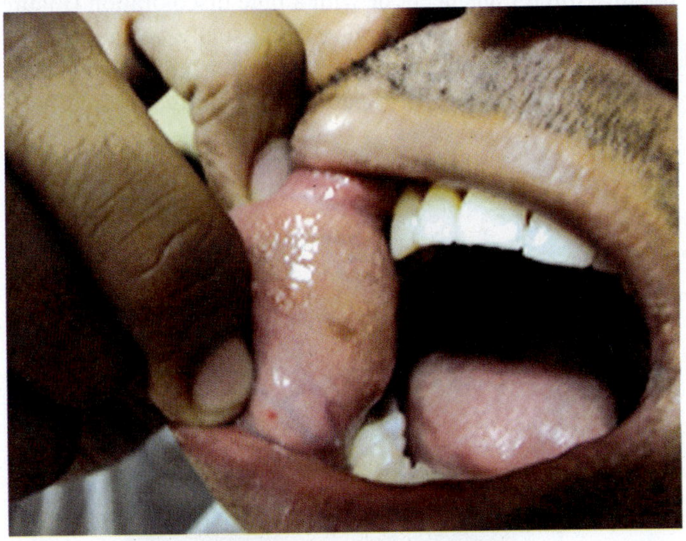

Figure 16.1: Fordyce's spots

Natal and Neonatal Teeth

Natal teeth are present at birth. Neonatal teeth are less common and erupt during the first month of life. A positive family history is noted in 8% to 46% of patients with natal and neonatal teeth. The teeth are frequently mobile because of poor root development and often have poorly calcified enamel secondary to their premature eruption. They frequently occur in pairs, most commonly in the mandibular incisor region. Ulceration of the sublingual aspect of the tongue, can result from trauma from these teeth. Extraction is recommended, if the tooth is extremely loose and poses an aspiration risk. Natal and neonatal teeth have been associated with a number of syndromes including chondroectodermal dysplasia and pachyonychia congenita.

Congenital Epulis of Newborn

Also known as gingival granular cell tumor of the newborn, it is a rare, benign tumor most commonly seen in female neonates. Clinically, the lesions appear as pedunculated, firm growths arising from the alveolar ridge. Histologically, tightly packed granular cells are seen surrounded by a fibrovascular stroma. Although these tumors can resolve spontaneously, they may interfere with feeding and respiration and can create anxiety for parents. Surgical excision is often preferred and is curative.

Melanotic Neuroectodermal Tumor of Infancy

This is a rare tumor usually occurring within the first 6 months of life. It appears as a smooth surfaced, rapidly enlarging, blue to black tumor most commonly located on the maxillary alveolar ridge. The tumor is most likely of neural crest origin suggested by high levels of vanillylmandelic acid (VMA) in some patients' urine. On histology, characteristic alveolar spaces lined by cuboidal cells filled with dark staining, neural-like cells are seen. Surgical excision is the therapy of choice.

Hemangioma (Also See Chapter 22)

Hemangiomas are the most common benign tumor of the oral mucosa in children. These are benign vascular growths, which typically appear as red to blue, poorly circumscribed, spongy tumors most commonly involving the lips, tongue, buccal mucosa and palate. They characteristically undergo a period of rapid growth over the first several months of life, followed by stabilization and gradual spontaneous involution over a period of years. Complications include cosmetic deformity and ulceration, which can be associated with bleeding, pain and risk of secondary infection. Hemangiomas may also interfere with respiration, speech and ability to suck.

Management is determined by the size and location of the lesion, complications and cosmetic concerns of the patient and family. Because many spontaneously regress without sequelae, close observation with parental reassurance is a frequent plan of action. Thin or ulcerated hemangiomas may respond to pulsed dye laser. Lesions that interfere with vital functions require aggressive therapy with intralesional or systemic corticosteroids. Proponolol is a non selective beta blocker which is given in dose of 1-2 mg/kg/day. It is known to inhibit the proliferation of endothelial cells and promote regression of these lesions during the proliferative phase. It is recommended to admit the children in the hospital as a day case for base line investigations before the start of therapy, with strict monitoring of blood pressure, pulse and blood glucose.

One percent Timolol eye drops also show excellent results in the treatment of uncomplicated hemangiomas.

Lymphangioma

The lymphangioma, or lymphatic malformation, is a relatively uncommon tumor of the mouth usually presenting at birth. It is a malformation of lymphatic vessels, and in contrast to hemangiomas, does not spontaneously regress. They most commonly occur on the tongue but may also arise on the lips, buccal mucosa, soft palate, and floor of the mouth. Superficial lesions have a papillated surface that can appear vesicular in nature. Deeper lesions are nodular and can result in macroglossia when the tongue is involved. Although often asymptomatic, lymphangiomas may enlarge leading to difficulty and pain with speech and feeding. They also can become secondarily infected. Circumscribed, smaller lesions can be surgically excised.

Congenital Fistulae

Congenital pits, also known as congenital fistulae of the lower lip, are rare developmental anomalies. Clinically, a pair of bilaterally symmetric indentations on the vermilion aspect of the lower lip is seen. A single pit may also occur. The lumen of the fistula is lined by stratified squamous epithelium similar to lip mucosa with scattered ducts and acini of mucinous glands. Saliva may be excreted spontaneously from the pits or may occur with mastication. Surgical correction of the pits is undertaken only if there is a visible deformity or if there is significant salivation from them.

Congenital Ranula

The congenital ranula presents as a soft tissue swelling in the anterior floor of the mouth lateral to the lingual frenulum. The overlying mucosa may have a blue discoloration or may be normal in appearance. The ranula results from obstruction, perforation or atresia of the sublingual or submandibular salivary gland duct. Although it resembles the mucocele clinically, a ranula is actually a pseudocyst as opposed to the mucocele, which is a true cyst. Treatment with marsupialization of the obstructed duct should be performed early to prevent the possibility of sialadenitis.

Sucking Pads

Sucking pads, also known as sucking calluses, are not congenital but occur frequently in the neonatal period. It occurs in almost all neonates in varying degrees of severity. Clinically, hyperkeratotic thickening is seen at the closure line of the upper and lower lips that extends inward to involve the mucosal surface. The lesions may be white or pigmented and may be smooth or become hyperkeratotic. These pads are adaptive response to the mechanical effects of sucking. They usually disappear after 3 to 6 months of age.

Genodermatoses

Multiple oral papules can be observed as a clinical feature in a number of genodermatoses like Cowden's disease, tuberous sclerosis, neurofibromatosis, lipoid proteinosis, Goltz syndrome etc.

ACQUIRED DISORDERS OF ORAL MUCOSA

Mucocele

The mucocele represents a mucous extravasation cyst resulting from trauma to salivary glands. They are common in childhood, and girls are more commonly affected than boys. The lower lip is the most frequent site, but mucoceles may occur on the palate, upper lip, and on the buccal mucosa. Mucoceles typically present as localized fluid-filled papules or nodules often translucent or with a blue discoloration (Figure 16.2). The lesion may rupture but usually recurs leading to fibrosis. If simply unroofed, the lesion generally recurs; surgical excision or electrocautery is usually required.

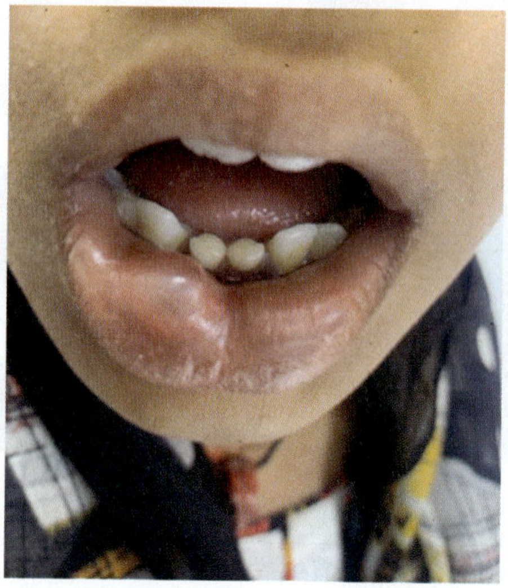

Figure 16.2: Mucocele

Oral Abscess

In the oral cavity, abscesses are almost always the result of a non vital tooth. This may result from dental caries, trauma or periodontitis. Abscesses present as painful, fluctuant soft tissue swellings of the gingiva, palate, or buccal sulci. **Parulis** is a term used to describe an abscess of the gingiva adjacent to a non vital tooth. Dental abscesses may be complicated by cellulitis, facial swelling, fever and systemic complaints. Use of systemic antibiotics is helpful, but definitive treatment requires therapy of the devitalized tooth (root canal therapy or extraction) or gingival surgery when periodontitis exists.

Squamous Papilloma

The squamous papilloma is a benign, common intraoral neoplasm that presents as a pink to white verrucous papule. They are caused by human papilloma virus infection. The most common location is the junction of the hard and soft palate, although lesions may occur anywhere. Treatment options include destruction modalities, such as cryotherapy, electrodesiccation or surgical excision.

Retrocuspid Papilla

This is a common, benign, soft tissue enlargement affecting most children under the age of 10 years. It affects girls more commonly than boys. Clinically, it is seen as a 2-3 mm, soft, sessile papule posterior to the mandibular canine tooth, frequently bilateral. A biopsy specimen reveals normal mucosa and connective tissue. Most lesions regress spontaneously with age.

Epulis

The term epulis is used to refer to a localized overgrowth that is not a neoplasm, but instead a non-specific hyperplastic inflammatory reaction. It presents as a local, red brown, sessile or pedunculated growth over the buccal mucosa, which may or may not bleed. The lesions presenting as epulis may be pyogenic granuloma, peripheral ossifying fibromas or fibroepithelial polyps. All of them appear similar on clinical examination but are distinguishable by histologic study. Local excision is the preferred treatment but recurrence is possible.

Malignancy

Lymphoma may very rarely present as an intraoral soft tissue enlargement, a non healing ulcer, or with loosening of the teeth. A radiograph may reveal bone resorption.

Histiocytosis X may cause lytic lesions of the skull and mandible with associated oral soft tissue swelling, ulceration, or disruption of teeth.

It is imperative that any growth or enlargement of soft tissue of unclear cause should undergo biopsy for a definitive diagnosis.

STOMATITIS AND ULCERATIONS OF ORAL MUCOSA

Stomatitis is an inflammation of the oral mucosa. It is frequently associated with oral ulcerations and significant pain. There are multiple disorders that may cause stomatitis and oral ulcers (Table 16.2).

Table 16.2: Differential diagnosis of oral ulcers

Trauma	
Infections	Herpes simplex, herpes zoster, coxsackie virus, echovirus, HIV, syphilis, candidiasis, deep fungal infections, Bacterial infections
Oro-genital syndromes	Behçet's syndrome, Reiter's syndrome
Nutritional disorders	Scurvy, Vitamin B12 and folic acid deficiency
Autoimmune bullous disorders	Pemphigus vulgaris, pemphigus vegetans
Drug induced	SJS/TEN
Systemic diseases (Table 16.3)	
Others	Aphthous ulcers, Sweet's syndrome, Genetic disorders

Trauma

Although any type of trauma can lead to ulceration, the most common cause is generally self-induced, such as involuntary chewing or biting on the oral mucosa. Accidental traumatic ulcers can also occur including punctures induced by pencils or pens, toothpicks and fish bones. Trauma from braces, other dental appliances and jagged teeth is also possible. Unless complicated by secondary infection, traumatic erosions and ulcers should heal in a period of days to a few weeks.

Infections

Bacterial Infections

Acute necrotizing ulcerative gingivitis mainly affects adolescents and young adults but can rarely also be seen in children. It is characterized by the abrupt onset of extremely painful, hyperemic gingivae with sharply demarcated ulcerations of the interdental papillae. Severe oral pain, profuse salivation with a distinct metallic taste, headache, malaise and low grade fever may also occur. A gram-negative spirochete, *Borrelia vincentii* and a gram-positive bacillus, *Fusobacterium dentium* are found on smears from the gingiva and grow on anaerobic culture. Poor oral hygiene, inadequate nutrition, and dental caries are predisposing factors. Children with leukemia or other blood dyscrasias are also more likely to

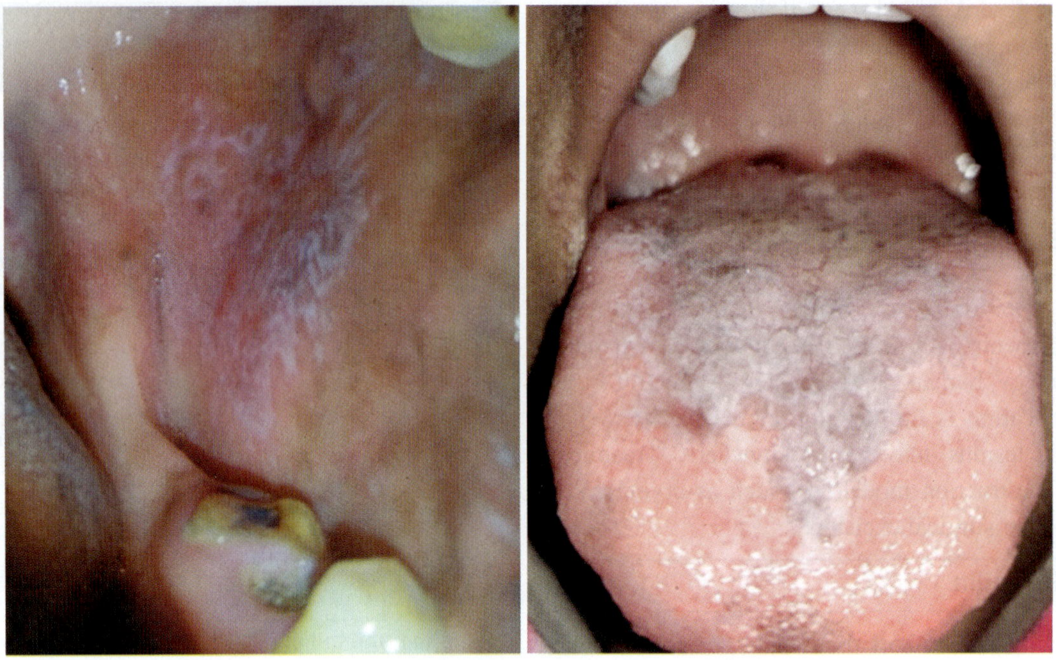

Figure 16.3: Lichen planus

develop acute necrotizing ulcerative gingivitis. Treatment includes antibiotic therapy and the care of a dentist.

Viral Enanthems

A number of viral infections are characterized by acute stomatitis, vesicles, erosions and ulcerations of the oral mucosa. These include herpetic gingiva stomatitis, varicella, hand foot mouth disease, herpangina and infectious mononucleosis. A careful examination of the oral mucosa in the acutely ill child can sometimes provide helpful clues toward making a diagnosis.

Fungal Infections

Although rare in immunocompetent children, fungal infections always need to be considered when evaluating oral ulcerations in immunocompromised children and adults. The possibilities in the differential diagnosis include disseminated candidiasis, histoplasmosis, blastomycosis paracoccidioidomycosis, cryptococcosis, aspergillosis and mucormycosis. A biopsy is often needed for definitive diagnosis because the oral lesions may be indistinctive.

Autoimmune Disorders

Autoimmune disorders include diseases like erythema multiforme, lichen planus (Figure 16.3), pemphigus vulgaris (Figure 16.4), cicatricial pemphigoid (Figure 16.5), linear IgA disease and dermatitis herpetiformis etc. These conditions are discussed in detail in their respective chapters.

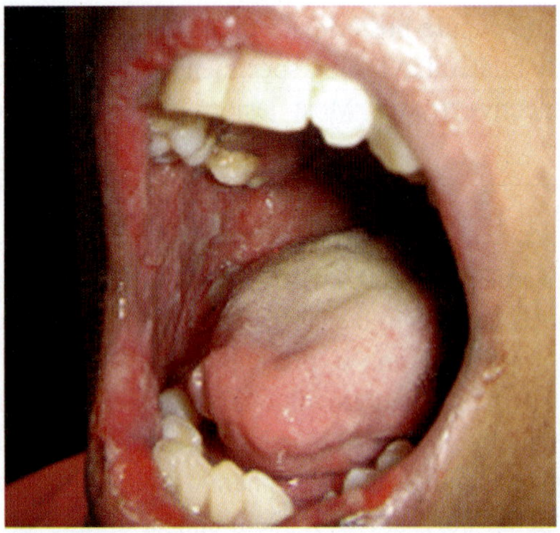

Figure 16.4: Pemphigus vulgaris

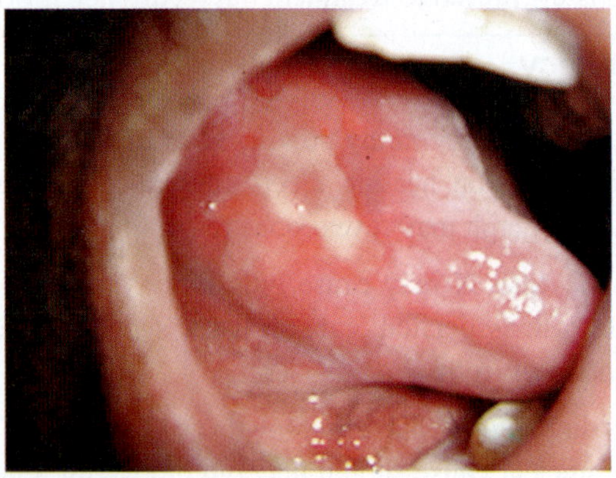

Figure 16.5: Cicatricial pemphigoid

Genetic Diseases

Epidermolysis bullosa (chapter 14) represents a large group of inherited disorders characterized by development of blisters following minor or insignificant trauma or traction to the skin. There are three major forms (Simplex, Junctional and Dystrophic). The various subtypes of epidermolysis bullosa result from a variety of defects in the proteins responsible for adherence of the epidermis to the dermis. Mucosal blistering may occur in all subtypes of epidermolysis bullosa, although with varying degree of severity. Patients with epidermolysis bullosa who have oral blistering are also at risk for dental problems. The painful erosions make dental hygiene more difficult leading to gingivitis and decay. Teeth also may be irregular in shape and have enamel hypoplasia leading to more caries.

Bullae and ulcerations of the mucosae which are usually present in infancy, are secondary to suckling and can be quite painful.

Management of patients with oral involvement should include regular visits to a dental specialist. Special nipples, such as those used in patients with cleft palate, also can be helpful in patients where intraoral blisters interfere with feeding.

Systemic Diseases

Many systemic diseases can lead to oral ulceration which are described in Table 16.3.

Recurrent Aphthous Stomatitis

Recurrent aphthous stomatitis is the most common inflammatory ulcerative condition of the oral mucosa. It is frequently encountered in the pediatric age group as well as adults. It is estimated that 20% of the general population has recurrent aphthous stomatitis during their childhood or early adult life.

Recurrent aphthous stomatitis can be classified according to the morphology of the lesions into three types (Table 16.4):

- **Minor aphthous ulcers.**
- **Major aphthous ulcers.**
- **Herpetiform ulcers.**

Seventy-five to 85% of patients who suffer from recurrent aphthous stomatitis have minor aphthous ulcers. This form is characterized by the infrequent development of one or more small (<1 cm) oval or round, shallow ulcers with a gray fibro

Table 16.3: Oral manifestations of systemic disorders

System	*Common oral manifestations*
Endocrine disorders	Microdontia, delayed tooth eruption, dental hypoplasia
Gastrointestinal disorders	Ulcers, glossitis, angular stomatitis, jaundice, bleeding tendency
Renal disorders	Xerostomia, halitosis, leukoplakia, dental hypoplasia
Cardiovascular disorders	Cyanosis, telangiectasia, referred pain
Hematological disorders	Glossitis, ulcers, angular stomatitis, infections, purpura

Table 16.4: Types of recurrent aphthous ulcers

Feature	*Minor aphthous ulcers*	*Major aphthous ulcers*	*Herpetiform ulcers*
Gender predilection	M=F	M=F	F>M
Age of onset	5-19 years	10-19 years	20-29 years
Number of ulcers	1-5	1-10	10-100
Size of ulcers (mm)	<10	>10	1-2 (larger if coalesced)
Duration (days)	4-14	>30	<30
Recurrence rate (months)	1-4	<1	<1
Site predilection	Lips, cheeks, tongue, floor of mouth	Lips, cheeks, tongue, palate, pharynx	Lips, cheeks, tongue, palate, pharynx, floor of mouth, gingiva
Permanent scarring	Unusual	Common	Unusual

membranous slough surrounded by a peripheral zone of erythema (Figure 16.6). They are moderately painful and usually heal without scarring in 1 to 2 weeks. Most patients suffer two to four episodes per year.

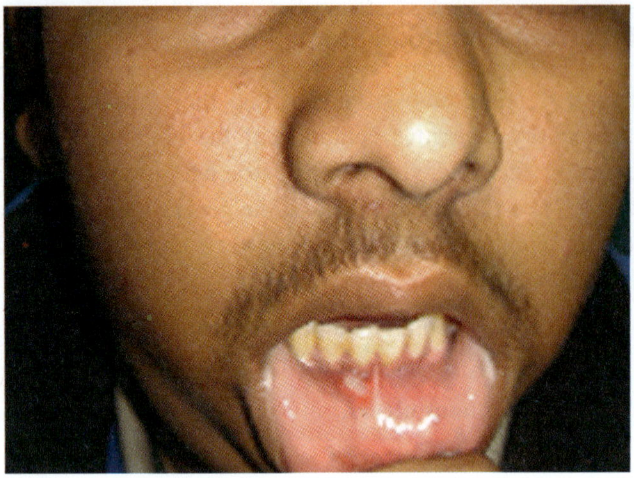

Figure 16.6: Aphthous ulcer

Major aphthous ulcers account for 10% to 15% of sufferers of recurrent aphthous stomatitis. The ulcers are larger (>1 cm) and deeper. They heal slowly and characteristically heal with scarring. The lesions of major aphthous ulcers cause significant discomfort, oral pain, fever and malaise.

Herpetiform ulcers account for the remaining 5% to 10% of patients with recurrent aphthous stomatitis. This variant presents with multiple, grouped, 1-2 mm papules that evolve into papulovesicles and subsequently into ulcers, which may coalesce. Lesions heal in 7 to 30 days sometimes with scarring.

Recurrent aphthous oral ulcers may be associated with many systemic diseases like cyclic neutropenia, severe combined immunodeficiency disease, chronic granulomatous disease, Chediak-Higashi syndrome, gluten sensitive enteropathy, inflammatory bowel disease, Behçet's syndrome, juvenile rheumatoid arthritis, HIV infection, nutritional deficiencies like iron, zinc, vitamin B_{12}, folic acid deficiencies, chemotherapy or radiotherapy.

Treatment

Recurrent aphthous ulcerations are most often treated with palliative agents, such as bland diet, avoidance of irritating agents, use of antiseptic mouthwash, local antiseptic and local anaesthetics. Local steroid paste is quite useful. For more severe disease systemic corticosteroids are effective.

WHITE PLAQUES OF ORAL CAVITY (Table 16.5)

Table 16.5: Oral white lesions

Hereditary or Developmental	Leukoedema White sponge nevus Hereditary benign intraepithelial dyskeratosis Pachyonychia congenita Dyskeratosis congenita
Reactive	Frictional keratosis Nicotine stomatitis Contact desquamation
Infectious	Candidiasis Oral hairy leukoplakia Mucous patches of secondary syphilis
Immunologic	Lichen planus, Discoid lupus erythematosus, Graft versus host disease
Systemic diseases	Uremic stomatitis
Premalignant and malignant	Leukoplakia, Squamous cell carcinoma

Leukoplakia

It is a term used to describe a chronic white lesion (Figure 16.7) that cannot be rubbed off and for which there is no known cause. Leukoplakia is a common finding in tobacco chewers. Leukoplakia is most commonly found in the buccal and labial sulcus where the tobacco is held. Smokeless tobacco users of all ages are at risk of dysplastic change and squamous cell carcinoma. Biopsy of leukoplakia should be done to rule out malignant changes.

Candidiasis

Candidiasis or thrush, is an opportunistic fungal infection of the oral mucosa caused by *candida albicans*. It is frequent in infants and children as well as adults and can be precipitated by broad-spectrum antibiotic therapy, oral corticosteroids or by compromised immune system. The condition presents with superficial white curd-like plaques on the mucous membranes, which can be wiped off (Figure 16.8).

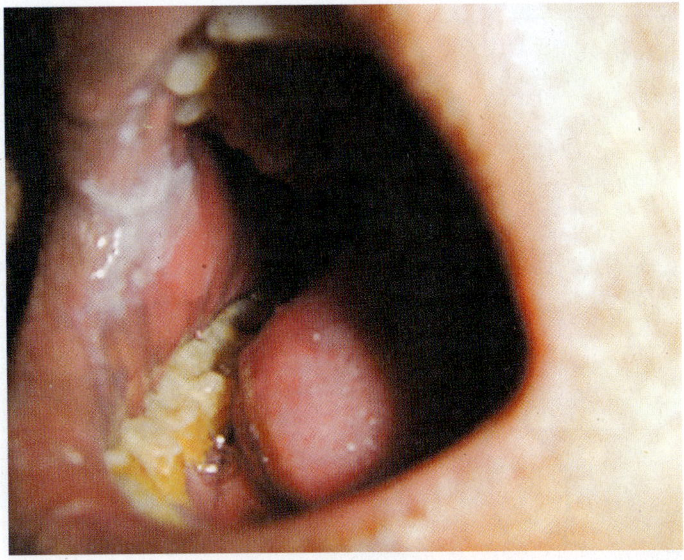

Figure 16.7: Leukoplakia

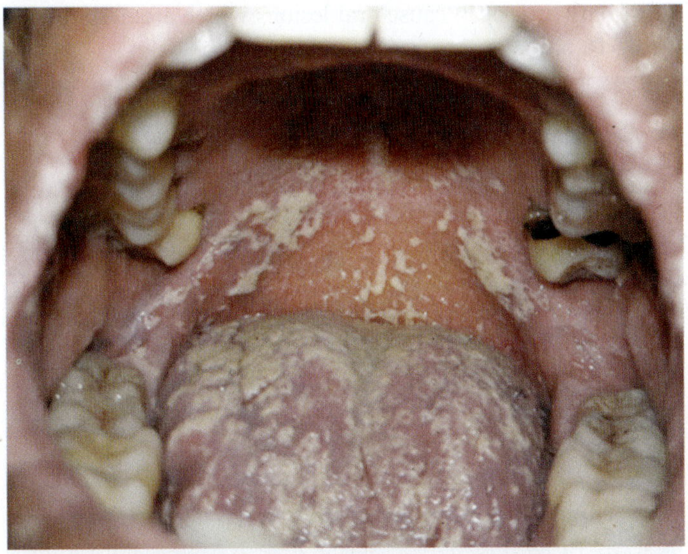

Figure 16.8: Oral mucocutaneous candidiasis

Treatment

Nystatin suspension applied to a gauze and held on the affected surfaces can be an effective treatment. Topical application of azoles like clotrimazole is widely used. A child may be able to swish and expectorate a nystatin solution or use a clotrimazole lozenge. Systemic therapy with oral fluconazole may be required in unresponding cases.

Koplik's Spots

Koplik's spots, an oral manifestation of measles, appear as small white lesions resembling grains of salt on the buccal mucosa opposite the second molar tooth, are pathognomonic. Because they often occur during the prodrome of measles, they frequently go unnoticed.

Oral hairy leukoplakia (Chapter 29)

PIGMENTED LESIONS OF THE ORAL MUCOSA

Melanocytic Nevi

Melanocytic nevi of the oral mucosa are relatively uncommon in children but can occur. Although intraoral melanoma is extremely rare in childhood, many advocate prophylactic excision of all intraoral pigmented nevi.

Peutz-Jeghers Syndrome

Peutz-Jeghers syndrome is an autosomal dominant condition with gastrointestinal polyposis and mucocutaneous hyperpigmented macules. More than 95% of patients have distinctive hyperpigmented macules involving the lips (Figure 16.9) and buccal mucosa. Pigmented macules may be noted in infancy, long before polyps are diagnosed. Hyperpigmented macules may also be noted on the digits or on periorbital, perianal or vulvar skin.

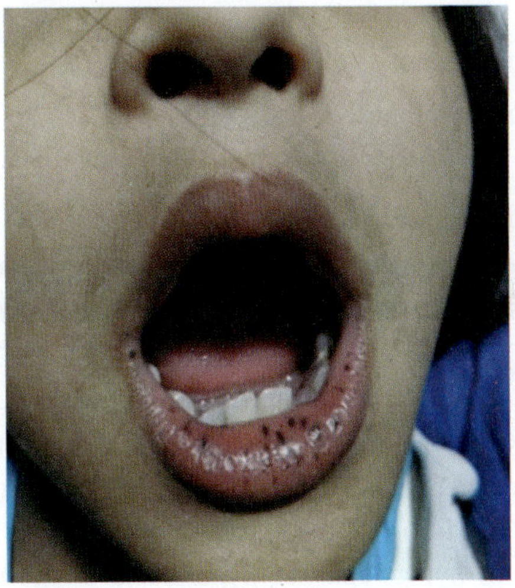

Figure 16.9: Hyperpigmented macules in Peutz-Jeghers syndrome

Generalized Hyperpigmentation

Generalized hyperpigmentation of the oral mucosa can be seen in a number of conditions. It can be drug-induced related to use of anticonvulsants, adrenocorticotropic hormone therapy, cytotoxic agents, oral contraceptives, antimalarial drugs and minocycline etc. Other rare causes include systemic diseases such as hemochromatosis, neurofibromatosis, incontinentia pigmenti, Addison's disease and Albright's syndrome etc.

Many drugs can cause oral lesions which are described in Table 16.6.

Table 16.6: Oral lesions due to drugs

Drug involved	*Effects*
Tetracyclines	Teeth discolouration
Phenytoin, cyclosporin, nifedipine	Gingival swelling
Metronidazole, penicillamine	Disturbed taste
Cytotoxic drugs	Oral ulcers
Corticosteroids	Oral thrush
Sulphonamides, barbiturates, NSAIDs	Erythema multiforme
Lithium, tricyclic antidepressants, phenothiazines	Dry mouth

DISORDERS OF TONGUE

Congenital

- Macroglossia.
- Ankyloglossia.
- Lingual tonsil.
- Lingual thyroid.

Acquired

- Benign migratory glossitis.
- Strawberry tongue.
- Furred tongue and hairy tongue.
- Smooth tongue.

CONGENITAL DISEASES OF THE TONGUE

Macroglossia

Macroglossia is defined as a tongue that protrudes beyond the teeth or alveolar ridge during rest and can be caused by a number of conditions. Most cases in children are congenital and represent hypertrophy or hyperplasia of the muscles of the tongue. Syndromes associated with macroglossia include Down syndrome (Figure 16.10), Beckwith-Widemann syndrome, Hurler's syndrome and cretinism etc.

Secondary macroglossia may result from hypothyroidism, amyloidosis, sarcoidosis and congenital malformations such as lymphangiomas and hemangiomas. Macroglossia can lead to psychologic distress, other maxillofacial abnormalities, impaired swallowing and speech, and even airway obstruction. Medical management may be beneficial if the macroglossia is caused by an underlying systemic disease as in hypothyroidism.

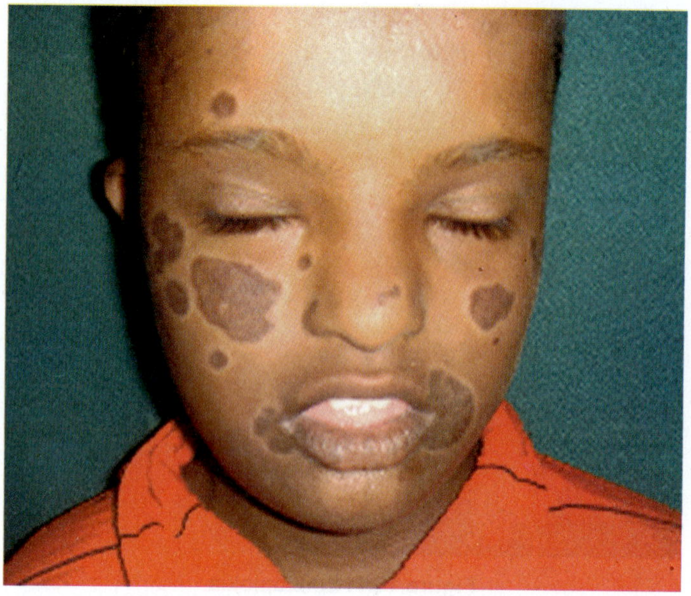

Figure 16.10: Macroglossia in Down syndrome (unable to close mouth properly), also showing actinic lichen planus

Surgical removal of a causative neoplasm or reduction glossectomy is another therapeutic option.

Ankyloglossia

Ankyloglossia, also known as tongue-tie, results from an abnormally short lingual frenulum. This congenital anomaly is relatively common in newborns. Although many believe that ankyloglossia is rarely of medical significance, it may lead to breastfeeding difficulties and neonatal frenulectomy is advised.

Lingual Tonsil

The lingual tonsil is a developmental anomaly found on the posterior third of the tongue between the epiglottis posteriorly and the circumvallate papillae anteriorly. It is a mass of lymphoid tissue usually divided through the midline by a ligament. Although often small and asymptomatic, lingual tonsils can become enlarged, creating dyspnea, dysphonia, and the sensation of a lump in the throat. Lingual tonsillitis can result in a painful swollen tongue and fever. The diagnosis can be confirmed by histopathology, which reveals lymphoid tissue. Treatment of symptomatic lesions is possible by lingual tonsillectomy.

Lingual Thyroid

Another developmental malformation is the lingual thyroid, a smooth-surfaced mass of ectopic thyroid tissue found at foramen cecum. Although usually asymptomatic, dysphagia, coughing or pain may occur. Other benign or malignant tumors should be excluded by biopsy. Surgical removal can be performed for symptomatic lesions, if thyroid gland present in the neck is functioning normally.

ACQUIRED DISEASES OF THE TONGUE

Benign Migratory Glossitis/Geographic Tongue

It is a benign tongue condition affecting 2% of the population. In children, it is one of the most common conditions of the oral mucosa clinically observed. The cause is unknown. The condition may be hereditary. An association with atopy, fissured tongue, and psoriasis has also been noted. Clinically, the dorsum of the tongue has well-defined erythematous regions of depapillation, each surrounded by a raised white edge. This can lead to a geographic configuration or map-like appearance (Figure 16.11), hence the name geographic tongue. The appearance may change daily. Although usually asymptomatic, soreness sometimes occurs, especially with salty or spicy foods. Reassurance is usually all that is needed.

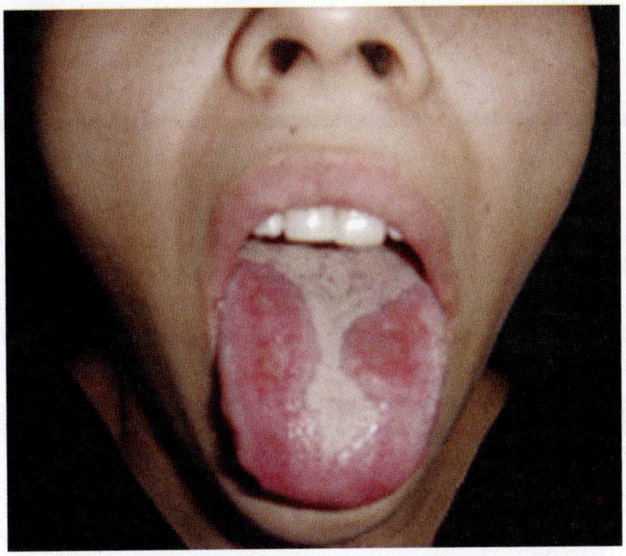

Figure 16.11: Geographic tongue

Strawberry Tongue

Both scarlet fever and Kawasaki's disease have been associated with a strawberry tongue. The strawberry tongue is a red inflamed tongue with a white exudate that covers the entire dorsum of the tongue. In scarlet fever, this white coating quickly resolves leaving a smooth, deep red tongue. Dramatic hyperemia of other oral mucosal surfaces and the oropharynx is also characteristic of both diseases.

Furred Tongue and Hairy Tongue

A furred tongue is the result of accumulation of keratin and hypertrophy of the filiform papillae. In children, it is most commonly seen with a febrile systemic illness and is caused by lack of mechanical debridement and changes in the oral flora. The furred tongue has also been associated with smoking and a diet low in fiber. In contrast, a hairy tongue is the result of excessive elongation of the filiform papillae. This may be idiopathic or caused by chronic irritation. Regular brushing of the tongue may be beneficial in improving the appearance of both conditions.

A brown or black discoloration may also occur with both the furred and the hairy tongue. Antibiotic use leading to a local excess of chromogenic bacteria may be responsible. It may also result from iron supplementation, coffee consumption or tobacco use. If aesthetically displeasing, brushing with 1% to 2% hydrogen peroxide solution can be tried.

Smooth Tongue

Atrophy of the filiform papillae leads to a smooth or bald tongue. Although seen in unusual genetic conditions, such as Riley-Day syndrome, the most common cause is nutritional deficiency. In children, nutritional deficiencies are usually caused by malnutrition or malabsorption, like in celiac sprue and Crohn's disease. Mostly, atrophic glossitis results from deficiencies of folate, iron or Vitamins.

CHAPTER 17

Vasculitis

Contents

Vasculitis refers to a heterogeneous group of disorders, characterized by immune mediated inflammatory destruction of blood vessel wall affecting both arteries and veins. Arteries and veins of any size may be affected, leading to ischemic damage to organs. Most of patients with vasculitis have variable clinical presentation based on the systems involved. Systemic involvement can vary from pulmonary, cardiac, CNS, GIT and most commonly renal involvement. Etiology includes mainly infections, drugs and autoimmune connective tissue diseases.

The cutaneous features may vary from palpable purpura, petechiae and ulcers to acral gangrene depending on the size of the vessel affected.

Large vessel vasculitis: Common presenting features of large vessels vasculitis are claudication, abnormal peripheral pulses, stroke, etc.

Medium vessel: It presents with livedo-reticularis, tender subcutaneous nodules, small ulceration and necrotic lesions.

Small vessels: Palpable purpura, erythema multiforme like lesion or urticarial lesions.

However, certain conditions can present with similar clinical picture as vasculitis, which is known as "pseudovasculitis". Histopathology helps to distinguish between the two. Two most common causes of vasculitis in children are, Henoch-Schönlein purpura and Kawasaki disease.

According to the Revised Chapel Hill classification (2012), vasculitis is to be classified on the basis of the size of vessel involvement (Table 17.1). It is the most widely used classification of vasculitis worldwide for adults as well as for pediatric patients.

Table 17.1: Revised Chapel Hill classification (2012)
CLASSIFICATION OF VASCULITIS
• Large vessel vasculitis
• Temporal arteritis
• Takayasu's arteritis
Medium vessel vasculitis
• Polyarteritis nodosa
• Kawasaki disease
Small vessel vasculitis
Immune complex mediated
• Henoch-Schönlein purpura
• Essential cryoglobulinemic vasculitis
• Associated with collagen vascular disease
• Hypocomplementaemic urticarial vasculitis
• Goodpasture's syndrome
ANCA associated (Pauci immune vasculitis)
• Wegener's granulomatosis

Contd.

- Churg-Strauss syndrome
- Microscopic polyangiitis

Single organ small vessel vasculitis (Skin)

- Cutaneous small vessel vasculitis
- Granuloma faciale
- Erythema elevatum diutinum
- Acute hemorrhagic edema of infancy

HENOCH-SCHÖNLEIN PURPURA

Henoch-Schönlein purpura (HSP) or anaphylactoid purpura is an IgA-mediated small vessel vasculitis characterized by involvement of skin, gastrointestinal system and joints with or without renal involvement. Clinically, it is a triad of palpable purpura, abdominal pain and arthritis. Renal involvement can also be present and is a serious complication. Although it can occur in adults, HSP is much more common in childhood; 75% of cases occur in children under 6 years and 90% in children under 10 years old.

Etiopathogenesis

HSP is a small vessel vasculitis characterized by immunoglobulin A (IgA), C3, and immune complex deposition in arterioles, capillaries, and venules. The circulating complexes become insoluble and are deposited in the walls of small vessels of skin, gastrointestinal system and renal glomeruli. Some infections such as those caused by group A β haemolytic streptococci are implicated as the cause of HSP, although evidence for streptococcal infection is only found in approximately 30% children. Additionally other pathogens have been implicated (including *Bartonella henselae,* parvovirus B_{19}, *Staphylocococcus aureus,* Mycobacterium tuberculosis, mycoplasma, coxsackie viruses, adenovirus hepatitis A and B viruses). Familial clustering has been reported, which may support an infectious etiology. MEFV Gene mutations have been observed in IgA vasculitis in some cases. HSP is associated with familial Mediterranean fever and is more common in such patients than general population.

Histopathology

Biopsy of purpuric lesions show polymorphonuclear cells or cell fragments around small dermal blood vessels (i.e., capillaries and post capillary venules). Immune complexes containing IgA, C_3 and fibrin have been found in skin, kidneys, intestinal mucosa and joints.

Clinical Features

- HSP manifests with the classic findings of purpura, arthralgia and abdominal pain.
- Cutaneous lesions are typically erythematous urticarial papules, which may evolve within 24 hours into palpable purpura with haemorrhage. They are mostly present over extensor aspects of limbs (especially elbow and knees, Figure 17.1) and buttocks (Figure 17.2) in a symmetrical fashion. HSP may also affect face and trunk. Additional features such as subcutaneous edema, vesicles, bullae and necrotic ulcers may be seen. A retiform pattern within a lesion is characteristic.

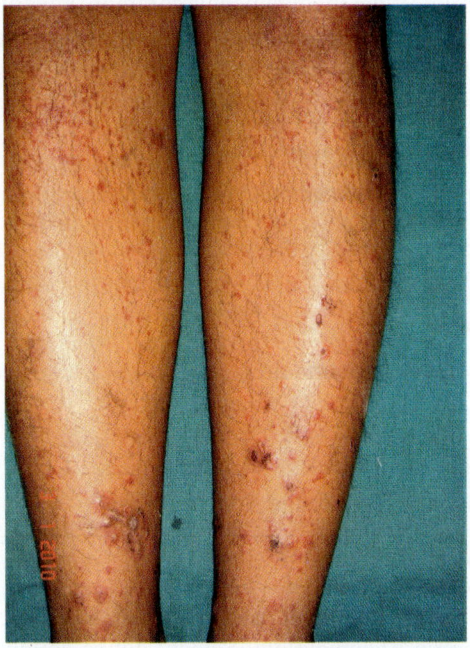

Figure 17.1: Henoch-Schönlein purpura

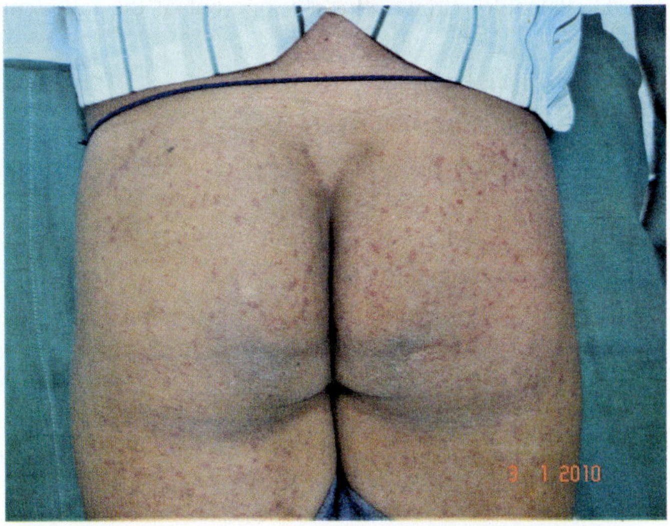

Figure 17.2: Henoch-Schönlein purpura showing purpuric lesions on buttocks

- Rash usually fades within 5-7 days. Crops of new lesions can recur for a few weeks to several months.

- Cutaneous involvement lasts for 6-16 weeks and then subsides.
- The spread of purpura to upper parts of trunk is a predictive factor for renal involvement.
- Renal involvement occurs in approximately 40-50% of patients; 25% have gross hematuria and the remainder microscopic hematuria. Proteinuria is seen in 60% of cases.
- Gastrointestinal involvement is common, affecting 65% of children with HSP. Frank gastrointestinal bleeding is seen in 30% of patients with HSP.
- Painful arthritis is seen in about 75% of patients, primarily affecting knees and ankles.

Less common manifestations of HSP include:

- Orchitis (10-20% of boys)
- Intussusceptions
- Pancreatitis
- Neurological abnormalities
- Uveitis
- Carditis
- Pulmonary hemorrhage

Diagnosis

- EULAR (European League Against Rheumatism) and Paediatric Rheumatology Society define childhood onset vasculitis as:
  - Palpable purpura plus any one out of the following four:
    - Acute arthritis.
    - Diffuse abdominal pain.
    - Biopsy from any organ involved showing IgA deposition.
    - Renal involvement in form of hematuria/ proteinuria.
- Diagnosis is based on clinical features and may be confirmed by histopathology from purpuric lesions. Biopsy with direct immunofluorescence shows perivascular IgA deposits.
- No laboratory test is specific for HSP, but urine and stool examinations may be helpful in its diagnosis.

Differential Diagnosis

- Thrombocytopenic purpura.
- Hypersensitivity vasculitis (CSVV).
- DIC (Purpura fulminans).

Treatment

- HSP is a self-limiting disease; most of the patients recover fully within months, so requiring mainly supportive treatment.
- For treatment of arthritis, abdominal pain and early resolution of mild nephritis, systemic corticosteroids, prednisolone (1 mg/kg/day for 2 weeks, tapering over a further 2 weeks) may be used.
- For severe nephritis, high dose methylprednisolone at a dosage of 30 mg/kg once daily for 3 days followed by oral corticosteroids and an immunosuppressive agent such as azathioprine or cyclophosphamide is used.
- Rapidly progressive nephritis can be halted with the use of intravenous immunoglobulin.
- Rituximab has been found to be effective in resistant cases of HSP.
- Dapsone (1-2 mg/kg/day) seems to shorten the duration of HSP as well as has a beneficial effect on the cutaneous lesions.
- For supportive therapy, antihistamines may be used. NSAIDs have minimal role and should not be used if child has nephritis.
- All cases of HSP should be followed up for 6 months for renal involvement.

CRYOGLOBULINEMIC VASCULITIS (CV)

- Cryoglobulins are circulating immunoglobulins that precipitate at temperatures below 37°C.
- They may be associated with infections, autoimmune disorders or malignancies. They form immune complexes, which are deposited in the walls of blood vessels which activate complement, and result in cryoglobulinemic vasculitis.
- Cryoglobulins have been classified into three types based on the presence or absence of monoclonality and their association with rheumatoid factor.
  - Type I (monoclonal cryoglobulinemia) – Monoclonal antibody and is usually associated with a hematologic malignancy.
  - Types II and III – Mixed antibody response – Mixed cryoglobulinemia.
- The most common infectious disease associated with CV is Hepatitis C virus infection, which is associated with mixed cryoglobulins. The term essential mixed cryoglobulinemia is used to describe mixed cryoglobulinemia in the absence of infections, immune conditions, or malignancies.
- Cryofibrinogen is a cryoprotein, which precipitates only in plasma and not in the serum.

- Cryofibrinogenemia may be primary (essential) or secondary to other underlying disorders, such as connective tissue disorders, carcinoma, infections, vasculitis or can be associated with cryoglobulinemia.
- The clinical presentation includes, papules, nodules, urticaria, purpura, skin necrosis, livedo reticularis, and bullous or ulcerated lesions. The classic triad called the Meltzer's triad of CV is palpable purpura, weakness and arthralgia.
- It is treated by treating the underlying cause. The main goals of therapy for mixed cryoglobulinemia are to treat the HCV infection, delete the underlying B-cell clonal expansions that occur, and deplete the cryoglobulins. A variety of immunosuppressive, anti-inflammatory and antiviral agents (pegylated interferon-α, ribavirin) have been used for treatment.

URTICARIAL VASCULITIS

Urticarial vasculitis is a cutaneous small vessel vasculitis characterized clinically by urticarial lesions. Although, it is a disease of adult women, but it has also been reported in children. It is characterized clinically by generalized erythematous, oedematous wheals which persist for more than 24 hours and is frequently associated with angioedema. Hypocomplementaemia, particularly C1q and other early complement components (C2-C4), is a frequent finding. Hypocomplementaemic urticarial vasculitis (HUVS) is also known as Mac Duffie syndrome.

Etiopathogenesis

- Urticarial vasculitis is strongly associated with some connective tissue diseases, like Sjögren's syndrome and SLE. Other associations are physical urticarias, hepatitis B or C, IgM or IgA gammopathies and serum sickness. It is considered to represent a type III hypersensitivity reaction, as circulating immune complexes are present in majority of patients.
- In hypocomplementaemic urticarial vasculitis, the anti-C1q IgG antibodies may be pathogenic, producing antigen antibody complexes with C1q.

Histopathology

Lesions of urticarial vasculitis typically show leukocytoclastic vasculitis. Hypocomplementaemic urticarial vasculitis shows a large number of interstitial neutrophils, rather than eosinophils. Some cases of urticarial vasculitis may have a lymphocytic vasculitis.

Clinical Features

- Urticarial vasculitis may involve other organs like joints, kidneys, lungs, eyes and gastrointestinal system.
- Cutaneous lesions of urticarial vasculitis are painful erythematous indurated wheals (Figure 17.3) which may contain purpuric foci. Angioedema. macular erythema, livedo reticularis, nodules and bullae may also be evident.
- Hypocomplementaemic urticarial vasculitis may have constitutional symptoms, such as fever, malaise and myalgia as well as signs and symptoms, such as lymphadenopathy, hepatosplenomegaly, abdominal pain, nausea, diarrhoea, laryngeal edema, dyspnoea, glomerulonephritis, conjunctivitis, uveitis and episcleritis etc. Microscopic hematuria may be present.

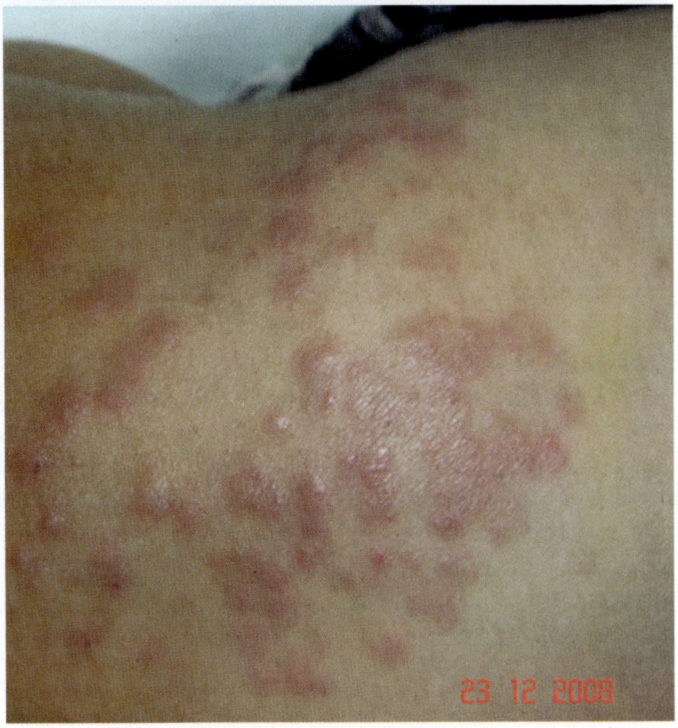

Figure 17.3: Urticarial vasculitis

Diagnosis

History, physical examination, skin biopsy and laboratory studies, including C3, C4 estimation and antinuclear body (ANA) help in establishing the extent of disease and to exclude underlying diseases. Other investigations may be done if required.

Differential Diagnosis

- Urticaria.
- Collagen vascular disorders, especially SLE.

Treatment

- The treatment includes corticosteroids (prednisolone 1 mg/kg/day followed by tapering in 2-3 weeks), antihistamines and antineutrophilic agents like dapsone (1-2 mg/kg), colchicine, sulphapyridine etc.
- NSAIDS (indomethacin), hydroxychloroquine and immunosuppressive agents like azathioprine, cyclophosphamide and methotrexate may be used.
- For life threatening edema subcutaneous adrenaline may be needed.
- Other modes of therapy include plasmapheresis and immunoglobulin G administration.

CHURG-STRAUSS DISEASE

Churg-Strauss syndrome (CSS, Allergic granulomatosis) is a rare disorder characterized by a granulomatous vasculitis involving small and medium sized arteries along with atopic manifestations. It is rare in children, and occurs primarily in males between 30 and 40 years of age. The three distinct phases of this disorder are – prodromal, eosinophilic and vasculitic.

Patients with CSS often experience a prodromal phase which is characterized by allergic rhinitis and asthma, and occasionally sinusitis and nasal polyps. After several years, they develop peripheral eosinophilia, eosinophilic tissue infiltration, worsening of their asthma, eosinophilic gastroenteritis, and diffuse pulmonary infiltrates (second phase). The third, or vasculitic, phase presents with fever, weight loss and widespread vasculitis and inflammation. If left untreated, this phase may result in death. Clinical manifestations include arthralgias, myositis, peripheral neuropathy, eosinophilic pneumonitis (Löffler syndrome), and occasional renal, cardiac, CNS or ocular involvement.

Cardiac involvement occurs in roughly half of the patients and which manifests as pericarditis, myocarditis, and tamponade. Skin involvement may occur in up to 70% of patients and includes palpable purpura, subcutaneous nodules, livedo reticularis, petechiae, urticaria and papulo-necrotic lesions. Digital ischemic ulcers and Raynaud's phenomenon may also be seen.

The ACR criteria for the diagnosis of CSS support the diagnosis when four of the following six criteria are met:

- Asthma.
- Eosinophilia (Greater than 10%).
- Nonfixed pulmonary infiltrates.
- Paranasal sinus abnormality.
- Mononeuropathy/polyneuropathy.
- Biopsy showing vasculitis with extra-vascular eosinophils.

Laboratory studies may be useful in diagnosis. Approximately 70% of adult patients with CSS have a positive ANCAs, usually perinuclear with anti-myeloperoxidase specificity (MPO-ANCA). However, in contrast to adult patients, pediatric patients with CSS may be negative for ANCA.

CSS is treated with glucocorticoids with or without the addition of other immunosuppressive agents (i.e., cyclophosphamide, azathioprine), with mostly favorable prognosis.

WEGENER'S GRANULOMATOSIS

Wegener's granulomatosis, also known as GPA (Granulomatosis with polyangiitis) is a necrotizing granulomatous vasculitis of small to medium sized arteries involving the upper and lower respiratory tract, kidneys and variable degree of vasculitis in other organ systems. The incidence rate is noted to be higher in adults than in the pediatric age group. It has a peak incidence of 64-75 years of age.

It usually presents with constitutional symptoms (malaise, fatigue, fever, weight loss), cough, rhinorrhea, nasal stuffiness, nasal mucosal erosions or ulcers, ear ache, or sinusitis. Conjunctival injection, arthralgias, myalgias, hemoptysis and renal involvement are some other presenting features. The nose, nasal sinuses, nasopharynx, glottis, trachea, bronchi, and lungs may all be affected by the necrotizing vasculitis. Subglottic stenosis and nasal deformity may result, the former occurring more commonly in children. End stage renal failure may occasionally result. Skin involvement occurs in up to 53% of patients with GPA. The manifestations are variable but most commonly consist of palpable purpura, necrotic papules and plaques, subcutaneous nodules, vesicles, pustules and ulcers resembling pyoderma gangrenosum. c-ANCA positivity is corelated with kidney involvement.

The most commonly used treatment is a combination of immunosuppressive agents, most often glucocorticoids and cyclophosphamide and occasionally azathioprine. Less commonly utilized therapies include plasmapheresis, extracorporeal membrane oxygenation, intravenous immunoglobulin (IVIG), mycophenolate mofetil and rituximab.

KAWASAKI DISEASE (KAWASAKI SYNDROME OR KS)

Kawasaki disease is a mucocutaneous lymph node syndrome, predominantly affecting young children.

It is discussed briefly here as the systemic component includes a multisystem medium vessel vasculitis, however, the exanthem it causes is not vasculitic. Children with KS who do not receive appropriate treatment within first 10 days of onset of fever have a 20% to 25% increased risk of developing coronary artery anomalies. Kawasaki disease is one of the leading causes of acquired heart disease of young children in developed countries. The case fatality rate of KS is approximately 0.4%.

Epidemiology

- KS is an illness of young children, with approximately 80% of patients being younger than 5 years of age. The ratio of males to females is about 1.5:1.
- Rate of recurrence is highest within the first 12 months after the first episode.

Etiopathogenesis

- KS results from immune activation. The acute phase is characterized by increased number of activated helper T cells and monocyte/macrophages, as well as a marked polyclonal B-cell activation.
- At present, however, there is no consensus regarding the etiology of KS, but it is widely hypothesized that it represents immune activation in response to an infectious agent based on acute, self-limiting nature of the disease, seasonal incidence, geographic clustering of outbreaks and the unique susceptibility of young children.
- Possible causes are a novel human corona virus infection and certain bacterial toxin which acts as super antigens, such as TSST-1 (toxic shock syndrome toxin-1 of *Staphylococcus aureus)* and streptococcal pyrogenic exotoxin B (SPEB) and C (SPEC).

Clinical Features

Skin manifestations

- KS is a triphasic illness beginning with an acute phase of 7-14 days, followed by a subacute phase of approximately 25 days and a convalescent phase that lasts for nearly 70 days.
- The cardinal feature of acute phase is prolonged *high fever* that frequently spikes to 40ºC (104ºF) and associated with a toxic appearance in virtually all patients. It is often accompanied by irritability, anorexia, vomiting and diarrhea.
- Approximately 90% of children develop an *exanthem* involving trunk and proximal extremities, but can be generalized. This exanthem usually develops in the first days of acute febrile illness. It can be quite variable, having been described as macular, papular, morbilliform, scarlatiniform, urticarial and even target like resembling erythema multiforme. It is rarely pustular, vesicular or bullous.
- In approximately 67% children with KS, characteristic *perineal eruption* develops within the first 6 days of illness and presents as diffuse macular or plaque type erythema involving part or all of the perineal skin. Within 48 hours, the erythematous areas begin to desquamate, earlier than desquamation of palms and soles.
- **Erythema and edema of distal aspects of hand and feet** with fusiform swelling of fingers are also noted within a few days of the start of illness in almost all cases. These hyperemic areas are subject to desquamation within 2 to 3 weeks after onset of fever during the subacute phase.
- In 90% of patients, a *bilateral non-exudative, conjunctival injection* begins shortly after onset of fever and generally involves the bulbar conjunctiva more severely. Conjunctival injection is associated with anterior uveitis in approximately 83% of patients examined within first few weeks of illness. There is a characteristic perilimbal sparing in these cases.
- Oral mucosal finding are present in almost all cases. The lips become "cherry" red, dry and often cracked, producing small haemorrhagic fissures. The *tongue* has been described as *"strawberry"* with hypertrophied papillae and hyperemia that is indistinguishable from that seen with streptococcal scarlet fever (But only 50% of cases seem to have this feature).
- Diffuse erythema is also common.
- Generalized fine desquamation, especially in the areas of the skin that had previously been erythematous, is seen.
- **Lymphadenopathy** is seen in less than 75% of patients which generally consists of a single, enlarged, non-suppurative cervical node measuring at least 1.5 cm, either non-tender or only slightly tender.
- Another unique finding in the patients of Kawasaki disease is the reactivation at the site of BCG vaccination or BCGitis.

Diagnostic criteria for Kawasaki syndrome

Fever of 5 or more days without other explanation and at least four of the five following criteria:

1. Bilateral painless bulbar non exudative conjunctival injection.
2. One of the following changes in the oropharynx: injected or fissured lips, injected pharynx or strawberry tongue.
3. One of the following extremity changes: erythema of the palms of soles, edema of the hands or feet or periungual desquamation.
4. Polymorphous exanthem.
5. Acute non-suppurative cervical lymphadenopathy (>1.5 cm in diameter).

A diagnosis of atypical Kawasaki syndrome can be made when less than four criteria are present if coronary artery aneurysms are present.

Systemic manifestations

- Arthralgia and arthritis seen in approximately 1/3rd of patients, typically involving small joints, such as interphalangeal joints in acute phase, whereas involvement of large weight bearing joints is more likely to occur in the second and third weeks of illness.
- Urethritis associated with sterile pyuria is a frequent finding.
- Aseptic meningitis may be present.
- Swelling of gallbladder may be present with or without obstructive jaundice.
- Diarrhea, vomiting, abdominal pain, cranial nerve palsies, tympanitis and infarction of organs may be presenting signs.
- Hepatic dysfunction may be seen.

Cardiac manifestations

- Abnormal cardiac findings are hallmark of KS. The subacute stage presents the greatest risk for developing coronary artery aneurysms.
- Myocarditis is frequently observed in first week after onset of fever. Pericardial effusion may also be present.
- Coronary artery aneurysms occur in nearly 25% of patients with KS who are not treated with IVIG.
- A minority of patients (around 5%) may suffer from aortic or mitral regurgitation.
- On examination, tachycardia and gallop rhythms may be found.

Diagnosis

- **In acute phase:** Leukocytosis with predominant neutrophils.
- **Anemia:** Normocytic normochromic.
- ESR is raised and persists even after resolution of fever.
- Thrombocytosis with marked hypercoagulability.
- C-reactive protein and serum α_1-antitrypsin are raised.
- Elevated liver transaminases, bilirubin and alkaline phosphatase, low serum albumin levels.
- Sterile pyuria (75% of patients).
- **Electrocardiography:** Prolonged PR interval, left ventricular hypertrophy, abnormal Q waves, non-specific ST-T wave changes.
- MRI of proximal coronary artery segments may show aneurysm.
- Angiography of coronary artery is also useful and gives evidence about stenosis and extent of collateral artery formation.

Histopathology

Cutaneous vasculitis is not a prominent feature of KS. There is vasculitis and perivasculitis of small blood vessels. The endothelial cell damage is associated with the infiltration of both neutrophils and mononuclear cells in small to medium size vessels.

Differential Diagnosis

- Stevens Johnson syndrome/Erythema multiforme.
- Staphylococcal scalded skin syndrome.
- Drug reaction.
- Scarlet fever.
- Toxic shock syndrome.
- Bacterial exanthem.
- Other causes of conjunctivitis.

Treatment

- The combined use of intravenous immunoglobulin G (IVIG) and acetylsalicylic acid (ASA or Aspirin) is mainstay of treatment.
- High dose ASA (80-100 mg/kg/day in four divided doses) is recommended during acute phase. It decreases the intensity of vasculitis and inhibits platelet aggregation thus reducing the risk of thrombosis.
- After the child becomes afebrile for 48 to 72 hours, a switch to low dose ASA (3-5 mg/kg/day) can be made and continued till 6-8 weeks after onset of illness in the absence of coronary artery abnormalities.
- ASA therapy is continued indefinitely if coronary artery aneurysm develops and persists.
- For skin manifestations symptomatic management with emollients and antihistamines is sufficient.
- IVIG in dosage of 2 mg/kg plus salicylate before tenth day of fever should be used, which reduces the risk of coronary artery disease from about 20% to <5%. The mechanism of action of IVIG is unknown. Approximately 0.5% of children show prompt defervescence and resolution of signs of inflammation.
- If fever persists after two or three doses of IVIG, intravenous methylprednisolone (pulse doses of 30 mg/kg for 3 days) can be considered, but the role is controversial.

- Other interventions that have been used in acute KS, refractory to more than one dose of IVIG include plasma exchange, ulinastatin (human trypsin inhibitor), abciximab (platelet glycoprotein IIb/IIIa receptor inhibitor), infliximab and cyclophosphamide etc.
- For the KS patients with obstructive changes in one or more coronary arteries, anticoagulant therapy may be required.
- For more severe cardiovascular symptoms, the options include the use of intravenous streptokinase or urokinase when a thrombus is present, balloon angioplasty, and/or coronary artery bypass grafting.

Prognosis

- The major long-term morbidity in KS is related to cardiovascular complications from this disease.
- It is generally recommended that children with KS be followed over the long-term by a cardiologist to rule out the development of myocardial dysfunction, late onset valvular regurgitation or premature coronary artery disease.

CUTANEOUS SMALL VESSEL VASCULITIS (CSVV)

- CSVV is also known as 'cutaneous leukocytoclastic vasculitis' or 'hypersensitivity angiitis or cutaneous necrotizing venulitis'. Features of CSVV include palpable purpura, urticaria or ulcers on the legs.
- It affects both children and adults and is seen more commonly in females. Extracutaneous manifestations are uncommon and should prompt a search for other pathology.

Etiopathogenesis

A history of drug exposure or recent infection is frequently present in cases of CSVV. About 50% of cases of cutaneous vasculitis are 'idiopathic', 15-20% due to infections, 15-20% related to inflammatory diseases such as collagen vascular diseases, 10-15% due to drugs and less than 5% are associated with malignancy. CSVV mainly affects postcapillary venules.

Clinical Features

Lesions typically occur on ankles and lower legs (Figure 17.4) and are often asymptomatic. The major cutaneous feature is palpable purpura, ranging in size from 1 mm to several centimetres. Sometimes macular in early stages, but the purpuric lesions may progress to form papules, nodules, vesicles, plaques, bullae or pustules, with secondary finding of ulcerations and necrosis (Figure 17.5). Sometimes macular or purpuric lesions on palms (Figure 17.6) and forearms may occur. Pruritus, pain or burning may be experienced, as well as systemic symptoms like fever, arthralgia, myalgia and anorexia may occur.

Involvement of other organ systems should raise the suspicion of other vasculitis such as HSP, mixed cryoglobulinaemia, or CSVV associated with polyarteritis nodosa or with Wegener's granulomatosis.

The American College of Rheumatology criteria for the diagnosis of CSVV include:

1. Age >16 years.
2. Use of a possible offending drug in temporal relation to the symptoms.
3. Palpable purpura.

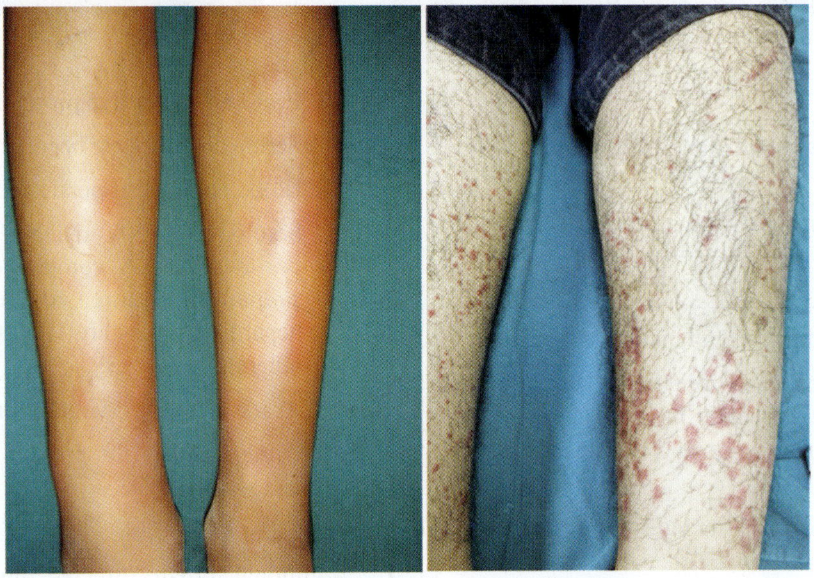

Figure 17.4: CSVV on legs

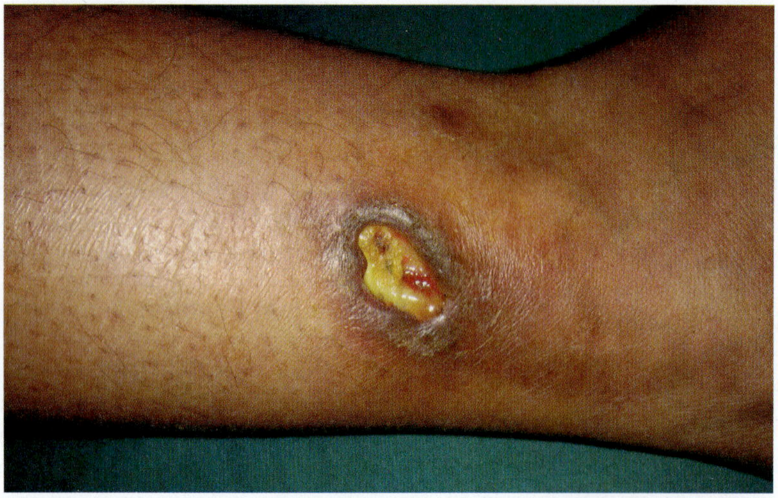

Figure 17.5: CSVV showing necrotic ulcer on medial side of lower leg

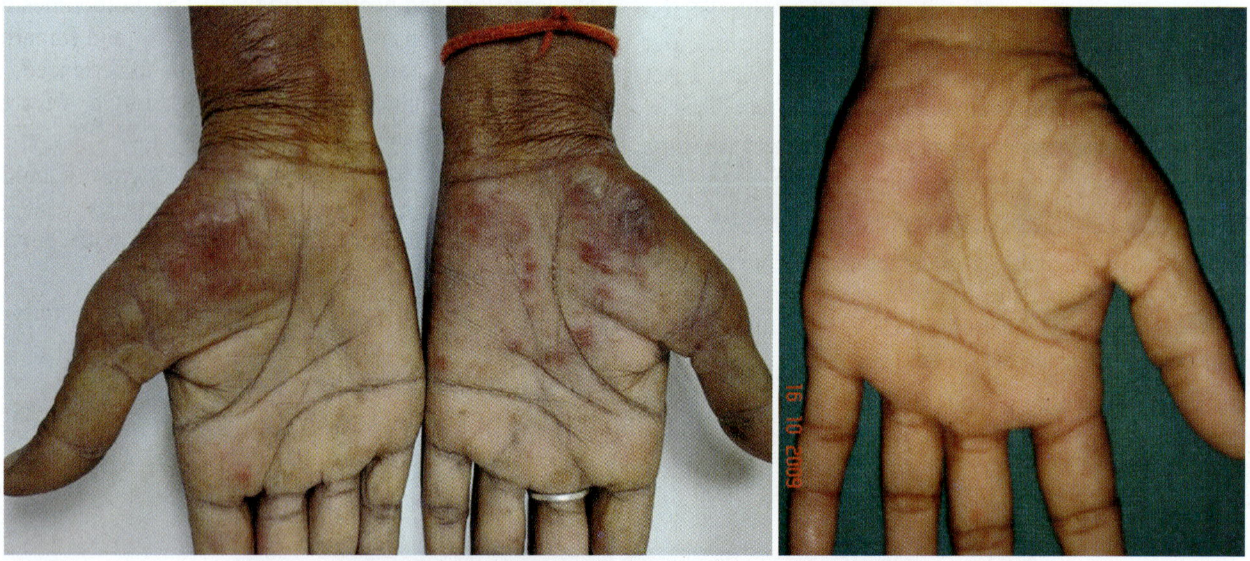

Figure 17.6: Cutaneous small vessel vasculitis on hands

4. Maculopapular rash.
5. Biopsy of skin lesion showing neutrophils around arterioles or venules.

Presence of 3 or more criteria is suggestive of CSVV.

Diagnosis

- Thorough clinical examination and history is essential.
- Screening for infections, e.g., sore throat, urinary tract infection, dental infections, otitis media etc, connective tissue diseases, medication usage and malignancy should be done.
- Reasonable initial test might include (along with skin biopsy).
  - Full blood count with differential while cell count.
  - ESR and C-reactive protein.
  - Serum electrolytes; hepatic transaminases.
  - Blood cultures (if persistent fever).
  - Serology – ANA, dsDNA (if ANA is found to be positive), ANCA, complement C3 and C4 level, anti-streptolysin-O titre, viral titres for hepatitis B and hepatitis C, possibly HIV, CMV, parvovirus B_{19} and others).
  - Assessment for cryoglobulins (also electrophoresis).
  - Urine analysis for protein and RBCs, urine culture and sensitivity.
  - Chest radiograph.
- Additional organ directed investigation as necessary (renal, bone marrow biopsy, arteriography etc.).

- Baseline tests should be done for planning possible corticosteroid and immunosuppressive therapy, e.g., blood glucose, thiopurine methyltransferase test –TPMT for azathioprine, Glucose-6 phosphate dehydrogenase-G-6PD status for dapsone etc.

Histopathology

Leukocytoclastic vasculitis with segmental inflammation in an angiocentric pattern, swelling of endothelium, fibrinoid necrosis of vessel walls, extravasation of erythrocytes and an infiltrate of neutrophils with karyorrhexis of nuclei (i.e., leukocytoclasia) are major features of CSVV. In superficial dermal papillary vessels, IgM or complement C3 perivascular deposits are demonstrated in over 80% of fresh lesions.

Treatment

- Any triggering factors, such as drug or infection, should be removed or treated.
- Supportive treatment such as compression hosiery may be required.
- Elevation of dependent areas is advised.
- Use of NSAIDs and antihistamines for symptomatic relief.
- Oral corticosteroids at a dosage of 1-2 mg/kg/day tapered over 2-3 weeks, give effective symptom control.
- Use of dapsone is found to be beneficial.
- For skin lesions, colchicine in the dose of 0.6 mg twice a day may be used. Its anti-inflammatory and immunosuppressive effects make it quite an effective choice of drug.
- Pentoxyphyllin, indomethacin or sulphapyridine are also effective.
- In patients who are refractory to the above therapies, agents like azathioprine (2 mg/kg/day), methotrexate at low dose of less than 25 mg/week (15-25 mg), cyclosporine, cyclophosphamide, infliximab and rituximab may be considered.

GRANULOMA FACIALE

It presents with asymptomatic cutaneous nodules occurring primarily on face with occasional extrafacial involvement. It is limited to the skin without any systemic symptoms.

Etiopathogenesis

It is an uncommon condition with unknown etiology.

Clinical Features

Granuloma faciale presents with soft red brown nodules and plaques with prominent follicular orifices and telangiectasia. The lesions never ulcerate.

Histology

Granuloma faciale is a misnomer as there is absence of granuloma. Characteristic histological findings include, mixed infiltrates with prominent eosinophils and plasma cells mainly in upper dermis. Nuclear dusting is present near blood vessels. Presence of grenz zone is the characteristic features of granuloma faciale.

Differential diagnosis: Differential includes sarcoidosis, tuberculosis and cutaneous lupus.

Management

First line treatment is calcineurin inhibitors. Other treatment includes topical or intralesional steroid, dapsone and PUVA.

ERYTHEMA ELEVATUM DIUTINUM (EED)

Erythema elevatum diutinum is a rare disease generally considered to be a chronic, localized, fibrosing variant of cutaneous small vessel vasculitis. EED is a disease of middle age with a peak incidence in the sixth decade and a small peak in childhood with a female preponderance.

Etiopathogenesis

EED is thought to be related to an arthus type reaction with immune complex deposition.

It has been associated with autoimmune diseases like rheumatoid arthritis, coeliac disease, inflammatory bowel disease and type I diabetes mellitus as well as with infections including streptococcus, hepatitis, syphilis and HIV. Hematological malignancies are also associated with EED.

Clinical Features

- Early lesions typically start as reddish brown to purple (purpuric) papules occurring symmetrically over acral and extensor surface, with a predilection for skin overlying joints (Figure 17.7). Common sites of involvement are hands, feet, elbows, knees, buttocks and achilles tendons. Trunk is universally spared. The lesions are soft, but eventually become fibrosed and later leave atrophic scars.
- EED is usually asymptomatic, but pain and to a lesser extent, pruritus has been described. Relapse after menses may occur. Constitutional symptoms are variable characterized by arthralgia and fever.

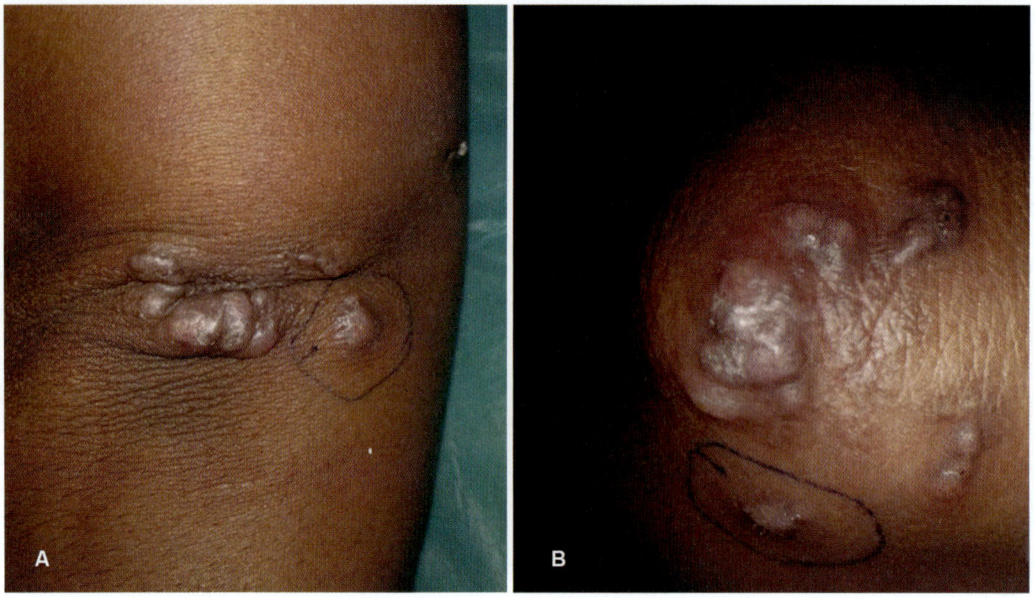

Figure 17.7: Brown to reddish papule and nodule over bilateral elbow area in erythema elevatum diutinum

Diagnosis

Clinical features and skin biopsy establish the diagnosis of EED.

Histopathology

EED is believed to be a part of the spectrum of cutaneous small vessel vasculitis. The histopathological features show at different stages, leucocytoclastic vasculitis, a nodular neutrophilic infiltrate and dermal fibrosis.

Differential Diagnosis

- Cutaneous small vessel vasculitis (Histologically).
- Sweet's syndrome.
- Granuloma annulare.
- Xanthomas.
- Multicentric reticulohistiocytosis.
- Hypertrophic lichen planus.
- Cutaneous sarcoidosis.

Treatment

Dapsone is considered to be the treatment of choice for EED. Dapsone is suppressive rather than curative. Treatment of associated disease is helpful. Surgical excision has been reported to be beneficial in older lesions.

Other therapies which have been used with good result are niacinamide sulphapyridine, colchicine, tetracycline, chloroquine, clofazimine and corticosteroids.

Prognosis

EED may last from 5 to 35 years, with crops of new lesion developing every few weeks to months.

ACUTE HAEMORRHAGIC EDEMA OF CHILDHOOD (AHEC)

Acute haemorrhagic edema of childhood/infancy (AHEC), also known as Finkelstein's disease is a rare benign leucocytoclastic vasculitis, whose manifestations are almost exclusively cutaneous.

Etiopathogenesis

Infections, drugs or immunization may trigger AHEC. Infections associated with AHEC are streptococcal, staphylococcal, *Escherichia coli,* CMV, adenovirus, coxsackie, or rotavirus infections.

AHEC shows leucocytoclastic vasculitis which has been linked pathologically to immune complex deposition, complement activation and chemotaxis of neutrophils.

Clinical Features

AHEC affects children between 4 months and 2 years of age. Cutaneous findings include non tender asymmetrical facial oedema, mainly affecting eyelids and sudden development of tender, oedematous lesions with petechiae and ecchymosis on the head and distal extremities. Large annular, arciform, coin shaped or targetoid lesions (Figure 17.8) may develop which may lead to bullae formation and necrosis.

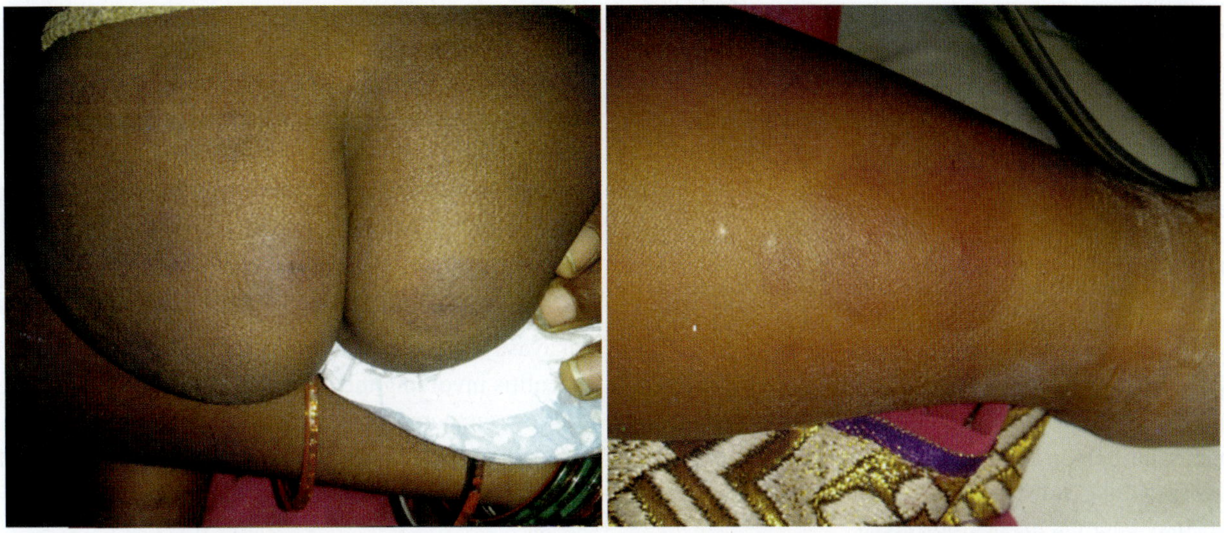

Figure 17.8: Coin shape targetoid lesion with edema of extremities in a child of AHEI

The general health of child remains good with mild fever usually. Spontaneous and complete resolution occurs within 1-3 weeks (mean 12 days) after 1-3 outbreaks of new lesions.

Differential Diagnosis

- HSP.
- Necrotic purpuras (e.g., purpura fulminans).
- Erythema multiforme.
- Urticaria.
- Kawasaki disease.
- Child abuse.

Treatment

There is no specific treatment for AHEC. Underlying cause should be treated first. Supportive treatment should be given. Steroids and antihistamines do not seem to improve course of disease, but can be used. Visceral involvement should be sought out and treated accordingly.

NODULAR VASCULITIS (Erythema Induratum of Bazin and of Whitfield)

Nodular vasculitis (NV) is a chronic relapsing lobular panniculitis with septal vasculitis, which is characterized by vasculitis of subcutaneous arteries and veins, with subsequent ischaemia of subcutaneous tissue, which results in clinical suppuration. It occurs primarily in middle-aged women, but cases have been reported in children.

Etiopathogenesis

Trigger factors for NV may be bacterial infections, such as streptococcal or mycobacterial infections and drugs. The pathogenesis may be similar to that of CSVV, but with septal vessels in the panniculus as the primary target.

Clinical Features

Typical lesions present as tender, dusky, often suppurative, nodules (Figure 17.9) or plaques, mainly on the posterolateral aspect of the legs, less common sites are anterior aspect of the thighs and legs. There may be erythrocyanosis and perifollicular erythema. Lesions may be unilateral and ulceration may occur. The lesions of NV heal slowly, sometimes leaving an atrophic scar. The course of NV is chronic, with relapses typically occurring over several years.

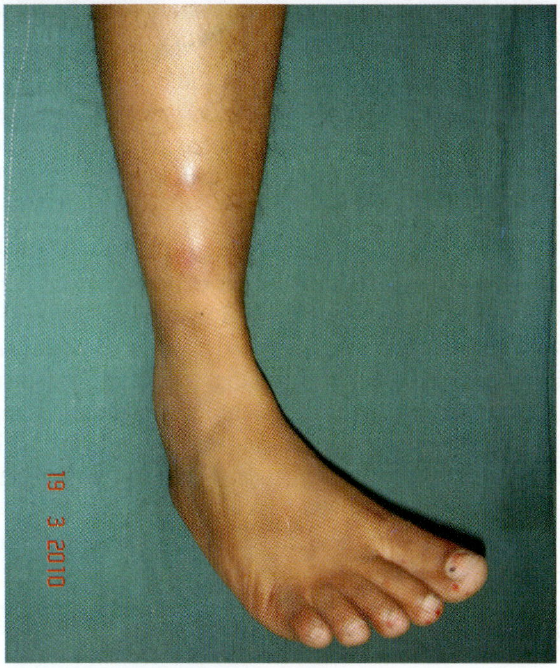

Figure 17.9: Nodular vasculitis

Diagnosis

- Nodular vasculitis is a clinicopathological diagnosis.
- Tuberculin skin test, chest X-ray, anti-tubercular antibodies (IgM and IgG) to rule out tubercular pathology.
- Other tests as for CSVV.

Histopathology

Regardless of the type of vessel involved, the early changes are of leukocytoclastic vasculitis of vessels in the subcutaneous tissue leading to ischaemic changes, followed by inflammation and injury to lipocytes. The necrotic subcutaneous fat demonstrates fat cysts bordered by a finely granular eosinophilic substance with pyknotic nuclei. Foamy histiocytes may encircle the necrotic areas.

Treatment

- Antitubercular therapy in the form of daily doses schedule or DOTS should be given if evidence of tuberculosis is found. Appropriate antibiotics may be used.
- In other cases, supportive treatment is recommended such as NSAIDs, dapsone, compression hosiery and bed rest.
- Systemic corticosteroids may also be considered.
- Other treatments outlined for CSVV is also helpful.

CUTANEOUS POLYARTERITIS NODOSA (CPAN, Benign Cutaneous Periarteritis Nodosa; Livedo with Nodules)

Cutaneous polyarteritis nodosa (CPAN) is a variant of polyarteritis nodosa (PAN) in which the disease is limited to the skin primarily. Infections such as Streptococcus, parvovirus B_{19}, HIV and hepatitis B virus, as well as inflammatory bowel disease (IBD), have been associated with CPAN; although the exact etiology is unknown.

The disease usually occurs between 20 and 60 years of age and is only occasionally seen in children. Some patients may report constitutional symptoms as well as chronic mild involvement of both muscles and nerves but cutaneous manifestations are the most striking feature of the disease. Dermal or subcutaneous nodules are most commonly located on the lower legs near the ankles and may extend proximally to the thighs, buttocks, arms or hands. There may be tenderness associated with the nodules, which may ulcerate and livedo reticularis may be seen. Sometimes necrosis and gangrene of fingers and toes may occur.

Treatment

NSAIDs may be used to relieve pain and compression hosiery may help symptomatically. High dose corticosteroids may be required to control the disease. Antibiotics against streptococcal infection can be given as it may be associated with CPAN. Other treatment modalities are immunosuppressants like methotrexate, azathioprine etc.

TAKAYASU'S ARTERITIS (Aortic Arch Syndrome, Pulseless Disease, Occlusive Thromboarteriopathy, Aortitis Syndrome)

Takayasu's arteritis is a rare chronic recurrent inflammatory vasculitis involving the aorta and the great vessels. Takayasu's arteritis is uncommon in males, the majority of cases occurring in females between the ages of 15 and 30 years. In children, it has a more aggressive course than in adults.

The exact pathogenesis of Takayasu's arteritis is unknown. The condition is characterized by segmental and patchy granulomatous inflammation of the aorta and major derivative branches. Infections (such as tuberculosis, viral infections), autoimmunity and genetic factors have been associated with Takayasu's arteritis.

Clinical Features

- Early, in the pre pulseless disease phase, patients may have constitutional symptoms.
- Later, in the pulseless disease phase, they may present with bruits, blood pressure inequality between the arms or with actual loss of pulses. Other signs and symptoms from ischemia caused by the vessel inflammation include hypertension, transient ischemic attacks, headaches, angina and seizures.
- Cutaneous lesions are present in 15–20% of patients with Takayasu's arteritis. In the early phase, erythema nodosum like nodules or lesions of erythema induratum are present, whereas in the late pulseless phase there may be pyoderma gangrenosum like lesions, or lesions related to necrotizing or granulomatous vasculitis.

Investigations

Takayasu's arteritis is identified by its clinical features. Vascular study is essential; angiography is gold standard.

Treatment

Takayasu arteritis, in acute phase, should be treated with corticosteroids (1mg/kg/day), and it should be tapered in 6 months to 2 years. Other agents like cyclophosphamide can be added. For vascular lesions surgical procedure like patch angiography or bypass grafting may be required.

CHAPTER 18 Exanthems

Contents

Exanthem is a medical **term, derived from the word "exanthema" meaning breaking out.** It refers to a widespread rash that is usually accompanied by systemic symptoms such as fever, malaise and headache. It is usually caused by an infectious agent such as a virus or bacteria and represents damage to the skin by the organism or its toxin, or an immune response. Exanthems may also be due to a drug (especially due to antibiotics).

Table 18.1: The six diseases causing exanthems in childhood

Number	*Name*	*Etiology*
First disease	Measles	Measles virus
Second disease	Scarlet fever	*Streptococcus pyogenes*
Third disease	Rubella	Rubella virus
Fourth disease	Duke's disease	No longer accepted as a separate entity. Similar to scarlet fever
Fifth disease	Erythema infectiosum	Parvovirus B19
Sixth disease	Roseola infantum	HHV-6, HHV-7

Causes (Table 18.1)

1. **Viral infections**
   - Chickenpox (varicella).
   - Rubella (German measles, Third disease).
   - Fifth disease (Erythema infectiosum).
   - Roseola infantum (Sixth disease).
   - Measles (First disease).
   - Respiratory viruses and enteroviruses.

- Dengue hemorrhagic fever.
- Infectious mononucleosis.

2. **Bacterial infections and other causes**
   - Toxic shock syndrome (TSS).
   - Staphylococcal scalded skin syndrome (SSSS).
   - Streptococcal toxic shock like syndrome (STSS).
   - Scarlet fever (Second disease).
   - Meningococcal disease.
   - Kawasaki disease.
   - Rickettsial diseases.
3. **Drug induced**

General Features of Exanthem

- Viral exanthems often occur in small epidemics, so there may be other children affected at the same time.
- Viral exanthems are non-specific rashes appearing as spots or blotches which may or may not be itchy.
- In most cases of viral rash, before development of rash, patients may have prodromal symptoms which include fever, malaise, headache, loss of appetite, abdominal pain, irritability, myalgia etc.
- Most commonly, childhood viral exanthems have distinct patterns of rashes and prodromal (pre-rash) symptoms.
- When there are no characteristic lesions and/or distinctive prodromal signs and symptoms, diagnosis of a specific cause is more difficult.
- Etiological diagnosis of some of the exanthems is very important as some of these conditions can become life-threatening, if not treated urgently with appropriate medications, e.g., meningococcal disease, Kawasaki disease etc.

Treatment of Exanthems

- For most patients with non-specific exanthems, no treatment is required, as the condition is usually short-lived and resolves spontaneously.
- If necessary, symptomatic treatment with paracetamol to reduce fever and/or with topical/oral antihistamines or preparations such as calamine lotion to relieve itch may be given.
- Treatment of specific viral or bacterial exanthems will depend on the cause and is discussed in detail under each individual cause.

RUBELLA (German measles/Third disease)

Rubella is caused by a single-stranded RNA togavirus. It affects both sexes equally. The peak incidence is in children aged 5-14 years. In developed countries where rubella vaccination is commonly done, most cases occur in teenagers or young adults.

Clinical Features

- The incubation period is 14-23 days.
- The prodrome is characterized by malaise, fever, anorexia, headache, mild conjunctivitis, rhinorrhea etc.
- The rash (Figure 18.1A) develops within 1-5 days of onset of symptoms. It begins on the face and forehead and spreads caudally to involve the trunk and extremities.
- The rash tends to clear in the same order as it appeared. It may be pruritic, but usually resolves within 3 days. Therefore, it is also known as three days measles.
- The rash consists of pink macules and papules, which may become confluent, resulting in a scarlatiniform eruption.
- Tiny red macules or petechiae of the soft palate known as Forchheimer sign, may be present (Figure 18.1B).
- Lymphadenopathy may be present, particularly in the posterior auricular, posterior cervical and suboccipital chains.
- Infection during early pregnancy may lead to miscarriage or a child born with congenital rubella syndrome. It may present as cataracts, glaucoma, salt-and-pepper retinopathy, microphthalmia, nerve deafness, diabetes mellitus, thyroid dysfunction and neuritis.
- The classical triad of congenital rubella syndrome includes: Cataract, sensorineural hearing loss and congenital heart disease.
- Neonatal manifestations of congenital infection include: Growth retardation, interstitial pneumonitis, radiolucent bone disease, hepatosplenomegaly, thrombocytopenia, and dermal erythropoiesis "blueberry muffin lesions".
- Standard and droplet precautions are recommended for patients with rubella for 7 days after rash onset.
- Neonates with congenital rubella syndrome require supportive care as well as appropriate attention to significant health issues.

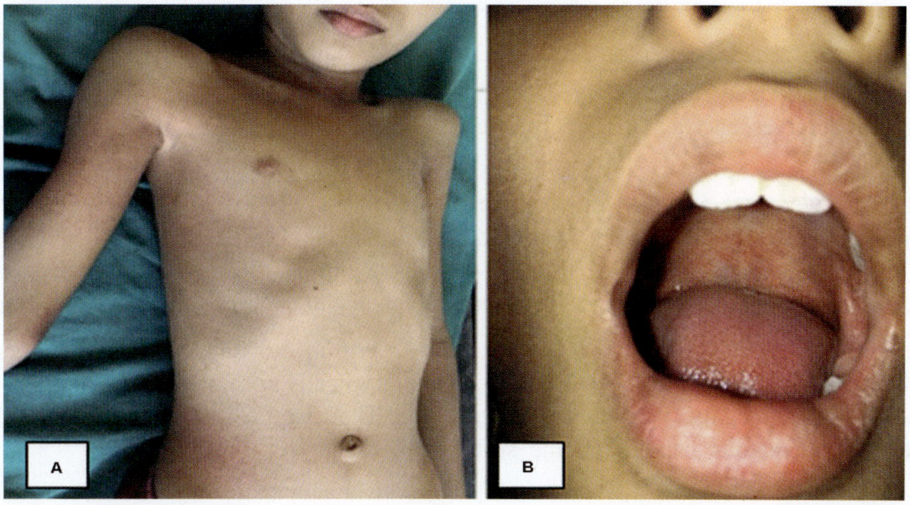

Figure 18.1: (A) Maculopapular rash in rubella and (B) Forchheimer sign (Courtesy– Dr. Bhumesh K Katakam)

ERYTHEMA INFECTIOSUM (Fifth Disease)

- Erythema infectiosum is caused by Parvovirus B_{19} (PV-B_{19}), which is a single stranded DNA virus.
- Males and females are affected equally.
- It is primarily a disease of children aged 3-15 years, but it can occur in several members of family and classmates may be affected. PV-B_{19} infection can lead to the classic symptoms of erythema infectiosum in adults but more often manifests as an acute arthropathy without cutaneous eruption.

Clinical Features

- Erythema infectiosum has an incubation period of 4-14 days and spreads primarily via aerosolized respiratory droplets.
- Transmission also occurs through blood products and from mother to fetus.
- The prodromal phase is often milder and is noticed only rarely but may include headache, coryza, low-grade fever, pharyngitis and malaise.
- Infrequently, nausea, diarrhea, arthralgia and abdominal pain may occur.
- Pertinent physical findings of erythema infectiosum predominantly are limited to the skin and joints.
- **First stage:** The exanthem begins with the classic slapped cheek appearance. The bright red erythema appears abruptly over the cheeks and is marked by nasal, perioral, and periorbital sparing. The exanthem may appear like a sunburn, occasionally is edematous, and typically fades over 2-4 days.
- **Second stage:** Within 1-4 days of the malar rash, an erythematous, macular to morbilliform eruption occurs primarily on the extremities. While the eruption tends to favor the extensor surfaces, it can also involve the palms and soles. Pruritus is rare. These characteristic rash appear in **fish net pattern**.
- **Third stage:** After several days, most of the second stage eruption fades into a lacy pattern, mostly on the proximal extremities. This reticulate pattern is distinctly characteristic for erythema infectiosum and may be the only manifestation of the illness. The third stage lasts from 3 days to 3 weeks.

In immunocompromised patients, it can cause serious, prolonged anemia from persistent lysis of red blood cell precursors. Parvovirus related chronic anemia has been reported in HIV infected patients, as well as in transplant recipients and those with congenital immunodeficiencies, acute leukemias, lupus erythematosus.

ROSEOLA INFANTUM (Sixth disease/ Exanthem subitum)

Roseola infantum is caused by *human herpesvirus type 6 (HHV-6)*. Respiratory secretions of asymptomatic individuals transmit the virus. The child is most likely to spread the infection during the febrile and viremic phase of the illness. Most cases present within the first 2 years of life, with peak occurrence in infants aged 9-21 months. Both sexes affected equally. The term *exanthem subitum* describes the sudden "surprise" appearance of the rash after the fall of the fever.

Clinical Features

- Roseola is typically characterized by a history of high fever followed by rapid defervescence and a characteristic rash.
- The rash begins as the fever goes away. Maculopapular or erythematous rash, typically beginning on the trunk, may spread to involve the neck and extremities. It is non-pruritic, pale pink, almond-shaped macules and blanches on pressure. The rash fades within a few hours to 2 days.
- Conjunctival erythema, lymphadenopathy, facial edema, seizures, diarrhea, splenomegaly, encephalopathy, **"Nagayama spots"** (erythematous papules on the soft palate and uvula) may be seen.
- **Treatment:** No active intervention required. Topical moisturizers.

MEASLES (FIRST DISEASE)

Measles is caused by *singlestranded RNA paramyxovirus.* The disease is transmitted by respiratory droplets produced by sneezing and coughing. Humans are the only known reservoir for this viral infection. There is no sex predilection for the disease. In developing countries, measles most commonly affects children of < 2 years of age.

Clinical Features

- Approximately 10 days after the initial exposure to the virus, the classic viral prodrome, i.e., fever, non-productive cough, coryza, conjunctivitis etc. occurs.
- Additional prodromal symptoms may include malaise, myalgia, photophobia and periorbital edema.
- Within 2-3 days, the pathognomonic *Kolpik spots* may typically arise on the buccal, gingival, and labial mucosae. They are 1-2 mm, blue-gray macules on an erythematous base.
- Maculopapular erythematous rash (Figure 18.2A) begins behind the ears and forehead and spreads caudally over the next 3 days as the prodromal symptoms resolve. It may involve the palms and soles also.
- The rash lasts for 4-6 days and then fades from the head downward. Desquamation may be present (Figure 18.2B) but is generally not severe.
- Complete recovery from the illness generally occurs within 7-10 days from the onset of the rash.

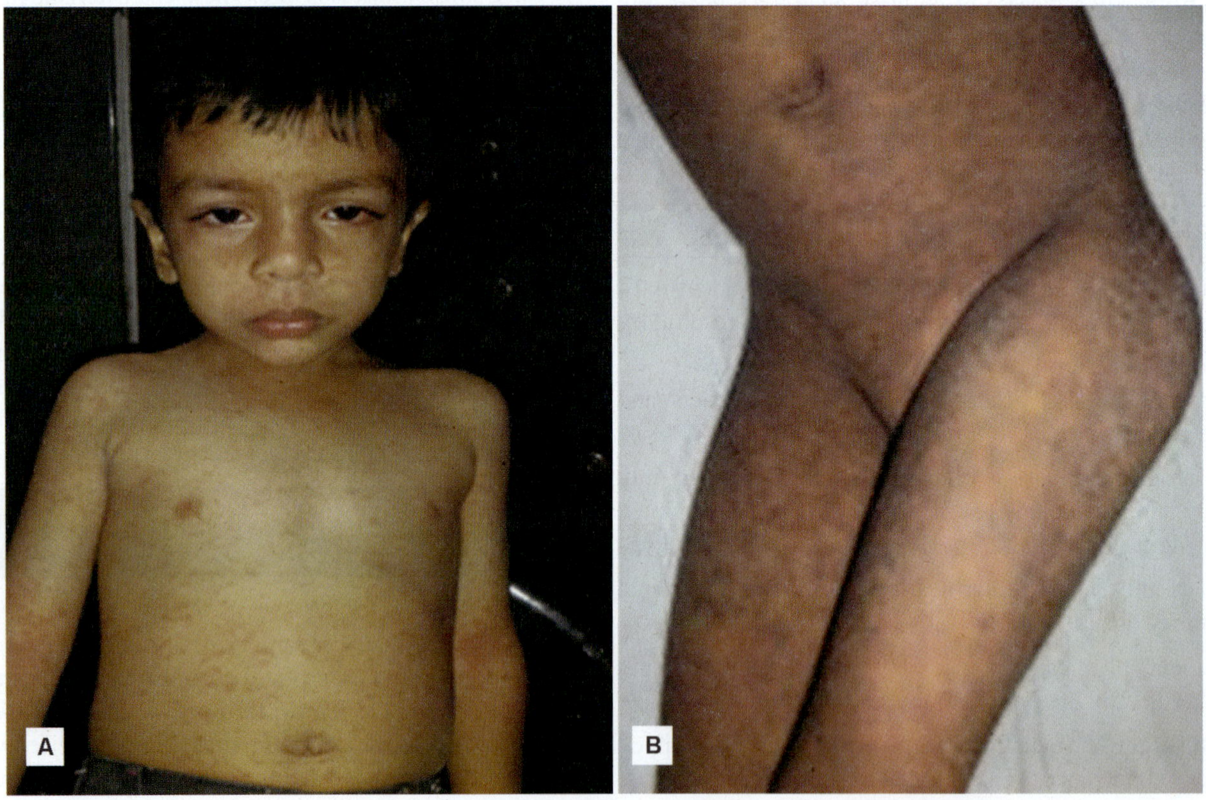

Figure 18.2: (A) Maculopapular rashes with 3 Cs (Cough, coryza and conjunctivitis) in measles and (B) Desquamative rash in measles (Courtesy– Dr. Bhumesh K Katakam)

Complications

- Complications may occur in adults and in children who are undernourished, who have Vitamin A deficiency, no previous vaccination, or who are immunocompromised.
- Croup, pneumonia and encephalitis are the common causes of death associated with measles.
- Clinically apparent encephalomyelitis occurs in about 1 of 1000-2000 patients with measles. This condition is fatal in about 10% of patients.
- Other complications are otitis media, thrombocytopenia with purpura and bleeding, myocarditis, hepatitis, pericarditis, and severe keratitis which may progress to blindness.
- Subacute sclerosing panencephalitis (SSPE), a disease with a latent period of several years is seen in children who have had measles when they were younger than 2 years.

SCARLET FEVER (Second Disease)

Scarlet fever is caused by Group A streptococcal infections. The disease occurs mostly in children aged 4-8 years because by the age of 10 years, upto 80% of children develop lifelong protective antibodies against streptococcal toxins. Males and females are affected equally. Incubation period is 1-4 days.

Clinical Features

- The disease starts usually with sudden fever associated with sore throat.
- Prodromal symptoms, e.g., headache, nausea, vomiting, loss of appetite, swollen and red *strawberry tongue,* (Figure 18.3B), abdominal pain, malaise etc. may be seen. Lymphadenopathy may also be seen during prodrome.
- The characteristic rash appears 12-48 hours after the start of the fever. The rash usually starts below the ears, neck, chest, armpits and groin before spreading to the rest of the body within 24 hours with perioral pallor (Figure 18.4A).
- Scarlet spots or blotches, giving a boiled lobster appearance, are often the first sign of rash.
- As skin lesions progress and become more widespread, they start to look like sunburn with goose pimples. The skin may have a rough sandpaper/cigarette paper like feel (Figure18.3C).
- Strawberry tongue may be seen (Figure 18.3B).
- In body folds, especially the armpits and elbows, fragile blood vessels (capillaries) can rupture and causes classic red streaks called **Thompson's sign or** *Pastia lines.* These may persist for 1-2 days after the generalized rash has gone.
- In the untreated patient, the fever peaks by the second day and gradually returns to normal in 5-7 days. When treated with appropriate antibiotics, the fever usually resolves within 12-24 hours. Patients recover after 4-5 days. The skin lesions may take several weeks for complete clearance.

Complications

- Rheumatic fever
- Otitis media
- Pneumonia
- Septicemia
- Glomerulonephritis
- Osteomyelitis
- In complicated cases the disease may be fatal.

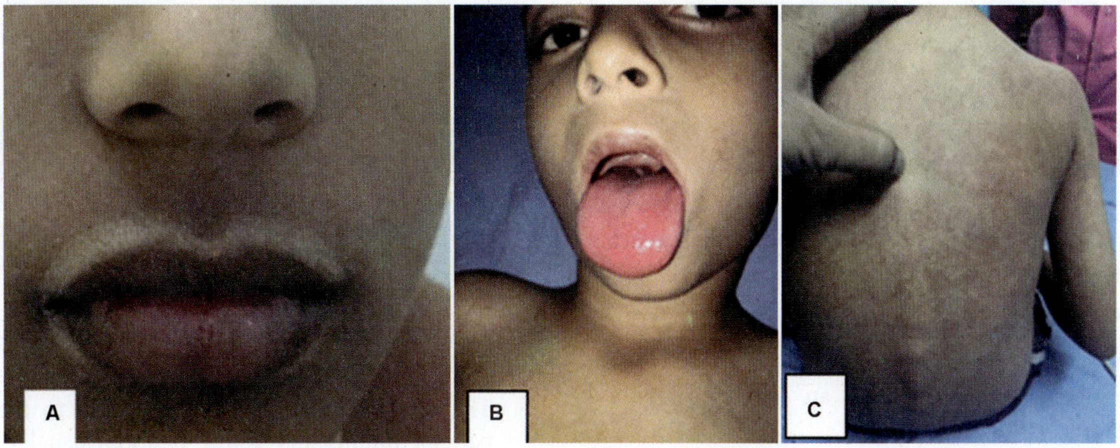

Figure 18.3: (A) Perioral pallor (B) Strawberry tongue with (C) Cigarette paper like rash in scarlet fever (Courtesy – Dr. Bhumesh K Katakam)

KAWASAKI DISEASE

See **Chapter 17.**

INFECTIOUS MONONUCLEOSIS

- Caused by HHV 4, Epstein-Barr virus.
- Transmitted by saliva through close contact – called kissing disease.
- Cutaneous findings are observed in 5% of patients.
- It includes pruritic copper colored macular, papular, urticarial, petechial, scarlatiniform, or erythema multiforme like eruptions.
- Palatal petechiae may be present.
- Around 90% of patients with infectious mononucleosis who receive antibiotics like ampicillin or amoxicillin develop a maculopapular eruption, 7-10 days after the initial administration of antibiotics.
- The rash is thought to be a result of EBV induced antibodies which are produced in response to the administered drug; these antibodies subsequently form immune complexes, which fix complement.
- Resolves, typically in 1-6 days.
- Periorbital and eyelid edema may be seen in up to 50% of patients.
- Painful lymphadenopathy is characteristic, particularly involving posterior cervical chain.
- Genital ulcers may occur, if bilateral, they are often **symmetric with a "kissing" pattern**, called LIPSCHUTZ ulcers.

PRIMARY HIV INFECTION

The generalized morbilliform exanthem of 'acute retroviral syndrome' which typically spares the palms and soles.

It usually lasts for 4-5 days.

SWINE FLU

- It is an infection caused by any one of several types of swine influenza A virus (H1N1 Swine flu virus), a strain of the influenza family of viruses that is endemic in pigs.
- The H1N1 influenza virus is an orthomyxo RNA virus.
- Swine flu causes upper and potentially, serious lower respiratory tract infection with an incubation period ranging from 1-4 days.
- Symptoms such as nasal secretions, chills, fever, malaise, decreased appetite may also be seen.
- Cutaneous manifestations include a diffuse erythematous, dusky red, non-pruritic confluent maculopapular rash over feet, legs and arms, usually sparing the axilla, groin, palms, soles, trunk and face.

COVID-19

- The SARS-CoV-2 is a β-coronavirus, which is enveloped non segmented positive sense RNA virus (subgenus sarbecovirus, Orthocoronavirinae subfamily). Incubation period is 1-14 days, mostly 3-7 days. It has four major categories α, β, γ and δ. The α and β are known to infect humans.
- 30 January 2020, World Health Organization (WHO) officially declared the COVID-19 epidemic as a public health emergency of international concern.
- World Health Organization (WHO) on March 11 declared COVID-19 a pandemic, pointing to over 118,000 cases of the coronavirus illness in over 110 countries and territories around the world and the sustained risk of further global spread.
- Bats are the reservoir of a wide variety of coronaviruses, including severe acute respiratory syndrome coronavirus (SARS-CoV) like viruses.
- Cutaneous manifestation includes:
    - Viral exanthem or maculopapular rashes and peri flexural exanthem.
    - Widespread urticaria.
    - Dermatitis like reaction specially over bilateral hands.
    - Chickenpox-like vesicles.
    - Petechiae or tiny bruises and transient blanching livedoid eruptions.
    - Acrocyanosis and chilblain like or pernio like lesions.
    - Pseudo-frost bite reaction.

DENGUE FEVER (DF)

- It is a severe, flu-like illness that affects infants, children, adolescents, and adults which is caused by dengue virus (DEN 1-4), a singlestranded RNA virus transmitted mainly by the mosquito *Aedes aegypti.*
- The incubation period of DF after the mosquito bite is between 3 and 8 days.
- The clinical features vary according to the age of the patient. Infants and young children usually have only a nonspecific febrile illness, with a rash that is hard to distinguish from other viral illnesses.

- The more severe cases usually occur in older children and adults and are characterized by a rapidly rising temperature (> 39° C) that lasts approximately for 5 to 6 days and sometimes may be biphasic.
- During the febrile period, the patient may have severe headache, retro-orbital pain, myalgia, arthralgia, nausea, and/or vomiting.
- The initial rash is a transient flushing erythema of face which typically occurs within the first 24-48 hours of the onset of symptoms and is due to capillary dilatation.
- The subsequent rash usually occurs 3-6 days after the onset of fever and is characterized by asymptomatic maculopapular or morbilliform eruption.
- In some cases, individual lesions may coalesce and are then seen as generalized confluent erythema with petechiae and rounded islands of sparing, "white islands in a sea of red" and is thought to be due to an immune response to the virus (Figure 18.4).

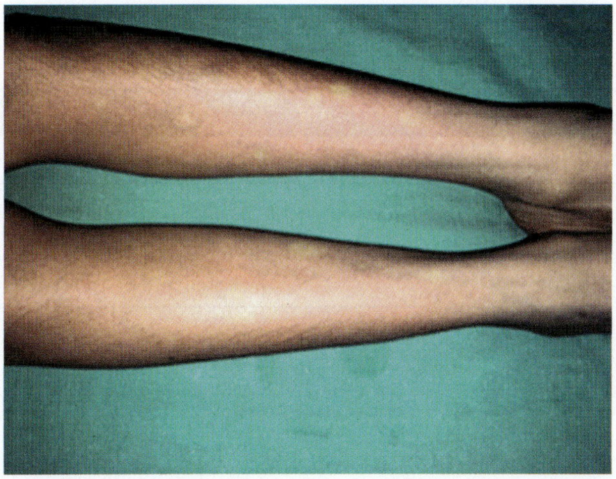

Figure 18.4: "White islands in a sea of red" in dengue fever (Courtesy– Dr. Bhumesh K Katakam)

GIANOTTI CROSTI SYNDROME (Papular Acrodermatitis of Childhood)

- It affects children between 1 and 6 years of age.
- Many viruses have been implicated to cause this disease, namely hepatitis B, EBV, cytomegalovirus and coxsackievirus.
- The rash that follows a prodrome of fever and respiratory symptoms is composed of symmetric, homogenous, flat topped pink brown papules distributed classically on cheeks, extensor extremities and buttocks.
- Hemorrhagic or moist eczematous papules may also be seen.
- The rash lasts for around 15-20 days, sometimes longer.

PAPULAR PURPURIC GLOVES AND SOCKS SYNDROME (PPGSS)

- Papular purpuric gloves and socks syndrome is usually caused by Parvovirus B_{19}.
- It is characterized by, itchy, painful, symmetric edema and erythema of the distal hands and feet. Purpuric papules appear on the hands and feet with abrupt demarcation at the wrists and ankles. Mild prodromal symptoms e.g. fatigue, low grade fever, myalgias and arthralgias may also be present. It generally affects teenagers and young adults, and resolves in 2 weeks.

TYPHOID FEVER

- The characteristic cutaneous sign is the 'rose spot'.
- It is a 2-8 mm, pink, blanching papule that is usually found on the anterior trunk in groups of 5-15 lesions.
- They occur in up to 50% of patients with typhoid fever and less often in non typhoidal enteric fever.
- Rose spots often occur in crops during the second to fourth weeks of the illness.

DRUG EXANTHEM

Drug exanthem or maculopapular drug rash is most common type of drug reaction. It occurs within 2 weeks of use of offending drug. The pattern of rash may be of any type, e.g., morbilliform, scarlatiniform, rubeliform, gyrate, reticulate, polycyclic or small papular eruptions etc. It may be associated with fever, eosinophilia and other constitutional symptoms. The rash usually starts over trunk and extremities and is symmetrical in distribution (Figure 18.5A). Face and pressure areas are usually spared (Figure 18.5B). Palms and soles may be involved. Commonly implicated drugs are penicillins, NSAIDs, gentamicin, gold, sulphonamides, allopurinol, phenytoin and carbamazepine, disorders of oral cavity etc. (Table 18.2).

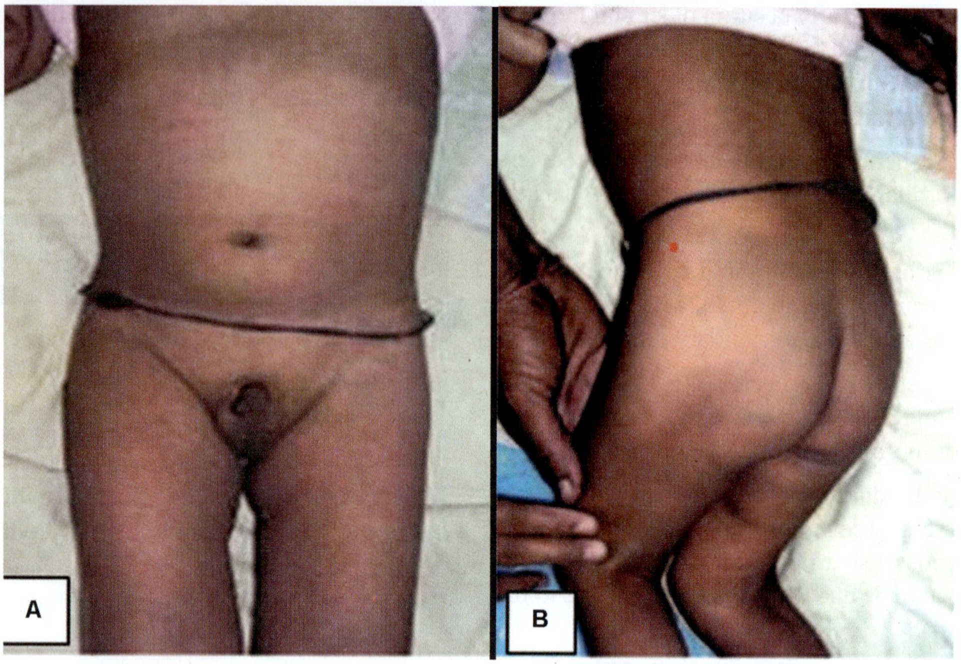

Figure 18.5: (A) Maculopapular rash due to ceftazidime and (B) Same child showing sparing of pressure areas

Table 18.2: Differences among viral, bacterial and drug exanthems

S.No.	*Differentiating features*	*Viral exanthem*	*Bacterial exanthem*	*Drug rash*
1.	Fever	Fever usually appears before rash	Fever presents with rash	Uncommon
2.	Pruritus	Uncommon	Uncommon	Significant
3.	Distribution of rash	Either centripetal or centrifugal Characteristic in many viral exanthems	Starts usually from trunk and flexures	May involve whole body symmetrically with predominant acral lesions. Face and pressure areas are usually not involved
4.	Constitutional symptoms	Appears before onset of rash	Usually appears with appearance of rash	Uncommon
5.	Rhinorrhea and conjunctivitis	Significant	Uncommon	Uncommon
6.	Drug history	–	–	Present
7.	Eosinophilia and raised IgE level	–	–	Usually present
8.	Treatment	Symptomatic and antiviral agents	Antibiotics and supportive	Rash resolves on discontinuing the offending drug
9.	Course	Usually self limiting. Sequel are rare	May involve other organ system with consequent poor prognosis if untreated	May progress to erythroderma

19 CHAPTER Pigmentary Disorders

Contents

In humans, melanin, is produced by the melanocytes in a specialized structure called as melanosomes, which impart unique colour to skin. Melanocytes are dendritic, pigment producing cells present in the basal layer of epidermis. About 2 billion melanocytes exist in the human body, with a density of 800-3000/mm^2. The melanocyte density is almost the same in all individuals of different ethnic groups and skin pigmentation does not depend on the melanocyte number. The difference in skin colour among different races exists due to the size and number of melanosomes and amount of melanin produced. It also depends on type of melanin (eumelanin or pheomelanin) and its transfer and distribution in keratinocytes.

Melanocyte development, migration and synthesis of melanosomes and melanin: The process of melanisation involves the following:

1. Migration of melanoblasts from neural crest to differentiate into epidermal melanocytes.
2. Development and maturation of melanosomes and formation of melanin by enzymatic processes.
3. Movement of melanosomes to dendritic processes of melanocytes.
4. Transfer of melanosomes to keratinocytes.
5. Transfer of melanin to superficial layers of skin.

Abnormality in any of the above process may lead to pigmentary disturbances, which may result into hypo-pigmentary or hyperpigmentary disorders.

Melanocytes are dendritic cells, which originate from neural crest. Melanoblasts have two different pathways of migration, dorsolateral pathway (major pathway) and dorsoventral pathway (minor pathway). These cells migrate to basal layer of epidermis, hair follicle, retina, uveal tract, inner ear and leptomeninges. Migration and development of melanoblasts from neural crest to basal layer is regulated by different factors e.g. c-KIT, PAX 3, SOX 10, MITF, EDN3, EDNRB, endothelin-1, endothelin-3, hepatocyte growth factors, fibroblast growth factor.

Melanosome, which is the metabolic unit of melanin formation, is a membrane bound vesicle with tyrosinase activity. Melanosomes are the main site for synthesis and storage of melanin. It contains parallel fibrillar glycoprotein network made of PMEL/PMEL17 protein. They are divided into two types, eumelanosomes (larger and elliptical) and pheomelanosomes (smaller and spherical). Stages of maturation of melanosomes:

- **Stage 1:** Spherical shaped without melanin deposition.
- **Stage 2:** Oval shaped with minimal melanin deposition and high tyrosinase activity.
- **Stage 3:** Oval shaped with moderate melanin deposition and high tyrosinase activity.
- **Stage 4:** Oval shaped with heavy melanin deposition and low tyrosinase activity.

Melanin synthesis (Figure 19.1): Two types of melanin are synthesized inside melanosomes:

1. **Eumelanin**
   - Polymers of Dihydroxy indole and Dihydroxy indole carboxylic acid.
   - Brown-black in color.
   - Insoluble in strong alkali.
   - Provides shield against UV radiation.
   - Scavenges UV induced reactive oxygen species (ROS).
2. **Pheomelanin**
   - Complex macromolecule formed by oxidation and polymerization of Sulphur containing cysteinyl dopa.
   - Red-yellow in color.
   - Soluble in alkali.

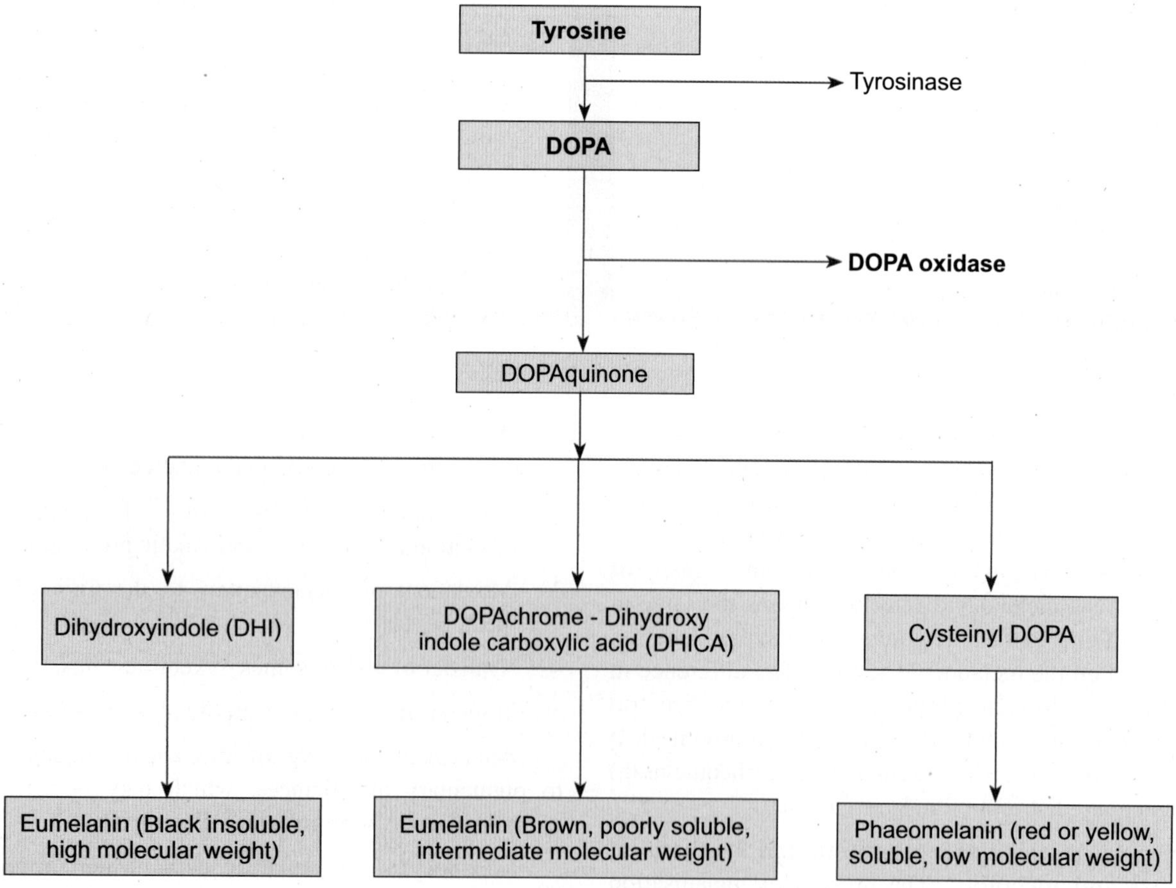

Figure 19.1: Showing melanin synthesis pathway (Raper- Mason pathway)

- Lesser shielding against UV radiation, may act as a prooxidant.

Melanosomes transfer melanin to keratinocytes by different mechanisms e.g. cytophagocytosis, membrane fusion, shedding phagocytosis or by exocytosis-endocytosis. Approximately 36 keratinocytes coexist functionally with a single melanocyte, forming an epidermal-melanin unit. Diseases having defects of melanocytes development, migration and defects in synthesis of melanosomes and melanin are given in Table 19.1.

HYPOPIGMENTARY DISORDERS

Common Disorders

1. **Non-infectious inflammatory disorders:** Vitiligo, pityriasis alba, pityriasis rosea.
2. **Infectious disorders:** Pityriasis versicolor, leprosy, leishmaniasis (Post kala azar dermal leishmaniasis).

Uncommon Disorders

1. **Post-inflammatory:** Post herpes zoster, trauma, burns.
2. **Non-infectious inflammatory:** Morphea, lichen sclerosus et atrophicus.
3. **Developmental:** Nevus depigmentosus.
4. **Genetic:** Albinism, Chediak-Higashi syndrome, Hermansky-Pudlak syndrome, piebaldism, neurocutaneous disorders like tuberous sclerosis, ataxia telangiectasia, Waardenberg's syndrome, Tietz's syndrome, Wolff's syndrome, Ziprkowski-Margolis syndrome.
5. **Inborn errors of metabolism:** Homocystinuria, phenylketonuria.
6. **Nutritional:** Malabsorption syndromes, kwashiorkor.
7. **Others:** Progressive macular hypomelanosis.

Hypopigmentary disorders can be arranged as per age of their appearance (Table 19.2).

Table 19.1: Showing diseases having defects of melanocyte development, migration and defect in synthesis of melanosomes and melanin

Melanocyte development and migration defect associated diseases	• Piebaldism -cKIT • Waardenburg syndrome (WS): o WS 1- PAX 3 o WS 2- MITF o WS 3- PAX3 o WS 4- SOX 10, EDN3, EDNRB
Defect in melanosomes packaging	• Chediak-Higashi syndrome (LYST) • Hermansky-Pudlak syndrome (BLOC, AP3)
Defect in transfer of melanosomes	• Gricelli syndrome: o MYO5A o RAB27A o MLPH
Defect in production of melanin	• Oculocutaneous albinism (TYR, OCA-2, TYRP-1, SLC 45 A5) • Prader-Willi syndrome and Angelman syndrome (OCA -2)

Table 19.2: Clinical classification of disorders of hypo/depigmentation

	Focal	*Segmental*	*Diffuse*
Birth/infancy	Tuberous sclerosis, Piebaldism, Waardenburg syndrome	Achromic nevus, Hypomelanosis of Ito	Oculocutaneous albinism, Phenylketonuria
Childhood	Vitiligo, Postinflammatory hypopigmentation, Nevus depigmentosus, Nevus anemicus	Segmental vitiligo	Generalized vitiligo, Postinflammatory hypopigmentation

HYPERPIGMENTARY DISORDERS

Common Disorders

1. **Post-inflammatory melanosis:** Acne, lichen planus, systemic lupus erythematosus, healed lesions of bullous disorders, healed lesions of psoriasis.
2. **Melasma.**
3. **Tanning:** Immediate pigment darkening (IPD), Persistent pigment darkening (PPD), Delayed tanning or melanogenesis (DT).
4. **Freckles, lentigenosis.**
5. **Mongolian spots.**

Uncommon Disorders

1. **Developmental:** Becker's nevus, nevus of Ota, nevus of Ito, blue nevus.
2. **Genetic:** Café-au-lait macules, incontinentia pigmenti, punctate and reticulate pigmentation (Dowling-Degos disease, Dermatopathia pigmentosa reticularis, Franceschetti-Jadassohn syndrome, Acro-pigmentation of Kitamura, dyskeratosis congenita), Dyschromatosis (Dyschromatosis symmetrica hereditaria, Dyschromatosis universalis hereditaria), xeroderma pigmentosum, Bloom's syndrome, Rothmund-Thomson syndrome.
3. **Nutritional:** Malabsorption, kwashiorkor, vitamin B_{12} deficiency, hemochromatosis, bronze baby syndrome, porphyria.
4. **Endocrine:** Addison's disease, Cushing's syndrome, acromegaly, hyperthyroidism, acanthosis nigricans.
5. **Others:** Schamberg's disease, AIDS, chronic renal failure, adrenoleukodystrophy, universal acquired hypermelanosis, phototoxic reactions etc.
6. **Acquired:** Lichen planus pigmentosus, Mastocytosis, Systemic sclerosis.
7. **Drug induced:** Fixed drug eruption, lichenoid eruptions, minocycline induced pigmentation, anti-cancer drug induced.

HYPOPIGMENTARY DISORDERS

Vitiligo

Vitiligo is an acquired pigmentary disorder of the skin and mucous membranes characterized by circumscribed depigmented macules and patches. In vitiligo some or all of the melanocytes in the affected skin are selectively destroyed.

Epidemiology

Vitiligo affects 0.5-2% of the world population. Approximately 30% of cases occur with a familial clustering of cases. A female preponderance has been reported, but it has been attributed to more cosmetic concerns by female patients. Vitiligo may appear at any time from birth to senescence, although the onset is most commonly observed in persons aged 10-30 years. It rarely begins in infancy or old age. Nearly all cases of vitiligo are acquired relatively early in life.

Pathophysiology

Vitiligo is a multifactorial disorder with a complex pathogenesis. It is related to both genetic and non-genetic factors. Although several theories have been proposed about the pathogenesis of vitiligo, the precise cause remains unknown. Generally agreed upon principles are an absence of functional melanocytes in vitiligo skin and a loss of histochemically recognized melanocytes, owing to their destruction. However, the destruction is most likely a slow process resulting in progressive decrease of melanocytes. Theories regarding destruction of melanocytes include autoimmune mechanisms, cytotoxic mechanisms, and an intrinsic defect of melanocytes, oxidant-antioxidant mechanisms and neural mechanisms.

- **Autoimmune and cytotoxic hypothesis:** Aberration of immune surveillance results in melanocyte dysfunction or destruction (best supported theory).
- **Neural hypothesis:** A neurochemical mediator destroys melanocytes or inhibits melanin production.
- **Oxidant-antioxidant mechanisms:** An intermediate or metabolic product of melanin synthesis causes melanocyte destruction.
- **Intrinsic defect of melanocytes:** Melanocytes have an inherent abnormality that impedes their growth and differentiation in conditions that support normal melanocytes.
- **Convergence theory:** All of the above factors together contribute to the pathogenesis.
- **Newer theories:** Decreased melanocyte survival, auto-cytotoxic theory, biochemical theory.

A genetic factor is definitely involved in vitiligo, 30-40% cases show positive family history in first or second grade relatives. Inheritance may be polygenic or determined by an autosomal dominant gene with partial penetrance. Human leukocyte antigens (HLAs) may be associated, but not in a consistent manner. HLA-DR4, HLA-B13 and HLA-B35 are found more frequently in patients with vitiligo.

Clinical Features

Vitiligo manifests as acquired depigmented macules or patches. They are chalk or milk-white in color. The lesions are usually well demarcated, and are round, oval or linear in shape. They enlarge centrifugally over time at an unpredictable rate and range from few millimeters to centimeters in size. Initial lesions occur most frequently on sun exposed areas or over sites of trauma and friction or over areas which are normally hyperpigmented, e.g., bony prominences, extensor surface of forearm, ventral aspect of wrist, digital phalanges, etc. Other preferred sites are face, axillae, groin, areola, nipples, dorsa of hands, face, neck, scalp, and periocular and periorbital area. Involvement of the mucous membranes is frequently observed in patients of generalized vitiligo. Vitiligo often occurs around body orifices such as the lips and genitalia.

Vitiligo lesions may be localized or generalized, with the latter being more common than the former. Localized vitiligo is restricted to one general area with a segmental or quasidermatomal distribution. Generalized vitiligo implies more than one general area of involvement. In this situation, the macules are usually found on both sides of the trunk, either symmetrically or asymmetrically arrayed. Patients of generalized vitiligo who show involvement of lips, ventral aspect of wrist, periungual areas, bony prominences usually respond poor to treatment.

Body hair in vitiliginous macules may be depigmented (leukotrichia). Vitiligo of the scalp usually appears as a localized patch of white or gray hair, but total depigmentation of all scalp hair may occur. Leukotrichia may indicate a poor prognosis in regard to repigmentation. Spontaneous repigmentation of depigmented hair in vitiligo does not occur.

Koebner phenomenon is observed in patients of active vitiligo. New lesions develop at the site of minimum injury, e.g., cut, burn or abrasion.

Vitiligo and Ocular Disease

The uveal tract, choroid and retinal pigment epithelium contain pigment cells. Uveitis is the most significant ocular abnormality associated with vitiligo. The most severe form of uveitis is seen in **Vogt-Koyanagi-Harada syndrome**. This syndrome is characterized by vitiligo, uveitis, aseptic meningitis, dysacusis, tinnitus, poliosis and alopecia. Choroidal abnormalities have been reported in upto 30% of patients, and iritis has been reported in approximately 5% of patients.

Alezzandrini syndrome consists of facial vitiligo, poliosis, deafness, and unilateral visual changes. The affected eye has decreased visual acuity and an atrophic iris.

Vitiligo and Autoimmune Disorders

Vitiligo is frequently associated with disorders of autoimmune origin, e.g., thyroid disease, diabetes mellitus, pernicious anemia, Addison's disease, alopecia areata, with thyroid abnormalities being the most common. Vitiligo usually precedes the onset of thyroid dysfunction. This association supports the autoimmune theory of vitiligo pathogenesis. Patients with autoimmune polyendocrinopathy have an increased prevalence of vitiligo. In this genetic syndrome, autoantibodies cause destruction of endocrine cells.

Clinical Classification of Vitiligo

The classification system is important because of the special significance assigned by some authorities to each type of vitiligo. The most widely used classification of vitiligo is localized, generalized and universal types. It is based on the distribution of lesions and is as follows:

Localized

- **Focal:** It is characterized by one or more depigmented macules in any one area of body.
- **Segmental:** This type manifests as one or more depigmented macules in a dermatomal or quasidermatomal pattern. It occurs most commonly in children. More than half the patients with segmental vitiligo have patches of white hair or poliosis. This type of vitiligo is not associated with thyroid or other autoimmune disorder (Figure 19.2).
- **Mucosal:** Mucous membranes alone are affected.

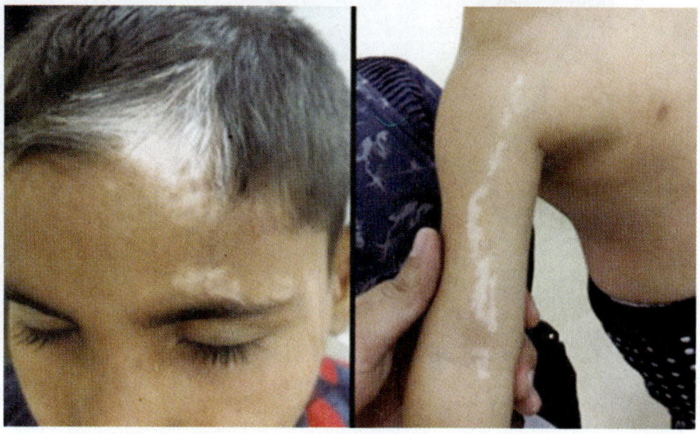

Figure 19.2: Segmental vitiligo

Generalized

- **Acrofacial:** Depigmentation occurs on the distal fingers and periorificial areas.
- **Vitiligo vulgaris:** This is characterized by scattered patches that are widely distributed (Figure 19.3).

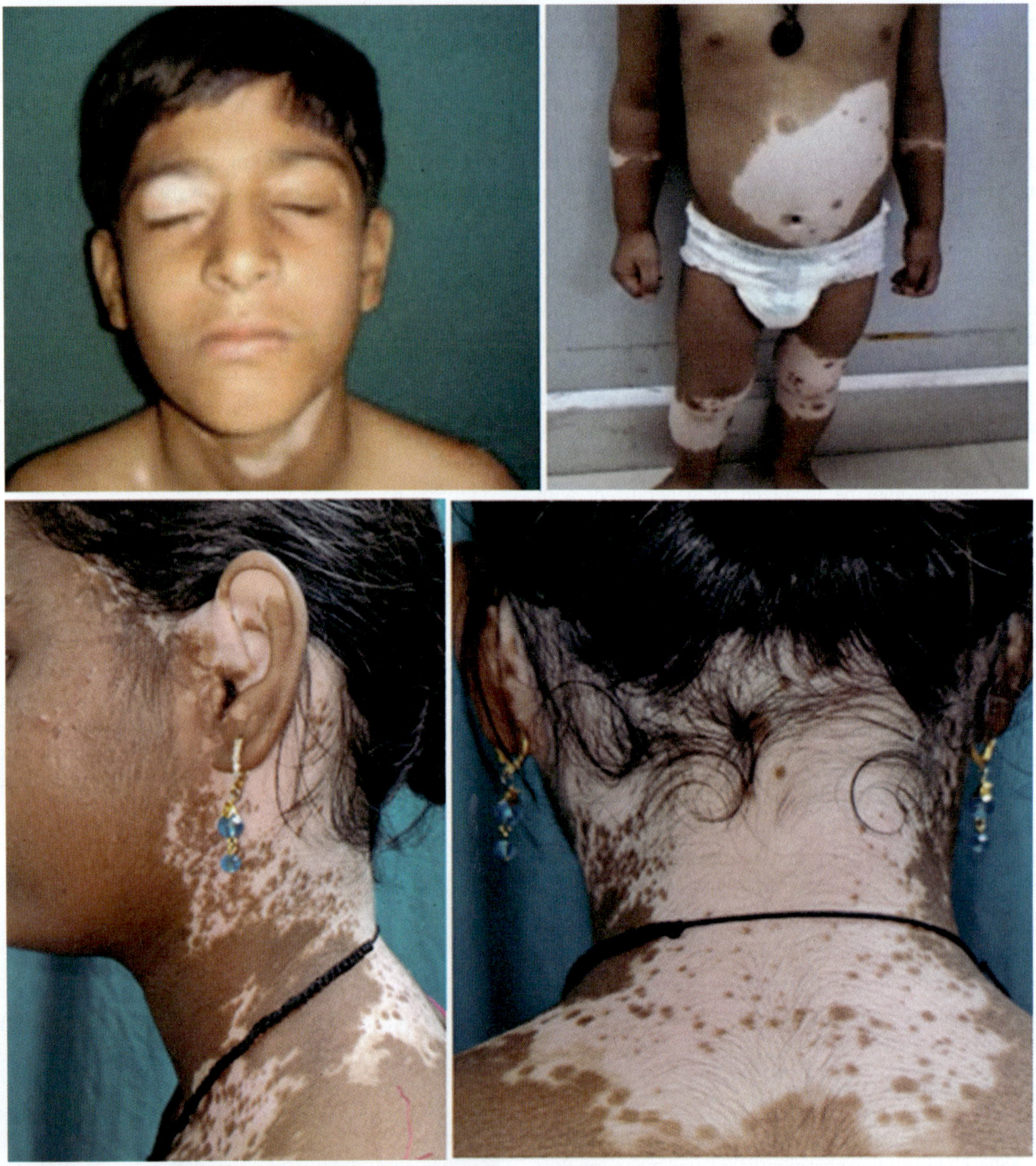

Figure 19.3: Vitiligo vulgaris

- **Mixed:** Acrofacial and vitiligo vulgaris may occur in combination, or segmental vitiligo and acrofacial vitiligo and/or vitiligo vulgaris pattern may be seen in combination.

Universal

There is complete or nearly complete depigmentation. It may be associated with multiple endocrinopathy syndrome.

UNSTABLE VITILIGO IN CHILDREN

Clinical indicators of unstable vitilgo are:

- Appearance of new lesions.
- Increase in size of old lesions.
- Hypomelanotic lesions with ill-defined borders.

- Confetti like depigmentation.
- Trichrome vitiligo.
- Inflammatory vitiligo.
- Koebner phenomenon present.
- Perifollicular pigmentation by dermoscopy.
- Histopathological features suggestive of unstability–spongiosis, epidermal lymphocytes, >100 dermal lymphocytes in lesions and perilesional skin.

Vitiligo European Taskforce (VETF) Consensus Classification 2012

1. NSV.

   Acrofacial.

   Mucosal (more than one mucosal site).

   Generalized.

   Universal.

   Mixed (associated with segmental vitiligo).
2. Segmental Vitiligo–Uni-, bi-, or plurisegmental.
3. Undetermined/Unclassified Vitiligo–Focal, Mucosal (one site in isolation).

Differential Diagnosis

- Pityriasis versicolor.
- Leprosy.
- Idiopathic guttate hypomelanosis.
- Nevus anemicus.
- Post-inflammatory depigmentation.
- Morphea.

Investigations

Although the diagnosis of vitiligo generally is made on the basis of clinical findings, biopsy is occasionally helpful for differentiating vitiligo from other hypopigmentary disorders.

Vitiligo may be associated with other autoimmune diseases, especially with thyroid disease, diabetes mellitus, pernicious anemia, Addison's disease, and alopecia areata. Patients should be investigated for these disorders if they show any signs and symptoms related to these disorders.

In doubtful cases vitiligo may be diagnosed by means of inspection with a Wood's lamp.

Treatment

No single therapy for vitiligo produces predictably good results in all patients; the response to therapy is highly variable. Treatment must be individualized, and patients should be made aware of the risks associated with therapy. During medical therapy, pigment cells arise and proliferate from the following 3 sources:

- The pilosebaceous unit, which provides the highest number of cells, migration occurs from the external root sheath into the adjoining epidermis.
- Spared epidermal melanocytes not affected during depigmentation.
- From the border of lesions, melanocytes may migrate upto 2-4 mm from the edge.

Following treatment modalities are generally used for treatment of vitiligo:

Topical Therapy

i. Topical PUVA (Psoralens + Ultraviolet A).

ii. Topical corticosteroids.

iii. Topical immunomodulators and Vitamin D analogues.

Systemic Therapy

i. Systemic PUVA.

ii. Systemic corticosteroids.

iii. Adjuvant therapy with antioxidants.

Phototherapy

i. Broad band UVB.

ii. Narrow band UVB.

Lasers

Surgical Modalities

Topical PUVA

Psoralens are applied topically followed by exposure to UVA. Topical psoralens are available as lotions or creams/ointment of 8-Methoxypsoralen (0.1-0.3%), which should be appropriately diluted before use and should be applied at night initially. They may cause erythema, burning, itching and even vesiculation if applied without dilution. Patients should be educated about these side effects and should be advised to stop topical psoralens if they occur. Topical and systemic steroids are used as per requirement if irritant contact dermatitis develops. Diluted topical psoralens can be used in daytime, once patient starts tolerating topical psoralen at night. Exposure to sunlight or UVA (0.1-0.3 J/cm^2) for few minutes, 30 minutes after topical psoralen application hastens repigmentation in patches of vitiligo. It should be done twice or thrice a week. Topical

PUVA is particularly useful in localized vitiligo. Another practical method of topical psoralen is to mix it with topical steroids (5 gm of mometasone cream may be mixed with 10 drops of psoralen lotion). It reduces possible local side effects as well as hastens repigmentation.

Topical Steroids

Topical steroid (e.g., clobetasol, triamcinolone or hydrocortisone) preparations are usually used to treat localized vitiligo. The results of therapy have been reported as moderately successful.

Topical Immunomodulators

Topical tacrolimus ointment (0.03% or 0.1%) is an effective alternative therapy for vitiligo, particularly when the disease involves the head and neck. In children only 0.03% ointment should be applied and is recommended after 2 years of age. They have advantage over topical steroid therapy as they have minimal local side effects. The topical calcipotriene can also be used, which should be applied with care, avoiding eyelids and mucosal surfaces.

Other topical therapies like bFGF decapeptide and pseudo catalase are variably effective. Topical tacrolimus can be used as maintenance therapy.

Systemic Photochemotherapy (Systemic PUVA)

Systemic photochemotherapy induces cosmetically satisfactory repigmentation in upto 70% of patients with early or localized disease.

It involves the use of psoralens combined with UVA light. Treatment with 8-methoxypsoralen, 5-methoxypsoralen, and trimethylpsoralen plus UV-A (PUVA) is most widely used treatment, especially in patients with widespread vitiligo. Oral PUVA is not recommended for children under 12 years.

Oral psoralens are given in a single dose of 0.3-0.4 mg/kg/day usually early in the morning. After 1.5-2 hours, the patches of vitiligo are exposed to sunlight (PUVASOL) or UVA for 10-15 minutes. It is usually given on alternate days till repigmentation is seen. Repigmentation starts from perifollicular areas and from the edges of lesions which gradually merges. The total number of treatments required may be 50-300. The best results from PUVA are obtained on the face, trunk, and proximal parts of the extremities.

Physicians who prescribe PUVA therapy should be thoroughly familiar with the risks associated with the treatment. Additional UVA exposure should be avoided by using appropriate sunscreen to prevent sunlight induced damage of PUVA treated skin. Patients receiving PUVA should be advised to use sun-protected glasses to prevent UVA induced damage to lens of eyes.

Systemic Steroids

Oral steroids are useful in vitiligo as it is considered an autoimmune disease. Different regimens including daily doses, oral pulse or oral mini pulse has been advocated. They are particularly useful to halt the disease when it is progressive. Oral mini pulse with methyl prednisolone 0.8 mg/kg 2 days a week for 6 months is safe and effective in active disease. Usually oral prednisolone is given in dose of 10-15 mg/day or oral deflazacort 12 to 18 mg per day for 8-12 weeks which usually stops the disease progression. Methyl prednisolone and deflazacort have lesser side effects. Low dose methotrexate, low dose dexamethasone (2.5 mg) and minocycline can be used to control unstable vitiligo in adults but the studies are lacking in children.

Phototherapy

Narrow-band UV-B phototherapy is widely used and produces good clinical results. It is better than broad-band UVA. Narrow-band fluorescent tubes (Philips TL-01/100W) with an emission spectrum of 310-315 nm and a maximum wavelength of 311 nm are used. Treatment frequency is 2-3 times weekly, but never on consecutive days. Short-term adverse effects include pruritus and xerosis. Several studies have demonstrated the effectiveness of narrow-band UV-B therapy when used as monotherapy.

In UV-B narrow-band microphototherapy small lesions are targeted. Selective narrow-band UV-B (311nm) is used with a fiber optic system to direct radiation to specific areas of skin. Narrow-band UV-B has become the first choice of therapy for children under 12 years of the age with generalized vitiligo where systemic PUVA is contraindicated.

The advantages of narrow-band UV-B over PUVA include shorter treatment times, avoidance of systemic side effects of psoralens and no need for subsequent photoprotection.

Laser Therapy

Another innovation is therapy with an excimer laser, which produces monochromatic rays at 308 nm to treat limited, stable patches of vitiligo. This new treatment is an efficacious, safe and well-tolerated treatment for vitiligo when limited to less than 30% of the body surface. However, therapy is expensive. Localized lesions of vitiligo are treated twice weekly for an average of 24-48 sessions.

Surgical Modalities

Patients who do not respond to conventional therapy may be treated with surgical procedures. Patients who have small areas of stable vitiligo, e.g., localized or segmental vitiligo are best candidates for surgery. The disease should be stable for at least

1-2 years and should have negative Koebner's phenomenon. Surgery is not useful for patients with progressive and generalized vitiligo. The donor skin or melanocytes are taken from the normally pigmented skin of the patients and is transplanted over surgically denude areas of vitiliginous skin. Transplanted melanocytes start proliferating and spreading. Satisfactory repigmentation is usually achieved in properly selected patients.

Various methods for repigmentation surgery are as follows:

1. **Tissue grafting**
   - **Thin dermoepidermal grafts:** The depigmented epidermis is removed by superficial dermabrasion, including the papillary dermis, and very thin dermoepidermal sheets of normal skin harvested with dermatome are grafted onto the denuded skin.
   - **Suction epidermal grafting:** Epidermal grafts can be obtained by vacuum suction, usually with 150 mm Hg. The recipient site can be prepared by suction, freezing, or dermabrasion. The depigmented blister roof is discarded, and the epidermal donor graft is placed on the vitiliginous area.
   - **Punch minigrafting:** Small donor punch grafts are inserted into the wells of recipient sites and held in place by a pressure dressing. The graft heals readily and begins to show repigmentation within 4-6 weeks. Some cobblestoning persists but is minimal, and the cosmetic result is excellent.
2. **Cellular grafting–suitable to treat larger area of vitiligo**
   - **Cultured epidermis with melanocytes or cultured melanocyte suspensions:** Depigmented skin is removed using liquid nitrogen, superficial dermabrasion or carbon dioxide lasers; very thin sheets of cultured epidermis are grafted or suspension is spread onto the denuded surface.
   - **Noncultured epidermal suspension:** After the achromic epidermis of vitilgo patch is removed, an epidermal suspension with melanocytes and keratinocytes previously prepared by trypsinization of normally pigmented donor skin is spread onto the denuded area and immediately covered with nonadherent dressing. Excellent cosmetic results are obtained in properly selected patients.

Depigmentation Therapy

If vitiligo is widespread and attempts at repigmentation do not produce satisfactory results, depigmentation may be attempted in selected patients to bring uniform appearance. The long-term social and emotional consequences of depigmentation must be considered. Depigmentation should not be attempted unless the patient fully understands that the procedure generally results in permanent depigmentation. A 20% cream of monobenzyl ether of hydroquinone is applied twice daily for 3-12 months. Burning, itching and allergic contact dermatitis may occur.

Oculocutaneous Albinism

Albinism is a group of congenital hypopigmentary diseases, that result from a generalized lack of pigmentation due to a defect in the melanin production, by melanocytes in the skin, eyes and the hair.

Classification

Albinism is classified as follows:

- **Oculocutaneous Albinism (OCA) Types 1, 2, 3 and 4:** Affects both eyes and skin and is autosomal recessive.
- **Ocular Albinism (OA):** Affects only eyes and is autosomal recessive.
- **Chediak-Higashi Syndrome (CHS):** Associated with defects of immunity due to leukocyte dysfunction.
- **Hermansky-Pudlak Syndrome (HPS):** Associated with platelet defects and defects in ceroid storage.
- **Griscelli Syndrome (GS):** Associated with defects in immunity and neurological defects.

Etiopathogenesis

These diseases present with a generalized, complete or partial loss in pigmentation of the skin, eyes and the hair. Mutations in genes that regulate the process of melanin synthesis and distribution of pigment by the melanocyte are the basis for these diseases.

- **OCA type 1** results from mutations in the tyrosinase gene, which maps to band 11q14-2 and is inherited as an autosomal recessive trait. Tyrosinase hydroxylates tyrosine to dihydroxyphenylalanine (DOPA) and subsequently dehydroxylates DOPA to DOPA-oxidase.
- **OCA type 2 results** from mutation in the P gene, which maps to band 15q11-13 and is inherited as an autosomal recessive trait.
- **OCA type 3** results from mutation in the tyrosinase-related protein-1 (Tyrp1) gene, which maps to band 9p23 and is inherited as an autosomal recessive trait.
- **OCA type 4** results from mutations in the membrane-associated transporter protein (MATP) gene, which maps to band 5p13.3 and is inherited as an autosomal recessive trait.
- **OA** results from mutation in a gene on the X chromosome, which maps to band Xp22.3-22.2 and is inherited as an X-linked recessive trait.

- **CHS** results from mutation in the LYST gene, which maps to band 1q 42-43 and is inherited as an autosomal recessive trait. The LYST gene encodes protein that putatively functions in the translocation of material from the Golgi apparatus to target sites in affected cells. As a result, the synthesis of melanosomes by the melanocyte, of delta granules by the platelet, and of lysosomes by some of the leukocytes (i.e., neutrophils and natural killer lymphocytes) is impaired.
- **HPS** is inherited as an autosomal recessive trait and exists with loci heterogeneity. The HPS type1 (HPS1), results from a gene that maps to band 10q23.1-23.3, HPS type 2 (HPS2) results from mutations in a gene that encodes the beta subunit of the adaptin 3 complex (AP3). AP3 is involved in trafficking specific glycoproteins from the Golgi apparatus to target sites in affected cells.
- **GS** is inherited as an autosomal recessive trait, due to mutations in the RAB27A gene and MYO5A gene located at band 15q21. In the melanocyte, these 2 gene products form a complex that facilitates the translocation of melanosomes along microtubules in the dendrites of the melanocyte. Griscelli syndrome is a rare autosomal recessive syndrome characterized by pigmentary dilution of skin and hair (silvery hair) with large clumps of pigment in hair shaft (Figure 19.4).

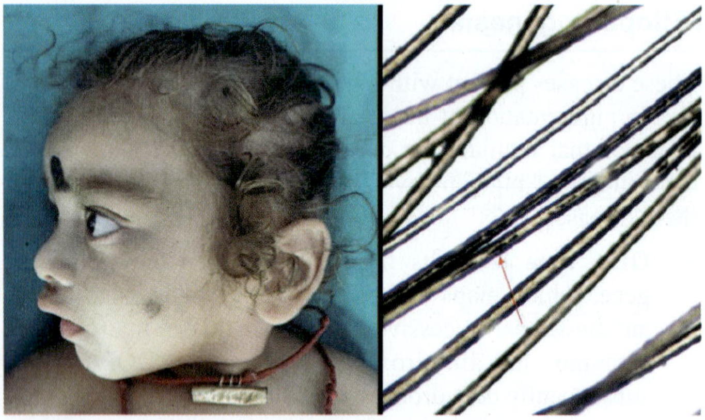

Figure 19.4: Griscelli syndrome showing pigmentary dilution of hair and skin with pigment clump in hair shaft

Epidemiology

The approximate incidences of these diseases are as follows:

- **OCA type 1 - One case per 40,000 population.**
- **OCA type 2 - One case per 15,000 population.**
- **OCA type 3 - Rare.**
- **OCA type 4 - Rare, except in Japan.**
- **OA - One case per 50,000 population.**
- **CHS, HPS, GS - Extremely rare.**

All races appear to be equally affected by the associated mutations. OCA type 2 is reportedly more common among Africans and African Americans. OCA 4 is common in Japanese. The incidence of these albino diseases is equal for men and women. In all of these patients, disease starts in neonatal period.

Clinical Features

The characteristic hypopigmentation of albinism is apparent at birth. An increase in the pigmentation of the skin and/or the hair may occur with age.

- **OCA type 1** primarily manifests with complete absence of pigment in skin, hair, eyes and this category is termed OCA type 1A. However, some patients can present with moderate pigmentation in these tissues (termed OCA type 1B). All forms of OCA type 1 also have photophobia, moderate to severe reduced visual acuity and nystagmus.
- **OCA type 2** presents with a minimal-to-moderate amount of pigment remaining in skin, hair and eyes. Many patients with OCA type 2 can develop pigmented freckles, lentigines, and/or nevi with age. The ocular involvement may occur (Figure 19.5).

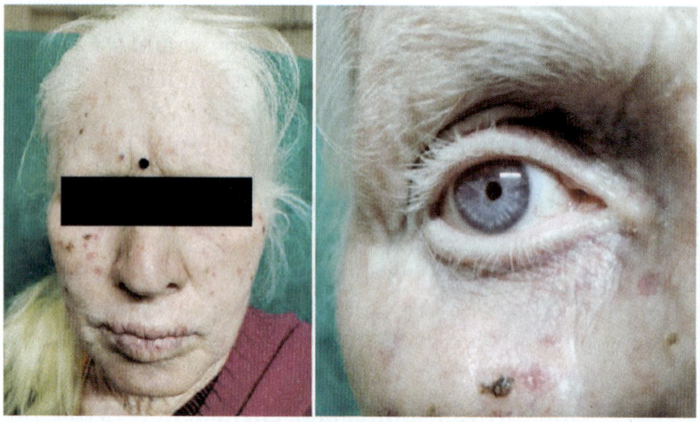

Figure 19.5: Albinism

- **OCA type 3** manifests with minimal pigment reduction in the skin, the hair and the eyes. This form of albinism was previously referred to as Red OCA or Brown OCA. The ocular involvement is less severe.
- **OCA type 4** manifests with a phenotype resembling OCA type 2.
- **OA** manifests with ocular depigmentation and iris translucency. In addition, patients with OA have congenital motor nystagmus, reduced visual acuity, refractive errors, fundus hypopigmentation, lack of foveal reflex and strabismus. Cutaneous depigmentation is not seen.

- Cutaneous malignancies, particularly squamous cell carcinoma (Figure 19.6) is frequent in all forms of albinism.

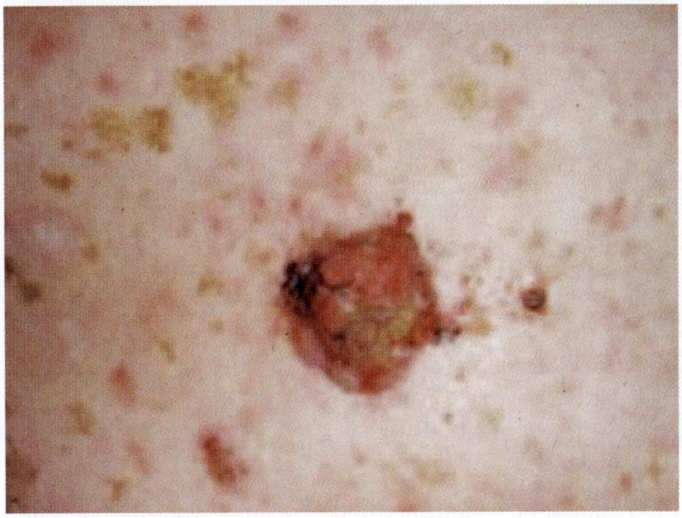

Figure 19.6: Squamous cell carcinoma in albinism

- **CHS** manifests with moderate to complete absence of pigment in skin, hair and eyes. Respiratory tract infections can occur within a few days of birth and recurrences increase with the age.
- **HPS** manifests with a variable amount of depigmentation in the skin, the hair, and the eyes with bleeding diathesis. The bleeding diathesis can occur within a few days of birth generally during circumcision. Throughout life, patients with HPS experience mild-to-moderate bleeding events, including bruising, epistaxis, gingival bleeding, and prolonged bleeding during menstruation or after tooth extraction. The respiratory system is affected and restrictive lung disease may occur. Ophthalmic findings are variable.
- **GS** manifests with a mild form of albinism (i.e., pale skin). Presence of silvery gray hair at birth is distinctive of GS. Immunodeficiency or neurological defects can occur shortly after birth.

Differential Diagnosis

- **Homocystinuria.**
- **Menkes kinky hair disease.**
- **Phenylketonuria.**

Investigations

- The hair bulb tyrosinase assay has been used to differentiate between OCA type 1 and the other forms of albinism. Scalp hair bulbs are gently plucked from the patient and placed in a 0.1% solution of L-DOPA for upto 4 hours. In OCA type 1 the hair bulbs remain white, but in all other forms of albinism, the hair turns dark during the incubation period.
- For CHS, analysis of a blood smear and the subsequent identification of neutrophils containing giant cytoplasmic granules are confirmatory.
- For HPS, prolonged bleeding time and electron microscopy of platelets showing the absence of dense bodies (delta granules) are diagnostic.
- For GS, confirmatory workup consists of immunologic function evaluation plus both CT and MRI for neurological abnormalities.

Treatment

- No treatment is available for hypopigmentation in skin, hair or eyes. The use of broad-spectrum sunscreens and clothing is recommended to prevent ultraviolet-induced damage to the skin. Visual impairment can be improved by using corrective lenses.
- Most therapy for CHS and GS is symptomatic in nature. Appropriate antibiotics should be administered to treat infections. Bone marrow transplantation can correct and improve hematologic and immunologic defects in persons with CHS and GS, respectively.
- In HPS if the bleeding diathesis is extreme, platelet and blood transfusions may be considered.

Nevus Depigmentosus

It is an asymptomatic, congenital, hypopigmented to depigmented macular lesion, which appears commonly on trunk (Figure 19.7), face and proximal limbs. It has a serrated border and does not cross the midline. Nevus depigmentosus may be segmental, focal or generalized in distribution. The most important differential is focal/segmental vitiligo, which can be differentiated by Wood's lamp examination. Nevus depigmentosus shows off white color on Wood's lamp while vitiligo shows chalky white color. Treatment, if required for cosmetic reasons, may be in the form of excision and skin grafting.

Piebaldism

- It is a form of patterned vitiligo, which usually presents at birth and have a depigmented patch on frontal scalp or upper face with a white forelock.
- It may be associated with heterochromic irides or deafness. There may be other areas of depigmentation over the body.
- Treatment consists of photoprotection and skin grafting.

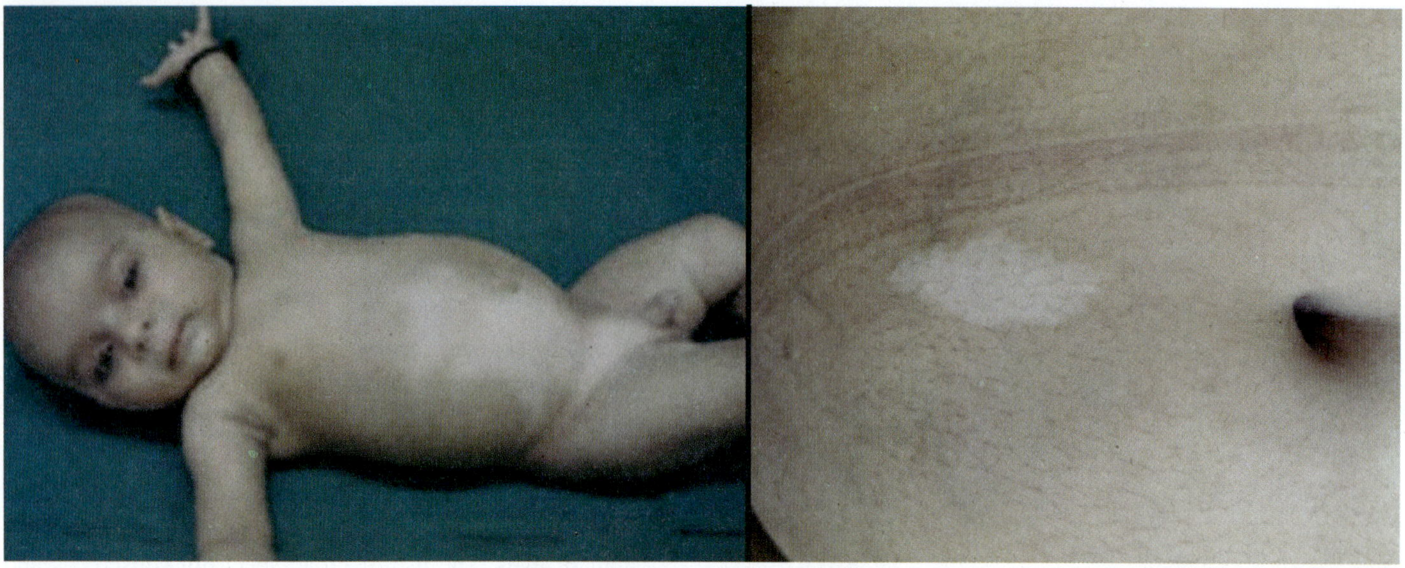

Figure 19.7: Nevus depigmentosus

Hypomelanosis of ITO

- Hypomelanosis of Ito (HI) is a syndrome characterized by presence of hypopigmented whorls along the Blaschko lines. Small, 0.5-1 cm hypopigmented or white macules (Figure 19.8) coalesce to form reticulated patches. The macules cover more than 2 dermatomes and are often asymmetrical and on both sides of the body.
- Congenital abnormalities, mental retardation, and seizures are the most commonly associated conditions. The associated anomalies may be seen in 30-50% cases.
- On examination other skeletal abnormalities like cleft palate, nail, hair and teeth abnormalities may be detected.
- Neurologic examination is essential to evaluate neural tumors, seizures and psychomotor delay.

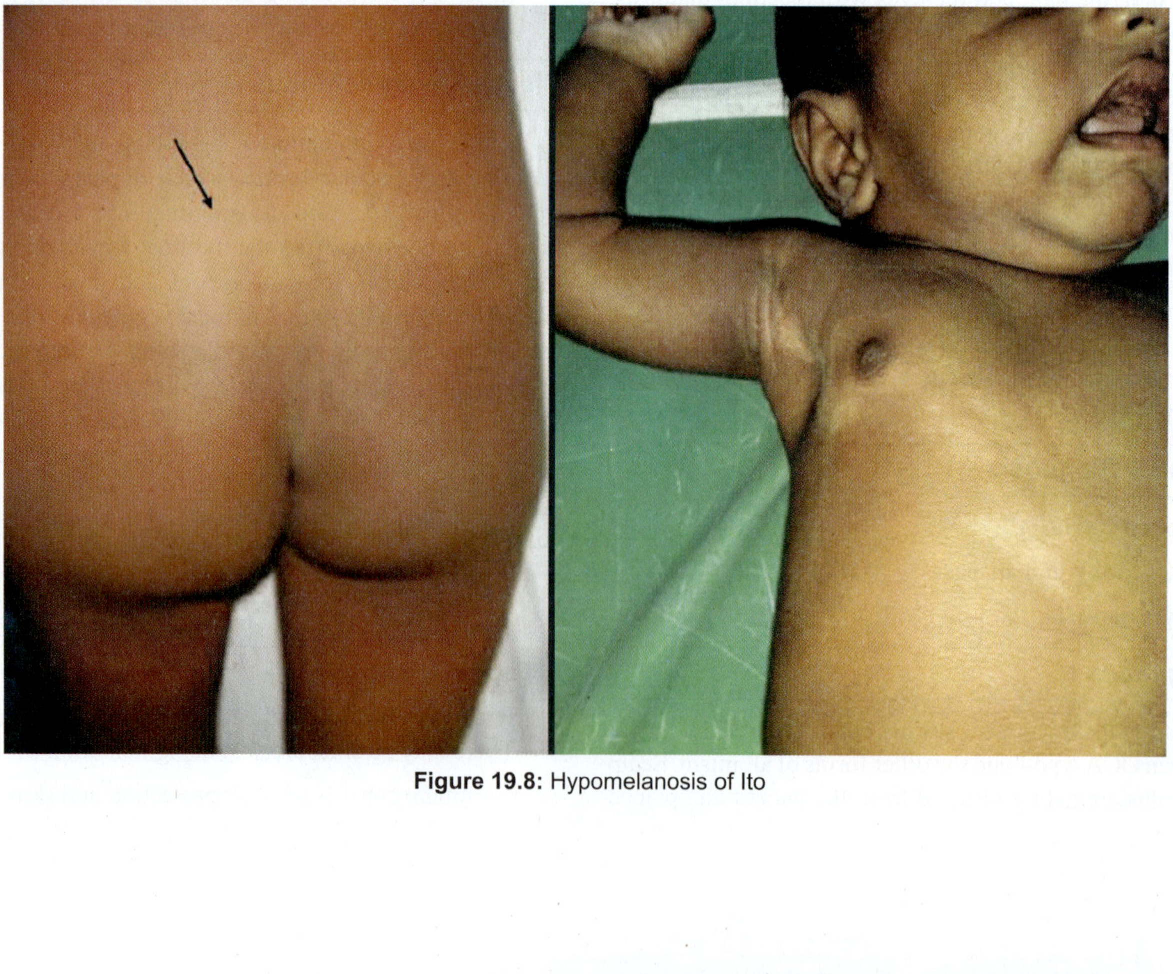

Figure 19.8: Hypomelanosis of Ito

- Wood's lamp enhances the pattern, especially in white patients.

Treatment

- No treatment is administered for the lesions of hypomelanosis of Ito (HI).
- Associated disorders like seizure, mental retardation, ear, eye, teeth, bone deformities require appropriate specialty care.

Clinical Pearls in Acquired Hypomelanosis in Children

1. Travel history in endemic regions–Leprosy, PKDL, yaws, pinta, oncocerciasis.
2. Weight loss–Neoplasm, nutritional deficiency.
3. Palpable lymph node–Neoplasm, infections.
4. Alopecia or Scarring–Leprosy, syphilis, mycosis fungoides, selenium deficiency.
5. Loss of sensation–Leprosy.
6. Chronic cough, dyspnea or uveitis–Sarcoidosis.

Idiopathic Guttate Hypomelanosis

Small flat pale or white spots are present on legs, upper chest and forearms due to abnormal or reduced transfer of melanin from melanocytes to keratinocytes. Proposed etiology is skin ageing, chronic sun exposure, trauma and autoimmunity.

Treatment includes topical steroids, tacrolimus, topical retinoids, 5-FU tattooing, phenol cautery, dermabrasion, CO_2 laser and cryotherapy.

HYPERPIGMENTARY DISORDERS

Mongolian Spots

Mongolian spot refers to a macular blue-gray pigmentation usually on the sacrococcygeal area of healthy infants. It is usually present at birth or appears within the first few weeks of life. Mongolian spot typically disappears spontaneously within 4 years but can persist for life.

Mongolian spot results from entrapment of melanocytes in the dermis during their migration from the neural crest into the epidermis.

Epidemiology

The prevalence of Mongolian spots varies among different ethnic groups. This condition is most common among Asians. Mongolian spots are observed in more than 90% of infants of the Mongoloid race (i.e., East Asians, Indonesians, Eskimos). No sex predilection is reported.

Clinical Features

- Typically, the Mongolian spot is few centimeters in diameter, although much larger lesions can also occur. Lesions may be solitary or numerous.
- Most commonly, Mongolian spot involves the lumbosacral area (Figure 19.9), but the buttocks, flanks and shoulders may be affected in extensive lesions.
- Generalized Mongolian spots involving large areas covering the entire posterior or anterior trunk and the extremities have been reported.
- The distinctive skin discoloration is due to the deep placement of the pigment in the dermis, which imparts a bluish tone to the skin from the Tyndall effect of scattered light.

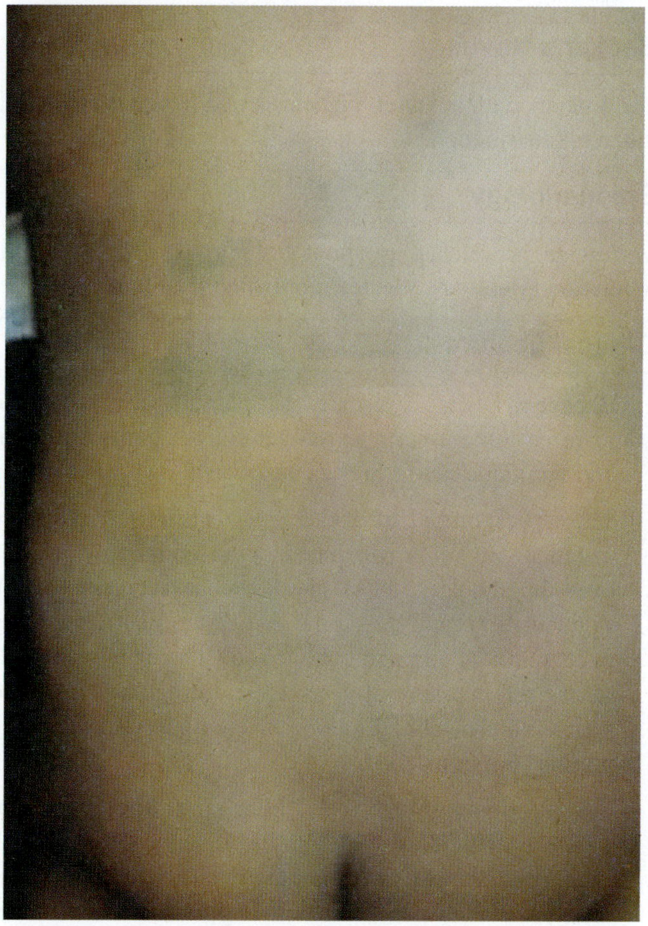

Figure 19.9: Mongolian spots

Differential Diagnosis

- Blue nevus.
- Nevus of Ota and Ito.
- Bruise marks (rule out child abuse).

Investigations

Investigations are not indicated, except when extensive Mongolian spots are present. In these circumstances, it is advisable to evaluate the patient for inborn errors of metabolism e.g. Lysosomal storage disease like GM1–gangliosidosis and Niemann-Pick disease, mucopolysaccharidosis like hurler's disease and hunter's disease etc., in order to avoid irreversible organ damage. (*See* Chapter 28). In extensive Mongolian spots involving the back, radiographic studies are needed to rule out a spinal meningeal tumor or anomaly.

Treatment

It is usually a self-limiting lesion so treatment is not required. In persistent cases, laser therapy with Q-switched Alexandrite laser has shown some benefit.

Becker's Nevus

It is a nevus with acquired melanosis and hypertrichosis in a unilateral distribution.

Epidemiology

Worldwide prevalence is about 0.25 to 0.52% in general population. Males are affected more often than females.

Clinical Features

- Becker's nevus is usually a sporadic condition that manifests in the peripubertal period, but both congenital and familial cases have been described.
- The earliest finding of Becker's nevus is an asymptomatic irregular tan to brown patch, most commonly located over the shoulder, upper chest, or back (Figure 19.10). Pigmentation may be subtle, and onset most commonly occurs in the peripubertal period. The patch expands during the first several years as new irregular pigmented macules and patches develop at the periphery and coalesce with the larger patch.
- Several months to years after the appearance of pigmentation, thick brown-to-black hairs develop both within and in close proximity to the patch. Hair density is highly variable and occasionally, hypertrichosis does not occur.
- The central area in the patch may thicken, and acne vulgaris may develop.
- Once present, the patch remains indefinitely, although minimal pigmentary fading may occur in adulthood.
- Associated findings:
  - Occasionally, Becker's nevus may be associated with smooth muscle hamartoma.
  - Other associations seen with Becker's nevus include ipsilateral developmental abnormalities like pectoralis major aplasia, ipsilateral limb shortening, ipsilateral foot enlargement, spina bifida, scoliosis, pectus carinatum, breast hypoplasia, supernumerary nipples etc, collectively termed as Becker's nevus syndrome.

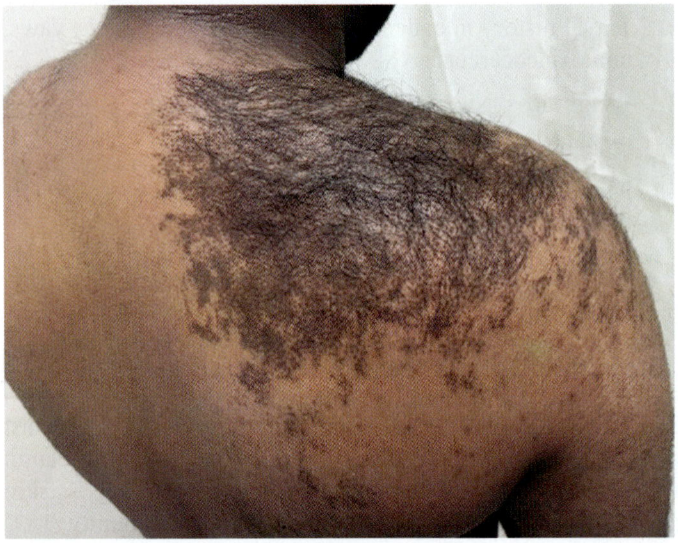

Figure 19.10: Becker's nevus

Differential Diagnosis

- Café-au-lait patch.
- Congenital melanocytic nevus: Giant congenital melanocytic nevus in an infant.
- Post-inflammatory hyperpigmentation.

Treatment

Therapeutic intervention for Becker's nevus is primarily for cosmetic reasons for complaints related to hypertrichosis and/or hyperpigmentation.

- Surgical removal of lesion with grafting is the best treatment.
- Laser therapy: Q-switched ruby laser (694 nm) has been used with variable success in the treatment of both the

hypertrichosis and hyperpigmentation of Becker's nevus. Er:YAG laser has showed complete clinical clearance in few cases.

Café-Au-Lait Macules

Café-au-lait macules (CALMs) are well-circumscribed, tan brown/light brown macules (Figure 19.11), oval to round in shape and of various sizes. It is derived from French word meaning "coffee with milk". They appear at birth or in early childhood. They are caused by increased number of melanosomes in keratinocytes with usually normal number of melanocytes. Only CALMs, which are small in size and few in number are a common occurrence. Multiple and large CALMs are associated with various syndromes like tuberous sclerosis, neurofibromatosis, McCune Albright syndrome, etc.

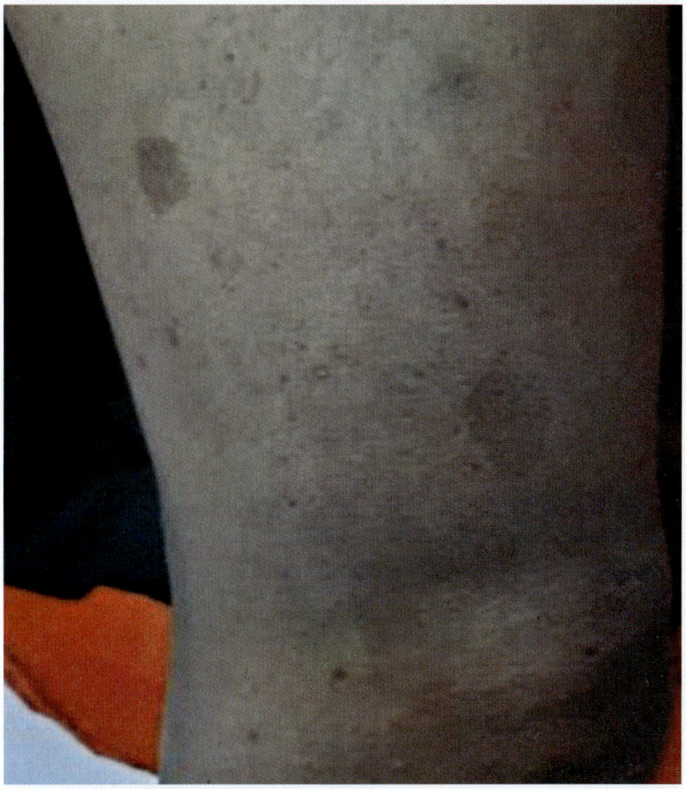

Figure 19.11: Café-au-lait macules

Freckles (Ephelides)

Freckles are small, circumscribed, multiple and symmetrical, light brown macules seen on sun exposed areas, usually in fair skinned individuals.

They are seen in genetically predisposed individuals, with sun exposure causing an increase in the melanin production temporarily. Freckles may be associated with other disorders like neurofibromatosis in which axillary freckling is known as Crowe sign (Figure 19.12), progeria, etc.

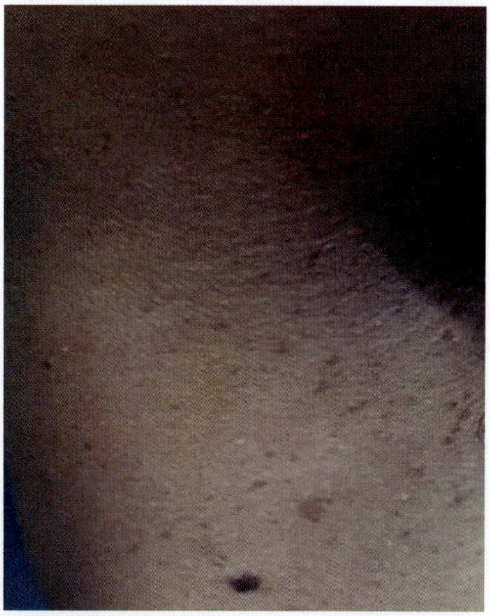

Figure 19.12: Axillary freckles with CALM

Treatment involves photoprotection and topical depigmenting agents like hydroquinone.

LENTIGO

It is a circumscribed macular lesion, associated with an increase in the number of melanocytes at the dermo-epidermal junction. It may occur in both sun exposed and unexposed areas, including mucosa.

Lentigo simplex is the most common form, which develops in childhood. It can affect the body, mucous membranes and even nails. Lesions are small in size (1-5 mm).

Solar lentigo occurs on sun exposed areas and lesions are larger (around 1 cm) in size.

Treatment consists of photoprotection, sunscreens or cryotherapy.

Peutz-Jeghers Syndrome (PJS)

Peutz-Jeghers syndrome is a rare autosomal dominant disease, characterized by gastrointestinal polyps in association with pigmentation affecting skin and mucous membranes. The most common cutaneous feature of PJS is the appearance of melanocytic macules. These are tan, dark brown, or bluish black flat patches 1 to 5 mm in size, seen around the mouth, lips, gums, inner lining of the mouth (Figure 19.13), eyes, hands and feet, fingers and toes, anus and genital areas. Mucous membrane pigmentation primarily appears on the buccal mucosa (66%) but rarely in the intestinal mucosa. Pigmentation usually appears before 5 years of age and may fade after puberty. Gastrointestinal features include gastrointestinal polyps which occur later in life. The polyps may cause bleeding and abdominal pain. The overall risk of Peutz-Jeghers syndrome patients developing a cancer in adulthood is around 93%. Cancers are not only located on the gastrointestinal tract but can occur on many other sites including the breast, ovary, testis, pancreas, uterus, oesophagus and lungs. There is no specific treatment for PJS but the main goal is to manage and prevent associated problems of intestinal obstruction, intussusception and cancer development. The freckling may be less obvious with careful sun protection. In some cases, the pigmentation may be lessened by cosmetic treatment. Cosmetic camouflage may also be useful.

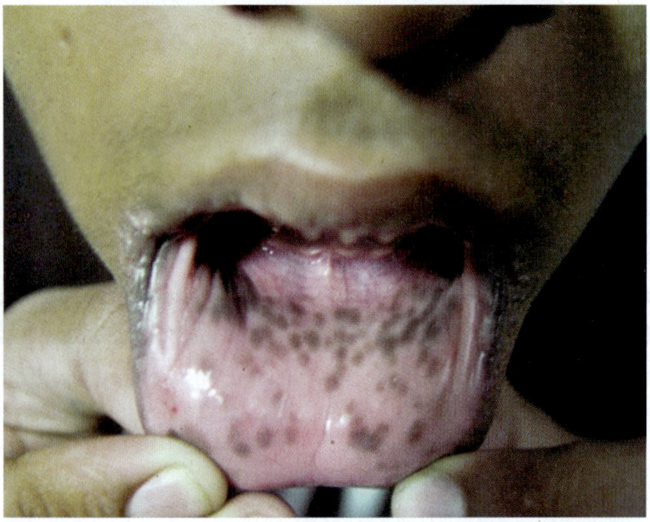

Figure 19.13: Mucosal lentigen in Peutz-Jeghers syndrome patient

Cronkhite-Canada Syndrome (CCS)

Cronkhite-Canada syndrome is a rare non-familial syndrome characterized by marked epithelial disturbances in gastrointestinal tract and epidermis. The gastrointestinal changes are generalized hamartomatous polyposis with abnormal intervening mucosa. The mucosal proliferation leads to fluid and electrolyte abnormalities, malabsorption, malnutrition, GI bleeding and surgical complications. The prevalence of GI malignancy in patients with Cronkhite-Canada syndrome is about 10%. Dermatological manifestations include alopecia, onychodystrophy and hyperpigmentation. Alopecia is initially patchy which rapidly progresses and leads to complete hair loss. Hair loss typically involves the scalp, eyebrows, face, axillae, pubic areas and extremities. Nail changes involve thinning, splitting, and color changes in all fingernails and toenails. Onycholysis and onychomadesis (the loss of all finger and toenails) can also be seen. Hyperpigmented light-to-dark brownish macules and plaques are diffusely distributed. These are most commonly found on the hands and arms. Patchy vitiligo is relatively common. Pigmentation can persist or resolve after treatment. Other symptoms such as hypoguesia and xerostomia have also been described.

The optimal treatment of CCS is currently unknown because of its rarity. Nutritional support aimed at improving electrolytes, vitamin, and mineral deficiencies can rarely induce complete remission as seen in some patients.

Centro-facial Lentiginosis

It is an autosomal dominant uncommon disorder. It usually starts in first year of life with small brown or black macules which increase in number upto the age of 8 or 10 years. Their distribution is restricted to a horizontal band across the centre of the face (Figure 19.14). The mucous membranes are not involved. The condition can be associated with mental retardation, seizures, coalescence of the eyebrows, high-arched palate, absent upper median incisors, sacral hypertrichosis, spina bifida and scoliosis.

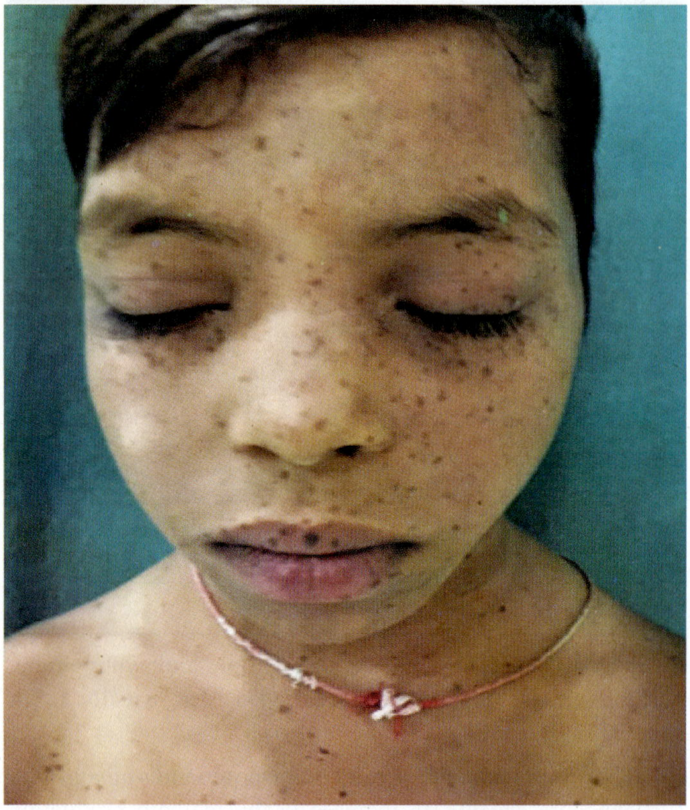

Figure 19.14: Centro facial lentiginosis

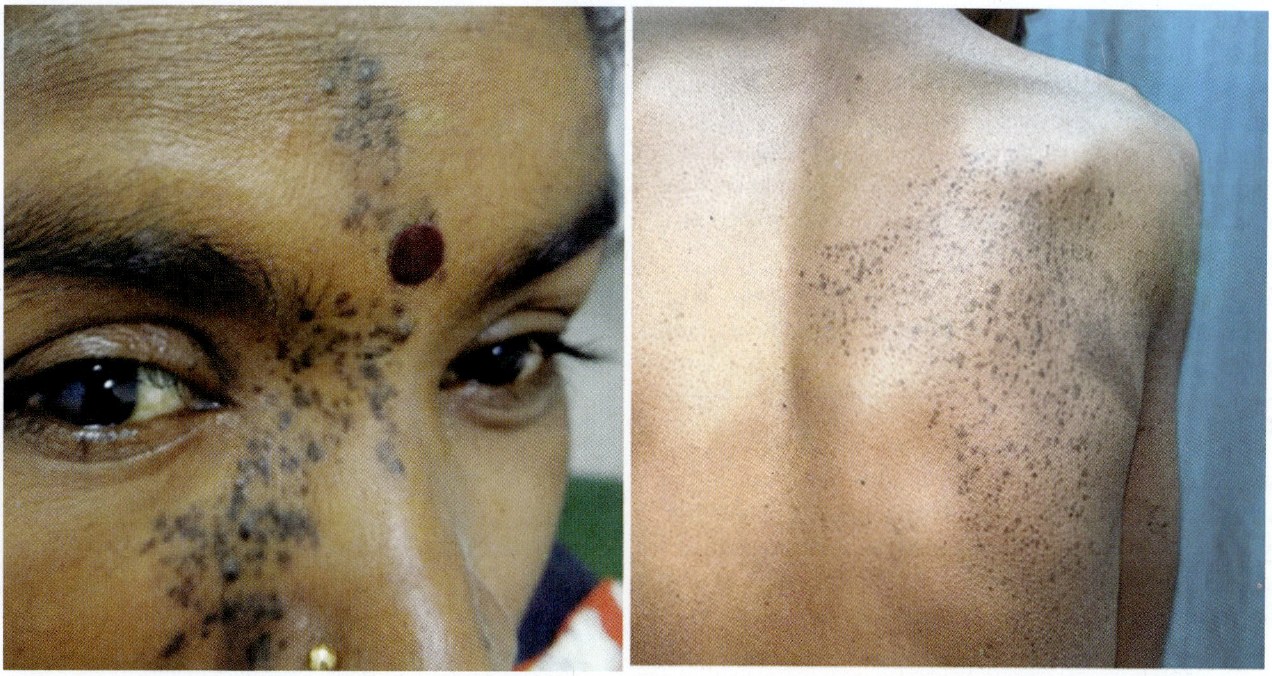

Figure 19.15: Segmental lentiginosis

Segmental Lentiginosis

Segmental lentigines is characterized by numerous small lentigenes grouped within an area of normal skin (Figure 19.15).

Acanthosis Nigricans

Acanthosis nigricans is marked by distinctive, velvety, warty hyperpigmentation in intertriginous areas. Although brown-to-black pigmentation and thickening of the skin is most intense in skin creases of the neck (Figure 19.16), axilla (Figure 19.17) and groin, skin over bony prominences, including the knuckles, elbows, knees and ankles may be affected.

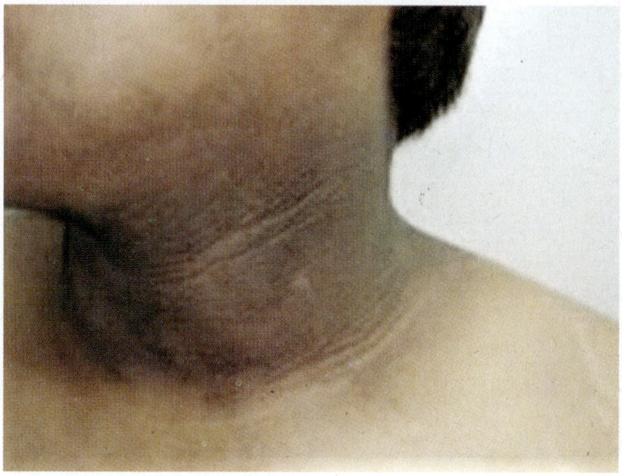

Figure 19.16: Acanthosis nigricans over neck

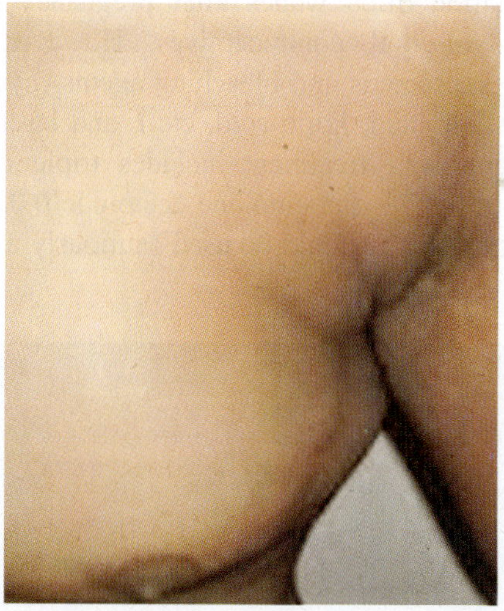

Figure 19.17: Acanthosis nigricans in axilla in same patient

A number of clinical variants are recognized. The inherited type usually erupts during infancy or childhood, but occasionally at puberty. Lesions tend to intensify in adolescence and may fade somewhat during adulthood. The inheritance is usually autosomal dominant and cutaneous findings may be associated with insulin resistance.

The endocrine type is usually associated with a pituitary tumor or polycystic ovary syndrome and insulin resistance. Obesity is a variable feature. Malignant acanthosis nigricans can often be differentiated from the other types by its extensive and more florid lesions, progressiveness, and onset in middle age. The malignant type is only rarely seen in childhood.

Associated tumors include gastric carcinoma, lymphoma, Hodgkin's disease, and osteogenic sarcoma. Idiopathic acanthosis nigricans is the most common type. Although there is no specific associated endocrine disorder, affected individuals are often obese, demonstrate insulin resistance, and are at significant risk for type II diabetes. Pigmentation may decrease after puberty, particularly in patients who experience a weight reduction.

Drug-induced acanthosis nigricans may occur with nicotinic acid, diethylstilbestrol, oral contraceptives and exogenous glucocorticoids.

Melasma

Melasma occurs primarily in pubertal girls and women, but also occasionally in adolescent boys. Although this symmetric, patchy, facial melanosis (Figure 19.18) may be idiopathic, it is often associated with pregnancy or with ingestion of oral contraceptives. Lesions tend to increase after sun exposure.

Clinically, melasma must be differentiated from post-inflammatory hyperpigmentation.

Pigmentation often wanes after pregnancy or the discontinuation of oral contraceptives. However, treatment with topical sunscreens and bleaching agents (hydroquinone, tretinoin, azelaic acid, kojic acid, etc.), and laser may help. The FDA approved treatment includes triple combination with tretinoin 0.05%, fluocinolone acetonide 0.01% and 2% hydroquinone, which should be used cautiously and for short period only.

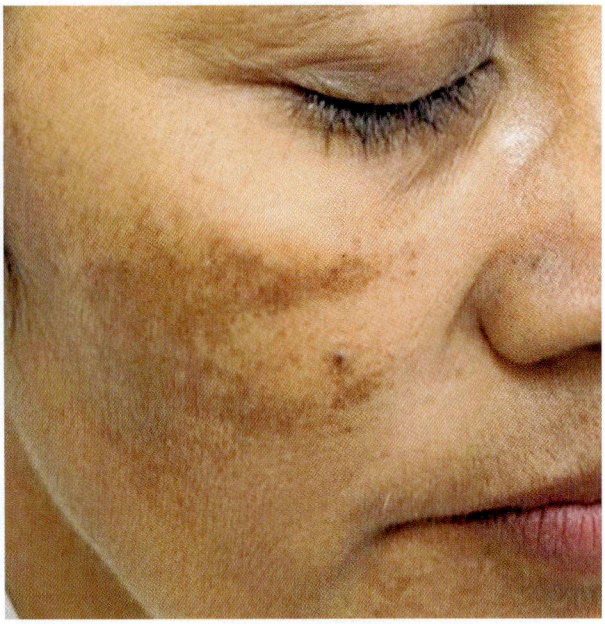

Figure 19.18: Melasma

LICHEN PLANUS PIGMENTOSUS (LPP)

Lichen planus pigmentosus is an uncommon variant of lichen planus characterized by hyperpigmented, dark-brown/slate grey coloured macules (Figure 19.19) commonly in sun-exposed areas. The palms and soles, are usually not involved, but involvement of mucous membranes has been observed. It may or may not be associated with typical lesions of lichen

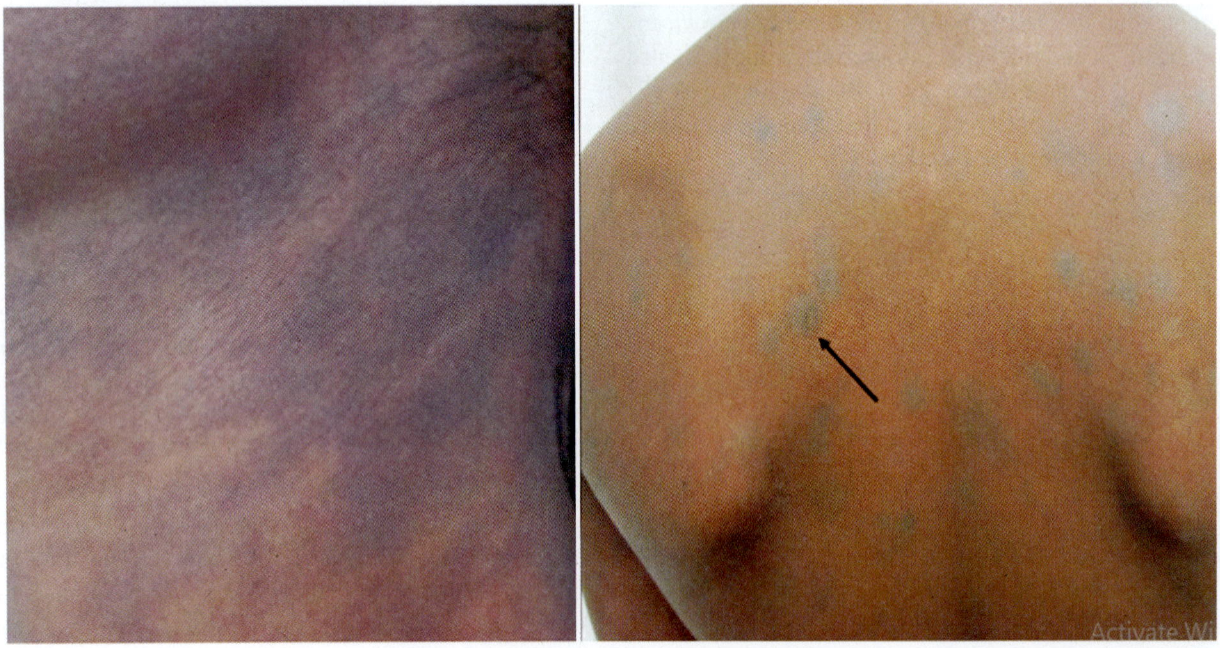

Figure 19.19: Lichen planus pigmentosus

planus. Topical application of mustard oil, which contains allyl isothiocyanate, a potential photosensitizer and Amla oil, has been proposed as possible causes in some patients..

Treatment

Avoidance of exacerbating factors should be advised. Topical steroids are of doubtful efficacy but topical tacrolimus is considered a reasonable treatment option. Systemic treatment modalities include systemic corticosteroids and Vitamin A. The use of dapsone may halt the progression of pigmentation. Combining it with topical tacrolimus may be beneficial in extensive involvement. The use of lasers [low-fluence Q-switched Nd-YAG (1064 nm) in 3 weekly sessions] or their combination with topical agents can be considered.

Linear and Whorled Naevoid Hypermelanosis

Linear and whorled nevoid hypermelanosis (LWNH) is a rare sporadic disease, characterised by hyperpigmented streaks or whorled patterns allowing the lines of Blaschko without any preceding inflammation. It usually occurs in first 2 years of life. Extracutaneous manifestations include neurological, ocular, hearing and skeletal abnormalities. Histology shows increased pigmentation in the basal layer and vacuolization of melanocytes. Treatment options include laser therapy (Q-switched Nd: YAG and Q-switched Ruby).

POST INFLAMMATORY HYPER-PIGMENTATION/MELANOSIS

Post-inflammatory melanosis (PIM) is a frequently encountered problem and represents the sequelae of skin disorders or therapeutic interventions. This acquired excess of pigment can be attributed to various preceding disease processes that affect the skin; like infections, allergic reactions, mechanical injuries, reactions to medications, phototoxic eruptions, trauma (e.g., burns) and inflammatory diseases. Common inflammatory diseases that result in post-inflammatory hyperpigmentation include acne, lichen planus, systemic lupus erythematosus, chronic dermatitis, etc.

Etiopathogenesis

Post-inflammatory hyperpigmentation is caused by either of these two mechanisms that result in either epidermal melanosis or dermal melanosis. The epidermal inflammatory response (i.e., dermatitis) results in the release and subsequent oxidation of arachidonic acid to prostaglandins, leukotrienes and other products. Specifically, these inflammatory products stimulate epidermal melanocytes, causing them to increase the synthesis of melanin, which results in epidermal hypermelanosis. On the contrary, dermal melanosis occurs when inflammation disrupts the basal cell layer, causing melanin pigment to be released and subsequently trapped by macrophages in the papillary dermis, also known as pigmentary incontinence.

Epidemiology

Post-inflammatory hyperpigmentation is more common in pigmented, darker skin. It is more apparent in photo-induced dermatoses and is more severe in lichenoid dermatosis. Although post-inflammatory hyperpigmentation occurs in whites, it is more common in dark-skinned individuals (e.g., African Americans). It occurs with equal incidence in males and females; it has no sexual predilection and can occur in persons of any age.

Clinical Features

Diagnosis of post-inflammatory hyperpigmentation should be considered if a history of a preceding pathologic process or injury to the affected area of hyperpigmentation is present.

- The distribution of the hypermelanotic lesions depends on the location of the original inflammatory dermatosis.
- The color of the lesions ranges from light brown to black (Figure 19.20), with a lighter brown appearance if the pigment is within the epidermis (i.e., epidermal melanosis) and a darker gray appearance if lesions contain dermal melanin (i.e., dermal melanosis).

Differential Diagnosis

- Melasma.
- Tinea versicolor.
- Lichen planus pigmentosus.
- Amyloidosis.
- Acanthosis nigricans.
- Addison's disease.

Investigations

- **Wood's lamp examination** enables distinction of epidermal post-inflammatory melanosis from dermal post-inflammatory hyperpigmentation. Epidermal lesions tend to have accentuated borders under a Wood's lamp examination, which is not seen in dermal lesions.
- **Skin biopsy:** If a history of preceding inflammatory dermatosis is unclear or absent, skin biopsy may be done to exclude other underlying causes of hyperpigmentation.
- Staining of the biopsy specimen with Fontana-Masson silver stain for melanin enables localization of the melanin in the epidermis and/or the dermis.

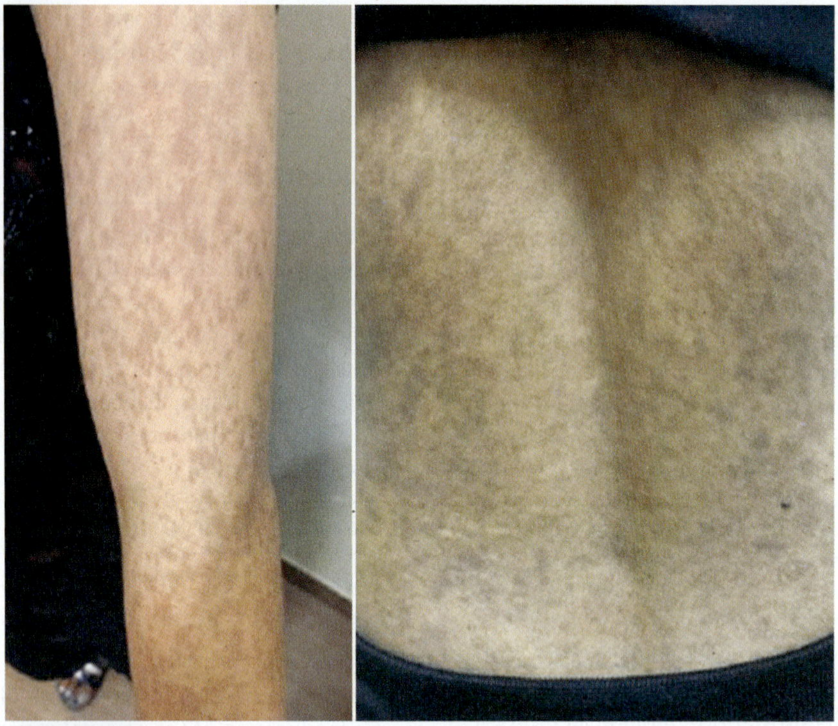

Figure 19.20: Post-inflammatory hyperpigmentation secondary to lichen planus

Treatment

The treatment of post-inflammatory melanosis tends to be a difficult and prolonged process that often takes 6-12 months to achieve the desired results of depigmentation. Each of these treatment options potentially improves epidermal hypermelanosis, but none has proven effective for dermal hypermelanosis. Daily use of a broad-spectrum sunscreen is an essential part of any therapeutic regimen.

- A variety of topical treatments have been used to treat epidermal post-inflammatory hyperpigmentation, with varying degrees of success. These agents include hydroquinone, tretinoin cream, corticosteroids, glycolic acid (GA) and azelaic acid. Chemical peels and sunscreens may be used for further improvement. They are only effective for epidermal hyperpigmentation.
- Topical tretinoin 0.1% with hydroquinone and corticosteroid combination has been shown to be beneficial, especially on the face.
- Carbon dioxide laser resurfacing may be helpful in dermal pigment deposition.

HEREDITARY RETICULATE PIGMENTARY DISORDERS

These are hereditary pigmentary disorders, which present with reticulate or net like arrangement of hyperpigmented and/or hypopigmented macules. Dyskeratosis congenita, Dowling Degos disease, acropigmentation of Kitamura, Naegeli Franceschetti Jadassohn (NFJ) syndrome, X-related reticulate pigmentary condition, dyschromatosis symmetrica hereditaria and dyschromatosis universalis are among the classically recognised true reticulate syndromes.

Dowling Degos Disease (DDD)

It is an autosomal dominant reticulate pigmentary disorder due to mutation in keratin protein. It presents with progressive symmetrical, flexural, reticulate hyperpigmented macules and comedone like papules in the groin, axilla, back and neck in 3rd to 4th decade of life. Acneiform perioral pits and comedones are the hallmark of the disease. It may be associated with hidradenitis suppurativa, keratoacanthoma and squamous cell carcinoma. Histology shows atrophic epidermis with narrow, long and branched rete ridges which intertwine at their bases ("antler-like" appearance) with increased melanin in basal layers. There is no effective treatment available for Dowling Degos disease. Topical azelaic acid, retinoic acid, hydroquinone and corticosteroids can be tried with variable response.

Dyskeratosis Congenita (Zinsser-Cole-Engman Syndrome)

It is an X-linked recessive disorder (most common inheritance), although AD and AR cases have also been reported. It is due to mutations in dyskerin (in X-linked), TERC, TERT, NHP2, and NOP10 genes. The disease presents with reticulate telangiectatic hyperpigmented macules with areas of hypopigmentation on the face, neck, trunk and upper thighs. Other features include acral cyanosis, atrophic skin, nail dystrophy and mucosal leukokeratosis. Extracutaneous manifestations include dental anomalies, aplastic anemia with bleeding tendencies, oesophageal diverticula with dysphagia, retardation of growth, hypogonadism and mental retardation. It may be associated with various malignancies e.g. Hodgkin's disease, GI tract, pancreatic carcinoma and squamous cell carcinoma. The prognosis is poor with mortality mainly due to malignant neoplasms, bone marrow failure or opportunistic infections.

Dermatopathia Pigmentosa Reticularis (DPR) and Naegeli Franceschetti Jadassohn syndrome (NFJ)

DPR is an autosomal dominant disorder due to mutations in keratin 14. It presents with the classical triad of reticulate hyperpigmentation, non cicatricial alopecia of the scalp, eyebrows, axillae and onychodystrophy. Generalized hyperpigmentation prominent on trunk and proximal extremities can also be seen. Other features include punctate palmoplantar keratoses, absent dermatoglyphics, non-scarring acral blisters and bulbar conjunctival pigmentated spots. NFJ syndrome presents with generalized pigmentation and dental defects with little or no nail dystrophy. Pigmentation may fade away by adolescence. Histology of both shows patchy clumps of melanophages in the papillary dermis without epidermal hyperpigmentation.

Reticulate Acropigmentation of Kitamura

It is an autosomal dominant disorder due to mutation in keratin 5, which occurs in first to second decade. It presents with slightly depressed, sharply demarcated brown freckle like macules on dorsal aspect of hands and feet. Other features include palmar pits and ridging on the palms. Histologically, hyperpigmented lesions show epidermal atrophy, elongation and increased melanin in of rete ridges. No definitive treatment is available.

DYSCHROMATOSIS

Dyschromatosis is defined as hyperpigmented macules of small size and irregular shape. It is of two types:

1. Dyschromatosis symmetrica hereditaria (Acropigmentation symmetrica of Dohi).
2. Dyschromatosis universalis hereditaria.

Dyschromatosis Symmetrica Hereditaria (Acropigmentation Symmetrica of Dohi)

It is an autosomal dominant disorder due to mutation in double stranded RNA specific adenosine deaminase gene. It presents in the first to second decade and lesions are classically non progressive. Clinical features include both hypopigmented and hyperpigmented macules on the dorsal and ventral aspects of the hands (Figure 19.21) and feet, which may extend to the proximal portions of the limbs (knees and elbows). Histology shows increased or decreased basal layer pigmentation. Q-switched laser treatment can be tried for hyperpigmented lesions.

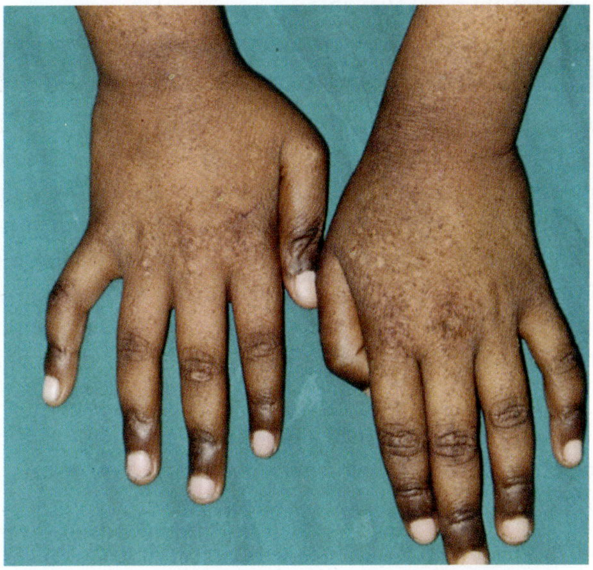

Figure 19.21: Acropigmentation symmetrica of Dohi

Dyschromatosis Universalis Hereditaria (Figure 19.22)

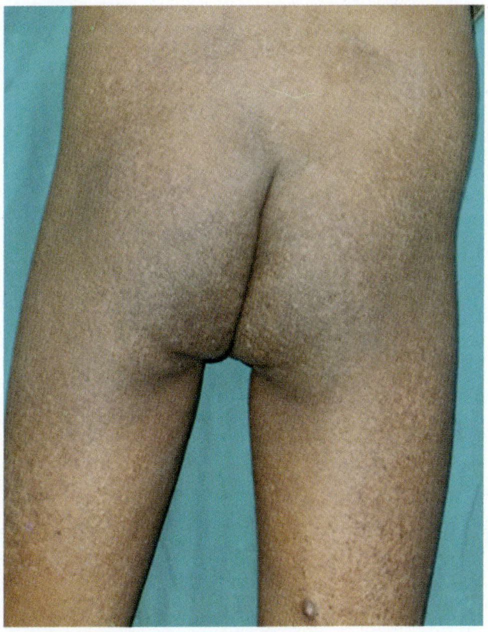

Figure 19.22: Dyschromatosis universalis hereditaria

Dyschromatosis universalis hereditaria (DUH) is an autosomal dominant disease. Onset is in early childhood and is characterized by both hyperpigmented and hypopigmented lesions, which initially appear on hands and gradually, progress to involve the trunk, extremities and the face. Pigmentation of mucosa, palms and soles can also be seen. Hyperpigmented dystrophic nails with pterygium formation is the characteristic feature of DUH. Short stature, sensory neural deafness, photosensitivity and coxa valga may also be associated. No specific treatment is available.

DRUG INDUCED PIGMENTATION

Drug induce pigmentation occurs either by direct stimulation of melanocytes or by non specific inflammation, which leads to hyperpigmentation. In dermis melanin is accumulated inside macrophages. Some of the drugs causing hyperpigmentation are minocycline, cyclophosphamide, hydroxychloroquine, clofazimine, hydroquinone, 5 fluorouracil, bleomycin, phenytoin, hydroxyurea, amiodarone, zidovudine, emtricitabine, imatinib, isoniazid, chlorpromazine, doxorubicin, paclitaxel etc.

Minocycline induced pigmentation: Minocycline induced pigmentation occurs due to accumulation of iron. The four patterns of pigmentation observed are:

- **Type I** – Dark blue-black macules over sites of previous inflammation
- **Type II** – Localized or diffuse hyperpigmentation away from the site of inflammation.
- **Type III** – Muddy skin syndrome which presents with diffuse brown- gray pigmentation.
- **Type IV** – Hyperpigmentation of vermillion area of lower lip.

Different patterns of drug induced pigmentation

Oval pattern: Fixed drug eruptions (FDE) after resolution leaves behind well-defined, round to oval pigmented macules. The common sites are lips and genitalia. Common drugs causing FDE are paracetamol, ibuprofen, Naproxen, Carbamazepine, phenytoin, cotrimoxazole and tetracyclines.

Serpentine supra venous pattern: It starts as an erythematous eruption over the venous network due to intravenous injection extravasation which resolves with supra venous pigmentation. It is seen with 5- fluorouracil and docetaxel based chemotherapy.

Flagellate pigmentation: It is a linear or streaked pigmentation seen classically with bleomycin. Trastuzumab and docetaxel have also been reported to cause flagellate erythema.

Melasma like pigmentation: Common drugs reported to cause melasma like pigmentation are oral contraceptive pills and phenytoin. Long-term imatinib therapy has also been reported to cause melasma like pigmentation. Drugs, which cause photoallergic or phototoxic reactions, can also produce pigmentation similar to melasma.

Reticulate hyperpigmentation: It can be seen over the face and neck e.g. due to therapy with diltiazem.

20

CHAPTER

Care of Skin in Infants, Children and Neonatal Skin Disorders

Contents

NEONATAL SKIN CARE

Maintenance of an intact skin barrier is the goal for all newborns who begin the process of **adaptation** to extrauterine life. Even healthy newborns can experience skin disruption and its consequences. Although the skin of the newborn has similar structural components as that of an adult, it differs in some characteristics from adult skin (Table 20.1). The most important anatomical differences are higher skin surface area to weight ratio, thinner and less elastic skin, higher permeability of the stratum corneum, underdeveloped epidermal barrier and lesser melanin production. Sebaceous glands are not fully functional until puberty and similarly, there are dense but less active sweat glands. In newborns and young infants, the pH of the skin surface is higher and the free fatty acid content is less than in adult skin. Certain principles of skincare have to be emphasized such as gentle cleansing, adequate hydration, moisturisation and protection from irritants and sunlight.

Table 20.1: Differences between neonatal and adult skin

	Neonatal skin	*Adult skin*
1.	Skin of infants is thinner and the body surface area to weight ratio of an infant is five times that of an adult.	The skin in adults is thicker and body surface area to weight ratio is less in adults.
2.	Epidermal thickness in term infant is same as that in adults but in preterm infants it is just half of that of adults.	Epidermis is 0.05 to 0.1 mm in thickness.
3.	Dermis is less thick than adults. Collagen and elastic fibers are immature and also the vessels and nerves are less organized.	Dermis is thicker with mature collagen fibers which are well organized and also the vessels and nerves are well organized
4.	Dermo-epidermal junction is flat without rete ridges.	DEJ is 200 micrometer in thickness with the presence of rete ridges.
5.	Melanosomes are less in both term and preterm infants.	Melanosomes are more as compared to skin of infants.
6.	Eccrine glands are immature in preterm infants resulting in poor thermal response on forehead and poor emotional sweating on palms and soles.	Eccrine glands are well developed and fully functional in adults.
7.	Thermoregulation is poor in preterm infants due to less fat, poor autonomic control of blood vessels and large surface area to body mass ratio.	Thermoregulation is well developed in adults.
8.	Sebum secretion is higher in neonates due to maternal hormones. However, it decreases by the end of first month and becomes stable at the end of first year.	Sebum secretion increases from puberty under the influence of androgens in adults.
9.	Skin is more fragile in preterm infants leading to increased chances of infection and sepsis.	Adult skin provides good physical, biological and biochemical barrier in adults.
10.	Neonatal skin is less hairy.	Well-developed hair in adults.
11.	High thermal conductance with an increased risk of heat loss.	Less
12.	Lipids–less	More
	Melanin–less	More
	Cell attachment and epidermal cellularity less	More
13.	Natural moisturizing factor is lower	Higher

Role of Vernix Caseosa

Vernix caseosa is a naturally occurring complex, lipid-rich substance clinging to the skin surface of the newborn and is produced partly by the fetal sebaceous glands. It consists of sebaceous secretions, shed epithelium and lanugo. At birth, the newborn's skin is covered with vernix caseosa, blood, meconium and cellular debris and it is better to clean this from the head and neck areas soon after birth. Excessive vernix may be removed but should probably not be eliminated entirely due to its other positive attributes. It reduces infection and heat loss, improve barrier function and healing.

Bathing

Bathing is an ideal way of cleansing the newborn to remove blood and vernix. Bathing should not be initiated until the newborn's temperature has stabilized and the baby is hemodynamically stable. Lukewarm water baths (temperature <37ºC) are given in the first few weeks of life. The bath is usually given 2-6 hours after birth in a healthy term baby weighing more than 2500 grams. Prolonged bath increases the hydration of the skin and reduces the threshold for friction thus the bath of the newborn should not last more than 5 minutes. For the initial bath, sterile or potable clean water is sufficient. Soaps and cleansers are best avoided in the first few weeks of life. The neonate should be given bath in a warm room, and should be dried quickly and thoroughly from head to toe, followed by wrapping in a warm dry towel and placing next to the mother. Only water should be used for bathing infants weighing less than 1000 grams. Bathing should not be done more than two to three times per week. Natural pH cleansing agents may be used, but should be rinsed off to avoid irritation or toxicity. Immersion bathing can be soothing and have other positive developmental effects.

Emollients

An emollient is an agent that softens and smoothens the skin. The use of emollients (without perfumes or dyes) such as petroleum ointment or coconut oil twice daily for newborns born after 32 weeks of gestation during first 2-4 weeks of life can counteract the dry skin surfaces and reduce friction and thereby decreases the risk for damage. These emollients do not seem to increase the risk of infection or cause burn from phototherapy and radiant warmers. The most common form of skin breakdown in a normal full term newborn is seen as diaper dermatitis. Use of irritants, adhesives and friction is the common cause of initiating diaper dermatitis. Besides diaper area, the skin of extremities, face, back and buttocks are most likely to be damaged.

Napkin Changes

Napkin should be changed frequently, at least at each nursing and feeding time. It should be washed in lukewarm water and then rinsed off and dried thoroughly.

The diaper area is specifically vulnerable because it is a closed environment suitable for microorganisms and with frequent wetting, it is more often moist therefore, the skin becomes prone to maceration, which increases its permeability to other irritants also.

Skin Disinfectant Solutions

The use of any disinfectant solution should be minimized. Povidone-iodine or chlorhexidine may be used but they should be completely irrigated off with sterile saline to prevent potential toxicity. Use of isopropyl alcohol is discouraged because it is less effective and more drying to skin.

Cord and Circumcision Care

Cleaning of the cord with sterile water is as effective and safe as the use of alcohol, antibiotic ointment, triple dye or povidone-iodine solution. In fact, separation of the cord occurs 2 to 3 days earlier and no umbilical infection occurs in those cleansed with sterile water. Prior to circumcision, skin disinfection is required. These solutions should be completely removed once the procedure is complete. Cleansing thereafter (3 to 4 days) with clear water is advised. Petrolatum or petroleum impregnated gauze can be used to promote healing and prevent adhesions to diaper. Antibiotic ointments are unnecessary.

SKIN CARE IN PREMATURE INFANTS

The stratum corneum of a premature newborn is thinner than that of full term newborn, leading to barrier dysfunction [trans epidermal water loss (TEWL)], heat loss, percutaneous absorption of toxins and increased vulnerability to injury and infection. Although epidermal development is complete *in utero* at 34 weeks of gestation age, those infants born after this time take at least an additional 2 to 4 weeks to attain competent barrier function. Those infants born at very early gestational age (23 to 25 weeks) may require more than 4 weeks (upto 9 weeks) to attain adequate barrier function.

In relation to above fact, there are certain management issues to be considered. The thinner stratum corneum of premature infants lead to increase TEWL and greater risk for volume depletion as well as electrolyte imbalance (usually hypernatremia). The fluid loss is accentuated by increased ambient temperature, radiant warmers, phototherapy and skin diseases that further interrupt the stratum corneum. Many strategies have been used to counter this problem including raising the humidity in incubators, use of plastic cover or blankets, semi-permeable occlusive dressings and topical ointments such as petrolatum.

Unfortunately, these are not without risks. Raising the humidity in incubator favors growth of *Pseudomonas,* a water-loving bacteria and puts the premature infant at risk for infection by the bacteria. Bacterial colonization is also a risk under any occlusive cover or dressing. Therefore, one must pay strict attention to keeping an antiseptic environment. There is further risk when these dressing are removed, because there may be damage to the epidermal barrier by the adhesive. Although topical ointments when applied every 4 to 6 hours seem to benefit premature infants (24 to 32 weeks of gestational age) by reducing TEWL, they increase the risk for infection. A further side effect of ointments is their interference with adhesive and conductive properties of monitoring devices.

Bathing of premature skin should be limited to no more than twice per week. Wait until body temperature has stabilized before initiating any bathing. Do not use cleaning agents in the first 2 weeks of a premature baby's life.

Prevention of Injury to Skin of Premature Infants During Medical Interventions

The premature infant's skin is more susceptible to injury. Due to their prematurity, intense monitoring, ventilation and intravenous support are frequently necessary for premature infants. All these interventions require the use of adhesive material for attachment to skin. The data suggests that gel adhesives are preferred for use on premature skin, except in very premature skin where adherence is less effective, and gel adhesives are not advisable for securing essential devices such as arterial lines and endotracheal tubes. Damage from adhesives may result from its chemical formulation or during its removal from skin. Repetitive application and removal of adhesives can produce skin stripping, tear and tension blisters. Maceration of skin is produced by prolonged occlusion by the adhesive material. Chemical irritation and sensitization may also occur. In an effort to minimize these effects the following measures have been suggested when adhesives are applied:

- Avoid alcohol cleaning.
- Use smallest amount of tape possible.
- Use a hydrocolloid or pectin based layer on the skin prior to heavy adhesive application.
- Avoid bonding agent such as benzoin.
- When adhesive is removed it has been suggested to:
  - Avoid adhesive removers or solvents.
  - Delay removal to intervals greater than 24 hours.
  - Use water soaked cotton balls to assist with removal.
  - Use mineral oil, petrolatum and emollients if reapplication is unnecessary.

Another consequence of skin injury (other than increased TEWL) is the potential for entry of microorganisms. Septicemia is a real concern. The use of topical emollients, which can reconstitute barrier function and minimize abrasive injury, may reduce the incidence of systemic infection. Central venous access in the ill neonate is another source of a blood stream infection. Prevention of invasion of microorganisms through the transcutaneous catheter is critical. Therefore, antisepsis and suppression of catheter site colonization becomes essential. Use of povidone-iodine, frequent dressing changes or application of chlorhexidine-impregnated dressings that are replaced weekly, helps in preventing this problem.

Routine Infant Skin Care

Generally, healthy skin tends to stay healthy as long as it stays intact. Damaged skin, however, is susceptible to a host of ills that have little if any effect on intact skin.

The goal of skin care in the early years of life, therefore, is to minimize skin irritation and maintain the integrity of the epidermal barrier. This goal can be achieved in a number of ways, many of which are inter-related, e.g.

- Avoid exposure to irritating or sensitizing agents such as harsh detergents and soaps.
- Reducing contact with environmental irritants.
- Maintaining a suitable degree of hydration.
- Reducing friction.
- Minimizing percutaneous absorption of toxic or irritating chemicals.
- Minimizing changes in the bacterial flora of skin.
- Avoiding excessive exposure to the sun.

As is true in another area of medicine, in matters of skin care, prevention is always the preferred route.

SKIN CARE IN CHILDREN

The skin, along with other organ systems, undergoes some degree of maturation during childhood, before transition to adulthood. School years bring exposure to a wide variety of infections such as measles, chickenpox, impetigo, warts, molluscum contagiosum, scabies and pediculosis. There is also a gradual increase in contact with potential irritants during outdoor sporting activities such as swimming and games. Following guidelines may be useful:

- Use gentle, fragrance free cleansers and soaps.
- To prevent dry skin and rashes, apply liberal amounts of moisturizer after bathing particularly in children suffering from atopic eczema.
- Initiate early sun protection behaviors, including:
  - The regular use of a broad-spectrum sunscreen that offers a Sun Protection Factor (SPF) of 15 or higher when going for prolonged outdoor activities.
  - If child is prone for skin irritation or allergic reactions, a physical or chemical-free sunscreen with the ingredients like zinc oxide or titanium dioxide should be advised.
  - Reapply sunscreen approximately every two hours, even on cloudy days, and after swimming or sweating.
  - Wear protective clothing, such as a long-sleeved shirt, pants, a wide brimmed hat, and sunglasses, whenever possible.
  - Seek shade when appropriate, and remember that the sun's rays are strongest between 10 a.m. and 4 p.m.
  - Use extra caution near water, snow and sand because they reflect the damaging rays of the sun, which can increase the chances of sunburn.

Use of Cosmetics in Children

Cosmetics are generally defined as products applied externally to improve appearance. In routine, cosmetics should be used less frequently as they may cause allergic reactions in children. Still, if they are used, cosmetics with natural ingredients should be preferred. Following points must be considered while using cosmetics in children:

Lotions and Oils

Always use a lotion prepared for infants and children. Natural ingredients are always best. Lotions with mineral oils should be avoided. Olive oil and coconut oil should be preferred over other oils including mustard oil and almond oil.

Soap

Soaps containing antibacterial substances should not be used in infants. If a soap is needed, do not use a harsh soap. A mild soap with natural ingredients should be advised. Soaps containing olive, coconut or palm oils are good. They help to keep the natural moisture of the skin.

Syndets or synthetic detergents do not have the theoretical disadvantages of soap but are subject to rapid disintegration. They can produce excessive dryness of skin, if moisturizers are not added to it. Antiseptic soaps are useful in preparation of an operative field, but are unsuitable for daily use in an infant as they can cause irritation to an infant's skin. Moreover, antiseptic soaps remove the commensal organism from the skin surface, thereby, making the skin prone to attack by virulent pathogenic organisms from outside.

Liquid cleansers are preferable to water alone, and liquid preparations are preferable to cleansing bars because the preparations often contain emollients.

Shampoos/Conditioners

Shampoos/conditioners specially formulated for infant's head should be used. As child gets older, use products that do not cause irritation to child's eyes. Same product should be continued if the child has no allergic to the ingredients. Products which contain perfumes, artificial colors, or preservatives which can cause allergic reactions in the child should be avoided. Products containing Diethanolamine (DEA) or Triethanolamine (TEA) should be avoided because they interact with nitrites, which are used as preservative in shampoos and may lead to allergic reactions. Products containing preservatives including citrus seed extracts, Vitamins A, E and C can be used.

Powder

Baby powder with no talc should be chosen. Baby powder can be used in the creases of the skin areas like underarms, genital areas and neck. Powders with cornstarch are the best for infant. They can prevent maceration over the skin folds in infants. However, too much of their use can lead to blockade of sweat duct pores resulting in miliaria formation.

Kangaroo mother care (KMC) defined as skin-to-skin contact between a mother and her newborn, frequent or exclusive breastfeeding, and early discharge from the hospital has been effective in reducing the risk of mortality among preterm and low birth weight infants. Research studies and program implementation of KMC have used various definitions.

NEONATAL SKIN DISORDERS

Neonatal skin differs from the skin of adults in the following ways:

- Presence of vernix caseosa.
- Thinner dermis.
- Smaller collagen bundles.
- Immature elastic fibers.
- Less organized vascular and neural elements.
- Increased ratio of surface area to weight (700 cm^2/kg) as compared to adults (250 cm^2/kg), thereby increased risk for toxicity.
- Decreased cohesion between the epidermis and dermis, therefore blisters can form easily.
- Increased permeability with a higher trans epidermal water loss content.
- Underdeveloped sweat glands and absence of sweating.

Most of neonatal skin disorders are transient and self-limiting. Broadly they may be classified as given in Table 20.2. A few important neonatal skin disorders are discussed below. Others are discussed in relevant chapters.

Vernix Caseosa

Skin of a full-term newborn at birth is covered with a white greasy, slippery substance called vernix caseosa. It is composed of dead epithelial cells, sebaceous secretion and lanugo hair. It facilitates the passage through birth canal. Vernix caseosa acts as a biofilm that has a number of antimicrobial peptides, proteins and lipids, giving it its two most important functions–mechanical protection and antibacterial action. Therefore, it should be left on the body till it sheds spontaneously.

Milia

Milia are one of the most common transient neonatal disorders, seen in upto 90% of neonates. They occur as 1-2 mm whitish-yellow papules on nose, cheeks, forehead (Figure 20.1 A and B) and chin, rarely on trunk and extremities. They are epidermal cysts derived from pilosebaceous unit. Epidermal cysts on the palate are termed as *Epstein's pearls* and similar lesions on alveolar margins are called Bohn's cysts. They regress spontaneously in a few weeks. Persistent or extensive milia may be seen in conditions like epidermolysis bullosa, orofacial-digital syndrome type 1, Marie-Unna type congenital hypotrichosis or the Bazex Dupre Christol syndrome and paronychia, hereditary trichodysplasia, etc.

Table 20.2: Broad classification of neonatal dermatoses	
Group	***Diseases***
Physiological	Vernix caseosa, milia, superficial cutaneous desquamation, Epstein pearls, physiological jaundice, sebaceous gland hyperplasia, acrocyanosis, harlequin color change, neonatal occipital alopecia and cutis marmorata
Transient noninfective	Erythema toxicum neonatorum, neonatal acne, miliaria, transient neonatal pustular melanosis, suckling blisters, eosinophilic pustulosis, infantile acropustulosis and subcutaneous fat necrosis of newborn, sclerema neonatorum
Naevi/Developmental defects	Mongolian spots, nevus simplex, congenital hemangiomas, congenital melanocytic nevi, supernumerary nipples, sebaceous naevi, naevus flammeus, nevus depigmentosus, nevus anemicus, familial lentiginosis syndromes, verrucous naevi, neural tube dysraphism, aplasia cutis congenital and accessory tragus
Genodermatoses	Ichthyosis, Epidermolysis bullosa, Incontinentia pigmenti, oculocutaneous albinism, café-au-lait macules, cutis laxa, Ehlers-Danlos syndrome, hereditary palmoplantar keratoderma, piebaldism and congenital erythropoietic porphyria and ectodermal dysplasia
Infections	Bacterial–Bullous impetigo, staphylococcal skin scalded syndrome (SSSS), congenital syphilis, necrotizing fasciitis, omphalitis, mastitis, listeriosis Viral–Cytomegalovirus, varicella zoster, enterovirus, herpes simplex, rubella and human parvovirus B19 Fungal–Candida and dermatophyte Parasitic–Toxoplasmosis, scabies and leishmaniasis Arthropods–Bites and stings
Eczema and Inflammatory disorders	Infantile seborrheic dermatitis, diaper dermatitis and psoriasis
Nutritional dermatoses	Acrodermatitis enteropathica and neonatal biotin deficiency
Erythroderma	Ichthyosis–Collodion baby, Lamellar ichthyosis, harlequin ichthyosis, congenital ichthyosiform erythroderma and Netherton syndrome Immunodeficiency disorders–Omenn syndrome, Graft vs host disease, severe combined immunodeficiency (SCID) Papulosquamous disorders–Congenital erythrodermic psoriasis, erythrodermic pityriasis rubra pilaris Others–Diffuse cutaneous mastocytosis and drugs
Immunodeficiency syndromes	AIDS, SCID, Omenn syndrome, DiGeorge anomaly, Wiskott-Aldrich syndrome and hyperimmunoglobulin E syndrome

(Sharma YK, Sadana DJ, Rizvi A, Dash K. A comprehensive classification and abbreviated update of neonatal dermatological entities. Indian J Paediatr Dermatol 2015;16:122-35)

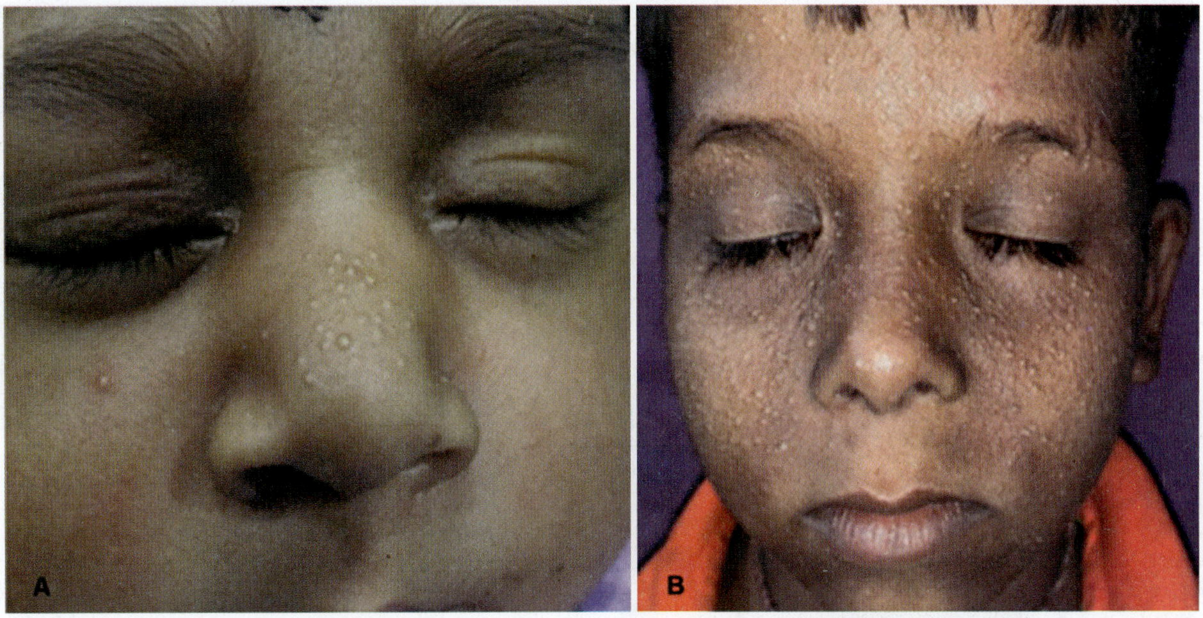

Figure 20.1: Milia over nose (A) and Milia all over face (B)

Cutis Marmorata

Cutis marmorata or "marbled skin" refers to mottled skin, typically seen in newborns in the first few months of life (Figure 20.2). This phenomenon is caused by instability or immaturity of the nerve supply to the superficial capillary blood vessels in the skin. This causes the blood vessels in some regions of the skin to dilate, producing erythema, while other regions are pale colored. It is most pronounced when the skin is cooled and disappears on rewarming. This condition is also a common finding in babies with Down's syndrome.

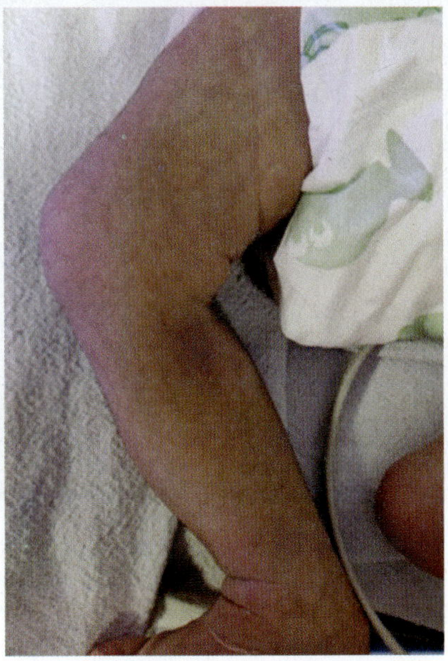

Figure 20.2: Cutis marmorata

A more pronounced form of this disorder is called cutis marmorata telangiectasia congenita (CMTC). It is an uncommon, congenital cutaneous vascular anomaly which presents as persistent cutis marmorata, telangiectasia and phlebectasia. The reticulated mottling does not disappear with rewarming. It has also been reported in association with a variety of other congenital anomalies like skin atrophy and ulcerations, capillary malformations, atrophy or hypertrophy of the affected extremity, macrocephaly and glaucoma.

Mongolian spot (See chapter 19)

Harlequin Colour Changes

Harlequin colour change is a rare condition of neonates showing transient erythema involving one half of the body, with blanching of the other half and a sharp demarcation at midline. It is a bizarre, gravity dependent, episodic color change, which is usually seen in low birth weight and sick babies. The face and genitalia are spared. It is believed to be due to transient autonomic dysregulation of cutaneous vasculature. The attacks may last from 30 seconds to 20 minutes, and may occur upto 12 times in 24 hours. It is a benign condition which generally subsides by the third week of life. No treatment is required.

Erythema Toxicum Neonatorum (ETN)

It is a self-limiting disorder of unknown etiology, clinically characterized by a macular erythematous eruption. It mostly presents as an asymptomatic condition. Erythema toxicum neonatorum may present any time after birth upto 4 days.

Lesions are distributed over trunk, face and proximal extremities (Figure 20.3). The macular erythema may subside or evolve into papules and pustules. Prolonged contact with meconium, enterotoxins, minor graft-versus-host reaction due to peri parturition materno fetal lymphocytic transfer, vaginal secretions during severe protracted labor and strengthened innate antimicrobial system during the first few days of life are possible etiological factors. Spontaneous recovery usually occurs within 2-3 days. No treatment is required, topical calamine lotion may be applied to involved areas.

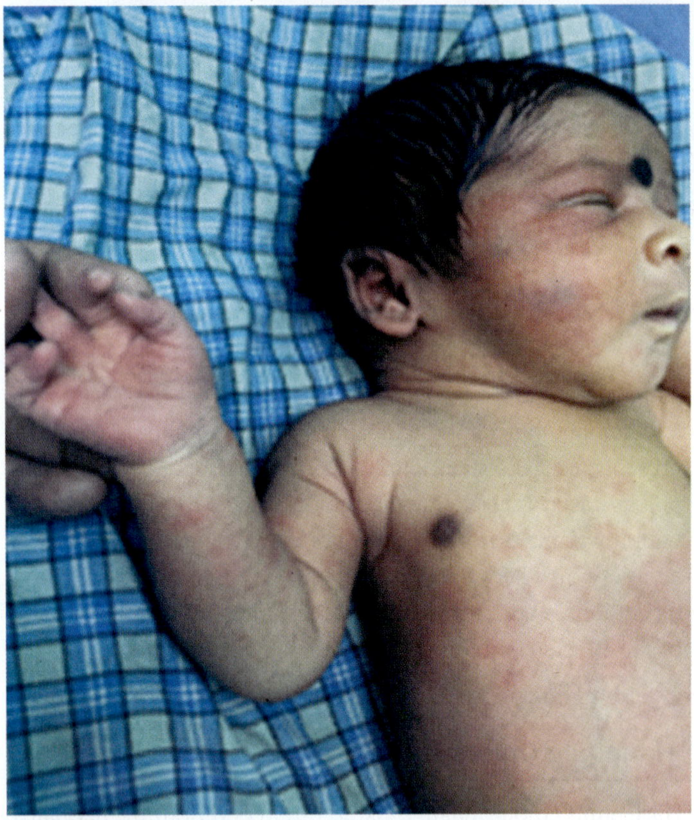

Figure 20.3: ETN (Rash appears 24 hours after birth. Palms and soles are spared (Courtesy– Dr. Bhumesh K Katakam)

Cradle Cap

It is the generalized scaling of the scalp seen in neonatal period. It is thought to be due to seborrheic dermatitis, caused by Pityrosporum ovale. It presents as erythematous, greasy scaly eruption of the scalp (Figure 20.4). Mild pruritus may be present. Face, eyebrows and ears may be affected. Persistence for a long period may suggest the diagnosis of atopic dermatitis. Treatment includes removal of scales by application of oil. Low potency topical steroids may be applied.

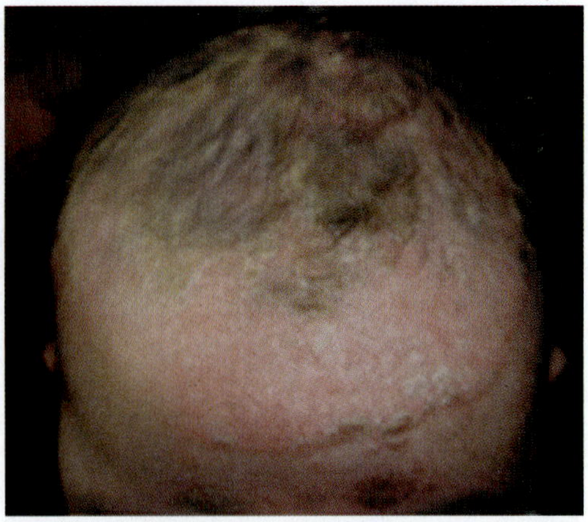

Figure 20.4: Cradle cap

Transient Pustular Melanosis of Neonates

Transient pustular melanosis (Figure 20.5) is an idiopathic benign condition, more commonly seen in black neonates. This condition presents at birth or on first neonatal day on face, back and buttocks as multiple asymptomatic superficial vesiculopustules of 1-3 mm size containing neutrophils and occasional eosinophils, which rupture easily leaving characteristic collarette of scales, crusting and eventually a pigmented macule that fade within 3-4 weeks. Affected sites are chin, neck, forehead, palms and soles. Sometimes the pustular stage may have occurred *in utero*, with only the pigmented lesions seen at birth. It is a self-limiting condition, and no treatment is required.

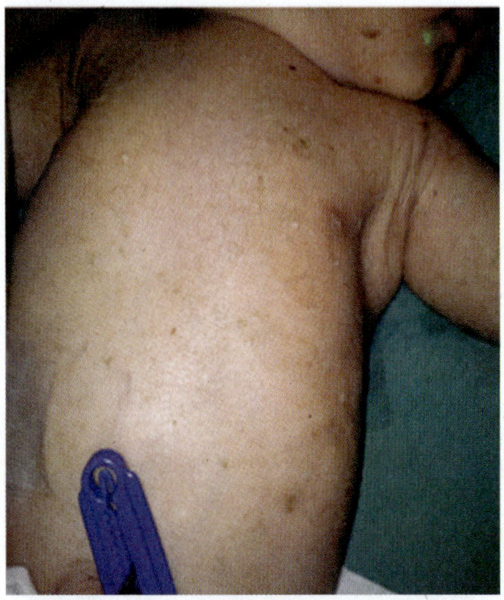

Figure 20.5: Transient pustular melanosis of neonates in a one-day old baby (Triad vesicle, collarette scale and hyperpigmentation) Courtesy– Dr. Bhumesh K Katakam

Eosinophilic Pustulosis

The lesions appear as itchy, 1-3 mm sized pustules with erythematous bases. (Figure 20.6) It is seen predominantly on scalp and face with onset in early infancy. It is possibly regarded as a hypersensitivity reaction to the dust mite, Dermatophagoides pteronyssium, or due to secretion of a chemokine in response to increased sebum. No treatment is required, oral antibiotics and topical steroids may have suppressive effect on the lesions.

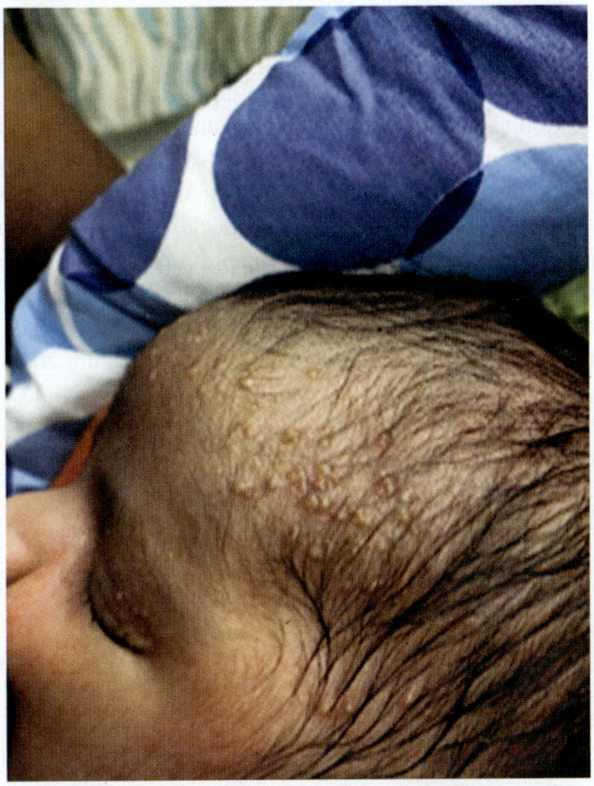

Figure 20.6: Eosinophilic pustulosis (Courtesy– Dr. Bhumesh K Katakam)

Infantile Acropustulosis (Figure 20.7)

Infantile acropustulosis is characterized by itchy, vesiculo-pustular lesions, which are predominantly present on palms and soles. They occur in recurrent crops, lasting for 7-14 days. The classic history of infantile acropustulosis is an infant aged 2-12 months developing pruritic erythematous macules or papules that progress into non coalescing vesicles and then pustules. The hands and the feet are always involved in infantile acropustulosis, usually on the palms, the soles, and the lateral surfaces. Lesions may occur on the dorsal aspects of the hands and the feet as well as on the trunk, the scalp and the face. Healing may leave macular hyperpigmentation.

No other organ systems are involved in infantile acropustulosis. Dapsone is an effective treatment, oral antihistamines may be given for symptomatic relief.

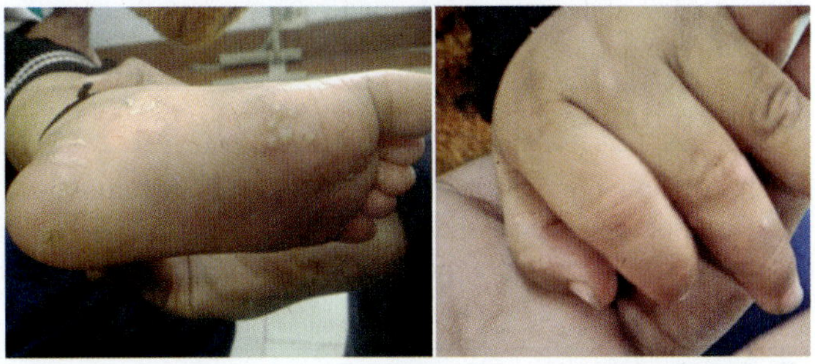

Figure 20.7: Infantile acral pustulosis

Sucking Blisters

Sucking blisters may be present at birth due to prenatal in utero sucking by the baby on its body parts. It presents as single or multiple non-inflammatory vesicles or bullae. They are mostly oval, thick-walled, and contain sterile fluid. Sometimes they only appear as well-demarcated erosions. The size varies between 0.5 and 2 cm (Figure 20.8). The lesions are located mainly at the dorsal or radial aspect of the wrists, hands, or fingers. Both unilateral or symmetrical bilateral distribution has been observed and has occasionally been accompanied by blisters or callus formation at the lips (sucking pads). Typically, the neonate is noted to suck excessively on the involved areas. No treatment is required.

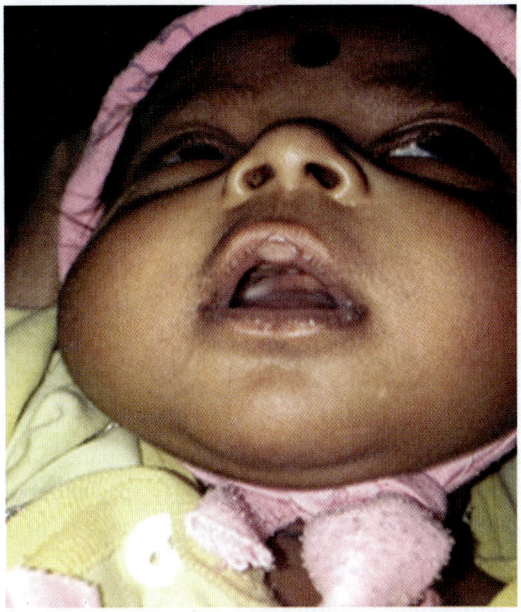

Figure 20.8: Infantile sucking blister (Courtesy– Dr. Bhumesh K Katakam)

Bronze Baby Syndrome

Infant who develops a greyish brown discoloration of the skin, serum and urine while undergoing phototherapy for hyperbilirubinemia.

Lanugo Hair

Fine soft non pigmented and unmedullated immature hair. First coat of lanugo hair shed in the third trimester. These are important consideration in preterm infants. These are replaced by vellus hair in first month of life.

Bohn Nodules and Epstein Pearls

These are keratin filled cyst derived from remnant of odontogenic epithelium over the dental lamina or may be remnant of minor salivary glands. Bohn nodules occur on alveolar ridge and more common on maxillary than mandibular. Epstein pearls are also keratin filled cyst occurs due to epithelial entrapment during palatal development.

Natal Teeth

The presence of teeth at birth or within a month of birth is an uncommon neonatal oral change. It can be classified into two groups:

1. **Mature natal teeth:** Fully developed natal teeth and it has good prognosis.
2 **Immature natal teeth:** Substandard or incomplete developed teeth and it has poor prognosis.

Most common location for natal teeth is mandibular incisors followed by maxillary incisors. This condition may associate with various syndromes like Ellis van Creveld syndrome, pachyonychia congenita, Rubinstein-Taybi syndrome, Hallerman-Streiff syndrome and ectodermal dysplasia. These natal teeth may cause inhalation of teeth due to it great motility, ulceration on tongue, painful feeding, and ulceration of nipple of mother.

Sebaceous Hyperplasia

Sebaceous hyperplasia occurs when maternal androgen hormones causes enlargement of sebaceous glands in newborn resulting in small yellow-white regularly spaced papules seen on node and cheeks. Usually occurs in about 50 % of newborn and resolves by 3-4 months of age.

Hemangiomas (chapter 22)

Diaper Dermatitis

Diaper dermatitis is caused by over hydration of the skin, maceration and prolonged contact with urine and feces. The incidence of this disorder is more in higher socioeconomic groups where diapers are used.

The precise etiology of most of the diaper rashes is not clearly defined. They likely result from a combination of factors that include wetness, friction, urine and feces, and the presence of microorganisms. Anatomically, skin in diaper area has numerous folds and creases, which presents a problem with regard to both efficient cleansing and control of the microenvironment.

The main irritants in infants are fecal proteases and lipases, whose activity is increased greatly with elevated pH. An acidic skin surface is essential for the maintenance of the normal microflora, which provides innate antimicrobial protection against invasion by pathogenic bacteria and yeasts. Fecal lipase and protease activity is also greatly increased by acceleration of gastrointestinal transit; this is the reason for the high incidence of irritant diaper dermatitis observed in babies who have had diarrhea in the previous 48 hours. Diaper dermatitis tends to spread to concave (i.e., skin folds) as well as convex surfaces, and often presents as central red, beefy erythematous plaques with satellite pustules (Figure 20.9).

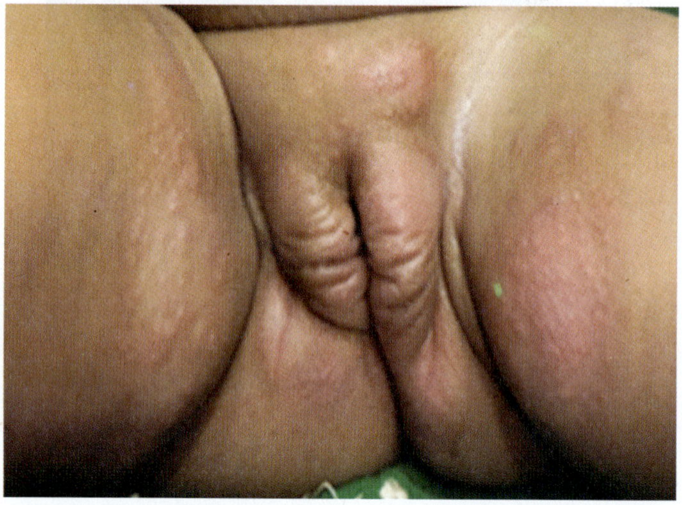

Figure 20.9: Diaper dermatitis: Primary irritant diaper dermatitis –rash on the convexities (If it persists beyond 72 hours, commensal candida will multiply and may produce clinical manifestations with the involvement of intertriginous groin spaces with or without satellite lesions) Courtesy– Dr. Bhumesh K Katakam

Irritant contact dermatitis most likely develops from a combination of intertrigo and miliaria. In addition, it has been shown to result from the irritating effects of mixing urine with feces. Urine in the presence of fecal urease becomes more alkaline due to the production of ammonia. This alkaline urine causes activation of fecal lipases, ureases and proteases. These, in turn, irritate the skin directly and increase its permeability to other low molecular weight irritants.

The wearing of diapers causes a significant increase in skin wetness and pH. Prolonged wetness leads to maceration (softening) of the stratum corneum, the outer protective layer of the skin, with extensive disruption of intercellular lipid lamellae. Weakening of its physical integrity makes the stratum corneum more susceptible to damage by (1) Friction from the surface of the diaper and (2) Local irritants. The dampness, lack of air exposure, acidic or irritant exposures, and friction begin to break down the skin barrier.

The normal pH of the skin is between 4.5 and 5.5. When urea from the urine and stool mix, urease breaks down the urine, decreasing the hydrogen ion concentration (increasing pH). Elevated pH levels increase the hydration of the skin and make the skin more permeable.

The pH of cleansing products can also change the microbiological spectrum of the skin. Soaps with high pH values encourage growth of Propionibacterium on skin.

Candidal Diaper Dermatitis

Once the skin is compromised, secondary infection by candida is common. Between 40 and 75% of diaper rashes that last for more than 3 days are colonized with candida albicans. Candida is a fecal origin and is not an organism commonly found on the perianal skin. Amoxicillin was found to increase the colonization by candida and worsen the diaper dermatitis.

Bacterial Diaper Dermatitis

Bacteria may play a role in diaper dermatitis through reduction of fecal pH and the resultant activation of enzymes. Additionally, fecal microorganisms probably contribute to secondary infections when they occur. Secondary infection presents as impetigo in which flaccid bullae are seen, but sometimes tense due to *Staphylococcus aureus* infection, or a cellulitis due to cutaneous streptococci, or even a folliculitis due to *S. aureus* infection.

Polymicrobial growth is documented in at least half of diaper rash cultures. *Staphylococcus* species are the most commonly grown organisms, followed by *Streptococcus* species and organisms from the family Enterobacteriaceae. Nearly 50% of isolates also contain anaerobes.

Clinical Features

Patients with diaper dermatitis present with an erythematous scaly diaper area often with papulovesicular or bullous lesions, fissures and erosions. The eruption may be patchy or confluent, and may spread up to the abdomen from the umbilicus down to the thighs and encompassing the genitalia, perineum and buttocks. Gluteal folds are spared in irritant dermatitis, but often involved in primary candidal dermatitis. Children with diaper dermatitis have marked discomfort from intense inflammation.

Treatment

Treatment should involve correcting the underlying cause such as overhydration of the skin, maceration, prolonged contact with urine and feces, avoidance of retained diaper, soaps or irritant topical preparations. Occlusive plastic diapers should be avoided. Topical preparations which are used, should be hypoallergic. Application of emollients, Vitamin E, aloe vera or zinc preparations may be done. In case of a secondary bacterial infection, oral and topical antibiotics are to be prescribed. If candidiasis is suspected or proven by potassium hydroxide (KOH) preparation or by culture, an antifungal agent effective against yeast is indicated. Topical creams like miconazole, ketoconazole, luliconazole etc are effective. In resistant cases, oral fluconazole 3-5 mg/kg/week may be used. If significant inflammation is obvious, a mildly potent steroid like mometasone can be used. It is best to avoid higher strength topical steroids as they may be systemically absorbed.

Intertrigo

Intertrigo occurs when wet skin, which is more fragile and has a higher coefficient of friction, becomes damaged from maceration. It is seen in the skin folds, most often in the groin region (Figure 20.10). Most cases of cutaneous candidiasis occur in skin folds where occlusion by clothes produces abnormally moist, favorable conditions for the growth of the fungus. Sites such as the perineum and anus, in which Candida organisms may be carried normally, are at further risk of infection. Erythema and inflammation with serous or seropurulent discharge is noticed in the skin folds.

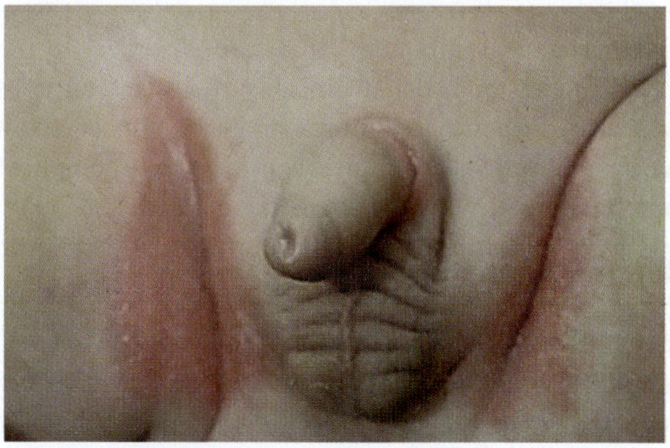

Figure 20.10: Candidal intertrigo

Perianal Dermatitis

Perianal dermatitis presents as erythema with erosion (Figure 20.11) and bleeding around the anal opening. It may occur due to formula feeding and resultant abnormal fecal PH. It is observed during the first week of life and commonly seen in premature babies. Application of emollients and change in feeding habits may cure the condition.

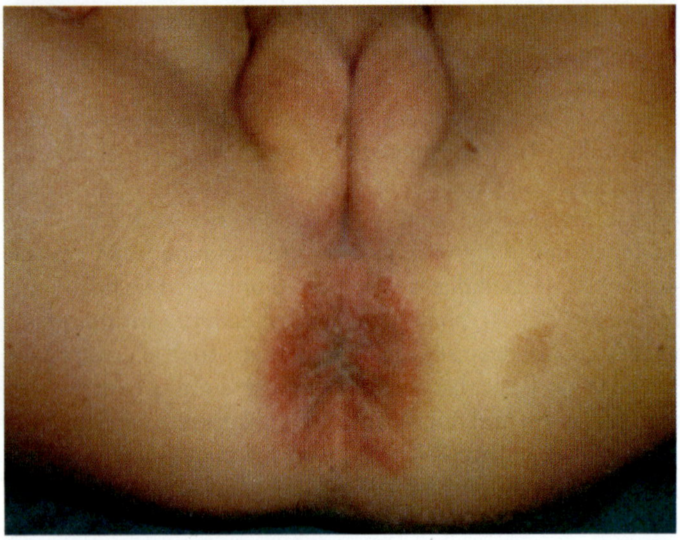

Figure 20.11: Perianal dermatitis

Jacquet's Erosive Dermatitis

Punched out or crateriform lesions over gluteal region seen in older infants or children. It is an irritant contact dipper dermatitis, occurs due to combined effect of friction, moisture, urine faces and secondary infection. Treatment includes frequent change of diaper, barrier creams, low potent topical steroid and topical antibiotics or antifungal in secondarily infected cases.

Granuloma Gluteal Infantum

Granuloma gluteal infantum is a rare disorder. It is not very well understood, but it probably represents an unusual inflammatory response to long-standing irritation, candidiasis, or fluorinated corticosteroids. It is considered as a complication of long standing primary irritant diaper dermatitis.

Sclerema Neonatorum

Sclerema neonatorum is a disorder of the subcutaneous fat in debilitated preterm neonates. In an infant, fat has a higher saturated-to-unsaturated fatty acid ratio compared to adult fat and thus, a higher melting point. Prematurity, hypothermia, shock, and metabolic abnormalities have been postulated to further increase this ratio. This leads to solidification of adipose tissue after a circulatory collapse.

Half the infants affected by sclerema neonatorum are premature, and the others are full term but have a serious underlying illness. They are often of low birth weight (< 2500 g) and have cyanosis and low Apgar score.

Induration in sclerema neonatorum appears suddenly, first on the thighs and buttocks and then, spreading rapidly, often affecting all parts of the body except the palms, soles, and genitalia. The involved skin is pale, waxy, and firm on palpation. The skin cannot be pitted or pinched up because it is bound to the underlying tissues. The affected infant often displays flexion contractures at the elbows, knees and hips; temperature instability, restricted respiration, difficulty in feeding, and decreased spontaneous movement.

Associated underlying conditions include pneumonia, septicemia, hypothermia, metabolic acidosis, respiratory distress syndrome, congenital heart defects, gastroenteritis and intestinal obstruction.

Recognition and the prompt institution of therapy specific for the underlying disease are mandatory.

- Careful monitoring, correction of electrolyte abnormalities, respiratory support, correction of hypovolemia, and control of hypothermia are important in sclerema neonatorum patients.
- Antibiotics: Prophylactic broad-spectrum antibiotic therapy should be instituted for possible associated sepsis.
- Systemic steroids: The value of systemic steroids is controversial. No controlled studies have demonstrated improved survival with the use of systemic steroids in sclerema neonatorum, although they are often used.
- Infants with sclerema neonatorum are best cared for in a neonatal intensive care unit.
- Medical therapy of the skin is not beneficial; successful treatment of the underlying disorder improves the skin.

Subcutaneous Fat Necrosis

It is a transient disorder of neonates presenting with multiple nodular lesions due to focal necrosis of fat. It may be associated with hypercalcemia. Exact cause is unknown but may be associated with maternal diabetes, preeclampsia, neonatal hypoxia and hypothermia.

Clinically single or multiple nodules are seen on buttocks, thighs, shoulders, back and arms. They may present at birth or from second day to third week of neonatal period. Nodules are rubbery in consistency and are red or bluish red in color. They disappear in few months. No treatment is required.

CHAPTER 21

Dermatosis of Pregnancy

Contents

Pregnancy is associated with many physiological changes affecting the skin, hair and nails. Three main factors cause skin changes which are commonly seen in pregnancy. These changes include an increase in hormone levels, intravascular volume expansion and skin compression from the pregnant uterus. There are several pathological dermatosis, which are specific to pregnancy. These will be discussed briefly in this chapter.

PHYSIOLOGICAL SKIN CHANGES IN PREGNANCY

1. **Cutaneous changes**
   - Diffuse hyperpigmentation
   - Selective hyperpigmentation (genitalia, axilla, areolae, recent scars)
   - Linea nigra
   - Melasma (chloasma/mask of pregnancy)
   - Darkening of ephelides and melanocytic nevi
   - Striae distensae
2. **Hair**
   - Hirsutism
   - Thickening of scalp hair
   - Postpartum telogen effluvium
   - Postpartum androgenetic alopecia
3. **Nails**
   - Subungual hyperkeratosis
   - Distal onycholysis
   - Transverse grooving
   - Brittle nails
   - Accelerated growth
4. **Glandular changes**
   - Increased eccrine function (except palms)-Miliaria, dyshidrotic eczema, hyperhidrosis
   - Elevated thyroid activity with resultant relative iodine deficiency
   - Increased sebaceous function- Montgomery tubercles, acne gravidarum
   - Decreased apocrine function
5. **Vascular changes**
   - Palmar erythema
   - Spider nevi
   - Pyogenic granulomas
   - Varicose veins of legs and DVT
   - Pregnancy epulis/granuloma gravidarum- small vascular lesions of gingival similar to pyogenic granuloma
   - Gingival hyperemia and hyperplasia

6. **Mucosa**
   - **Chadwick's sign:** Bluish-purple coloration of the vagina.
   - **Goodell's sign:** Bluish-purple coloration of the cervix.
   - Nasal congestion
7. **Immune system changes**

   There is a shift from Th1 to Th2 profile which results in increased susceptibility to autoimmune disorders and reduced cell mediated immunity posing an increased risk of skin infections.

SPECIFIC PREGNANCY DERMATOSIS

Specific skin conditions occur during pregnancy or in the postpartum period and range from benign and transient to more severe and chronic. These dermatological manifestations can cause discomfort, distress, or pose potential risks to both the mother and the developing fetus. The dermatosis specific to pregnancy include the following:

- Polymorphic eruption of pregnancy (PEP)
- Intrahepatic cholestasis of pregnancy (ICP)
- Atopic eruption of pregnancy (AEP)
- Pemphigoid gestationis (PG)
- Pustular psoriasis of pregnancy (PPP)

Polymorphic Eruption of Pregnancy (PEP)

- It is benign and self-limiting condition, occurring at the end of pregnancy (between the 36th and 39th weeks) and, rarely, in the immediate puerperium.
- It is considered to be most frequent specific dermatosis, with an estimated incidence of 1:200 pregnancies, the vast majority occurring in primigravidae.
- Although exact pathogenesis is not yet elucidated, however it is related to an inflammatory process triggered by rapid abdominal distention, which may explain its association with excessive weight gain, twin pregnancy and a large fetus for gestational age. Upregulated Th2 cytokine profile, including IL-9 and IL-33 and the reaction against bacteria and fungi residing in the skin, may be involved in the pathogenesis.
- It typically presents with urticarial papules along the abdominal striae which extend to the limbs, trunk, and buttocks sparing periumbilical area, palms and soles, face and mucus membrane. Papules may coalesce to form plaques which may exhibit small vesicles, target lesions and polycyclic lesions. Generally, the condition persists for 4–6 weeks. Recurrence in subsequent pregnancies is rare.
- Pruritic eruption of pregnancy (PEP) is not associated with any adverse maternal or fetal outcomes.
- Polymorphic eruption of pregnancy (PEP) has non-specific histopathology findings. It variably shows scattered stromal mast cells, polymorphous mononuclear infiltrates with eosinophils and dermal edema. Superficial and deep perivascular mononuclear infiltrate with eosinophilia may be seen in half of the cases.
- **Treatment:** The main goal of treatment is to decrease itching. The lesions frequently resolve on their own in 4 to 6 weeks. Oral antihistamines (chlorpheniramine maleate, cetirizine and hydroxyzine hydrochloride are safe in pregnancy) and topical steroids are commonly used for treatment. Topical hydrocortisone 2.5% ointment or cream, desonide 0.05% ointment or cream, triamcinolone acetonide 0.1% ointment or cream, mometasone furoate 0.1% cream, or fluocinolone acetonide 0.025% ointment may be used. Systemic corticosteroids may be used as a short course if topical treatment is not satisfactory. Common regimens include prednisolone or prednisone 0.5 mg/kg daily for a week which are tapered over the subsequent 1 to 2 weeks.

Intrahepatic Cholestasis of Pregnancy (ICP)

- It is the only specific dermatosis of pregnancy which initially presents with pruritus without primary cutaneous lesions. Its prevalence ranges between 0.3 and 5.6% of pregnancies, depending on geographic and ethnic factors.
- The family history is positive in 50% of the cases and it is more frequent in twin pregnancies.
- Intrahepatic cholestasis of pregnancy (ICP) presents as generalized pruritus in the late second or third trimester, frequently starting on the palms and soles. The itching is worse at night. There are no visible primary skin lesions. Secondary lesions like excoriations, erosions, and scabbing are seen. Jaundice, pale stools, and steatorrhea may or may not be present.
- ICP may recur in subsequent pregnancies in 70% of cases and with the use of oral contraceptives.
- It is associated with elevated serum total bile acid levels >11 micromoles/L. If bile acids are >40 micromoles/L, the disease is considered severe. Direct or indirect bilirubin and liver transaminases may be elevated. Ultrasound of the liver may help exclude other causes of transaminitis.
- Intrahepatic cholestasis of pregnancy (ICP) shows abnormal placental histopathology, including increased terminal villous and capillary surface area, increase in the number of syncytial knots, as well as decidual arteriopathy,

delayed villous maturation, choriangiosis and decidual arteriopathy.

- The disease may result in poor outcomes for the fetus. Prematurity, respiratory distress, and meconium-stained amniotic fluid are all fetal risks associated with ICP. Stillbirth is an additional fetal risk, especially when bile acid levels are >100 micromoles/L.
- **Treatment:** Ursodeoxycholic acid (UDCA) is currently the most effective pharmacologic treatment for ICP. However, the Society for Maternal-Fetal Medicine states that UDCA therapy does not improve fetal outcomes with ICP. It significantly improves maternal pruritus. A starting dose of UDCA of 10 -15 mg/kg per day can be divided into 2 or 3 daily doses. After 1 week, the dose can be increased to a maximum of 21 mg/kg per day to control symptoms. A dose in the range of 450 - 1200 mg/day reduces total bile acids in cord blood, colostrum, and amniotic fluid. Alternative treatment options include oral antihistamines, S-adenosyl-l-methionine and rifampin. Cholestyramine has a high side effect profile and does not improve itching but does reduce bile acid resorption. Delivery is recommended at 36 weeks gestation when bile acid levels are ≥100 micromoles/L to reduce risk of stillbirth. Delivery between 36 and 39 weeks of gestation is recommended when bile acid levels are <100 micromoles/L.

Atopic Eruption of Pregnancy (AEP)

- It is usually seen in pregnant women with a history of atopy and most likely occurs due to a change in the maternal immune response during pregnancy, including the downregulation of T-helper 1 cytokine production and cell-mediated immune function. There is an increase in T-helper 2 cytokine production and humoral immune response. This shift in the immune response, which is specific to pregnancy, exacerbates the imbalance already seen in people with atopy, resulting in the itching and skin lesions seen with atopic eruption of pregnancy.
- In 75% of patients, AEP begins before the third trimester, which is earlier in pregnancy than the other dermatoses specific to pregnancy.
- There are two clinical presentations: the eczematous type (E-type) with a classic distribution of lesions, including eczematous eruption on the face, neck, pre-sternal region, and flexors, and the prurigo type (P-type) with the presence of small, pruritic, erythematous papules, often clustered, distributed predominantly on extensor surfaces of extremities and trunk.
- There is no associated maternal or fetal risk.
- Histopathology shows subepidermal pustules and perifollicular neutrophilic infiltration. Epidermal hyperplasia, spongiosis, and parakeratosis may also be seen.
- **Treatment:** Topical therapies to improve skin hydration to prevent dryness and relieve itching is primarily needed. Urea and 1% to 2% menthol are recommended. Antihistamines such as chlorpheniramine, loratadine, and cetirizine may also be used. Topical medium to high potency steroids in the amount of 200 mg/month are considered safe in pregnancy. Fluticasone propionate should not be used in pregnancy because the placenta does not metabolize it and can, therefore, reach the fetus in higher concentrations. Oral corticosteroids may be needed when initial treatment is not successful. Prednisone or prednisolone at a maximum dose of 0.5 mg/kg/day for 2 to 3 weeks may be necessary to control symptoms. Broad and narrowband UVB and UVA-1 light therapy have also been utilized. Cyclosporin A and azathioprine (off-label use) may be used in pregnancy when the benefits to the mother are deemed to outweigh any potential risk to the fetus. Use of methotrexate and mycophenolate mofetil is contraindicated during pregnancy. Janus kinase inhibitors, baricitinib, upadacitinib, and abrocitinib are also contraindicated for use in pregnancy.

Herpes Gestationis or Pemphigoid Gestationis (PG)

- It is a rare, pruritic autoimmune bullous disease with clinical and pathological features similar to bullous pemphigoid (BP). Its incidence varies from around 1:50,000 to 1:60,000 pregnancies, and it is more common in multiparous women.
- It may rarely occur with hydatiform moles or choriocarcinoma. The immune response begins in the placenta and stimulates maternal antibody production. These antibodies to the placenta then cross react with collagen XVII antigens in the skin causing splitting of the dermis and epidermis resulting in tense bullae formation.
- PG develops most commonly (34% of the time) in the second and third trimester of pregnancy. However, it may occur in the first trimester (18%) and during postpartum (14%).
- Clinically, there is an initial phase in which erythematous and urticarial papules and plaques predominate, followed by vesicles and blisters. Itching is intense and can be disabling. In 90% of the cases, the lesions are initially located in the periumbilical region and then spread to the abdomen and limbs. The oral mucosa is rarely affected (15–20%). The skin lesions frequently resolve in the last few weeks of pregnancy. However, 10% of women have a

recurrence of lesions with the use of oral contraceptives, and 75% of women have recurrences postpartum.

- It may be associated with fetal growth restriction and preterm delivery. Neonatal pemphigoid gestationis occurs in 10% to 13% of neonates.
- **Histopathology:** Initial lesions show papillary edema with lymphocyte infiltration and a variable number of eosinophils in the dermis. Recent intact blister shows subepidermal cleavage without acantholysis. DIF of perilesional skin biopsies reveals linear deposition of C3 in all cases and approximately 30% of cases show IgG along the BMZ. IIF in patient's serum is positive in most cases and immunoblotting studies show that 90% of patients have antibodies against collagen XVII. Detection of the NC16A domain of collagen XVII by ELISA has a sensitivity and specificity of 96%.
- **Treatment:** The main goals of treatment are to minimize itching and decrease blister formation. The first line treatment is topical steroids such as fluocinonide 0.05% cream or ointment or clobetasol propionate 0.05% cream or ointment. Oral antihistamines, like 10 mg of loratadine daily, may help treat itching. Systemic corticosteroids may be necessary if topical therapy does not achieve an adequate response. Intravenous immune globulin, azathioprine and dapsone have also been used as therapy. Rituximab has been used for the treatment of postpartum flares.

Pustular Psoriasis of Pregnancy (PPP) or Impetigo Herpetiformis

- It is a very rare dermatosis of pregnancy which is seen most commonly in third trimester patients. It frequently occurs in primigravidas.
- The underlying pathophysiology is poorly under-stood but hypocalcemia, low vitamin D, hyper-parathyroidism, genetic susceptibility or hormonal changes may be responsible.
- Patients present with circumferential rings of non-itchy, erythematous plaques covered with sterile pustules on periphery, mainly in flexural areas which may spread to the trunk and extremities. Hands, feet, and face are generally spared but onycholysis may occur. The plaques may become centrally crusted and eroded. Systemic symptoms like nausea, vomiting, diarrhea, fever, anorexia, lymphadenopathy, malaise and seizures may be seen.
- Maternal electrolyte imbalances, especially low calcium, can lead to delirium, seizures, or tetany. Fluid loss may result in dehydration and systemic infections can lead to sepsis. Other complications include fetal growth retardation, premature rupture of membranes, intrauterine fetal death due to placental insufficiency, preterm labor and neonatal demise.
- In subsequent pregnancies, PPP may occur at an earlier stage of pregnancy with a more severe clinical presentation. It can also recur during menstruation or on taking birth control pills.
- Pustular psoriasis of pregnancy (PPP) is usually diagnosed by clinical findings rather than by microscopic examination.
- **Treatment:** Prednisolone 15 mg to 30 mg daily which may be increased to 60 mg to 80 mg daily if needed, is the most common treatment for PPP. Topical betamethasone 0.05%, 15 g/day to 30 g/day may also be used. Dapsone, H1-receptor antagonists and colchicine have been tried. Cyclosporine or tumor necrosis inhibitors, infliximab and adalimumab, may be used in very severe cases. Acitretin has been successfully used in postpartum women. Several other medications have been used in pregnancy to treat PPP, but since this disease is so rare, there is limited data on the efficacy and safety in pregnancy. Delivery is curative, so this may be considered, especially when close to term and with refractory disease.

ANTIHISTAMINES IN PREGNANCY (Table 21.1)

Table 21.1: Antihistamines in pregnancy

FDA approved first generation antihistamines in pregnancy	
Drug name	***Pregnancy category***
Chlorpheniramine	B
Cyproheptadine	B
Hydroxyzine	C
Promethazine	C
FDA approved second generation antihistamines in pregnancy	
Cetirizine	B
Levocetirizine	B
Loratadine	B
Desloratadine	C
Fexofenadine	C

CHAPTER 22 Naevi and Other Development Defects

Contents

NAEVI

Definition

Naevus in simple term is any congenital growth or mark on the skin, such as a mole or birthmark. More specifically it is defined as a type of hamartoma representing a circumscribed stable malformation of the skin or of the oral mucosa, which may involve epidermal, connective tissue, adnexal, nervous, or vascular tissue. Naevi usually follow lines of Blaschko.

Lines of Blaschko

The lines of Blaschko were described and drawn in 1901 by Alfred Blaschko (1858-1922), a private practitioner of dermatology in Berlin. They represent a pattern assumed by many different nevoid and acquired skin diseases on the human skin and mucosa. These lines do not correspond to any known nervous, vascular or lymphatic structures but represent the developmental growth pattern of the skin. In Blaschko's lines there is a V-shape over the upper spine, an S-shape on the abdomen, and an inverted U-shape from the breast area onto the upper arm (Figure 22.1). There are perpendicular lines down the front and back of the lower extremities. Mosaicism remains the most widely accepted theories to explain Blaschko's lines.

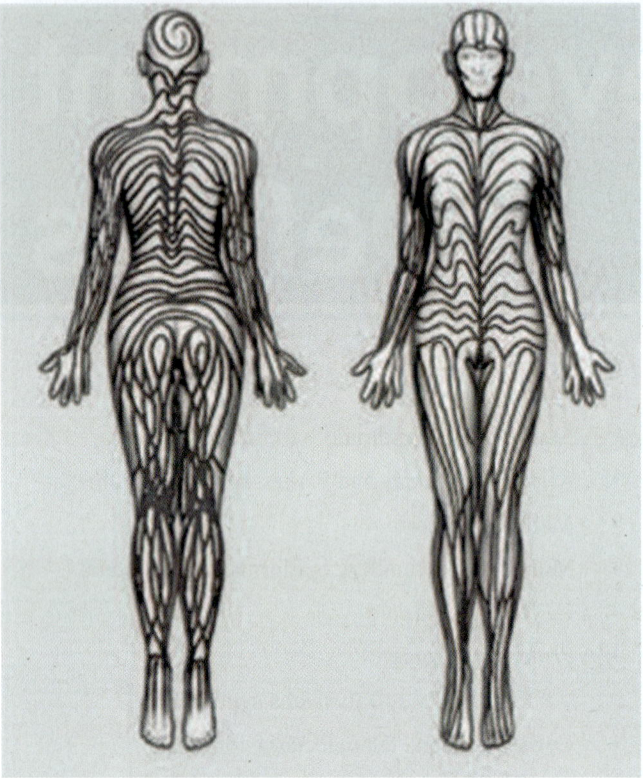

Figure 22.1: Lines of Blaschko

Epidermal Naevi

Epidermal naevi are hamartomatous lesions derived from epidermal components originating in pluripotential cell mutations during early embryonic stages. Their location and extension are variable, following Blaschko lines, and reflect embryonic migration patterns of the skin. The incidence is approximately 1 in 1000 live newborns.

There are two major types of epidermal naevi: non-organoid (keratinocytic) and organoid (sebaceous, follicular and sweat gland). The type of epidermal naevus is determined by its predominant components; keratinocytes or epidermal appendages, both of which originate from embryonic ectoderm.

Verrucous Epidermal Naevi (VEN)

The term verrucous epidermal naevus (Figure 22.2 A, B and C) refers to a benign hyperplasia of the epidermis. It may either be of epidermolytic or non-epidermolytic type. VEN are often present at birth but may develop as late as adolescence. They are usually asymptomatic in contrast to inflammatory linear verrucous epidermal naevi, which are pruritic. The characteristic VEN is a linear, hyperpigmented plaque, which can vary from skin colored to black, velvety to verrucous, subtle to thick, and limited to extensive. VEN typically occurs on the trunk or extremities along the lines of Blaschko but may occur on the face and neck. Many syndromes with cutaneous manifestations have mosaic properties at the cellular level.

VEN can be a part of syndromes. Well defined epidermal naevus syndrome includes congenital hemidysplasia with ichthyosiform erythroderma and limb defects (CHILD), Proteus syndrome, Schimmelpenning syndrome, naevus comedonicus syndrome, phacomatosis pigmentokeratotica and Becker naevus syndrome. Rarely, squamous cell carcinoma, basal cell carcinoma, and keratoacanthoma can arise in VEN.

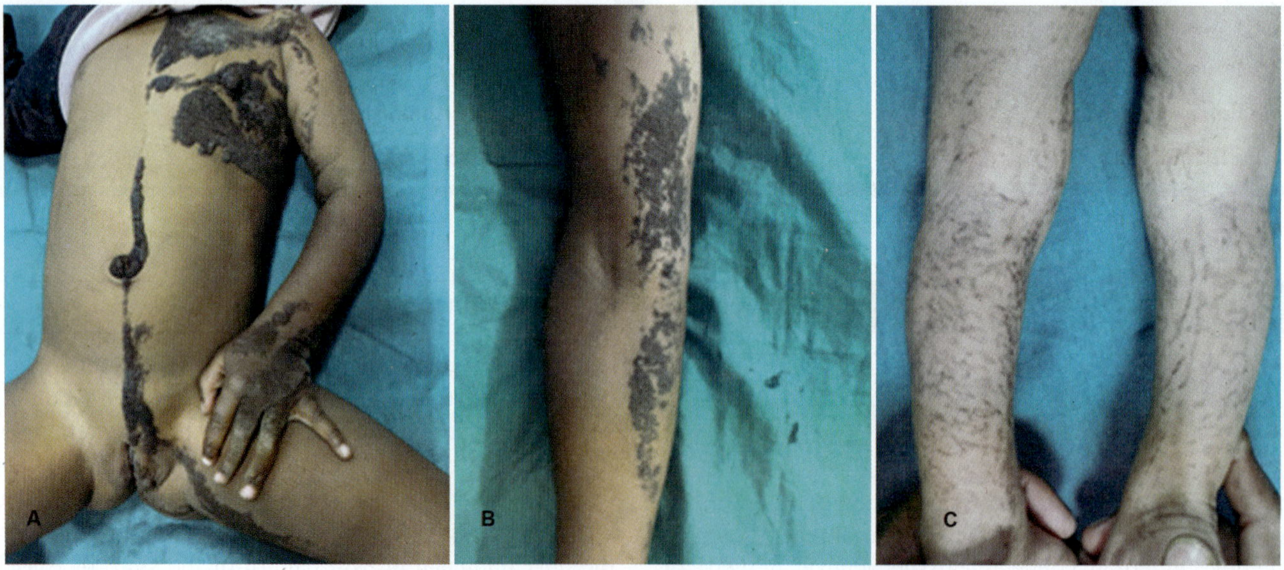

Figure 22.2: Verrucous epidermal naevus (A, B and C)

Management of epidermal naevi is challenging. Therapies include topical and intralesional glucocorticoids, topical and systemic retinoids and topical 5-fluorouracil. Ablative measures include dermabrasion, electrocautery, cryotherapy, laser therapy and surgical excision.

Inflammatory Linear Verrucous Epidermal Naevus (ILVEN)

It presents as erythematous and verrucous papules arranged in a linear fashion. The lesions are characteristically pruritic. ILVEN is usually unilateral and is frequently located on an extremity (Figure 22.3).

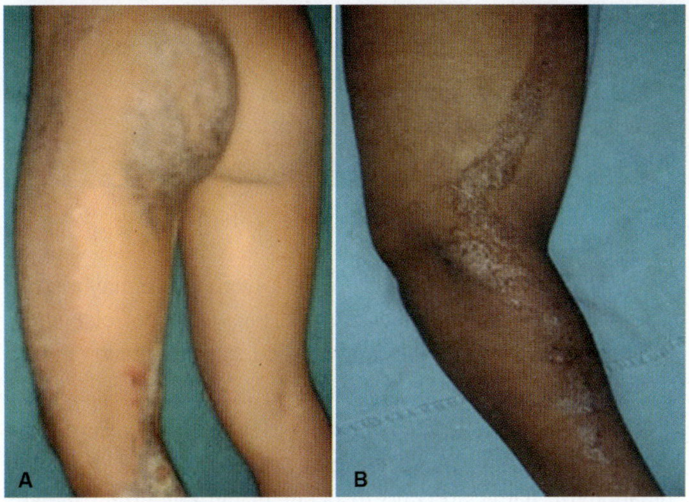

Figure 22.3: Inflammatory linear verrucous epidermal naevus

ILVEN is difficult to treat. Therapeutic options include topical and intralesional glucocorticoids, topical retinoids, excision, cryotherapy, electrocautery and laser therapy with CO_2 or Er:YAG.

Naevus Sebaceous

First described by Jadassohn in 1895, naevus sebaceous (NS) is a circumscribed hamartomatous lesion predominantly composed of sebaceous glands. It is better designated as an 'organoid naevus', as proliferative changes also involve sweat glands and hair follicles.

Naevus sebaceous is usually present at birth and its most common location is head and neck area. Its morphologic appearances vary with the age of the lesion. During infancy and childhood, it is manifested by a well-defined area of alopecia with smooth surface and yellow to orange discoloration. In this stage, the epidermis is only slightly acanthotic and may be hyperpigmented. The hair follicles are small, incompletely formed, and are often represented by solid cords of undifferentiated basaloid cells.

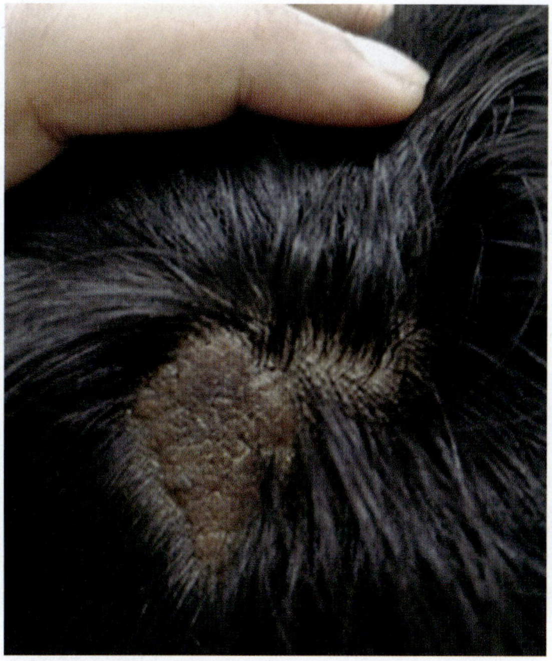

Figure 22.4: Naevus sebaceous

The sebaceous glands are not prominent. During adolescence there is increase in the thickness of the lesion, which may then show smooth surface nodularities or verrucous hyperkeratosis (Figure 22.4). At this stage there is epidermal hyperplasia, large sebaceous glands, and ectopic apocrine glands dominate the histologic findings. The hair follicles remain primordial.

A variety of benign and malignant adnexal tumors can arise in NS. The incidence of these tumors increases with age, particularly after puberty. Benign tumors are much more common as compared to the malignant ones. Benign adnexal tumors include trichoblastoma, syringocystadenoma papilliferum, trichilemmoma, sebaceoma, nodular hidradenoma, hidrocystoma, and eccrine poroma. Malignant cutaneous neoplasms include basal cell carcinoma, squamous cell carcinoma, trichilemmal carcinoma, sebaceous carcinoma, porocarcinoma and apocrine carcinoma.

Due to the concern regarding the occurrence of malignant neoplasms, prophylactic surgical removal in all cases is not recommended, unless there is clinical suspicion. However, lesion may be removed for cosmetic concerns.

Congenital Melanocytic Naevi

A melanocytic naevi is considered congenital if it is seen at birth or within 2 years of life. Melanocytic naevi are normal, benign proliferations of melanocytes. They are generally considered to be present in between 1 and 2% of newborns. Small congenital naevi are defined as under 1.5 cm in diameter, large as having a diameter between 1.5 and 20 cm and giant

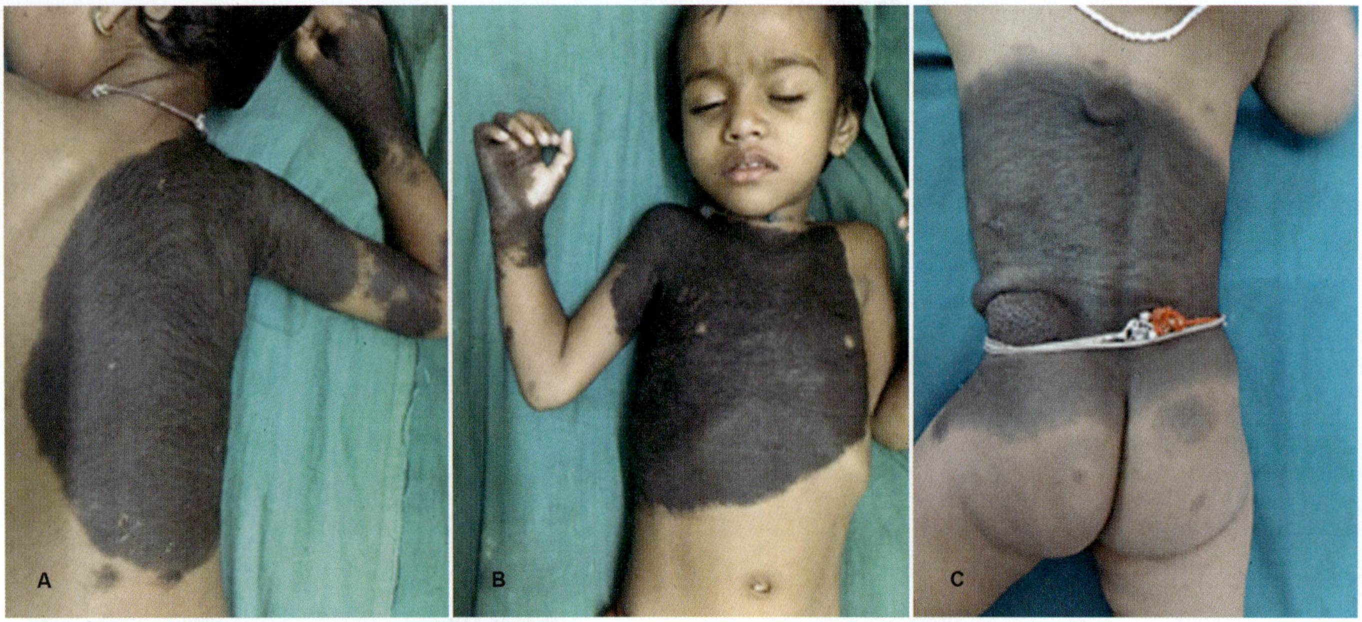

Figure 22.5: Giant melanocytic naevus (A, B and C)

naevi (Figure 22.5A, B and C) as having a diameter of 20 cm or more. There is no sex predilection for melanocyctic naevi development. Congenital naevi are one of several known risk factors for the eventual development of melanoma.

Melanocytic naevi most commonly are tan to brown, but color can be variable, ranging from skin-colored (non-pigmented) to jet black. The majority are macular at birth. As the child grows the naevus usually grows in proportion. The giant or bathing trunk naevus is very rare. The common site is the lower back and thigh area and a very large proportion of the infant's surface area may be involved. There may also be large numbers of smaller congenital naevi present elsewhere on other areas of skin which are called satellite naevi (Figure 22.6).

The lesions tend to become warty or rugose and may have hair (Figure 22.7) components later on. Congenital melanocytic naevi are said to occur in the epidermal naevus syndrome. Melanocytic naevi can be surgically removed for cosmetic considerations and also for their doubtful malignant potential.

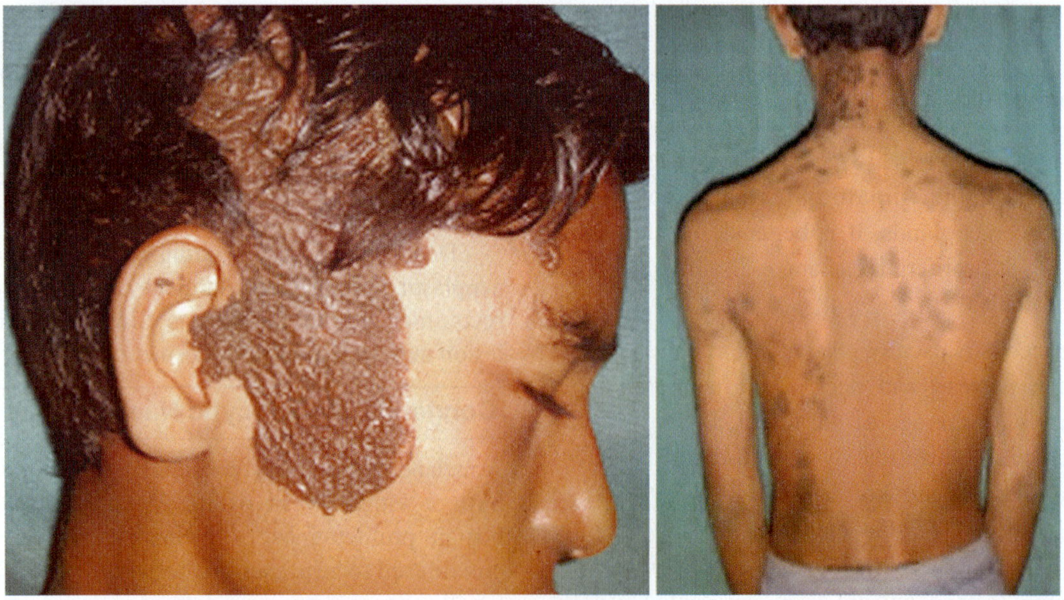

Figure 22.6: Segmental congenital melanocytic nevus with satellite lesions

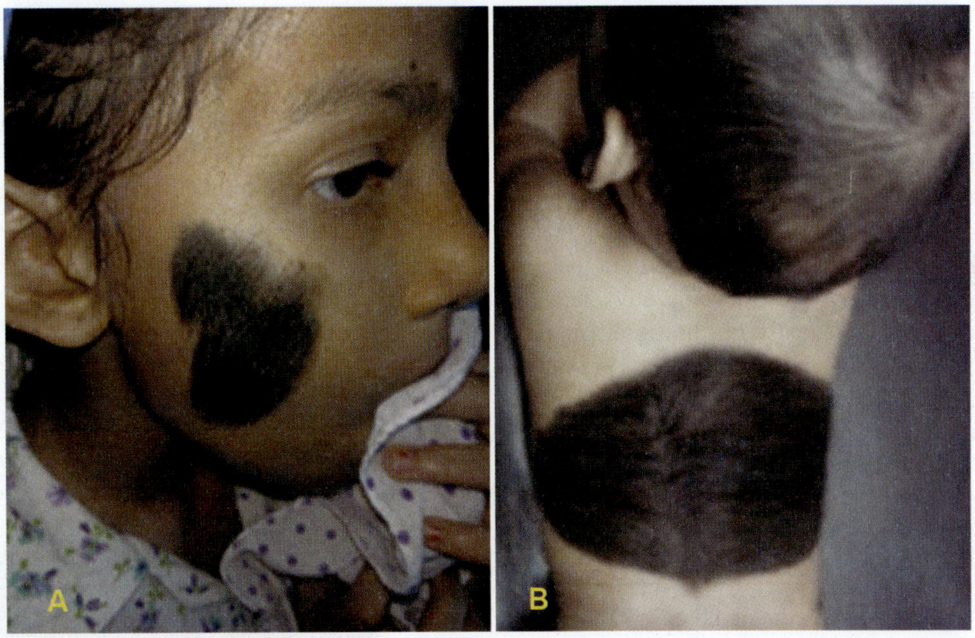

Figure 22.7: Giant melanocytic naevus with abundant hair growth

Naevus Spilus OR Speckled Naevus

Speckled naevus or lentiginous naevus has lentiginous components in childhood which later on progresses to develop palpable components. Speckled naevus is comprised of variable number of black, brown, or red-brown macules and papules within a patch of tan-to-brown hyperpigmentation (Figure 22.8). The lesions are around 3-6 cm or more in size and usually oval, but they can be linear. Some follow the lines of Blaschko or have a sharp demarcation at the midline. An extensive amount of body surface area may be involved.

The macules (speckles) and papules lying within the background patch range from lentigines to junctional, compound, or dermal naevi. The speckles range from 1-9 mm; most commonly, they are 2-3 mm in diameter. Though, the risk for malignant transformation is very low, regular examination

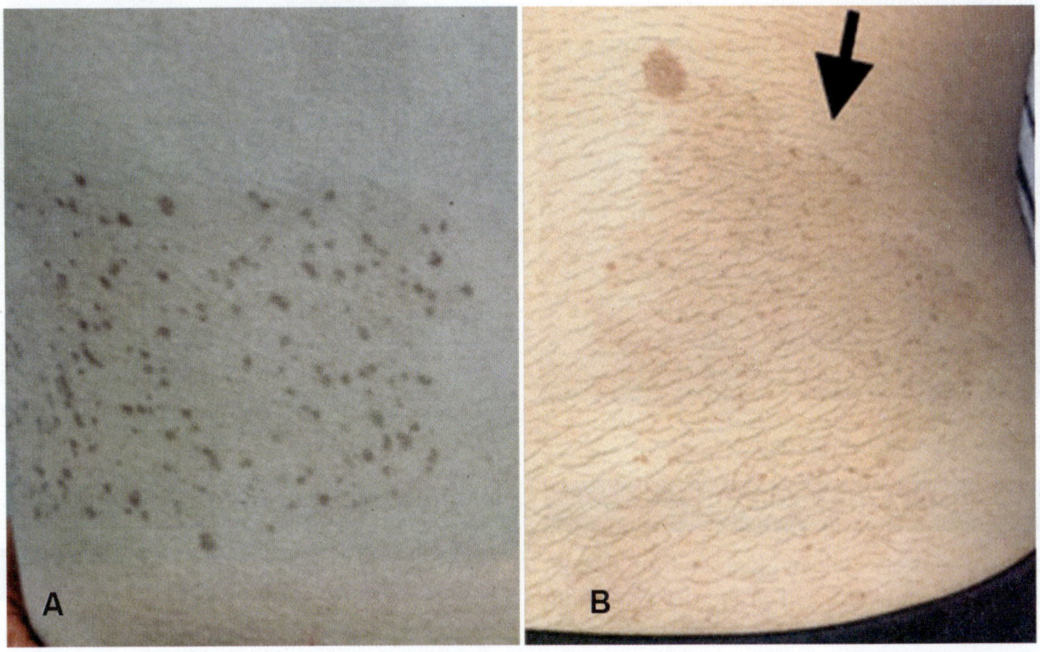

Figure 22.8: Speckled naevus

is required to check for any atypical melanocytic proliferation. For cosmetic purpose laser therapy may be useful.

Halo Naevus OR Sutton's Naevus

Halo naevi are common benign skin lesions that represent melanocytic naevi in which an inflammatory infiltrate develops, resulting in a zone of depigmentation surrounding the naevus. The average age of onset is 15 years. Halo naevi are usually single but may be multiple. They can develop anywhere on the body but are seen most frequently on the trunk (mainly back). Over the next few months, the central naevus gradually disappears leaving a macular area of non-pigmented skin. This hypopigmented area may or may not regain its color. It must be differentiated from superficial spreading type of melanomas. Surgical resection can be done for cosmetic concern.

Nevus Lipomatosus

Nevus lipomatosus superficialis is a rare and benign idiopathic condition characterized by the presence of ectopic mature adipose tissue in the dermis. The proportion of fatty tissue varies from 10% to 50% of the volume of dermis.

Two clinical types have been described: (i) Classical type and (ii) Solitary type. Classical type consists of multiple, soft, nontender, pedunculated, cerebriform, yellowish or skin-colored papules or nodules commonly situated on the pelvic girdle area in a zonal pattern (Figure 22.9) and occur at birth or during first three decades of life. Solitary form usually occurs after the age of 20 years and presents with a single nodular lesion on any area over the body.

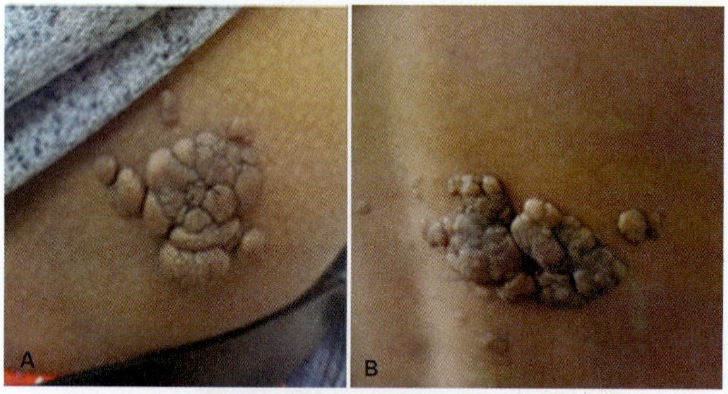

Figure 22.9: Nevus lipomatosus

DERMAL MELANOCYTIC LESIONS

Dermal melanocytic lesions are believed to arise from dermal melanocytes that have become arrested in the dermis during fetal life and tissue modeling and have not reached their normal site in the basal layer of the epidermis.

Naevus of Ota (Figure 22.10)

Naevus of Ota is a hamartoma of dermal melanocytes. Clinically, naevus of Ota presents as a blue or gray patch on the face, which is congenital or acquired and is within the distribution of the ophthalmic and maxillary branches of the trigeminal nerve. The naevus can be unilateral or bilateral, and, in addition to skin, it may involve ocular and oral mucosal surfaces. It is seen in less than 1% pediatric population. Naevus of Ota most frequently presents as blue-to-gray speckled or mottled coalescing macules or patches affecting the forehead, temple, malar area, or periorbital skin. In addition to skin, pigmentation of naevus of Ota may involve oral mucosa and ocular structures such as the sclera, retrobulbar fat, cornea and retina. Treatment is laser therapy with pulsed Q-switched laser or Q-switched ruby laser.

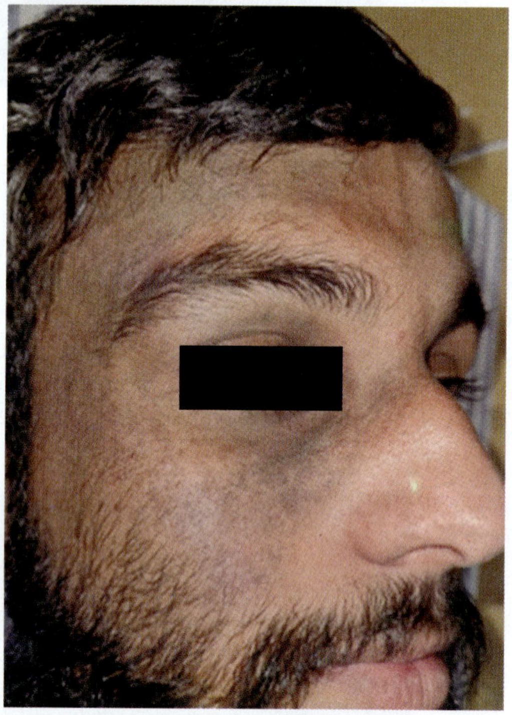

Figure 22.10: Naevus of Ota

Naevus of ITO

Naevus of Ito is a dermal melanocytic condition, like naevus of Ota, affecting the acromioclavicular region and the upper chest.

Mongolian Spot (*See Chapter 19*)

VASCULAR TUMOURS

Vascular tumors are classified in different types given in Table 22.1. Important vascular tumors are described below:

Table 22.1: Vascular tumors classification	
Benign	• Infantile hemangioma • Congenital hemangioma • Lobular capillary hemangioma (Pyogenic granuloma) • Tufted angioma • Epithelioid hemangioma
Locally aggressive or Borderline	• Kaposiform hemangioendothelioma • Papillary intralymphatic angioendothelioma (Dabska tumor) • Kaposi sarcoma
Malignant vascular tumors	• Angiosarcoma • Epithelioid hemangioendothelioma

INFANTILE HEMANGIOMA (IH) OR HEMANGIOMA OF INFANCY

It is also called *strawberry naevus or capillary hemangioma.* Infantile hemangiomas are benign vascular neoplasms that have a characteristic clinical course marked by early proliferation and followed by spontaneous involution. During the proliferative phase in the neonatal period or early infancy, a rapidly dividing endothelial cell proliferation is responsible for the enlargement of infantile hemangiomas. Finally, an involutional phase occurs, whereby most infantile hemangiomas are clinically resolved by the age of 9 years. Hemangiomas are the most common tumors of infancy and most infantile hemangiomas are medically insignificant. Occasionally infantile hemangiomas may impinge on vital structures, ulcerate, bleed, cause high output cardiac failure or significant structural abnormalities or disfigurement. Rarely, a cutaneous infantile hemangioma may be associated with one or more underlying congenital anomalies.

Eighty percent of infantile hemangiomas are focal and solitary. More than 50% of cutaneous hemangiomas occur on the head and neck, around 25% on the trunk, and 15% on the extremities. Hemangiomas also can occur in extracutaneous sites, including the liver, gastrointestinal tract, larynx, CNS, pancreas, gallbladder, thymus, spleen, lymph nodes, lung, urinary bladder, and adrenal glands. Multiple hemangiomas (Figure 22.11 A and B) may be associated with internal organ hemangioma, five or more cutaneous hemangiomas require an ultrasound abdomen to screen to rule out liver hemangioma. The earliest sign of infantile hemangioma is blanching of the involved skin. This may be followed by fine telangiectasias and then a red or crimson macule. As proliferation ensues, the infantile hemangioma becomes elevated and may be dome shaped, lobulated, plaque like, tumoral, or any combination of these morphologies. Fifty percent of infantile hemangiomas undergo complete involution by the age 5 years and 70% by age 7 years; the remainder may take an additional 3-5 years to complete the process. Of the lesions that which have involuted by age 6 years, around 38% have residual evidence in form of scar formation, telangiectasia, or redundant or anetodermic skin.

If the infantile hemangioma is located in the subcutaneous tissue, the overlying skin may be completely normal (Figure 22.12 A). Color varies with the depth from the surface and can be bright red or crimson (superficial dermis), purple, blue, or flesh colored with predominant involvement of the deeper tissues. Telangiectasias and large superficial veins

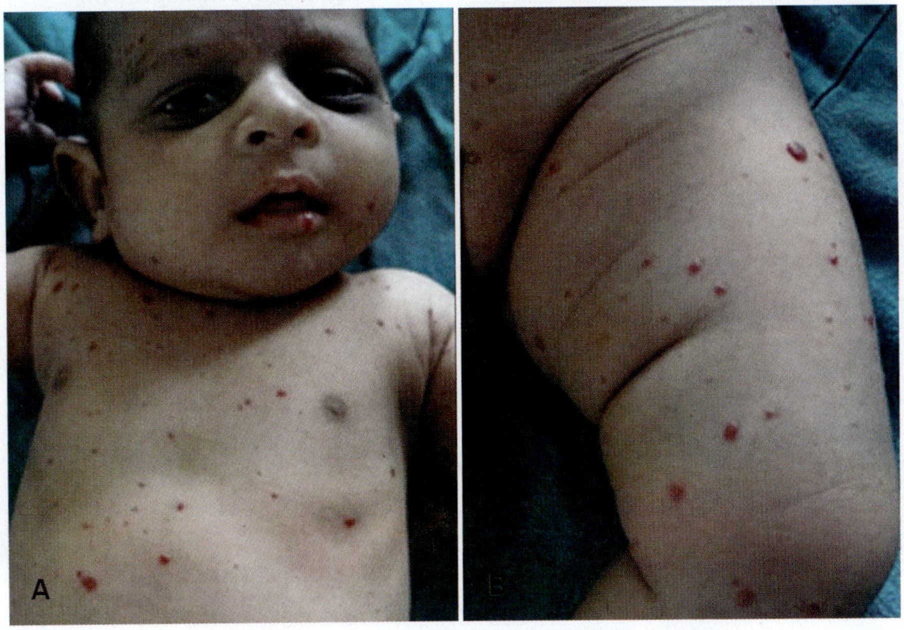

Figure 22.11: Multiple hemangiomas (Both A and B)

radiating from the infantile hemangioma are often associated. The consistency is firm, rubbery, and tense and expands with increased intravascular pressure (e.g., with crying when on the head and neck). Most infantile hemangiomas reach a maximum size of 0.5-5 cm (Figure 22.12 B), but they can range from the size of a pinhead to greater than 20 cm in diameter and remain well circumscribed and focal. A minority may be segmental in nature, covering a larger portion of the cutaneous surface. This variant has more superficial than deep involvement, as is seen with extensive facial lesions. Large capillary hemangioma of the face has also been termed as 'field fire hemangioma'. Initially these lesions show sudden increase in size for about 6 to 8 months, followed by an arrest in growth and thereafter, regression and involution sets in, which is completed by 3 to 5 years of age.

Complications

- **Ulceration:** It is seen in around 13% of cases, commonly in IH located at head and neck as well as over perineal areas (Figure 22.12 C).
- **Heart failure:** e. g. in hepatic hemangiomas.
- **Visual impairment and other ocular complications:** Astigmatism, amblyopia, lacrimal duct obstruction, exposure keratitis, strabismus, mostly associated with periocular hemangiomas.
- **Breathing difficulty:** In upper airway hemangiomas.
- **Auditory canal obstruction:** Hearing problems.
- **Disfigurement:** Cosmetic problems.

Associated Syndromes

'PELVIS' consists of the association of large perineal haemangiomas (P) with the following congenital abnormalities: External genitalia malformations (E), lipomyelomeningocoele (L), vesicorenal abnormalities (V), imperforate anus (I) and skin tags (S) and 'SACRAL' for a similar association of perineal haemangiomas and spinal dysraphism (S), anogenital anomalies (A), cutaneous anomalies (C), renal and urologic anomalies (R), associated with angioma (A) of lumbosacral localization (L). LUMBAR syndrome consists of lower body hemangiomas (L), urogenital anomalies/ulceration (U), myelopathy (M), bony deformities (B), anorectal malformations/arterial anomalies (A) and rectal anomalies (R).

PHACES syndrome: Posterior fossa defects, hemangiomas, arterial anomalies, cardiac defects (coarctation of the aorta is the most common), eye abnormalities, sternal clefting or supraumbilical raphe.

Diagnosis

MRI or CT scan is useful to delineate the extent of lesions and response to treatment. Immunohistochemical analysis for IH is GLUT1 positive (as well as merosin, Fcg receptor II and Lewis Y antigen positive). Other benign vascular lesions are GLUT1 negative.

Management

There are wide varieties of vascular lesions of different etiology. Hence, no single form of medical or surgical treatment can be applied uniformly to all the vascular lesions (hemangiomas). The most important aspect to remember about hemangiomas is that, these lesions are rarely seen in adults, as most involutes during early childhood and thereafter regress spontaneously. This fact should always be taken into consideration prior to planning invasive management.

1. **Local wound care for ulcerated lesions:** Topical antibiotic, non-sticking wound dressings, compresses.

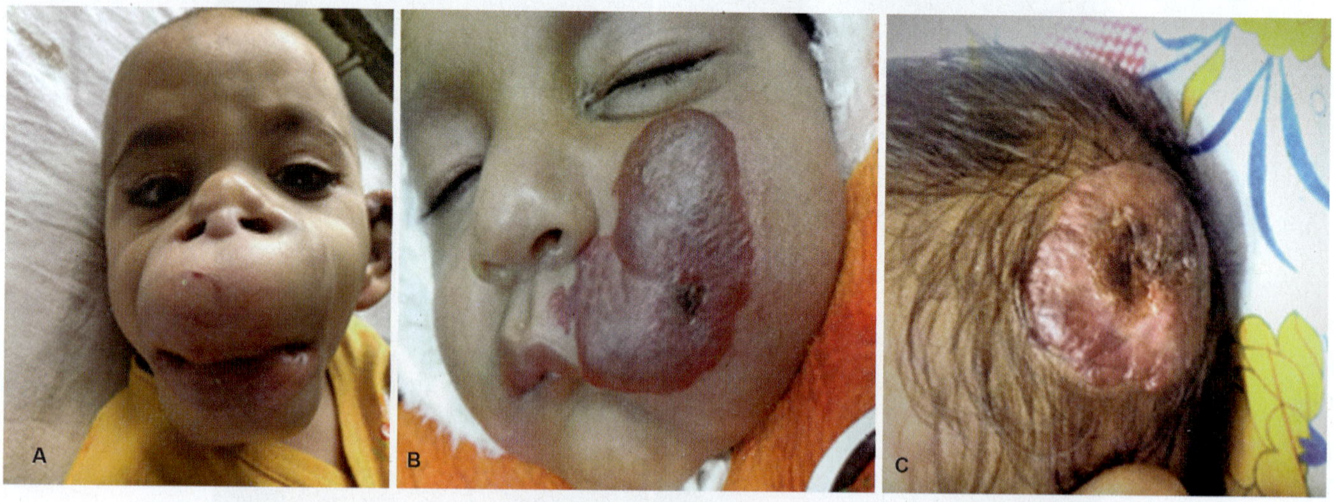

Figure 22.12: (A) Deep or subcutaneous type of infantile hemangioma, (B) Infantile hemangioma, (C) Infantile hemangioma with ulceration

2. Oral antibiotics for secondary infections.
3. Pain control.
4. **Topical corticosteroids:** Potent topical steroids are useful for localized and superficial hemangiomas.
5. Intralesional corticosteroids (triamcinolone) for localized lesions.
6. Oral corticosteroids are traditionally gold standard treatment for systemic therapy. Prednisone or prednisolone, 2-4 mg/kg per day is advised as single oral dose and maintained for 1-3 months followed by a gradual taper. Deflazacort in equivalent doses may be used which has lesser side effects.

   Indication of oral steroids:

   - Large periocular infantile hemangioma with complete visual axis occlusion.
   - Problematic hemangioma or rapidly proliferating hemangiomas.
   - Large airway hemagioma with respiratory difficulty.
7. Topical β-blockers in the form of timolol gel ophthalmic solution, 0.1%-0.5%, can be applied 2-4 times daily. It is useful for smaller, localized and/or superficial IH.
8. **Oral β-blockers:** Newer innovation for IH is propranolol, a non-selective beta-blocker. The drug is given at a starting dose of 2 mg/kg/day, in 2 divided doses, for 3 to 9 months depending on the severity of the clinical condition. If the optimal dose exceeds 3 mg/kg/day, gradual tapering of propranolol after 4 weeks should be considered as soon as clinically indicated. Proper cardiac monitoring should be done in a pediatric care unit. Side effects include bradycardia, hypotension, hypoglycemia, bronchospasm, hypothermia and nightmares, which should be properly monitered.
9. Interferon α subcutaneous injection can be used for severe, treatment-resistant, or life-threatening IH. Its disadvantage is the risk of spastic diplegia.
10. **Laser therapy:** Long pulsed dye laser (PDL) seems safer and more efficient. Currently, there are no optimal laser systems for treatment of deep IH. Because PDL can only penetrate to a depth of around 1.2 mm, so it is not effective in treating deeper components of IH, which may continue to grow even as the superficial component recedes. Other lasers, such as Nd: YAG or KTP, can reach the deeper parts of the lesion but carry significantly greater risks of post therapy scarring, dyspigmentation, or textural abnormalities.
11. Vincristine can be considered only in severe, treatment-resistant or life-threatening IH. Its risks include myelosuppression, peripheral neuropathy and extravasation necrosis.
12. In most cases of hemangiomas, there is no urgency to undertake surgical procedures. However, there are certain indications where surgery may be considered necessary; some of these include atypical growth, cardiopulmonary decompensation, large hemangiomas with thrombocytopenia, obstruction to vision, luminal obstruction and rarely, uncontrollable hemorrhage.

KASABACH-MERRITT PHENOMENON

- Kasabach-Merritt phenomenon (or syndrome) is characterized by thrombocytopenia, coagulopathy, and microangiopathic hemolytic anemia associated with a rapidly enlarging vascular lesion. The mortality rate ranges from 10% to 30%.
- It occurs most often within the first few weeks of life and manifests as sudden enlargement of the vascular lesion, ecchymosis, prolonged bleeding, epistaxis, hematuria, or hematochezia. The cutaneous manifestations include purpura, edema, induration, and an advancing ecchymotic margin.
- Thrombocytopenia, anemia, hypofibrinogenemia, elevated D-dimers, fragmentation of erythrocytes on manual smear, and prolonged coagulation studies are observed.

VASCULAR MALFORMATION

Simple vascular malformation is classified into four main subtypes (Table 22.2):

- Capillary malformation
- Lymphatic malformation
- Venous malformation
- Arteriovenous malformation

Table 22.2: Classification of simple vascular malformation

Capillary malformation	Lymphatic malformation	Venous malformation	Arteriovenous malformation
1. Nevus simplex /Salmon patch 2. Port wine stain (Non syndromic) 3. Syndromic capillary malformation • Sturge Weber syndrome • Klippel Trenaunay syndrome • Parkes Weber syndrome • Maffucci syndrome • Microcephaly-CM syndrome • Macrocephaly-CM syndrome • CLOVES syndrome • Proteus syndrome • Bannayan Riley Ruvalcaba syndrome 4. Cutis Marmorata Telangiectasia Congenita (CMTC) 5. Hereditary Hemorrhagic Telangiectasia (HHT)	1. Common lymphatic or cystic malformation • Macrocystic lymphatic malformation like cystic hygroma • Microcystic lymphatic malformation like lymphangioma circumscriptum 2. Lymphedema • Primary lymphedema – Congenita (Nonne-milroy syndrome) – Lymphoedema praecox – Lymphoedema tarda • Secondary lymphedema	1. Common venous malformation 2. Blue rubber bleb syndrome 3. Glomuvenous malformation	

SALMON PATCH/ NEVUS SIMPLEX

Salmon patch or stork mark (found on nape of neck) or nuchal stain is a common capillary malformation with incidence of more than 50% in newborns. It usually fades in infancy, so also called 'fading macular stains'. But some of them may persist without significant fading.

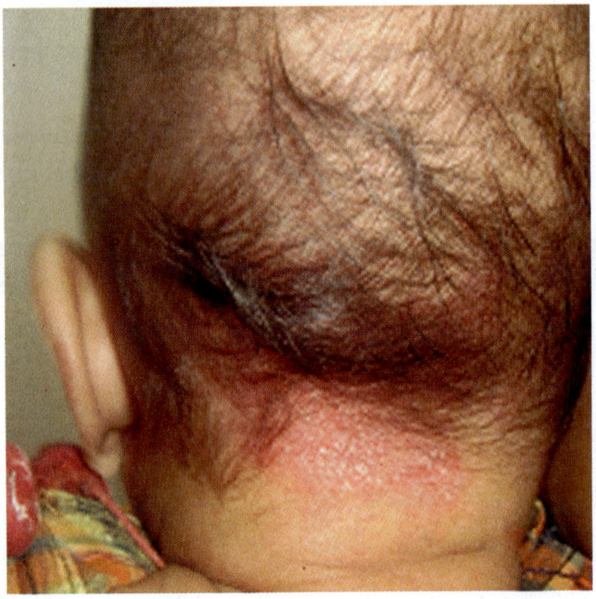

Figure 22.13: Salmon patch

'Angel kiss' represents a subset of capillary malformations that occupies the midline location in glabellar region. Common sites for salmon patch are occipital scalp, nape of neck (Figure 22.13) and forehead upto upper eyelids. The less common site includes the sacral region. The sacral lesions are of concerns as they may be associated with an occult spinal dysraphism. Autosomal inheritance is found in number of cases.

PORTWINE STAIN

At birth, 0.2-0.3% of newborns have portwine stains (PWS). Unlike salmon patches, PWS represents a capillary malformation in form of macular telangiectatic patch (Figure 22.14) that tends to persist unchanged during childhood and to darken and thicken in adolescence and adulthood. Progressive angiomatous papules and nodules and underlying soft tissue hypertrophy develop gradually over years. Although unilateral lesions on the head and neck are most common, particularly in the distribution of trigeminal branches (V1, V2 or V3), but any part of the body surface and mucous membranes may be involved.

Children with involvement of the first division of the trigeminal nerve may have a vascular malformation of the ipsilateral meninges, cerebral cortex, and eye **(Sturge-Weber syndrome).** Superficial vascular lesions associated with

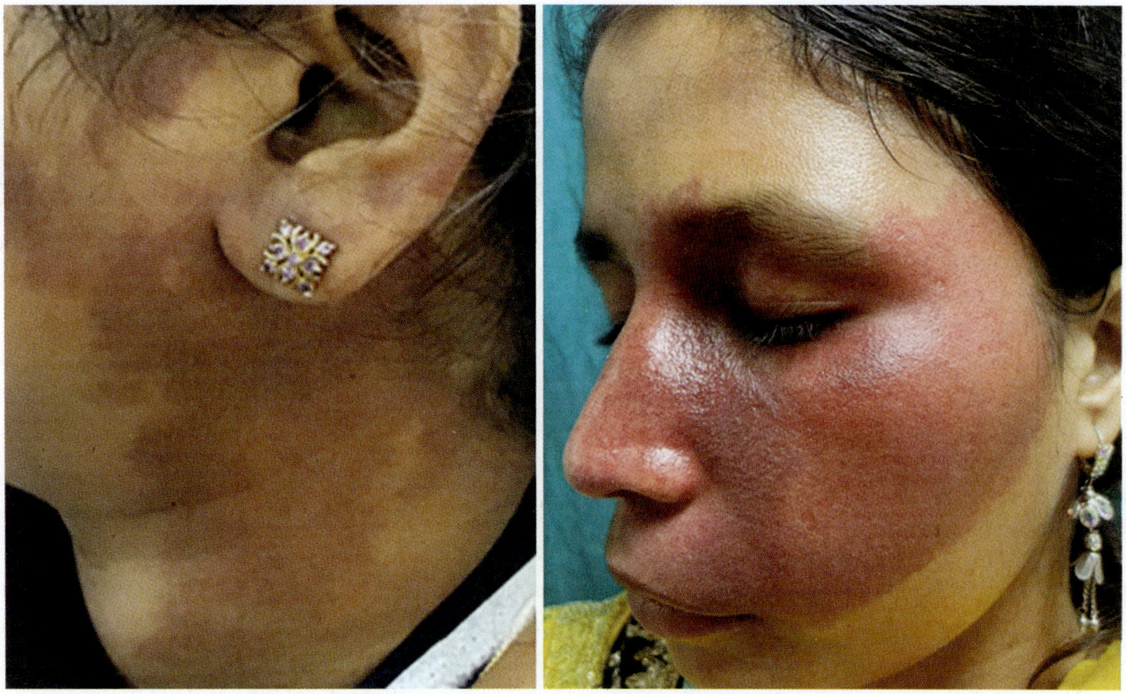

Figure 22.14: Portwine stain

limb or segmental trunk hypertrophy is typical of **Klippel-Trénaunay-Weber syndrome** (Figure 22.15). These patients may have underlying malformations of the deep venous system as well (discussed later).

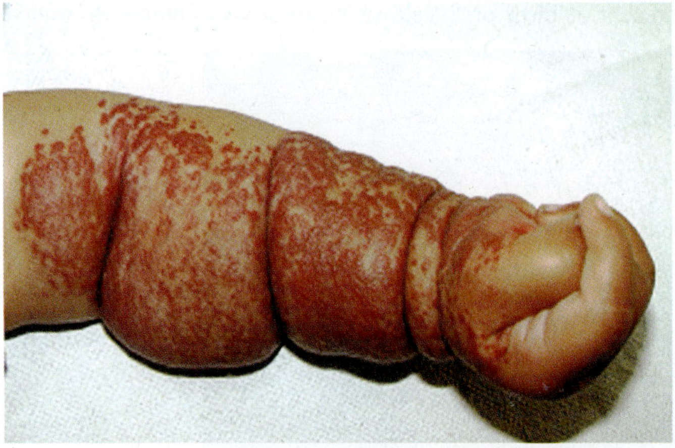

Figure 22.15: Klippel-Trénaunay-Weber syndrome

Management

Infants with PWS deserve a thorough physical examination for signs of systemic disease. Children with forehead and periorbital involvement require careful neurodevelopmental follow up, regular eye examinations to exclude glaucoma, and further neurologic studies as indicated.

Cosmetic camouflage is quite useful. Pulsed dyed laser therapy is quite safe and painless procedure. Maximal improvement of PWS requires an average of five to ten treatments separated by a 2-3 months healing period. The laser penetrates only 1.5-2 mm deep into the skin, which results in little improvement in those naevi with a deep component. Other lasers such as the Nd: YAG (longer wavelength 1064 nm) have achieved good results compared with the second generation PDL. Early treatment in childhood produces the best outcome with the fewest number of treatments and the least cost.

STURGE–WEBER SYNDROME (SWS)

Sturge-Weber syndrome is a neuroectodermal syndrome characterized by a portwine stain in the area of distribution of ophthalmic branch of trigeminal nerve along with leptomeningeal angiomatosis and glaucoma.

A somatic activating mutation in GNAQ has been identified as etiological cause of SWS.

Clinical Presentation

1. The port wine stain may be multi dermatomal or may have more extensive cutaneous involvement. When PWS lesion is unilateral, there is usually a sharp demarcation at the midline. Involvement of the other trigeminal dermatomes may be useful in predicting the risk of SWS. In one study, involvement of V1, V2 and V3 or bilateral trigeminal

involvement was associated with an increased incidence of SWS. There is a higher incidence of glaucoma and leptomeningeal angiomatosis with bilateral or complete involvement of V1.

2. In CNS component, seizures are the most common feature and often starts during the first year of life and may lead to future developmental and cognitive delay. Headache, emotional and behavioral problems including depression, violent behavior, and self-inflicted injury are also common. Leptomeningeal angiomatosis is a classic component of the syndrome, and lesions are commonly ipsilateral to the cutaneous vascular stain. Cerebral atrophy is a common radiologic finding and MRI is the modality of choice for identifying these changes, although CT scans are better at detecting the classic cortical calcifications, characterized by double-contoured parallel streaks of calcification ("tram lines"). EEG can be done for brain activity in young children.
3. Ocular involvement occurs in around 60% of patients. Glaucoma is the most common ocular finding, and it may present at any time from birth to the fourth decade. It may be unilateral or bilateral. Vascular malformations of conjunctiva, episclera, choroid and retina may also be seen.

Management

Care of the child with SWS should be multidisciplinary. Dermatologic, neurologic and ophthalmologic follow up care is indicated. For seizures surgical therapy may become necessary (visually guided lobectomy with excision of the angiomatous cortex).

KLIPPEL–TRÉNAUNAY AND PARKES WEBER SYNDROMES

Klippel-Trénaunay (KT) syndrome is characterized by the triad of vascular malformation, venous varicosity and hyperplasia of soft tissue and bone (Figure 22.16). It is often confused with *Parkes-Weber Syndrome (PWS)* which is characterized by limb overgrowth, capillary malformations (portwine stains) and diffuse arteriovenous malformations.

The difference between these two entities is that PWS occurs because of vascular malformation that may or may not be because of genetic mutations, whereas Klippel-Trénaunay syndrome is a condition in which blood vessels and/ or lymph vessels do not form properly due to genetic defect. PWS and KTS almost have the same symptoms, except PWS patients are seen with both AVMs and AVFs occurring with limb hypertrophy.

Clinical Presentation

The lower extremity is the most common site affected. Capillary malformation may vary from fairly localized, faint lesions to extensive, bright red or purple stain, which is usually present at birth or develops during early infancy. Prominent

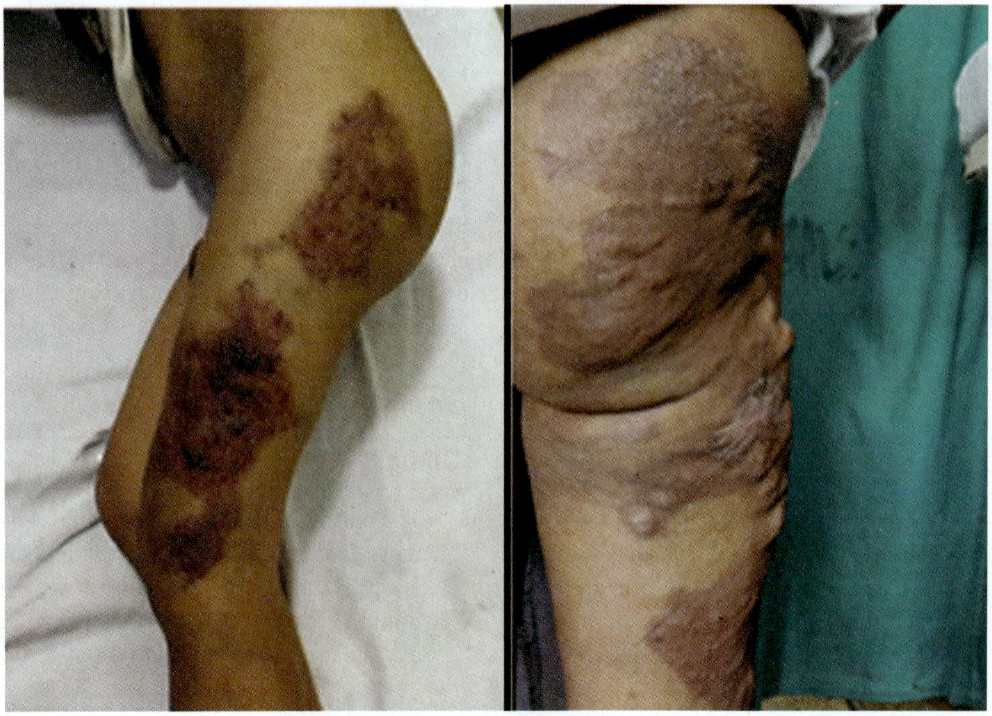

Figure 22.16: Klippel-Trenaunay syndrome

superficial veins or venous varicosities develop at later age. Hypertrophy of the affected body part is another manifestation of the syndrome and usually presents with increased limb girth and length.

Lymphatic abnormalities in the form of lymphangiectasia, large lymphatic malformations, lymphedema, vascular blebs and pseudoverrucous papules may be present.

Treatment

Supportive treatment includes compression garments, chronic pain therapy, laser therapy and vascular/orthopedic surgical procedures. Surgical therapy is required for correction of leg length discrepancy.

MAFFUCCI SYNDROME

Maffucci syndrome is a rare, congenital, nonhereditary disorder characterized by dyschondroplasia and vascular malformations. The cutaneous lesions are compressible, red blue papules and nodules, consistent with vascular malformations (VMs). They are mostly present on the hands and feet. Presence of enchondromas is another important feature, which is the result of a developmental abnormality in cartilage formation (dyschondroplasia). A significant risk in patients with Maffucci syndrome is of malignancy, especially chondrosarcoma.

MICROCEPHALY CAPILLARY MALFORMATION SYNDROME (MC-CAP)

It is an autosomal recessive disorder characterized by severe congenital microcephaly, early onset refractory epilepsy, developmental delay and multiple cutaneous vascular malformation.

CLOVES SYNDROME

It occurs due to PI3KCA abnormalities. It is characterized by congenital lipomatous overgrowth, vascular malformation, epidermal nevi and skeletal abnormalities.

PROTEUS SYNDROME

It is a sporadic disease due to lethal mutation in AKT1 gene. Clinical characteristics includes asymmetric distorting overgrowth of the skeletal architecture primarily lower limbs, cerebriform connective tissue nevi, linear verrucous epidermal nevus, lipomatous overgrowth and lipoatrophy. Epidermal nevus follows the lines of blaschko and they can be present anywhere on the body.

Diagnostic criteria

All of the following are general criteria:

- Lesions follow a mosaic distribution or pattern
- Problems follow a progressive course
- The disorder appears to be sporadic (i.e. not inherited)

Specific criteria include:

Category A

- Connective tissue nevus

Category B (2/3)

- Epidermal nevus
- Disproportionate overgrowth of one or more of the following: limbs, digits, cranium, vertebrae, external auditory meatus, spleen, thymus etc.
- Bilateral ovarian cystadenomas or parotid monomorphic adenoma (<20 years).

Category C (3/3)

- Dysregulated adipose tissue
- Vascular malformation
- Characteristic facial features or facial dysmorphism: dolichocephaly, long face, down slanting palpebral fissures.

BANYAN–RILEY–RUVALCABA SYNDROME

It is an autosomal dominant disorder associated with PTEN Mutation.

It is characterised by triad of macrocephaly, genital lentigines and intestinal hamartomatous polyps. Other clinical features include lipomas, haemangiomas, benign thyroid neoplasms, thyroid carcinoma, gastrointestinal malignancy, breast carcinoma.

CUTIS MARMORATA TELANGIECTASIA CONGENITA (CMTC)

It is characterised by persistent reticulate mottling with telangiectasia over lower extremities, with occasional ulceration and atrophy. It may be associated with various congenital anomalies like body asymmetry in the form of hypertrophy and atrophy, lymphangioma and haemangioma.

HEREDITARY HAEMORRHAGIC TELANGIECTASIA (Osler Weber Rendu Syndrome)

It is an autosomal dominant disorder due to mutation in endoglin gene (ENG), ACVRL1, SMAD4, GDF2, HHT3,

HHT4 genes, presents with mucocutaneous and gastrointestinal telangiectasia with arteriovenous malformation of brain, lungs and liver. Clinical features include epistaxis, telangiectasia, fast flow vascular malformation in viscera.

VENOUS MALFORMATION

Venous malformation is a common type of vascular malformation may associate with pain, discomfort, serious local and systemic complication. These are the common type of low-flow vascular lesions.

1. **Common venous malformation**
2. **Blue rubber bleb syndrome**
3. **Glomuvenous malformation**

Common Venous Malformation

These patients present in early childhood. This may be associated with a loss of function mutation of angiopoietin receptor gene TIE2/TEK. Clinically these patients present with stagnate blood flow, purplish, soft compressible, swelling and may associated with pain, phleboliths and thrombi formation. Absence of hyperaemia, thrill and pulsatility are differentiating feature from high flow malformation. Malformation can occur anywhere in body but predominantly seen on head and neck region. Treatment includes, surgical resection, sclerotherapy and laser therapy.

Blue Rubber Bleb Nevus Syndrome

Blue rubber bleb nevus syndrome is a rare disorder characterized by the presence of cutaneous and gastrointestinal vascular malformations (VMs). It is an autosomal dominant disorder in which numerous blue to purple, soft, compressible nodules are present at birth or soon after birth. The lesions keep increasing in both size and number. One of the diagnostic features is the ability to compress the nodules, which leaves an empty wrinkled sac that refills rapidly upon withdrawal of the pressure. GI involvement is characterized by hematemesis or melena with chronic anemia. CT, MRI, barium studies, skin biopsy, and upper and lower GI tract endoscopy may be needed for diagnosis.

Treatment of the condition is primarily supportive and includes iron replacement, transfusions, endoscopic sclerotherapy, band ligation or laser photocoagulation.

GLOMUVENOUS MALFORMATION

This is an uncommon venous malformation also known as glomangioma or glomenagiomatosis, occurs due to mutation in glomulin gene. Clinically it presents with localized collection of soft red blue nodules or plaques. These lesions are less compressible than common venous malformation. Later in life lesion may become more widespread and deeper with tenderness. On histology, clusters of alpha actin positive glomus cells in venous spaces are the characteristic finding. Treatment includes surgical excision.

ARTERIOVENOUS MALFORMATION

Arteriovenous malformations (AVMs) are vascular malformations consisting of both arterial and venous components with AV shunting. These lesions may range from macular erythema or thin vascular plaques to larger pulsating nodules with an audible bruit. AVMs grow and change over time. AVMs are often arranged by using a scale called the Schöbinger staging system, though, not all AVMs go through every stage.

- **Stage I (quiescence):** The AVM is "quiet". The skin on top of the AVM may be warm and pink or red.
- **Stage II (expansion):** AVM gets larger. A pulse can be felt or heard in the AVM.
- **Stage III (destruction):** Causes pain, bleeding or ulcers.
- **Stage IV (decompensation):** Heart failure occurs.

Its major complications are functional or cosmetic deformity and in some patients, cardiovascular compromise related to increased blood flow. Ultrasound with Color Doppler study, CT or MRI evaluation, or arteriography can be done for diagnostic confirmation. Treatment is difficult, the options include surgical excision, embolization and amputation. Multidisciplinary management is advised.

LYMPHATIC MALFORMATIONS

Lymphangioma (cystic lymphatic malformation) refers to a group of localized congenital malformations of the lymphatic system, most of which become clinically evident at birth or during infancy. These lesions may represent lymphatic structures that failed to link with the rest of the lymphatic or venous system. Clinically similar lesions may result from lymphedema secondary to tumor infiltration, surgical or accidental injury to normal lymphatics. Small superficial lesions can be referred as microcystic lymphatic malformations and larger deeper lesions as macrocystic lymphatic malformations. Combined microcystic and macrocystic lesions can occur.

Superficial lymphatic malformations (microcystic lymphatic malformation, lymphangioma circumscriptum) consists of one or several patches of thick-walled skin colored to gray vesicles that resemble fish eggs or frog spawn (Figure 22.17). Thrombosis or bleeding into vesicles after trauma may result in purple or black discoloration. Lesions may be associated with an underlying soft-tissue fullness or extensive

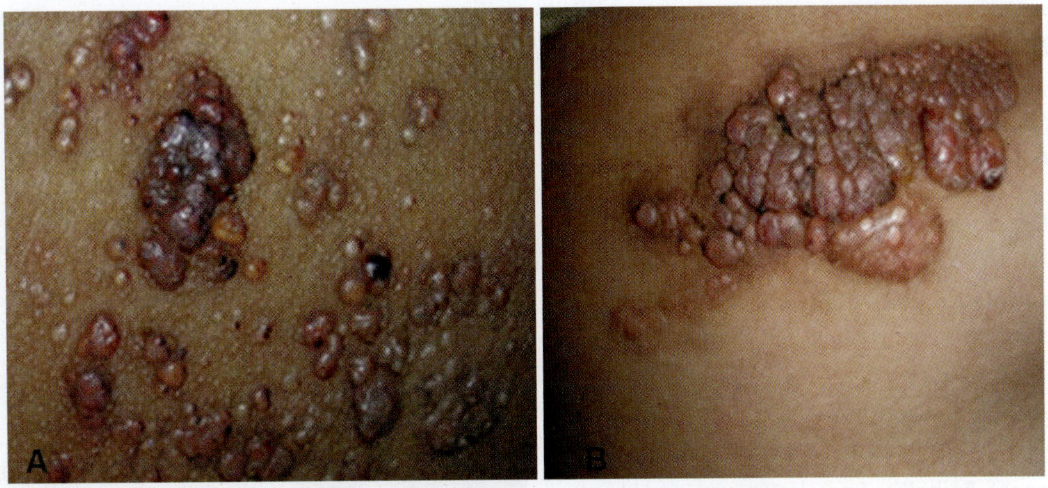

Figure 22.17: Lymphangioma circumscriptum

swelling of the involved area. Although there is a predilection for involvement of the proximal extremities and limb girdle regions, lesions may occur at any cutaneous or mucous membrane site.

Deep lymphatic malformations (macrocystic lymphatic malformations, cavernous lymphangiomas, cystic hygromas) develop as localized, subcutaneous, cystic swellings, most commonly in the head and neck (Figure 22.18). These lesions may surround and compress vital structures in the anterior neck. Their presence may be marked by overlying superficial lymphatic malformations or capillary vascular malformations such as a portwine stain.

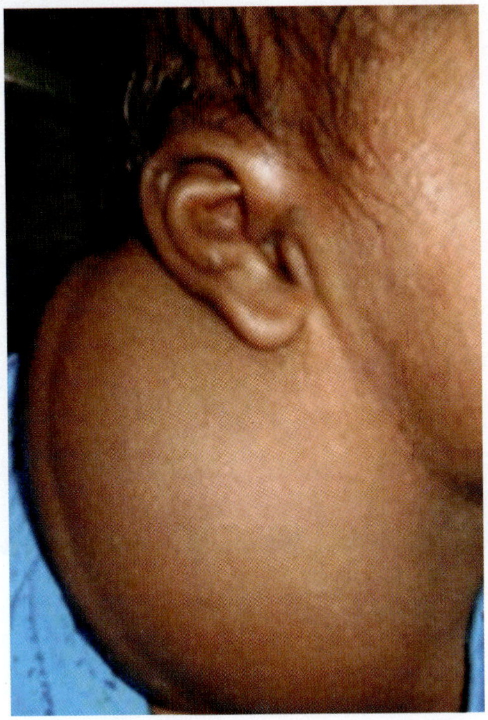

Figure 22.18: Cystic hygroma

Lymphatic malformations may be associated with complex congenital vascular malformations. In the proteus syndrome, extensive dermal and subcutaneous lymphatic and venous malformations are associated with cutaneous PWS, soft tissue tumors and epidermal naevi.

Surgical management of lymphangiomas is difficult, because they often extend around vital structures, and recurrence rates are high. Superficial lesions may be ablated with the carbon dioxide laser, and deeper malformations may improve with sclerotherapy.

LYMPHEDEMA

Lymphedema is a chronic disease which occurs due to progressive accumulation of lymphatic fluid in body leading to swelling of involved part. Signs of lymphedema include distal swelling in extremities like hands, feet which is associated with heaviness, pain and skin discoloration. Lymphedema is classified into two categories:

Primary lymphedema: Primary lymphedema occurs due to hyperplasia, hypoplasia and aplasia of lymphatics. It is further divided into three types:

1. Congenital lymphedema (onset within 2 year of life)
2. Lymphedema praecox (2 year to 35 years of age)
3. Lymphedema tarda (begins after 35 years of age)

Secondary lymphedema: It occurs due to obstruction, injury of lymphatics due to infection, malignancy and post irradiation.

Lymphedema can be diagnosed clinically. Confirmation is done by lymphoscintigraphy. Management includes, decongestive lymphedema surgery, manual lymph node drainage, compression therapy and surgical intervention (vascularized lymph node transfer, lymphaticovenous anastomoses, suction assisted protein lipectomy).

ANGIOKERATOMAS

Angiokeratomas are characterized by ectasia (dilation) of superficial vessels of the dermis along with hyperkeratosis of the overlying epidermis. Clinically they present as hyperkeratotic, dark red to purple or black papules ranging from 1 mm and 10 mm in diameter. Several types of angiokeratomas are recognized:

1. **Solitary or Multiple Angiokeratomas:** Usually occur on the lower extremities of young adults and are blue black in colour.
2. **Angiokeratoma Circumscriptum:** Multiple, clustered red to purple papules forming a plaque (Figure 22.19).
3. **Angiokeratoma of Mibelli:** Angiokeratomas occurring on dorsal fingers or toes or in interdigital spaces.
4. **Angiokeratoma of Fordyce:** It consists of numerous red to purple papules on the scrotum or vulva of adults (Figure 22.20).
5. **Angiokeratoma Corporis Diffusum:** This term is used to denote numerous dark red to black papules distributed primarily on the abdomen, genitals, buttocks and thighs ("bathing trunk" distribution) (Figure 22.21). Most common disorder associated with this condition is Fabry's disease.

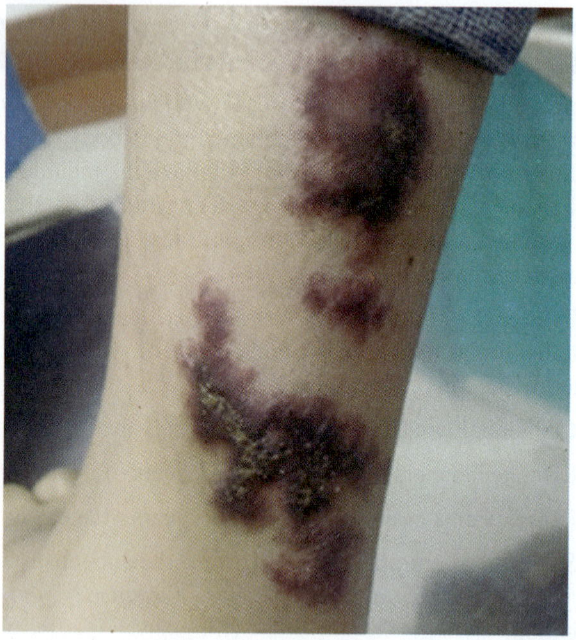

Figure 22.19: Angiokeratoma circumscriptum

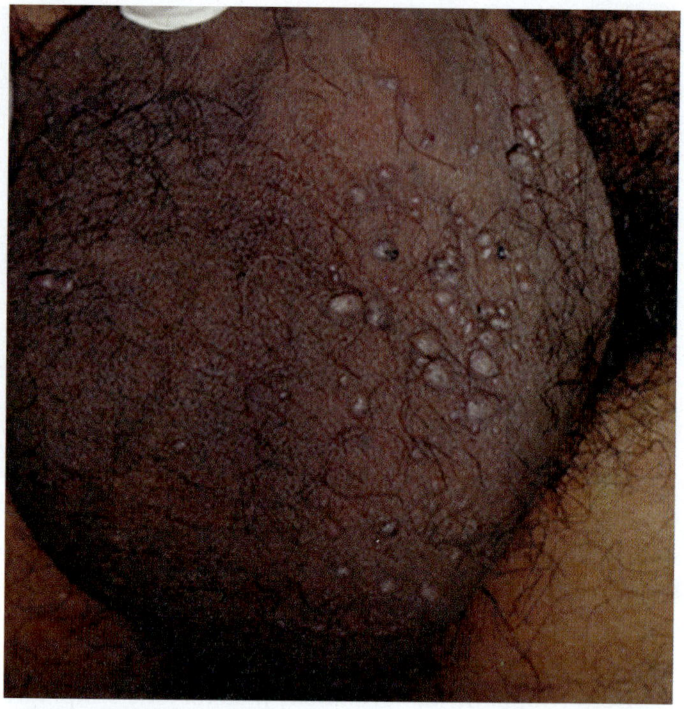

Figure 22.20: Angiokeratoma of Fordyce

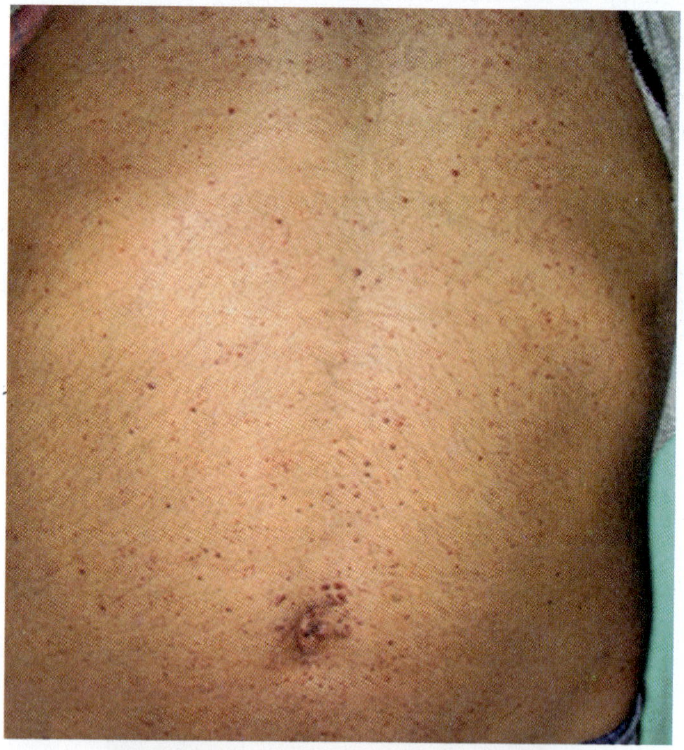

Figure 22.21: Angiokeratoma corporis diffusum

23 CHAPTER Genodermatosis

Contents

Genodermatosis is a cutaneous phenotype caused by a single mutation that may be a point mutation, deletion, or chromosomal aberration.

Irvine and Mellerio, in 2010, classified genodermatoses into following categories:

1. **Inherited immunobullous disorders**
   - Epidermolysis bullosa (EB) of different groups.
2. **Disorders of keratinization**
   - Ichthyosis.
   - Palmoplantar keratoderma.
   - Erythrokeratoderma.
   - Follicular keratosis.
3. **Hereditary disorders of pigmentation**
   - Carney complex.
   - Chediak-Higashi syndrome (CHS).
   - Griscelli syndrome.
4. **Familial multiple tumor syndrome**
   - Neurofibromatosis Type 1 and 2.
   - Tuberous sclerosis complex (TSC).
   - Gardner syndrome.
   - Cowden syndrome.
   - Peutz-Jeghers syndrome.
5. **Ectodermal dysplasias (EDAs) and disorders of ectodermal appendages**

6. **Disorders with defects in DNA repair and chromosomal instability**
   - Bloom syndrome.
   - Xeroderma pigmentosum.
   - Cockayne syndrome.
7. **Poikilodermatous disorders**
   - Rothmund-Thomson syndrome.
   - Dyskeratosis congenital (DKC).
   - Acrokeratotic poikiloderma of Weary.
   - Kindler syndrome.
8. **Connective tissue disorders**
   - Ehlers-Danlos syndrome (EDS).
   - Pseudoxanthoma elasticum.
   - Marfan syndrome.
   - Cutis laxa.
   - Fabry disease.
   - Williams syndrome.
   - Menkes kinky hair syndrome.
9. **Vascular and lymphatic disorders**
   - Osler-Rendu-Weber syndrome Type 1 and 2.
   - Lymphedema distichiasis syndrome.
10. **Porphyrias**
11. **Disorders associated with immunodeficiency**
    - Wiskott-Aldrich syndrome.
    - Omenn syndrome.
12. **Miscellaneous disorders**
    - Bazex syndrome.
    - Goltz syndrome.
    - Pachydermoperiostosis.
    - Nail-Patella syndrome.
    - Apert syndrome.

NEUROCUTANEOUS SYNDROMES (PHAKOMATOSES)

Phakomatoses are neurocutaneous conditions with frequent involvement of the skin, eyes, and the nervous system.

Neurofibromatoses

Classification of neurofibromatosis (Table 23.1):

Table 23.1: Riccardi's classification

NF-1	Von Recklinghausen disease
NF-2	Acoustic schwannoma
NF-3	Mixed
NF-4	Variants
NF-5	Segmental café au lait macule, neurofibroma or both, affecting one or more dermatomes
NF-6	Café au lait macule only
NF-7	Late onset
NF-8	Not otherwise specified

It is an autosomal dominant disorder with population prevalence of 1 in 5000. There is a high rate of mutation and up to 50% patients may not have family history. The genetic locus of NF-I gene is located on the long arm of chromosome 17, which encodes for a protein neurofibromin, which is found in neurons, oligodendrocytes and in non-myelinating schwann cells. Neurofibromin is involved in cell growth and differentiation. The cutaneous manifestations include café au lait macules (CALMs), which are flat brown pigmented macules (Figure 23.1 A and B) occurring due to focal hyper pigmentation in basal layer. Upto 53% patients have > 6 CALMs by 3 years and 97% will have > 6 CALMs by 6 years. Intertriginous freckling is commonly seen in axilla (Figure 23.2 A and B) and inguinal region, under breasts and is not related to sun exposure. It is considered virtually pathognomonic of NF-I (Crowe Sign). A characteristic palmar freckling known as the Patrick Yasudian sign, is also seen in a few patients (Figure 23.2 C). Discrete neurofibromas (Figure 23.1 A and C) are benign nerve sheath tumors that appear as discrete masses arising from peripheral nerves and generally start after puberty (<20% have neurofibroma before 10 years age). Plexiform neurofibromas (Figure 23.2 D) are like discrete neurofibromas but involve single or multiple nerve fascicle of the branches of major nerves. They elicit a "bag of worm" sensation on palpation and often there is overlying hyperpigmentation (giant café au lait spot) or hypopigmentation.

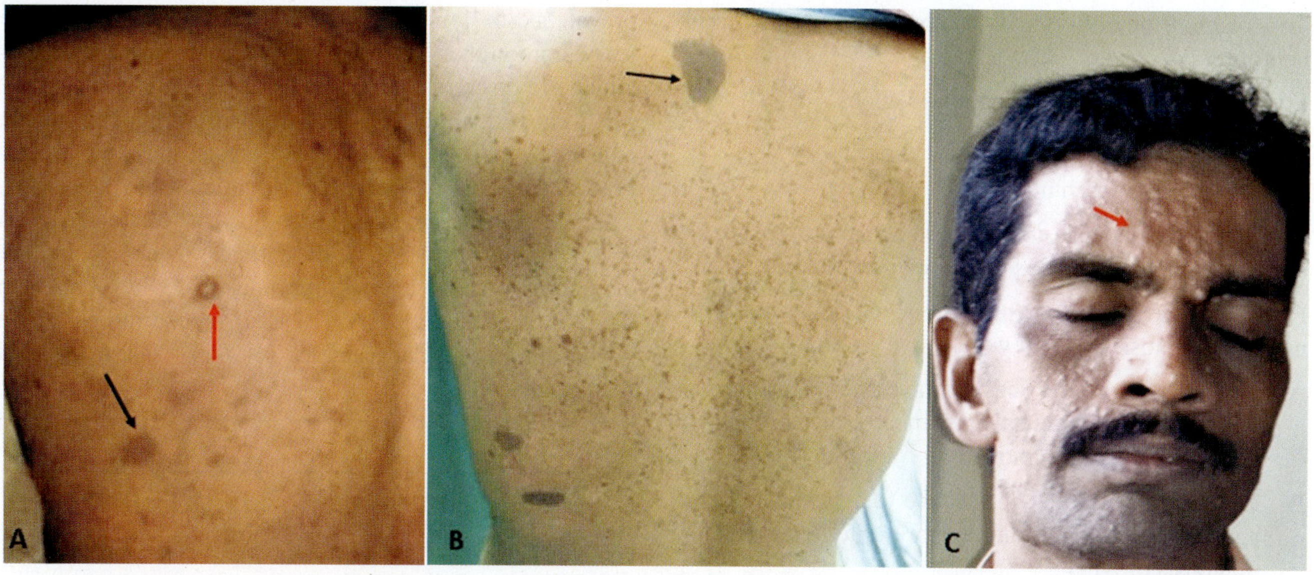

Figure 23.1: Neurofibromatosis showing CALMs (Black arrow A and B) and neurofibromas (A and C Red arrow)

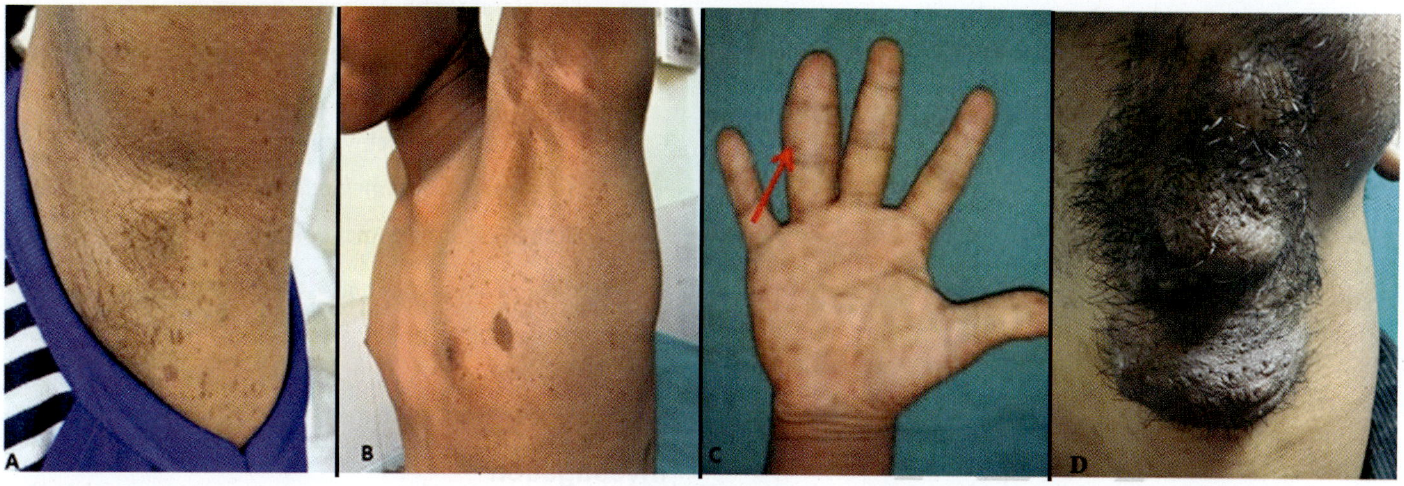

Figure 23.2: Axillary freckling or Crowe sign (A and B), palmer freckling on hand with neurofibroma of ring finger (C) and plexiform neurofibroma (D)

Neurofibromatosis Type I (SYN:Von Recklinghausen's Disease, Peripheral NF)

The extracutaneous manifestations include Lisch nodules, which are slightly raised well circumscribed melanocytic hamartomas of the iris thought to be virtually pathognomic of NF-I. They are found in 90% adult patients and 30% children (< 6 years age) with NF-I. The osseous lesions include dysplasia of wing of the sphenoid bone and dysplasia of long bone characterized by congenital thinning and bowing (tibia is most affected). Scoliosis is the most common skeletal manifestation seen in up to 10-30% patients. The IQ is almost normal but 30-60% patients have learning disabilities.

There is 10-13% lifetime risk of developing malignant peripheral nerve sheath tumors, which exclusively arise from pre existing plexiform neurofibromas (Figure 23.2 D). There is also risk of pheochromocytoma as in 1.4% of cases and increased risk of CML and ALL. The optic pathway tumors (OPTs) develop in 15% of children with NF-I.

National Institute of Health Diagnostic Criteria for Neurofibromatosis Type 1

- Six or more café au lait macules larger than 5 mm in greatest diameter in prepubertal individuals, and larger than 15 mm in greatest diameter in post pubertal individuals.

- Two or more neurofibromas of any type or 1 plexiform neurofibroma.
- Freckling in the axillary or inguinal regions.
- Optic glioma.
- Two or more iris Lisch nodules.
- A distinctive osseous lesion such as sphenoid dysplasia or thinning of long bone cortex with or without pseudarthrosis.
- First degree relative (parent, sibling, or offspring) with neurofibromatosis Type 1 by the above criteria.
  A. In an individual who does not have a parent diagnosed with NF-1, then patient must meet 2 or more of the listed criteria for diagnosis.
  B. If a patient parent meets the diagnostic criteria specified in A, only one or more criteria require for diagnosis of NF-1.

Investigations

The diagnosis is clinical. Prenatal and presymptomatic diagnosis can be made by exon sequencing and/or mutation analysis with 95% sensitivity. Routine radiological screening and neuroimaging is not recommended and should be undertaken only in symptomatic patients.

Treatment

For Café-au-lait spots, Q switched ruby laser (694 nm), continuous mode copper vapour laser (511 nm) and Erbium: Yttrium-aluminium garnet laser (2940 nm) are useful but there is recurrence in up to 67% of patients. Cutaneous neurofibromas can be removed surgically or by CO_2 laser in general anaesthesia. Plexiform NFs need surgical excision, but recurrences are common. Trials are going on in phase I and II with **Pirfenidone**, which is a farnesyl transferase inhibitor that decreases Ras oncogene expression. It is an antifibrotic agent that decreases proliferation of fibroblasts and collagen synthesis. Peg IFN-2b is also under consideration. Optic nerve sheet tumors need chemotherapy with methotrexate and vinblastin.

Besides, all primary relatives should be examined for cutaneous lesions and Lisch nodules. Children <10 years of age should undergo yearly ophthalmological examination for ophthalmic tumours (OPTs). Regular BP measurement should be done to look for signs of renovascular hypertension. A yearly spine examination is enough to detect scoliosis.

Neurofibromatosis Type II (SYN-Bilateral Acoustic Neurofibromatosis, Central Neurofibromatosis)

It is also an autosomal dominant disorder with population prevalence of 1 in 33000. The cutaneous manifestations are less common than NF1, but include cutaneous schwannomas, which are discrete, well circumscribed, slightly raised lesions of <2 cm with slightly rough surface, mild hyperpigmentation and hypertricosis. Café au lait spots may be present in upto 43% patients but only 1% patients have >6 CALMs. The extracutaneous manifestations are bilateral vestibular schwannomas in 85-92% of patients, which gives rise to symptoms such as deafness, tinnitus or vertigo. Patients may develop meningiomas (45% cases), ependimomas, juvenile posterior subcapsular cataract (60-80% cases) and retinal hamartomas.

Diagnosis

Manchester clinical diagnostic criteria for NF type 2 (>1 should be present).

1. Bilateral vestibular schwannomas.
2. A first degree relative with NF2 and
   - Unilateral vestibular schwannoma or
   - *Any two of the following:* Meningioma, Schwannoma, Glioma, Neurofibroma, Posterior subcapsular cataract.
3. Unilateral vestibular schwannoma and
   - *Any two of the following:* Meningioma, Schwannoma, Glioma, Neurofibroma, Posterior subcapsular cataract
4. Multiple meningiomas and
   - Unilateral vestibular schwannoma or
   - *Any two of the following:* Schwannoma, Glioma, Neurofibroma, Cataract.

Investigation

MRI (acoustic), CT scan and slit lamp examination, whenever necessary.

Treatment

Surgery for acoustic neuromas and cataracts. Annual clinical screening including skin and ophthalmologic examination.

TUBEROUS SCLEROSIS COMPLEX (SYN: Bourneville's Disease, Pringle's Disease) EPILOIA (Epilepsy, Low Intelligence, Adenoma Sebaceum)

It is an autosomal dominant disorder caused by mutations in a tumor suppressor gene, either TSC1 or TSC2 on chromosome 9p and 16q respectively. TSC1 encodes hamartin and TSC2 encodes tuberin. TSC1 and TSC2 form a complex that inhibits signaling through the mammalian target of Rapamycin (mTOR) pathway.

The cutaneous manifestations include hypomelanotic macules (Ash leaf macules, Figure 23.3) that are present in over 90% of children with tuberous sclerosis complex (TSC) at birth and may fade in adulthood. They are usually present over buttocks. This may be the earliest finding and the disease may develop later. In a child with convulsions without any other findings of TSC, it may suggest the correct diagnosis. A less common type of lesion is a confetti like skin lesion. Adenoma sebaceum or facial angiofibromas appear at 2-5 years of age on centrofacial area of face and are concentrated on nasolabial folds with relative sparing of upper lip and lateral face and affect 75% to 90% of patients. They appear as firm, red brown or skin colored discrete papules (Figure 23.4A and B).

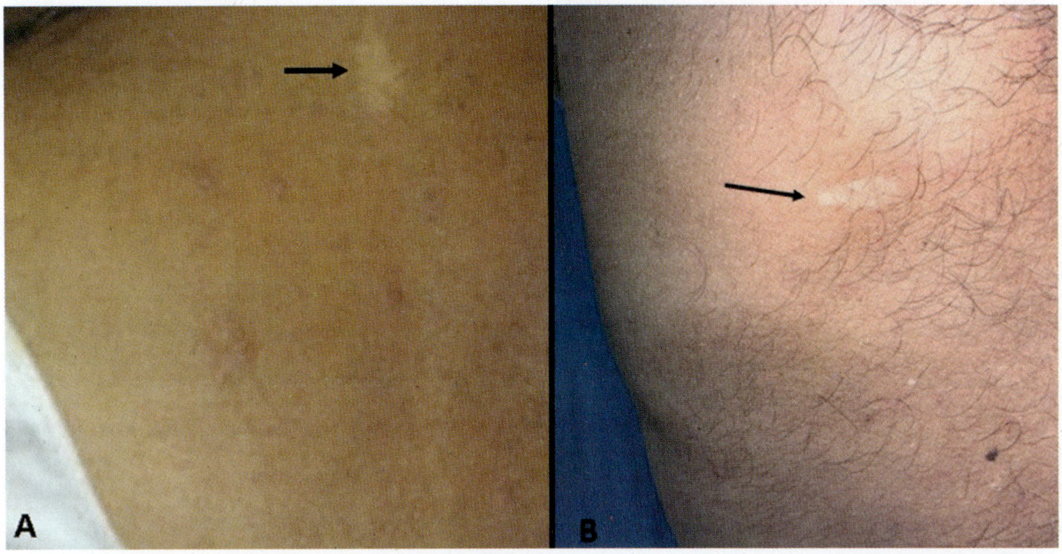

Figure 23.3: Hypomelanotic macule or ash leaf macule over upper back in tuberous sclerosis

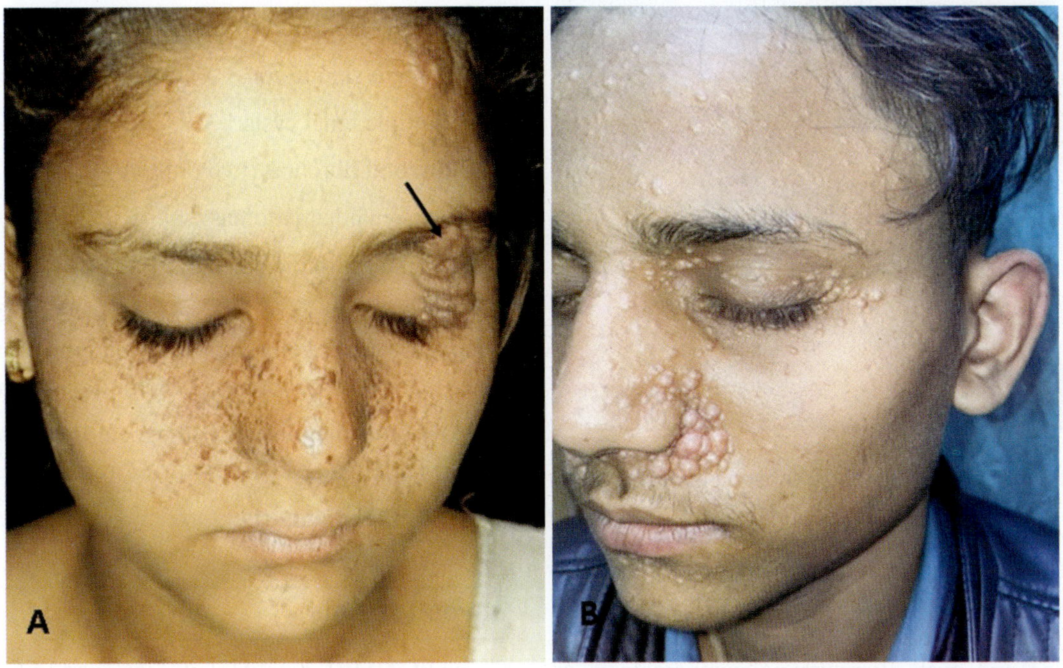

Figure 23.4: Facial angiofibroma (A and B) with fibrous facial plaque (A -Black arrow)

Fibrous facial plaques are irregular soft to firm skin colored to hyperpigmented connective tissue nevus (Figure 23.4 A). Shagreen patch (Figure 23.5) is a firm or rubbery irregular plaque which may have bumpy surface with coalescing papules and nodules or orange peel like surface. Ungual fibromas (Koenen's tumor) usually appear after 10 years of age and are periungual or subungual (Figure 23.6).

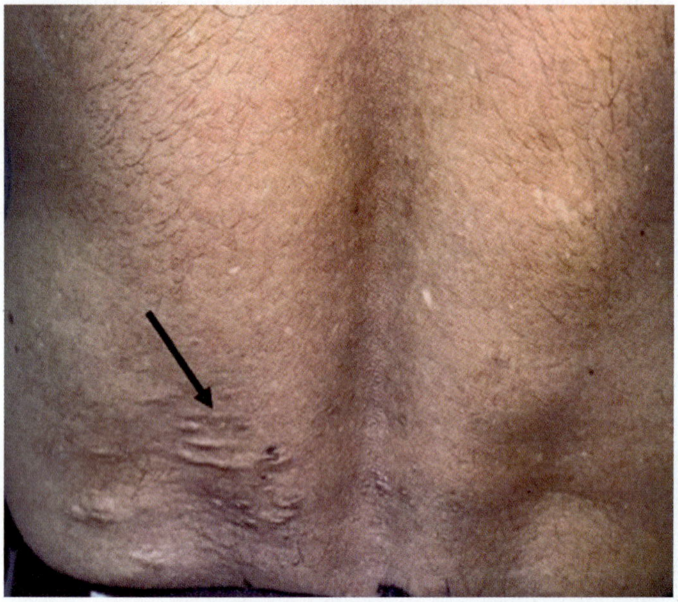

Figure 23.5: Shagreen patch over lower back

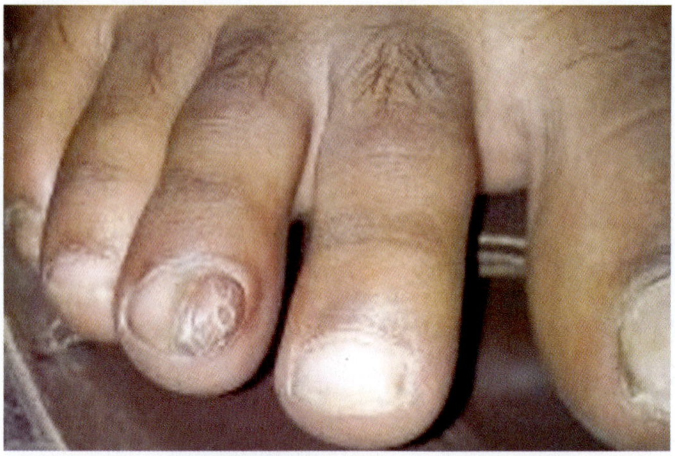

Figure 23.6: Periungual fibromas (Koenen tumour)

Extracutaneous manifestations include seizures, mental retardation, dental pitting, cortical tubers, subependymal nodules and subependymal giant cell astrocytomas in the brain, cardiac rhabdomyomas – mostly asymptomatic, renal angiomyolipomas and cysts, lymphangioleiomyomatosis in lungs, retinal astrocytic hamartomas and rectal polyps.

Diagnosis

The diagnosis is clinical.

The Criteria for Diagnosis of TSC are:

Genetic Criterion:

- Pathogenic mutation in TSC1 or TSC2 in DNA from normal tissue.

Major Features:

- Angiofibromas (three or more) or fibrous cephalic plaque.
- Ungual fibromas (two or more).
- Hypomelanotic macules (three or more, at least 5 mm diameter).
- Shagreen patch.
- Multiple retinal hamartomas.
- Cortical dysplasia.
- Subependymal nodules.
- Subependymal giant cell astrocytoma.
- Cardiac rhabdomyoma.
- Lymphangiomyomatosis.
- Angiomyolipomas (two or more).

Minor Features:

- Dental enamel pits (three or more).
- Confetti skin lesions.
- Multiple renal cysts.
- Intraoral fibromas (two or more).
- Non-renal hamartomas.
- Retinal achromic patch.

A combination of only two major clinical features (e,g, lymphangioleiomyomatosis and angiomyolipomas) without other features does not meet criteria for a definite diagnosis.

Definite diagnosis: Pathogenic mutation or 2 major features or 1 major feature with ≥2 minor features.

Possible diagnosis: One major feature or ≥2 minor features.

Investigations

Cranial CT/MRI, renal USG/CT/MRI and ECG may be done, as indicated.

Management

A multidisciplinary approach for CNS and CVS manifestations is required. Skin tumors may be removed surgically or by lasers like PDL and CO_2 laser. Rapamycin is an mTOR inhibitor, which is used in TS. It has been found to result in regression of pulmonary, renal and cutaneous lesions. Imatinib is a tyrosinase kinase inhibitor which blocks the signals of Akt pathway.

Both rapamycin and Imatinib are FDA approved drugs and well tolerated.

INCONTINENTIA PIGMENTI (Bloch–Sulzberger Syndrome)

It is inherited as an X-linked dominant trait and a single affected unpaired gene on X-chromosome is lethal for males. The disorder results from mutations in nuclear factor kappa B (NF-κB) essential modulator (NEMO; IKBKG).

Epidemiology

IP has a worldwide distribution. IP appears to be more common among white patients, but it has also been reported in blacks and Asians. More than 95% of reported cases of IP occur in females.

Clinical Features

The skin, eyes and central nervous system (CNS) are primarily affected. It usually presents at birth or within two to six weeks of infancy and has the following clinical stages:

- **Vesicular stage (Figure 23.7):** Inflammatory vesicles and pustules appear on the skin of the trunk and limbs and spontaneous resolution occurs within few months.

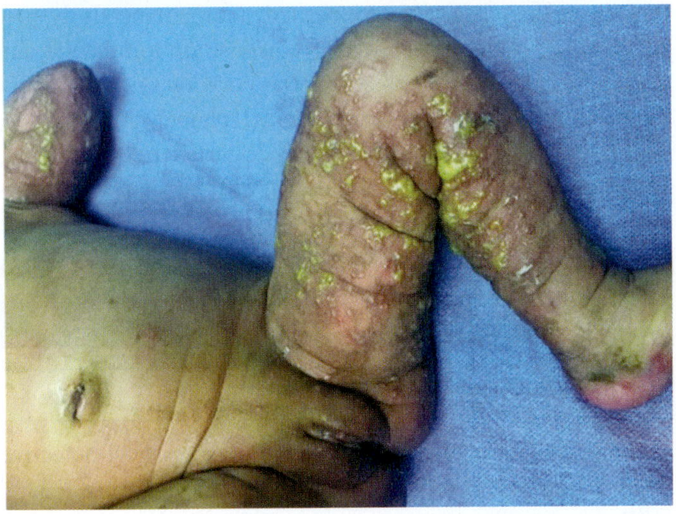

Figure 23.7: Vesicular form of incontinentia pigmenti

- **Verrucous stage (Figure 23.8):** Characterized by irregular warty papules and plaques linearly present over the limbs.
- **Hyperpigmentation stage (Figure 23.8):** Macular, brown to grey thin bands of coloration in swirling pattern along the lines of Blaschko over extremities and trunk. Resolution of this stage occurs by adolescence.
- A fourth **phase of atrophy and hypopigmentation** has been observed where atrophic streaks and hypopigmentation of the skin ultimately occurs (Figure 23.9).

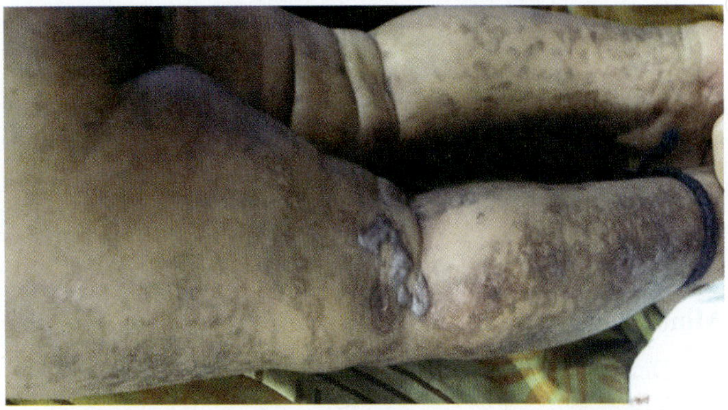

Figure 23.8: Verrucous and hyperpigmented form of incontinentia pigmenti

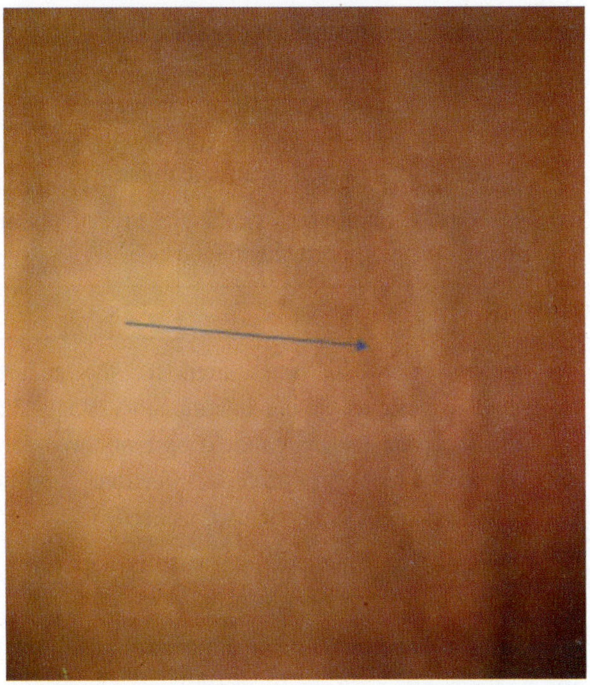

Figure 23.9: Incontinentia pigmenti showing splashed pattern of hypopigmentation

- Central nervous system abnormalities like mental retardation, seizure disorders, neurocognitive and motor difficulties can occur. Eye involvement in the form of strabismus, cataracts, optic nerve atrophy or retinal vascular abnormalities can accompany skin lesions. Both the primary and permanent dentitions are affected with characteristic missing or malformed small, cone shaped teeth.

The proposed diagnostic criteria for IP are as follows:

- In the absence of a family history, the presence of at least one major criterion is necessary. The presence of minor criteria supports the diagnosis of IP.

Major criteria:

- Typical neonatal vesicular rash with eosinophilia.
- Typical splashed pattern or Chinese letter pattern hyperpigmentation on the trunk (Figure 14.13), fading in adolescence.
- Linear, atrophic hairless lesions.

Minor criteria:

- Dental anomalies.
- Alopecia.
- Wooly hair.
- Abnormal nails.

Other suggestive features are:

- Vertex alopecia.
- Retinal disease.
- History of multiple male miscarriage in mother.
- With a definitive family history, the presence of any major criterion strongly supports the diagnosis of IP.

Treatment

- Treatment is not usually required for the cutaneous lesions. The vesicles of the inflammatory stage should be left intact, and the skin should be monitored for the development of secondary bacterial infections. Emollients and topical antibiotics may be used as needed.
- Oral hygiene and regular dental care is necessary and dental restoration may be indicated.
- Seizures should be treated with anticonvulsants.
- Frequent ophthalmologic evaluations are required, especially during the first year of life, in order to diagnose and treat potential ophthalmologic complications.
- Genetic counseling and genetic testing should be done for the patient and family members.

ATAXIA TELANGIECTASIA (SYN: Louis-Bar Syndrome, At)

It is inherited as an autosomal recessive disorder with incidence of 1 in 40,000. It results from mutations in ATM gene that plays a central role in activating apoptotic and cell cycle responses to DNA damage. The cutaneous manifestations include telangiectasias that usually appear at 3 to 6 years of age, and begin near the ocular canthi and progress across the bulbar conjunctivae. The cutaneous telangiectasias subsequently may develop on the malar prominences, ears, eyelids, anterior chest, popliteal, antecubital fossae, and on the dorsal aspects of the hands and feet, may be related to sun exposure. Progeric changes of the skin such as xerosis and gray hair occur in 90 percent of patients.

Facial skin may become atrophic, causing a mask like appearance. Mottled hyper and hypopigmentation commonly occur and, together with the telangiectases and atrophy, can resemble the poikiloderma. The extracutaneous manifestations include progressive cerebellar ataxia (median age of onset 1.2 years), recurrent bacterial and viral sinopulmonary infections (upto 80% patients) – the most common cause of death. Growth retardation is common and malignancies such as lymphomas and leukemias may develop in 40% of cases.

Treatment

The therapy for AT is supportive and includes administration of antibiotics for infection, physiotherapy for pulmonary bronchiectasis, sunscreens and sun avoidance to diminish actinic like changes. Patients should be aggressively screened for malignancy.

VON HIPPEL-LINDAU SYNDROME

It is an autosomal dominant, inherited, neurocutaneous dysplasia complex characterized by a predisposition to bilateral and multicentric retinal angiomas, central nervous system hemangioblastomas, renal cell carcinomas, pheochromocytomas, islet cell tumors of the pancreas, endolymphatic sac tumors, and renal, pancreatic and epididymal cysts. Cutaneous manifestations may include CALMs.

DISORDERS OF GENOME INSTABILITY AND DNA REPAIR DISORDERS

Xeroderma Pigmentosum (XP)

It is inherited as an autosomal recessive disorder of defective DNA repair on exposure to UVR due to abnormalities in NER (nucleotide excision repair) pathway. It manifests as acute sunburn reaction on minimal UV exposure. Numerous freckle like hyperpigmented macules (Figure 23.10) appear predominately on sun exposed skin. Continued sun exposure causes the patient's skin to become dry and parchment like, with increased pigmentation, atrophy, mottled hypopigmentation and hypopigmentation (Figures 23.11 A and 23.12). Premalignant actinic keratosis develop at an early age. Patients with XP younger than 20 years of age have a greater than 1000 fold increased risk of cutaneous basal cell carcinoma, squamous cell carcinoma (Figure 23.11 B) or melanoma.

The patients develop photophobia, conjunctival injection, keratitis, and corneal opacity (Figure 23.11 B). CNS abnormalities include mild to severe mental retardation, deafness and seizures. The most severe form is known as **DeSanctis-Cacchione syndrome**.

The diagnosis is clinical. Prenatal diagnosis is possible by measuring UV induced unscheduled DNA synthesis in cultured amniotic fluid cells, DNA studies of trophoblast cells obtained in early pregnancy.

Treatment

Sun protection–Full clothes, avoidance of sun exposure and sunscreens. Premalignant lesions such as actinic keratoses should

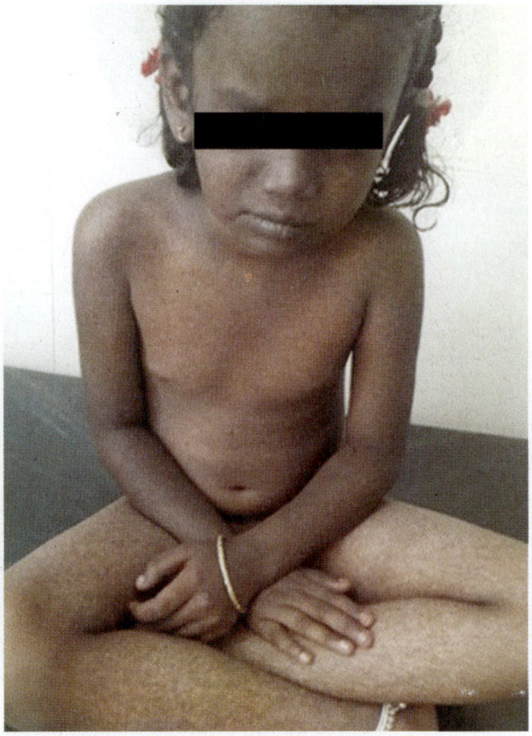

Figure 23.10: Progressive freckling, hyperpigmentation and photosensitivity in XP

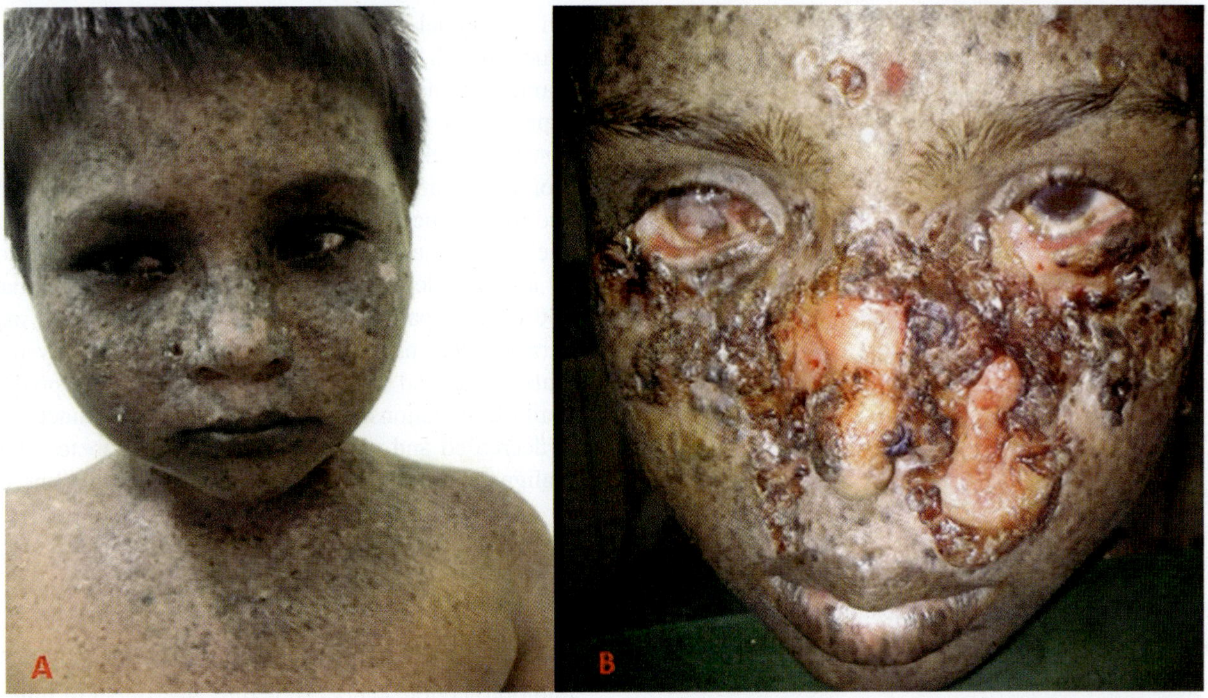

Figure 23.11: Xeroderma pigmentosum showing photophobia, mottled pigmentation (A) Freckling, scarring of cornea, conjunctiva with SCC in XP (B)

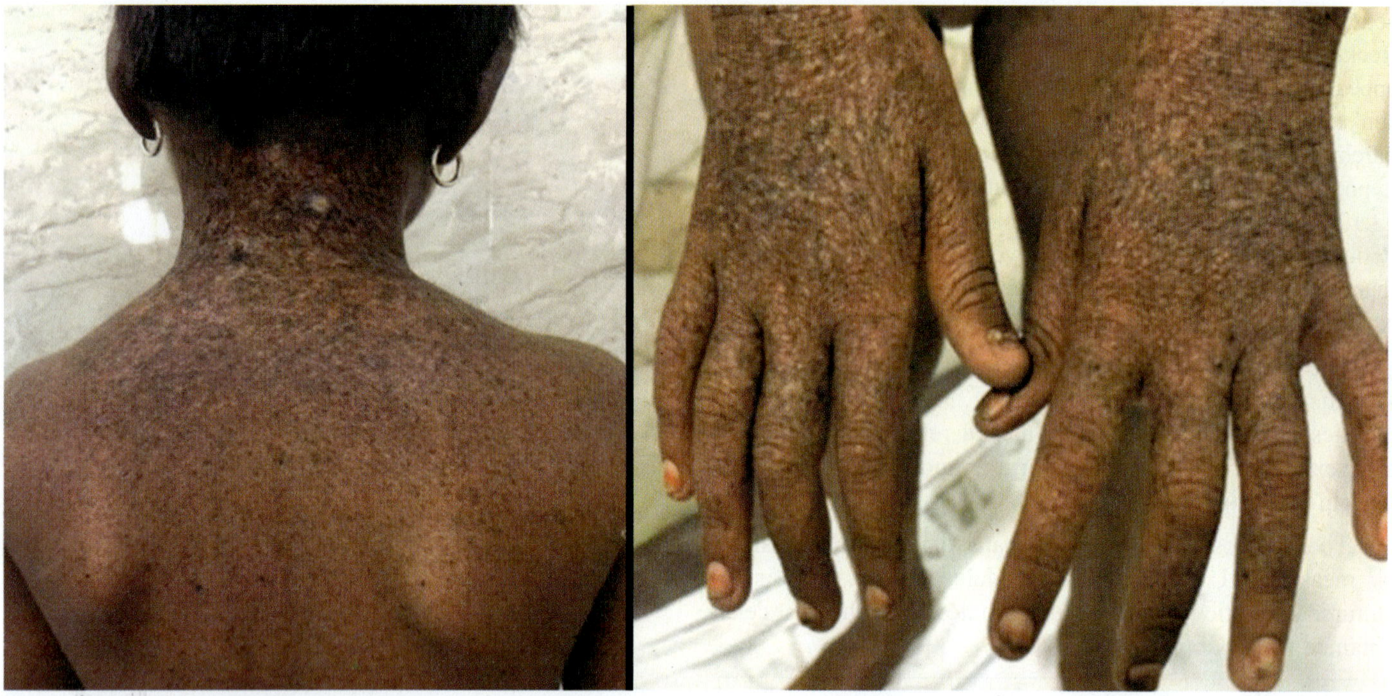

Figure 23.12: Photodermatitis, mottled pigmentation with atrophy in xeroderma pigmentosum

be treated with liquid nitrogen cryotherapy, topical 5-FU and imiquimod. Cutaneous malignancies require electrodissection, curettage, surgical excision or Mohs micrographic surgery.

TRICHOTHIODYSTROPHY (SYN: Amish Brittle Hair Syndrome, Sabinas Brittle Hair Syndrome, Pollat Syndrome,TTD)

It is an autosomal recessive disorder that manifests as photosensitivity and brittle hair shafts, due to reduction of high sulfur matrix proteins (Figure 23.13 A). Patients may have ichthyosis (Figure 23.13 D), intellectual impairment, short stature, microcephaly, cataract, immunodeficiency, characteristic facial features (protruding ears, micrognathia), and decreased fertility. There are no increased chances of malignancy. BIDS (Brittle hair, intellectual impairment, decreased fertility, short stature), IBIDS (BIDS with ichthyosis), PIBIDS (IBIDS with photosensitivity) are some associated conditions.

The diagnosis of TTD is based on examination of hair shafts under polarizing microscopy that display tiger tail banding (Figure 23.13 C). In addition, they show a spectrum of typical hair shaft abnormalities, including trichoschisis, trichorrhexis nodosa like fractures, surface irregularities, ribboning and pili torti (Figure 23.13 B). Amino acid analysis of hair shafts can confirm reduced levels of cysteine and cystine. The treatment involves sun protection, ophthalmological evaluation and treatment of infections.

BLOOM'S SYNDROME

An autosomal recessive disorder due to mutations in BLM gene, which encodes a RecQ helicase. The cutaneous manifestations include facial erythema and telangiectasia, superficially resembling lupus erythematosus seen within the first few weeks after birth in the malar area, on the nose, and around the ears. Sun exposure accentuates these abnormalities and may induce bullae, bleeding, and crusting of the lips and eyelids. Café au lait spots are common at times accompanied by adjacent depigmented areas. Adult height is usually under 150 cm and patients have a characteristic facies with a long narrow head, narrow prominent nose, relatively hypoplastic malar areas and a receding chin. Patients are predisposed to multiple infections, as there is immune dysfunction. Fertility is decreased and patients may develop diabetes mellitus and malignancies. Diagnosis is clinical which may be confirmed by genetic analysis (observation of quadriradial chromosomes and the approximately 10-fold increased frequency of spontaneous sister chromatid exchanges).

Treatment

Photoprotection, cancer screening, treatment of infections and malignancies.

HERITABLE DISORDERS OF THE CONNECTIVE TISSUE

They are caused by genetic mutations affecting individual

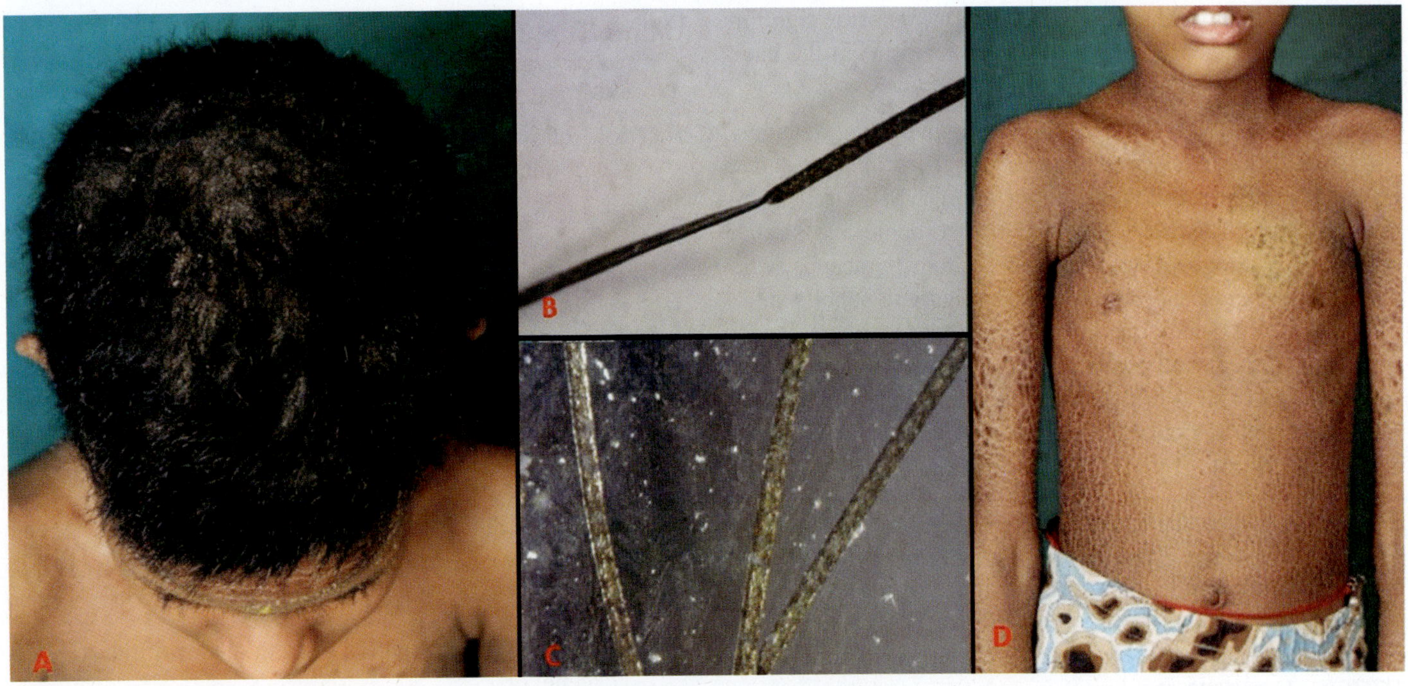

Figure 23.13: Trichothiodystrophy showing brittle hair (A), Pili torti on dermoscopy (B), Tiger tail appearance of hair shaft on polarized microscopy (C) and ichthyosis (D)

components like collagen and elastin or enzymes regulating their metabolism. The important disorders in this group include Ehlers-Danlos syndrome, pseudoxanthoma elasticum, cutis laxa and Marfan syndrome. Cardiovascular, skeletal and ophthalmic manifestations are frequently seen. Often, the cutaneous features provide the initial clue to the diagnosis.

Ehlers-Danlos Syndrome (EDS)

It is a group of heterogeneous connective tissue disorders of collagen with characteristic tissue fragility, joint hypermobility, skin hyperextensibility and easy bruising.

The International Nosology of Heritable Disorders of Connective Tissue, in 1986, defined EDS into subtypes I–VIII and X, which has been replaced by a newer, the Villefranche classification. According to Villefranche classification, it is classified into:

- **Classical (Type I and II):** Soft velvety hyperextensible skin; easy bruising; atrophic scars; hypermobile joints; pseudotumours.
- **Hypermobility (Type III):** Hypermobile joints; minimal skin abnormality.
- **Vascular (Type IV):** Thin skin; easy bruising; small joint hypermobility; vascular and bowel ruptures.
- **Kyphoscoliosis (Type IVA):** Soft hyperextensible skin; hypermobile joints; scoliosis; ocular fragility; keratoconus.
- **Arthrochalasis (Type VII A, B):** Floppy infant; congenital hip dislocation; hypermobile joints; soft skin; normal scarring; short stature.
- **Dermatosparaxis (Type VII C):** Markedly hypermobile joints; very soft and extremely fragile skin; easy bruising.
- **Other forms:** Resembles mild classical type, bruising more pronounced (Type V); Severe periodontitis, pigmented pretibial plaques and scarring. (Type VIII); Similar to mild classical type with prominent easy bruising (Type X).

The skin in patients with EDS is soft, velvety and hyperextensible (Figure 23.14). If pulled out in a fold, it rapidly retracts following release. This feature is responsible for the origin of the name "India rubber man" in circuses in earlier days. Gorlin sign refers to the ability to touch the tip of the nose with the tongue, which is present in 50% of patients.

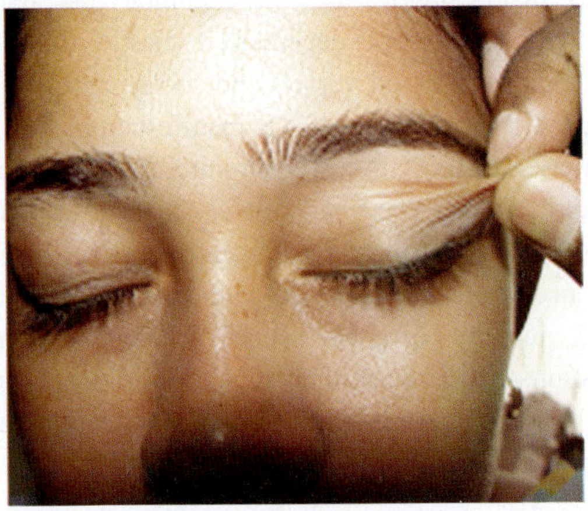

Figure 23.14: Hyperextensibility of skin in Ehlers-Danlos syndrome

Reverse Namashkar sign is a new diagnostic sign, in which the patients are able to fold their forearms at the back and oppose his/ her palms facing each other.

Hyperextensibility of the skin may give rise to gaping "fish- mouth wounds" over bony prominences like the shins, knees, and elbows following minor trauma. Scars following trauma or surgical procedures are thin, atrophic and stretch considerably after healing. Such wide, thin, papyraceous scars over the knees and elbows are called "cigarette paper scars". Therapy for EDS involves a triad of anticipatory guidance, pain management and physical therapy. Avoidance of injury and sun protection is critical to prevent the skin thinning and loss of dermis associated with ultraviolet radiation induced damage.

Pseudoxanthoma Elasticum (PXE) (SYN: Gronblad-Strandberg Syndrome)

PXE is an autosomal recessive disorder of elastic tissue, in which there is mutation of ABCC6 gene on chromosome 16. It predominantly has cardiovascular and ophthalmologic involvement. Cutaneous signs are subtle and present as yellow, flat-topped, discrete or confluent papules resembling xanthomas on the sides of the neck, axillae, periumbilical area and perineum. This "plucked chicken skin" or "Moroccan leather" appearance is quite characteristic of PXE. This clinical feature is exaggerated with advancing age with the appearance of redundant skin folds over the involved areas.

The ophthalmic manifestations include angioid streaks of retina (slate gray to reddish brown linear bands, resembling vasculature, radiating from the optic papilla), irregular retinal epithelial mottling (*peau d'orange*) and ultimately loss of central vision due to retinal hemorrhage and choroidal neovascularization.

CVS manifestations can be common and potentially serious: calcification of degenerated elastic tissue of the internal lamina of blood vessels and subsequent hemorrhage is often the most common CVS manifestation. The middle sized arteries of extremities, gastrointestinal tract and renal vasculature are involved early. It can lead to hypertension (from renal artery stenosis) and gastrointestinal bleeding in adolescence. Late sequelae of cardiovascular involvement in PXE include cerebrovascular accidents, intermittent claudication, and myocardial infarction. Severe coronary artery disease and generalized arterial calcification have also been reported.

Revised diagnostic criteria for pseudoxanthoma elasticum (PXE) (Plomp *et al.*).

Minor Diagnostic Criteria

1. **Skin**
   (a) Yellowish papules and/or plaques on the lateral side of the neck and/or flexural areas of the body; or
   (b) Increase of morphologically altered elastin with fragmentation, clumping and calcification of elastic fibres in a skin biopsy taken from clinically affected skin.
2. **Eye**
   (a) Peau d'orange of the retina; or
   (b) One or more angioid streaks, each at least as long as one disk diameter.

   When in doubt, fluorescein or indocyanine green angiography of the fundus is needed for confirmation.
3. **Genetics**
   (a) A pathogenic mutation of both alleles of the ABCC6 gene; or
   (b) A first-degree relative (parent, sibling, child) who meets independently the diagnostic criteria for definitive PXE.

Minor Diagnostic Criteria

1. **Eye**
   (a) One angioid streak shorter than one disk diameter; or
   (b) One or more 'comets' in the retina; or
   (c) One or more 'wing signs' in the retina.
2. **Genetics**

   A pathogenic mutation of one allele of the ABCC6 gene.

Requirements for the Diagnosis of PXE

1. **Definitive diagnosis**

   The presence of two (or more) major criteria not belonging to the same (skin, eye, genetic) category.
2. **Probable diagnosis**
   (a) The presence of two major eye or two major skin criteria; or
   (b) The presence of one major criterion and one or more minor criteria not belonging to the same category as the major criterion.
3. **Possible diagnosis**
   (a) The presence of a single major criterion; or
   (b) The presence of one or more minor criteria.

Diagnosis is confirmed by histopathology of skin that shows swollen, clumped, fragmented elastic fibers and calcium deposits in the mid and deep reticular dermis. These alterations are easily visualized with calcium (Von Kossa) and elastin (Verhoeff-van Giesonororcein) stains.

The treatment is directed towards minimizing complications.

Marfan Syndrome

It is an autosomal dominant disorder occurring due to mutations in the *FBN1* gene that encodes fibrillin-1. It presents with unusually tall habitus, long, thin extremities, arachnodactyly, joint hypermobility, kyphoscoliosis, pectus excavatum, and flat feet. The cutaneous manifestations include striae distensae (more prominent during adolescence and on the buttocks, thighs, breasts, abdomen and thighs), inguinal or incisional hernia and elastosis perforans serpigenosa. The arm span (fingertip to fingertip when expanded) is usually longer than the height by several centimeters; the thumb when propped across the palm extends well beyond the ulnar margin of the hand (Steinberg's sign) and wrist sign denotes thumb overlapping the fifth finger as they grasp the opposite wrist. These can be used as screening tests for the joint hypermobility of Marfan syndrome. The most common ocular abnormalities are lens displacement and myopia. Cardiovascular abnormalities occur in almost 70% of children and include dilatation of aorta, aortic regurgitation and mitral valve prolapse. Patients should avoid vigorous exercise and heavy weight lifting.

Osteogenesis Imperfecta

Osteogenesis imperfecta (OI) is a group of inherited disorders of bone fragility in which the skin may be thin, atrophic and translucent.

Most patients have mutations in type I collagen, composed of two alpha1 (*COLIA1*) and one alpha2 (*COLIA2*) polypeptide chains,

Patients commonly show hyperlaxity of ligaments and hypermobility of joints, but joint dislocation does not occur. Blue sclera is a distinctive feature in almost 90% of patients. Otosclerosis and fragile, discoloured teeth may be seen in these patients.

Supportive orthopedic therapy and bisphosphonates are used for treatment.

Cutis Laxa

Cutis laxa (generalized elastolysis) occurs due to mutation in elastin, leading to abnormal or absent elastic fibers. It can be acquired or congenital, with the genetic forms inherited as autosomal dominant or autosomal recessive. Clinical findings include loose inelastic redundant skin sagging and hanging as pendulous folds (Figure 23.15).The eyelids are drooping and ectropion can be present, which along with sagging facial skin and accentuated nasolabial folds produce a 'blood hound' or 'aged appearance'.

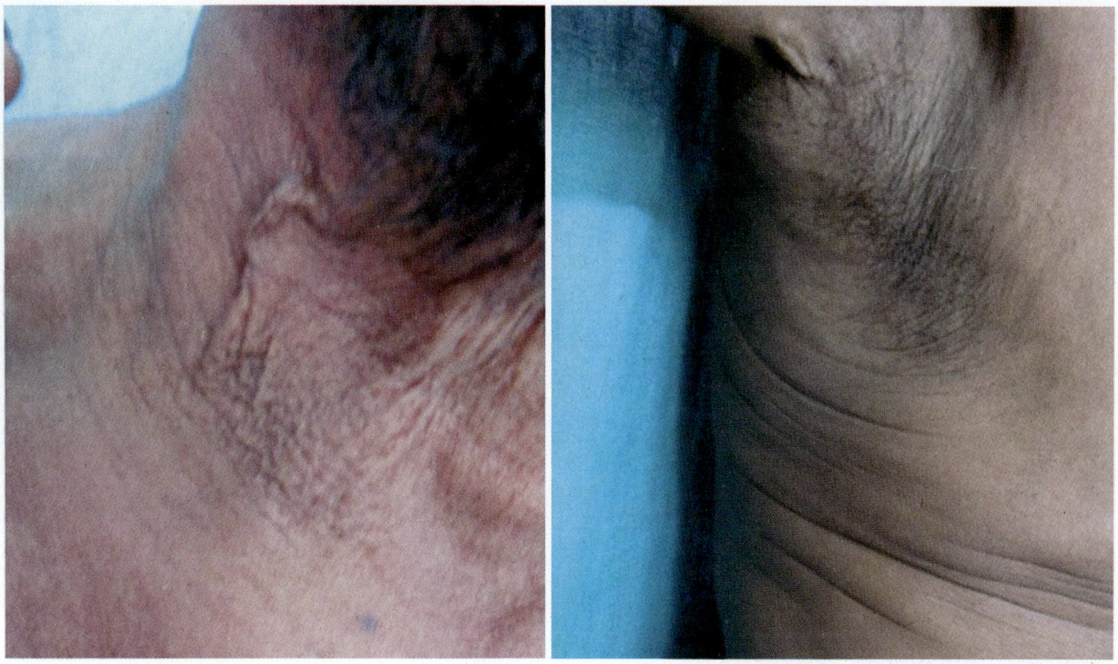

Figure 23.15: Cutis laxa

Other common findings are facial dysmorphism, aortic dilatation, pulmonary artery stenosis, pulmonary emphysema, diverticulae, uterine or rectal prolapse, ventral, hiatal and inguinal hernias.

Therapy for cutis laxa is limited. Surgery can correct diverticulae, rectal prolapse, or hernias, and plastic surgery can make a dramatic improvement in patients by procedures like facelift.

PREMATURE AGEING SYNDROMES

Poikilodermatous-like changes with prominent hyper- and hypopigmented macules from childhood are visible. Child has typical 'Bird-like' facies with sharp, thin nose and micrognathia with hydrocephalus-like appearance (Figure 23.16).

Premature ageing syndromes include mainly:

- Pangeria (Werner's syndrome).
- Acrogeria (Gottron's syndrome).
- Progeria (Hutchinson-Gilford syndrome).

Pangeria or Werner's Syndrome

It usually starts between 14 and 18 years of age with graying of hairs and progressive alopecia. But other signs and symptoms of ageing usually appears after 18 years of age. Clinical features are short stature, senile appearance, premature cataracts, joint contractures, premature arteriosclerosis, various skin changes (including scleroderma like features, canities, alopecia and ulceration) and an increased risk of malignancy.

Acrogeria (Gottron's Syndrome)

The term 'acrogeria' refers to premature ageing of the extremities, but face and less commonly trunk may be involved in this disorder. Clinical features appear soon after birth. Skin becomes thin, dry, transparent and wrinkled particularly over extremities and face. Face becomes pinched with beaked nose, thin lips, hollow cheeks and typical owl eye appearance of eyes. Micrognathia is also present.

Progeria (Hutchinson Gilford Syndrome or HGS)

Age of onset is infancy. There is atrophic, scleroderma like skin (Figure 23.16) with progressive loss of subcutaneous fatty tissue. Epidermis has cigarette paper like appearance. Venous network becomes clearly visible, especially on the upper trunk, scalp and face. Hairs are sparse from birth, but worsen within the first years of life to almost complete alopecia in next 2-3 years. There is bird like facies, beaked nose, micrognathia, and hydrocephalus like head (Figure 23.17).

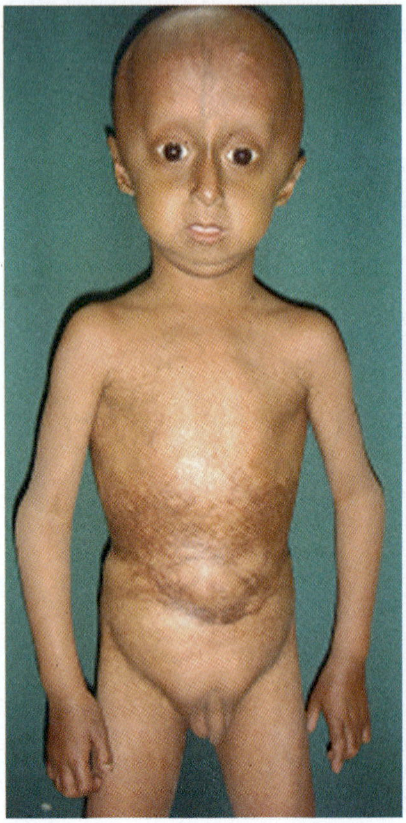

Figure 23.16: HGS showing sclerodermatous changes over trunk

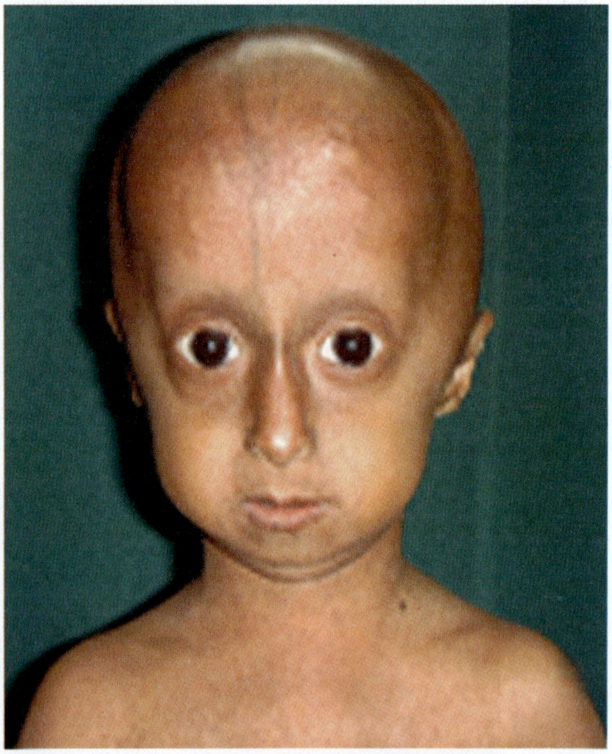

Figure 23.17: HGS showing dilated prominent veins, diffuse alopecia, 'Bird-like' facies, beaked nose, micrognathia and hydrocephalus like head

Extracutaneous Findings

- Cardiovascular anomalies (rapidly progressive atherosclerosis, early myocardial infarction and strokes, hypertension, congestive heart failure).
- Low weight and stature and general growth failure.
- Coxa valga is frequent, as well as flexural contractures in major joints ('horse-rider' gait).
- Aseptic necrosis of bones, acro-osteolysis and osteoporosis.
- Delayed and abnormal dentitions.

ECTODERMAL DYSPLASIA

Ectodermal dysplasias are group of inherited disorders which have developmental abnormalities of two or more of the structures i.e., hairs, teeth, nails, sweat glands and other ectodermal derived elements (eye, brain, mammary glands, melanocytes). It can be classified into two groups:

Group 1

- NF-kB signaling pathway defect (Ectodysplasmin)
- p63 transcription factor pathway defect
- DLX 3 transcription factor pathway defect

Group 2

- Wnt-beta-catenin pathway defect
- Connexin/ Gap junction defect
- Cytoskeletal and adhesive molecules (keratin, plakophilin, corneodesmosin, cadherin) defect

Approach in a patient of ectodermal dysplasia (Table 23.2):

NF-kB Signaling Pathway Defect (Ectodysplasmin)

Christ Siemen Touraine syndrome (Hypohidrotic ectodermal dysplasia)

X-linked hypohidrotic ectodermal dysplasia is most common of the ectodermal dysplasias. However, autosomal dominant and autosomal recessive forms have also been described. The disorder is characterized by hypotrichosis with fine, slow growing scalp and body hair, sparse eyebrows, hypohidrosis, and hypodontia. Peg shaped primary and secondary teeth are typical. decreased sweating leads to heat intolerance and enhanced dryness of the skin. Collodion like membrane at birth, ichthyosis like skin, periorificial wrinkling, milia and characteristic facies (frontal bossing, saddle nose, everted lips, perioral and periorbital pigmentation and wrinkling). X-linked hypohidrotic ectodermal dysplasia 1 is caused by a mutation in the eda gene, which encodes ectodysplasin.

p63 Transcription Factor Pathway

Ankyloblepharon-ectodermal dysplasia-clefting / Hay-Well syndrome (AEC syndrome)

It is an autosomal dominant form of ectodermal dysplasia caused by mutations in the TP63 gene. The most common feature is missing patches of skin (erosions) on the scalp, neck, hands and feet. Skin erosions can lead to infection, scarring and hair loss. Other features include changes in skin coloring, dystrophic or absent nails, malformed or missing teeth, increased sensitivity to heat, hearing loss, cleft lip and/or palate, filiform ankyloblepharon adnatum (congenital adherence of the eyelids), dental changes and hypohidrosis. These patients need care like epidermolysis bullosa.

Table 23.2: Approach in a patient of ectodermal dysplasia

Absent or severely reduced sweating	**With severe immunodeficiency (NEMO gene mutation)**	**Without immunodeficiency** Christ Siemen Touraine syndrome
Normal or minimally reduced sweating	**Normal teeth** • Clouston syndrome • Ectodermal dysplasia with skin fragility	**Abnormal teeth** **With facial cleft and limb abnormality** • EEC syndrome (Ectrodactyly-Ectodermal dysplasia-Clefting) • Limb mammary syndrome • ADULT syndrome (Acro-Dermato-Ungual-lacrimal- Tooth syndrome) **With facial cleft without limb abnormality** • AEC (Ankyloblepharon-Ectodermal dysplasia-Clefting) • Rapp-Hodgkin syndrome **Without facial cleft** • Tricho-Dento-Osseous syndrome (TDO)

Ectrodactyly-Ectodermal Dysplasia-Clefting (EEC)

EEC syndrome is characterized by abnormalities affecting the limbs including ectrodactyly (split hand and feet syndrome, lobster claw hand), a condition in which part or all of the central digits (fingers or toes) are missing. Other features include cleft lip, cleft palate, genitourinary tract abnormalities (megaureter most common) and increased risk of lymphoma. The ectodermal dysplasia component affects the hair, teeth, nails, skin and sweat glands.

DLX 3 Transcription Factor Pathway

Tricho-dento-osseus syndrome (TDO Syndrome)

This autosomal dominant ectodermal dysplasia due to defect in DLX 3 gene, affects the hair, bone, teeth, nails and skin. It may be apparent at birth as kinky curly hair which are present in all affected newborns. Besides kinky curly hair, enamel hypoplasia, hypocalcification, splitting of nail plate, osteosclerosis of base of the skull, mastoid, long bones and premature closure of fibrous bones may be present.

WNT-Beta-Catenin Pathway Associated Ectodermal Dysplasia (Table 23.3)

Table 23.3: WNT-Beta-catenin pathway associated ectodermal dysplasia
WNT 10A gene
• Odonto-onycho-dermal dysplasia (OODD)
• Schopf-Schulz-Passarge syndrome (SSPS)
HR gene (human hairless gene)
• Atrichia with papular lesions
• Alopecia universalis congenita
APCCDD1 gene
• Hereditary hypotrichosis complex

Schopf-Schulz-Passarge syndrome (SSPS)

It is due to mutations in the WNT10A gene on chromosome 2 transmitted by autosomal recessive mode. Cutaneous features do not appear in childhood, which start appearing in the early teenage and become more obvious with age. Multiple eyelid cysts (apocrine hidrocystomas) are seen which is a cardinal feature, but often does not appear until middle age. Other cutaneous features are eccrine tumors (poroma and syringocystadenoma), palmoplantar keratoderma, hypotrichosis, onychodystrophy (nail fragility or hypoplastic nails). Non cutaneous features include abnormal development of the teeth (hypodontia, – abnormal deciduous teeth), bilateral early senile cataract, optic atrophy and myopia.

Odonto-Onycho-Dermal Dysplasia (OODD)

It presents with severe oligodontia, absent or dystrophic nail, palmoplantar keratoderma. Other clinical manifestations include smooth tongue, malar telangiectatic atrophic plaque and keratosis pilaris.

Connexin/ Gap Junctions

Clouston syndrome

This autosomal dominant hidrotic ectodermal dysplasia is caused by mutations in the gap junction β-6 (GJB6) gene encoding connexin 30, which is a potential target of p63. It presents with small dystrophic nails, hypotrichosis, papillomatous or warty fissured transgradient keratoderma, but the presentation may resemble pachyonychia congenita, oral leukokeratosis. This autosomal dominant ectodermal dysplasia is caused by mutations in the gap junction β-6 (GJB6) gene encoding connexin 30, which is a potential target of p63.

Focal dermal hypoplasia/ Goltz syndrome (FDH)

Goltz syndrome synonymously known as focal dermal hypoplasia (FDH), is an extremely rare genetic disorder characterized by distinctive skin manifestations like linear hypoplastic streaks following Blaschke lines or fat herniation, telangiectasia, pyogenic granuloma like lesions, warty papilloma of mucus membrane, overgrowth of palmoplantar skin, alopecia, hyperhidrosis and a wide range of abnormalities affecting the eyes, teeth, skeletal, urinary, gastrointestinal, cardiovascular and central nervous system. The disease is inherited as a X-linked dominant condition due to PORCN gene mutation.

GENE THERAPY IN SKIN

Gene therapy is a promising approach for prevention and cure of rare genodermatoses. It has been an unexplored arena in the past but recent developments and research in this field have given way to future prospects. Major obstacles in its development are: hindered absorption of macromolecules due to skin barrier; and relatively small number of affected cells in genetic disorders of skin.

Gene therapy in skin can be defined as introduction of nucleic acid into the skin cells using a vector, with the aim of altering its gene expression to ultimately prevent or stop a pathological disease process.

There are two primary approaches for gene transfer:

1. In vivo gene therapy, where genetic material is transferred directly into the patient's skin using a vector.

2. Ex vivo gene therapy, where cells collected from the patient are cultured, genetically modified, and then re-administered to the patient.
3. An effective gene therapy requires a genodermatosis with a well identified gene, a therapeutic gene and a gene delivery system with a viral or non-viral vector.

Vectors in Gene Therapy

1. **Viral vectors:** Oncoviral and lentiviral retroviruses, adenoviruses and adeno-like viruses are the commonly used vectors. These viral vectors can effectively alter the skin cells because of their innate ability to transfect them. Retroviruses are most frequently used. They convert their genetic material from RNA to DNA using reverse transcriptase and then integrate with host DNA using integrase. They are also effective in ex vivo techniques by producing altered therapeutic response in cultured keratinocytes for multiple epidermal turnover cycles. Other virus vectors for gene delivery are under research.
2. **Non-viral vectors:** They are cost effective, safe, non-toxic and nonimmunogenic as compared to viral vectors, but the duration of desired gene expression is short. Non-viral vectors include: Plasmid DNA, microRNA, and more recently developed genetically engineered nucleases which break and repair the desired loci on gene. There are several methods to induce this break in genetic material:
    - Zinc finger nucleases, clustered regularly interspaced short palindromic repeats (CRISPR) or transcriptor activator like effector nucleases (TALEN).
    - Other methods of mechanical gene delivery like ultrasound mediated gene transfer and magneto or electroporation are being used.
    - Lipid based nanoparticles and polymer nanoparticles have also been developed as vectors.

Currently, gene therapy is being used to target severe genodermatoses like epidermolysis bullosa, ichthyosis, melanoma, pachyonychia congenita, xeroderma pigmentosum and for transient effect in wound healing.

CHAPTER 24

Disorders of Keratinization

Contents

ICHTHYOSIS

Introduction

The term *ichthys* means fish and *ichthyoses* means fish-like scales. It comprises a large group of scaling disorders with diverse etiology. To date, more than 25 genes have been identified that encode a wide spectrum of epidermal proteins, including enzymes of lipid metabolism and of peptide cross-linking, proteases and their inhibitors, epidermal structural proteins, and proteins involved in cellular communication, signaling and gene transcription. Abnormalities in any of these components result in a rather stereotypic epidermal response with epidermal hyperplasia and the formation of excess stratum corneum accompanied by abnormal (delayed and/or disordered) desquamation, with visible accumulation of squames (scales) on the skin's surface – the clinical hallmark of all the ichthyoses. In certain instances, there is at least transiently increased skin fragility or blistering, as in Netherton syndrome and epidermolytic hyperkeratosis (EHK). The term isolated ichthyosis refers to ichthyoses which are not part of a disease syndrome. Isolated ichthyosis are clinically distinguished in two subclasses: ichthyoses with an age of onset after birth (IV and XLRI) and rare ichthyoses presenting at birth (congenital ichthyoses).

The Ichthyosis group of disorders are classified on the basis of clinical picture and distinguishes inherited ichthyosis into syndromic and non-syndromic forms (Table 24.1.

Ichthyosis Vulgaris (IV)

Ichthyosis vulgaris represents the least severe and most common type of ichthyosis. It is transmitted as an autosomal semidominant trait with variable penetrance. Genetic

Table 24.1: Classification of non-syndromic ichthyosis			
	Disease	***Mode of inheritance***	***Gene/Locus***
Common ichthyoses (often delayed onset)	Ichthyosis vulgaris X-linked recessive ichthyosis (XLRI)	Autosomal semidominant X-linked recessive	FGL 1q21-22 STS Xp22.3
Autosomal recessive congenital ichthyoses	• Harlequin ichthyosis • Lamellar ichthyosis • Non-bullous congenital ichthyosiform erythroderma	AR AR AR	ABCA12 TGM1, NIPAL4 TGM1 14 q11 ABCA12 2q34 ALOX12B, ALOXE3
Keratinopathic icthyosis	**Major types:** • Bullous ichthyosiform erythroderma/ Epidermolytic hyperkeratosis (BIE/EI) • Superficial epidermolytic ichthyosis (SEI) **Minor variants:** AEI, ICM, AREI	Autosomal dominant Autosomal dominant	KRT1 17q21-q22 KRT10 12q13 KRT2

AEI: Annular type of Epidermolytic Icthyosis; ICM: Icthyosis Hystrix Curth-Macklin;
AREI: Autosomal Recessive Epidermolytic Icthyosis

variations in the gene encoding for filaggrin (FLG), located in the epidermal differentiation complex (EDC) on chromosome 1q21 have recently been proposed to cause ichthyosis vulgaris.

IV manifests usually 3-6 months after birth, usually in childhood and becomes more severe with age. Its prevalence appears to vary with geographical region but is roughly 1 in 250. Individuals with ichthyosis vulgaris commonly display rather mild generalized fine scaling with a "pasted on" appearance and are larger and more prominent on the lower extremities (Figure 24.1). The extensor surfaces of the extremities are usually most affected and flexural areas such as axillae, groins are spared. Involvement of palms and soles (hyperlinearity) is common as is the association with keratosis pilaris and atopic dermatitis.

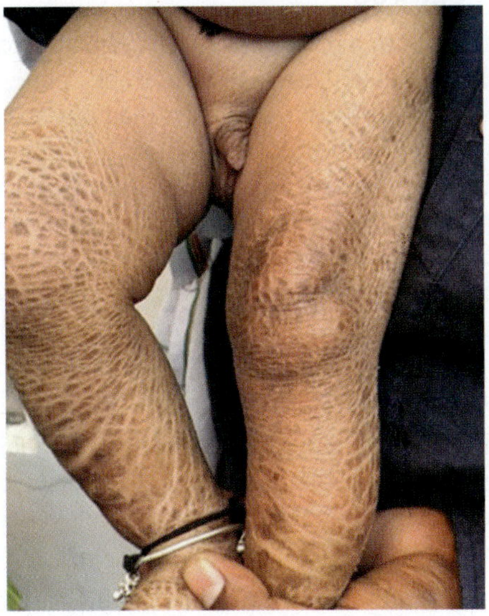

Figure 24.1: Ichthyosis vulgaris

It is difficult clinically to differentiate between mild ichthyosis vulgaris and the xerosis that accompanies atopic dermatitis, which is not surprising in view of the common mutations found in these disorders.

Treatment involves explaining the nature and course of the skin condition to the patients. Soap is best avoided. Application of emollients such as vegetable oils, liquid paraffin, or Vaseline will prevent further scaling and dryness. 10-15% urea in a cream or ointment is effective along with other topical agents like propylene glycol and ammonium lactate lotions.

Systemic treatment with acitretin or isotretinoin is an option in severe conditions.

X-Linked Recessive Ichthyosis (XLRI)

It is an inherited disorder of keratinization due to steroid sulfatase enzyme (STS) deficiency, affects approximately 1 in 6000 boys and men. Females are carriers.

The gene encoding STS is located in the distal portion of the short arm of the X chromosome. STS enzyme is responsible for hydrolysis of cholesterol sulfate to cholesterol in the epidermis. Accumulation of the cholesterol sulfate in the epidermis leads to skin barrier instability.

Patients present during the first few weeks of life with generalized desquamation of large, loosely adherent, translucent scales. This phase is followed by the appearance of tightly adherent, dark brown, polygonal scales that are distributed symmetrically on the preauricular areas of the cheeks, neck, lateral areas of the trunk, and extremities, with relative sparing of flexural surfaces (Figure 24.2). Extracutaneous manifestations of XLRI include corneal opacities that do not affect vision (found in 25-50% of adult patients), cryptorchidism (10-20%

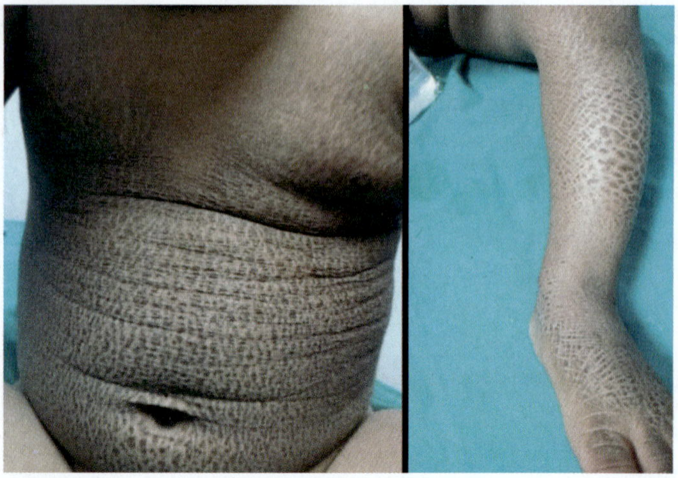

Figure 24.2: X- linked ichthyosis showing dark brown polygonal tightly adherent scales

of patients), and an increased risk of testicular cancer, which is independent of testicular maldescent.

Pathogenesis

The STS enzyme is responsible for hydrolysis of cholesterol sulfate (CS; a serine protease inhibitor) to cholesterol in the epidermis. In patients with XLRI, accumulation of CS in the epidermis leads to barrier instability and inhibits the desmosomal degradation, which is required for normal desquamation, thereby leading to corneocyte retention. Detection of increased serum levels of CS can confirm the diagnosis of XLI.

The gene encoding STS is mapped to the distal portion of the short arm of the X chromosome (Xp22.3). This region escapes lyonization (random inactivation of one of the two X chromosomes), which explains the absence of skin lesions in female carriers of XLI. In addition, this portion of the X chromosome is particularly susceptible to deletions. More than 90 percent of patients with XLI have complete deletion of the STS gene and flanking sequences, which represents one of the highest incidences of chromosomal deletions among all genetic disorders. Deletions that extend to neighboring genes can result in contiguous gene syndromes of XLI in association with Kallmann syndrome (hypogonadotropic hypogonadism and anosmia), ocular albinism type 1, X-linked recessive chondrodysplasia punctata, short stature, and mental retardation.

Application of emollients such as vegetable oils, liquid paraffin, or Vaseline will prevent further scaling and dryness. 10-15% urea in a cream or ointment is effective along with other topical agents like 40-60% propylene glycol and ammonium lactate lotions.

Systemic treatment with acitretin or isotretinoin may be considered.

Harlequin Ichthyosis (HI)

It is the most severe form of keratinizing disorders, usually lethal in the neonatal period. It is believed to be inherited in an autosomal recessive manner. "Harlequin" refers to the resemblance of the facial features and diamond-shaped scales in affected neonates to the costume of the comic servant character named Harlequin.

Pathogenesis

Mutations in lipid transporter encoding gene ABCA12 cause HI. In the granular layers of healthy skin, the ABCA12 coded lipid transporter transfers lipids from the cytosol into lamellar granules where lipid-processing enzymes, proteases, and protease inhibitors are also concentrated. At the granular layer–stratum corneum interface, the lamellar granules fuse with the cell membrane and discharge their content into the intercellular lamellae. Complex enzymatic reactions lead to modifications of the lipid composition of the intercellular space (cholesterol, ceramides, free fatty acids) that provide a very effective water permeability barrier. Corneocytes detach from each other in the superficial layers of the stratum corneum as a result of finely regulated proteolytic cleavage of corneodesmosomes.

However, in the skin of HI patients, the absence of ABCA12 prevents the transfer of lipids into lamellar granules, which themselves are abnormally shaped, reduced in number, or absent. As a result, exocytosis of lamellar granule content is reduced and intercellular lipid lamellae are absent. Abnormal lipid containing vacuoles form in the cytoplasm of the corneocytes. The stratum corneum is remarkably thickened and does not desquamate. This defect in the lamellar granules results in thickening of the stratum corneum and the accumulation of armor like scales in HI (Figure 24.3).

Clinical Features

There is still birth or a preterm delivery. The affected newborn is encased in dense "armor" like thick plates of scales measuring up to 4 or 5 cm that covers the body like the suit of a harlequin clown with deep red fissuring (Figure 24.4). The skin is pulled tight to such an extent that the face loses its normal appearance and appears frog like, with eversion of the eyelids (ectropion) and lips (eclabion) and flattening of the ears and nose. Eyelashes and eyebrows are usually absent. The extremities are swollen due to constriction by massive thickening of the skin. Due to massive constricting skin bands, autoamputation occurs.

Complications include sepsis, electrolyte imbalances, heat intolerance, ocular problems related to persistent ectropion, chronic constipation, joint contractures, delayed growth and development.

Death is usually from respiratory failure, infections, and/or dehydration related complications.

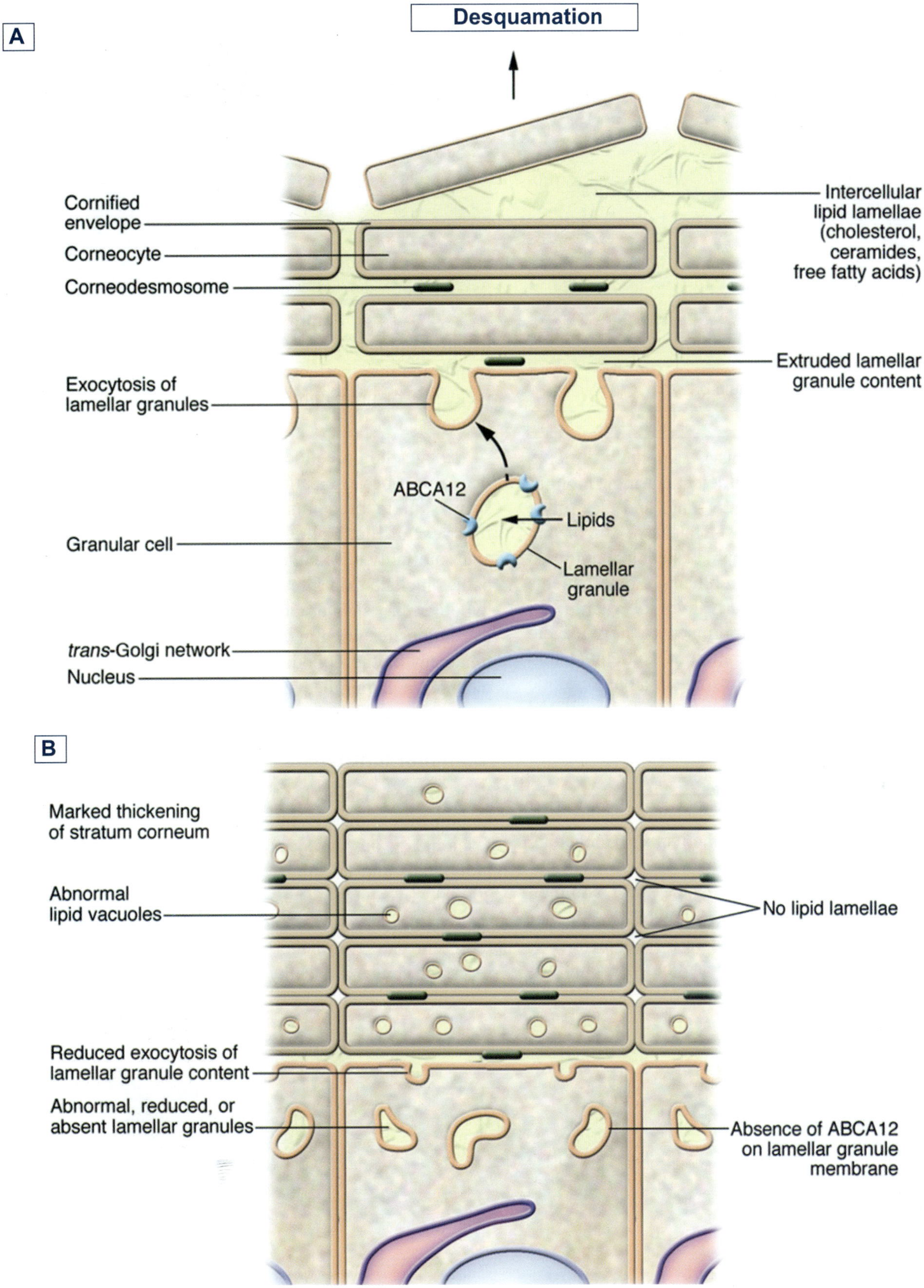

Figure 24.3: (A) Normal formation of cornified envelope (B) Pathogenesis of Harlequin ichthyosis

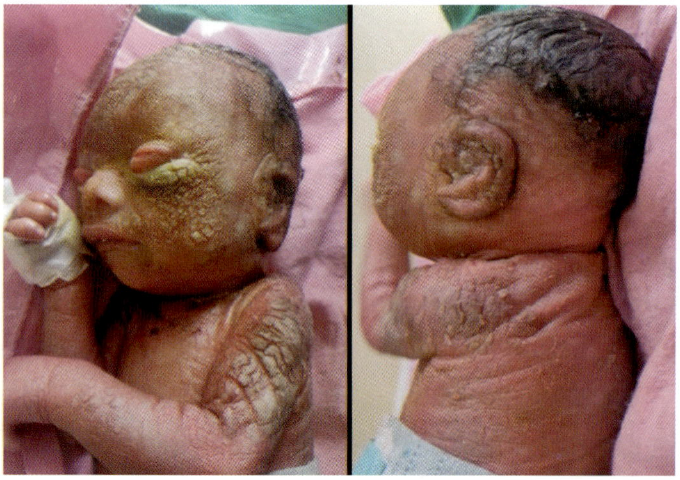

Figure 24.4: Harlequin baby

Management

The management of live born infants is extremely difficult. Intensive care is needed to provide sufficient nutrition, monitor and manage body temperature, correct fluid and electrolyte imbalances, and prevent and treat sepsis. Intensive care of skin and eyes is very essential. Infants should be kept in humidified incubators and treated with bland emollients. Some patients treated with retinoids (synthetic derivatives of vitamin A) have survived and subsequently continued to have severe ichthyosis. However, early administration of Acitretin (1 mg/kg/day) has been shown to result in shedding of large, keratotic plates within weeks as well as improvement in ectropion and eclabium.

Collodion Baby

It is a common presentation of several congenital ichthyoses, mostly with autosomal recessive inheritance. Congenital ichthyosiform erythroderma, previously known as non-bullous ichthyosiform erythroderma, is the most common condition resulting in collodion baby, followed by lamellar ichthyosis. The entire body is encased in a parchment like, shiny, taut membrane (Figure 24.5). The collodion membrane

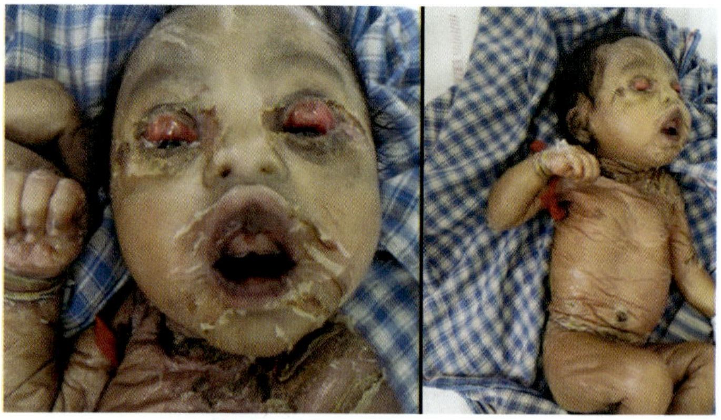

Figure 24.5: Collodion baby

usually completely peels off in 2 weeks; however, a prolonged membrane may not completely peel off until 12 weeks. The incidence of premature birth is more common among these neonates.

Diagnosing a collodion baby can sometimes take longer than a year because patients may change from predominantly scaly skin to predominantly erythematous skin during the first year of life. Collodion babies have increased morbidity and mortality. Documented complications for collodion babies include skin infections, fissures, conjunctivitis, sepsis, hypothermia, dehydration, and constrictive bands of the extremities resulting in vascular compromise and edema. The treatment of the collodion baby during the neonatal period includes a humidified incubator, hydrophilic ointment, and supportive care.

Lamellar Ichthyosis (LI)

It is a genetically heterogeneous group of disorders of keratinization that is inherited in an autosomal recessive fashion. LI has an equal incidence in male and female individuals and is estimated to occur in approximately 1 in 300,000 live births. The large, dark, plate like quadrilateral scales (Figure 24.6 A and B) that characterize classic LI represent one end of the phenotypic spectrum of autosomal recessive congenital ichthyosis.

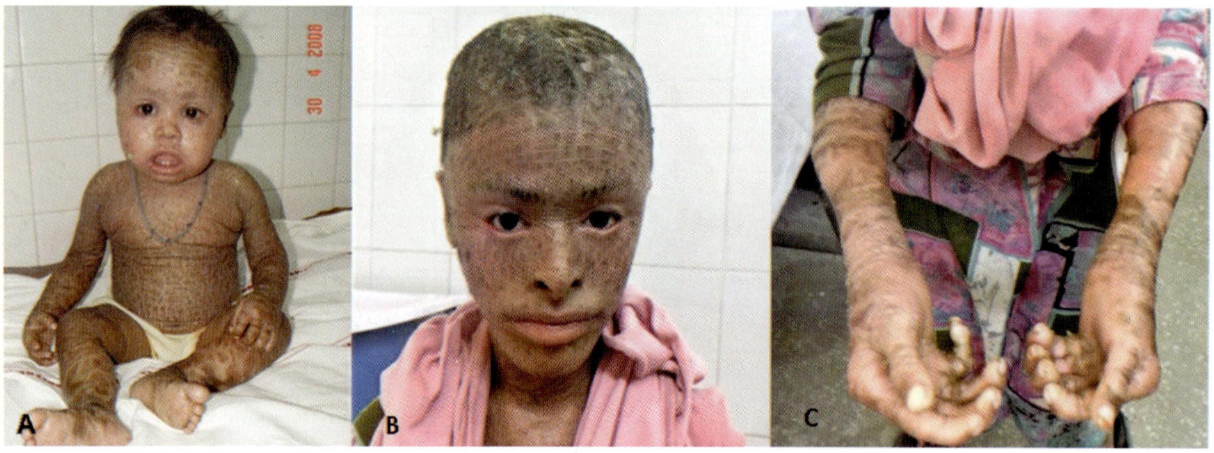

Figure 24.6: Lamellar ichthyosis (A, B & C)

The erythroderma and fine, white scales, which typify non-bullous congenital ichthyosiform erythroderma (NBCIE, Figures 24.7 and 24.8), lie at the opposite end of this spectrum, and various intermediate phenotypes have been observed.

Patients with LI are typically born encased in a translucent collodion membrane, which is replaced over the first month of life with generalized scale that is accentuated in flexural areas as well as on the forehead and lower extremities. Sometimes, there is maceration of the thick scales, leading to malodor. Eclabium, ectropion, and scarring alopecia at the periphery of the scalp are often observed as sequel of excessively taut skin, and heat intolerance frequently occurs due to obstruction of the sweat ducts by plates of scale. Patients may also develop palmoplantar keratoderma, pseudo ainhum (Figure 24.6 C) and nail dystrophy. Lamellar ichthyosis is more prone to develop nutritional or Vit D deficiency rickets (Figure 24.9).

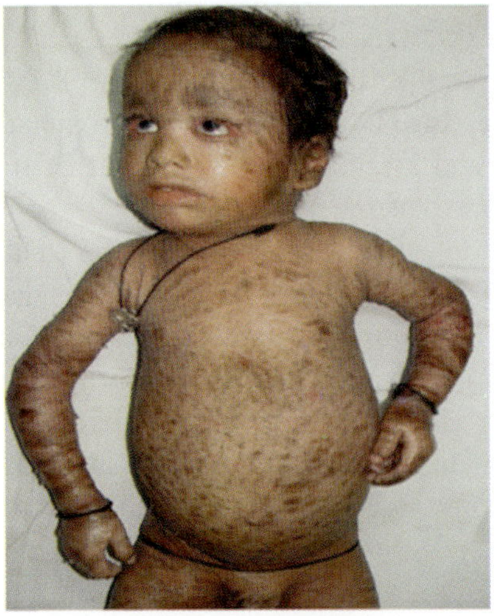

Figure 24.9: Lamellar ichthyosis with rickets

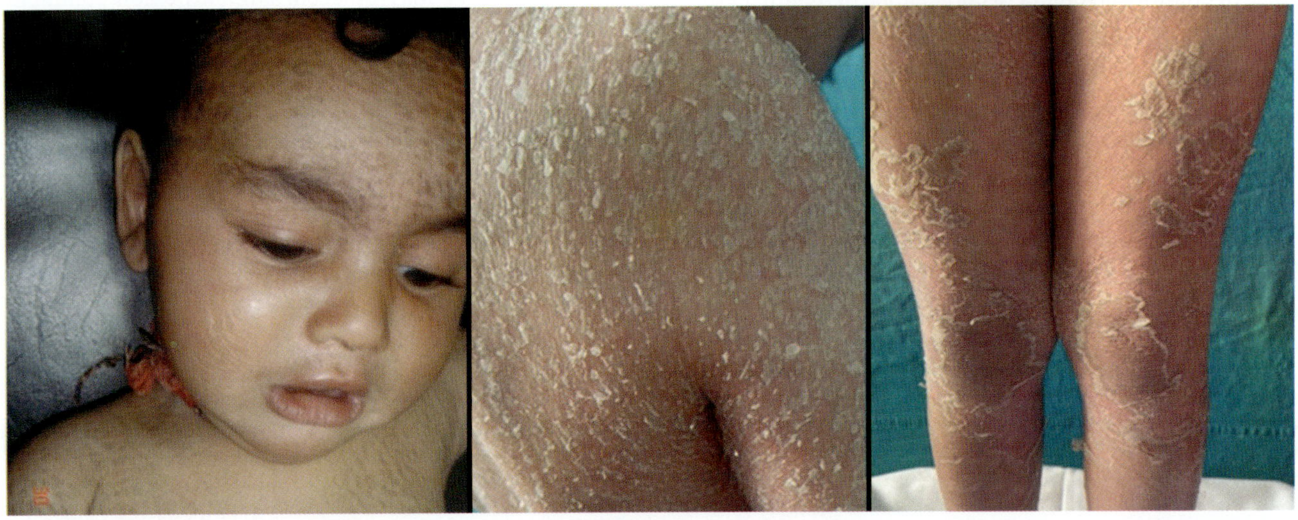

Figure 24.7: Non bullous congenital ichthyosiform erythroderma

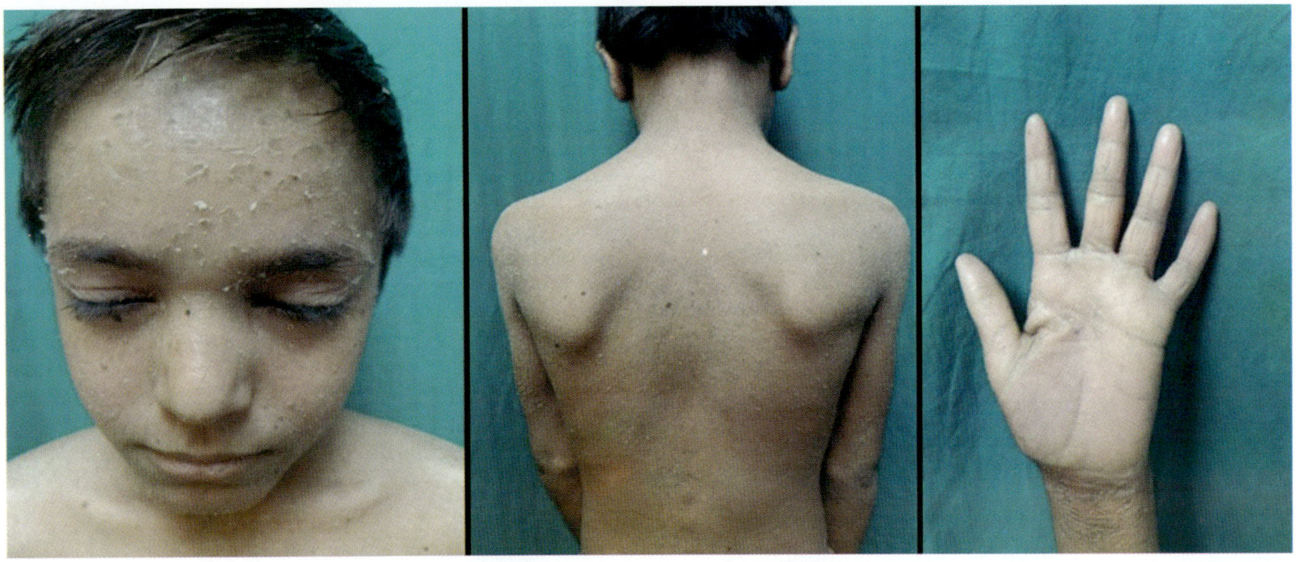

Figure 24.8: Non bullous congenital ichthyosiform erythroderma

Pathogenesis

Mutations in the transglutaminase-1 (TGM1) gene on chromosome 14q11 account for approximately half the cases of LI and a minority of cases of NBCIE. The TGM1 mutations are heterogeneous (including point mutations, deletions, truncations, and splice-site mutations), and consistent genotype-phenotype correlations have not been observed. A lack of transglutaminase 1 activity impairs cross-linking of proteins and lipids in the cornified cell envelope of the upper epidermis and leads to defective cornification and desquamation. Recently mutations in the ABCA12 gene on chromosome 2q35 has been found to account for a LI phenotype.

Management

The use of emollients remains a cornerstone of treatment for LI. The use of keratolytics in children with LI is limited due to skin irritation and the risk of systemic absorption. Lactic acid 5% and propylene glycol 20% in a lipophilic base have been shown to be particularly effective in reducing scale. Topical retinoids and vitamin D3 derivatives may also be helpful, and topical application of the antioxidant N-acetylcysteine was reported to result in marked improvement. Oral retinoids are particularly effective in reducing the amount of scales in LI patients, but this alteration may expose underlying erythroderma. Patients should be counseled to avoid overheating and those with ectropion should receive ophthalmologic care.

CONGENITAL ICTHYOSIFORM ERYTHRODERMA (CIE) OR NON-BULLOUS CONGENITAL ICTHYOSIFORM ERYTHRODERMA (NBIE)

CIE is a rare AR ichthyosis. Till date, mutations in at least 5 genes have been shown to cause CIE: ALOX12B, ALOXE3, TGM1, ABCA12 and NIPAL 4.

Clinical Features

Also known as non-bullous congenital ichthyosiform erythroderma (NBCIE). CIE usually presents at birth with a collodion membrane. After shedding of the membrane, erythroderma becomes evident and it persists. The scales are thin, superficial and "powdery" (Figures 24.7 and 24.8). The palms and soles show diffuse, fissuring keratoderma. Nail dystrophy may be seen. Digital flexion contractures are commonly seen. Pityriasis amiantacea on the scalp, ectropion with resultant exposure keratitis are also not uncommon. Hypohidrosis due to sweat gland duct obstruction by hyperkeratotic horny layer is common.

Management

Topical treatment consists of application of emollients after hydration of skin. Keratolytics and retinoids are avoided. Oral retinoids are often effective.

Various differentiating features for commonly seen ichthyotic conditions have been shown in Table 24.2.

Table 24.2: Showing differentiating features of common ichthyotic conditions

Features	Ichthyosis vulgaris	X-linked recessive ichthyosis	Lamellar ichthyosis	Congenital ichthyosiform erythroderma (CIE)
Inheritance	AD	XLR, affects only males	AR	AR
Genes	Filaggrin	STS	TGM/ABCA12	ALOX12B/ALOXE3
Severity	Mild	Moderate	Severe	Severe
Age of onset	Infancy/childhood (in between 3-12 months of age)	Infancy (before 3 months of age)	Birth (collodion membrane)	Birth
Cutaneous features	Fine, adherent scales all over body sparing flexures and face. Hyperlinearity of palms and soles. Back is more affected than abdomen.	Large, coarser and darker adherent scales all over the body except palms and soles. Abdomen is more affected than back	Black to brown quadrangular, thick generalized plate-like scales	Fine, white scales, erythroderma
Associated features	Keratosis pilaris, Atopic dermatitis	Corneal opacities, cryptorchidism, history of prolonged labor	Heat intolerance, scarring alopecia, ectropion, eclabium	Heat intolerance, scarring alopecia, ectropion, eclabium
Treatment	Emollients	Emollients	Retinoids	Retinoids
Prognosis	Good	Good	Severe	Moderate to severe disability

Epidermolytic Hyperkeratosis (EHK) Or Bullous Icthyosis Erythroderma (BIE)

Due to the blistering phenotype of the newborn, EHK was previously termed bullous congenital ichthyosiform erythroderma (BCIE) to distinguish it from the autosomal recessive, non-bullous group. EHK is caused by mutations in the epidermal keratin 1 or keratin 10 genes. A characteristic feature in many EHK patients is a phenotypic shift from widespread blistering at birth to prominent hyperkeratosis during later life. Erythroderma is prominent in some patients but absent in others. The hyperkeratosis in EHK often is generalized, and it may either involve or spare the palms and soles. Depending on the presence or absence of PPK, six phenotypes of EI have been identified (PS1,2,3 and NPS-1,2,3).

In the generalized variants, typically, involvement of flexural and extensor surfaces of large joints (elbows, knees) is accentuated, sometimes with massive hyperkeratosis, giving a peculiar, ridged appearance (Figures 24.10 and 24.11). Flexural scales often become secondarily colonized by bacteria, producing a foul odor. Variants with particularly widespread and thick, porcupine like (hystrix) hyperkeratosis (but lack of an early blistering phase) have been termed ichthyosis hystrix of Curth and Macklin. A milder variant of EHK, ichthyosis bullosa of Siemens (IBS), is characterized by peeling as well as annular, hyperkeratotic plaques preferentially over joints, shins and the periumbilical region. There are also localized forms, which are more limited to acral and flexural surfaces plus the palms/soles, or distributed in a linear pattern along the lines of Blaschko; i.e., as epidermal nevi. Epidermolytic hyperkeratosis strictly limited to palms and soles has been termed Vörner's palmoplantar keratoderma (PPK).

Mutations in keratin 1 (chromosome 12q13) and keratin 10 (chromosome 17q21-q22) have been identified as the cause of the classic generalized form of EHK. Localized forms are due to chromosomal mosaicism.

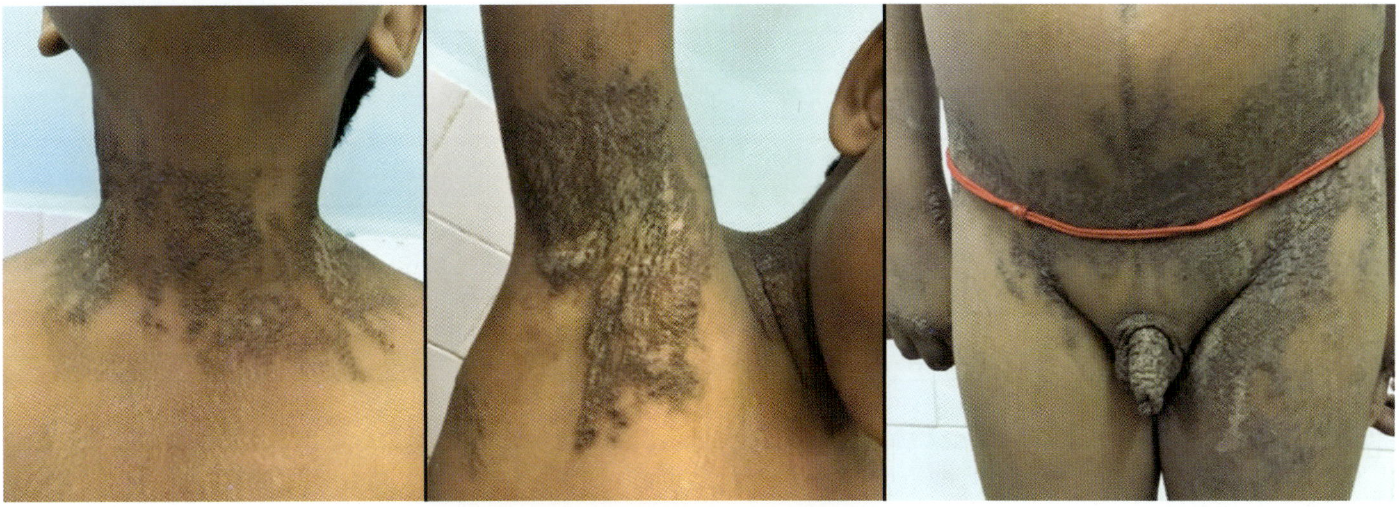

Figure 24.10: Epidermolytic hyperkeratosis

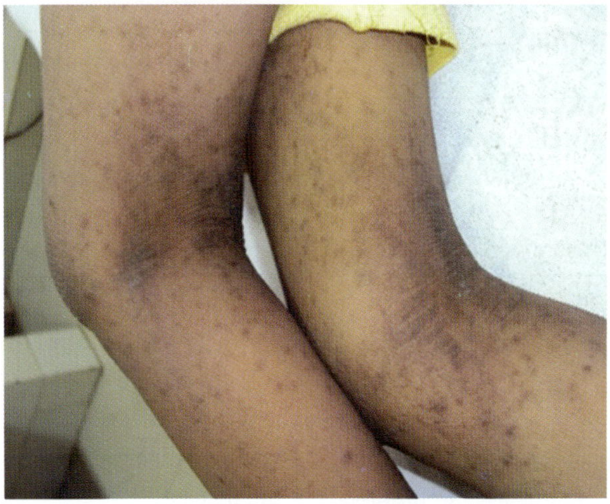

Figure 24.11: Epidermolytic hyperkeratosis

ICHTHYOTIC SYNDROMES

Various types of syndromic ichthyosis have been shown in Table 24.3.

Table 24.3: Syndromic ichthyosis

	Disease	Mode of inheritance	Gene
X-linked ichthyosis syndrome	Recessive X-linked ichthyosis	XLR	STS
	Conradi-Hunerman Happle Syndrome	XLD	EBP
	Ichthyosis Follicularis Alopecia Photophobia (IFAP)	XLR	MBTPS2
	CHILD syndrome	XLD	NSDHL
Associated with prominent hair abnormalities	Netherton syndrome	AR	SPINK5
	Ichthyosis with hypotrichosis	AR	ST14
	Neonatal ichthyosis-Sclerosing cholangitis	AR	CLDN1
	Severe dermatitis multiple allergies metabolic wasting	AR	DSG1
Prominent neurological deficit	Refsum syndrome	AR	PHYH, PEX7
	Chanarin dwarfman syndrome (Neutral lipid storage disease	AR	ABHD5
	Multiple sulphatase deficiency	AR	SUMF1
	Sjögren-Larsson syndrome	AR	ALDH3 A2
	Gaucher syndrome type 2	AR	GBA
	Trichothiodystrophy	AR	ERCC2, ERCC3, C7ORF11
	(ARC)-Arthrogryposis-Renal dysfunction-Cholestasis	AR	VPS33B
	(CEDNIK)-Cerebral dysgenesis-Neuropathy-Ichthyosis-Keratoderma	AR	SNAP29
Deafness	Keratitis ichthyosis deafness	AD	GJB2
	(MEDNIK)-Mental retardation-Enteropathy-Deafness-Neuropathy-Ichthyosis, Keratoderma	AR	AP1S1
Transient neonatal respiratory distress	Ichthyosis prematurity syndrome	AR	SLC27A4

Here we are describing some of the commonly seen ichthyotic syndromes.

NETHERTON SYNDROME (Syn: Ichthyosis Linearis Circumflexa, Comèl-Netherton Syndrome)

Netherton syndrome is a triad of Ichthyosis linearis circumflexa (ILC), atopic diathesis and trichorrhexis invaginata. It is caused by autosomal recessive mutations in the SPINK5 gene, coding for the serine protease inhibitor lymphoepithelial-Kazal- type 5 inhibitor (LEKTI), and presumably resulting in unopposed serine protease activity.

Patients display generalized scaling with marked inflammatory features, often with similarities to atopic dermatitis. At or shortly after birth, infants commonly present with generalized erythroderma. In older children and adults, a unique scaling pattern, termed ichthyosis linearis circumflexa, may develop in which serpiginous areas of double edged scale are present. The plaques are usually distributed on the trunk and extremities. These lesions are pruritic and many patients develop eczematization or lichenification. Patients with Netherton syndrome are at risk for excessive systemic absorption of topical medications as a result of a severe barrier abnormality. The skin changes are typically accompanied by pathognomonic hair shaft defects, called bamboo hair or trichorrhexis invaginata, in which the distal hair segment is telescoped into the proximal part. Only 20–50% of hair may be affected, and this feature may be absent in some patients.

Another feature of NS, is immune imbalance. serum IgE levels are markedly elevated. Eosinophilia and allergic reactions to various foods like nuts, eggs and fish are common. Atopy with anaphylactic reactions to food is another feature of the disease.

Keratitis-Ichthyosis-Deafness (Kid) Syndrome

It is a rare ectodermal disorder characterized by clinical triad of progressive vascularizing keratitis, sensorineural hearing impairment, and erythrokeratoderma/ichthyosis. First described by Burns in 1915, and the KID acronym was coined by Skinner and colleagues in 1981.

Affected individuals may present at birth with a transient erythroderma. Later in infancy and during childhood, most patients develop well demarcated, keratotic plaques with an erythematous base and a stippled, verrucous, or ridged surface. These plaques favor the extremities, scalp, ears and face; perioral plaques with radial furrows are a common finding. Diffusely thickened skin with a rough or ridged appearance, deep facial grooves, and follicular keratoses may occur. Palmoplantar keratoderma, which is usually diffuse with a grainy or reticulated texture, is almost invariably present. Angular cheilitis frequently develops, and chronically fissured lips and gingival hyperemia have been described. Sparse hair, hypohidrosis, dystrophic nails, and abnormal dentition represent additional features. Patients with KID syndrome are predisposed to mucocutaneous infections with bacteria, fungi (especially Candida spp.) and viruses. Ocular findings, which may develop by early childhood or have a delayed onset, are progressive and include vascularizing keratitis, dry eyes, blepharitis and conjunctivitis. Non-progressive, congenital, sensorineural hearing loss is consistently present with variable degrees of compromise.

Pathogenesis

KID syndrome is an autosomal dominant condition caused by mutations in the GJB2 gene, which encodes connexin 26. Connexin 26 is a gap junction protein that is expressed in ectoderm-derived epithelia of the inner ear and cornea as well as in the epidermis and its appendages, which explains the constellation of findings in KID syndrome.

Management

Multidisciplinary is required care by dermatology, ophthalmology, and otolaryngology services. Topical retinoids and keratolytics have limited benefits. There are several reports of substantial improvement in hyperkeratosis with acitretin therapy. Oral antibiotics and antifungal medications are necessary when infections develop, and prolonged courses are occasionally required. Close monitoring of the skin and oral mucosa for the development of malignancy is essential. Lubricating and anti-inflammatory agents have variable success in managing ocular disease, and cochlear implants have restored hearing in several affected individuals.

Child Syndrome

The CHILD syndrome is a congenital disorder characterized by congenital hemidysplasia, ichthyosiform erythroderma, and limb defects. The hallmark of the disorder is the sharp midline demarcation and its largely unilateral cutaneous and skeletal features. It is an X-linked dominant condition which occurs almost exclusively in girls and is lethal in affected males.

The inflammatory ichthyosiform skin lesions of CHILD syndrome may be present at birth or develop during the first few months of life. They are characterized by yellow and waxy scaling and/or streaks of inflammation and scaling that is often patchy but follow Blaschko lines. Unilateral alopecia and severe nail dystrophy with claw like nails have also been described. The face is typically spared. With increasing age, lesions may improve or even clear spontaneously, but lesions in intertriginous areas tend to persist and be the most severely affected sites. Rarely, a localized hyperkeratotic plaque with a sharp demarcation at the midline is the sole manifestation of the CHILD syndrome (CHILD nevus).

Ipsilateral skeletal hypoplasia, ranging in severity from hypoplasia of the fingers to complete agenesis of extremity, is an important feature of CHILD syndrome.

Punctate epiphyseal calcifications may be demonstrable by radiography but tend to disappear after the first few years of life. Cardiovascular and renal abnormalities are the major visceral manifestations of CHILD syndrome.

Refsum Disease

Refsum disease is an autosomal recessive neurocutaneous disorder caused by deficiency in oxidation of phytanic acid, a branched, long chain fatty acid. It results from mutations in one of two genes, either PHYH which encodes the peroxisomal enzyme phytanoyl-CoA hydroxylase, or PEX7, which encodes the PTS2, resulting in disturbance in cholesterol and lipid metabolism. The clinical features are due to accumulation of phytanic acid and usually develop in late childhood or early adult life and progress slowly during months to several years. Neurologic manifestations are most prominent and include sensorineural deafness, anosmia, failing vision, night blindness owing to retinitis pigmentosa and a progressive weakness, foot drop, and loss of balance caused by a mixed sensorimotor neuropathy and cerebellar involvement. Delayed diagnosis may result in severe neurologic impairment, wasting and depression. The associated ichthyosis, resembles ichthyosis vulgaris or in severe untreated cases, lamellar icthyosis.

Sjögren-Larsson Syndrome

It is an autosomal recessive disorder. It results from mutations in the fatty aldehyde dehydrogenase gene (FALDH or

ALDH3A2), a component of fatty alcohol, fatty alcohol oxidoreductase (FAO),which converts fatty alcohol to fatty acid. The defective lipid metabolism results in abnormal lamellar bodies and lipid droplets in epidermal cells of affected individuals.

The ichthyosis of the Sjögren-Larsson syndrome (SLS), usually manifests in the neonatal period as fine, white scaling, accentuated in flexural areas. Erythema is occasionally present at birth but clears within months. Presentation as a collodion baby is rare. By 1 year of age, the affected baby shows generalized velvety lamellar thickening on the trunk and neck with minimal desquamation. The skin is characteristically pruritic.

The neurologic disease usually presents within the first year with failure to reach normal developmental milestones and the onset of spasticity.

Prenatal diagnosis of SLS is possible by measurement of FAO activity in cultured amniotic or chorionic cells, histologic analysis, and/or analysis of fetal deoxyribonucleic acid (DNA) if the gene defect is known.

Few other ichthyosis syndromes are:

- CHIME syndrome (coloboma, heart defects, ichthyosiform dermatosis, mental retardation, and ear anomalies).
- Neu–Laxova syndrome (congenital ichthyosis, marked intrauterine growth retardation, microcephaly, short neck, central nervous system anomalies, limb deformities, hypoplastic lungs, oedema and abnormal facial features including severe proptosis with ectropion, hypertelorism, micrognathia, flattened nose and malformed ears).
- CEDNIK (Cerebral dysgenesis, enteropathy, neuropathy, ichthyosis and keratoderma) and MEDNIK (mental retardation, enteropathy, deafness, neuropathy, ichthyosis, keratoderma) syndrome.
- Conradi–Hünermann–Happle syndrome (mosaic presentation of linear ichthyosis, chondrodysplasia punctata, asymmetrically shortened limbs, unilateral, sometimes sectorial cataracts and short stature).

ACQUIRED ICHTHYOSIS

Acquired ichthyosis or secondary ichthyosis is clinically indistinguishable from hereditary ichthyosis. However, acquired ichthyosis is associated with various systemic diseases.

The appearance of ichthyosis in child can occur before or after the diagnosis of a systemic condition. Acquired ichthyosis is associated with many systemic diseases, e.g., lymphoma, sarcoidosis, leprosy, thyroid diseases (Figure 24.12), hyperparathyroidism, nutritional disorders, bone marrow transplantation, HIV infection, autoimmune diseases, including systemic lupus erythematosus and dermatomyositis. Ichthyosis may occur with chronic metabolic disorders such as malnutrition, malabsorption (including Coeliac disease and Crohn's disease, essential fatty deficiency, and pancreatic insufficiency. **Ichthyosis** may be a presenting feature of inborn errors of metabolism, such as methylmalonic acidaemia, holocarboxylase and biotinidase deficiencies.

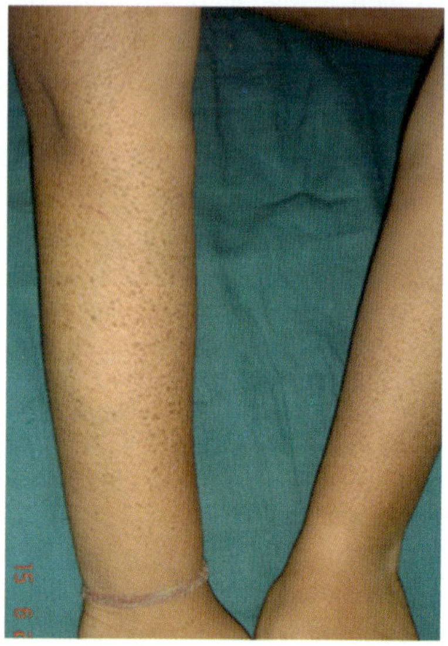

Figure 24.12: Secondary ichthyosis in a patient with hypothyroidism

The use of certain medications has been linked to acquired ichthyosis, namely nicotinic acid, triparanol, butyrophenones, cimetidine and clofazimine.

MANAGEMENT OF ICHTHYOSIS (IN GENERAL)

Management should be directed at both the skin and other sites. There is no specific treatment at this time. Moisturizers and keratolytics are the mainstay of topical therapy. Calcipotriene, retinoids, and for select types, anti-inflammatories such as topical steroids and calcineurin inhibitors have also been used. Systemic therapy is limited to retinoids. Superinfection of the skin should be anticipated and treated. Pruritus can be disabling. Failure to sweat normally may result in heat intolerance. Eye care should seek to prevent corneal changes resulting from ectropion and more specific changes associated with specific disorders. Hearing can be impaired by the accumulation of material in the external auditory canal. Severely affected children may require caloric supplementation, especially of vitamin D to avoid growth retardation. Affected individuals and their family should be counseled about the long-term outlook and the genetic nature of their disorder.

ERYTHROKERATODERMAS (EK)

They are a heterogenous group of inherited cornification disorders characterized by widespread erythematous and hyperkeratotic plaques which are either migratory or stationary.

They can be classified as:

i. Confluent and reticular EK of Gougerot and Carteaud.

ii. Variable EK (EKV) of Mendes da Costa.

iii. Symmetric progressive EK.

EKV is a rare autosomal dominant disorder that usually appears within the first year of life but may arise later in childhood. There is a defect in the GJ connexin proteins Cx31 and Cx30.3 expressed in stratum granulosum.

Children display sharply demarcated erythematous patches of bizarre geographical configuration that appear, change in shape or size, or regress over minutes to hours. Concomitantly, there are persistent, well-demarcated, brown, hyperkeratotic plaques, which are scattered on the face, buttocks, trunk and extremities (Figure 24.13). In some instances, the hyperkeratosis may be generalized. The course of the disease is chronic with remissions and exacerbations throughout life. Approximately 50 percent of patients display a palmoplantar keratoderma associated with peeling. The transient erythematous patches develop independently of the hyperkeratotic plaques, and lesions may either sting or be asymptomatic.

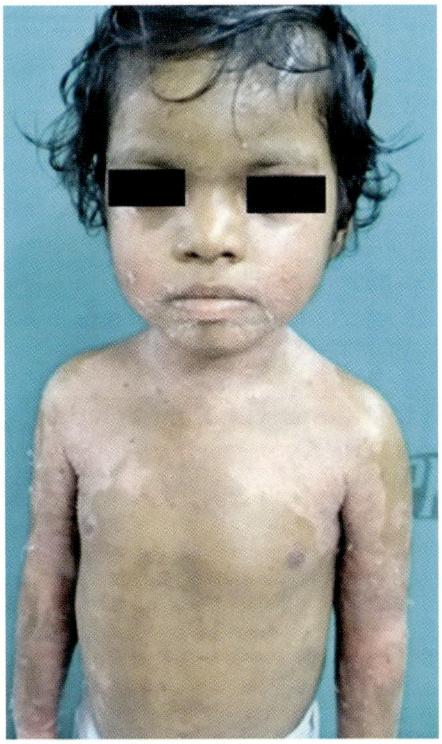

Figure 24.13: Erythrokeratoderma variabilis

PROGRESSIVE SYMMETRIC ERYTHROKERATODERMA (PSEK)

Progressive symmetric erythrokeratoderma (PSEK) is an autosomal dominant genodermatosis that shares many clinical features with EKV. The disease causes fixed, slowly progressive, symmetric, and well-defined hyperkeratotic plaques, which predominantly appear on the extensor surface of the extremities (Figure 24.14), trunk and face. In contrast to EKV however, the independent migrating red patches are absent, and the hyperkeratosis develops on an erythematous base and more often affects palms and soles (Figure 24.15).

Treatment with systemic retinoids such as acitretin can be very effective but is limited by long-term toxicities. Agents such as urea, salicylic acid, or lactic acid are effective as topical therapy for the hyperkeratotic plaques. Stinging and pruritus might be ameliorated with mildly sedating antihistamines.

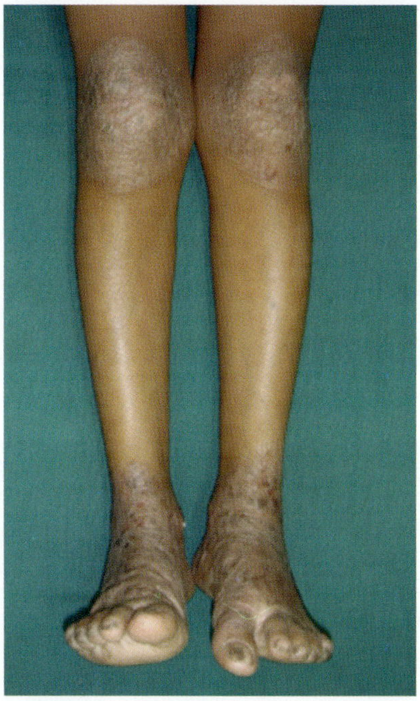

Figure 24.14: Progressive symmetric erythrokeratoderma

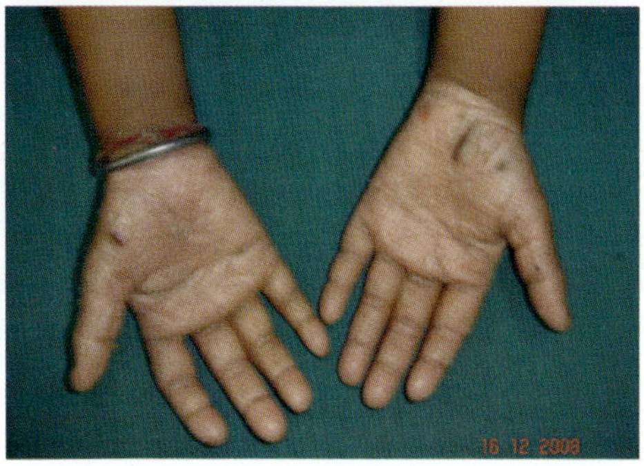

Figure 24.15: Progressive symmetric erythrokeratoderma involving palms

DARIER-WHITE DISEASE (KERATOSIS FOLLICULARIS)

It is an autosomal dominant form of blistering anomaly of the skin caused by mutations in the gene ATP2A2 located on 12q23-24.1 which encodes the sarcoplasmic/endoplasmic reticulum Ca2+ ATP isoform 2 protein (SERCA2), which is a calcium pump. It is characterized by greasy warty papules (Figures 24.16 and 24.17) and plaques distributed predominately at the seborrheic sites involving scalp, forehead, retroauricular folds, flexures and front and back of the central trunk and distinctive nail abnormalities.

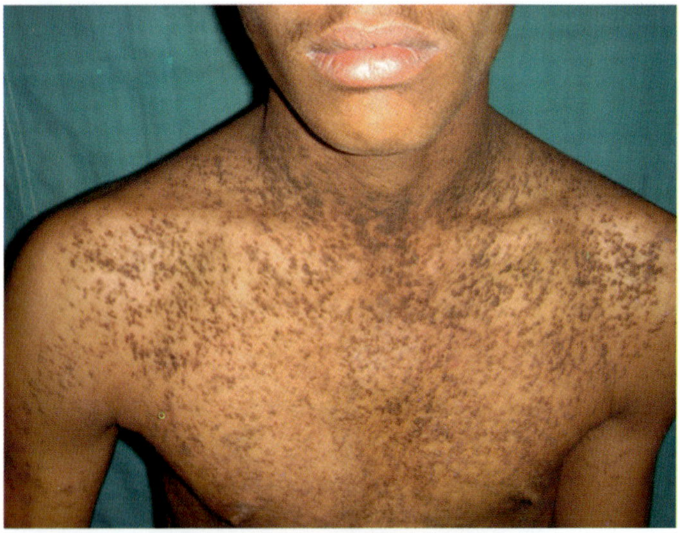

Figure 24.16: Darier's disease

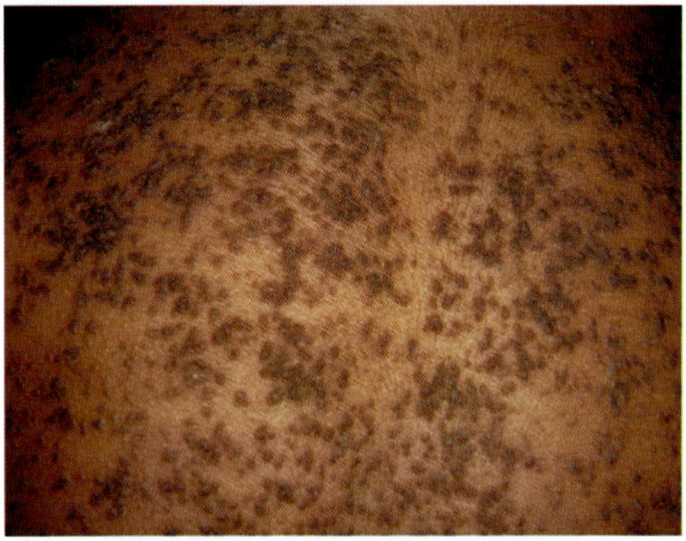

Figure 24.17: Darier's disease showing hyperpigmented warty papules

Nail changes include white and red longitudinal bands with a V-shaped nick at the free margin of the nail (pathognomonic), longitudinal nail ridges, longitudinal splitting and subungual hyperkeratosis.

White papules with central depressions appearing as cobblestones are commonly seen on the palate in oral mucosa. Diagnosis can be made clinically and confirmed by histopathology, which shows distinct histopathological findings that include dyskeratosis (abnormal keratinization of keratinocytes) with corps ronds (apoptotic hallmark) and acantholysis (focal areas of separation between suprabasal epidermal cells).

Treatment

The purpose of treatment is to reduce severity and symptoms, thereby improving the quality of life. Patients should be advised to protection from sunlight. Sunscreens, moisturizers, topical steroids and topical retinoids should be used in mild cases. Oral retinoids (isotretinoin or acitretin) are effective when the involvement is severe or extensive.

PALMOPLANTAR KERATODERMAS

PPK are a heterogeneous group of disorders characterized by hyperkeratosis of palms and soles. Majority of the disorders in this group are hereditary, and a few are acquired. Hereditary PPK's are due to defects of the genes that encode intracellular proteins, desmosomal proteins and other intercellular adhesion molecules.

Depending on the pattern of involvement, inherited PPKs can be further classified into Diffuse PPK (uniform involvement), focal PPK (localized involvement) and punctate (multiple, small, hyperkeratotic discrete round lesions on the entire palmoplantar surface or localized to certain locations. Diffuse PPK which extends beyond the palms and soles on to their dorsal aspects and to the flexor aspect of the wrist is called as transgradient keratoderma.

Approach to Patient with Palmoplantar Keratoderma (PPK)

Ask age of onset: Decide if PPK is hereditary or acquired.

If hereditary, decide if PPK is predominant finding non-syndromic (Table 24.4) or part of syndrome (Table 24.5), focal (Table 24.6), Striate (Table 24.7), Punctate (Table 24.8) or miscellaneous (Table 24.9).

Table 24.4: Diffuse Non-syndromic PPK

Transgradient		*Non Transgradient*	
Grether's keratoderma	**Sybert' keratoderma**	**Vorner keratoderma**	**Unna-Thost syndrome**
K1 mutation, Transgradient, progressive, non epidermolytic, involves tendoachillis, hyperhidrosis	More severe and hyperkeratotic type with involvement of natal cleft and groin	K1/K9 mutation, Epidermolytic PPK, dirty appearance,hyperhidrosis, dermatophyte infections common	K1/K2 mutation, waxy appearance, hyperhidrosis, hermatophyte infections common, nail thickening, pitted keratolysis, maceration
Gamborg-Nielsen Syndrome	**Mal de meleda**		
Diffuse PPK, Knuckle pads	SLURP gene mutation, gloves and stocking with erythematous border, hyperhidrosis,dermatophyte infections, nail abnormalities, perioral erythema, high arch palate, pseudoainhum, amputation of digits, psoriasiform plaque over knee and elbow		
Nagasima	**Bothnia**		
SERPINB-7 gene mutation, diffuse PPK perioral erythema, white spongy keratosis on water exposure is classical	Aquaporin 5 mutation, curved nail and ragged cuticle, white spongy keratosis on water exposure is classical		

Table 24.5: Syndromic diffuse PPK with associated features

Ectodermal Dysplasia	*Deafness*	*Cancer*
Olmsted syndrome	**Vohwinkel syndrome**	**Huriez syndrome**
TRPV-3 mutation, mutilating PPK, periorificial hyperkeratosis, alopecia, hyper-IgE with eosinophilia, bone deformity	Honeycomb pattern PPK, starfish hyperkeratosis on knuckles, pseudo-ainhum, sensorineural hearing loss	SLURP 1 mutation, scleroatrophy of extremities, risk of developing squamous cell carcinoma (SCC), severe nail changes
Papillon-Lefèvre Syndrome	**Bart Pumphrey syndrome**	**Palmoplantar keratoderma, sex reversal and cancer**
Cathepsin C mutation, periodontitis and gingivitis, loss of teeth, floating in air appearance of teeth, recurrent pyogenic infections, ectopic calcification (e.g., dural calcification)	Connexin 26 mutation, sensory neural hearing loss, knuckle pads, cystic lesion, leukonychia	RSPO1 gene mutation, mild PPK, sclerodactyly, true hermaphroditism
Haim-Munk syndrome	**Keratitis ichthyosis deafness (KID)**	
Cathepsin C mutation, arachnodactyly, acro-osteolysis, onychogryphosis, joint contracture, pes planus, arthralgia of multiple joint	Keratitis, Ichthyosiform erythroderma, Deafness, Acrofacial, Verrucous plaque, Increased risk of SCC	
Clouston Syndrome	**Mitochondrial PPK with deafness**	
Connexin 30, alopecia, nail dystrophy, pigmentation over joints		
Schopf-Schulz-Passarge syndrome		
Hyperhidrosis, cystic lesion around the eyes		

Table 24.6: Focal keratoderma

Pachyonychia congenital (PC) type I and II	*Howel Evans syndrome (AD)*	*Focal keratoderma with oral leukokeratosis*	*Oculocutaneous tyrosinemia/ Richner Hanhart Syndrome*
Autosomal dominant, KRT 6a, 6b,16,17 gene mutation, toenail dystrophy, plantar keratoderma and plantar pain, oral and laryngeal, leukokeratosis resulting in hoarseness of voice, Natal teeth, pilosebaceous cyst like steatocystoma	PPK with deep, painful fissures, oral leukokeratosis, risk of oesophageal squamous cell cancer	KRT 16 mutation	Painful PPK, photophobia, progressive mental retardation, corneal scarring

Table 24.7: Striate palmoplantar keratoderma

Non-Syndromic	*Syndromic*
SPPK 1 (Brunauer-Fuh-Siemens syndrome)	**Carvajal syndrome**
Desmoglein 1 mutation, striate PPK, hyperhidrosis	Desmoplakin mutation, striate keratoderma, woolly hair, predominantly left ventricular cardiomyopathy
SPPK 2	**Naxos syndrome**
Desmoplakin mutation, striate keratoderma, woolly hair without cardiomyopathy	Plakoglobin mutation, arrhythmogenic right ventricular cardiomyopathy, woolly hair, high arch palate, hyperextensibility of joint
Striate PPK 3	
K1 v1 domain mutation, striate PPK	

Tablet 24.8: Punctate palmoplantar keratoderma

Bushcke-Fischer-Brauer keratoderma	*Spiny keratoderma or Music box keratoderma*	*Marginal papular keratoderma/Linear or paving stone PPK*
Pinpoint keratotic papule which coalesce over pressure point, late childhood or adolescence onset, increase gradually with age, worsening with water exposure	Filiform, minute, digitate PPK, star under moonlight appearance, onset in early childhood	**Focal acral hyperkeratosis**
		Cornified umbilicated Papule over border of hands and feet, without elastorrhexis
		Acrokeratoelastoidosis
		Cornified papular keratoderma with elastorrhexis

Table 24.9: Miscellaneous

Loricrin	*Transient aquagenic keratoderma*	*Cole disease*
Loricrin mutation, honeycomb appearance, pseudoainhum, congenital ichthyosiform erythroderma	Keratoderma appears when immersing the hands and feet in water, lesion disappear shortly after drying leaving minimal hyperkeratosis	ENPP mutation, early onset punctate PPK, sharply demarcated irregular hypopigmented macules over extremities, calcific tendinopathy or calcinosis cutis

LORICRIN KERATODERMA

The disease is caused by mutations in the gene encoding loricrin, a glycine rich cornified envelope protein. Clinically there is combination of honeycomb keratoderma (Figure 24.18) with mild ichthyosis. Generalized desquamation may be evident at birth, and history of collodion baby may be present. No associated extracutaneous features have been reported.

A rugose keratoderma develops during childhood, gradually extending to the confluent 'honeycomb' pattern. The edges of the keratoderma are diffuse. Cicatricial bands may form at digits causing pseudoainhum. Knuckle pads and warty keratoses may be found.

Treatment with isotretinoin has been to be useful.

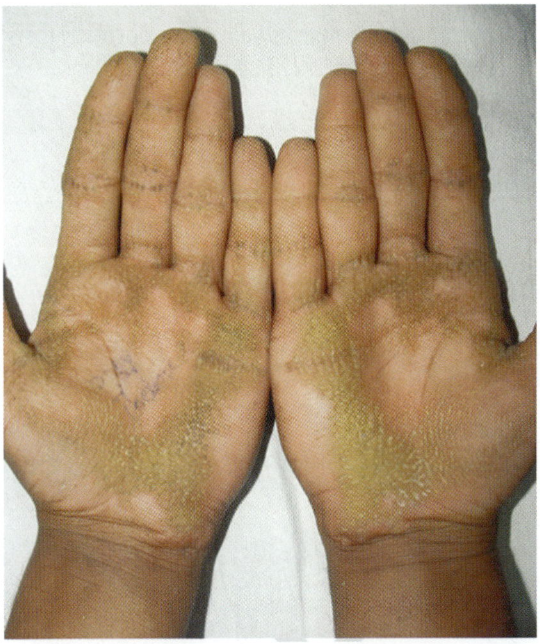

Figure 24.18: Loricrin keratoderma

ACQUIRED PALMOPLANTAR KERATODERMAS

There are various causes of acquired PPK (Table 24.10) which include certain dermatosis (e.g. psoriasis, hyperkeratotic eczema (Figure 24.19), chronic eczema, lichen planus, pityriasis rubra pilaris, lupus erythematosus etc.), infections (e.g., dermatophyte infections, crusted scabies, secondary syphilis etc.) certain drugs (e.g., beta-glucan, lithium, dioxin, chemotherapy agents etc.), exposure to certain chemicals (e.g., arsenic, chlorinated hydrocarbons etc.), metabolic disorders (e.g., hypothyroidism, myxedema etc.) and malignancy associated (e.g., Hodgkin's lymphoma, solid organ tumors etc.). Contact allergy, toxic irritants, atopic dermatitis and psoriasis are common causes of acquired palmoplantar keratoderma.

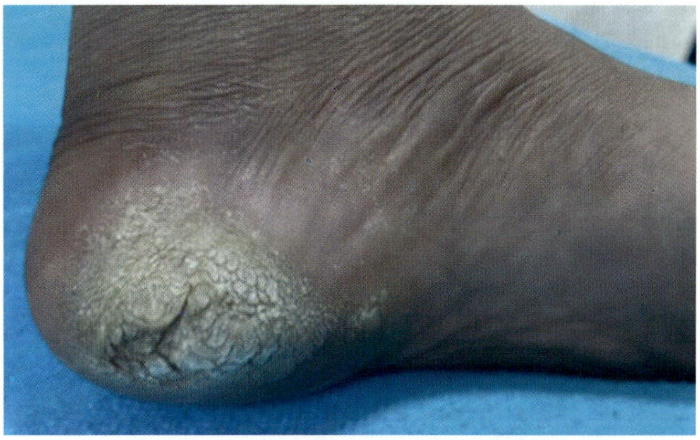

Figure 24.19: Acquired keratoderma

Table 24.10: Acquired causes of palmoplantar keratoderma
Dermatosis • Psoriasis • Pityriasis Rubra pilaris • Keratoderma blannorrhagicum in reactive arthritis • Lichen planus • Hand eczema • Atopic dermatitis
Infection • HPV • Crusted scabies • Dermatophytosis • Syphilis
Systemic disease • Hypothyroidism • Chronic lymphedema
Malignancy • Bazex syndrome or Acrokeratosis paraneoplastica • Tripe palms • Solid organ malignancy • Mycosis fungoides • Sezary syndrome
Drugs • Hydroxyurea • Bleomycin • Lithium • Verapamil • Venlafaxine • 5-fluorouracil • Glucan
Chemical • Arsenic
Miscellaneous • Keratoderma Climactericum • Malnutrition • Idiopathic

OTHER KERATINIZATION DISORDERS

Keratosis Pilaris

Keratosis pilaris (KP) is a common benign skin condition characterized by follicular based hyperkeratosis with mild erythema (Figure 24.20). It is most prominent on the lateral upper arms and thighs, but can also be seen on the cheeks of children. It is commonly seen in individuals with a personal or family history of atopy. Keratolytic emollient should be used for treatment.

Porokeratosis

Porokeratosis of Mibelli is a genetic disease transmitted as an autosomal dominant trait. Onset is usually in childhood, but the disease can occur at any age. It begins as a tiny keratotic papule that slowly enlarges peripherally to form an annular or serpiginous plaque with central hyperpigmentation, dryness and mild atrophy. Each lesion has a characteristic peripheral, slightly raised, keratotic wall, at the summit of which is a gutter like furrow. The sites of predilection are the dorsal portions of the extremities, face and neck.

The porokeratosis may appear in several forms:

1. Classic porokeratosis of Mibelli (Figure 24.21).
2. Linear porokeratosis (Figure 24.22).
3. Porokeratotic eccrine ostial and dermal duct nevus (PEODDN).
4. Punctate porokeratosis.
5. Porokeratosis palmaris et plantaris disseminata (PPPD).
6. Disseminated superficial actinic porokeratosis (DSAP) (Figure 24.23).

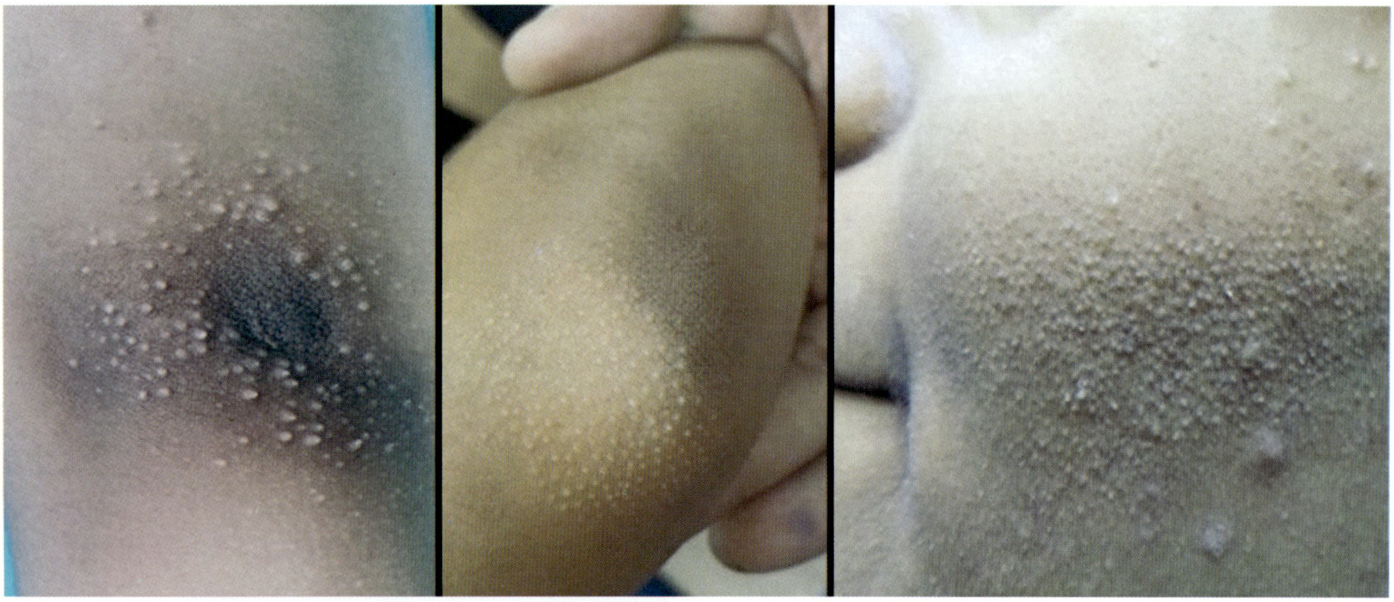

Figure 24.20: Keratosis pilaris

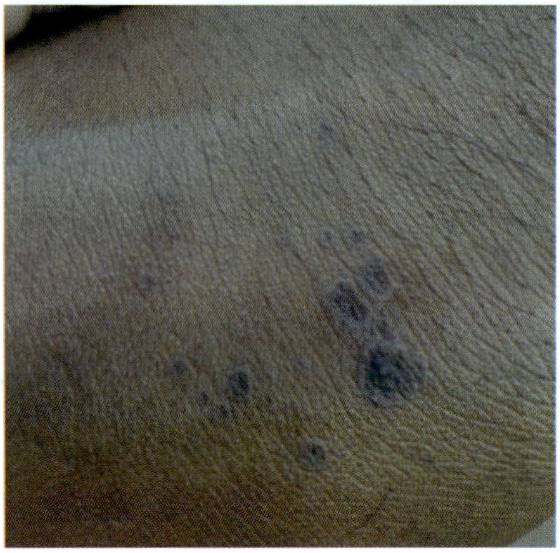

Figure 14.21: Classical porokeratosis or porokeratosis of Mibelli

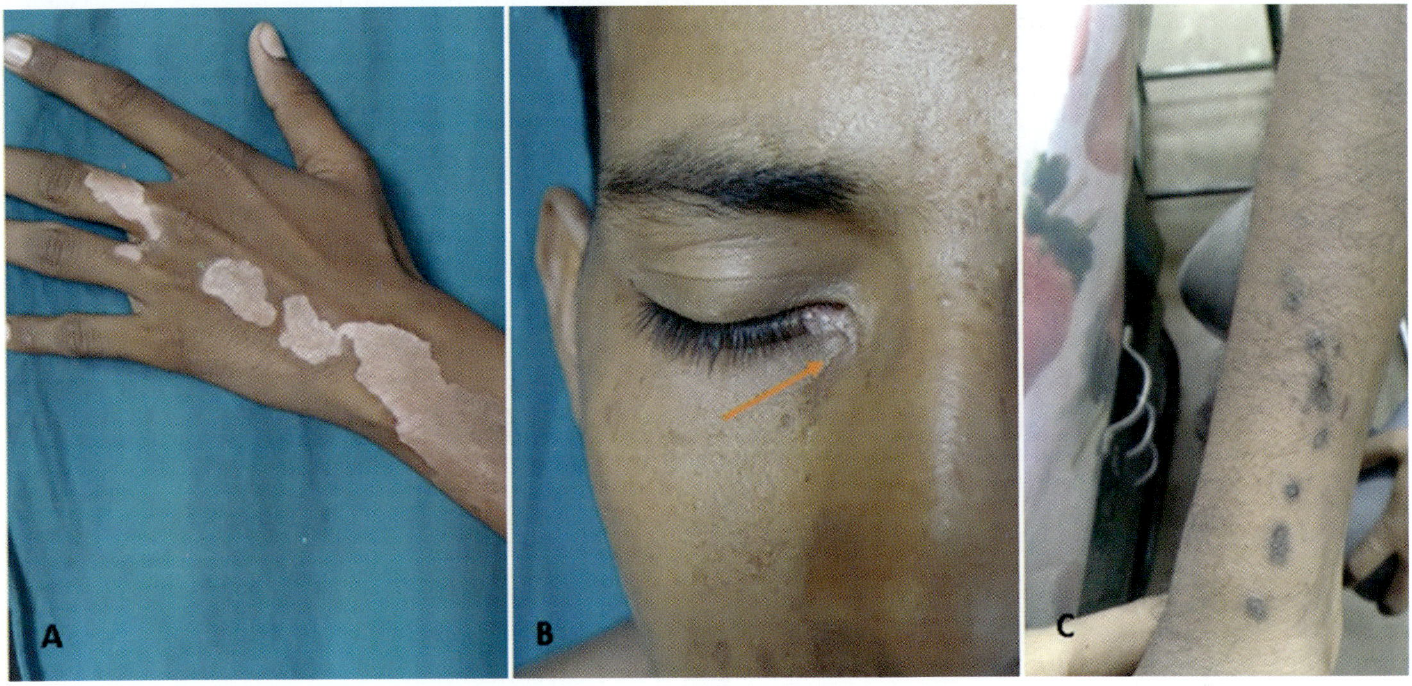

Figure 24.22: Linear porokeratosis (A,B and C)

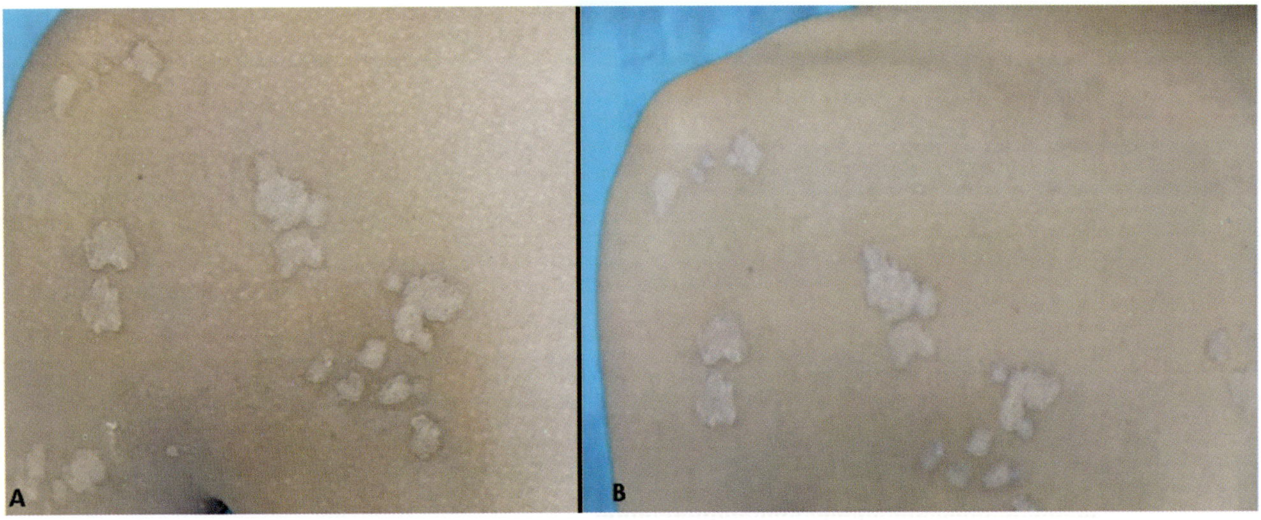

Figure 24.23: Disseminated superficial porokeratosis (A & B)

Most characteristic histologic feature is the cornoid lamella, a parakeratotic column in which the horny cells appear homogenous and have deeply basophilic pyknotic nuclei.

Treatment consists of local excision if there are only a few lesions. Carbon dioxide laser ablation and liquid nitrogen are also effective. Topical 5-fluorouracil solution or cream has also been used. Oral retinoids have been used in some cases but lesions tend to recur once the drug is discontinued.

Keratolysis Exfoliativa

It is characterized by the development of asymptomatic non-inflammatory, pinhead sized macules with white scales. Typically affects the skin of palms and soles. Neighbouring patches may coalesce, leading to widespread flaky scaling. Dyshidrosis is associated in some cases. Treatment consists of application of mild keratolytics like 3% salicylic acid ointment with emollients.

25

CHAPTER

Disorders of Sweat and Sebaceous Glands

Contents

ECCRINE SWEAT GLANDS

Eccrine sweat glands are the most abundant sweat producing glands. They are merocrine in nature, i.e., there is no loss of cytoplasm during their secretion. They develop from the epidermis and are not related to the hair follicle, hence also called 'atrichial'. They occur on almost all parts of the body, with different densities, the maximum being on the palms and soles. Structurally, they consist of 3 parts, the secretory coil, intradermal duct and the acrosyringium. The secretory coil is located at the junction of dermis and subcutis or in the lower third of the dermis. It consists of the clear cells, dark cells and myoepithelial cells. Functionally 50-60% of sweat secretion occurs in this part of the gland. The intradermal sweat duct consists of two layers of cells and like the secretory coil, it also has an active role in the formation of sweat. The acrosyringium is the intraepidermal spiral part of the duct which opens on the skin surface (Figure 25.1).

Functions of the eccrine sweat glands include thermo-regulation, moistening the palms and soles for added grip and excretion of certain drugs. The stimuli for sweat secretion are thermal, emotional and gustatory stimuli and they are innervated by sympathetic cholinergic fibres.

Sweat is a colourless, odourless fluid secreted by the eccrine sweat glands. It consists of electrolytes like sodium, potassium, chloride, bicarbonate, its pH is mostly alkaline (7.2-7.3) and specific gravity is about 1.005. Other constituents of sweat include glucose, lactate, urea, ammonia, proteins and amino acids.

APOCRINE SWEAT GLANDS

Apocrine sweat glands (Figure 25.1) are so-called because of a loss of apical cytoplasm, which is pinced-off during secretion. They develop from the hair follicle and are hence termed 'epitrichial'. Apocrine glands are found in the axillae, areolae, anogenital region and periumbilical skin. Modified apocrine glands exist in some parts of the body, like the ceruminous glands in the external ear, glands of Moll on eyelids and the mammary glands. Apo eccrine glands are present in the axillae and have combined feature of both apocrine and eccrine glands.

Structurally, apocrine glands have a secretory coil and a duct. The secretory coil lies in the lower dermis or subcutis and consists of secretory cells and myoepithelial cells. The duct is short, straight, tubular and opens into the infundibulum of the hair follicle. The apocrine glands become functional at puberty under the influence of circulating hormones.

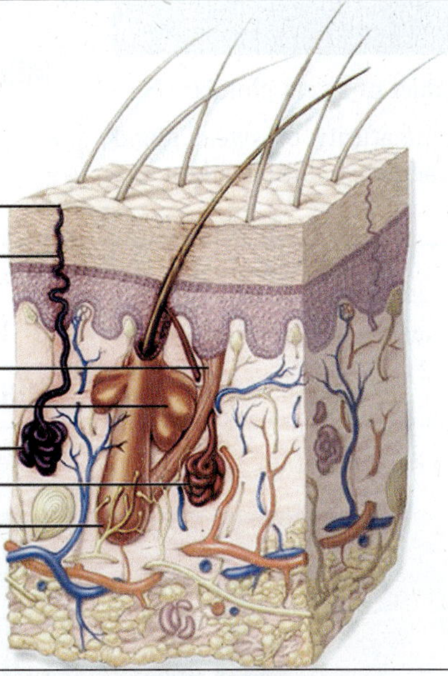

Figure 25.1: Structure of sweat and sebaceous glands

The secretion of the apocrine glands is a viscous colourless fluid, with a peculiar odour, which can be attributed to bacterial activity. Apocrine secretion occurs in response to emotional stimuli. The glands are supplied by sympathetic adrenergic and cholinergic fibres. The glands secrete pheromones in lower animals, but have no known function in humans.

SEBACEOUS GLANDS

Sebaceous glands are holocrine in nature, i.e., there is complete destruction of the cell before secretion. They originate from the hair follicle, at the junction of the infundibulum and isthmus.

The gland consists of many lobes or acini which have their ducts converging to form the main sebaceous duct opening into the canal of the hair follicle. The glandular cuboidal epithelium gradually transforms into squamous epithelium along the duct as it comes near the follicle.

Sebaceous glands are present all over the body except the palms and soles. They are more in number over the scalp, nasolabial fold, eyebrows, external auditory meatus, postauricular fold, chest and genital region. Modified sebaceous glands include the Montgomery's turbercles over areola, Meibomian glands over eyelids, Tysons glands over prepuce and ectopic glands over female genitalia and lips.

Sebum or secretion of the sebaceous glands contains lipids like triglycerides, fatty acids, cholesterol, cholesterol esters and squalene. Role of sebum includes barrier function, anti-bacterial and anti-fungal action and preventing transepidermal water loss. The sebum secretion occurs under the influence of hormones, predominantly androgens.

Common disorders of sweat and sebaceous glands (Table 25.1) are described below:

Table 25.1: Disorders of sweat and sebaceous glands

Eccrine sweat glands	*Apocrine sweat glands*	*Sebaceous glands*
Hyperhidrosis	Hidradenitis suppurativa	Acne
Hypohidrosis	Fox-Fordyce disease	Sebaceous hyperplasia
Anhidrosis	Bromhidrosis	Nevus sebaceous
Miliaria	Chromhidrosis	Sebaceous adenoma
Granulosis rubra nasi		
Neutrophilic Eccrine Hidradenitis		
Syringoma		Sebaceoma /Sebaceous epithelioma
Cylindroma		Sebaceous carcinoma

MILIARIA

- It occurs due to obstruction of duct of sweat glands.
- Predisposing factors include immaturity of sweat gland duct, warm and humid environmental conditions, tight and occlusive clothing.

Miliaria Crystallina

- Miliaria crystallina is clear, thin-walled superficial vesicles 1-2 mm in diameter (Figure 25.2).
- There is no associated erythema.
- Rupture of vesicles may lead to desquamation.
- Most often seen on head, neck and upper trunk.

Miliaria Rubra

- Typical lesions are papules and vesicles, 1-4 mm in diameter, with surrounding erythema (Figure 25.3).
- It is seen in flexural areas like neck, groin and axilla, scalp and face may be affected as well.
- Recurrent crops of lesions may be seen.

Miliaria Profunda

Lesions are large erythematous papules and plaques.

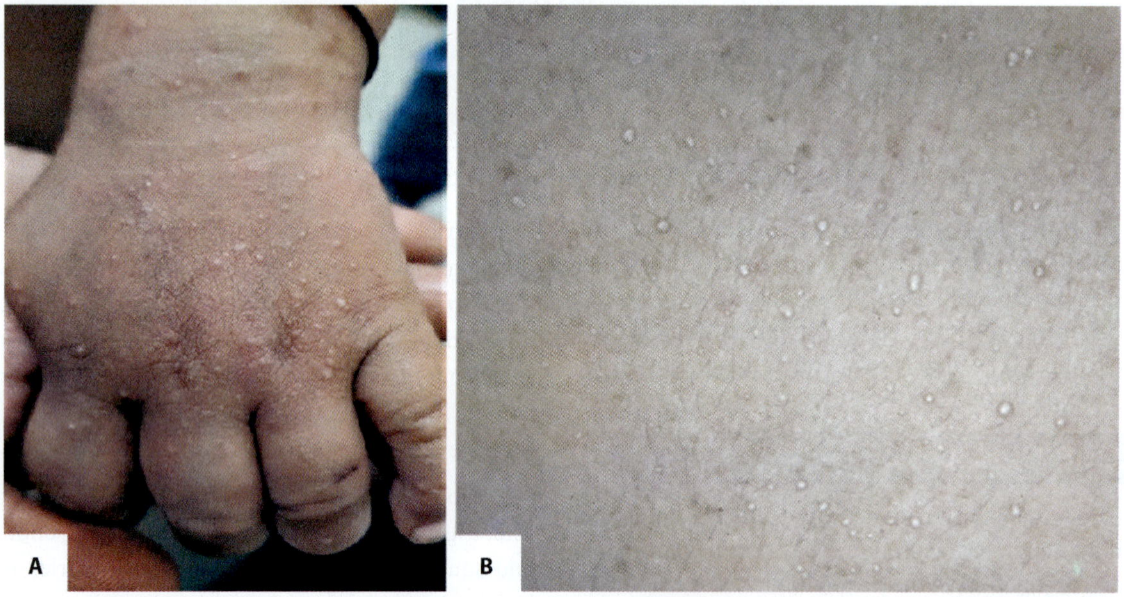

Figure 25.2: Miliaria crystallina

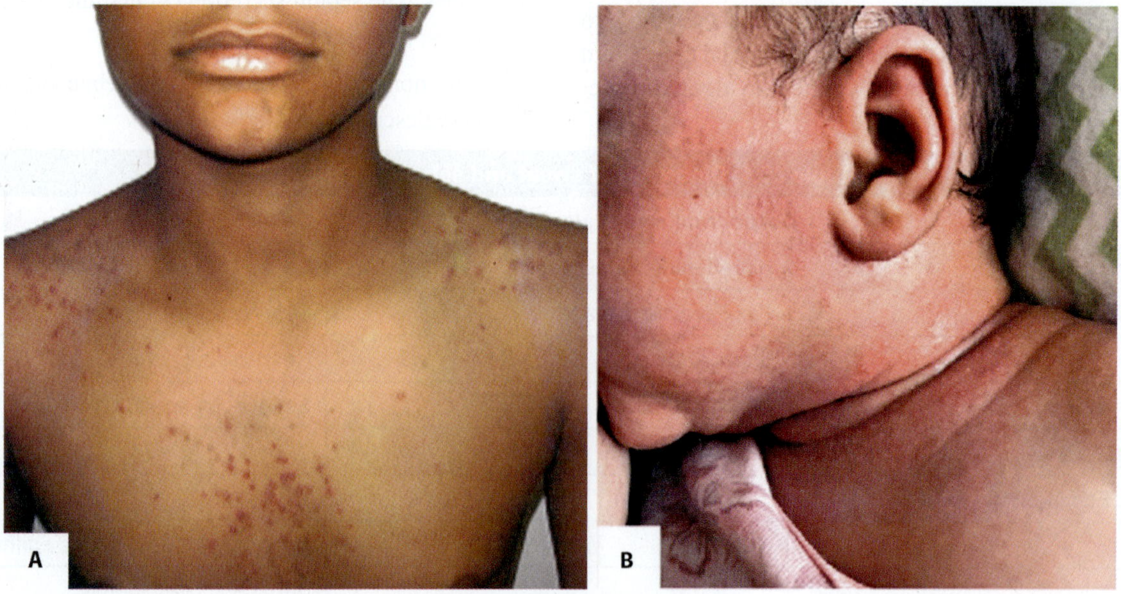

Figure 25.3: Miliaria rubra

Miliaria Pustulosa

- Pustules develop in the pre-existing lesions. The pustules are sterile and are not a sign of secondary infection.

Treatment

- Ice cold compresses.
- Change in environmental conditions.
- Application of soothing agents like calamine lotion.
- Antihistamines and antibiotics, if necessary.

GRANULOSIS RUBRA NASI (GRN)

GRN is an inflammatory condition involving sweat glands of central face and presents as erythema, hyperhidrosis, papules, pustules and vesicles over central face. Treatment options include topical indomethacin, oral corticosteroids, tetracycline, cryotherapy, botulinum toxin A.

NEUTROPHILIC ECCRINE HIDRADENITIS (NEH)

NEH is an uncommon disease affecting the eccrine glands, leading to eccrine unit necrosis. It is most commonly seen in adults receiving cytarabine as part of the induction chemotherapy for the treatment of hematological malignancy. It can present as quickly as 2 days or up to 2 years after chemotherapy initiation. Patient presents with fever along with solitary or multiple erythematous macules, papules, nodules or plaques most frequently over the face, trunk and extremities.

NEH is a self-limiting disease and does not require therapy, the use of steroids- topical or systemic is debatable.

HYPERHIDROSIS

Hyperhidrosis is excessive sweating, more than that is required for normal thermoregulation. The sites most commonly affected are the palms, soles and axillae. Hyperhidrosis occurs in 3 forms: emotionally induced hyperhidrosis, localized hyperhidrosis and generalized hyperhidrosis.

Classification

Most cases of hyperhidrosis can be classified as one of the following:

- Generalized:
    - Primary (idiopathic).
    - Secondary.
- Focal (palmar, plantar, axillary and craniofacial):
    - Primary (idiopathic).
    - Secondary.
- Localized nevoid.
    - Compensatory hyperhidrosis with extensive anhidrosis (Ross syndrome).

Epidemiology

In adolescents and young adults, an incidence rate of 0.6-1% is reported. Hyperhidrosis affects all races and both sexes. Persons of all ages can be affected by hyperhidrosis. Localized hyperhidrosis, unlike generalized hyperhidrosis, usually begins in childhood or adolescence.

Etiopathogenesis

Generalized hyperhidrosis may be the consequence of autonomic dysregulation, or it may develop secondary to a metabolic disorder, febrile illness, or malignancy. In its localized form, hyperhidrosis may result from a disruption followed by abnormal regeneration of sympathetic nerves or a localized abnormality in the number or distribution of the eccrine glands. Palmoplantar hyperhidrosis may be an inherited disorder.

Causes

Generalized hyperhidrosis may be secondary to numerous conditions including the following:

- Neurologic or neoplastic diseases.
- Metabolic disorders or processes (e.g., thyrotoxicosis, diabetes mellitus, hypoglycemia, gout, pheochromocytoma, menopause).
- Febrile illnesses.
- *Medications:* Agents such as propranolol, physostigmine, pilocarpine, tricyclic antidepressants and serotonin reuptake inhibitors, etc.
- Chronic alcoholism.
- Hodgkin's disease and tuberculosis (nocturnal hyperhidrosis).

Localized hyperhidrosis may also be associated with the following:

- Gustatory stimuli (associated with Frey's syndrome, syringomyelia, diabetic neuropathies, herpes zoster, parotitis and parotid abscess).
- Eccrine nevus.
- Glomus tumor.
- POEMS syndrome which includes **P**eripheral neuropathy, **O**rganomegaly, **E**ndocrinopathy, **M**onoclonal plasma-proliferative disorder and **S**kin changes.
- Pachydermoperiostosis.

Clinical Features

Patients note excessive sweating in affected areas, which ultimately prompts them to seek medical attention. Generally areas of hyperhidrosis are clearly seen. If confirmation of hyperhidrosis is desired, the iodine starch test may be used. This test requires spraying of the affected area with a mixture of 0.5-1 gm of iodine crystals and 500 gm of soluble starch. Areas that produce sweat turn black.

Localized unilateral or segmental hyperhidrosis is rare and of unknown origin. The condition usually presents on the forearm or forehead in otherwise healthy individuals, without evidence of the typical triggering factors found in essential hyperhidrosis. Unilateral hyperhidrosis with accompanying contralateral anhidrosis is also seen.

Localized hyperhidrosis, unlike generalized hyperhidrosis, usually begins in childhood or adolescence. Hyperhidrosis beginning later in life should prompt a search for secondary causes such as systemic diseases, adverse effects of medication use, or metabolic disorders.

Investigations

- Search for primary causes if generalized hyperhidrosis is noted.
- Important laboratory studies in the hyperhidrosis workup may include the following:
  - Thyroid function tests may reveal underlying hyperthyroidism or thyrotoxicosis.
  - Blood glucose levels may reveal diabetes mellitus or hypoglycemia.
  - Urinary catecholamines may reveal a possible pheochromocytoma.
  - Chest radiography may be used to rule out tuberculosis or a neoplasm.

Treatment

- Topical agents for hyperhidrosis therapy include topical anticholinergics, boric acid, 2-5% tannic acid solution, resorcinol, potassium permanganate, formaldehyde, glutaraldehyde and methenamine.
- 20% aluminum chloride hexahydrate in absolute anhydrous ethyl alcohol is more commonly used as the first-line topical agent. It should be applied nightly on dry skin with or without occlusion until a positive result is obtained, after which the intervals between applications may be lengthened.
- Systemic agents used to treat hyperhidrosis include anticholinergic medications. Anticholinergics such as propantheline bromide, glycopyrrolate, oxybutynin, and benztropine are effective because the pre glandular neurotransmitter for sweat secretion is acetylcholine. The use of anticholinergics may be unappealing because their adverse effects profile includes mydriasis, blurred vision, dry mouth and eyes, difficulty in micturition and constipation.
- Iontophoresis consists of passing a direct current across the skin. The mechanism of action remains unclear. In palmoplantar hyperhidrosis, the daily treatment of each palm or sole for 30 minutes at 15-20 mA with tap water iontophoresis is effective. Numerous agents have been used to induce hypohidrosis, including tap water and anticholinergics. However, treatment with anticholinergic iontophoresis is more effective than tap water iontophoresis.
- Botulinum toxin injections are effective because of their anticholinergic effects at the neuromuscular junction and in the postganglionic sympathetic cholinergic nerves in the sweat glands.
- Surgical treatments include surgical sympathectomy, surgical excision of the affected areas and sub-cutaneous liposuction. Sympathectomy involves the surgical destruction of the ganglia responsible for hyperhidrosis. The second (T2) and third (T3) thoracic ganglia are responsible for palmar hyperhidrosis, the fourth (T4) thoracic ganglia controls axillary hyperhidrosis, and the first (T1) thoracic ganglia controls facial hyperhidrosis.

ANHIDROSIS AND HYPOHIDROSIS

Anhidrotic and hypohidrotic disorders may be caused by lesions anywhere from the cerebral cortex to the eccrine sweat glands.

Anhidrosis can be classified as:

1. Congenital/genetic – e.g., hypohidrotic ectodermal dysplasia, congenital insensitivity to pain with anhidrosis and Fabry's disease.
2. Acquired (secondary anhidrosis)–Due to an underlying:
   - Neurological disorder.
   - Endocrine or metabolic disturbance.
   - Drugs.
   - Idiopathic.
3. Acquired idiopathic generalized anhidrosis (AIGA).
4. Idiopathic segmental anhidrosis.
5. Ross syndrome.

Central Nervous System Disease

- Generalized anhidrosis is a frequent manifestation of CNS lesions, with orthostatic hypotension and extrapyramidal or cerebellar impairment usually dominating the clinical picture. Global or patchy patterns of anhidrosis may also accompany Parkinson's disease or progressive supranuclear palsy. In these disorders preserved facial sweating is thought to be a compensatory response.
- Demyelinating lesions involving central thermoregulatory pathways frequently result in regional or global anhidrosis in patients with multiple sclerosis, particularly with more advanced disease. Hemibody anhidrosis has also been observed in patients following stroke or thalamotomy. Spinal cord transection typically impairs thermoregulatory sweating below the lesion.

Peripheral Nervous System Disease

- Diabetes mellitus, the most common cause of autonomic neuropathy in the developed world, typically impairs thermoregulatory sweating in 'gloves and stocking' distribution. As the neuropathy progresses, asymmetric truncal anhidrosis or global anhidrosis may develop.
- Hypohidrosis commonly occurs in the autonomic neuropathy associated with Sjögren's syndrome. Hypohidrosis also accompanies neuropathies due to amyloidosis, alcoholism, Tangier disease, vasculitis and Fabry's disease. Focal areas of hypohidrosis may be found in patients with leprosy.
- Anhidrosis is a prominent feature of hereditary sensory and autonomic neuropathies type IV and V (congenital insensitivity to pain with anhidrosis), in which there is absent skin innervation (See Chapter 30).

Ross Syndrome

- Ross syndrome is the clinical triad of progressive segmental anhidrosis with Adie's tonic pupils and areflexia. The anhidrosis is often asymmetrical, and there may be areas of compensatory hyperhidrosis elsewhere in the body.

Chronic Idiopathic Anhidrosis

- Chronic idiopathic anhidrosis refers to the syndrome of total or subtotal anhidrosis occurring either in isolation or without prominent accompanying autonomic signs or symptoms. These patients become hot, flushed, dizzy, dyspneic and weak in response to heating or exercise but do not sweat.

Dermatologic Disorders

- Hypohidrosis commonly occurs when sweat glands are injured by burns, irradiation, skin inflammation, scarring or trauma. Sweat gland necrosis may accompany the blistering disorders. Anhidrosis also occurs in primary dermatologic disorders such as psoriasis, exfoliative dermatitis, lichen sclerosis et atrophicus, ichthyosis, miliaria, scleroderma and cholinergic urticaria.

Anhidrotic Ectodermal Dysplasia

- Mutations in the ED-1 gene encoding for ectodysplasin result in X-linked anhidrotic ectodermal dysplasia, which is characterized by disrupted morphogenesis of eccrine sweat glands, hair and teeth. Affected children may experience life threatening hyperpyrexia caused by inability to sweat. Other accompanying features include frontal bossing, depressed nasal bridge, everted lips, fine wrinkling around eye, facial sebaceoma or milia like sebaceous papules, sparse hair, severe xerosis (Figure 25.4), nail dystrophy, cleft palate, conical teeth, extensive skin peeling , mammary gland hyperplasia and hyperkeratosis of the palms and soles.

Medications

Hypohidrosis is a common reversible side effect of anti-cholinergic medications such as oxybutynin, tricyclic antidepressants, phenothiazines and trihexphenidyl.

SWEAT GLAND TUMOURS

Syringoma

Syringomas are very common neoplasms presenting as small papules 1 to 3 mm in diameter. They may be yellow, brown or pink. They are virtually always multiple and most frequently occur on and around the eyelids (Figure 25.5) and upper cheeks. Other sites of involvement include the axillae, abdomen, forehead, penis and vulva. Familial cases of syringomas have been reported. Syringomas develop slowly and persist indefinitely without symptoms. Syringomas occur in adults with Down syndrome, particularly females. The lesions may be removed by superficial electrocauterization.

Cylindroma

Cutaneous cylindroma, also known as dermal eccrine cylindroma, occurs predominantly on the scalp and face as a solitary lesion. The tumor is firm, pinkish-blue, ranging from a few millimeters to several centimeters. The solitary cylindroma

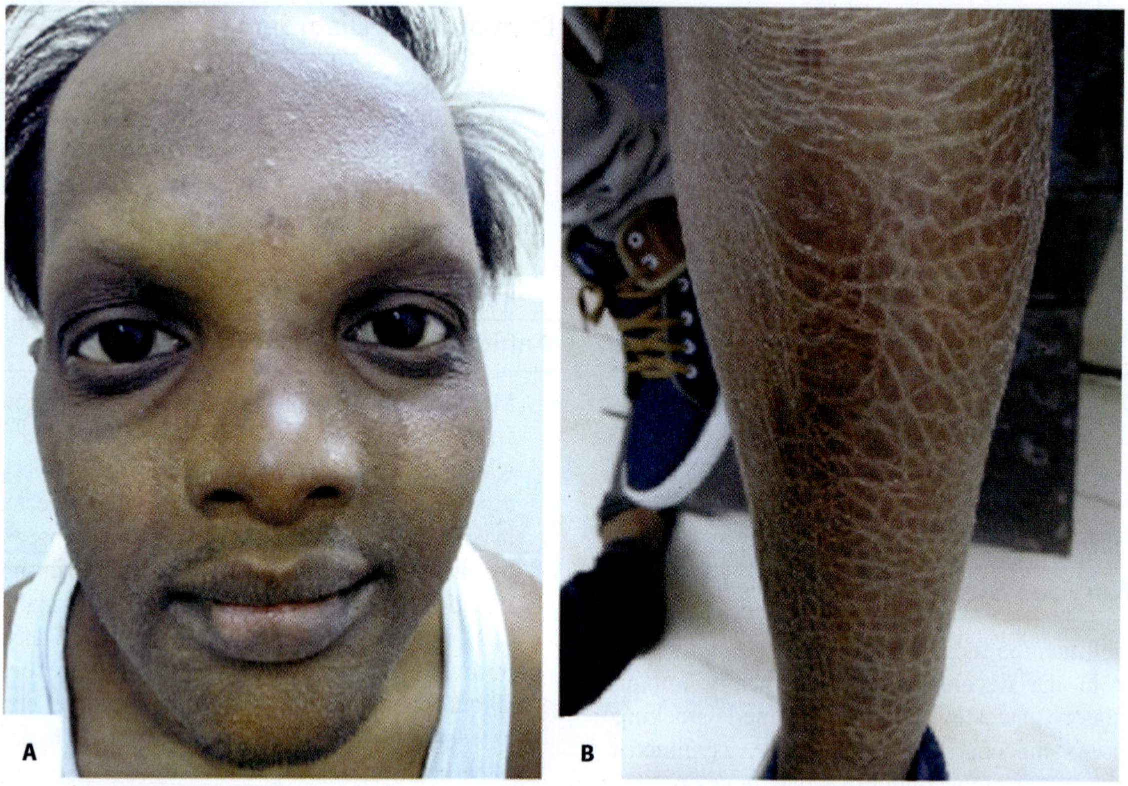

Figure 25.4: Anhidrotic ectodermal dysplasia

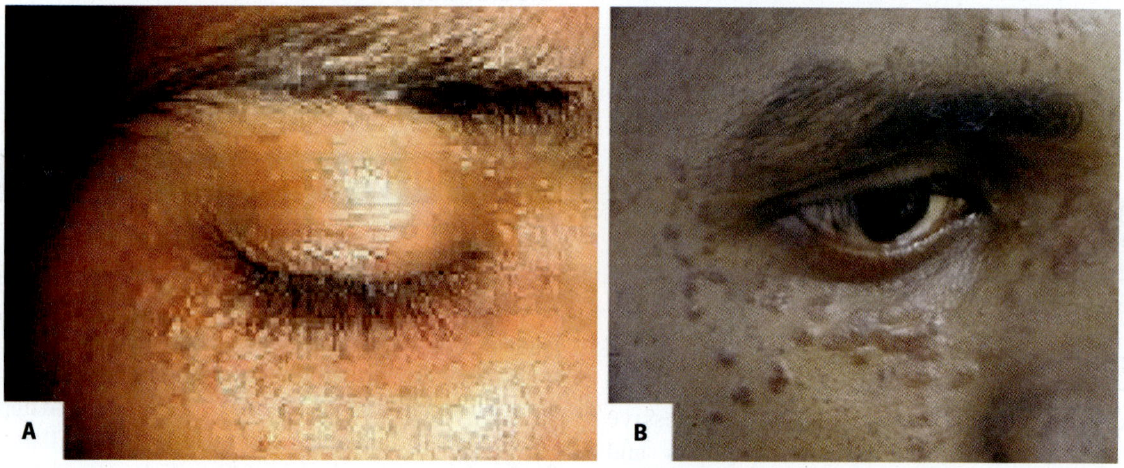

Figure 25.5: Syringoma

is considered to be non-hereditary and may at times be found in areas other than the head and neck. Women are affected more than men.

The autosomal dominantly inherited form, **Brooke-Spiegler syndrome**, appears soon after puberty as numerous rounded masses of various sizes on the scalp. The lesions resemble bunches of grapes. They are frequently associated with trichoepitheliomas and milia. This syndrome is due to a mutation in the CYLD1 gene on chromosome 16q12-13.

HIDRADENITIS SUPPURATIVA

Hidradenitis suppurativa (HS) is a disorder of the terminal follicular epithelium in the apocrine gland-bearing skin. It is characterized by comedone like follicular occlusion, chronic relapsing inflammation, mucopurulent discharge and progressive scarring.

Epidemiology

The prevalence of hidradenitis suppurativa appears to be 1-2%

in the general population. An increased incidence is observed in blacks, possibly because blacks have a greater density of apocrine glands compared with whites. It occurs more frequently in females than in males. The onset of hidradenitis suppurativa occurs in individuals aged 11-50 years.

Etiopathogenesis

The earliest change is follicular plugging, which obstructs the apocrine gland ducts and causes perifolliculitis around the ducts. Whether this initial inflammatory change is due to a bacterial infection or factors similar to those involved in acne formation is not known. In the later stages of hidradenitis suppurativa, bacterial infection seems to be a risk factor for the destructive scarring and extension of hidradenitis suppurativa lesions. Coagulase-negative staphylococci is the most commonly isolated bacteria.

The earliest inflammatory event in hidradenitis suppurativa is the rupture of the follicular epithelium. The rupture is followed by the spillage of foreign-body material into the dermis, which initiates an inflammatory response.

Clinical Features

The disease onset is insidious, with early symptoms of pruritus, erythema and local hyperhidrosis. The areas most frequently affected by hidradenitis suppurativa are the axillae and the groin. The extent and the severity of the disorder vary widely. Some patients have relatively mild forms of the disease that involve only one region. In many patients, more than one major site is involved. One or both axillae can be affected. In addition, the inguinal region can be involved, often with spread to scrotum, labia, mons pubis, mammary or perianal region and buttocks.

A firm pea-size nodule appears and may spontaneously rupture, yielding a purulent discharge. The lesion then heals with fibrosis and eventual recurrence in an adjacent area. The progression from non-inflamed nodules to painful, round, deep-seated lesions and subsequent scarring is highly diagnostic. The nodules tend to coalesce, and they may become infected, resulting in acute abscesses. These abscesses may temporarily resolve or alternatively, they may progress to multiple abscesses with persistent pain, fistula formation and scarring (Figure 25.6). Infected ruptured apocrine glands

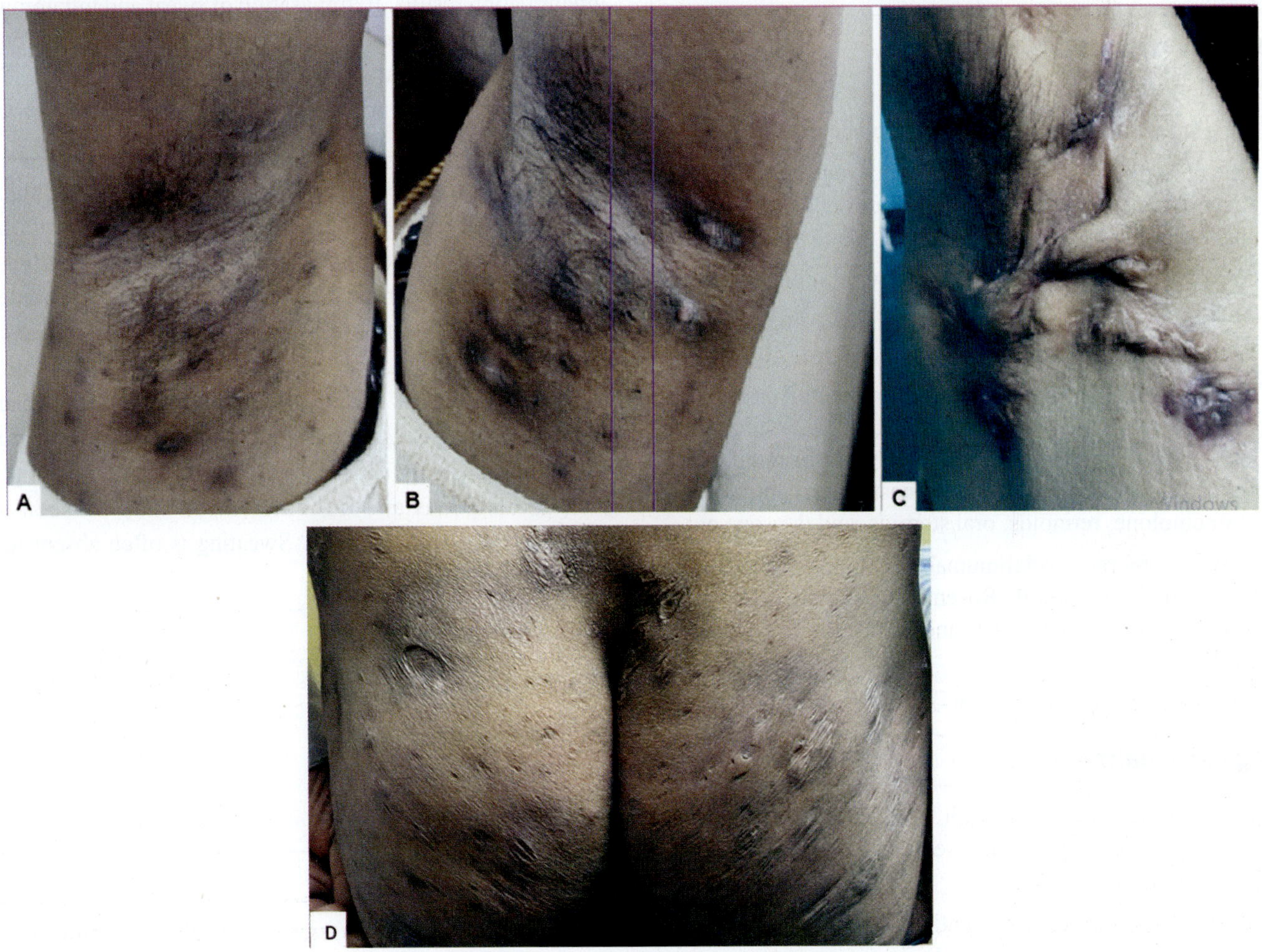

Figure 25.6: Hidradenitis suppurativa

coalesce, creating subcutaneous abscesses with discharge through multiple openings.

Differential Diagnosis

Actinomycosis, Erysipelas, Carbuncle.

STDs like syphilis, granuloma inguinale, LGV.

Staging (Hurley clinical staging)

Clinical staging of hidradenitis suppurativa has diagnostic value.

- The first stage is characterized by solitary or multiple, isolated abscess formation without scarring or sinus tracts.
- The second stage is characterized by recurrent abscesses, single or multiple widely separated lesions, with sinus tract formation and cicatrization.
- The third stage is characterized by diffuse or broad involvement, with multiple interconnected sinus tracts and abscesses.

Treatment

Treatment includes the following:

- Local hygiene.
- Weight reduction in patients who are obese.
- Use of ordinary soaps and antiseptic and antiperspirant agents (e.g., 6.25% aluminum chloride hexahydrate in absolute ethanol).
- Application of warm compresses with sodium chloride solution or burrow's solution.
- Wearing of loose-fitting clothing.
- Medical treatment includes anti-inflammatory, antibiotics (tetracycline, minocycline clindamycin, rifampicin, moxifloxacin, metronidazole, cotrimoxazole) or antiandrogen therapy (e.g., finasteride), intralesional triamcinolone, retinoids, oral steroids, and dapsone etc.
- Biologic therapy–Adalimumab is being used which has been found useful. Recently infliximab, etanercept, ustekinumab, secukinumab and anakinra are also being used.
- Phosphodiesterase 4 inhibitor–Apremilast.

Surgical Treatment

- Wide surgical excision, with margins well beyond the clinical borders of activity, remains the most definitive surgical therapy.
- More limited surgical intervention, consisting of unroofing abscesses and sinus tracts, with vigorous curettage of the base, and secondary-intention healing can be valuable in some cases. Electrosurgery is an alternative to be considered.

FOX-FORDYCE DISEASE

Fox-Fordyce disease is a chronic pruritic papular eruption that localizes to areas of apocrine glands.

Epidemiology

Fox-Fordyce disease is most common in women aged 13-35 years; it is rare before or after this age. A distinct predilection for women exists; the female-to-male ratio is 9:1. No racial predilection is evident.

Etiopathogenesis

The pathophysiology is formation of a keratin plug in the hair follicle infundibulum obstructing the apocrine acrosyringium and producing an apocrine anhidrosis. Histologically, a rupture of the apocrine excretory duct occurs and spongiotic inflammation results. Extravasation of sweat and inflammation is postulated to cause the intense itching. Heat, humidity and stress act as exacerbating factors.

Clinical Features

Fox-Fordyce disease frequently appears under conditions of heat, humidity and friction. Few patients are asymptomatic. Most patients have pruritus that disturbs sleep. Lesions are most often found in the axillae, where they tend to be bilateral. Lesions may also affect the periareolar, inframammary and pubic areas (Figure 25.7). The primary lesion is a flesh-colored to reddish, smooth, dome-shaped, discrete and follicular or perifollicular papule. Affected areas usually have many papules. The papules usually appear to affect every follicle in a given area. Excoriations and lichenification may be seen as a consequence of scratching. Sweating is often absent in the affected area.

Differential Diagnosis

- Acneiform eruptions.
- Folliculitis.
- Milia.
- Miliaria.

Treatment

Topical retinoids, topical steroids, antibiotics, clindamycin, ultraviolet light, dermabrasion, and surgical excision are the

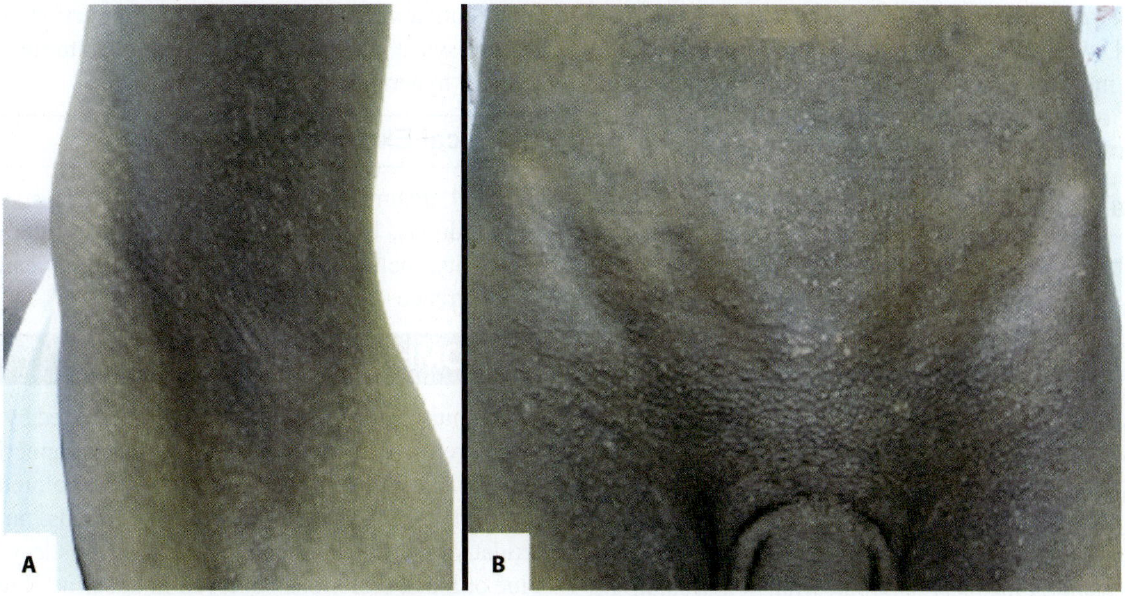

Figure 25.7: Fox-Fordyce disease

various treatments that have been used. Hormonal therapy for Fox-Fordyce disease with high estrogen oral contraceptives, estrogen creams, and testosterone creams has been reported.

BROMHIDROSIS (BAD SMELL IN SWEAT)

Apocrine Bromhidrosis

Apocrine bromhidrosis is the most prevalent form of bromhidrosis and should be differentiated from the less common eccrine bromhidrosis.

Axillary bacterial florae have been shown to produce the distinctive axillary odor by transforming non-odoriferous precursors in sweat to more odoriferous volatile acids. The most common of these are *Corynebacterium* species. Bacterial decomposition of apocrine secretion yields ammonia and short-chain fatty acids, with their characteristic strong odors.

Eccrine Bromhidrosis

In certain circumstances, eccrine secretion, which is typically odorless, assumes an offensive aroma and causes eccrine bromhidrosis. Ingestion of some foods, including garlic, onion, curry, alcohol, certain drugs (e.g., penicillin, bromides), metabolic disorders and toxins may cause eccrine bromhidrosis.

Epidemiology

Apocrine bromhidrosis is believed to be more common in patients in dark-skinned ethnic groups than in others.

Bromhidrosis exhibits a male predominance, which may be a reflection of greater apocrine gland activity in men compared with women. Axillary bromhidrosis depends on apocrine function and therefore manifests exclusively after puberty. It occurs only rarely in the elderly population.

Causes

- Inadequate hygiene and medical or dermatologic conditions associated with hyperhidrosis or overgrowth of bacteria may further contribute to its development, e.g., obesity, diabetes mellitus, intertrigo, etc.
- Nasal foreign body is a reported cause of generalized bromhidrosis in the pediatric population.
- Eccrine bromhidrosis may rarely be caused by metabolic disorders, primarily those with disturbances in amino acid metabolism (which include phenylketonuria, trimethylaminuria, isovaleric acidemia and hyper-methioninemia).
- Ingestion of certain foods, drugs or toxic materials may cause eccrine bromhidrosis.

Clinical Features

Patients present with particularly offensive body odor that most commonly originates from the axillary region. However, the condition may also occur as genital or plantar bromhidrosis. The odor has been described as pungent, rancid, musty or sour in character.

The skin appears normal, except when bromhidrosis is associated with concomitant skin conditions such as **erythrasma**, in which case a sharply marginated erythematous macular rash is seen, or **trichomycosis axillaris**, in which case concretions are visible on the hair in the affected area.

Differential Diagnosis

- Erythrasma.
- Trichomycosis axillaris.

Investigations

- If concomitant erythrasma, a chronic bacterial infection of *Corynebacterium minutissimum* is suspected, the skin has a characteristic coral-red fluorescence under Wood's lamp examination and a potassium hydroxide preparation is negative for fungal hyphae. In cases of trichomycosis axillaris, bacteria inside concretions from axillary hair are seen.
- If an underlying metabolic disorder is suspected as a cause of odor, specific testing of urine or sweat may be indicated to detect the aberrant amino acid product.

Treatment

Conservative measures, which aim to reduce bacterial florae and maintain a dry environment, include improved hygiene and topical therapy. Hygienic measures, such as adequate washing of the axillary vault, prompt removal of sweaty clothing, and the use of topical deodorant (which covers the odor and decreases bacterial counts) are beneficial in cases of apocrine bromhidrosis. Regular shaving of axillary hair prevents the accumulation of sweat and bacteria on the hair shafts. Use of topical antibiotics such as clindamycin and erythromycin and antiseptic soaps may yield clinical benefit by limiting the growth of the contributory bacteria.

Drying Agents

Measures to enhance drying and limit maceration, such as the use of antiperspirants including aluminum chloride, may improve bromhidrosis of either apocrine or eccrine origin, particularly if hyperhidrosis is a contributing factor. Iontophoresis, which disrupts sweat production, has a role in the treatment of eccrine bromhidrosis. Systemic anticholinergic agents decrease sweating, but they are not commonly used because of their significant adverse effect profile.

Lasers and Botulinum Toxin

A frequency-doubled, Q-switched Nd:YAG laser has been effective in axillary bromhidrosis. The inhibitory action of botulinum toxin A to decrease sweat production by denervating eccrine sweat glands has also been applied to successfully treat axillary hyperhidrosis.

Surgical Excision

Surgical treatment improves the long-term management of bromhidrosis, but it is associated with an increased risk of morbidity, including scarring, surgical complications and risk of recurrence.

CHROMHIDROSIS

Chromhidrosis is a rare condition characterized by the secretion of colored sweat. Chromhidrosis is usually apocrine in origin. Lipofuscin pigment is responsible for the colored sweat. This pigment is produced in the apocrine glands, and its various oxidative states account for the characteristic yellow, green, blue or black secretions observed in apocrine chromhidrosis.

In contrast, eccrine chromhidrosis is rare and occurs with ingestion of certain dyes or drugs. Pseudochromhidrosis occurs when clear eccrine sweat becomes colored on the surface of the skin as a result of extrinsic dyes, paints or chromogenic bacteria.

Epidemiology

Apocrine chromhidrosis appears to be more common in blacks than in whites, but facial chromhidrosis is described only in whites. No sexual predilection is reported. Chromhidrosis is noted after puberty, when the apocrine glands become active.

Clinical Features

Usually, patients report axillary staining of their undershirt and, less frequently, staining of the face or areola. Yellow is the most common color of axillary staining. An aura of warmth or a prickly sensation prompted by emotional or physical stimuli may precede the onset of colored sweat. Facial apocrine chromhidrosisis rarely described. It occurs most frequently on the cheeks and malar eminences. Clinically, odorless yellow, green, blue, brown or black and turbid secretion that can be manually expressed from apocrine-bearing skin, is seen.

Differential Diagnosis

- Hyperbilirubinemia.
- *Pseudomonas* infection Poisoning.
- Alkaptonuria.
- Contamination from *Corynebacteria*.
- Paint or clothing dye.

Treatment

Apocrine chromhidrosis has no fully satisfactory cure or treatment. Patients can manually or pharmacologically empty the glands to achieve a symptom-free period of about 48-72 hours or until the glands replenish the pigment.

A few reports have described successful treatment with capsaicin cream and botulinum toxin injections.

DISORDERS OF SEBACEOUS GLANDS

Sebaceous Hyperplasia

It is especially common in middle aged persons around 40 years of age with significant chronic sun exposure. Sebaceous hyperplasia is usually not seen in children. Premature sebaceous hyperplasia, also known as familial pre senile sebaceous hyperplasia presents with extensive sebaceous hyperplasia with onset at puberty and worsening with age. Familial patterns have been reported which is inherited in an autosomal dominant fashion. It involves the face, neck and upper thorax but spares the periorificial regions.

Treatment is solely for cosmetic purposes and employs electrosurgery, laser treatment, photodynamic therapy or even shallows have biopsy. Isotretinoin will reduce lesions, but they immediately recur when it is stopped.

SEBACEOUS NEVI

See Chapter 26.

ACNE

See Chapter 12.

Sebaceous Adenoma, Sebaceoma (Sebaceous Epithelioma), Sebaceous Carcinoma, Muir-Torre Syndrome

Sebaceous adenoma, sebaceoma (sebaceous epithelioma), sebaceous carcinoma, Muir-Torre syndrome (Sebaceous tumors of the skin associated with internal malignancy such as colonic adenocarcinoma) are the uncommon disorders of sebaceous glands of middle age and elderly people which are not commonly seen in children.

26

CHAPTER

Hair Disorders

Contents

- Congenital atrichia with papules
- Occipital neonatal alopecia
- Temporal triangular alopecia
- Aplasia cutis congenita
- Premature ageing syndrome
- Nevus sebaceous
- Traction alopecia
- Alopecia areata
- Tinea capitis
- Trichotillomania
- Telogen effluvium/anagen effluvium
- Morphea
- Folliculitis decalvans
- Pseudopelade of Brocq
- Hair shaft disorders
  - Trichorrhexis nodosa
  - Trichoschisis
  - Pili torti
  - Menkes syndrome
  - Trichorrhexis invaginata
  - Monilethrix
- Uncombable hair syndrome
- Woolly hair
- Hypertrichosis
  - Hypertrichosis lanuginosa
  - Circumscribed naevoid hypertrichosis
  - Hirsutism

Hair disorders are quite common both in childhood and adults. Many disorders are congenital and are attributed to inherited diseases or to defects of the ectoderm formation. The acquired disorders may be chronic or indicative of systemic disease. It is also important for both dermatologists and pediatricians to know the clinical pictures which although seem to be pathological, are normally present at infancy or in childhood. Hair disorders pose significant cosmetic problem with psychological implications for both parents and children and in adults suffering from them.

Hair can be divided into 3 regions: The lower segment (bulb and stem), the middle segment (isthmus), and the upper segment (infundibulum) (Figure 1.2). The lower segment extends from the base of the follicle to the insertion of the arrector pili muscle. The middle segment is a short section that extends from the insertion of the arrector pili muscle to the entrance of the sebaceous gland duct. The upper segment extends from the entrance of the sebaceous gland duct to the follicular orifice.

The follicular life cycle can be divided into 4 phases: Anagen, catagen, telogen and exogen (Table 26.1). The anagen phase is the phase of active growth. The catagen phase marks follicular regression, the telogen phase represents a resting period and exogen phase represents the shedding of hair. The length of anagen phase determines the length of hair and it differs according to heredity, age, sex, body region and follicular size. Both congenital as well as acquired causes can lead to hair loss (Table 26.2).

Table 26.1: Scalp hair cycle			
Phase	***Function***	***Scalp hair (%)***	***Average duration***
Anagen	Growth period	80-90	3 years (2-10 years)
Catagen	Transition phase	2-5	2 weeks (1-3 weeks)
Telogen	Resting period	10-20	3 months
Exogen	Shedding phase	-	-
Kenogen	Interval phase	-	-

Table 26.2: Causes of hair loss	
Congenital	***Acquired***
• Circumscribed hair loss • Aplasia cutis congenita • Epidermal naevus • Sebaceous naevus • Hair follicle hamartoma • Congenital triangular alopecia (Brauer naevus) • Vitamin D dependent rickets type II	• Circumscribed hair loss • Alopecia areata • Tinea capitis • Pyoderma • Lichen planus • Lupus erythematosus • Trichotillomania • Traction alopecia • Post traumatic alopecia (abrasions, burn) • Morphea • Keratosis pilaris atrophicans • Folliculitis decalvans • Dissecting cellulitis of scalp • Pseudopelade of Brocq
Diffuse hair loss	**Diffuse hair loss**
• Congenital atrichia • Ectodermal dysplasia • Photosensitivity disorders • Premature ageing disorders	• Telogen effluvium • Anagen effluvium • Nutritional: Hypervitaminosis A, zinc deficiency, marasmus • Endocrine: Hypothyroidism, hypopituitarism, hypoparathyroidism and diabetes mellitus • Androgenetic alopecia • **Chemical: Thallium poisoning, antithyroid drugs, heparin, coumarin, antimetabolites**

CONGENITAL ATRICHIA WITH PAPULES

Congenital atrichia or papular atrichia is a unique condition in terms of the hair loss pattern. Patients with congenital atrichia can be born with hair but shortly thereafter lose all their hair including eyebrows and eyelashes and it never regrows. Papular lesions are present over elbows and knees. These patients have normal physical and mental development with normal teeth and nails. It is due to mutation in gene present over chromosome 8p12, which plays a pivotal role in cellular transition from the natal to first postnatal hair cycle.

OCCIPITAL NEONATAL ALOPECIA (TRANSIENT NEONATAL HAIR LOSS)

Occipital neonatal alopecia (transient neonatal hair loss) is a common type of alopecia that develops in the occipital area in the first few months of life. It was previously wrongly attributed to friction of the head on the pillow but it is actually explained by an understanding of hair cycle patterns during the intrauterine life. The fetus normally undergoes synchronous shedding of scalp hair in the fifth month of fetal life. The regrown hair enters into the telogen phase in a wave from front to back, starting approximately 12 weeks before term. Most hair roots will have entered the anagen phase again before delivery. The occipital area is the last area in the scalp to enter the telogen phase and does not do so until birth.

Therefore, shedding of hair in occipital area during first few weeks of life is normal. Neonatal occipital alopecia regresses spontaneously.

TEMPORAL (CONGENITAL) TRIANGULAR ALOPECIA (BRAUER NAEVUS)

Temporal triangular alopecia is not a rare condition and is noted at 2-5 years of age as a well-circumscribed triangular or oval patch of alopecia that involves the temporal region. It is unilateral in most cases. Vellus, thin hairs are present in the affected area.

The condition is often mistaken for alopecia areata. However, histologic examination is not always necessary, because of the typical location, shape, presence of vellus hair and the absence of exclamation mark (dystrophic) hair. Temporal triangular alopecia is benign and there is no effective treatment.

APLASIA CUTIS CONGENITA

Aplasia cutis congenita is a rare condition, affecting newborns. There is a patch of hair loss with atrophic skin, usually occurring on the scalp. (Figure 26.1) Sometimes, in the affected area, vesicles or ulcers develop. Lesions range from a few millimeters to many centimeters in diameter. Aplasia cutis congenita has no clear cause and it can be associated with other developmental anomalies.

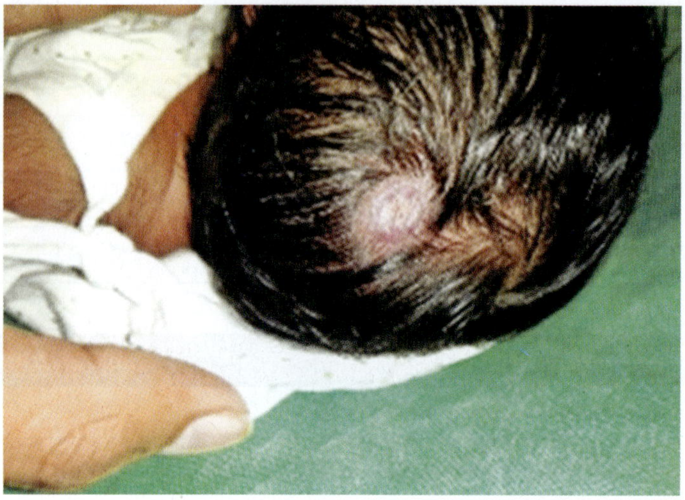

Figure 26.1: Aplasia cutis congenita

PREMATURE AGEING DISORDERS

Premature ageing disorders like progeria (Hutchinson-Gilford syndrome) and less commonly pangeria (Werner's syndrome) may show diffuse hair loss. Clinically, progeria (Figure 26.2) is characterized by a disproportionately large cranium with patent fontanelles and frontal bossing, prominent eyes and scalp veins, complete absence or very sparse, downy scalp hair, sparse or absent eyebrows and eyelashes, micrognathia, thin lips, a 'beaked' nose and mottled hyperpigmentation.

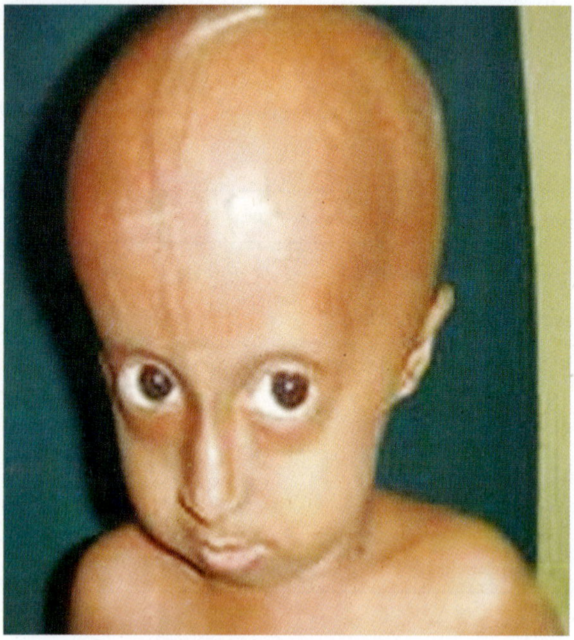

Figure 26.2: Progeria showing diffuse hair loss

NEVUS SEBACEOUS

Nevus sebaceous of Jadassohn is a common, solitary, benign congenital lesion that typically presents at birth or within the first few months of life. It occurs in approximately 3 in 1000 neonates. Most cases are sporadic, although rare familial cases have been reported. The pathogenesis is unknown and represents a hamartoma. The scalp is the most common location (50%), but other areas of the head and neck (45%) are also common. The trunk is involved in 5% or less of cases. Less common sites include the neck and extremities. It presents as a sharply circumscribed, yellow-orange, hamartoma varying from a few millimeters to several centimeters in size. Before puberty, it appears as an oval or linear, well-circumscribed hairless plaque of yellowish or orange papules on the scalp (Figure 26.3) or face. After puberty, the lesion enlarges, tends to show yellow-brown to brown colour, becomes verrucous and characteristic mature sebaceous glands are seen in the overlying epidermis. The lesions persist throughout life and usually cause alopecia. Numerous neoplasms, most of them adnexal, have been described arising in nevus sebaceous. The risk for tumor development increases with age.

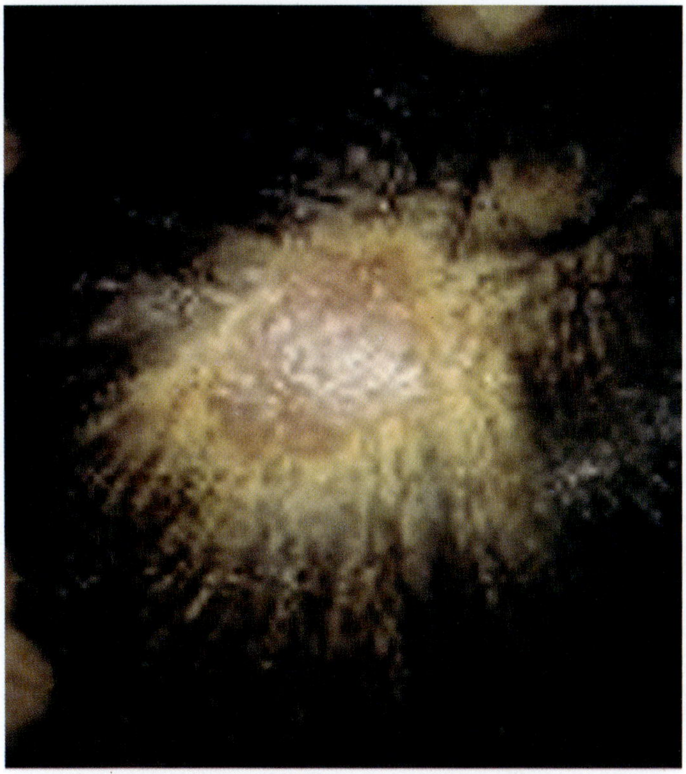

Figure 26.3: Nevus sebaceous

Prophylactic excision of a nevus sebaceous is controversial. Some investigators suggest surgical excision before puberty, because of the malignant potential and cosmetic considerations. Others suggest that prophylactic excision is not recommended.

TRACTION ALOPECIA

Traction alopecia is caused by prolonged traction of scalp hair by tight braids, pony tails and rollers. Although this condition is normally reversible, if the traction is continued over months to years, a chronic severe mechanical damage to hair follicles may result in permanent hair loss.

ALOPECIA AREATA (AA)

Alopecia areata is a localized loss of hair in circumscribed areas without any visible inflammatory signs. Almost all patients exhibit hair loss on the scalp, body and even on eyelashes and eyebrows. The disease onset in approximately 60% of patients is before the age of 18 years and affects both sexes equally. Approximately 1.7% of the population will experience an episode of alopecia areata during their lifetime.

Etiology

It is a chronic, organ-specific autoimmune disease, probably mediated by autoreactive T cells, which affects hair follicles. The exact cause is unknown. However, loss of immune privilege within hair follicles and subsequent immune dysregulation are central to its development. The following factors contribute significantly to its pathogenesis:

1. Heredity: Genetic factors play an important role in the etiology of AA and the genetic predisposition is polygenic in nature. There is a strong association with the genes of the HLA-DQ3, DR4 and DR11 regions. Approximately10-20% of patients give a family history of the disease.
2. Autoimmunity: There have also been reported associations between AA and classic autoimmune disorders, such as Hashimoto thyroiditis, vitiligo and/ or autoimmune polyglandular syndrome-I. AA is also common in Down's syndrome.
3. A variety of environmental factors, physical or psychological, has been suggested as 'trigger factors' such as emotional or physical stress, vaccinations, viral infection and medications.

Clinical Features

Patients present with a circumscribed area that is completely devoid of hair. The lesions are round or oval, bald, smooth without any signs of inflammation and may be singular (Figure 26.4A) or multiple (Figure 26.4B). The affected area is characterized in many cases by the intact hair and the pathognomonic **'exclamation-mark'** hair. Black dot or short hair, near margins of a patch of alopecia areata, represents the remaining tip/end of the broken hair. The

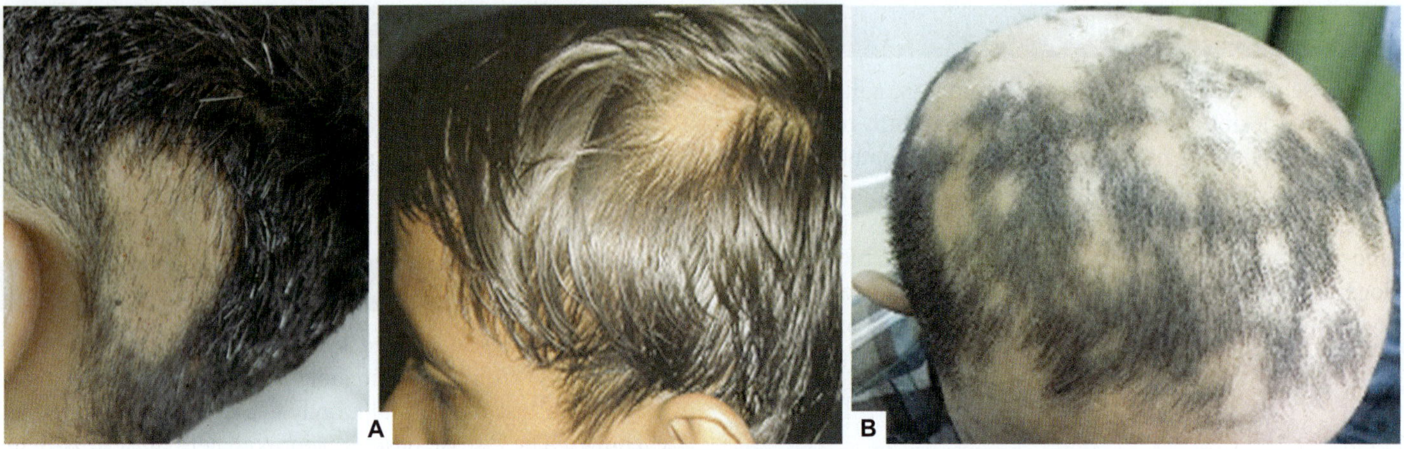

Figure 26.4: Alopecia areata (A and B)

dystrophic anagen or telogen hair has broader distal end than the proximal end.

Whenever a pull test at the margins of the lesion is positive, the disease is active. Clinical presentation of AA is subcategorized according to pattern as:

- **Patchy AA:** The most common form.
- **Ophiasis:** When the bald-like hair loss is located at margins of temporo-occipital area.
- **Diffused AA:** When an intense decrease in hair density is observed over the entire scalp.
- **Sisaipho:** Also called as ophiasis inversus, presents with alopecia involving the frontal, temporal, and parietal scalp but spares hair along the scalp periphery, mimicking androgenetic alopecia.

In addition, AA is subcategorized according to the extent of hair loss as alopecia totalis with complete loss of scalp hair, and alopecia universalis with total loss of all terminal hair on scalp and body.

Ikeda classification of AA is based on the associated conditions and on the course of the disease.

- **Atopic type:** It begins early in life and mostly (30-75%) progresses to AT.
- **Autoimmune type:** It is seen in middle-aged groups associated with autoimmune diseases, diabetes mellitus and progresses to AT in 10-50%.
- **Prehypertensive type:** It is seen in young adults whose parents were hypertensive and progress fastly to AT in 40% of cases.
- **Common type:** It affects adults aged 20-40 years and AT develops in 5-15% of cases.

Nail dystrophy often occurs with AA which is seen as fine pitting, red spotted lunula, trachyonychia, punctate or transverse leukonychia or onychomadesis.

Differential diagnosis includes tinea capitis, trichotillomania, triangular temporal alopecia, scarring alopecia (e.g., trauma), or circumscribed alopecia (e.g., nevus sebaceous and aplasia cutis congenita). Commonly it is to be differentiated from tinea capitis, which shows signs of inflammation, e.g., scaling, erythema, pustulation, swelling, etc. in most of the cases.

Management

Spontaneous remission is common in the majority of cases in patchy alopecia, although most patients experience recurrences.

Poor prognosis indicators are young age of onset (especially before puberty), a positive family history, extensive hair loss (ophiasis, alopecia totalis and alopecia universalis), atopy, the presence of other immune disorders and nail involvement.

In individuals with the usual type of AA (1-3 small patches) prognosis is fairly good and their hair are expected to regrow entirely within one year, even without treatment. However, approximately 30% of young patients will have a future episode of AA and 7-10% will have a severe chronic form of the disease.

There is no effective or specific treatment for AA. At present, all treatments are palliative and do not cure the disease. Many forms of local, systemic and combination therapies have been proposed. Topical, intralesional and systemic steroids, anthralin, minoxidil, psoralen and UVA treatment (photochemotherapy), cyclosporine and topical immunotherapy with contact sensitizers [diphenyl-cyclopropenone (DCP) and squaric acid dibutyl ester (SADBE)] are the main treatment modalities. Usually most of the patients respond to local corticosteroids in lotion form along with local 2% minoxidil. Patients with large number of patches, ophiasis pattern, recurrent disease will require systemic corticosteroids (8-16 mg of methylprednisolone in tapering dose) for 12-16 weeks.

The risks and benefits of all available treatments should be explained. Psychological support plays a crucial role in the overall therapeutic strategy. It is also of great importance to emphasize the probability of a spontaneous remission.

TINEA CAPITIS

Different patterns of hair loss in tinea capitis have been described in Chapter 5. It can lead to non-scarring (Figures 5.1 and 5.2) as well as scarring (Figures 5.4 and 5.5) alopecia.

TRICHOTILLOMANIA

Trichotillomania is classified as a compulsive disorder that commonly affects children, especially girls. The prevalence rate is between 0.5 and 3% of the population under 18 years of age.

Trichotillomania affects mainly the scalp. However, other terminal hairs of body can also be involved, especially of eyelashes and eyebrows. It is usually localized but sometimes widespread areas of alopecia are also seen. The clinical feature is most probably due to the common technique of twisting multiple strands of hair around fingers and pulling them simultaneously. This results in areas of alopecia that contain hair of varying length (Figure 26.5). Sometimes, skin of the involved area shows folliculitis and repeated trauma may result in small scars. The uninvolved areas appear completely normal.

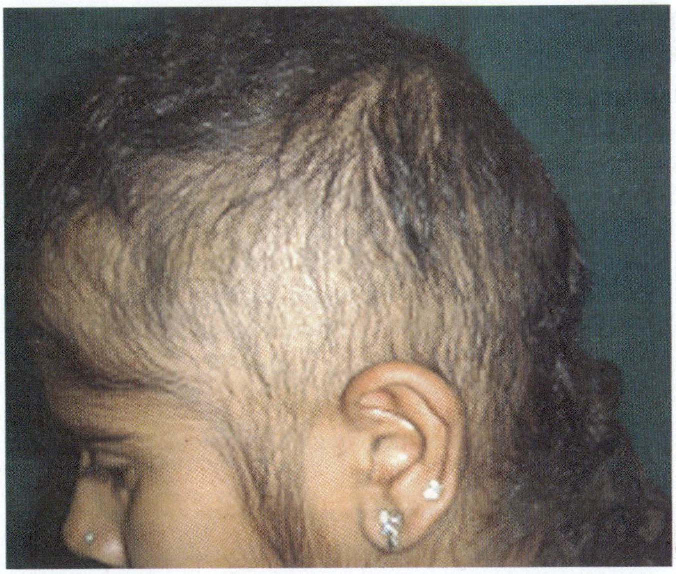

Figure 26.5: Trichotillomania

Differential diagnosis includes other conditions of non-scarring alopecia (Table 26.3). Shaving of a small area in the involved part of the scalp **('Hair window test')** and watching the normal regrowth of hair in this area, confirms the diagnosis of trichotillomania.

Typical histopathologic findings include pigment casts, catagen hair, deformed hair shafts (trichomalacia), perifollicular hemorrhage (in early lesions) and traumatized hair bulbs without significant inflammation or scarring.

On trichoscopy decreased hair density and broken hair at different length, short hair with trichoptilosis (split ends), irregular coiled hair, black dots, flame hair, V-sign, follicular hemorrhage, tulip hair and hair powder are seen.

Effective treatment of this obsessive-compulsive disorder is difficult. Psychotherapy with antipsychotic agents (e.g., selective serotonin reuptake inhibitors or clomipramine 100-200 mg/day) have been reported to be effective.

TELOGEN EFFLUVIUM/ANAGEN EFFLUVIUM

Telogen effluvium causes non-inflammatory, non-scarring, diffuse hair loss. There are five different functional types of telogen effluvium based on alternations in particular phases of the follicular cycle.

It has two clinical presentations:

1. **Acute Telogen effluvium:** It is defined as hair shedding lasting for less than six months. Generally, hair loss occurs two to three months after the trigger exposure and usually undergoes remission in around 95% of cases. A variant of acute telogen effluvium is telogen gravidarum, which is associated with pregnancy and usually occurs two to five months after childbirth
2. **Chronic Telogen Effluvium:** It is a condition lasting for more than six months. The disorder mostly affects middle-aged women, having a prolonged fluctuating course.

Pathogenesis: Telogen effluvium is caused by an abnormality in the normal hair cycle, which is triggered by numerous factors. The five proposed mechanisms by which shedding of the hair may occur in telogen effluvium are as follows:

- ***Immediate anagen release:*** This is due to an underlying cause. Follicles leave the anagen phase and enter the telogen phase prematurely, leading to increased shedding two to three months later.
- ***Delayed anagen release:*** This is due to prolongation of the anagen phase resulting in heavy telogen shedding.
- ***Short anagen syndrome:*** This is due to idiopathic shortening of the anagen phase, leading to persistent telogen effluvium. The pathogenesis behind most of the cases of chronic telogen effluvium is considered to be the short anagen syndrome.
- ***Immediate telogen release:*** This is due to the shortening of the telogen phase, resulting in a massive release of club hair.

- ***Delayed telogen release:*** This is due to a prolonged telogen phase and a delayed transition to anagen phase.

Causes of telogen effluvium: Various factors that can initiate disturbance in the normal hair cycle include:

1. ***Drugs:*** Numerous drugs can cause telogen hair loss and it usually starts after 12 weeks of dosage. Drugs that can cause telogen effluvium include oral contraceptive pills, androgens, retinoids, beta-blockers, ACE (angiotensin-converting enzyme) inhibitors, anticonvulsants, antidepressants, and anticoagulants (heparin).
2. ***Physiological Stress:*** Physiological stress during surgical trauma, high fever, chronic systemic illness, and hemorrhage can cause telogen effluvium. Childbirth can also cause excessive hair to enter the telogen phase.
3. Emotional Stress
4. ***Medical Conditions:*** Hyper- and hypothyroidism can cause telogen effluvium, and this is reversed once the euthyroid state is achieved. Chronic systemic disorders such as systemic amyloidosis, hepatic failure, chronic renal failure, inflammatory bowel disease, and lymphoproliferative disorders can also cause telogen effluvium. Some autoimmune diseases like dermatomyositis, chronic infections such as HIV and secondary syphilis and inflammatory disorders such as psoriasis and seborrheic dermatitis can also lead to diffuse telogen hair loss.
5. ***Dietary Triggers:*** Severe protein, fatty acid and zinc deficiency, chronic starvation, caloric restriction, reduced biotin, vitamin D and B12 levels can cause telogen effluvium.

Management: Acute telogen effluvium becomes self-limited if the triggering factor is identified and removed. The longer the duration of shedding, the more probable the involvement of multiple and repetitive triggers such as nutritional deficiencies, thyroid disease, systemic illnesses, or infections which should be identified and addressed.

Treatment includes correction of nutritional deficiencies, topical and oral minoxidil, topical and oral systemic steroids (especially if underlying disease like SLE is present, steroids can be used) and CNPDA comprises a combination of caffeine, niacinamide, panthenol, dimethicone, and an acrylate polymer.

In anagen effluvium, sudden loss of growing hair is caused by abnormal cessation of the anagen phase. Various toxins and antimetabolites trigger this diffuse process, which may involve upto 90% of scalp hair over several days to several weeks. The extent of hair loss is determined by the toxicity of the agent, and by the dose and length of exposure. In anagen effluvium, the hair shafts taper and loose adhesion to the follicle. This type of alopecia is most common after systemic chemotherapy.

Anagen effluvium must not be confused with loose anagen syndrome, an autosomal dominant disorder characterized by actively growing hair that are loosely anchored to the follicle and are pulled easily and painlessly from the scalp.

MORPHEA

Morphea can also progress in a linear pattern, particularly on the scalp, face and extremities. **En coup de sabre** describes a subset of linear morphea cases in which a furrow extends vertically from the scalp across the forehead and down the face. In the vicinity of en coup de sabre, scarring alopecia (Figure 26.6) ensues.

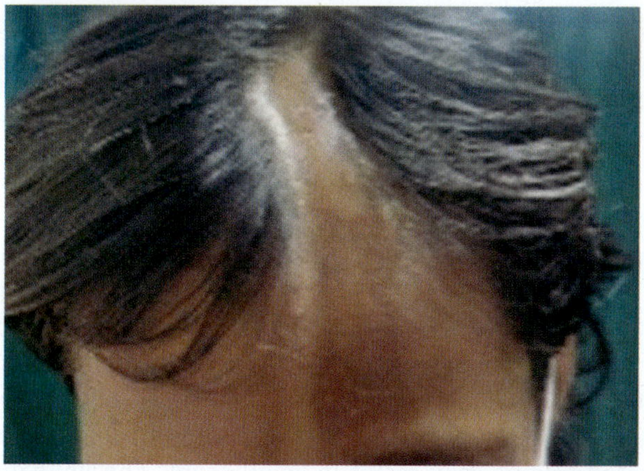

Figure 26.6: Linear morphea showing scarring alopecia

FOLLICULITIS DECALVANS

Folliculitis decalvans is characterized by progressive scarring (Figure 26.7) secondary to clinically evident chronic folliculitis. The cause of this condition is unknown. *Staphylococcus aureus* may be a possible etiological agent. The disease usually affects adolescent population. Clinically, following pustular folliculitis, rounded areas or patches of hair loss develop which are surrounded by crusting and pustular follicles. The condition should be differentiated from kerion type of tinea capitis.

Management includes topical clindamycin and prolonged courses of oral antibiotics, e.g., rifampicin, doxycycline, clindamycin, cipro-floxacin, etc.

PSEUDOPELADE OF BROCQ

Pseudopelade is chronic idiopathic cicatricial alopecia which is characterized by patchy hair loss with usually no evidence of inflammation. Pseudopelade of Brocq has been reported rarely in children, the onset most commonly occurs between ages 30 and 50 years. Females are affected by pseudopelade of Brocq more often than males.

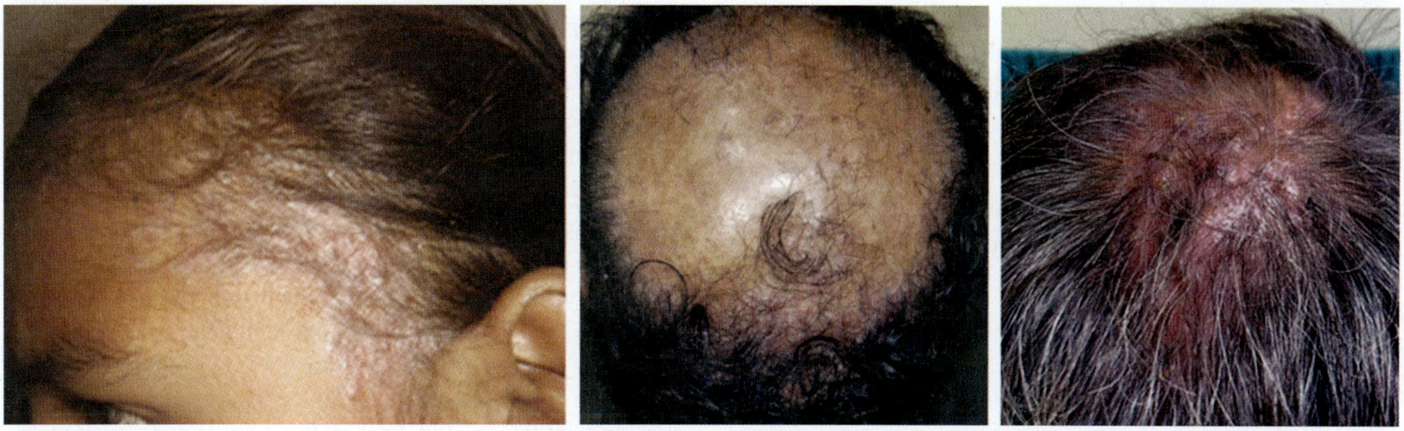

Figure 26.7: Folliculitis decalvans

The aetiology and pathogenesis are unknown. Some authorities believe that about 90% of cases of 'pseudopelade' are caused by lichen planus.

The typical pseudopelade of Brocq shows discrete asymptomatic areas of scalp hair loss (most commonly affecting the vertex and parietal scalp). Lesions of pseudopelade are randomly distributed, irregularly shaped, and often cluster in patches on the scalp. Cases with exclusive crown or vertex involvement actually may represent examples of burnt-out, central, cicatricial alopecia. The individual lesion is hypopigmented (porcelain white) and slightly depressed (atrophic). Pseudopelade of Brocq lesions often are shaped irregularly, as opposed to the round or oval patches usually seen in alopecia areata and most cases of central cicatricial alopecia. Pseudopelade of Brocq is slowly progressive disease. Disease progression in pseudopelade eventually ends spontaneously.

The alopecia is irreversible and does not respires to topical or intralesional corticosteroids. No treatment is known to arrest progression.

HAIR SHAFT DISORDERS

These abnormalities can be primary and hereditary or secondary. In table 26.3 causes of hair shaft defects are enumerated.

Table 26.3: Causes of hair shaft abnormalities

Increase fragility	*Without increase fragility*
Trichorrhexis nodosa	Pili annulati
Trichorrhexis invaginata	Woolly hair
Monilethrix	Acquired progressive kinking of hair
Pseudo monilethrix	Uncombable hair syndrome
Pili torti	
Pili bifurcati	
Trichothiodystrophy	
Marie-Unna hypotrichosis	
Mitochondrial disorders	

Trichorrhexis Nodosa

Trichorrhexis nodosa (Figure 26.8) is the most common defect of the hair shaft. Microscopically, affected hair develops a break in the cuticle with eventual separation and fraying of the exposed cortical fibers leading to a nodal swelling. The fibers then fracture and the shaft breaks.

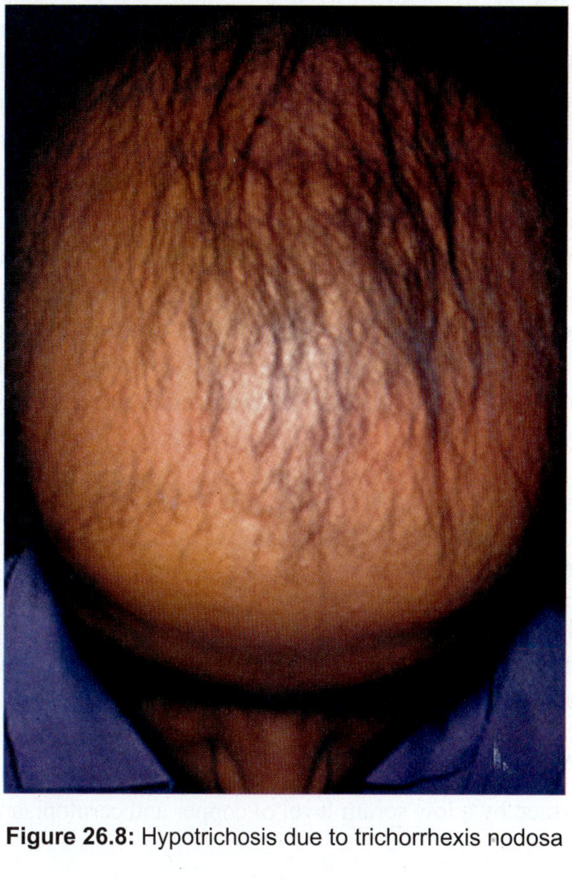

Figure 26.8: Hypotrichosis due to trichorrhexis nodosa

Congenital trichorrhexis nodosa may be present at birth or appear within the first few months following birth. The occurrence of congenital trichorrhexis nodosa should lead to an investigation of an underlying metabolic disorder (arginosuccinic aciduria and citrulinemia).

Acquired trichorrhexis nodosa is less common in childhood. Mechanical or chemical damage may trigger the response.

Trichoschisis or Trichothiodystrophy

Trichothiodystrophy is an autosomal recessive neuroectodermal disorder characterized by low sulfur content in hair and is caused by mutation of a regulatory gene involved in the repair and transcription of DNA. Clinically, brittle hair and trichoschisis are seen. Polarized light examination shows light and dark bands of hair shafts ('tiger tail' pattern), possibly due to the irregular sulfur content. The hair cystine and sulfur content is less than 50% of normal in both the cuticle and cortex. An amino acid analysis of the hair shaft confirms the diagnosis.

Pili Torti

Pili torti or 'twisting hair dystrophy' may occur as an isolated defect or in many different syndromes. Hereditary pili torti is usually autosomal dominant. It is present at birth or develops over the first few years of life. Patients have patchy alopecia with coarse, stubble or longer broken hair. Hereditary pili torti improve after puberty.

Children with this condition should have early testing for hearing loss. **Bjornstad syndrome** is an autosomal recessive disorder characterized by sensorineural hearing loss and pili torti. In addition, in **Crandall syndrome**, which is probably inherited as an X-linked recessive trait, congenital hypotrichosis with pili torti is associated with sensorineural deafness and hypopituitarism. Late onset pili torti presents after puberty and should be differentiated from patchy alopecia areata.

Menkes Syndrome

Menkes syndrome is an X-linked recessive disorder of copper metabolism. The defective gene is *ATP7A*, and the affected child has depigmented brittle hair, pili torti or trichorrhexis nodosa, pale lax skin, severe psychomotor retardation, neurologic abnormalities and growth failure. Diagnosis is confirmed by a low serum level of copper and ceruloplasmin.

Trichorrhexis Invaginata (Bamboo Hair)

Trichorrhexis invaginata is a distinctive hair shaft abnormality, characterized by the presence of nodes made up of 'ball and socket'.

If the shaft fractures, a golf tee-shaped distal end may occur. This deformity may be sporadic in normal hair or occur with other hair shaft abnormalities or, commonly, in association with ichthyosis linearis circumflexa in patients with Netherton's syndrome (NS). NS is a congenital ichthyosiform dermatosis caused by serine protease inhibitor SPINK5 mutations which contribute to the balance of serine protease inhibitors in the skin and influence skin barrier function and desquamation. Atopic manifestations are commonly present. The primary defect appears to be a disturbance of keratinization and the hair shafts of children are short, dry and fragile.

Monilethrix

Monilethrix is a rare inherited (autosomal dominant) condition with variable expression. This disorder is caused by mutations in the genes for type II hair keratins *hHb1* and *hHb6* on chromosome 12q13. Both *hHb1* and *hHb6* are largely co-expressed in cortical trichocytes of the hair shaft.

Monilethrix is characterized by dryness, fragility and sparseness of the scalp hair. Affected children usually have normal-appearing hair at birth, but within the first few months of life, this hair is replaced by brittle and fragile hair. Hair fibers have uniform elliptical nodes of normal thickness and intermittent constrictions. Microscopically, these elliptical nodes have a regular periodicity of 0.7-1 mm. The term 'regularly bended ribbon sign' has been suggested for describing the specific dermoscopic feature of monilethrix, that differentiates it from pseudomonilethrix and other causes of hair loss. Between nodes, the hair shaft usually fractures and hair rarely grows beyond 1-2 cm in length because of breakage. In most cases, the scalp is the only region involved and the disease is often associated with keratosis pilaris, physical retardation, cataract, syndactyly and nail/teeth abnormalities.

Monilethrix may improve spontaneously with age. Retinoids and topical minoxidil have been used in some cases.

UNCOMBABLE HAIR SYNDROME

Uncombable hair syndrome is noted any time from infancy to puberty, and may be autosomal dominant or sporadic.

Clinically, hair are dry, silvery, blond, shiny, slow growing, cannot be combed but not unduly fragile. On light microscopy, the hair shaft may appear quite normal but on scanning electron microscopy, the longitudinal grooves that make it abnormally rigid (triangular shape) and which accounts for the alternate term of 'pili triangulati et canaliculi', can be seen. In any event, this abnormality in the hair shaft is not specific, but can be seen in normal hair and in several types of ectodermal dysplasia.

Generally, there is no effective treatment for the syndrome. However, some cases improve spontaneously.

WOOLLY HAIR

Presence of tight curly hair on the scalp of non-Africans is a condition known as 'woolly hair'. It presents at birth or in infancy, being inherited either as autosomal dominant or recessive trait. A localized patch of woolly hair (Figure 26.9) woolly hair naevus, has an associated linear epidermal naevus in 50% of cases. Acquired curling can occur as a paraneoplastic manifestation or due to medications including antiretroviral therapy, etretinate, isotretinoin and interferons.

DISEASES HAVING INCREASED HAIR GROWTH

Hypertrichosis means growth of hair that is in excess for that age or site and is non-androgen dependent. Hypertrichosis may be congenital (hairy congenital naevi, hypertrichosis lanuginosa and familial hypertrichosis) or acquired. Acquired hypertrichosis may be due to medications or disease (Figure 26.10). Hirsutism is the result of the conversion of fine

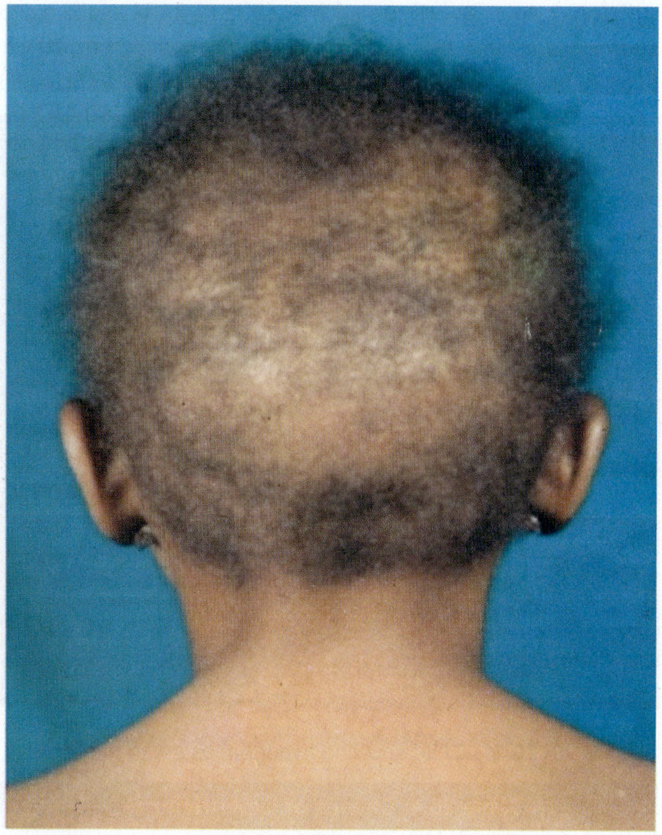

Figure 26.9: Woolly hair

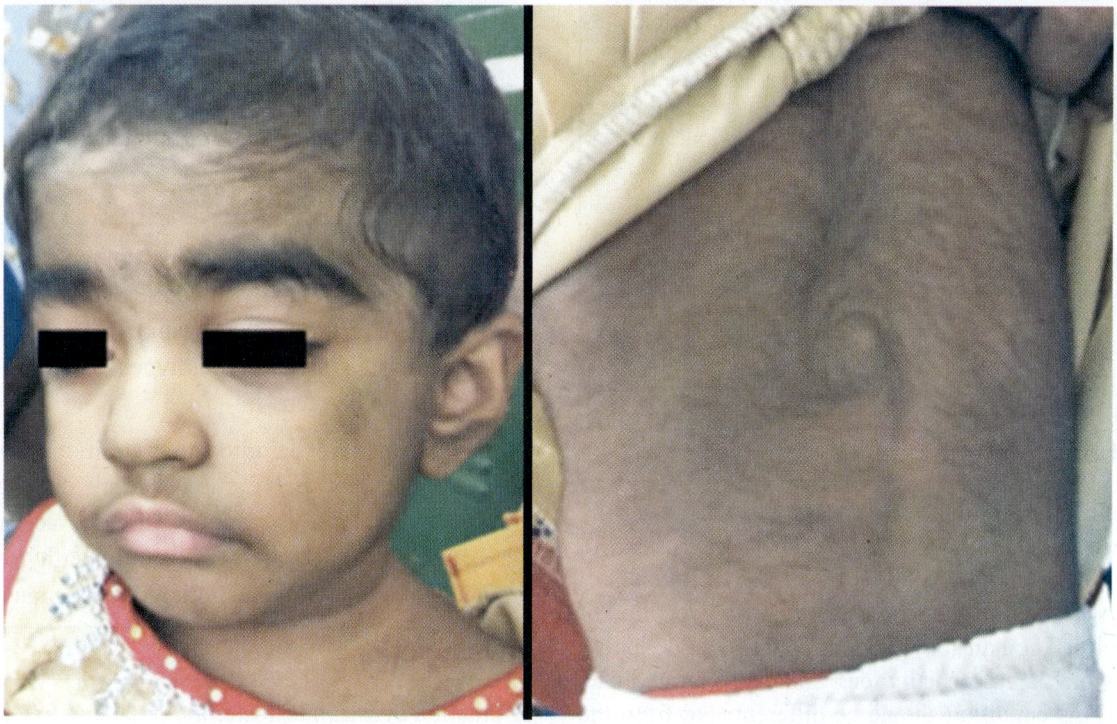

Figure 26.10: Cyclosporine induce hypertrichosis over face and back

vellus hair to coarse terminal hair (Figure 26.11) induced by androgens. These may be endogenous (adrenal, pituitary or ovarian origin) or exogenous (androgenic drugs) (Table 26.4).

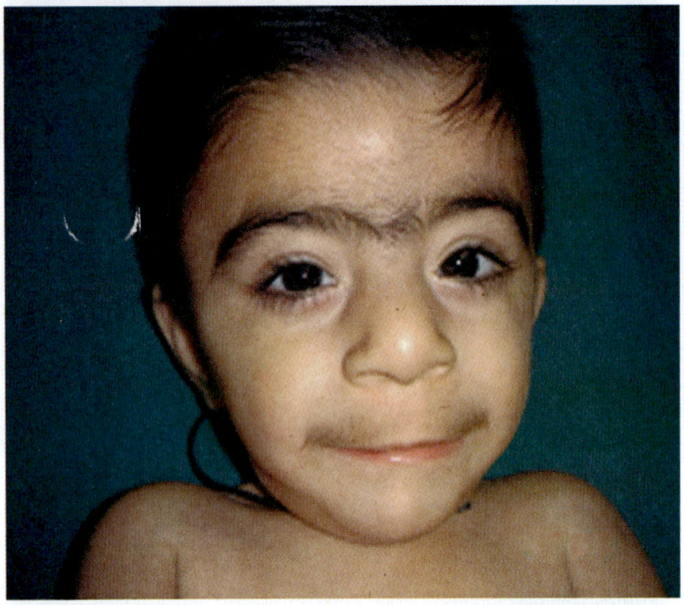

Figure 26.11: Child showing hypertrichosis with hirsutism

Table 26.4: Causes of hypertrichosis

Congenital hypertrichosis	*Acquired hypertrichosis*
• Congenital hypertrichosis lanuginosa • Ambras syndrome (Hypertrichosis universalis congenita) • Naevoid hypertrichosis • Congenital pigmented hairy naevi • Congenital smooth muscle hamartoma	• **Medications:** Minoxidil, corticosteroids (systemic and topical), ciclosporin, diazoxide, phenytoin, psoralens, acetazolamide, streptomycin, androgens, penicillamine • Hypothyroidism • Hypercorticism • Porphyria cutanea tarda • Acrodynia (mercury poisoning) • Juvenile dermatomyositis

Hypertrichosis Lanuginosa

This dominantly transmitted rare disorder is characterized by the persistence of fetal lanugo hair throughout life instead of replacement by vellus hair. Child is covered by profuse soft lanugo hair over most of the body surface, with exception of palms and soles. The hair may grow to a considerable length upto 10 cm which are especially long and dense around ears and nostrils. This condition should be differentiated from the normal lanugo hair of premature infant that are shed in a few weeks. Regular shaving, cutting, depilatories, electrolysis or laser helps to improve the appearance.

Circumscribed Naevoid Hypertrichosis (Faun Tail Nevus)

It is a developmental abnormality characterized by a tuft of long hairs in lumbosacral region, which may be associated with a spinal defect. It is characterized by long, coarse, darkly pigmented terminal hair present in the centre of lower back resembling animal's tail (Figure 26.12). The abnormality is important as it draws attention to the possibility of underlying spinal dysraphism.

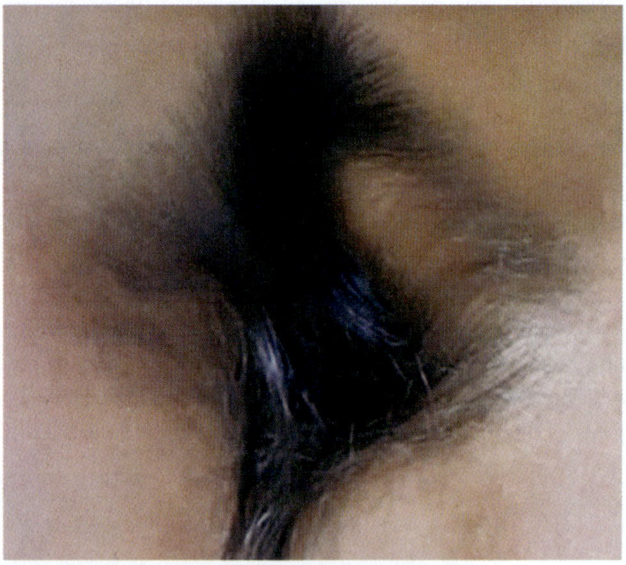

Figure 26.12: Faun tail nevus

Hirsutism (Figure 26.11)

Hirsutism is growth of terminal hair in male sexual pattern. It is observed predominantly in adolescent females. Along with increased hair growth other features of virilization such as increased muscle mass, clitoral hypertrophy and deepening of voice may also be seen.

Hirsutism may be idiopathic or it may be caused by diseases such as polycystic ovarian disease, congenital adrenal hyperplasia, Cushing's disease, adrenal adenoma, adrenal carcinoma, hypothyroidism, hyperthyroidism, hyperprolactinemia or by administration of exogenous androgens.

Investigations

Estimation of serum testosterone (total and free levels), serum cortisol (basal level and after dexamethasone suppression), serum17-hydroxyprogestrone, sex hormone binding globulin (SHBG), serum ACTH levels, serum androstenedione, serum 11-deoxycortisol, urinary 17-ketosteroids may be done, if indicated.

Treatment

Treatment of hirsutism depends on the underlying endocrine abnormality. Treatment options include decreasing androgen production by giving antiandrogens, spironolactone, combined contraceptive pills containing Ethinyl estrodiol and cyproterone or 50-200 mg cyproterone for days 1 to 10 of the menstrual cycle, finasteride, aldactone, flutamide and metformin in the setting of hirsutism associated with hyperinsulinaemia and insulin resistance.

Physical methods of hair removal are very popular which include:

- Shaving.
- Depilating cream.
- Waxing.
- Electrolysis.
- Lasers (Ruby, Diode, Alexandrite, Nd:YAG).

27 CHAPTER Nail Disorders

Contents

Nail disorders are not uncommon and may be due to physiological, congenital or acquired factors. There are several nail variants at birth, considered to be normal alterations. Although nail dystrophies are quite often a cosmetic problem, they may be important signs of congenital or systemic diseases.

MORPHOLOGICAL VARIATIONS IN NAILS

- Transverse depressions (Beau's lines).
- Fragile nails with transverse lamellar splitting at the free edge (Onychoschizia).
- Pits of the nail plate.
- Koilonychia (Spoon-shaped nails).
- Chevron nails (V-shaped ridging).
- Punctate leukonychia.

Transverse Depressions (Beau's Lines)

Normal infants between 8 and 9 weeks of age have a single transverse depression on the nail plate as a consequence of parturition. This depression grows out to the distal edge. Beau's line in all twenty nails presenting soon after birth appears to be associated with intrauterine distress. It is similar to hair loss due to telogen effluvium, commonly seen in newborns and their mothers.

Beau's lines are caused by temporary disruption in the growth of proximal nail matrix. Febrile illness, severe malnutrition, trauma, pemphigus, Raynaud's disease and anticancer therapy with drugs like vincristine, hydroxyurea, paclitaxel, etoposide, daunorubicin, bleomycin, cyclophosphamide, dacarbazine and methotrexate can be associated with Beau's lines. Thus a cause should be searched for and once it is removed, it resolves completely.

Fragile Nails with Transverse Lamellar Splitting at the Free Edge (Onychoschizia)

Onychoschizia is caused by the impairment of intercellular adhesive factors of the nail plate and thus the nail plate exfoliates into fine horizontal layers. Onychoschizia is common in the first few years and mostly noted on thumbs and big toes. Thumb sucking, nail biting and repeated trauma are thought to be the most common exacerbating factors in children. In adults, this type of nail fragility is almost exclusive to fingernails and it is typical of patients who wash their hands too frequently (e.g., homemakers, but also doctors and nurses). It may occasionally be observed in lichen planus or during etretinate or acitretin therapy.

Pits of the Nail Plate

Small and shallow or large and deep pits, involving few or all twenty nails may be normally seen in children. Pits of the nail plate may be caused by alterations in the proximal matrix.

Koilonychia (Spoon-shaped Nails)

Koilonychia is defined as concave dorsal surface of nail (Figure 27.1). This condition is common in neonates and early childhood, usually on the great toenails. It is caused by the fact that nails at this age are thin and soft. It resolves spontaneously in few years. There is a correlation between koilonychia and mild iron deficiency in infants. Although koilonychia is a temporary physiological condition in infants, it may also result from several congenital and acquired causes, such as ectodermal dysplasias, trichothiodystrophy, LEOPARD (lentigines, ECG abnormalities, ocular hypertelorism, pulmonary stenosis, abnormalities of genitalia, retardation of growth and deafness) syndrome, **nail-patella syndrome**, thyroid diseases, **Plummer-Vinson syndrome**, alopecia areata, psoriasis, lichen planus and Darier's disease, or may be idiopathic or traumatic.

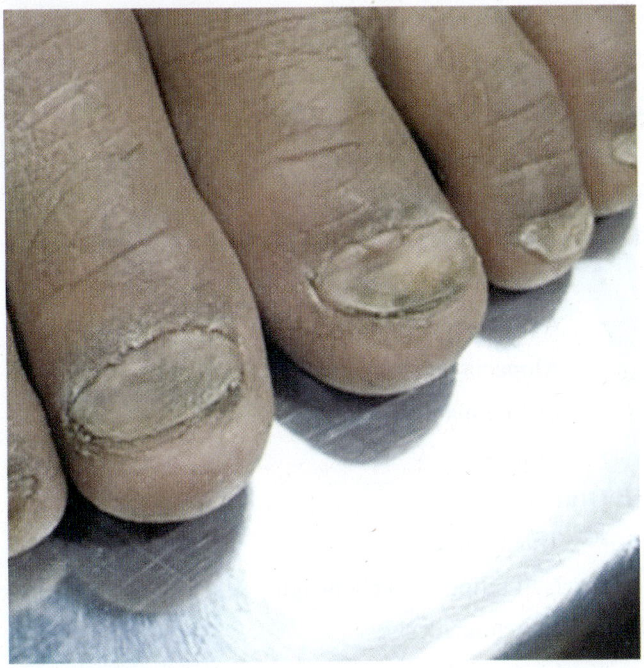

Figure 27.1: Showing koilonychia of toe nail

Chevron Nails (V-shaped Ridging)

Fingernails in early childhood often show superficial longitudinal oblique ridges, across the nail plate diagonally, from the matrix to the distal margin, forming a V-shaped pattern. Chevron nails remain of unclear significance and regress spontaneously in early adolescence.

Punctate Leukonychia

A few or numerous small white scattered opacities may be seen in nails. Trauma in the nail matrix area, is the most probable cause of this common condition.

NAIL DISORDERS IN NEWBORNS AND INFANTS

I. Deformities

- Anonychia
- Micronychia
- Polyonychia
- Congenital malalignment of the great toe nail
- Ingrowing toenail of infancy
- Racket nails

II. Nail changes associated with other cutaneous diseases

- Epidermolysis bullosa
- Pachyonychia congenita
- Dyskeratosis congenita
- Nail-patella syndrome

Anonychia

Anonychia refers to the absence of the nail plate and may be observed with autosomal dominant or recessive inheritance. Congenital anonychia of all nails is rare and is often associated with other ectodermal or mesodermal malformations (e.g., epidermolysis bullosa, DOOR [deafness, onychodystrophy, osteodystrophy and mental retardation] syndrome, Iso-Kikuchi syndrome [nail dysplasia involving index fingers. Nail changes include micronychia, polynychia, anonychia, malalignment or irregular lunula] etc.).

Micronychia

Micronychia is an unusual defect, characterized by a small nail plate, shorter or narrower than normal. When this deformity is congenital it is associated with syndromes or toxin exposure. The degree of micronychia may vary (e.g., Iso-Kikuchi syndrome, Zimmermann-Laband syndrome, Nail-Patella syndrome etc.).

Polyonychia

In this rare condition there are several nails on the same digit due to bifurcation of the distal phalanx. It may be seen also in polydactyly and syndactyly patients.

Epidermolysis Bullosa

Scarring (dystrophic) forms of epidermolysis bullosa may be accompanied by nail lesions. Abnormalities of collagen VII make the nail attachment vulnerable to mild trauma. Recurrent nail loss then leads to scarring and nail dystrophy, mainly of the great toes.

Pachyonychia Congenita

Thickening of the nail presents during the neonatal period with yellowish-brown discoloration. This condition is a consequence of subungual hyperkeratosis and is more evident on the distal part of the nails, which have an upward angling. Pachyonychia congenita is rare and diagnosis is based on family history and on other manifestations of the disease, such as foamy white mucosal plaques, symmetric thickening of the palms and soles, dry greyish spiny papules over the elbows, knees and other body surfaces.

Pachyonychia congenita has been classified into two variants:

- **Type I PC** has mutations in keratins 16 or 6a and show palmoplantar hyperkeratosis, extensive follicular hyperkeratosis and oral leukokeratosis.
- **Type II PC** has mutations in keratins 17 or 6b and show natal teeth, corneal dystrophy, hair abnormalities and steatocystoma multiplex.

Dyskeratosis Congenita

In dyskeratosis congenita, the nail plate is completely absent or hypoplastic. Pterygium formation may also be present. Other associated abnormalities are hyperpigmentation, leukoplakia, Fanconi-like anemia, blepharitis, keratoderma of the palms and soles and dental dystrophy.

Congenital Malalignment of the Great Toenail

The main characteristic of this condition is a lateral deviation of the nail plate from the longitudinal axis of the distal phalanx. The most important complication of this situation is an ingrowing painful toenail. Spontaneous improvement occurs in approximately 50% of patients. Treatment depends on the degree of malalignment and on the associated changes. Surgical procedures offer the best results.

Ingrowing Toenail in Infancy

Infantile ingrowing toenails are thought to have a congenital origin. It's a benign painless condition. The thin, sharp edge of the great toenail embeds into the hypertrophic lateral nail folds of the hallux, often bilaterally and usually appears at birth. This condition improves spontaneously with age.

Racket Nails

Racket nails are broad and shortened, and reflect an underlying disturbance in the formation of distal phalanx, which may be inherited.

Nail Patella Syndrome

This genodermatosis is an autosomal dominant disorder due to mutations in the LMX1B gene with variable expressivity, where nail abnormalities are associated with bone and renal disorders. The nail abnormalities are recognized at birth and include micronychia or anonychia, especially on the thumbs. The lunula can be triangular or V-shaped which may be pathognomonic for this condition. The patella is aplastic or luxated in 90% of patients. Other bone changes include scapular hypoplasia, scoliosis and hypoplastic lateral humerus epicondyle.

COMMON DISEASES CAUSING NAIL CHANGES

I. Infective

- Acute paronychia
- Chronic paronychia
- Herpetic whitlow
- Blistering distal dactylitis
- Onychomycosis

II. Cutaneous diseases with nail changes

- Eczema
- Acropustulosis
- Alopecia areata
- Lichen planus
- Psoriasis

III. Others

- Trachyonychia
- Nail biting (Onychophagia)
- Onychomadesis
- Leukonychia
- Melanonychia
- Tumors

Acute Paronychia

Acute paronychia may present as a symptom of nail biting or other local injuries. It is caused by *Staphylococcus aureus* less often by Gram-negative organisms *(Pseudomonas, proteus)* and herpes simplex virus (HSV). This condition presents with pain in distal phalanx followed by redness, swelling and abscess formation. Soft tissue changes subsequently may lead to onycholysis, Beau's lines or onychomadesis. Distal phalanx may also be involved in impetigo. Vesiculopustules with honey crusted lesions, usually due to β-hemolytic streptococci, is the pathognomonic clinical feature.

Infection by HSV is distinguished by grouped vesicles containing clear fluid that becomes turbid, although rarely purulent. Tzanck smear reveals multinucleated ballooned giant cells that establish the diagnosis. It is recurrent in nature.

Topical and systemic antibiotics or antiviral agents should be administered to treat each episode.

Chronic Paronychia (Figure 27.2)

Chronic paronychia is a difficult but very common problem, especially in children who are thumb suckers and nail biters. It presents as a dull-red swelling of the nail fold, which is indurated and raised, with loss of the cuticle margin. It is commonly caused by yeasts, *Candida albicans* being most common.

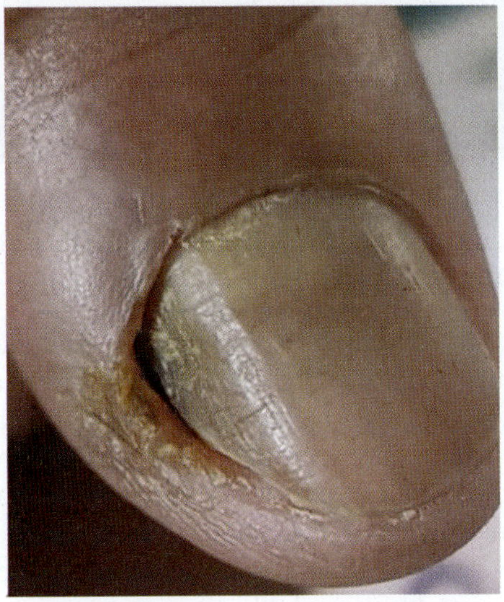

Figure 27.2: Chronic paronychia

Herpetic Whitlow

Herpes simplex infection, mainly due to HSV-1 in children, may affect the terminal phalanx of the finger and produce acute, painful paronychia with vesicular eruption, surrounded by an erythematous border. The vesicles often coalesce into large, honeycombed bullae and which may be located in the nail bed, sometimes leading to onycholysis.

In most cases, this condition is secondary to autoinfection with HSV gingivostomatitis, as a result of nail biting or finger sucking. Herpetic whitlow must be differentiated from other vesiculopustular eruption (e.g., impetigo, blistering distal dactylitis and Hallopeau's acrodermatitis). Oral acyclovir is the treatment of choice and may prevent recurrences.

Blistering Distal Dactylitis

Blistering distal dactylitis, which is caused by β-hemolytic streptococci, affects the fingers of children, aged 2-16 years. This condition is characterized by large painful tense blisters, with purulent content, at the tip of the digits. Topical antiseptics and systemic antibiotics (e.g., erythromycin, amoxicillin, flucloxacillin, dicloxacillin and cloxacillin) are the treatment of choice.

Nail Biting (Onychophagia)

Two-thirds of children under 12 years of age bite their nails. The causes suggested for nail biting include anxiety, stress, loneliness, imitation of a family member, hereditary, inactivity and transfer from a thumb sucking habit.

Nail biting involves one, many or all nails. Nail biters more often bite the periungual skin and, therefore, paronychia, distal ingrowing and periungual warts are the most frequent complications. The nails appear short and irregular. Longitudinal melanonychia due to activation of matrix melanocytes is a consequence of this habit. Application of distasteful topical preparations (solutions) discourages children from biting their finger nails.

Onychomadesis

Onychomadesis is the complete separation of the nail plate from the nail bed, beginning at the proximal nail fold that induces nail shedding. Severe intrauterine distress may be a cause of onychomadesis in infants, although idiopathic familial onychomadesis has also been reported.

When it is inherited as a dominant trait, shedding may be periodic. In addition, when this condition affects most or all nails, it usually results from generalized diseases, such as chicken pox bullous dermatoses, acrodermatitis enteropathica, Kawasaki disease, measles, hand foot mouth disease, Stevens-Johnson syndrome, Lyell's syndrome, high fever or due to drugs, etc.

Onychomadesis limited to one or few digits or the toenails is usually caused by trauma, eczema or paronychia.

Leukonychia

White nails (leukonychia) are the most frequent form of chromonychia. In this condition, nails are partially or totally milky, ivory or porcelain white (Figure 27.3) in color. This disorder can be temporary or permanent, depending on their etiology which may be idiopathic or caused by a large number of diseases, both congenital and acquired or drug induced (e.g., Leopard syndrome, Kawasaki disease, Darier's disease, anemia, zinc deficiency, alopecia areata, psoriasis, drugs like sulfonamides and retinoids, etc).

Leukonychia is classified into three categories, based on clinical characteristics and underlying pathology:

1. **True leukonychia,** since the nail plate is white and the white hue shifts towards distal end, as it grows. This occurs due to persistence of parakeratotic cells in nail plate because of defective distal nail matrix. True leukonychia has three different variants, diffuse, punctate and striate.

2. **Apparent leukonychia,** white discolouration fades away when pressure is applied because the abnormality is in the nail bed. It can be divided into several categories based on the clinical features:

   Terry's nails, a condition frequently seen in liver cirrhosis, congestive heart failure, and diabetes mellitus patients, affecting the whole nail, sparing 1-2 mm pink to brown distal band.

   Half and half nails (Lindsay's nails) are seen in chronic renal disease patients who are on haemodialysis. The nails appear proximally opaque white while distal portion is pink or reddish brown with clearly defined boundary.

   Muehrcke's lines, nails show several transverse white bands running parallel to the lunula. It is seen in patients with hypoalbuminemia and liver cirrhosis, but now it is also frequently observed following chemotherapy.

3. **Pseudoleukonychia**, a condition in which whitening of the nails has an external cause, such as white superficial onychomycosis (WSO).

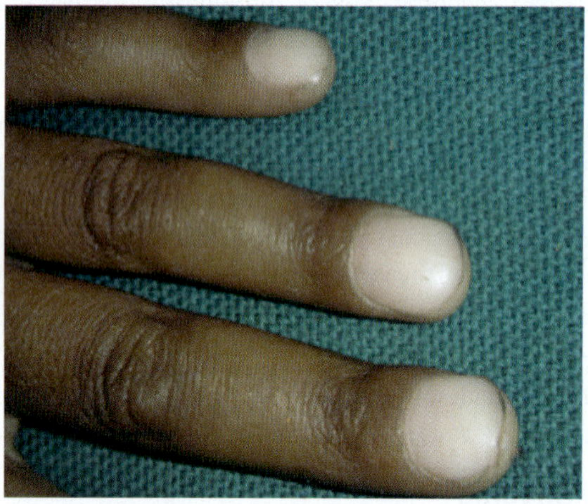

Figure 27.3: Total leukonychia

Melanonychia

Melanonychia is characterized by the presence of a brown or black color change of the nail plate. Many causes induce this discoloration, including nevi, drugs, hemorrhage, onychomycoses, dyes, Peutz-Jeghers-Touraine syndrome, Addison's disease and, the most serious, malignant melanoma.

Longitudinal melanonychia (Figure 27.4) may be caused by activation or hyperplasia of the nail matrix melanocytes. In children, the most common cause of longitudinal melanonychia is a nail matrix nevus. Most of the nevi in children are junctional. Hutchinson's sign, periungual soft tissue extension of brown black pigmentation from longitudinal melanonychia. Dermoscopy is a useful method for differentiating between nevi, melanoma and hemorrhages of the nail apparatus.

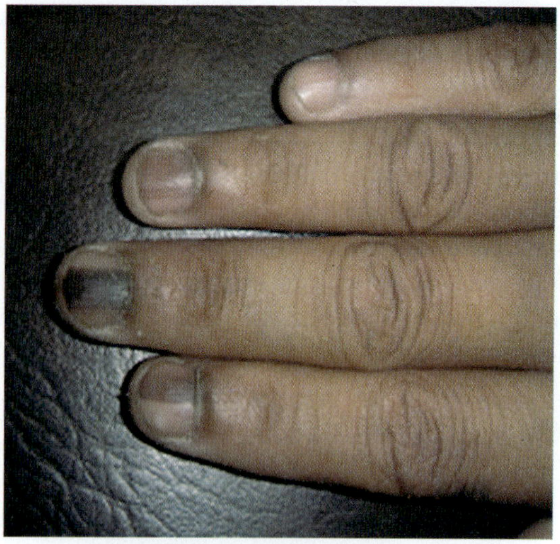

Figure 27.4: Melanonychia

Trachyonychia (Twenty Nail Dystrophy)

Trachyonychia describes a spectrum of nail-plate surface abnormalities that give the nail plate a rough appearance known as sand paper nails. This condition usually occurs sporadically, affects few or all twenty nails (Figures 27.5). It may be idiopathic or associated with alopecia areata, psoriasis, lichen planus, ichthyosis vulgaris and atopic dermatitis etc. It may present as a self-limiting condition in childhood or as a more chronic problem in adulthood.

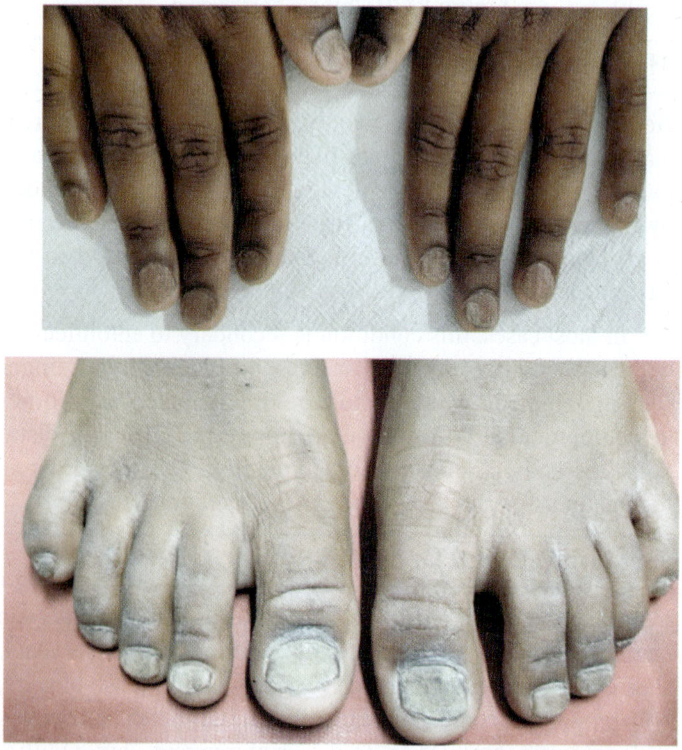

Figure 27.5: Twenty nail dystrophy

Two clinical varieties of trachyonychia have been described:

- **Opaque trachyonychia:** The nails are thin, opaque and give the impression of having been sand papered in a longitudinal direction. Some degree of koilonychia is often present.
- **Shiny trachyonychia:** The nail plate is shiny with opalescent longitudinal ridging. This variety is less severe.
- Trachyonychia is generally a benign condition which does not cause permanent nail damage and tends to regress spontaneously over the years. Associated skin lesion often guides to the diagnosis. Biopsy is not much helpful. No standard treatment protocol is there except frequent and generous application of emollients. Topical 5-fluorouracil and steroids have been tried.

Eczema

When eczema affects the phalanx and periungual skin, it causes inflammation of the nail matrix and therefore leads to pitting, Beau's lines and transverse ridges of the nail plate (Figure 27.6). The proximal and lateral nailfolds may be red and swollen. Small vesicles, loss of cuticle, acute or chronic paronychia may also be present.

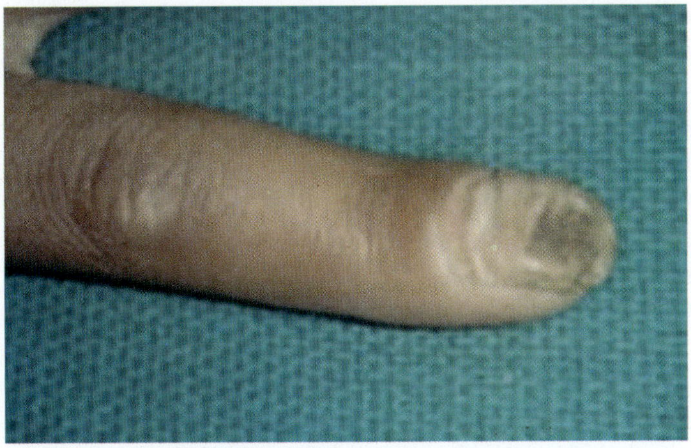

Figure 27.6: Nail changes in eczema

Psoriasis (Figure 27.7)

Psoriasis of the nails is quite common, seen in 7 to 40% of patients with psoriasis and varies in severity. Nail changes include pitting onycholysis, subungual hyperkeratosis, yellowish green-brown spots under the nail plate (oil spot), splinter hemorrhages, multiple transverse grooves, splits, atrophy, fragility and trachyonychia (roughened nail). Periungual involvement may be severe, giving rise to a disruption of the nail matrix. The nail fold may be scaly and the cuticle is lost.

Treatment of nail psoriasis is challenging. Topical calcipotriol or topical/intralesional steroids and topical calcineurin inhibitors with or without occlusion are, however, moderately effective.

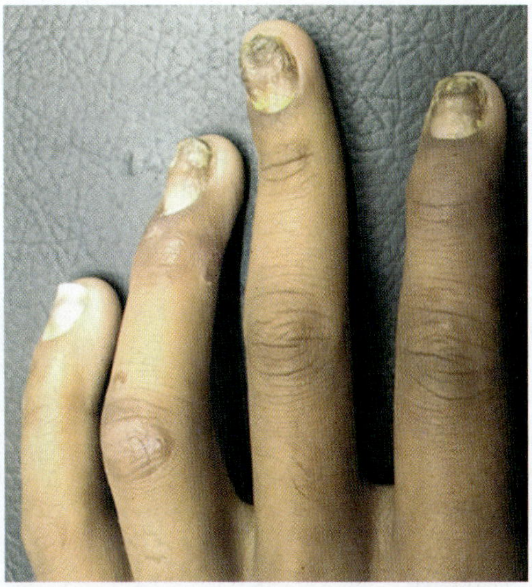

Figure 27.7: Psoriasis of nail showing deformity, onychodystrophy and color changes Psoriasis showing pitting of nails

Acropustulosis (Acrodermatitis continua of Hallopeau)

Acropustulosis is a clinical variant of psoriasis which affects few or only single digits, especially in young girls. It is characterized by relapsing pustular eruptions. Often suppurative process begins with the formation of crops of pustules on an erythematous base, particularly on the fingertips, rarely, on toes. Nails of the involved digits may show onycholysis, subungual hyperkeratosis or partial nail-plate destruction. Pustulation of the nail bed and nail matrix may lead to severe onychodystrophy or onychomadesis. The distal pulp in most of cases shows mild erythema and scaling. It is often misdiagnosed as onychomycosis. Acropustulosis usually regresses spontaneously, although some children may develop nail psoriasis later. Moderate to potent topical steroid is the treatment of choice but recurrences are common.

Alopecia Areata (AA)

Fine pitting, fragile distal edge, roughened surface ('sand paper nail' or trachyonychia), onychomadesis and loss of lunula are present in 10-66% of children with AA. Pits on the nail plate are finer and closely set than those in psoriatic nails. Nail involvement is generally considered a bad prognostic marker for alopecia areata.

Lichen Planus

Lichen planus of the nails is potentially scarring condition and may overlap with the twenty nail dystrophy. Lichen planus affects fingernails more frequently than toenails and the most common changes include slight thinning of the nail plate, longitudinal ridging of nail plate, brittleness, onychorrhexis, and transient or permanent longitudinal melanonychia. Rarely, a fibrotic band of tissue fusing the dorsal nail fold with the nail bed, causes irreversible partial destruction of the nail plate (Pterygium unguis, Figure 27.8). Onychoscopy and nail matrix biopsy can aid in diagnosis.

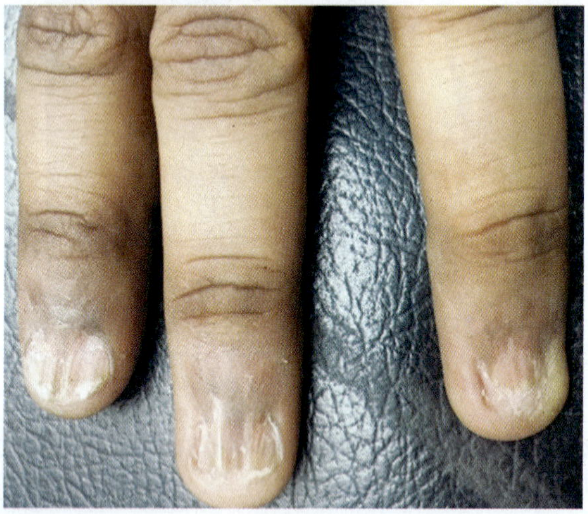

Figure 27.8: Pterygium unguis

Onychomycosis (OM)

Onychomycosis is rare in early childhood, with an estimated prevalence of 0.2% of all fungal infections in childhood. The age range for onychomycosis in children is 6-14 years of age. Older children and teenagers are affected more frequently.

Candidal onychomycosis: Biting or sucking of digits in the first few months of life can lead to maceration of the digits and exposure to *C. albicans*. The fingernails are usually affected and the nail-fold inflammation leads to deformity of the nail plate, appearing as irregular Beau's lines, opaque milky white or yellow-brown discoloration, thickening and onycholysis. The disease of newborns resolves spontaneously in majority, in a few months and rarely tends to be chronic. Chronic candidal OM involving all nails may be an indicator of chronic mucocutaneous candidiasis (CMC).

Dermatophyte onychomycosis: Dermatophyte OM which occurs in children after the age of 6 years, usually presents with distal thickening and yellowish white discoloration (Figure 27.9) of the free edge of the nail and subungual hyperkeratosis. Distal lateral subungual onychomycosis (DLSO) is due to infection with *Trichophyton rubrum*. This feature is attributed to the subungual accumulation of friable keratinous debris and entrapment of air between the nail plate and nail bed due to onycholysis.

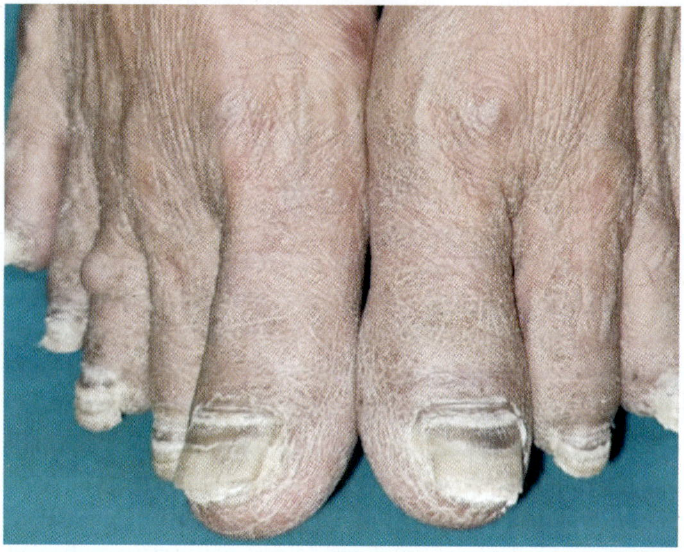

Figure 27.9: Onychomycosis

Proximal subungual onychomycosis occurs when the cuticle of the proximal nail fold is disrupted, and fungal invasion occurs. It is extremely uncommon in children.

Superficial white onychomycosis appears as a white, sharply outlined area on the nail plate and is more common. It is frequently due to *T. mentagrophytes* and usually involves one-to-two digits.

Total dystrophic onychomycosis is used to describe end stage nail onychomycosis. The entire nail unit becomes thick, crumbled, friable and dystrophic.

Endonyx onychomycosis is an unusual variant of onychomycosis with invasion of fungal elements or hyphae into nail plate without resulting nail bed hyperkeratosis ,onycholysis, or inflammatory changes. Endonyx onychomycosis is clinically present as diffuse milky white discoloration of nail plate due to invasion by T. soudanense.

A careful clinical examination is required, as a fungal skin infection can usually be detected elsewhere (tinea pedis or tinea of the scalp mostly). Potassium hydroxide (KOH) examination and culture of the subungual debris on Saboruad's Dextrose Agar medium, confirms the diagnosis. Demonstration of fungal hyphae in onycholytic nail plate histology by PAS staining is the most sensitive diagnostic test.

Extensive OM raises suspicion for immunosuppression, such as CMC or HIV infection. Psoriasis, lichen planus, twenty nail dystrophy, trauma and alopecia areata mimic OM and should be considered in the differential diagnosis.

Treatment of OM in childhood is similar to that in adults and usually requires systemic antifungal agents. However, as children appear to respond faster than adults, there is a tendency to use topical therapy, including ciclopirox 5% lacquer or imidazoles.

Itraconazole (5 mg/kg/day), terbinafine (3-4 mg/kg/day) and fluconazole (6 mg/kg/day), for 6 weeks for fingernail infection and 3 months for toenails, have been used.

NAIL TUMORS

Suspicion of a nail tumor should arise particularly when only one nail is involved. Dermoscopy and nail imaging are helpful in diagnosis. Histopathology remains as the gold standard method. Depending on origin and aggressiveness of lesion, different therapeutic approaches should be applied. Surgical exploration is the treatment of choice for most of the nail tumors.

1. Soft tissue tumor of nail	**Fibrous tumors** • Acquired ungual fibrokeratoma • Koenen tumour • Subungual filamentous tumor • Fibromas • Keloid **Vascular Tumors** **Benign:** • Pyogenic Granuloma • Glomus Tumor • Hemangiomas **Malignant:** • Kaposi Sarcoma **Tumor of Peripheral Nerves** • Neuroma • Neurofibroma • Swannoma **Osteocartilagenious Tumor** • Subungual Exostosis • Osteochondroma • Enchondroma **Synovial Tumor** • Giant Cell tumor • Ganglion **Lipomatous & Myxomatous Tumors** • Lipoma • Superficial Acral fibromyxoma
2. Epithelial Tumor	**Benign Tumors** • Onychopapilloma • Distal Digital Keratoacanthoma • Onychomatrichoma • Subungual Epidermoid Inclusions **Rare** • Syringoma • Eccrine Poroma • Eccrine Syringofibroadenoma • Ungual Seborrheic Keratosis • Subungual Warty Dyskeratoma **Malignant Tumors** • Squamous cell carcinoma • Bowen disease of the nail apparatus • Verrucous carcinoma (epithelioma cuniculatum) • Basal cell carcinoma • Sweat gland carcinomas • Sebaceous gland carcinoma
Pseudotumors	• Warts • Digital Myxoid Pseudocyst

Contd.

Few important nail apparatus associated tumors are described below.

Glomus Tumor

It is a benign vascular hamartoma which originates from neuromyoarterial cells of normal glomus apparatus in reticular dermis. It accounts for about 1-2% of soft tissue tumor of hands in women.

Patients may present with a triad of symptoms i.e. temperature sensitivity, severe localized pain and localized tenderness. Tumors are seen as painful small bluish to reddish spots through nail plate or as longitudinal erythronychia with distal notching. Subungual area is the most common site of glomus tumor.

Clinical tests for diagnosis of glomus tumor:

1. **Cold sensitivity test:** Most accurate test, performed by applying ice cube to the affected area.
2. **Love's pin test:** A pinhead is used to apply gentle local pressure to the painful area as indicated by patient subjectively, which usually increases the pain.

3. **Hildreth's test:** Applying a tourniquet to the upper arm can cause transient ischaemia, resulting in a temporary period of reduced pain that quickly returns after the tourniquet is removed.
4. **Transillumination test:** When light is thrown through finger pad in a dark room, an opaque red image is seen at the site of tumor and also allows assessment of the size of tumor.

   High resolution MRI and HVFUS (High variable frequency ultrasound) are used for assessment of preoperative location, size and depth of tumors. Histological examination shows cluster of glomus cells surrounding capillaries.

Treatment consist of complete surgical removal by trans-ungual or lateral approach.

Onychomatricoma

It is a rare benign tumour of nail matrix epithelium. It commonly affects single finger in 75% of cases. Clinically it presents with thickening of the nail plate, transverse and longitudinal over curvature of the affected portion and xanthonychia. Longitudinal ridging and splinter haemorrhages can also be associated. Woodworm cavities at the free edge of thickened nail plate is the characteristic finding. Dermoscopy shows woodworm perforation at distal end of nail plate.

Treatment: Complete surgical excision.

Onychopapilloma

It is a benign neoplasm which arises from distal matrix. Clinical characteristics include, localized longitudinal erythronychia, fissuring of nail plate and V shaped distal onycholysis. Nail clipping shows localized asymmetric keratotic thickening on the underside of the nail plate. Histology shows papillomatous nail bed with hyperkeratotic layer and absent granular layer. Treatment is complete surgical excision.

Subungual Exostosis

It is benign osteochondral proliferations from distal phalanx, which clinically presents as firm subungual growth at free margin of nail plate. Radiographic examination is cornerstone for diagnosis, which shows well circumscribed area lacking clear contiguity of both medullary cavity and cortex. For treatment complete resection of outgrowth is required.

Myxoid cyst

It is a common benign tumor of nail unit which presents as a small soft nodule between distil interphalangeal joint and proximal nail fold or in proximal nail fold. It occurs due to breach in joint capsule of distil interphalangeal joint resulting in leakage of synovial fluid.

Histology shows well circumscribed but unencapsulated cyst with spindle shape fibroblast and mucin filled spaces. Surgical excision is the mainstay of treatment.

CHAPTER 28

Nutritional and Metabolic Disorders

Contents

PROTEIN ENERGY MALNUTRITION (PEM)

Malnutrition is globally the most important risk factor for illness and death, contributing to more than half of the deaths in children worldwide. Kwashiorkor and marasmus are two forms of PEM. The distinction between the two forms of PEM is based on the presence of edema (kwashiorkor) or absence of edema (marasmus). Marasmus involves inadequate intake of protein and calories, whereas a child with kwashiorkor has fair-to-normal calorie intake without adequate protein intake. Although significant clinical differences between kwashiorkor and marasmus are noted, some studies suggest that marasmus represents an adaptation to starvation whereas kwashiorkor represents a dysadaptation to starvation. In addition to PEM, children may be affected by vitamin and micronutrient deficiencies, which also have a detrimental effect on growth and development. Overnutrition or excessive intake of specific nutrient is another form of malnutrition.

Classification of Malnutrition

A number of classifications including WHO classification are available for assessing different degrees of under nutrition. Although weight for age classification (Gomez, Indian Academy of Pediatrics [IAP]) is the most commonly used, weight for height classifications (McLaren, Waterlow's) have also been used. Each of these classifications uses different sets of reference data and each system uses different standards to demarcate mild, moderate and severe under nutrition. However, using different reference values and cut off points has caused problems in standardizing data across various studies in different countries.

1. IAP (Indian Academy of Pediatrics) classification of PEM (Table 28.1):

Table 28.1: IAP (Indian Academy of Pediatrics) Classification of PEM

Grade	*Weight for age (%)*
Normal	>80
Grade I	71- 80
Grade II	61- 70
Grade III	51- 60
Grade IV	<50

2. The WHO recommendation is to use the *z* score or standard deviation (SD) system to grade under nutrition. Children who are more than 2 SD below the reference median (a *z*

score of less than −2) are considered to be undernourished, i.e., to be stunted, wasted, or underweight. Children with measurements below 3 SD (a *z* score of less than −3) are considered to be severely undernourished (Table 28. 2).

Table 28.2: World Health Organization (WHO) Classification of Nutritional Status of Infant and Children

Nutritional status	Age: Birth to 5 years Indicator and cut-off value compared to the median of the WHO child growth standards[a]
Obese	Weight-for-length/height[b] or BMI-for-age >3 standard deviations (SD) of the median
Overweight	Weight-for-length/height[b] or BMI-for-age >2 SD and ≤3 SD of the median
Moderately underweight	Weight-for-age <−2 SD and ≥−3 SD of the median
Severely underweight	Weight-for-age <−3 SD of the median
Moderate acute malnutrition	Weight-for-length/height[b] or BMI-for-age ≤−2 SD and ≥−3 SD of the median or mid-upper arm circumference ≥115 mm and <125 mm
Severe acute malnutrition	Weight-for-length/height[b] or BMI-for-age <−3 SD of the median or mid-upper arm circumference <115 mm or bilateral pitting oedema
Moderately stunted (moderate chronic malnutrition)	Length/height-for- age[b] ≤−2 SD and ≥−3 SD of the median
Severely stunted (severe chronic malnutrition)	Length/height-for-age[b] <−3 SD of the median
Moderately wasted	Weight-for-length/height ≤−2 SD and ≥−3 SD of the median
Severely wasted	Weight-for-length/height <−3 SD of the median

a: WHO child growth standards: method and development, Length/height-for-age, weight-for-age, weight-for-length, weight -for-height and body mass index-for-age

b: Weight-for-length used in infant and young children aged 0-23 months and weight-for-height used for children aged 24 months and older

Clinical Features

Clinical signs and symptoms of protein energy malnutrition (PEM) include the following:

- Poor weight gain.
- Slowing of linear growth.
- Behavioral changes – Irritability, apathy, decreased social responsiveness, anxiety and attention deficits.
- In marasmus, severe wasting is present.
- There is 'pitting edema' of legs and feet in a kwashiorkor baby.

Skin Changes

- In kwashiorkor, desquamation and hyperpigmentation of skin occurs. If these hyperpigmented areas become confluent, they may show 'flaky paint' appearance (Figure 28.1).
- In marasmus, skin is thin, lax or wrinkled and loss of buccal fat results in 'monkey face' or an aged appearance.
- Dry peeling skin may leave raw exposed areas.
- Hyperpigmented plaques over areas of trauma.
- Other cutaneous manifestations are erythema, petechiae, ecchymosis, purpura, etc.

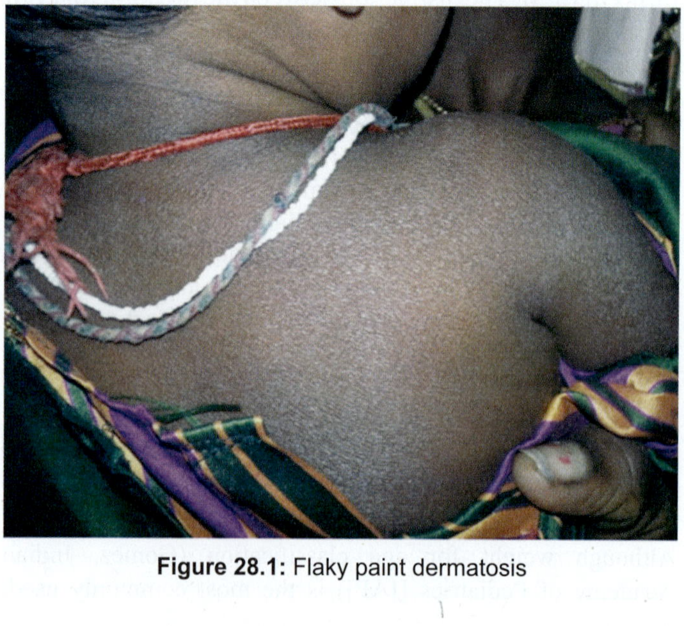

Figure 28.1: Flaky paint dermatosis

Mucous Membranes

- Glossitis, smooth tongue and cheilitis are common findings.
- Herpes labialis may be seen.

Nail Changes

- Nails become fissured or ridged.

Hair Changes

- Hair show gradual loss of pigmentation and become brown or light red. Loss of characteristic curls may occur. They become sparse, lose their luster and are easily pluckable.
- In intermittent periods of malnutrition, child may show alternate bands of depigmented and normal pigmented colour of individual hair, called 'flag sign' (Figure 28.2).

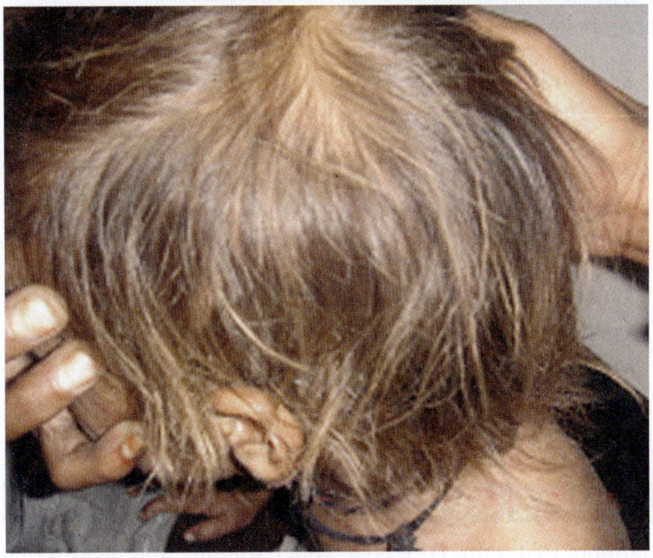

Figure 28.2: Flag sign

Orofacial Gangrene/Cancrum oris/NOMA: Found in conditions of extreme poverty, malnutrition and HIV. Presents as blackish necrotic ulcer followed by sequestration of exposed bone and teeth. Treatment requires systemic antibiotics, antiseptic wound care and debridement.

Clinical Signs and Symptoms of Micronutrient Deficiencies: The most common and clinically significant deficiencies include the following:

- ***Deficiency of iron:*** Fatigue, anemia, decreased cognitive function, headache, glossitis and nail changes.
- ***Deficiency of iodine:*** Goiter, developmental delay and mental retardation.
- ***Deficiency of Vitamin D:*** Poor growth, rickets and hypocalcemia.
- ***Deficiency of Vitamin A:*** Night blindness, Bitot's spots, xerophthalmia, phrynoderma, poor growth and hair changes.
- ***Folate deficiency:*** Glossitis, anemia (megaloblastic).
- ***Deficiency of zinc:*** Anemia, dwarfism, hepatosplenomegaly, hyperpigmentation and hypogonadism, acrodermatitis enteropathica, diminished immune response, poor wound healing.

Treatment

- Cutaneous changes regress as child receives adequate nutritional supplement.
- During acute phase, cutaneous lesions should be treated with emollients and topical antibacterial agents for superimposed bacterial infections.
- Children with chronic malnutrition may require caloric intakes more than 120-150 kcal/kg/day to achieve appropriate weight gain. Protein intake of 3 gm/kg/day is sufficient.
- Additionally, any micronutrient deficiencies must be corrected to attain appropriate growth and development.
- A patient with malnutrition may require hospitalization based on the severity and instability of the clinical situation. Hospitalization of patients is warranted in cases where dehydration and acidosis complicate the clinical picture. In moderate-to-severe cases of malnutrition, enteral supplementation via tube feedings may be necessary.
- In case of severe malnutrition, the child should be assessed for dietary intake and socioeconomic status, diarrhea, tuberculosis, HIV infection or any serious underlying disease.

VITAMIN A

There are essentially 3 forms of Vitamin A: Retinols, beta carotenes and carotenoids. Deficiency of Vitamin A is found among malnourished children especially after acute illnesses such as diarrhea, pneumonia and viral infections; it is more prevalent in developing countries.

Clinical Findings

Subclinical forms of Vitamin A deficiency (VAD) may not cause any symptoms, but the risk of developing respiratory and intestinal infections is increased, the growth rate is decreased, and bone development is slowed. Signs and symptoms of Vitamin A deficiency include the following:

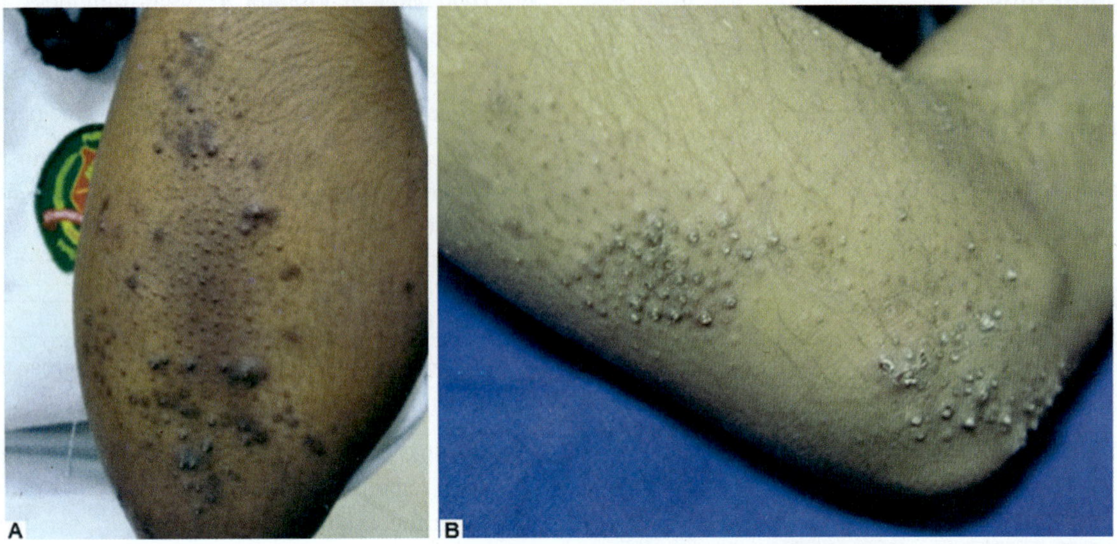

Figure 28.3: Phrynoderma

Skin Changes

- Dry, scaly or hyperkeratotic patches commonly on the arms, legs, shoulders and buttocks.
- Follicular hyperkeratosis (phrynoderma) secondary to blockage of hair follicles with plugs of keratin on dorsal and lateral areas of the extremities (Figure 28.3).
- Hair become sparse and fragile.
- Broken fingernails.

Other Changes

- As Vitamin A is required for effective barrier function, deficiency may lead to diarrhea, increased respiratory tract infections, urinary tract infections leading to pyuria and hematuria.
- **Ocular abnormalities:** Bitot spots (areas of abnormal squamous cell proliferation and keratinization of the conjunctiva), poor adaptation to darkness (nyctalopia), keratomalacia, xerophthalmia and corneal perforation etc.
- Other signs of VAD include excessive deposition of periosteal bone; secondary to reduced osteoclastic activity, anemia, keratinization of mucous membranes and impairment of the humoral and cell-mediated immune system.

Treatment

- Treatment for subclinical VAD includes the consumption of Vitamin A rich foods, such as liver, beef, chicken, eggs, fortified milk, carrots, mangoes, sweet potatoes and leafy green vegetables.
- For VAD syndromes, treatment includes daily oral supplements till clinical recovery, as follows:
  1. Children aged 3 years or younger – 600 µg (2000 IU).
  2. Children aged 4-8 years – 900 µg (3000 IU).
  3. Children aged 9-13 years – 1700 µg (5665 IU).
  4. Children aged 14-18 years – 2800 µg (9335 IU).
- A therapeutic dose for severe disease is 60,000 µg (200,000 IU) orally or intramuscularly, until recovery, which has been shown to reduce child mortality rates by 35-70%.
- Xerophthalmia is treated by giving 1,500 µg/kg body weight orally for 5 days followed by intramuscular injection of 7,500 µg of Vitamin A in oil, until recovery.

THIAMINE (VITAMIN B1)

Thiamine (Vitamin B1) is a water-soluble and heat-labile vitamin required for carbohydrate metabolism. Beriberi occurs because of deficiency of thiamine which is of two main types, depending on the system of maximum involvement. Wet (edematous) beriberi leads to cardiovascular dysfunction that is usually chronic but may have an acute presentation. Dry beriberi leads to multifocal peripheral and/or central neurologic dysfunction, which includes Wernicke encephalopathy and Korsakoff syndrome. Sometimes, patients present with involvement of both the systems.

Clinical Features

Thiamine deficiency has a wide range of clinical presentations. Although clinical overlap is common, the basic phenotypes are as follows:

Wet Beriberi

- This phenotype affects the cardiovascular system and is divided into acute and chronic forms.

- Presenting symptoms include tachycardia, low diastolic pressure, cardiomegaly, pulmonary edema and cyanosis. Wet beriberi is characterized by elevated lactic acid levels. This condition can be readily reversed with thiamine infusion, if administered early.
- Chronic wet beriberi with high output cardiac failure causes fluid overload resulting in peripheral edema and pleural effusion or pulmonary edema.

Dry Beriberi

- This phenotype affects the neuromuscular system.
- Polyneuritis and symmetric, ascending paralysis of the peripheral nervous systems predominate.
- The sensory system is affected first, followed by the motor and autonomic systems.
- Typically, tactile sensation is the first to be lost, followed by pain, and finally, temperature.
- Paresthesia and hyperesthesia usually begin from the lower extremities and gradually involve the upper extremities and perioral area.
- Deep tendon reflexes are lost, calf muscles become painful, and foot drop and, eventually, wrist drop occur.
- Encephalopathy is an alternative mode of presentation, with vomiting, disorientation, horizontal nystagmus, ophthalmoplegia, ataxia, and progressive loss of memory and mental impairment.
- No specific skin changes have been mentioned.

Treatment

Treatment of choice is thiamine hydrochloride (aneurine hydrochloride, Vitamin B_1). It is given as 2-3 mg three times daily till resolution of symptoms in mild cases. In severe cases, 25-50 mg/dose slow IV, followed by 10 mg/day intravenous for 7 days, then 3-5 mg/day orally for at least 6 weeks is given.

VITAMIN B2 (RIBOFLAVIN)

Riboflavin is a water soluble vitamin. It acts as a component of coenzymes which are involved in a number of metabolic pathways. Mucocutaneous changes related to riboflavin deficiency are cheilitis, angular stomatitis (perleche) and glossitis. The tongue is purplish red and smooth. A scaly seborrheic dermatitis-like eruption may be seen around the nose, eyes, ears and genital area. Ocular abnormalities are keratitis, conjunctivitis and photophobia. Treatment consists of 3-10 mg riboflavin daily by mouth till complete recovery.

VITAMIN B3 (NIACIN)

Vitamin B_3 is an essential component of several coenzymes. Pellagra is a systemic nutritional wasting disease caused by a deficiency of vitamin B_3. Drug induced pellagra may also occur, which is caused by azathioprine and AKT. In endemic cases, pellagra tends to be seasonal and occurs during spring and early summer. Early symptoms are non-specific. Patients express weakness, lassitude and anorexia.

Clinical Features

Skin Manifestations

- Affected skin lesions are initially well defined dry, erythematous patches and are associated with a burning sensation.
- The distribution of the cutaneous eruption is typically symmetrical and bilateral in areas of the body exposed to sun which include the dorsum of the hands, feet (Figure 28.4), forearms and legs. On face the lesions are seen in

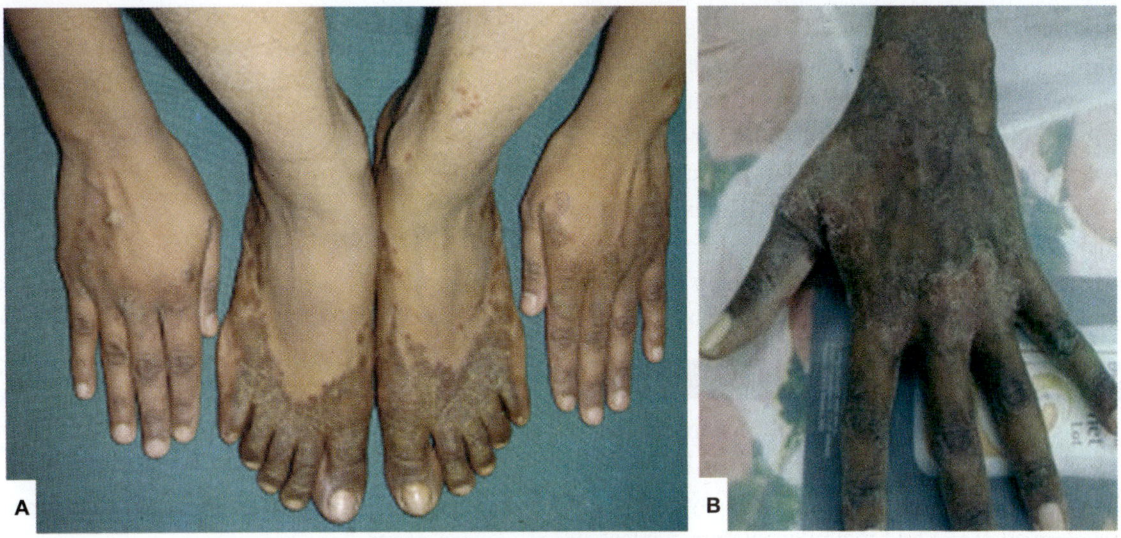

A B

Figure 28.4: Pellagrous dermatitis

butterfly distribution over the cheeks, forehead, tip of the nose and over V of the neck. The neck lesion is referred to as the *Casal's necklace*.

- As the dermatitis progresses, the affected skin becomes hyperpigmented and thickened.

Gastrointestinal Manifestations

- Poor appetite, nausea, epigastric discomfort, abdominal pain and increased salivation.
- Glossitis typically causes soreness of the mouth and dysphagia.
- Diarrhea is the manifestation of intestinal inflammation which is typically watery but is occasionally bloody and mucoid.

Neuropsychiatric Manifestations

- Early neuropsychiatric symptoms of pellagra include lethargy, apathy, depression, anxiety, irritability and poor concentration.
- As the disease advances, patients become disoriented, confused and delirious. Eventually, the patient becomes stuporous and comatose.
- Death may result from the depletion of the coenzyme required to generate sufficient energy to support vital body functions.

Treatment

- Nicotinamide or niacin taken orally is usually effective in reversing the clinical manifestations of pellagra. It is given in the dose of 10-50 mg orally four times a day until resolution of symptoms and signs.

VITAMIN B6 (PYRIDOXINE)

Pyridoxine is a pyridine derivative, participating as a coenzyme in transaminase and decarboxylase reactions and in the metabolism of cystein, tryptophan and essential fatty acids. Pyridoxine deficiency may follow therapy with isoniazid, hydralazine and penicillamine but it usually occurs in association with other deficiencies. Skin lesions consist of cheilitis, glossitis and periorificial seborrheic like dermatitis. Convulsions, anemia and acrodynia may develop in infants. Treatment includes 20-100 mg/day of pyridoxine by mouth.

VITAMIN B12 (COBALAMIN)

Vitamin B12 has crucial role in the normal functioning of the nervous system and formation of blood. It exists in 3 forms- cyanocobalamin (semisynthetic form), adenosylcobalamin (human physiological form) and methylcobalamin. Causes of deficiency include inadequate intake, malabsorption or due to inborn errors of transport or metabolism.

Clinical Features

The classic triad of Vit B12 deficiency consists of megaloblastic anemia, glossitis and neuropsychiatric symptoms.

Oral manifestations: Hunter's glossitis, glossodynia, recurrent ulcers, lingual paresthesia, cheilitis, burning, xerostomia and stomatitis.

Cutaneous manifestations: Generalized hyperpigmentation with accentuation in flexural areas, poliosis, vitiligo and alopecia areata.

Investigations

Hematological findings- macrocytic anemia, hypersegmented neutrophils.

Serum cobalamin levels <200 pg /ml are indicative of B12 deficiency.

Treatment

RDA- 1 mcg per day.

Therapeutic doses are 1000-1500 mcg of Vit B12 per week intramuscular for 1 month then monthly doses.

VITAMIN C (ASCORBIC ACID)

The human body lacks the ability to synthesize and make vitamin C and therefore depends on exogenous dietary sources to meet vitamin C needs. Consumption of fruits and vegetables or diet fortified with vitamin C is essential to avoid ascorbic acid deficiency or scurvy. Normal requirement of vitamin C are 30-40 mg/day for infants and 40-70 mg/day for children. Although scurvy is uncommon, it still occurs and can affect adults and children who have chronic dietary vitamin C deficiency. Scurvy can occur at any age. Most cases of infantile scurvy occur when the infant is aged 6-24 months. Scurvy is uncommon in the neonatal period.

Clinical Features

Skin Changes

- The initial skin change is follicular keratosis with coiled hair on the upper arms, back, buttocks and lower extremities.
- Later, perifollicular haemorrhage with discoloration due to haem especially on the legs, swollen bleeding gums, stomatitis and epistaxis occur.
- Petechial haemorrhage of the skin and mucous membranes can occur.

- Large skin haemorrhages may be seen.
- Chronic hypovitaminosis C sometimes causes 'woody' oedema and discoloration of the legs.
- Alopecia and positive hair pull test may be present.

Other Findings

- Irritability.
- Pain and tenderness of the legs (Pseudoparalysis).
- Swelling over the long bones and subperiosteal haemorrhages.
- Rarely, hematuria, hematochezia and melena are noted.
- Proptosis of the eyeball secondary to orbital haemorrhage is a sign of scurvy.
- Costochondral beading or **scorbutic rosary** may be seen.
- Low-grade fever, anemia and poor wound healing are usually present.

Treatment

- Ascorbic acid (vitamin C) 25 mg four times a day for a week administered orally or parenterally is effective in curing infantile scurvy.
- Daily intake of 3.4 oz of orange or tomato juice produces good recovery in children.
- Treatment for adults include upto 2g/day for initial 3 days, 500mg/day for 1 week and then 100mg/day for 1 to 3 months.
- Upon instituting dietary or pharmacologic treatment, the clinical recovery is impressive. The appetite of the infant is recovered within 24-48 hours. The symptoms like irritability, fever, tenderness upon palpation and hemorrhage generally resolve within 7 days.

VITAMIN D

Vitamin D deficiency causes rickets. Rickets is a disease of growing bone that occurs in children due to unmineralized matrix at growth plates. It is caused by a failure of osteoid to calcify in a growing person.

Causes

1. Vitamin D deficiency disorders.
2. Calcium deficiency.
3. Phosphorus deficiency.
4. Distal renal tubular acidosis.

Clinical Features

- Generalized muscular hypotonia is observed in most patients with clinical signs of rickets.
- Craniotabes (softening of cranial bones) manifests early in infants with vitamin D deficiency, although this feature may be normal in infants, especially for those born prematurely.
- If rickets occurs at a later age, thickening of the skull develops. This produces frontal bossing and delays the closure of the anterior fontanelle.
- Weight bearing produces deformities such as bowlegs and knock knees.
- In the chest, knobby deformities result in the **rachitic rosary** (Figure 28.5) along the costochondral junctions.

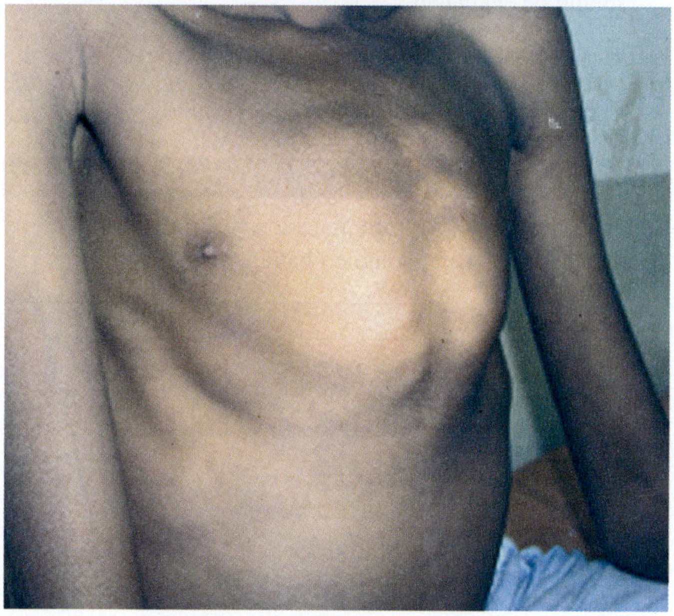

Figure 28.5: Rachitic rosary

- The weakened ribs pulled by muscles also produce flaring over the diaphragm, which is known as **Harrison groove**.
- The sternum may be pulled into a pigeon-breast deformity.
- In more severe instances in children older than 2 years, vertebral softening leads to kyphoscoliosis.
- Small papules and cysts representing abnormal, rudimentary hair structures characteristically developing on the face and scalp as well as alopecia are found in vitamin D-dependent rickets type II.

Investigations

- On posteroanterior radiographs of the wrist, characteristic rachitic changes can be seen. At metaphysis, there is sharp border, which is described as 'fraying'.
- Other changes are cupping, widening of metaphysis of distal ends of radius, ulna or fibula.

Treatment

- Treatment for rickets may be gradually administered over several months as 125-250 µg (5000-10,000 U) of vitamin D four times a day for 2-3 months or in a single day dose of 15,000 µg (600,000 U) of vitamin D.
- If the vitamin D dose is administered in a single day, it is usually divided into 4 or 6 oral doses. An intramuscular injection is also available. Vitamin D is well stored in the body and is gradually released over many weeks.
- In case of inadequate response, other causes of rickets should be evaluated.
- If severe deformities have occurred, orthopedic correction may be required after healing. Most of the deformities resolve with growth of child.

BIOTIN

Biotin deficiency is a rare nutritional disorder caused by deficiency of this water soluble vitamin.

Clinical Features

Skin Changes

Symptoms develop within 3-5 weeks of the onset of deficient biotin intake. It includes:

- Dry skin.
- Photosensitivity.
- Seborrheic dermatitis.
- Rashes, including erythematous periorificial macular rash and erythematous rash in intertriginous area.
- Fine and brittle hair.
- Hair loss or total alopecia.

Neurological Manifestations

Approximately1-2 weeks later, neurologic symptoms begin to develop. The most common neurologic findings include the following:

- Mild depression, which may progress to profound lassitude and eventually, to somnolence.
- Changes in mental status.
- Generalized muscular pains.
- Hyperaesthesias and paraesthesias.

Intestinal tract symptoms also develop and most commonly present as anorexia, nausea, occasionally severe vomiting.

Treatment

Profound biotinidase deficiency can be detected with newborn screening. The most important aspects of the medical care in patients with biotin deficiency include the early recognition of the condition and the prompt institution of therapy with adequate amounts. All cutaneous features rapidly respond to biotin 5-20 mg/day orally.

ZINC

Acrodermatitis enteropathica is an inborn error of zinc metabolism which is inherited as an autosomal recessive disorder. Symptoms in infancy typically include periorificial and acral dermatitis, behavioral changes and neurologic disturbances. In older children, failure to thrive, anorexia, alopecia, nail dystrophy, and repeated infections are most

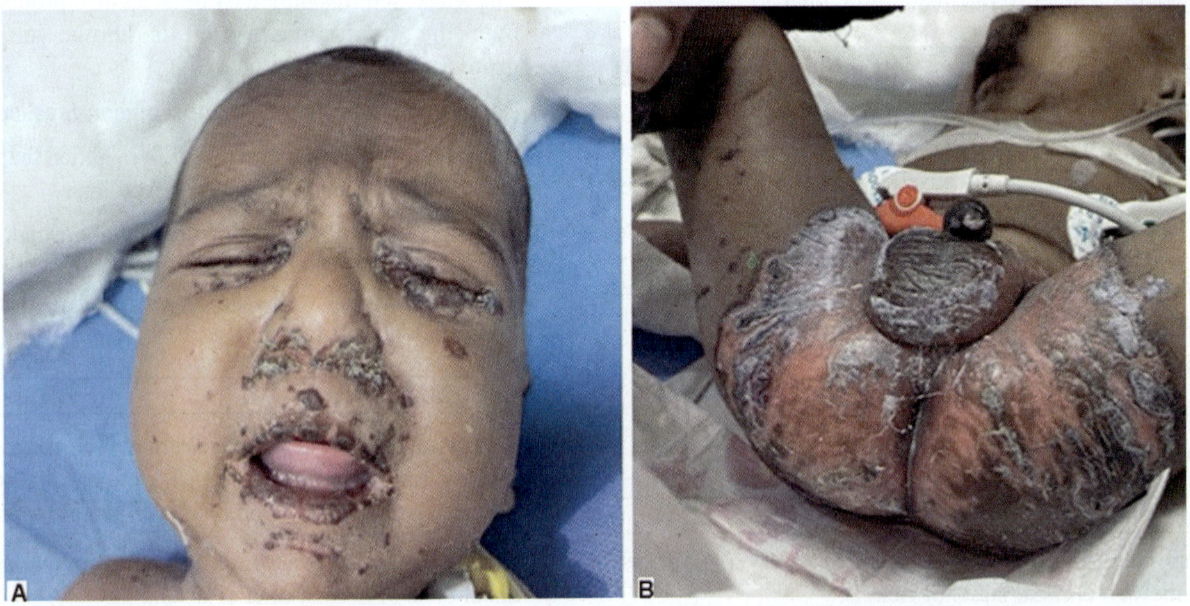

Figure 28.6: Acrodermatitis enteropathica showing erythematous erosive rashes around perioral perinasal and perianal area

common. Diarrheal illness in children is an important cause of zinc deficiency in developing countries.

Etiology

Defective gene SLC39A4 codes for a zinc transporter due to which there is less absorption of zinc from the gut. Breast milk has a protein which helps in absorption of zinc, hence the deficiency does not manifest until breast milk is discontinued.

Zinc deficiency may also be seen due to:

- Inadequate intake.
- Malabsorption.
- Excessive loss.
- Prolonged parenteral nutrition without zinc supplementation.
- Low birth weight, preterm babies.

Clinical Features

- Symptoms typically appear in the first few months of life, when an infant is weaned from breastfeeding. AE can also develop in full term breastfed infants as a result of zinc deficiency in breast milk and decreased maternal plasma zinc levels.
- **Dermatitis:** Erythematous, vesiculobullous, erosive (Figure 28.6) or pustular lesions that lead to dry, scaly, eczematous, psoriasiform (Figure 28.7A and B) or desquamating lesions (Figure 28.7C) distributed around periorificial areas, (e.g., mouth, anus, genitalia) and acral areas of the body are characteristic of AE. The borders of affected areas are sharply demarcated and have scaling at the periphery. Perioral eruption of zinc deficiency often spares the upper lip, resulting in a horseshoe shaped distribution. They may become secondarily infected with *Staphylococcus aureus* or *Candida albicans*.
- Other mucosal findings include angular cheilitis, glossitis, conjunctivitis, blepharitis, punctate keratopathy and photophobia etc.
- Paronychia and nail dystrophy may be present.
- **Alopecia:** Partial or total hair loss of scalp, eyebrow, eyelashes may be evident.
- Diarrhea.
- Growth retardation, bacterial and fungal infections and behavioral changes may also be seen.
- Patients are miserable and depressed. Infants are inconsolable and may withdraw from contact.
- Chronic zinc deficiency may cause dwarfism, hypogonadism and T-cell medicated immunodeficiency.
- Transient neonatal zinc deficiency is possible in exclusively breastfeeding fed infant whose mothers have inadequate secretion of zinc in breast milk.

Differential Diagnosis

- Atopic dermatitis.
- Biotin deficiency.
- Candidiasis.
- Epidermolysis bullosa.

Investigations

- In most patients with AE, plasma zinc concentrations is low (<50 μg/dL) but it is not diagnostic.
- Production of serum alkaline phosphatase depends on zinc; therefore, a low level of alkaline phosphatase may support a diagnosis of AE.

Treatment

- In patients with AE, zinc gluconate or sulfate is administered orally at a dosage of 1-3 mg/kg/day. Although

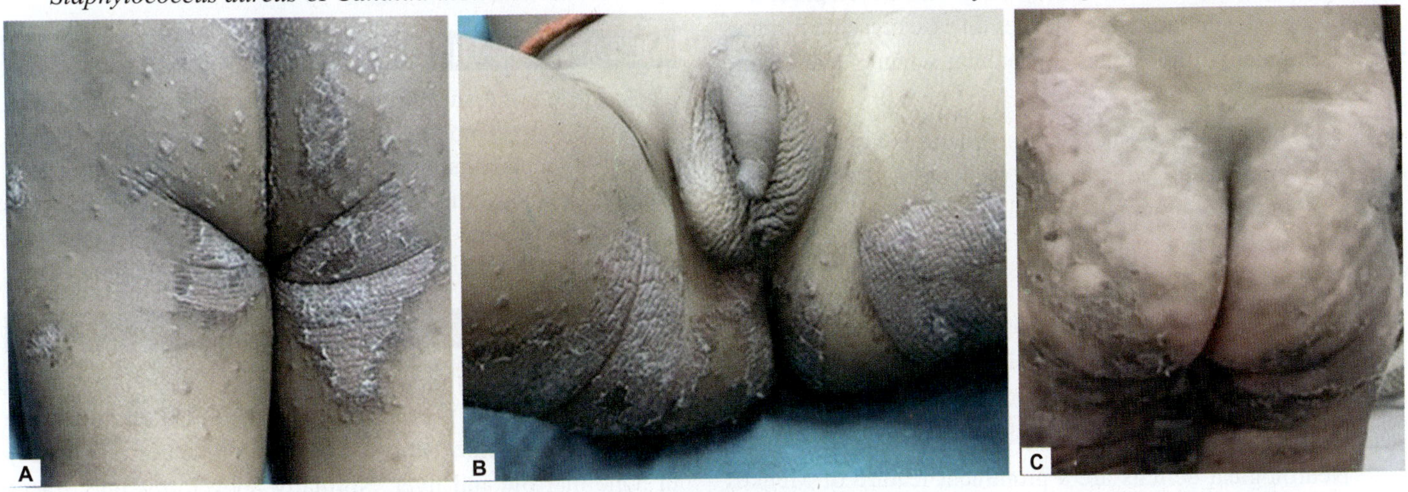

Figure 28.7: Acrodermatitis enteropathica showing psoriasiform lesions (A and B) and desquamating lesions (C)

the intravenous dosage have not clearly been estimated, amounts of 300-1000 μg/kg/day may be sufficient for rapid reversal of symptoms.

- Clinical response is observed within 5-10 days. Zinc therapy has to be maintained throughout the patient's life span, though periods of remission are reported. Exacerbation during pregnancy or the stress of disease may require an increase in dose. In acquired zinc deficiency, treatment can be stopped after the precipitating cause is resolved.
- Warm compresses and vaseline applied three times a day to areas of weeping or crusting is helpful.

ESSENTIAL FATTY ACID DEFICIENCY

Essential fatty acid deficiency (EFA) manifests as periorificial dermatitis and a generalized xerotic or eczematous dermatitis. Failure to thrive, alopecia with lightly colored hair, and thrombocytopenia are other signs that may occur. The condition occurs in patients receiving parenteral nutrition without lipid supplementation, severe fat malabsorption from gastrointestinal disorders, and in cases of surgery of the gastrointestinal tract.

Management

Decreased plasma levels of linoleic, arachidonic, icosatrienoic acid and an icosatrienoic/arachidonic acid ratio of greater than 0.4 confirms the diagnosis. The treatment consists of oral or parenteral administration of fat emulsions. Topical application of 2 to 3 mg/kg soybean or safflower oil may restore plasma levels of linoleic acids.

COPPER DEFICIENCY (MENKES DISEASE)

Hair changes can be the first sign of disease at 1–2 months of age. Scalp and eyebrow hair resemble steel wool, appearing short, sparse, lustreless, tangled and depigmented. Pili torti is a classic feature and monilethrix may also develop. At 2–3 months of age, children with Menkes disease present with loss of developmental milestones, hypotonia, seizures and failure to thrive.

The physical appearance in these infants is a characteristic cherubic appearance with a depressed nasal bridge, pudgy cheeks, 'cupids bow' upper lip and doughy skin. The skin at the nape of the neck, axillae and trunk is depigmented and feels soft and inelastic.

Bone abnormalities include osteoporosis, scalloping of the posterior aspects of the vertebral bodies, subperiosteal new bone formation, ossification of sutures, diaphyseal periosteal reaction, metaphyseal widening and lateral spur formation.

Neurological deficits are a prominent feature of Menkes disease. Infants have severe truncal hypotonia with poor head control, but increased tone in the extremities. Deep tendon reflexes are increased. Severe developmental delay occurs. Patient may be able only to smile and babble.

The primary manifestation of acquired copper deficiency is a myeloneuropathy that affects both sensory and motor nerves (progressive symmetrical sensory loss in addition to weakness of the upper and lower extremities). It may progress to optic neuropathy.

Treatment

The recommended daily intake of copper for infants up to 12 months of age is 200–220 μg/day. Children 1–13 years of age require 340–700 μg/day. RDA for adults is 8mg/day in females and 11mg/day in males.

Children with Menkes disease require lifelong supplementation with parenteral copper, usually cupric chloride.

SELENIUM DEFICIENCY

Selenium is an essential trace element vital for maintaining human health. Deficiency results in Keshan disease which is a type of congestive cardiomyopathy characterized by symptoms like heart failure, cardiac enlargement, ECG irregularities, gallop rhythm and cardiogenic shock. Other features include muscle pain and weakness.

Treatment: Selenium 2mg/kg/day is enough to treat selenium deficiency.

ANOREXIA NERVOSA AND BULIMIA

These are eating disorders that can lead to nutritional deficiencies. Affected individuals have psychiatric disturbances. Dermatological manifestations include dry skin, telogen effluvium, lanugo like hair, brittle nails, carotenoderma, cheilitis, calluses and enlarged salivary glands and erosion of tooth enamel.

METABOLIC DISORDERS

There are more than 300 metabolic disorders. Most of them, however, remain undetected or misdiagnosed. Most inborn errors of metabolism are autosomal recessive disorders. Patients develop symptoms in infancy or later in adolescence or adulthood. Some common metabolic disorders along with their cutaneous manifestations are summarized in Table 28.3.

PORPHYRIA

It is a group of rare disorders in which excessive amount of porphyrins or their precursors are produced. Porphyrins are byproducts of heme pathway. They are synthesized mainly in bone marrow and liver. Normally body forms only traces of porphyrins, which are excreted in urine and stool. Patients

Table 28.3: Common Metabolic Disorders with Cutaneous Manifestations

Metabolic disorder	*Skin manifestations*
Aminoacidopathies	
• Phenylketonuria	• Eczema, hypopigmentation, photosensitivity
• Tyrosinaemia	• Keratoderma
• Homocystinuria	• Malar rash, livido reticularis, skin ulceration
Organic Acidurias	
• Alkaptonuria	• Black-brown stained napkins, ochronosis
• Propionic acidemia	• Seborrheic dermatitis or SSSS like eruption
• Methylmalonic acidemia	• Erythematosquamous eruptions in periorificial and acral areas, scalded skin
• Biotinidase deficiency	• Photosensitivity, alopecia, erythema in periorificial and intertriginous areas
Transport Defects	
• Hartnup's disease	• Photosensitivity, malar rash
Lysosomal Storage Disease	
• Fabry's disease	• Angiokeratoma, erythematous pinpoint lesions, perioral erosions, alopecia, anhydrosis
• Fucosidosis	• Erythematous pinpoint lesions, coarse facial features
• Mucopolysaccharidoses	• Ivory coloured papules on back, coarse facies, skin infiltrations
• Farber lipogranulomatosis	• Nodular swellings on ankle, elbow, wrist and on friction sites
• GM type 1 gangliosidosis	• Thick, rough and hirsute skin. Hyperpigmented macules

of porphyria may present as acute attacks or with cutaneous disease or both. According to this, they may be classified as follows:

Classification

1. **Acute attacks only**
   - Acute intermittent porphyria (AIP).
2. **Cutaneous disease and acute attacks**
   - Hereditary coproporphyria (HC).
   - Variegate porphyria (VP).
3. **Cutaneous disease only**
   - Porphyria cutanea tarda (PCT).
   - Congenital erythropoietic porphyria (CEP).
   - Erythropoietic protoporphyria (EP).

Acute Intermittent Porphyria (AIP)

Acute porphyria attacks are brought about by uncontrolled upregulation of the ALA synthase enzyme. This can be precipitated by certain lipophilic drugs, hypoglycemia and by deficiency of heme, the end-product of the heme pathway that acts as a negative feedback mechanism in normal circumstances. Acute attacks result in neuronal dysfunction which may be due to:

- Disturbed metabolism of neurotransmitters.
- Direct neurotoxicity of accumulated ALA (which structurally resembles with GABA).
- Acute heme deficiency within neurons.

Hereditary Coproporphyria

Hereditary coproporphyria results in most cases from half than normal activity (50%) of coproporphyrin oxidase. It is an acute hepatic porphyria, which is characterized by abdominal pain, neuropsychiatric symptoms and cutaneous photosensitivity.

Variegate Porphyria

Variegate porphyria is an autosomal dominant inherited trait that results in decreased activity of protoporphyrinogen oxidase. It is characterized clinically by photosensitive skin disease and a propensity to acute neurovisceral crisis.

Porphyria Cutanea Tarda

Porphyria cutanea tarda (PCT) is characterized by the defective uroporphyrinogen III decarboxylase enzyme. Patients present with skin fragility, erosions, vesicles, bullae and milia in sun-exposed areas of the skin. Sometimes, there is the presence of periorbital mottled hyperpigmentation, sclerodermatous

Glycine + Succinyl-CoA

↓ Aminolaevulinic acid synthase

5-aminolaevulinic acid (ALA)

↓ Aminolaevulinic acid dehydratase **[Aminolaevulinic acid deficiency]**

Porphobilinogen (PBG)

↓ PBG deaminase **[Acute intermittent porphyria (AIP)]**

Hydroxymethybilane (HMB)

↓ Uroporphyrinogen cosynthase **[Congenital erythropoietic porphyria]**

Uroporphyrinogen III

↓ Uroporphyrinogen decarboxylase **[Porphyria cutanea tarda (PCT)]**

Coproporphyrinogen III

↓ Coproporphyrin oxidase **[Hereditary coproporphyria (HCP)]**

Protoporphyrinogen IX

↓ Protoporphyrinogen oxidase **[Variegate porphyria (VP)]**

Protoporphyrin IX

↓ Ferrochelatase **[Erythropoetic porphyria (EP)]**

Haem

Flowchart: Showing haem synthesis pathway

changes (Figure 28.8), hypertrichosis (Figure 28.9) and ulceration. Hemochromatosis gene (HFE gene) mutations and the hepatitis C virus (HCV) are both risk factors for PCT.

Congenital Erythropoietic Porphyria (Gunther's Disease)

Congenital erythropoietic porphyria or Gunther's disease (Figure 28.10) is one of the least common porphyrias. It results from a deficient activity of uroporphyrinogen III synthetase (URO-synthase). Hemolysis may be a feature in homozygous cases. Prolonged exposure to sunlight may precipitate a blistering rash, red urine and even blindness.

Erythropoietic Porphyria

In erythropoietic porphyria, the protoporphyrin molecule accumulates and can be excited by absorbing light energy. This causes the generation of free radicals and thereby, photosensitivity of all tissues exposed to light. When patient is

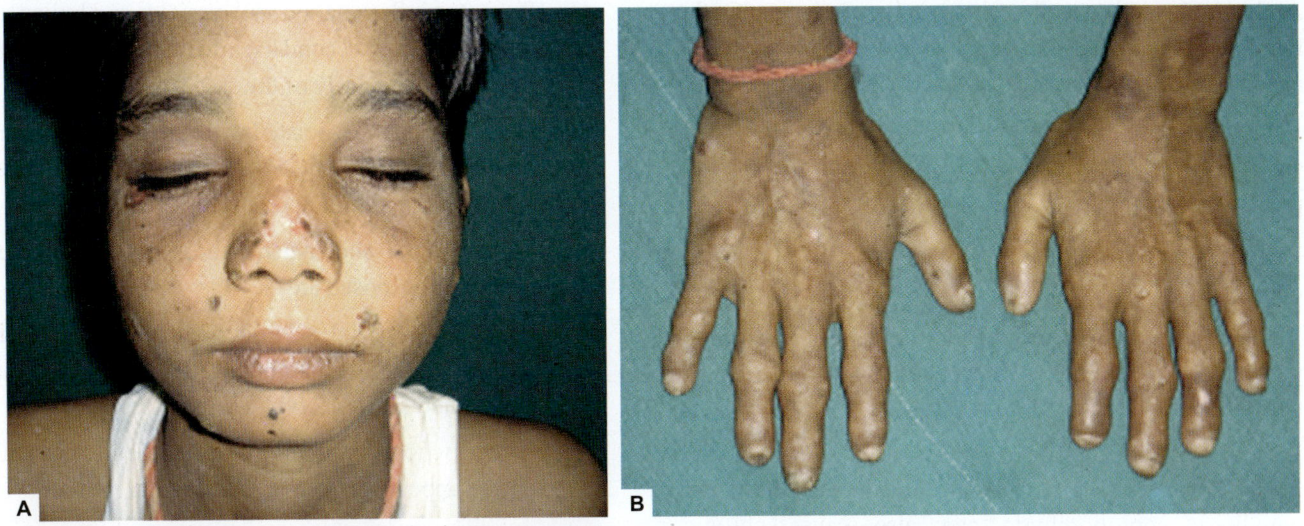

Figure 28.8: Porphyria cutanea tarda showing hyperpigmentation and sclerodermatous changes

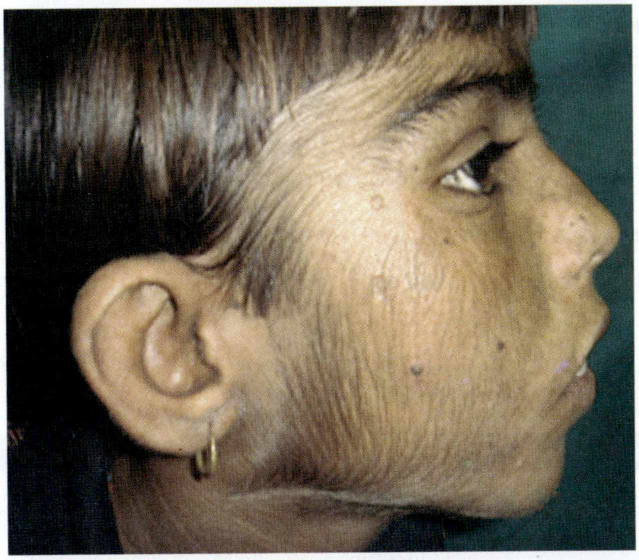

Figure 28.9: Porphyria cutanea tarda showing hypertrichosis

in dark, several other toxic mechanisms have been described, e.g., deposition of protoporphyrin crystals in hepatocytes and bile canaliculi, interference with redox systems and recently, formation of cytotoxic bile. Clinical manifestations of erythropoietic porphyria are photosensitivity, insignificant hematologic abnormalities, and liver disease.

GENERAL CLINICAL FEATURES OF PORPHYRIAS

Acute Attack

- Acute attacks are five times more common in females, and most frequently occur between the ages of 10 and 40 years.
- Severity of acute attack varies from mild abdominal pain, vomiting to severe attacks with bulbar palsy and respiratory paralysis.

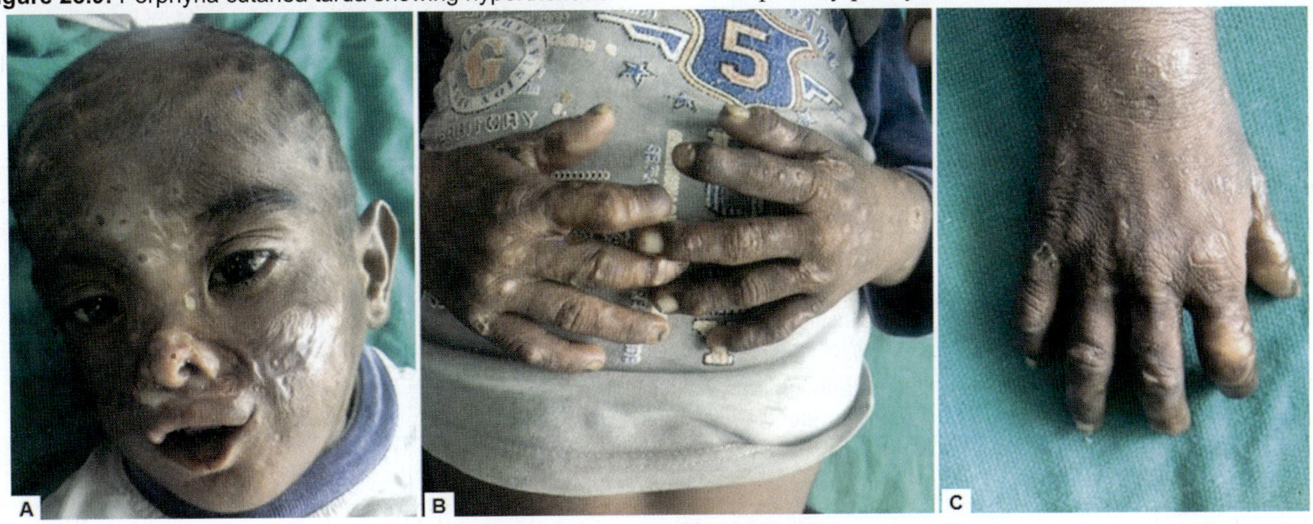

Figure 28.10: Gunther's disease

- Abdominal pain is usually colicky in nature, located in the left lower abdomen, and lasts hours to days. It is rarely accompanied by fever, leukocytosis or peritoneal signs.
- Jaundice may or may not be present.
- The pulse rate and blood pressure are often moderately raised.
- Dehydration is common and hyponatraemia may cause convulsions.
- A focused neurologic examination should be performed to identify motor and sensory deficits and peripheral neuropathy.
- In some but not all acute porphyrias, a skin rash may be seen. Variegate porphyria and, much less commonly, hereditary coproporphyria can also cause chronic, blistering lesions on sun-exposed skin that are identical to those in porphyria cutanea tarda, a much more common condition.

Cutaneous Features

- Features seen in various porphyrias are summarized in Table 28.4. The severity varies according to the type of porphyrias.
  - Severe photosensitivity begins in infancy, often in the neonatal period, with blisters developing in light-exposed skin on minimal light exposure.
  - Exposed (and sometimes non-exposed) skin is fragile.
  - Repeated inflammation with vesicles and bullae, often complicated by secondary infection, cause mutilating scarring particularly of the face and hands.
  - Sometimes it is associated with erosion of the terminal phalanges, onycholysis and destructive changes affecting the pinnae and nose.
  - Patchy hypo- and hyperpigmentation occur even in minimally exposed areas.
  - A diffuse pseudosclerodermatous thickening of exposed skin often gradually develops, with microstomia and sclerodactyly-like changes.
  - Hypertrichosis is found in most patients, particularly on the upper arms, temples and malar region.

Other System Involvement

Eyes

- In congenital erythropoietic porphyria and hepatoerythropoietic porphyria keratoconjunctivitis, blepharitis, cataracts, corneal ulcers, scars, cicatricial ectropion and scarring alopecia of eyelashes and eyebrows may occur.

Bones and Teeth

- Bones and teeth changes are seen in congenital erythropoietic porphyria and hepatoerythropoietic porphyria.
- When teeth emerge, they are almost always stained brown and fluoresce under Wood's light.

Table 28.4: Summary of major findings in the porphyrias

Type	*Major signs and symptoms*	*Results of laboratory tests*
1. ALA dehydratase deficiency	Abdominal pain, neuropsychiatric symptoms	Urinary ALA and coproporphyrin III increased
2. Acute intermittent porphyria	Abdominal pain, neuropsychiatric symptoms	Urinary ALA and PBG increased
3. Congenital erythropoietic porphyria	Photosensitivity, hypertrichosis, eyes, bones and teeth involvement, haemolytic anaemia, splenomegaly, patchy hypo and hyperpigmentation	Urinary, fecal and red cell uroporphyrin I increased
4. Porphyria cutanea tarda	Photosensitivity, hypertrichosis, mottled hyper or hypopigmentation, morphoea like changes	Urinary uroporphyrin I increased
5. Hereditary coproporphyria	Photosensitivity, hypertrichosis, abdominal pain, neuropsychiatric symptoms	Urinary ALA, PBG and coproporphyrin III and fecal coproporphyrin III increased
6. Variegate porphyria	Photosensitivity, hypertrichosis, abdominal pain, neuropsychiatric symptoms	Urinary ALA, PBG and coproporphyrin III and fecal protoporphyrin IX increased
7. Protoporphyria	Nonblistering photosensitivity, anaemia, gallstones, jaundice, liver failure	Fecal and red cell protoporphyrin IX increased
8. Hepatoerythropoietic porphyria	Photosensitivity, hypertrichosis, eyes, bones and teeth involvement, haemolytic anaemia	Urinary uroporphyrin increased, fecal isocoproporphyrin increased
Abbreviations: ALA δ-aminolevulinic acid; PBG-porphobilinogen		

- Decreased bone density, osteopenia and osteolytic lesions secondary to erosion by hyperplastic bone marrow are seen on X-ray and are associated with vertebral compression and collapse, and with pathological fractures.
- In the hands there is resorption of terminal phalanges with acro-osteolysis and cortical bone rarefaction.
- Occasionally, strict avoidance of the sun may impair Vitamin D metabolism.

Haematological Findings

- Congenital erythropoietic porphyria and hepatoerythropoietic porphyria may show hemolytic anemia.
- The high concentrations of porphyrins in red cells cause hemolytic anemia, severe enough to induce marrow hyperplasia often with visible expansion of the maxillary bones on the face.
- Hypersplenism is common.
- Very severe hemolytic anemia may even cause hydrops fetalis.

Investigations

Urine Examination

- Urine porphyrin studies are the mainstay in the diagnosis of acute porphyria attacks.
- Significantly increased ALA and PBG in urine have 100% specificity for acute intermittent (hepatic) porphyria, variegate porphyria and coproporphyria.

Stool Examination

Stool coproporphyrin and protoporphyrin are the most commonly measured porphyrins in faeces. The ratio of fecal coproporphyrin to fecal protoporphyrin varies among the porphyrias.

Bone Marrow Examination

It reveals normoblastic hyperplasia and under ultraviolet illumination most normoblasts have persistent red fluorescence localized to their nuclei, with heme-containing inclusion bodies being seen in the nuclei of these fluorescent cells.

Treatment

During acute attack following measures should be taken:

- Withdrawal of suspected medications, alcohol, drugs, toxins and chemicals is the key to therapy.
- Supportive treatment includes analgesia, sedatives and antiemetics (with drugs known to be safe in acute porphyria) and careful management of fluid balance with rehydration and correction of hyponatraemia.
- Monitor for hyponatremia or hypomagnesemia and treat vigorously if found.
- Aggressively treat respiratory failure, which may ensue once muscle weakness involves the diaphragm, and ventilate in an intensive care unit.
- Treat pain with parenteral meperidine or morphine. Complicated and debilitating chronic cases may require celiac plexus injection.
- Administer phenothiazines for nausea, vomiting, agitation, etc.
- Treat tachycardia and/or hypertension with propranolol or nadolol, which can be safely used for beta blockade.
- Treat acute porphyria attacks with **hemin** (intravenous heme) 3-4 mg/kg/day for 3-5 days which is the definitive treatment and mainstay of management.
- Heme arginate is more effective when given earlier during an attack, increasing the importance of early diagnosis.

Management of Cutaneous Lesions

- Avoidance of sunlight is the key in treating cutaneous porphyrias. Use of sun protective clothing and hats are essential. Sunscreens containing titanium dioxide or zinc oxide, sometimes with added iron oxide and filter films for car and home windows, play an important role in controlling symptoms.
- Prompt treatment of secondary infection is important.
- β-carotene may help cutaneous disease in some patients.
- HCQS.

Allogeneic bone marrow transplantation from a human leukocyte antigen (HLA)-compatible sibling has emerged as the treatment of choice in severe congenital erythropoietic porphyria. Gene therapy has been successfully used in various studies.

Drugs Considered as Safe in Patients with Acute Porphyria

- **Antiemetics:** Cyclizine, domperidone, promethazine, prochlorperazine.
- **Antihistamines:** Trimeprazine, chlorpheniramine, diphenhydramine, ketotifen.
- **Antibacterial drugs:** Aminoglycosides, amoxiclav, ethambutol, penicillins, vancomycin.
- **Lipid lowering drugs:** Clofibrate, gemfibrozil, bezafibrate

- **Local anaesthetic drugs:** Bupivacaine, lignocaine, procaine, prilocaine, tetracaine.
- **Immunization:** IV IgG, vaccines.
- **Antidepressants:** Fluoxetine, amitryptiline.
- **Antipsychotics:** Chlorpromazine, haloperidol, mianserin.
- **Antivirals/antifungals:** Acyclovir, amphotericin B, ganciclovir, zalcitabine.
- **Analgesics:** Aspirin, codeine, alfentanil, dextropropoxyphene, fenbufen, fentanyl, ibuprofen, morphine, indomethacin, paracetamol.

Hartnup's Disease

Hartnup's disease is an autosomal recessive disorder caused by impaired neutral (i.e., monoamino monocarboxylic) amino acid transport in the apical brush border membrane of the small intestine and the proximal tubule of the kidneys. Patients present with pellagra like skin eruptions, cerebellar ataxia and gross aminoaciduria. Cutaneous signs usually precede the neurologic manifestations.

Clinical Features

Skin Findings

- The skin reddens after exposure to sunlight. Further exposures lead to the development of dry, scaly, well-marginated eruptions, sometimes resembling chronic eczema. This eruption preferentially affects the forehead, the cheeks, the periorbital regions, the dorsal surfaces of the hands, and other light-exposed areas.
- Lesions on the face may resemble the malar rash of lupus erythematosus.
- A vesiculobullous eruption with exudation may occur.
- Skin changes leave long-lasting hypopigmentation and/or hyperpigmentation, which are intensified with further sunlight exposure.

Neurological Findings

- Mental development is normal in most patients, but mental retardation (intelligence quotient of 50-70) is described in a few patients.
- Neurologic symptoms may vary and are fully reversible. Intermittent cerebellar ataxia, a wide-based gait, spasticity, delayed motor development, and tremulousness are the most frequent findings. Headaches and hypotonia may also occur.
- Ocular manifestations include double vision, nystagmus, photophobia and strabismus.

Treatment

- A high protein diet can overcome the deficient transport of neutral amino acids in most patients.
- Advise all patients who are symptomatic to use physical and chemical protection from sunlight. Avoiding excessive exposure to sunlight, wearing protective clothing, and using physical and chemical sunscreens are mandatory. Recommend sunscreens with a skin protection factor of 15 or greater.
- Advise patients to avoid other aggravating factors, such as photosensitizing drugs, as much as possible.
- Neurologic and psychiatric treatment is needed in patients with severe CNS involvement.
- Nicotinic acid or nicotinamide (50-300 mg/day) provides relief from both the skin manifestations and the neurologic manifestations.
- Administration of tryptophan ethyl ester (a lipid-soluble tryptophan metabolite) in children with Hartnup's disease at a dose of 20 mg/kg every 6 hours results in normalization of serum and cerebrospinal fluid tryptophan levels.

Hyperlipoproteinemia

This group of diseases is caused by defects in structural components of lipoproteins or receptors that affect the formation and removal of lipoproteins. They are characterized by elevated serum cholesterol and triglyceride levels.

Classification

Hyperlipidemias may be classified basically as either familial or primary caused by specific genetic abnormalities, or acquired (also called secondary) when resulting from another underlying disorder that leads to alterations in plasma lipid and lipoprotein metabolism.

Familial (Primary)

1. **Hyperlipoproteinemia type I:** Type I hyperlipoproteinemia is a form of hyperlipoproteinemia associated with deficiencies of lipoprotein lipase.
2. **Hyperlipoproteinemia type II:** Hyperlipoproteinemia type II, the most common form, is further classified into type IIa and type IIb, depending mainly on whether there is elevation in the triglyceride level in addition to LDL cholesterol.
    a. *Type IIa:* This may be sporadic (due to dietary factors), polygenic, or truly familial as a result of a mutation either in the LDL receptor gene on chromosome 19 (0.2% of the population) or the Apo B gene (0.2%).

b. *Type IIb:* The high VLDL levels are due to overproduction of substrates, including triglycerides, acetyl CoA, and an increase in B-100 synthesis. They may also be caused by decreased clearance of LDL.

3. **Hyperlipoproteinemia type III:** Also known as broad beta disease or dysbetalipoproteinemia. This form is due to high chylomicrons and IDL (intermediate density lipoprotein).
4. **Hyperlipoproteinemia type IV:** This form is due to high triglycerides. It is also known as hypertriglyceridemia.
5. **Hyperlipoproteinemia type V:** This type is very similar to type I, but with high VLDL in addition to chylomicrons.

Unclassified Familial Forms

Non-classified forms are extremely rare, e.g.:

- Hypo-alpha lipoproteinemia.
- Hypo-beta lipoproteinemia.

Acquired (Secondary) Hyperlipidemias

Acquired hyperlipidemias (also called secondary dyslipoproteinemias) may mimic primary forms of hyperlipidemia and can have similar consequences. The most common causes of acquired hyperlipidemia are:

- Diabetes mellitus.
- Drugs: Diuretics, beta blockers and estrogens.
- Hypothyroidism
- Renal failure
- Nephrotic syndrome
- Some rare endocrine disorders and metabolic disorders

Cutaneous Manifestations of Hyperlipidemia

Cutaneous xanthomas associated with hyperlipidemia can be clinically subdivided into:

- **Tuberous xanthomas** are firm, painless, red-yellow nodules. The lesions can coalesce to form multilobulated tumors. They usually develop on pressure areas, such as the extensor surfaces of the knees, the elbows and the buttocks (Figure 28.11). **Tendinous xanthomas** appear as slowly enlarging subcutaneous nodules related to the tendons or the ligaments. The most common locations are the extensor tendons of the hands, the feet and Achilles tendon.

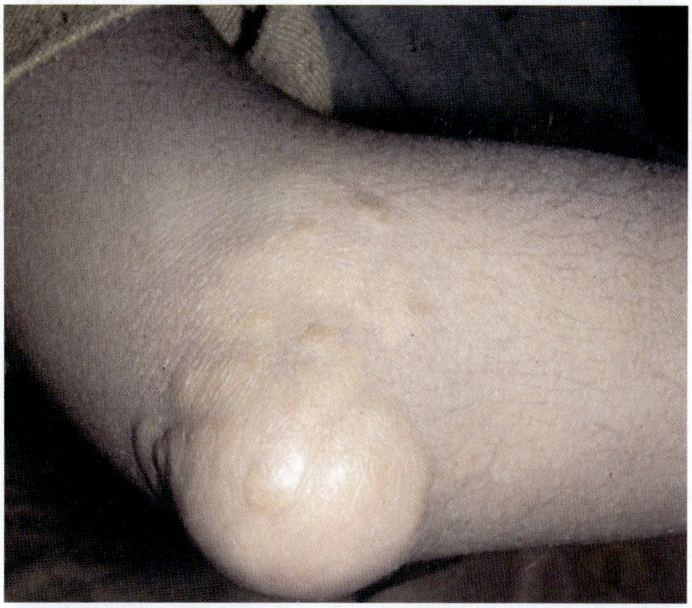

Figure 28.11: Tuberous xanthoma

- **Eruptive xanthomas** most commonly arise over the buttocks, the shoulders, and the extensor surfaces of the extremities. Rarely, the oral mucosa or the face may be affected. The lesions typically erupt as crops of small, red-yellow papules on an erythematous base (Figure 28.12) and they may spontaneously resolve over weeks.

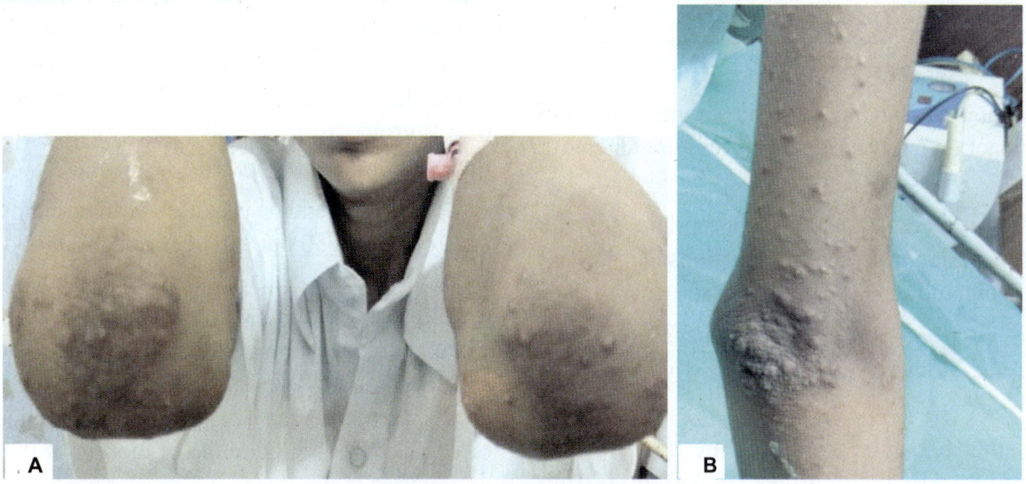

Figure 28.12: Eruptive xanthoma

- **Plane xanthomas** are mostly macular and rarely form elevated lesions. They can occur in any site. Generalized plane xanthomas can cover large areas of the face, the neck, thorax; the flexures can also be involved.
- **Xanthoma disseminatum and verruciform xanthoma** are particular forms of xanthomas that occur in normolipemic patients. Xanthoma disseminatum develops in adults as red-yellow papules and nodules with a predilection for the flexures. Verruciform xanthoma predominantly occurs in the oral cavity of adults as a single papillomatous yellow lesion (Figure 28.13).

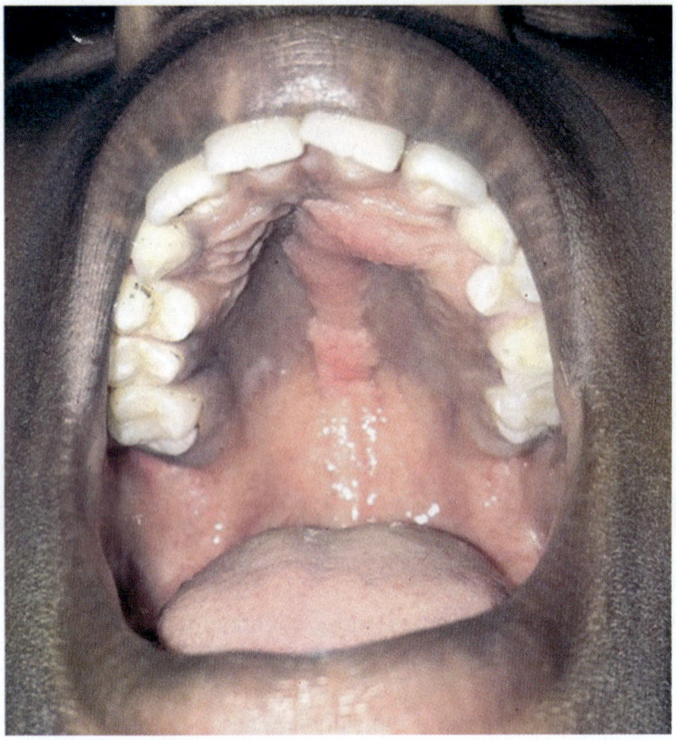

Figure 28.13: Verruciform Xanthoma

Treatment

- Total fat intake should be restricted.
- Exercise, particularly sustained aerobic activity, can have a dramatic impact on triglyceride levels and may increase HDL slightly.
- Three classes of medications are appropriate for the management of major triglyceride elevations: fibric acid derivatives, niacin and omega-3 fatty acids.
- High doses of a strong statin (simvastatin, atorvastatin, rosuvastatin) also lower triglycerides, by as much as approximately 50%.
- Patients with the metabolic syndrome are often treated with metformin, which improves impaired fasting glucose levels, frequently causes weight loss and can lower triglyceride levels.

GRANULOMA FACIALE

Granuloma faciale (GF) is a benign, inflammatory disease. It was first described as 'eosinophilic granuloma'. Although most commonly seen in middle aged white males (between the second and seventh decades of life), but it has been reported in childhood too. Etiology may be related to actinic damage or trauma.

Clinical Features

Granuloma faciale typically presents as a chronic, progressive, asymptomatic, isolated, well defined reddish brown to a violaceous asymptomatic papule, nodule or plaques showing follicular accentuation and telangiectasia. The most common sites are the face and other sun-exposed areas. Dermoscopic features include: linear, arborizing vessels, dilated follicular openings and brown dots/globules.

Treatment

Treatment modalities reported to be useful in granuloma faciale include:

- **Topical treatment:** Considered as first-line therapy which includes topical corticosteroids. topical tacrolimus or topical dapsone.
- Intralesional corticosteroids have been reported to be effective in some cases.
- **Systemic treatment:** Systemic corticosteroids, dapsone.
- Phototherapy, psoralens plus ultraviolet A (PUVA) therapy.

  Other therapeutic modalities like lasers, cryotherapy and surgical excision.

SCLEROMYXEDEMA

Scleromyxedema is a rare disorder causing papular and sclerodermoid lesions due to abnormal accumulation of mucin in the skin, increased production of fibroblasts (in the absence of a thyroid disorder) and monoclonal gammopathy. It often involves internal organs also.

Scleromyxedema is a disease affecting people between the ages of 30 and 50 but can occur in childhood also.

Clinical Features

The papules may be dome shaped, firm, skin colored, or red and approximately 3 mm in diameter (Figure 28.14). Extensive areas of the skin may be involved. Face, knees and elbows are often affected and the range of motion of the face, fingers and extremities is decreased. Other symptoms include esophageal aperistalsis, hoarseness of voice, inflammatory polyarthritis, proximal myopathy, neurologic dysfunction, ophthalmic abnormalities, breathing difficulty caused by restrictive and obstructive pulmonary dysfunction and cardiac involvement.

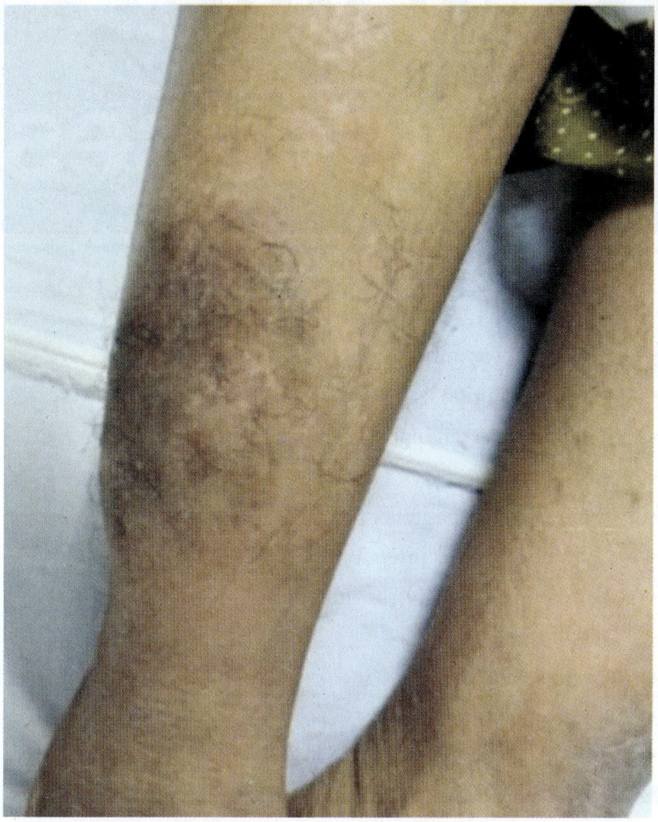

Figure 28.14: Scleromyxedema

Treatment

Thalidomide and systemic glucocorticoids may be used as oral therapy. In resistant cases autologous bone marrow transplantation, melphalan or bortezomib with dexamethasone can be tried. Intravenous immunoglobulins and plasmapheresis are effective to prevent relapses.

LIPOID PROTEINOSIS

Lipoid proteinosis is an autosomal recessive disorder characterized by hoarseness of voice which begins in infancy followed by appearance of yellowish, beaded papules and nodules in the skin. These manifestations are due to the abnormal deposition of hyaline material at the dermoepidermal junction, in microvascular basement membrane and in papillary dermis. There is underlying mutation in extracellular matrix protein 1 (ECM1), which plays a role in skin adhesion and protein interactions near the basement membrane.

Clinical Features

Vocal cord involvement causes hoarseness and this feature is seen in almost every case. The voice may be hoarse from birth or may develop within the first few years of life. It becomes progressively worse during early childhood. Initially, the lesions are discrete or confluent, 2 to 3 mm yellowish white to yellowish brown papules, found most commonly on the face, eyelids, neck and hands. The flexures often show a yellow waxy appearance with diffuse thickening of the skin. Adults develop hyperkeratotic plaques on elbows, knees and palms. Young children commonly show vesicles or bullae that rapidly erode and become crusted. Electron microscopy reveals "free-floating" intact desmosomes. Characteristic linear or discrete varioliform scars subsequently develop, particularly on the face, trunk and upper extremities.

Other manifestations are eversion of the lips, hypertrophic or vegetative lesions at the corners of the mouth, round papules just below the lip on the midline of the chin and radiating fissures at the corners of the mouth. Partial alopecia of the scalp, eyebrows, eyelashes, or bearded area may develop later in childhood. Other features like hypohidrosis, hypertrichosis, hypoplasia or aplasia of permanent teeth, parotid pain and recurrent parotid swelling have been described. The tongue becomes thick, firm and woody due to hyaline deposition. Pharyngeal infiltration and respiratory obstruction are serious complications. CNS involvement can occur in form of seizures.

Management

Diagnostic confirmation can be done with histopathological examination showing thick homogeneous bands of eosinophilic, periodic acid–Schiff-positive, hyaline like amorphous material in the upper dermis with a patchy distribution surrounding blood vessels, sweat glands and arrector pili muscles.

Treatment consists of surgical or laser removal of laryngeal nodules or tracheostomy for laryngeal obstruction. Cosmetic measures such as laser resurfacing or dermabrasion can be done. Acetretin has been tried.

CHAPTER 29 Sexually Transmitted Diseases

Contents

- Syphilis
- Non venereal treponematoses
- Chancroid
- Lymphogranuloma venereum
- Donovanosis
- Herpes genitalis
- Neonatal herpes
- Urethritis
- Non gonococcal urethritis
- Vaginal discharge
- Candidial vaginitis
- Bacterial vaginosis
- Trichomonas vaginalis
- Cervicitis
- Syndromic management of STI
- Cytomegalavirus infection
- Human papilloma virus infection
- HIV infection/AIDS
- Child sexual abuse
- Point of care tests in sti
- Sexual disorders

INTRODUCTION

Sexually transmitted diseases (STDs) (Table 29.1) is a significant health problem because of medicolegal, social and psychological consequences. STDs are becoming increasingly common in pre-adolescent age group as well. Early sexual maturity, increased promiscuity and sexual offences/assault are the probable causes. If not treated promptly and adequately, it results in significant physical and psychological consequences.

Epidemiology

- Every day, over a million treatable STIs (sexually transmitted infections) are contracted in individuals aged 15 to 49 worldwide; the vast majority of these infections are asymptomatic. There has been a steady rise in the STDs in recent years. It is estimated that reported cases represent only 50-80% of STDs, may be due to limited screening or low disease reporting as many STDs are asymptomatic and also because clinical expertise and diagnostic facilities are lacking in most of the places. Bacterial STDs appear to be more frequent than viral STDs.

Transmission

STDs are transmitted by following routes:

1. Sexually active individuals.
2. Transplacental and intrapartum transmission.
3. Postnatal transmission (during breastfeeding, accidental and sexual abuse).
4. In pre pubertal children transmission is due to sexual abuse.

SYPHILIS

It is an infectious treponematosis caused by *Treponema pallidum*, affecting most of the organs. In children it may be congenital or acquired.

Table 29.1: Classification of sexually transmitted diseases

Bacterial, Chlamydial and Mycoplasmal	
Common:	**Pathogen:**
Syphilis	*Treponema pallidum*
Gonorrhoea	*Neisseria gonorrhoeae*
Chlamydial infections	*Chlamydia trachomatis*
Chancroid	*Haemophilus ducreyi*
Less common:	
Granuloma inguinale or Donovanosis	*Calymmatobacterium granulomatis*
Bacterial vaginosis	*Gardnerella vaginalis, Mobiluncus, Mycoplasma hominis*
Non-gonococcal urethritis	*Chlamydia trachomatis, Ureaplasma urealyticum, Staphylococcus saprophyticus, Mycoplasma genitalium*
Viral	
Common:	
Anogenital warts	Human papilloma virus
Herpes genitalis	HSV 2 and less commonly HSV1
Less common:	
Molluscum contagiosum	Molluscum contagiosum virus
Viral hepatitis	Hepatitis A, B, C, D viruses
Cytomegalovirus infection	Cytomegalovirus
Epstein-Barr virus infection	Epstein-Barr virus
Fungal	
Candidiasis	*Candida albicans*
Protozoal	
Trichomoniasis	*Trichomonas vaginalis*
Giardiasis	*Giardialamblia*
Amoebiasis	*Entamoeba histolytica*
Ectoparasite	

Pathophysiology

- When untreated, syphilis is a lifelong infection that progresses in 3 characteristic stages. After initial invasion through mucous membranes or skin, primary lesion develops at the site of inoculation. This is called as primary sore. At the same time organism spreads through the perivascular lymphatics to regional lymph nodes causing lymphadenopathy. Further spread of infection to systemic circulation causes spirochaetemia which leads to development of secondary stage.
- Secondary stage occurs 6-12 weeks after inoculation and during this period of rapid spirochetal multiplication, invasion of most of the tissues of body specially skin, mucous membrane, lymph nodes and CNS occurs.
- Secondary stage becomes latent within 1-2 months after the onset of rash. Relapses with manifestations of secondary stage may be seen between 1-2 years of latency, a period referred to as early latent syphilis. After 2 years syphilis enters into late latent stage.

Different clinical stages and classification of congenital and acquired syphilis is given in Figure 29.1.

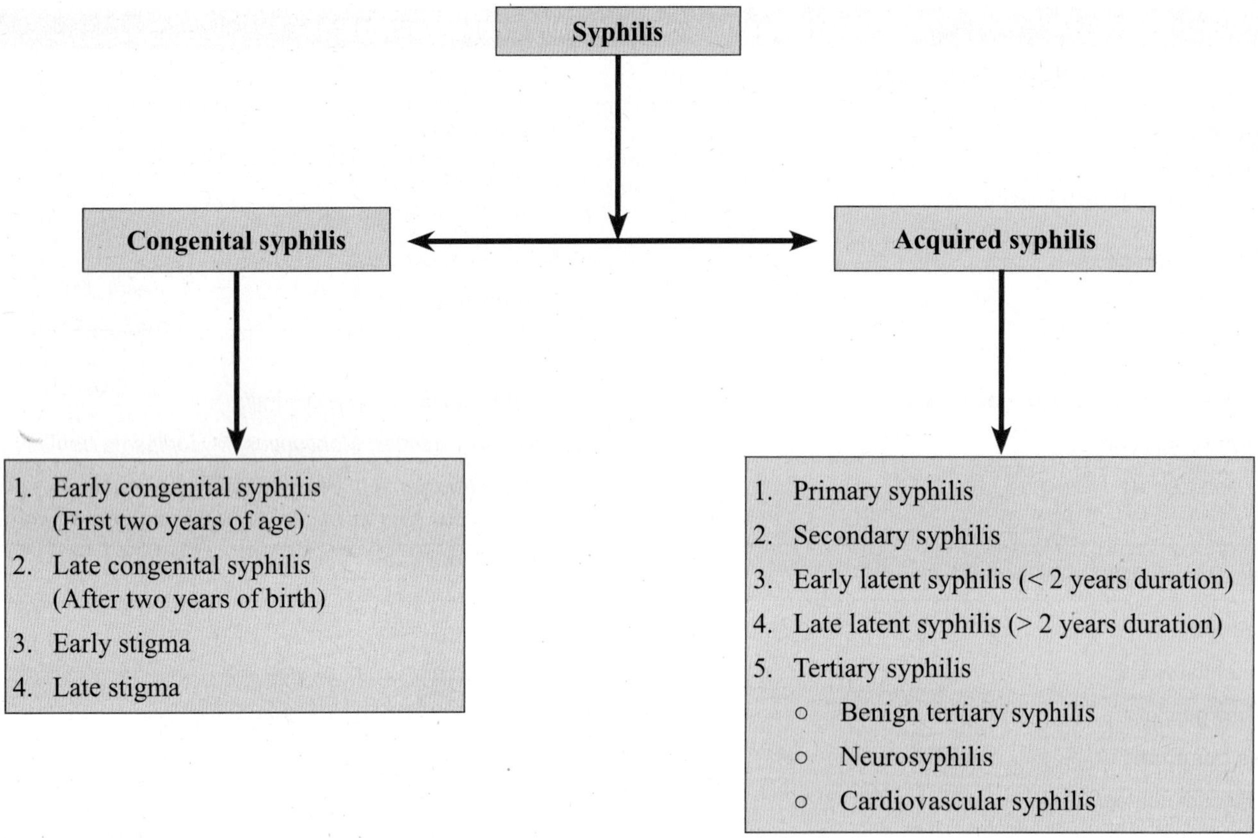

Figure 29.1: Classification of syphilis

Congenital Syphilis

Out of all the patients of congenital syphilis only 30% patients are born with symptoms of congenital syphilis. In many children the clinical evidence of disease is subtle or non-specific at the time of birth hence, cannot be diagnosed.

Congenital syphilis can be divided into following stages:

- Early congenital syphilis: Features appearing within first 2 years of life.
- Late congenital syphilis: Features appearing later than 2 years of life.
- Stigmata.

Transmission

Congenital syphilis occurs due to transplacental spread from affected mother to foetus.

Early Congenital Syphilis

Child may be normal or born with cutaneous manifestations of disease. Baby may be born full term or premature. A period of 2-6 weeks may elapse after birth before the signs of congenital syphilis appear.

Clinical Features

- Rash (symmetrically distributed vesicobullous eruptions over body including palms and soles and multiple superficial erythematous erosion (Figure 29.2) over palms, soles and buttocks).
- Condyloma lata (flat topped, broad based, hypertrophic, grayish white moist papules over angle of mouth, nose, perianal region, vulvar area, Figure 29.3A).
- Syphilitic rhagades (linear radiating fissures at the angle of mouth and anus).
- Syphilitic paronychia due to involvement of nail bed and folds.
- Follicular lesions resulting in patchy alopecia.
- Fever.
- Failure to thrive.
- Hepatosplenomegaly.
- Lymphadenopathy.
- Central nervous system involvement.
- Pseudoparalysis.
- Pneumonitis.
- Ascites.
- Osteitis (Figure 29.3B).

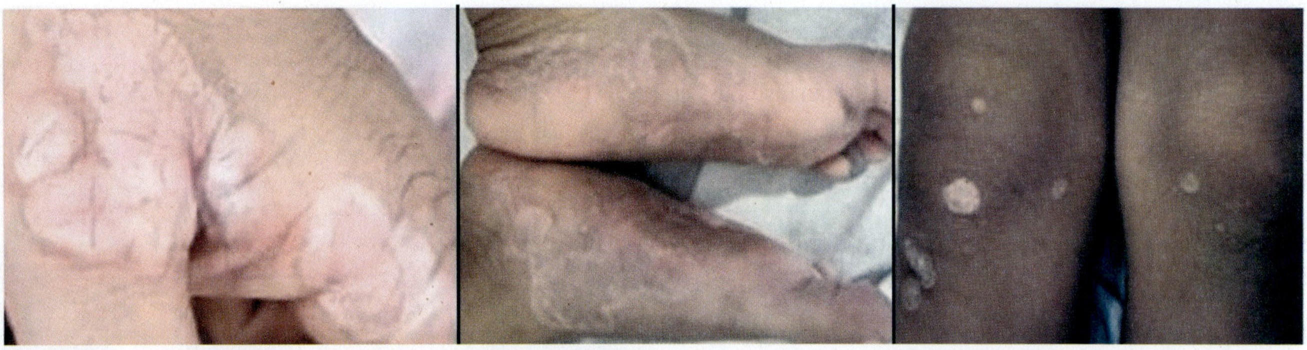

Figure 29.2: Multiple well-defined erosion with erythematous base with scaling on bilateral hands, soles and knee

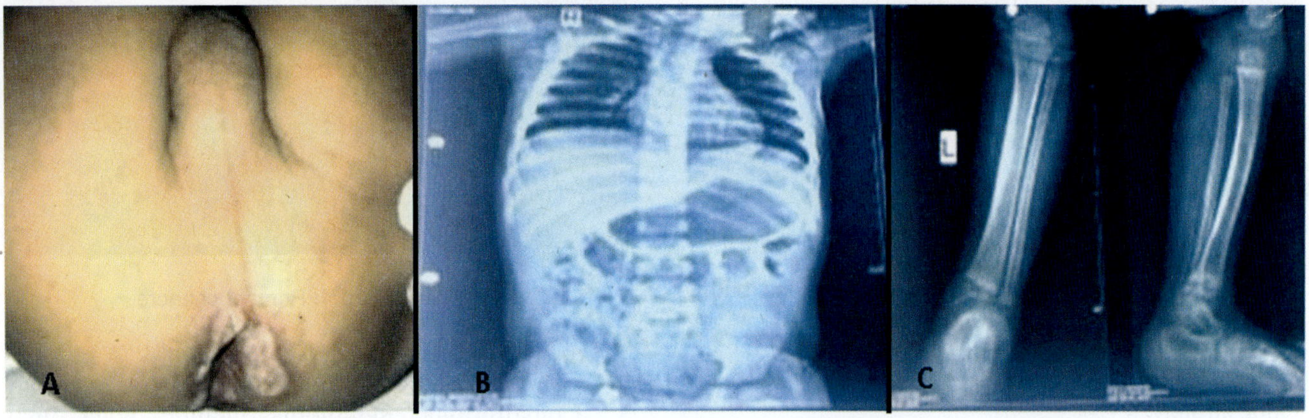

Figure 29.3: Flat topped moist erythematous plaques in perianal area (A), Osteitis of ribs on CxR (B), Marked cortical thickening and periosteal reaction noted in the lateral aspect of left tibia with sabre tibia deformity (C)

Late Congenital Syphilis

Treatment of neonates with congenital syphilis has nearly eliminated these consequences in developed countries, but late manifestations occur in approximately 40 percent of untreated survivors. Many of these manifestations are the destructive residua of early lesions, and, therefore, are not reversible with antibiotic treatment.

Clinical Features

- **Gumma:** Manifests as nodules or nodulo ulcerative lesions affecting skin, mucous membrane, bones and viscera.
- Nasal cartilage destruction resulting from snuffles can lead to a saddle-nose deformity.
- Prolonged periostitis can lead to frontal bossing **(Olympian brow).**
- Thickening of the sternoclavicular portion of the clavicle **(Higouménakis sign).**
- Anterior bowing of the mid tibia (sabre shins, Figure 29.3 C) and scaphoid scapula.
- Clutton joints are symmetric, painless, sterile, synovial effusions, usually localized to the knees.
- Perforation of the hard palate can be seen.
- Syphilitic vasculitis around the time of birth can damage the developing tooth buds and lead to dental anomalies called Hutchinson's teeth (peg shaped, notched central incisors) and mulberry molars (multi-cuspid first molars).
- Deciduous teeth are largely unaffected except for a possible predisposition to dental caries.
- Eye involvement can lead to interstitial keratitis (usually between 5 and 20 years of age), secondary glaucoma or corneal scarring. Keratitis may respond to corticosteroids but not to antibiotic therapy.
- Eighth nerve deafness develops in approximately 3 percent of untreated cases and often starts with high frequency hearing loss when the child is between 8 and 10 years of age.

- Together, Hutchinson's teeth, interstitial keratitis, and eighth nerve deafness comprise **Hutchinson's triad.**
- Other findings of early congenital syphilis can also persist and progress.

Stigmata

These are the scars or deformities resulting from congenital syphilis.

Early Stigmata

- Syphilitic facies: Saddle nose, syphilitic rhagades, small maxillae, high arched palate, prominent mandible (bull dog jaw).
- Hutchinson's teeth.
- Salt and pepper fundus.

Late Stigmata

- Tissue paper scars over skin and mucous membrane.
- Ghost vessels or network of empty blood vessels extending from sclera into deep layers of cornea.
- Perforation of palate.
- Optic atrophy.
- Bony deformities: Parrot nose, craniotabes and sabre shin.

Acquired Syphilis

- Clinical features in children are almost similar to that of adults. Incubation period is 9-90 days (average 3 weeks).

Transmission

- Acquired syphilis is almost always associated with sexual abuse excluding transmission through breastfeeding in children. In adolescents and adults, it is acquired by sexual indulgence.

Primary Syphilis

- Primary lesion, called a chancre (hard chancre), is usually a painless ulcer but may be slightly tender. It is raised with smooth surface, firm and without exudate (Figure 29.4). It usually develops at the site of the inoculation after an average period of 3 weeks. Patients may ignore a visible lesion because it is painless and small in size unless it becomes secondarily infected.
- Painless non-suppurative enlargement of inguinal lymph nodes accompanies the chancre and can persist for months.

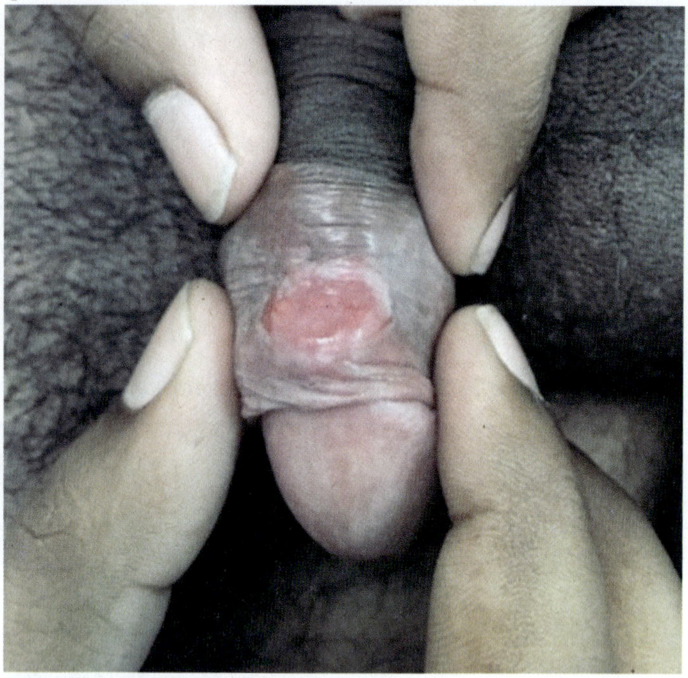

Figure 29.4: Primary chancre

Secondary Syphilis

- Constitutional symptoms include fever, malaise, pharyngitis, rash, anorexia, arthralgia, and generalized painless lymphadenopathy.
- Mucocutaneous lesions are the most frequent manifestation of disease and strongly suggest the diagnosis. Initially discrete, evanescent, macular, pink to red lesions, 3-10 mm in size appear and may spread to involve the entire body, including the palms, soles, and other locations. It disappears in few days and evolve into papular rash. Papular lesions are asymptomatic, usually discrete symmetrically distributed over trunk and extremities. They may be arranged in few cases in linear, circinate or corymbose pattern. Linear pattern along the hairline is known as corona veneris. Deep tenderness can be observed on pressing with a blunt object which is known as Buschke Ollendorf sign. Papules in warm, moist, intertriginous areas, e.g., in groin, perianal region may enlarge and coalesce together to form broad greyish plaques called condyloma lata (Figure 29.5). Condyloma lata at angle of the mouth may be fissured. Syphilitic alopecia may be diffuse or in mouth eaten pattern (Figure 29.6A).
- Secondary syphilis may mimic psoriasis specially guttate psoriasis. Lichenoid presentation of syphilis is a very rare form, which may present with lichenoid macule papules (Figure 29.6B), or plaques. Malignant syphilis is

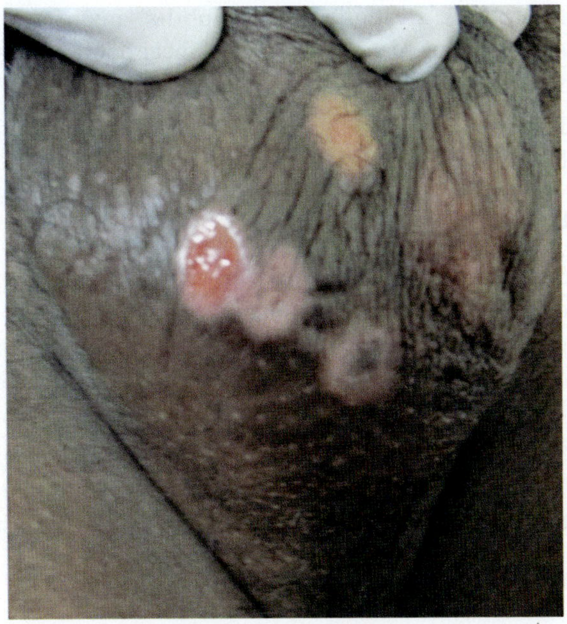

Figure 29.5: Condyloma lata over scrotum (Grey white moist erythematous plaque)

an uncommon feature which presents as pustule necrotic lesions with ulceration due to end arteritis obliterans. It also has systemic manifestations.

- Symmetrical papules, plaques with collarette of scales or keratotic rim (Figure 29.7A) or coppery ham coloured macules (Figure 29.7B) may be present over the palms and soles which is a characteristic feature of secondary syphilis.
- Nails may show paronychia, brittleness, splitting, fissuring, pitting, beau's line, onychomadesis erosive changes (Figure 29.7) and nail loss. Periungual violaceous plaques can be seen in secondary syphilis (Figure 29.8). In oral mucosa slightly raised greyish white lesion with irregular margin (Figure 29.9) may be seen. Large coalescing superficial ulcers can lead to the formation of snail tract ulcers.
- Renal, hepatic and ophthalmologic manifestations may be present.
- Meningitis occurs in 30% of patients with secondary syphilis but may be asymptomatic. Symptomatic

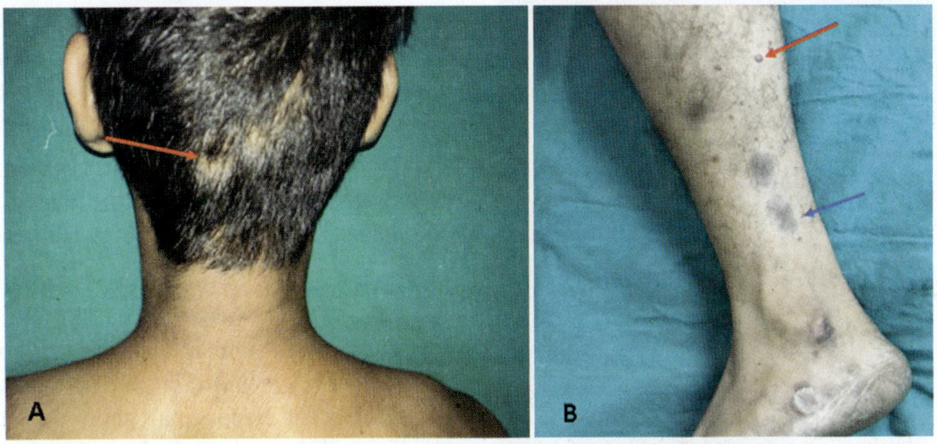

Figure 29.6: Syphilitic alopecia (A) and lichenoid macules (blue arrow) with 'Papular Syphilid' over legs (red arrow)(B)

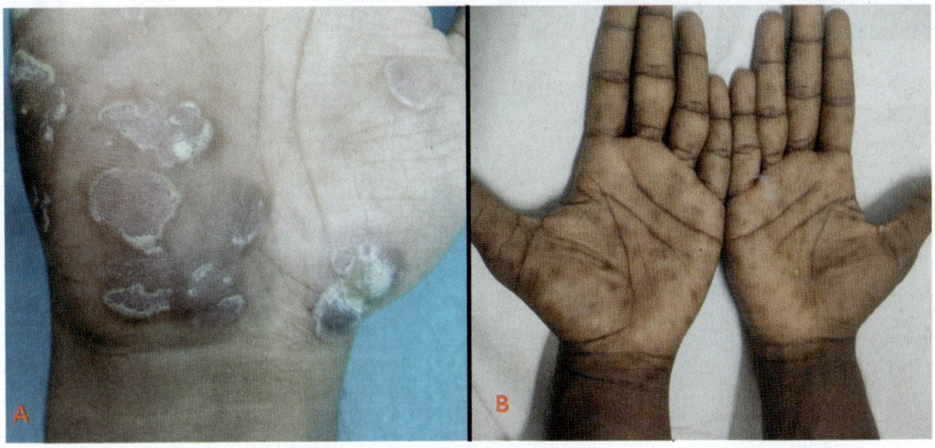

Figure 29.7: Erythematous papules and plaques with surrounding keratotic rim (A) and coppery ham coloured palmer lesion in secondary syphilis (B)

aseptic meningitis occurs in 1-2% of patients and is characterized by headache, stiff neck, nausea and vomiting.

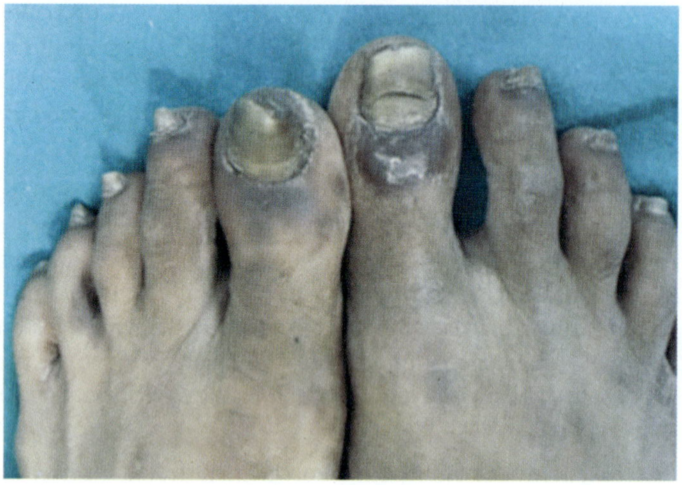

Figure 29.8: Erosive nail changes with periungual violaceous plaque

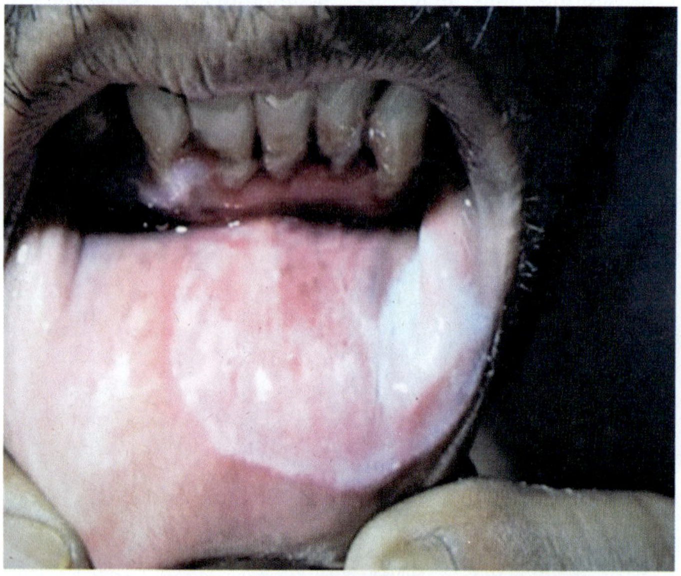

Figure 29.9: 'Mucosal patch' in syphilis well defined corrugated white plaque over oral mucosa

Tertiary Syphilis

- In benign tertiary syphilis, gummatous lesions are found in skin and bones but rarely in other organs. Gummas are considered benign because they rarely involve vital body structures.
- Cardiovascular tertiary syphilis can cause aortitis, aortic aneurysm, coronary stenosis, aortic insufficiency and myocarditis.
- Meningitic tertiary neurosyphilis manifests with symptoms of meningitis or with focal deficits consistent with stroke.
- Prevention of late syphilis can be adequately achieved by treating early syphilis.

Diagnosis

- Serologic testing is commonly used to confirm a diagnosis of syphilis. Direct examination for spirochetes by dark ground illumination is a definitive evidence of syphilis. The organism cannot be cultured on artificial media. Simple laboratory stains fail to demonstrate the spirochetes.
- Serology has the primary role in confirming the diagnosis. The two types of serologic tests for syphilis are non-treponemal reaginic tests and treponema specific tests.

Non-Treponemal Reaginic Serologic Tests

- A positive non-treponemal reaginic test must be confirmed by a treponema specific test.
- Non-treponemal reaginic tests include the rapid plasma reagin (RPR), Venereal Disease Research Laboratory (VDRL) and the automated reagin test (ART), all of which are useful in routine screening and are equally sensitive, inexpensive, simple to perform and rapid.
- These tests are also useful for measurement of ongoing disease activity by estimating them in serial dilutions (e.g., assessment of response to treatment or reinfection).

Treponema Specific Tests

- These tests, which measure antibodies specific for *T. pallidum*, include *T. pallidum* immobilization (TPI), fluorescent treponemal antibody absorption (FTA-Abs), T. pallidum hemagglutination assay (TPHA) and microhemagglutination assay for antibodies to T pallidum (MHA-TP).
- Use these tests in all cases to confirm a positive non-treponemal reaginic test.
- Usually a combination of VDRL and TPHA or MHA-TP are used to confirm the diagnosis.

Traditional and Reverse Algorithm for Diagnosis of Syphilis

- **Traditional Algorithm:** Begins with screening non-treponemal test such as VDRL or RPR followed by confirmatory treponemal test such as fluorescent treponemal antibody test or treponema pallidum particle agglutination (TPPA) or treponemal pallidum hemagglutination (TPHA) test.

- **Reverse Algorithm:** First screen with treponemal test enzyme immune assay (EIA) or Syphilis IgG, followed by non-treponemal test for disease activity assessment by measuring the titer. Discordant treponemal and non-treponemal test results are resolved by a second treponemal test (TPPA or TPHA).

Direct Examination of Spirochetes

- Dark ground illumination (DGI).
- Direct fluorescent antibody tests.

Other Tests Useful in Syphilis

Cerebrospinal Fluid (CSF) Analysis

Indications:

- Signs of neurosyphilis.
- Ocular syphilis.
- Auditory symptoms.
- Tertiary syphilis.
- Treatment failure.
- All infants suspected of prenatal syphilis.
- >1:32 titer in late syphilis.

CSF examination in syphilis will show pleocytosis (>5 WBC/µl), increased protein concentration and positive VDRL test.

Complete Blood Count

- Congenital syphilis is characterized by anemia, thrombocytopenia and either leukopenia or leukocytosis.
- Monocytosis is common.
- Evidence of Coomb's negative hemolytic anemia or a leukemoid reaction may be present.

Liver Function Tests

- Syphilitic hepatitis is characterized by a disproportionately high alkaline phosphatase level and a normal or moderately elevated serum bilirubin level but no cholestasis.
- SGOT and SGPT levels are often elevated.
- Prothrombin time may be increased.

Imaging Studies

- **Chest radiography:** Syphilitic pneumonia may occur in congenital syphilis and appears as fluffy diffuse infiltrate.
- **Long bone radiography:** Radiologic abnormalities are common in early congenital syphilis and are found in 95% of symptomatic infants and in as many as 20% of infants with asymptomatic disease. Bone involvement includes multiple sites of osteochondritis at the wrists, elbows, ankles and knees, and periostitis of long bones and, rarely, the skull.
- Lesions are symmetric and involve multiple bones. The lower extremities are almost always affected.
- Metaphyseal lesions (i.e., osteochondritis) vary from punctate lucencies to more destructive changes.

Histological Findings

- The presence of obliterative endarteritis, which consists of concentric endothelial and fibroblastic proliferative thickening, strongly suggests syphilis. These pathologic changes are found in all stages of syphilis.
- In biopsy specimens, the spirochete may be visualized with specific immunofluorescence (Fontana stain, Levaditi Warthin starry stain, silver stain) or immunoperoxidase staining.

Treatment

In congenital and acquired syphilis upto early latent syphilis:

- Benzathine penicillin G 50,000 units/kg IM after sensitivity test, upto adult dose of 2.4 million units in a single dose.

In late latent syphilis:

- Benzathine penicillin G 50,000 units/kg IM after sensitivity test, upto adult dose of 2.4 million units administered as three doses at weekly interval.

If patient is allergic to penicillin:

- For children <14 years of age: Erythromycin 12.5 mg/ kg orally four times a day for 14 days.
- For chidren >14 years of age: Doxycycline 100 mg orally twice a day for 14 days.

Skin test reagents to identify patient at risk for adverse drug reaction:

Major determinants:

- Benzylpenicilloyl polylysine injection (Pre pan).

Minor determinants:

- Benzylpenicillin G injection.
- Benzylpenicilloate injection.

NON-VENEREAL TREPONEMATOSES

Yaws, endemic syphilis (Bejel) and pinta are caused by treponema which are morphologically and antigenically similar to venereal treponema, treponema pallidum they are differ in their mode of transmission and clinical presentation.

YAWS

Yaws is a chronic, contagious, highly infectious, nonvenereal treponemal disease which is caused by spirochaete, Treponema pallidum pertenue. It is common in Africa, South east Asia and Central America. In India, it reported from tribal communities living in hilly areas. Source of infection for yaws is exudate from skin lesion. It commonly occurs in early childhood. Incubation period is 3-6 weeks. It has three clinical stages:

Primary Stage

- Classical lesions seen in primary stage is mother yaw or framboesia. Lesion initially start as small erythematous papules which enlarge to form raspberry like lesion having central ulceration and yellow crust. At this stage the disease is highly infectious. These lesions heal spontaneously in 3-6 months , leaving atrophic depressed scar with hypopigmented center, surrounded by dark halo. Other features include fever and joint pain with regional lymphadenopathy. Perioral papilloma may occurs in few cases.
- **Decapitated yaws:** When mother yaws is absent ,disease progress directly into secondary stage which is seen in 10 % of the cases.

Secondary stage

Secondary stage has three different clinical manifestations:

1. Cutaneous manifestations
2. Palmoplantar manifestations
3. Bone and joint manifestations

1. **Cutaneous manifestations (Daughter yaws or Pianomas):** Patient have ulcerated lesions, located around periorificial areas. Circinate, annular and condylomatous lesions may also be seen.
2. **Palmoplantar manifestations:** Hyperkeratotic plaques with cracks and fissures are seen on soles (worm eaten sole), which result in painful crab like gait (crab yaws). Nail fold papilloma (Painic onychia) may occur in few cases.
3. **Bone and joint manifestations:** Painful periostitis, polydactylitis and fusiform swelling of metatarsals and metacarpals is seen.

Tertiary Stage (Late yaws)

Tertiary stage is seen in 10 % of affected patients. Tertiary stage has three different clinical manifestations:

- Cutaneous manifestations
- Bone and joint manifestations
- Neurologic and ophthalmic manifestations.

1. **Cutaneous manifestations:** Skin manifestations include subcutaneous nodules, abscess, ulceration which heal with scarring, keloid formation and contractures. Squamous cell carcinoma may develop in long standing ulcerated lesions of late yaws. Keratoderma and hyperkeratosis of palms and soles may also be seen.

   Hormiguillo: Painless minute craters surrounded by hyperkeratotic papules similar to keratoderma punctatum, seen in late yaws.
2. **Bone and joint manifestations:** Hypertrophic periosteitis (painic osteoperiosteitis), gummatous periosteitis and osteomyelitis are seen in this stage. Other features include sabre shins, **gondou** (exostoses of nasal bones resulting in thickened bony masses with prominence of nasal bridges), **gangosa** (mutilation of central part of face which results in destruction of nasal mucosa, cartilaginous and osseous structures of nasal septum, palate and posterior aspect of pharynx with foul smelling discharge).
3. **Neurologic and ophthalmic manifestations:** Optic atrophy and myeloneuropathies may occur in few patients.

Investigation

Dark field microscopy of early lesions and skin biopsy of late lesions can be done for diagnosis. Other investigations include Treponema pallidum particle agglutination (TPPA) and rapid plasma reagin (RPR) tests.

Treatment

- Azithromycin (single oral dose), 30 mg/kg (maximum 2 gm) is the preferred choice as per the WHO "Yaws Eradication Strategy" (the Morges Strategy).
- Benzathine penicillin (single intramuscular dose), 1.2 million units.
- For patients allergic to penicillin and azithromycin, doxycycline 100mg (1 tab) orally, twice daily for 7 days may be used.

Chancroid (Ulcus Mole /Soft Chancre)

It is a caused by Haemophilus ducreyi, a gram negative, facultative anaerobic, fastidious coccobacilli which require factor x (hemin) for growth. Haemophilus releases cytolethal distending toxin (CDT) and increases expression of CXCR 4, CCC5 chemokines which results in increased susceptibility to HIV infection.

Clinical Features

After entering through abraded skin and completion of incubation period (2-7 days), small erythematous papules or pustules develops which converts into multiple, painful ulcers having undermined, ragged margins and soft yellow necrotic material on base, which usually bleeds on touch (Figure 29.10). Ulcers usually occur on prepuce, frenulum , shaft of penis in male and labia majora, labia minora, fourchette or vestibule in females. Due to autoinoculation kissing ulcer can be seen. They may spontaneously heal within 4-6 weeks. Inguinal bubo develops in 50% of cases in 1-2 weeks after ulceration which is unilateral, unilocular and tender and may rupture to form fistulas.

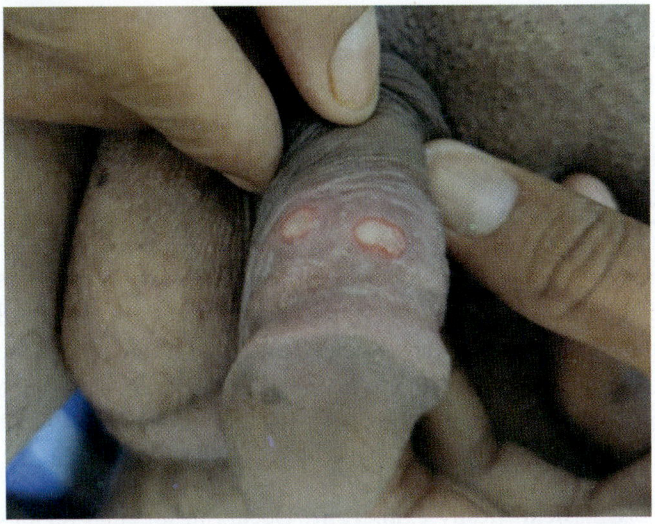

Figure 29.10: Chancroid, painful soft ulcer with ragged edge over penile shaft

Complication

There is no systemic spread of Haemophilus. Balanoposthitis, phimosis, paraphimosis and urethral stricture are the common complications of chancroid.

Clinical variants of Chancroid:

- Papular
- Transient
- Follicular
- Giant
- Dwarf/pustular
- Serpiginous
- Pseudo-granuloma inguinale
- Phagedenic type
- Mixed type

Investigation

Gram stain from edges of ulcer or bubo aspirate shows the **'school of fish'** or **'railroad track appearance'** of gram negative coccobacilli. Culture is gold standard by using Mueller Hinton agar. Serological tests may detect surface antigen (haemoglobin receptor A). Ito Reenstierna test, an intra dermal test may aid to the diagnosis. PCR is confirmatory test. Skin biopsy from ulcer shows three layer with different stage of changes;

- **Top layer:** RBC, fibrin, and neutrophils
- **Middle layer:** Vascular proliferations
- **Lowest layer:** Lymphocytic infiltrates.

Treatment

Macrolides:

- Azithromycin 1 g orally in a single dose or Erythromycin base 500 mg orally TDS for 7 days

Cephalosporine:

- Ceftriaxone 250 mg in a single dose or

Fluoroquinolones:

- Ciprofloxacin 500 mg orally bd for 3 days

  For inguinal bubo Incision and drainage is preferred over aspiration and these patients need longer duration of treatment.

LYMPHOGRANULOMA VENEREUM (LGV, Climatic, Tropical Bubo, Durand Nicolas Favre Disease)

Lymphogranuloma venereum is a caused by Chlamydia trachomatis serotype L1, L2, or L3, which is a gram negative , obligate intracellular pathogen. This organism has two stages of development:

- Elementary body (Metabolically inactive , infective stage)
- Reticulate body (Metabolically active stage or growing stage)

Incubation period: 3-30 days

Clinical Features

- **Incubation period**: 3-30 days. Clinically it has three stages:
- **Primary stage:** Primary stage is usually unnoticed by patients, as transient erosion, ulcer, transient herpetiform vesicle may occur. It may be followed by lymphangitis over dorsal surface of penis and may be seen as cord like swelling of lymphatics, known as **bubonulus.**
- **Secondary stage (inguinal bubo syndrome):** Second stage develops few weeks to months after primary stage. It is characterised by unilateral prominent inguinal lymphadenopathy. In few cases, femoral lymph nodes may also be involved resulting in groove sign. In one third of cases, multilocular abscesses and sinuses discharging purulent material may be seen.
- **Tertiary stage (Genito-anorectal syndrome):** It is a late feature due to destruction of lymphatics causing lymphedema and genital elephantiasis (ram-horn or saxophone penis in male and esthiomene or vulval elephantiasis in female). Due to involvement of anorectal lymphatics, patients may present with multiple fissures, fistulae and stricture in the perianal region.

Complications

- **Acute complications:** Pneumonitis, hepatitis, endocarditis, uveitis, aseptic meningitis, erythema multiforme, erythema nodosum etc.
- **Chronic complication:** Genital elephantiasis, fistula, fissure, strictures etc.

Investigation

- Giemsa stain helps to identify the characteristic inclusion bodies. Cell Culture medium like McCoy cell line can be used for culture. Frei's test, an intradermal test may also be used. Serological tests include complementary fixation test and immune fluorescent test.

Treatment

Primary Treatment

- Doxycycline 100 mg twice a day for 21 days.

Secondary Treatment

- Azithromycin 1 g orally once a week for 3 weeks
- Erythromycin base 500 mg four times a day for 21 days
- Tetracycline 500 mg four times a day for 21 days
- Surgical interventions are required for esthiomene and strictures.

Mnemonic: LGV is the infection of lymphatics

- **A:** Asymptomatic
- **B:** Bubo
- **C:** Chlamydia trachomatis L1, L2, L3
- **D:** Doxycycline
- **E:** Esthiomene
- **F:** Frei's test
- **G:** Groove sign

DONOVANOSIS (Granuloma Inguinale/ Infective Granuloma & Serpiginous Ulceration of Groin)

It is caused by Klebsiella granulomatis (Calymmatobacterium granulomata), a gram negative capsulated intracellular bacilli. The disease is endemic in Orissa, Andhra Pradesh and Tamil Nadu. It is commonly seen in humid climate and in people having low socioeconomic status.

Clinical Features

Incubation period: 8-80 days. Lesion start as painless erythematous firm papule which ulcerate. The ulcer is well defined with beefy red appearance, having red granulation tissue at base, which bleeds on touch (Figure 29.11). Pseudo bubo formation may occur due to subcutaneous autoinoculation.

It has four types:

- **Classical /fleshy exuberant:** Occurs in inguinal regions with classical ulceration.
- **Hypertrophic type:** Presents with pale warty granulation tissue without exudation.
- **Sclerotic or cicatricial:** Early and extensive fibrosis results in deformity of genitalia.
- **Destructive or phagedenic:** Presents with rapidly proliferative necrotic ulcers with abundant foul smelling discharge.

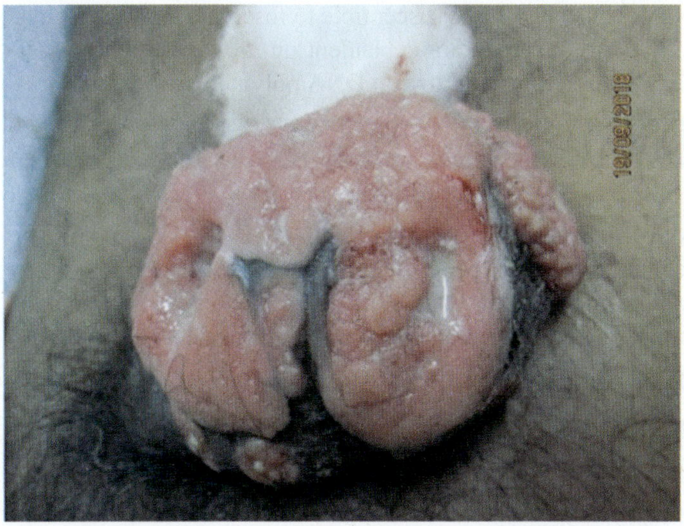

Figure 29.11: Beefy red ulcer of donovanosis

Complications

- Lymphedema
- Pseudo elephantiasis
- Vulval stenosis
- Bone and joint invasion
- Perinephric and psoas abscesses
- Rarely squamous cell carcinoma can develop in ulcer.

Investigation

- Smear should be prepared from tissue obtained from the margin of the ulcer. On staining with Giemsa or Leishman stain, Donovan bodies are seen in clumps of 20-30 bacilli inside monocytes and histiocytes, having safety pin appearance. Histology reveals granulomas where the organisms are occasionally identifiable using silver or Giemsa stains.
- Culture can be done on Hep2 cells, yolk sack of check embryo or on human peripheral blood monocytes.

Treatment

Primary Treatment

- Azithromycin 1 g orally once a week for 3 week or until all lesions have completely heal.
- Doxycycline 100 mg twice daily for 21 days.

Secondary Treatment

- Trimethoprim sulfamethoxazole, double strength once daily for 2 weeks.
- Erythromycin base 500 mg once daily for 3 weeks.

HERPES GENITALIS

It is the most common sexually transmitted disease in world. Causative organism are Herpes simplex virus 1 and 2 (HSV 2 > HSV 1). It can be acquired through genital or orogenital contact. Majority of the patients acquire infection by asymptomatic shedders.

Clinical Features

- **Incubation period**: 2 days -14 days.

Primary Herpes Genitalis

- Patients present with grouped vesicular lesions with surrounding erythema which soon ulcerate into multiple, small superficial painful ulcerations with polycyclic margins (Figure 29.12). It may be associated with fever and malaise. Inguinal lymph nodes may become painful and tender. It heals in 2-3 weeks without scarring. Chronic non healing herpetic ulcer (>1 month duration) raises the suspicions of HIV infection.

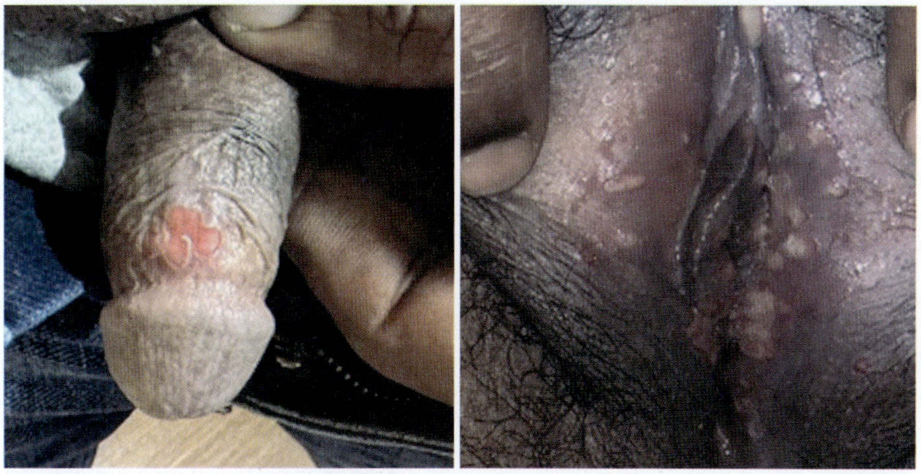

Figure 29.12: Herpes genitalis showing multiple superficial grouped erosion

Complications

- Secondary infections
- Acute urinary retention
- Aseptic meningitis

Recurrent Herpes Genitalis

Recurrence is unpredictable and occurs due to reactivation of virus which is present in the sacral dorsal root ganglia. The common trigger factors are physical or psychological stress and immunosuppression. Clinically recurrent episodes are milder, lesions are less extensive and heal earlier.

Asymptomatic Shedding

It is defined as detection of herpes virus in the absence of visible lesion. Transmission of herpes usually occurs during asymptomatic viral shedding phase.

Investigation

Tzanck smear by using Leishman stain or Giemsa stain shows multinucleate giant cells (page no.) Serological tests are not type specific, although they may be positive during recurrent genital or oral episodes of herpes, these tests are not recommended or are of little diagnostic value. HSV culture (on Hep-2 cells) is highly specific test but less sensitive. Polymerase chain reaction (PCR) is highly sensitive test.

Treatment

Primary Episode

- Acyclovir 400 mg orally three time a day for 7-10 days.
- Famciclovir 250 mg orally three time a day for 7-10 days
- Valacyclovir 1 g orally twice a day for 7-10 days

Recurrence Episodes

Recurrence treatment:

- Acyclovir 800 mg twice a day for 5 days
- Famciclovir 125 mg twice a day for 5 days or
- Valacyclovir 1 g once daily for 5 days

Suppressive Therapy: Indicated if > 6 episodes/year

- Acyclovir 400 mg twice daily for 12 months
- Famciclovir 250 mg orally twice daily for 12 months
- Valacyclovir 1 gm once a day for 12 months

Acyclovir resistant: Resistance occurs due to mutation in HSV thymidine kinase gene.

- Resistant virus is susceptible to foscarnet and cidofovir as these drugs are not dependent on viral thymidine kinase. These drugs inhibit viral DNA polymerase.

NEONATAL HERPES

Neonatal herpes is a severe life threatening disease acquired through birth passage of infected mother. Infection can also be acquired in utero, peripartum and postpartum, through either active infection or asymptomatic viral shedding. Asymptomatic mothers transmits about 70 % cases of neonatal HSV.

Risk factors:

- Active herpes genitalis (primary or recurrent)
- Vaginal delivery increases risk of transmission
- Prolonged duration of rupture of membranes
- Use of fetal scalp electrode or other invasive instrumentation

Neonatal herpes presents with following clinical patterns:

- **Skin, Eye and Mouth (SEM) disease**
- **Central Nervous System (CNS) disease**
- **Disseminated disease**

SEM disease: It presents 9-11 days after birth with characteristic vesicular or ulcerative skin lesions which can turn into pustular, bullous and necrotic lesions.

Central nervous system (CNS) disease: Clinically these patients presents with lethargy, irritability, poor oral intake. Due to CNS infection patient may develop CNS focal encephalitis and meningoencephalitis, which are associated with fever, seizures and coma. CSF analysis shows lymphocytic pleocytosis.

Disseminated disease: This type of neonatal HSV is most life threatening, due to widespread dissemination of virus to vital organs like liver, brain, lungs and kidney.

Investigations

Material for skin smear can be collected from mouth, conjunctival or skin lesions and from CSF. The collected material may be used for Tzanck smear, culture and PCR examination. Skin biopsy shows intraepidermal bulla, with large multinucleated cells.

Preventive measures:

- Treat the mother if she has history of HSV infection during pregnancy
- Avoid invasive monitoring and blood sampling
- During delivery if active lesions are present, Caesarean section is preferred mode of delivery.

- If mother develops active herpes after delivery, isolate the foetus.
- Prophylactic suppressive therapy can be given to HSV 2 seropositive pregnant mother, from 36 weeks of gestation.

Treatment

Recommended dose of acyclovir is 20 mg/kg IV 8 hourly.

- For SEM-14 days
- For CNS and disseminated infection -21 days

URETHRITIS

Urethritis is inflammation of the urethra, commonly seen in adolescent age group. It usually resolves without any complication but may be associated with peri urethral abscess formation and urethral stricture. Recurrent urethritis may occur due to reinfection or therapeutic failure. Untreated urethritis may lead to epididymitis, orchitis, prostatitis, proctitis, hepatitis, reactive arthritis, uveitis, pneumonia etc.

Aetiology

Infectious:

Gonococcal:

- Neisseria gonorrhoea (50-90%)

Non gonococcal:

- Chlamydia trachomatis (serotype-D-K) (most common)
- Ureaplasma urealyticum
- Mycoplasma genitalium
- Trichomonas vaginalis
- Yeast
- Herpes simplex

Non-Infectious:

- Trauma
- Urethral stricture
- Catheterization
- Chemical irritants
- Dehydration

Symptoms

Patient presents with yellowish pus discharge from urethra (sometimes blood discharge) burning micturition, increased urinary frequency, urinary urgency, irritation around the penis and painful sexual intercourse in women. It may be asymptomatic in few patients.

Examination

Examination should be done in morning or at least 2 hours after the last micturition in standing or supine position in male and in lithotomy position in female. Underwear should be examined for dried discharge. If a foreskin is present, it should be retracted for adequate evaluation of the meatus for discharge, crusting, and redness. If no discharge is seen, the urethra should be gently milked.

GONOCOCCAL URETHRITIS

It is caused by Neisseria gonorrhea, a gram negative, non-motile, non-spore forming diplococci, predominantly seen intracellularly in the polymorphonuclear leucocytes (PMN). It affects urethra in both sexes.

Transmission of Gonorrhea

- Perinatal transmission.
- Direct or indirect contact with infected fomites.
- Sexual indulgence.
- Sexual abuse.
- Rarely, accidental infections.

Incubation period is 2-5 days

In male: Patient presents with intense burning sensation in anterior urethra with profuse purulent discharge (Figure 29.13). In 15 % of patients, it may be asymptomatic. It can lead to posterior urethritis, epididymitis, acute or chronic prostatitis. If left untreated for long time, periurethral abscess and water can perineum can occur.

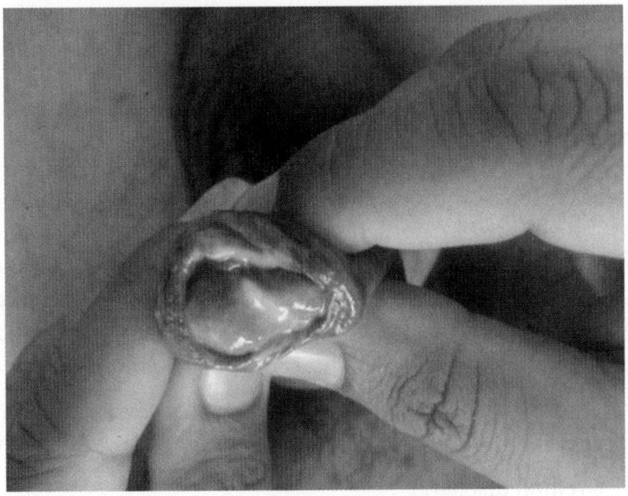

Figure 29.13: Purulent urethral discharge

In females: It presents with scanty mucopurulent urethral discharge, vaginal pruritus and dysuria. Fifty percent of infected females may be asymptomatic. Complications include pelvic inflammatory disease, tubo-ovarian abscess, ectopic pregnancies, chronic pelvic pain, Bartholin gland abscess, infertility and inflammation of liver capsule (Fitz-Hugh-Curtis syndrome).

Complications like disseminated gonococcal infection, acute arthritis-dermatitis syndrome, pustular skin eruptions, gonococcal arthritis, meningitis, proctitis, pharyngitis and endocarditis may occur in both sexes.

Complications in Infants Due to Gonorrhea

Ophthalmia neonatorum

A child with purulent discharge from the eyes within 30 days of birth is diagnosed to have ophthalmia neonatorum.

Aetiology of Ophthalmia Neonatorum: The etiology can be chemical or microbial. Several non- infectious and infectious agents can inflame the conjunctiva in a child within 30 days of birth. Chemical conjunctivitis maybe caused due to use of silver nitrate drops. Among infectious agent's chlamydia, gonococci, staphylococci and herpes virus may cause conjunctivitis in this age group.

Clinical Presentation of Gonococcal Conjunctivitis

Gonococcal conjunctivitis tends to be more severe than other causes of ophthalmia neonatorum, which presents as purulent conjunctivitis, usually bilateral. Corneal involvement leads to diffuse epithelial edema and ulceration that may progress to perforation of the cornea and endophthalmitis. Patients may also have systemic manifestations (e.g., rhinitis, stomatitis, arthritis, meningitis, anorectal infection and septicemia). The organism can cause permanent injury to the eye in a very short time so prompt recognition and treatment are essential to avoid blindness.

Investigations

Smear should be prepared from the pus coming out from urethral meatus. If no sample can be expressed even after milking, specimen should be collected by inserting a small dacron swab 2 cm into the urethra and rotated for 5-10 seconds to obtain the specimen. Neisseria gonorrhoeae are seen as gram negative intracellular diplococci in polymorphonuclear cells (Figure 29.14).

Criteria for clinical diagnosis of urethritis (CDC guideline)

- Urethral discharge
- ≥ 2 polymorphonuclear leukocytes/oil immersion field or
- ≥10 PMNs/High power field in sediment from first void urine

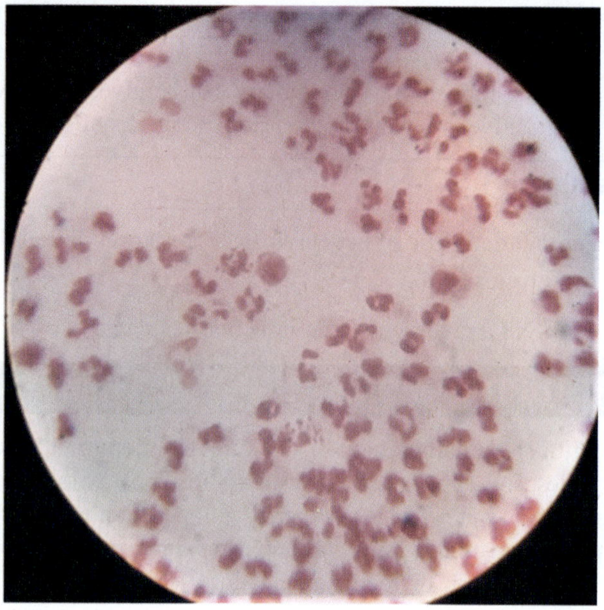

Figure 29.14: Gram stain showing bacteria inside neutrophils

NACO guideline

- Urethral discharge
- >/= 5 PMNs/oil immersion field in smear examination

Culture for gonorrhea: Culture is gold standard for diagnosis of gonorrhea. Direct plating has better results but if direct plating is not available then swab can be transport to laboratory in transport medium. It gives fermentation reaction with glucose.

- **Transport medium:** Non-nutritive medium: Stuart's or Amie's medium
- **Nutritive medium:** Transgrow, Jembec, Gono Pak, In Tray Gc system
- **Selective medium:** Modified Thayer martin or New York city medium
- **Non selective medium:** Chocolate agar with NADP and hemoglobin

POCTs (point of care tests) for Gonorrhea: Bio Star OIA, PATH GC-check, One Step one strip.

Treatment

Uncomplicated Infection

- Single dose ceftriaxone 500 mg intramuscular
- Single dose 400mg oral
- Single dose Ciprofloxacin 500 mg oral
- Single dose Ofloxacin 400 mg oral

Disseminated Gonococcal Infection

- Ceftriaxone 1 gm IM or IV every 24 hours for 2 days or
- Cefotaxime 1 gm IV 8 hourly for 2 days or
- Ciprofloxacin 400 mg IV 12 hourly for 2 days or
- Ofloxacin 400 mg IV 12 hourly for 2 days or
- Levofloxacin 250 mg IV daily for 2 days or

Followed by Cefixime 400 mg twice daily for 7 days or ciprofloxacin 500 mg twice daily or ofloxacin 400 mg twice daily or levofloxacin 500mg twice daily.

Cefixime and ceftriaxone are recommended for pregnant women as well as for HIV positive patients.

Partner Treatment

- Should be done in suspected or confirmed urethritis patients
- Decreases risk of reinfection in patient and interrupts disease transmission
- All sexual contacts within 60 days of onset of symptoms should be treated.
- If last sexual contact >60 days before onset of symptoms, treat the most recent sexual partner.

Gonococcal Ophthalmia Neonatorum

- Single dose Ceftriaxone 25-50 mg/kg IV or IM, up to a maximum of 125 mg.

Disseminated gonococcal infection in infants:

- Ceftriaxone 25-50 mg/kg/day IM or IV, daily for 7 days or cefotaxime 25 mg/kg IM or IV every 12 hours for 7 days
- If documented meningitis then treatment is Ceftriaxone 25-50 mg/kg/day IM or IV for 10-14 days or Cefotaxime 25 mg/kg IM or IV every 12 hours for 10-14 days.
- Alternate drugs are gentamicin, azithromycin, cefixime if ceftriaxone and cefotaxime is not available.

NON GONOCOCCAL URETHRITIS

It presents with clear creamy white urethral discharge with or without urethritis. Chlamydia and Mycoplasma genitalium are the commonest cause for non-gonococcal urethritis. Discharge of NGU is less purulent and have longer incubation period as compared to gonococcal urethritis.

Complications of NGU:

- Epididymo-orchitis
- Sexually acquired reactive arthritis
- Pelvic inflammatory disease
- Infertility
- Reactive arthritis

Chlamydial infection in neonates and children:

- In neonates, *Chlamydia trachomatis* is mainly transmitted by infected mother during vaginal delivery.

Clinical Features

- Incubation period is 1-3 weeks.
- **Neonatal conjunctivitis:** Most common presentation, reported in 50% of infants born to infected mothers. Clinical findings are variable, ranging from mild conjunctivitis with scanty mucoid discharge to copious purulent discharge.
- Nasopharynx is the second most common site of perinatally acquired chlamydial infections. Some patients may develop pneumonia.
- Vaginitis.
- Proctitis, non-specific urethritis, otitis media, pelvic inflammatory disease (PID) can also be seen in older children who acquire chlamydial infections by sexual activity.

Investigation

- Gram-stained urethral smear shows absence of diplococci and ≥ 5 PMNs per oil immersion field should be present on microscopy and/ or positive urinary leukocyte esterase in first voided urine or ≥10 PMNs/High power field in sediment from first void urine.
- Other tests for diagnosis of chlamydia are Nucleic acid amplification test (NAAT) and POCTs (Bio Star OIA, Clearview chlamydia, Quick Vue, CRT, etc).
- NAAT for Mycoplasma genitalium and Ureaplasma urealyticum is also available but not approved.
- Diagnosis of chlamydial conjunctivitis is made by examining Giemsa-stained conjunctival scraping for characteristic basophilic intracytoplasmic inclusions.
- Culture on McCoy cells, enzyme immunoassay (EIA), direct fluorescent antibody (DFA) test may also be done.

Treatment

- Doxycycline 100 mg twice daily for 7 days or
- Azithromycin 1gm oral single dose
- Alternative regimen
- Erythromycin 500 mg four time a day for 7 days

VAGINAL DISCHARGE

Normal physiological vaginal discharge is white, odourless, floccular/granular, variable in quantity and acidic in pH (3.5-4.5). Microscopic examination usually shows abundant lactobacilli and clue cells ≤ 20%. Excessive physiological discharge is seen in pregnancy and during sexual arousal.

Abnormal vaginal discharge – Any one of the following may be present:

1. Excessive vaginal discharge not associated with menstruation
2. Offensive or malodorous discharge
3. Yellowish or muco-purulent discharge

Etiology of abnormal vaginal discharge:

Infective:

Due to cervicitis (details describe in cervicitis)

Vaginitis:

- Candidial vaginitis
- Trichomonas vaginitis
- Bacterial vaginitis

Non infective:

- Chemical irritants
- Foreign body
- Radiations
- Medications

Summary of different types of infective vaginitis showing in Table 29.2.

CANDIDIAL VAGINITIS

Risk factors:

- Over use of antibiotics
- Uncontrolled diabetes mellites
- Local irritants application
- Estrogens (Cyclical candidiasis)
- Immunosuppression
- **Drugs:** Tamoxifen (C. glabrata)
- High sugar diet

Uncomplicated vulvovaginal candidiasis:

- Sporadic or infrequent infections
- Mild to moderate symptoms
- Suspected C. albicans infection
- Non-pregnant, non-diabetic women

Complicated vulvovaginal candidiasis:

- 4 or more recurrences in 12 months OR
- Severe symptoms or signs OR
- Suspected or proven non albicans infection
- Impaired host immunity

C. albicans is the most common species causing vulvovaginal candidiasis. Rarely it may be caused by *C. glabrata, C. tropicalis.* Recurrence after 3 months of previous episode is most likely due to infection with a different strain of C. albicans. Patient usually presents with moderate, white, clumpy or cheesy adherent exudative discharge with itching, erosion, oedema of external genitalia and dyspareunia.

Table 29.2: Summary of different types of infective vaginitis

	Candidial vaginitis	*Trichomonas vaginitis*	*Bacterial vaginitis*
Causative organism	Candida species	Trichomonas vaginalis	Gardnerella vaginalis, Bacteroides, Prevotella, Mobiluncus
Symptoms	Itching of external genitalia, erosion and oedema of genitalia	Genital pruritis and irritation Vulval dermatitis, cervical petechiae	Asymptomatic discharge
Discharge characteristics	Moderate white clumpy or **cheesy adherent** exudate	Profuse, malodorous, **greenish, frothy,** homogenous	Moderate, malodorous, **grey white, homogenous** with coating of vaginal wall
pH	< 4.5	> 5	> 4.5
Whiff test or amide odour with 10% KOH	No	Usually present	Present

Investigation

Examination should be done by using Sim's speculum or Cusco's self-retaining bivalved vaginal speculum. Wet mount and KOH examination of vaginal discharge shows budding yeast, hyphae, and pseudo yeast.

Culture can be done in some cases on Sabouraud Dextrose Agar (SDA). In recurrent cases, antifungal susceptibility testing can be done by using disk diffusion in Muller-Hinton agar with 2% glucose and methylene blue. When human or sheep serum is added to culture, germ tube formation occurs which is known as Reynolds- Braude Phenomenon. Different species of candida can be identified by culture on CHROM agar medium.

Treatment

For uncomplicated

Short course of topical clotrimazole or miconazole intravaginally for 7-14 days. Vaginal suppositories (clotrimazole, terconazole, miconazole, fenticonazole) can also be used. Oral treatment includes single dose of fluconazole.

For Complicated

Suppressive

- Topical miconazole, clotrimazole cream for 14 days (preferred in pregnancy)
- **Oral treatment:** Three doses of fluconazole (100mg/150mg/200mg) on day 1, day 4 and day 7

Maintenance

- Oral fluconazole 150mg per week for 6-12 months OR
- Oral fluconazole 200mg per week for 8 weeks, biweekly for 4 months, monthly for 6 months.

Non-albicans treatment

- **First line:** Long term non-fluconazole azole
  - ***Topical:*** Clotrimazole or miconazole intravaginally for 14 days.
  - ***Oral:*** Itraconazole 200 mg daily for 14 days
- **Recurrence:** Following may be used in addition to topical or systemic antifungals
  - Intravaginal boric acid 600 mg od × 14 days
  - Intravaginal nystatin ovules
  - Gentian violet paint

BACTERIAL VAGINOSIS

Risk factor:

- Vaginal douching
- Use of intrauterine contraceptive device
- Multiple sexual partners
- Use of high dose spermicidal
- Use of excessive vaginal antiseptic

Aetiology

Bacterial vaginosis is caused due to change in normal vaginal flora. There is increased levels of Gardnerella vaginalis, Bacteroides, Prevotella, Mobiluncus and other anaerobic bacteria and decreased levels of Lactobacillus (i.e imbalance in good and harmful bacterial flora's).

Clinical features: Common symptoms include abnormal moderate, malodorous, grey white homogenous vaginal discharge, which also coats the vaginal wall.

Recurrent Bacterial Vaginosis

When three or more documented episodes in a period of 12 months occur, it is called recurrent bacterial vaginosis. The recurrence occurs in 30-50% patients within 2-3 months of clinical cure of prior episode. It may occur due to development of vaginal bacterial biofilm or antibiotic resistance in Gardnerella vaginalis. Biofilm is temporarily suppressed with standard metronidazole therapy and typically reoccurs in 10-12 weeks.

Diagnosis

Amsel's criteria:

1. Homogenous grey adherent vaginal discharge
2. Whiff test with 10% KOH- fishy/amine odour
3. pH > 4.5
4. > 20% clue cells in wet mount examination

Three out of four criteria must be present to confirm the diagnosis of bacterial vaginosis. Nugent's score based on gram staining for bacterial vaginosis described in Table 29.3.

Point of care tests for bacterial vaginitis:

OSOM BV Blue is an FDA approved point of care test for bacterial vaginosis. It detects elevated sialidase enzyme activity in vaginal fluid. AFFIRM VPIII is a DNA hybridization assay for gardenalia vaginalis.

Management

Primary Regimen

Metronidazole 500 mg twice daily for 7 days or Metronidazole gel 0.75 % (5 gm once a day intravaginally for 5 days) or clindamycin 2% (5 gm once a day intravaginally for 5 days).

Table 29.3 : Nugent's score based on gram staining for bacterial vaginosis

Score I	*Score II*	*Score III*
Lactobacillus: Gram positive rods / HPF	**Gardnerella:** Small gram negative variable rods / HPF **Bacteroides:** Small gram variable rods / HPF	**Mobiluncus:** Curved gram negative rods / HPF
0 if >30	0 if 0	0 if 0
1 if 5-30	1 if < 1	1 if <5
2 if 1-4	2 if 1-5	2 if >5
3 if <1	3 if 5-30	
4 if 0	4 if >30	
Total score I+II+III 0-3: Negative for bacterial vaginosis 4-6: Intermediate >7 : Bacterial vaginosis		

Alternate Regimen

- Tinidazole 2 gm once daily for 2 days
- Clindamycin 300 mg bd for 7 days

Probiotics in Bacterial Vaginosis

Probiotics promote growth of Lactobacillus, resulting in restoring of normal vaginal microenvironment. Commonly used probiotics are Lactobacillus reuteri R-14 and Lactobacillus rhamnosus GR-1. These probiotics can be given as supplementary treatment with standard therapy.

Treatment of Recurrences Bacterial Vaginitis

- Standard therapy followed by maintenance regimen
- Maintenance regimens:
  - 0.75% metronidazole gel intravaginally twice weekly for 4-6 months
  - Intravaginal boric acid 600mg OD for 21 days and then suppressive 0.75% metronidazole gel twice weekly for 4-6 months
  - Monthly oral metronidazole 2g with fluconazole 150mg
- Metronidazole resistance: In metronidazole resistance cases clindamycin 300mg BD 7 days is recommended.

TRICHOMONAS VAGINALIS

Risk factors:

- Multiple sexual partners
- Lack of barrier contraception
- Smoking

It usually presents with profuse, malodorous, greenish, frothy, homogeneous discharge with genital pruritis and vulval dermatitis. Cervical petechiae can also occurs in few cases.

Recurrent Trichomoniasis

Common causes for recurrent trichomoniasis are:

- Reinfection from the untreated partner
- Antimicrobial resistance
- Treatment failure

Partner infection rates is very high in trichomoniasis (70-80%), so in recurrent trichomoniasis partner treatment is required in spite of negative diagnosis. Even after adequate partner management, recurrence may be due to nitroimidazole resistance or metronidazole resistance. 5% of all clinical trichomoniasis is resistant to metronidazole

Diagnosis

Wet mount from vaginal discharge shows motile trichomonas vaginalis. It can be cultured on Kupferberg's, Diamond or Modified Diamond by Klaas medium. Culture is gold standard test for trichomoniasis, which takes upto 5 days. FDA approved point of care tests are OSOM Trichomonas rapid test and APTIMA test, which detect species specific 16S ribosomal RNA. Nucleic acid amplification test can also be done to identify trichomonas.

Treatment

Primary Treatment

- Metronidazole 2g stat or tinidazole 2g stat

Recurrence

- Metronidazole 500mg BD × 7days or
- Metronidazole 2g or Tinidazole 2g OD × 7days or
- Tinidazole 1g BD × 7days or
- Others treatment options include intravaginal boric acid or 5% intravaginal paromomycin.

CERVICITIS

Cervicitis is inflammation of cervix due to the infection or irritation.

Aetiology

Infectious:

- Trichomonas vaginalis
- Chlamydia trachomatis
- Neisseria gonorrhoeae
- Herpes simplex virus infection
- Human papilloma virus infection

Non infectious:

- Local trauma/irritation
- Malignancy
- Radiation

Risk factors: Risk factor for cervicitis includes high-risk sexual behavior, history of STDs, multiple sexual partners, sexual intercourse at an early age.

Symptoms

Cervicitis may be asymptomatic or it may present with abnormal mucopurulent vaginal discharge, abnormal bleeding especially post coital, dysuria, or dyspareunia. On examination, erythema of cervix, friability, petechia, strawberry cervix and cervical motion tenderness is seen.

Investigation

Gram stain from cervical discharge to look for white blood cells and Nisseria gonorrhea and wet mount for trichomonas. NAAT for Chlamydia trachomatis or Neisseria gonorrhoeae, rapid tests for trichomonas like OSOM trichomonas and AFFIRM VP III can also be done. Pap smear should be done in patients suspected for cervical cancer.

Treatment

- NACO: Cefixime 400mg stat + Azithromycin 1g stat
- Concurrent treatment of vaginitis if present: Secnidazole 2g stat + fluconazole 150mg stat
- CDC: Azithromycin 1g + Ceftriaxone 500 mg intramuscular stat

Syndromic management of sexually transmitted infection (Table 29.4)

CYTOMEGALOVIRUS (CMV) INFECTION

CMV infection can also be transmitted through transplacental, perinatal and sexual route.

Clinical Features

Ninety percent of infants with congenital CMV infection are asymptomatic. Approximately 5-15% of them are at risk of developing developmental abnormalities including sensorineural hearing loss, microcephaly, mental retardation, chorioretinitis and dental defects. Symptoms become apparent within 2 years of life.

Treatment

Ganciclovir 8-12 mg/kg/day given in divided doses at 12 hourly interval for 6 weeks.

Table 29.4: Syndromic management of sexually transmitted infection (NACO guidelines)

Clinical features	*STI kit*	*Color of std kit*	*Drugs included in kit*
Urethral or cervical or anorectal discharge	Kit -1	Grey	Tab. Azithromycin 1gm (single tablet) Tab. Cefixime 400 mg (single tablet)
Vaginal discharge	Kit -2	Green	Tab. Fluconazole 150 mg (single tablet) Tab. Secnidazole 2 gm (single tablet)
Non-herpetic genital ulcer	Kit -3	White	Injection benzathine penicillin 2.4 mIU (single vial) Tab. Azithromycin 1 gm (single tablet)
Non-herpetic genital ulcer allergic to penicillin	Kit -4	Blue	Tab. Doxycycline 100mg BD for 14 days Tab. Azithromycin 1 gm (single tablet)
Herpetic genital ulcer disease	Kit-5	Red	Tab. Acyclovir 400 mg TDS for 7 days
Pelvic inflammatory disease or lower abdominal pain	Kit-6	Yellow	Tab. Cefixime 400 mg (single tablet) Tab. Metronidazole 400 mg BD for 14 days Tab. Doxycycline 100 mg BD for 14 days
Inguinal bubo	Kit-7	Black	Tab. Azithromycin 1 gm (single tablet) Tab. Doxycycline 100 mg BD for 21 days

HUMAN PAPILLOMA VIRUS (HPV) INFECTION (VENEREAL WARTS/ ANOGENITAL WARTS / CONDYLOMA ACUMINATA)

Genital wart (Figure 29.15) is a sexually transmitted disease caused by human papillomavirus (HPV) types 6, 11, 16, and 18. It has a low transmission rate, ninety percent of individuals exposed to this HPV, will not develop the disease. Disease spreads by direct skin to skin with an infected person, during sexual intercourse. New born may be infected during delivery if mother has venereal warts in birth passage. Children having genital warts in genital or anal area, may point toward sexual abuse.

They commonly occurs on penile shaft, glans penis, scrotum, perianal or labia majora, but can also be found on internal surfaces of the vagina, cervix and the anus. Sometimes bleeding, discomfort, redness, or itching may occur.

High risk HPV types including 6, 11, 16, 18, 31, 33, 45, 52 and 58 infection appears to be the cause of most cases of anal, cervical, vulvar and vaginal cancers. In men, Bowen disease of the penis and all penile cancers are associated with HPV infection.

Differential Diagnosis

- Condyloma lata
- Familial benign pemphigus
- Benign nevi
- Vulvar neurofibromatosis

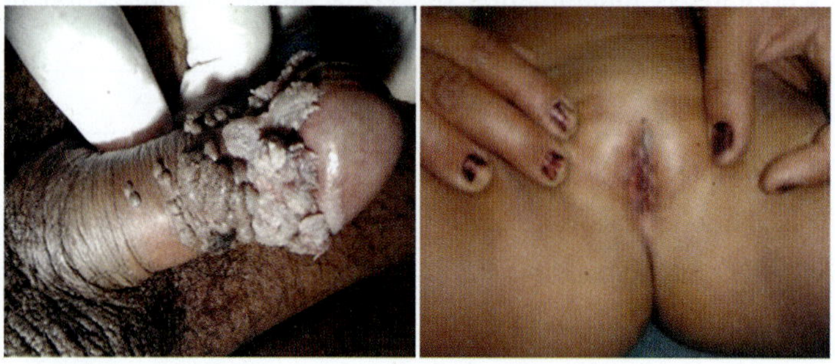

Figure 29.15: Genital warts

Diagnosis

The diagnosis of genital warts is usually made clinically, although a biopsy may be necessary for confirmation. On histology, epidermis is hyperplastic, which shows koilocytes, which are squamous epithelial cells with an acentric, hyperchromatic nucleus displaced by a large perinuclear vacuole. After application of acetic acid solution, genital warts are seen as white area, which helps to identify small warts.

Treatment (Table 29.5): Genital wart may occasionally subside spontaneously. Topical agents are very effective and less traumatic then surgical intervention.

Table 29.5: Showing treatment option for Genital warts

Topical treatment	*Mechanism of action*	*Application*	*Side effects*
Podophyllin solution in tincture of benzoin (20%)	It works by binding to microtubular subunits.	Once or twice weekly for 4-6 application	Irritation, burning ulceration, Sometimes neurotoxicity, bone marrow suppression, tachycardia, tachypnoea
Podophyllotoxin solution 0.15% to 0.5% in a gel or cream (can be applied by patient at home)	Anti mitotic drug, appears to be safer than podophyllin. It works by binding to microtubular subunits.	Twice daily for three days followed by four days off, then repeat application for 3 cycles.	Burning, itching, pain and inflammation.
Imiquimod 5% or 3.75% cream (can be applied by patient at home)	Immune enhancer and increases cytokines (tumor necrosis factor- alfa and interferon - alfa).	Three times per week (alternate day) at bed time (left for 6-8 hours) Maximum upto 16 weeks	Local side effects such as pain, burning, inflammation, itching and erythema
Sinecatechins 15% ointment (catechins extracted from green tea) (can be applied by patient at home)	Immuno enhancers, antiproliferative and antitumor properties	Three times daily application for upto 16 week	Local redness, inflammation, and pain.
Trichloroacetic acid	Chemical coagulation of protein	Once a week up to six applications	Ulceration pain and scarring
Cryotherapy	Ice crystal formation leads to membrane disruption	Two freeze-thaw cycles, every 2 weeks for 6-10 week by spray or cotton bud method	Burning and pain blistering dyspigmentation , scarring
Electrosurgery	Thermal destruction of tissue	Single session	Pain, dyspigmentation and scarring

In pregnancy cryotherapy, electrocautery and trichloroacetic acid application are safe options.

Other treatment options include 5-fluorouracil, cantharidin, laser vaporization (for extensive warts), topical and intralesional cidofovir and oral isotretinoin.

Immunotherapy in Genital Warts (Table 29.6)

Immunotherapy is a biological therapy, which stimulate the immune system to help the body to fight the infection. For recalcitrant, recurrent, extensive warts and difficult to treat areas (periungual and palmoplantar sites) immunotherapy may be used.

Table 29.6: Showing immunotherapy in genital warts

Intralesional Immunotherapy	*Doses/ route of administration / sessions*
Mycobacterium Indicus Pranii (MIP)/ Mycobacterium Welchii	0.1 ml intralesional, 2-4 weekly, maximum 10 sessions
Measles Mumps Rubella (MMR)	0.3-0.5 ml into single largest wart fortnightly for up to 5 sessions
Purified Protein Derivative (PPD)	0.1 ml/week intradermal injection in the forearm for 12 weeks
Trichophyton antigen	0.3 ml into largest wart every 3 weeks, maximum of 5 sessions
Interferon alpha 2B	1-2 million units 3 days/ week for 3 weeks
BCG vaccine	0.1ml intralesional injection in largest wart, in 2 weeks interval in 5 sessions
Candidial extract	0.3 ml injected into the largest wart at first session, then 3 weekly intralesional.

Vaccinations (Table 29.7)

Vaccines are preventative and should not be considered therapeutic. According to the Advisory Committee for Immunization Practices (ACIP), routine HPV vaccination is recommended for women of 9 to 26 years of age, but it has shown high efficacy up to age 45. Most common use vaccine is Gardasil, which protect against human papillomavirus types 6, 11, 16 and 18 infection. Gardasil 9 vaccine has been recommended for both males and females.

Table 29.7: Vaccines for HPV

Vaccine	*HPV Strain*
Cervarix	16, 18
Gardasil	6,11,16,18
Gardasil 9	6,11,16,18,31,33,45,52, 58

HIV INFECTION/AIDS

Human immunodeficiency virus (HIV) is an infection that attacks body's immune system particularly CD 4 type of lymphocytes. HIV infection leads to destruction of these cells leading to decrease immunity against opportunistic infections e.g., tuberculosis, pneumocystis carinii pneumonia (PCP), deep fungal infections and some cancers. WHO has classified this disease into four stages (Table 29.8). HIV is mainly transmitted by unsafe sexual activity, though it can also be transmitted by blood transfusion, sharing of needle by drug addicts, mother to child transmission and breast milk. As sexual activity is less practiced in children, incidence of HIV infection is less than in adults.

Table 29.8: WHO clinical staging of HIV

Stage 1
Asymptomatic
Persistent generalized lymphadenopathy
Stage 2
Unexplained persistent hepatosplenomegaly
Papular pruritic eruptions
Extensive wart virus infection
Extensive molluscum contagiosum
Recurrent oral ulcerations
Unexplained persistent parotid enlargement
Lineal gingival erythema
Herpes zoster
Recurrent or chronic upper respiratory tract infections (otitis media, otorrhoea, sinusitis, tonsillitis)
Fungal nail infections
Stage 3
Unexplained moderate malnutrition not adequately responding to standard therapy
Unexplained persistent diarrhoea (14 days or more)
Unexplained persistent fever (above 37.5 °C, intermittent or constant, for longer than one month)
Persistent oral Candidiasis (after first 6 weeks of life)
Oral hairy leukoplakia
Acute necrotizing ulcerative gingivitis/periodontitis
Lymph node TB
Pulmonary TB
Severe recurrent bacterial pneumonia
Symptomatic lymphoid interstitial pneumonitis
Chronic HIV-associated lung disease including bronchiectasis
Unexplained anaemia (<8.0 g/dl), neutropenia (<0.5×109/L3) or chronic thrombocytopenia (<50 × 109/L3)

Contd.

Stage 4
Unexplained severe wasting, stunting or severe malnutrition not responding to standard therapy
Pneumocystis pneumonia
Recurrent severe bacterial infections (e.g., empyema, polymyositis, bone or joint infection, meningitis, but excluding pneumonia)
Chronic herpes simplex infection (orolabial or cutaneous of more than one month's duration, or visceral at any site)
Extrapulmonary TB
Kaposi sarcoma
Oesophageal candidiasis (or candidiasis of trachea, bronchi or lungs)
Central nervous system toxoplasmosis (after the neonatal period)
HIV encephalopathy
Cytomegalovirus (CMV) infection; retinitis or CMV infection affecting another organ, with onset at age more than 1 month
Extrapulmonary cryptococcosis including meningitis
Disseminated endemic mycosis (extrapulmonary histoplasmosis, coccidioidomycosis, penicilliosis)
Chronic cryptosporidiosis (with diarrhoea)
Chronic isosporiasis
Disseminated non-tuberculous mycobacterial infection
Cerebral or B cell non-Hodgkin lymphoma
Progressive multifocal leukoencephalopathy
HIV-associated cardiomyopathy or nephropathy

CUTANEOUS MANIFESTATIONS OF HIV/AIDS

Available data suggest that cutaneous manifestations of HIV in children and adults are more or less same. Skin diseases may be the first presenting sign of HIV infection or may serve as a prognostic marker and ominous sign of the deteriorating immunodeficiency (Table 29.9).

Children may pose difficulty as they may have multiple problems complicated by nutritional dermatitis, diaper dermatitis, superadded fungal infections and drug rash. Some skin diseases, e.g., cutaneous cryptococcosis and Kaposi sarcoma are highly suggestive of HIV/AIDS. Other conditions which are seen in immunocompetent children also, may lead to suspicion of HIV/AIDS by their severity, frequency of recurrence or recalcitrant nature. Patients who have progressed to AIDS may show following skin manifestations:

1. **Infections**
   - ***Bacterial infection***
     - Impetigo and folliculitis may be recurrent and persistent in HIV disease, particularly in children.
     - Disseminated furunculosis, gingivitis, gangrenous stomatitis and abscess formation can occur in patients with HIV infection.
     - *Mycobacterial Infections: Mycobacterium tuberculosis; Mycobacterium avium intra-cellular* complex; and, rarely, *Mycobacterium kansasii* may present as acneiform papules and indurated crusted plaques.
   - ***Spirochaetes infection***
     - *Syphilis:* Patients with HIV infection with primary syphilis tend to present more frequently with multiple ulcers compared with patients who are not infected with HIV. Rapid progression of secondary syphilis to tertiary syphilis has been reported in patients infected with HIV. Syphilis seroconversion may be delayed, and standard serologic tests that aid in diagnosing syphilis may be unreliable.

Table 29.9: Mucocutaneous manifestation in HIV infection with CD4 count

CD4 >500	*CD4 < 500 and >250*	*CD 4< 250*
Acute retroviral syndrome	Recurrent or persistent dermatophyte infection	Invasive fungal infection
Herpes zoster	Oral candidiasis	Cutaneous tuberculosis
Seborrheic dermatitis	Oral hairy leukoplakia	Chronic herpes simplex >1 month
	Disseminated herpes zoster	Large molluscum contagiosum
		Hyperkeratotic scabies
		Bacillary angiomatosis
		Eosinophilic folliculitis
		Kaposi sarcoma
		Papular pruritic eruption of HIV
		Idiopathic pruritis

- ***Viral infections***
  - *Herpes Virus:* In patients infected with HIV, several viruses of the herpes viridae family may lead to cutaneous disease, including chronic and recurrent, genital, perianal (Figure 29.16) and perioral herpetic ulcers caused by HSV. Recurrent typical dermatomal zoster caused by herpes zoster virus (HZV) along with atypical features like multi dermatomal distribution, widespread dissemination may be seen.

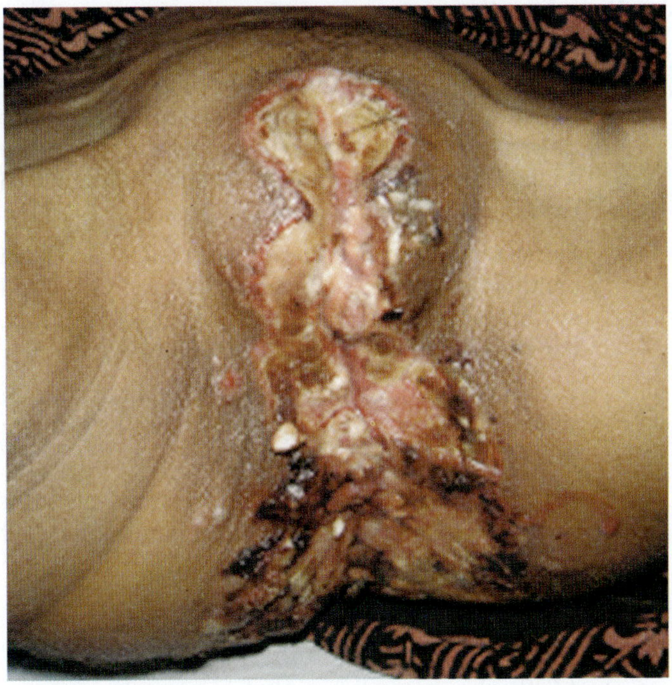

Figure 29.16: Genital herpes infection in HIV positive girl

  - *Human Papilloma Virus (HPV):* Widespread or recalcitrant warts may be observed on oral mucosa, face, perianal region, and genital tract in patients infected with HIV.
  - *Epstein-Barr virus (EBV):* It has been implicated in the pathogenesis of oral hairy leukoplakia, characterized by filiform white papules localized on the sides of the tongue (Figure 29.17).
  - *CMV Infection:* Ulcers in the perineal region are the most common presentation for CMV infection in patients infected with HIV. Disseminated CMV infections may be seen.
  - *Molluscum Contagiosum:* Lesions of Molluscum Contagiosum in HIV infected patients may be widespread and atypical. They may be observed on unusual sites, such as face, neck and scalp; the lesions may be of unusual morphology and size (Figure 29.18).

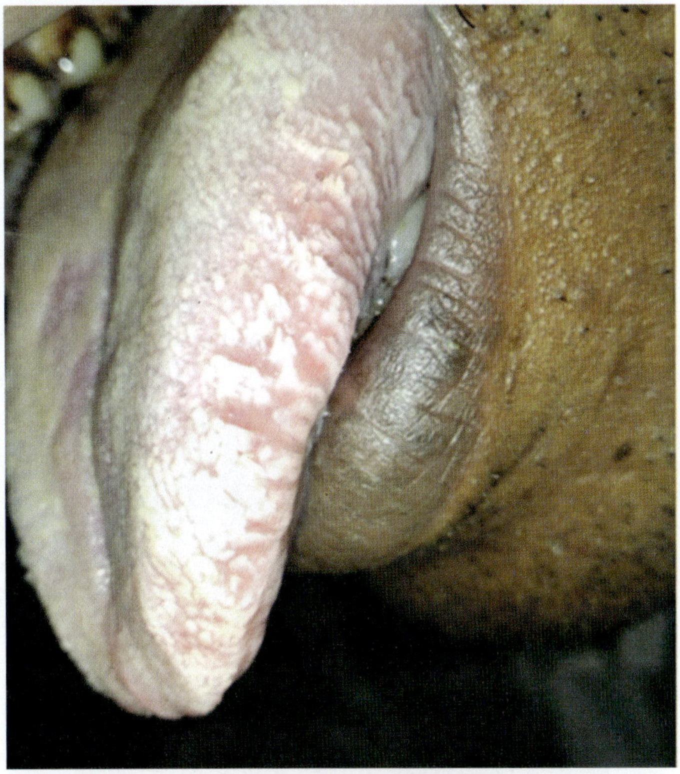

Figure 29.17: Oral hairy leukoplakia

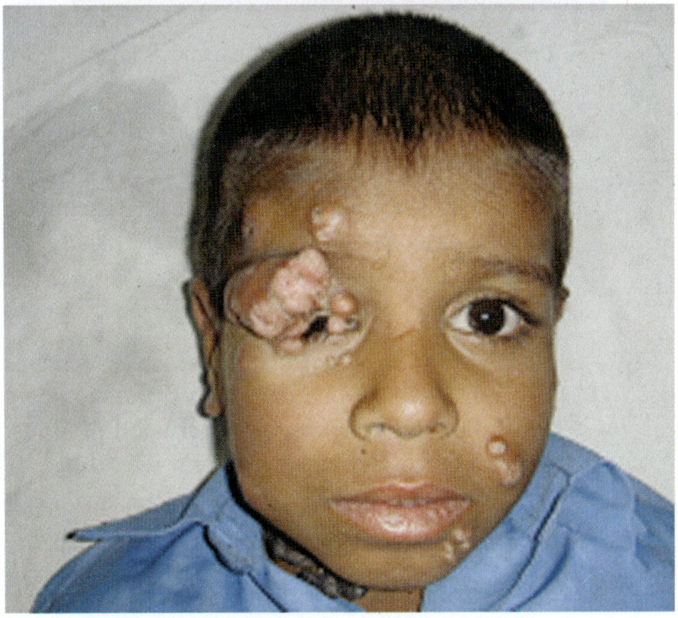

Figure 29.18: Molluscum contagiosum infection in HIV positive child

- ***Fungal infections***
  - Recurrent and persistent mucocutaneous candidiasis is common.
  - Generalized dermatophytosis, or tinea capitis, which is typically caused by *Trichophyton rubrum*, may suggest HIV infection.

- Pityriasis versicolor may be persistent and recurrent.
- Rarely, cutaneous cryptococcosis may be observed. Clinical manifestations include cellulitis, papules, plaques, ulcers or translucent dome shaped papules with central umbilication, resembling molluscum contagiosum.
- Cutaneous histoplasmosis may lead to red papules, a cellulitis like eruption, ulcerations, acneiform papules, or molluscum like lesions (Figure 29.19).

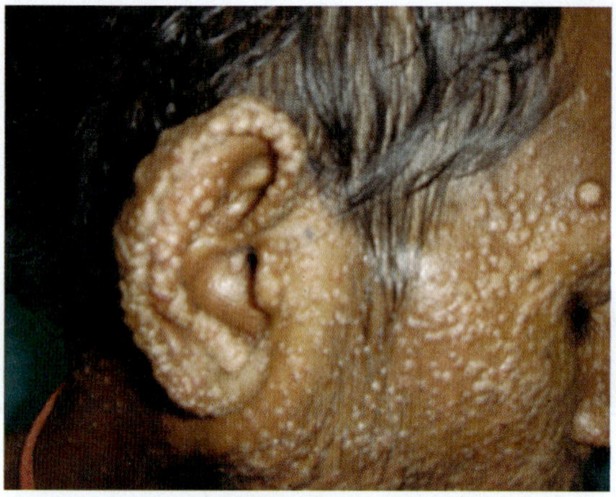

Figure 29.19: Disseminated histoplasmosis in an HIV positive boy

- North American blastomycosis may present as a disseminated maculopapular eruption.
- Systemic coccidioidomycosis may disseminate to the skin, usually as hemorrhagic papules or nodules.

- ***Others:***
  - *Scabies:* Atypical or Norwegian scabies, which is characterized by widespread hyperkeratotic, scaly maculopapular eruptions or crusted plaques, can occur in patients with HIV infection.
  - *Leishmaniasis:* Atypical disseminated leishmaniasis has been reported in HIV-infected patients.

2. **Inflammatory Conditions**

- ***Seborrheic dermatitis:***
  - The eruption, which is characterized by widespread erythematous plaques with greasy scales, may progress to erythroderma in some patients.
  - Incidence of seborrheic dermatitis may be increased in patients with AIDS-associated dementia or CNS disease.
- ***Eosinophilic folliculitis:***
  - It manifests as an idiopathic, highly pruritic, papulopustular eruption of sterile pustules involving the face, neck, trunk and extremities.
- ***Pruritic papular eruption (PPE):***
  - PPE is a common cutaneous manifestation in patients infected with HIV. It manifests as small, itchy, red or skin-colored papules on the head, neck and upper part of the trunk.

3. **Drug Eruptions**

- Morbilliform drug eruptions can occur in as many as 65-70% of patients who are treated by trimethoprim-sulfamethoxazole (TMP-SMZ) for *Pneumocystis carinii (or P. jeroveci)* pneumonia within 7 days of starting the therapy. Generalized reddish macules and papules may be seen.
- Sulfonamides may cause urticaria, erythema multiforme, toxic epidermal necrolysis and systemic reactions, including fever, leukopenia, thrombocytopenia, hepatitis and nephritis.
- Toxic epidermal necrolysis has been reported with antibiotics, fluconazole, phenobarbital in patients with HIV.
- Drug eruptions have been reported as the most common cause of erythroderma in patients infected with HIV.

4. **HIV-associated Malignancies**

- Kaposi sarcoma.
- AIDS related B cell non-Hodgkin lymphomas may lead to skin nodules.
- Anal carcinoma and cervical intraepithelial neoplasia are papilloma virus-associated tumors. These tumors tend to be more progressive and aggressive.
- An increase in incidence of squamous cell carcinoma of the anal mucosa has been reported, especially in young homosexual men with HIV infection.
- Intraoral or multiple squamous cell carcinoma, Bowen's disease, and metastatic basal cell carcinoma have occasionally been reported in patients infected with HIV.
- Malignant melanoma in patients with HIV appears to be more aggressive than in individuals without HIV.
- Children with AIDS have a higher risk of developing leiomyosarcoma.

5. **Miscellaneous**

- Acute primary HIV infection may lead to a transient, generalized, morbilliform eruption on the trunk and the arms.

- In the early asymptomatic stage of HIV disease, no signs of infection other than lymphadenopathy are present. This stage may last for 10 years or longer.
- Generalized dry skin syndrome is frequently observed in patients with HIV infection. Xerosis may be the initial clinical manifestation of AIDS and is often a cause of pruritus.
- ***Hair and nail disorders***
  - Diffuse alopecia or alopecia areata and telogen effluvium may be associated with HIV disease and may be inflammatory and permanent.
  - Beau's line and pallor of the nail beds are the general effects of the chronic illness.
  - Proximal subungual onychomycosis is usually a sign of HIV disease.
  - Long eyelashes may be seen.

Management

For diagnosis of HIV in an infant born to HIV infected mother until 18 months of age, NACO recommends (National Guidelines for HIV Care and Treatment 2021) nucleic acid amplification test because maternal HIV antibodies passively transfer through the placenta to infant, and persist till 18 months of age. The breastfed children should be tested 3 months after cessation of breastfeeding as there is ongoing risk of HIV transmission through breast milk. Risk of HIV transmission from parent to child is given below (Table 29.10).

ARV Intervention Risk of HIV Transmission from Mother to Child

Table 29.10: Risk of HIV transmission from parent to child (PTCT) with or without intervention

Intervention	*Risk of HIV transmission from mother to child*
No ARV, breastfeeding	30-45%
No ARV; no breastfeeding	20-25%
Short course with one ARV; breastfeeding	15-25%
Short course with one ARV; no breastfeeding	5-15%
Short course with two ARVs; breastfeeding	5%
3 ARVs (ART) with breastfeeding	2%
3 ARVs (ART) with no breastfeeding	1%

ARV: Antiretroviral, ART: Antiretroviral therapy

Exclusive breastfeeding is recommended for infant born to HIV infected mother in India.

When to start ART?

Recommendations by WHO (2016)

- ART should be initiated for all people living with HIV regardless of WHO clinical stage and at any CD4 cell count.
  - Adults
  - Pregnant and breastfeeding women
  - Adolescents
  - Children living with HIV one year old to less than 10 years old
  - Infants diagnosed in the first year of life
- The antiretroviral prophylaxis recommended as given in Table 29.11. Low-risk infants shall receive single ARV prophylaxis whereas those with high risk should receive dual ARV prophylaxis.

Table 29.11: Recommended nevirapine doses for infant

Age of infant	*Dose*
Birth to 6 weeks	
Birth weight 2 – 2.5 kg	10 mg once daily (1ml)
Birth weight > 2.5 kg	15 mg once daily (1.5 ml)
>6 week, upto 6 months	20 mg once daily (2 ml)
>6 month, upto 9 months	30 mg once daily (3 ml)
>9 month, upto 12 months	40 mg once daily (3 ml)

NACO has published beautiful booklet (National Guidelines for HIV Care and Treatment 2021) regarding detailed HIV care and management. For ready reference ART regimen for infants and children is given in Tables 29.12 and 29.13.

Table 29.12: First-line ART regimens for infants and children with HIV-1 and HIV-2 infection

Age and weight	*Recommended regimen*
Age less than 6 years and body weight less than 20 kg	Abacavir + Lamivudine + Lopinavir/ritonavir (AL+LPV/r)
Age between 6 and 10 years and body weight between 20 kg and 30 kg	Abacavir + Lamivudine + Dolutegravir (ALD)
Age more than 10 years and body weight more than 30 kg	Tenofovir + Lamivudine + Dolutegravir (TLD)

Note: On every visit, check body weight of the infant/child before writing the prescription. Even though the drug regimen remains the same, drug dosages have to be modified according to change in body weight.

<table>
<caption>Table 29.13: Preferred and alternative first-line ART regimens for adults, adolescents, children and neonates</caption>
<tr><th>Populations</th><th>Preferred first-line regimen</th><th>Alternative first-line regimen</th><td rowspan="4">TDF- Tenofovir disoproxil fumarate
3TC- Lamivudine
DTG- Dolutegravir
AZT- Zidovudine
EFV- Efavirenz
RAL- Raltegravir
ABC- Abacavir
LPV/r- Lopinavir/ritonavir
TAFe-Tenofovir alafenamide
NVP- Nevirapine</td></tr>
<tr><td>Adults and adolescents</td><td>TDF + 3TC (or FTC) + DTG</td><td>TDF + 3TC + EFV 400 mg</td></tr>
<tr><td>Children</td><td>ABC + 3TC + DTG</td><td>ABC + 3TC + LPV/r
TAF + 3TC (or FTC) + DTG</td></tr>
<tr><td>Neonates</td><td>AZT (or ABC) + 3TC + RAL</td><td>AZT + 3TC + NVP</td></tr>
</table>

CHILD SEXUAL ABUSE

Sexual abuse of children is a harsh fact of life in our society. It is more common than most people realize. Some surveys say at least 1 out of 5 adult women and 1 out of 10 adult men report having been sexually abused in childhood.

"Child sexual abuse is any sexual act with a child performed by an adult or an older child. This might be fondling the child's genitals, getting the child to fondle an adult's genitals, mouth to genital contact, rubbing an adult's genitals on the child or actually penetrating the child's vagina or anus."

Physical findings of sexual abuse are often not present. The most important determinant for child abuse is the child's (ora witness's) account of the incident. Physical indicators may be present, such as bruises to the skin (e.g., on the arms and legs from pinch marks or force), abrasions on wrists and ankles (e.g. from tethering), bruises on genital area and mucosa, palatal bruises and/or petechiae and rectal abnormalities. Hymenal abnormalities may be present from chronic abuse or acute injury. Sexually transmitted diseases (STDs) may be present in sexually abused children and teenagers.

Besides increasing the risk of STDs and teenage pregnancy, sexual abuse also has been linked to cause impaired psychological well being, suicidal ideation and alcohol abuse and prostitution. Thus it is essential to develop strategies to prevent sexual abuse and to have adequate counselling measures.

Clinical Presentation

History

Children suspected of being sexually abused require a behavioral, social, gynecologic and general medical history. In addition to information obtained from the child, details about the abuse should be obtained from other reliable sources including from parents and caretaker. The history should include following questions:

I. **Behavioral Indicators:**
   - *Abrupt behavioral changes:* Aggression, depression, suicidal behaviors, withdrawal, low self-esteem, nightmares, phobias, regression, school problems, etc.
   - *Self-destructive behaviors:* Substance abuse, sleep disorders, prostitution, cutting or other self-mutilation.
   - Sexualized behavior inappropriate for developmental level (e.g., excessive masturbation, forcing sexual acts on other children).
   - Runaway behavior in teens, loss of memory for events following a social gathering, intimate partner violence, etc.

II. **Physical complaints:**
   - Genitourinary complaints, e.g., painful defecation or urination, vaginal discharge, bleeding or itching, grasp or rope marks, oral complaints, etc.
   - General complaints including headaches, abdominal pain, constipation, diarrhea and general fatigue.

III. **In adolescents, the gynecologic history should always include the following:**
   - Date of last menstrual period, number of pregnancies, possible gynecologic surgery or traumatic injury to the genital area.
   - Date of the last consensual intercourse and use of contraceptives.
   - Prior STDs.

IV. **Family and social histories are vital in understanding the environment in which the abuse occurred. A brief developmental history may be critical in legal aspects of a child's case and should be documented.**

Physical Examination

Complete physical examinations in prepubertal children should include an examination of the external genitalia. Children who are suspected of being sexually abused need an examination by physician. If the child and family are adequately prepared for this examination, it will improve the diagnostic capability of the examiner.

- Preparation of the child and family should be a part of every examination for sexual abuse.

  The discussion should include the following:
  - Information regarding the need for an external examination of the genitalia.
  - The fact that almost all prepubertal children do not need a speculum or internal examination.
  - Information on the use of cotton-tipped swabs to check for infections (if determined that these will be needed).
- The examination of the external genitalia should occur as part of the natural progression of the complete head to toe pediatric examination.
- Abnormal findings that are suspicious for sexual abuse are rare. In most cases, children who are sexually abused are not physically injured (as in fondling), and the abuse does not leave physical evidence.
  - Findings of sexual abuse in boys may include injuries to the glans, shaft of the penis or scrotum. Anal findings are unusual but may include scars (most apparent if located off the midline), distorted or irregular folds, flattening of the anal folds and poor anal tone.
  - Most cases of suspected or substantiated sexual abuse of prepubertal girls have normal examination findings. This may be due to elasticity of the hymenal tissue and genital mucosa and rapid healing of any injury.
- Foreign bodies may be found in vagina or rectum.
- Child should also be examined for STDs or for possible pregnancy.
- Other areas of the body should be inspected for signs of injury, including the oral mucosa for bruises to the hard or soft palate and grasp, rope or tie marks on the extremities.

Management

- According to the clinical manifestations abused child should be thoroughly investigated and treated accordingly. Prophylactic antibiotics in prepubertal sexually abused children are indicated in rare cases. Prophylactic antibiotics may be given to pubertal sexually abused children after an acute assault. Use of post-assault pregnancy prevention options should be discussed with the pubertal sexual assault
- **Prognosis:** Sexually abused children have significantly higher occurrences of the following:
  - Eating disorders.
  - Suicidal behaviors.
- Children who are sexually abused may be at increased risk of re-abuse.
- Sustained emotional/psychological problems may be indicative of abused children's false beliefs about themselves and the sexual abuse experience.

POINT OF CARE TESTS IN SEXUALLY TRANSMITTED INFECTION

"Tests designed to be used at or near the site where the patient is located, that do not require permanent dedicated space, and that are performed outside the physical facilities of clinical laboratories".

POCT should be "ASSURED" **A**ffordable, **S**ensitive, **S**pecific, **U**ser friendly, **R**apid and robust, **E**quipment free, **D**eliverable to end users. Difference between rapid test and point of care test are given in Table 29.14.

Table 29.14: Showing difference between rapid test and point of care test

Rapid test	*Point of care test*
Simple	Simple to perform, even at PHC level
Results take only 20-40 mints	Results will be ready in less than 15 mints
May require equipment's like electricity, centrifuge.	Equipment free
Often required well trained staff	Minimal training sufficient to perform test
Usually no internal quality control with test	Have built in control and results are more reliable
Example: Gram stain, wet mount pH testing, whiff test	Example: lateral flow test, dipstick test

AIM

- Improve specificity of syndromic management
- Reduce over treatment
- Screen for asymptomatic STIs

Types of POCT in STIs:

1. **Agglutination/Precipitation Reactions**
   - E.g., Latex agglutination

2. **Immunochromatography (ICT)**
   - Lateral flow format
   - Multiplex ICT
   - Flow through format
   - Optic immune assay
3. **Emerging technologies**
   - Microfluidic assays
   - Rapid Molecular assays

Different STI and their related point of care test are given in Table 29.15.

Table 29.15: Showing different STI and related point of care test

Disease	*Point of care test*
Syphilis	• Syphi-check • SD BIOLINE syphilis • VISITECT Syphilis • Determine Syphilis TP • Espiline TP • Syphilis Fast
Chlamydia	• Clear view • Quick Vue • Bio Star OIA • CRT
Gonorrhoea	• Bio Star OIA • PATH GC • One Step strip test
Trichomoniasis	• XenoStrip TV • OSOM TV • Affirm VPIII
Herpes	• HSV-2 IgG LFIA • BioKit HSV-2 • Herpes Select Express (CLIA waived)

SEXUAL DISORDERS

Erectile Dysfunction

"The inability to attain and/or maintain penile erection sufficient for satisfactory sexual performance" or "the consistent or recurrent inability to attain and/or maintain penile erection sufficient for sexual satisfaction" are the definitions of erectile dysfunction (ED), formerly known as impotence. The causes of ED are psychological or physical or combination of psychological and physiological.

Causes of ED are vascular (atherosclerosis, hypertension) ,neurological (Alzheimer disease), endocrinological, penile (peyronie disease, epispadias, priapism), psychiatric (depression), haematological (anaemia and leukaemia) , surgical (neurological and urogenital surgery) and medical (antihypertensives).

Investigations

Common investigation includes, fasting blood sugar levels, lipid profile and early morning testosterone estimation. Other investigations are based on history and examination.

Treatment

Treatment principles is to identifying and treating any treatable causes of ED, initiating lifestyle change and risk factor modification and providing education and counselling to patients and their partners.

- **First line:** Psychotherapy, PDE-5 inhibitors
- **Second line:** Vacuum erection devices, Intra-cavernous injection therapy and Medicated Urethral System for Erection (MUSE)
- **Third line:** Penile prostheses

Premature Ejaculation

Commonest male sexual dysfunction, affecting around 20-30% of men below 40 year of age. It is described by inability to control ejaculation for a 'sufficient' length of time, most commonly used definition includes 'an intravaginal latency time of less than 60 seconds'. Premature ejaculation can be primary or secondary:

- **Primary:**
  - Psychological difficulties
  - Deep anxiety about sex that relates to one or more traumatic experiences encountered during development
- **Secondary:**
  - Erectile dysfunction
  - Performance anxiety
  - Psychotropic drug use
- Higher free and total testosterone levels have been demonstrated in men with premature ejaculation. Many men with premature ejaculation have low serum prolactin levels.
- Group of nerves in the lumbar spinal cord has been identified as the possible generator of ejaculation. Decreased nerve conduction and somatosensory latency times have been demonstrated in premature ejaculation.

Management

- Both male and female partner counselling and sex therapy needs to be done. Other treatment includes stop-start or squeeze-pause technique of Masters and Johnson. Pharmacotherapy includes topical local anaesthetic cream or spray applied 15-20 minutes before coitus, SSRIs and TCAs (on demand or daily) and PDE-5 inhibitors.

30 CHAPTER Autoinflammatory Syndrome

Contents

Autoinflammatory disorders are due to aberrant activation of the innate immune system. Clinical features include recurring inflammation, fever and urticarial rash. Other clinical features may include pyoderma gangrenosum, erysipelas like lesions, oedema and pustulosis. Acute phase reactants, neutrophils, erythrocyte sedimentation rate and C reactive protein level are usually raised. Biopsy shows neutrophilic infiltrate in perivascular and interstitial area of dermis without vasculitis.

MONOGENIC AUTOINFLAMMATORY SYNDROMES (Table 30.1)

These syndromes present in early childhood with recurrent inflammation of skin, joints, eyes, and serous membrane. Environmental factors may responsible for flare up of disease.

Cryopyrin Associated Periodic Fever Syndrome (CAPS)

1. **Familial cold autoinflammatory syndrome (FCAS)**

   It is an autosomal dominant disorder occurring in early childhood and is triggered by cold exposure. Clinical feature include recurrent episodes of fever, fatigue, conjunctival erythema, arthralgia and non-itchy symmetrical urticarial rashes without angioedema on trunk and extremities. The flare last upto 24 hours.

2. **Muckle wells syndrome (MWS)**

   Sensorineural hearing loss and polyarthritis are the characteristic feature of MWS. There is also increase risk of amyloidosis.

3. **Chronic infantile neurological and articular syndrome / neonatal onset multisystem inflammatory diseases (CINCA/NOMID)**

This is the most severe form of CAPS characterised by aseptic meningitis, mental retardation, sensory neural deafness, deforming polyarthritis with characteristic facies (frontal bossing, midfacial hypoplasia and saddle nose). It may associated with renal amyloidosis.

Table 30.1: Classification of monogenic autoinflammatory syndrome

Hereditary periodic fevers
- Cryopyrin associated periodic fever syndrome (CAPS)
  - Familial cold autoinflammatory syndrome (FCAS)
  - Muckle wells syndrome (MWS)
  - Chronic infantile neurological and articular syndrome / neonatal onset multisystem inflammatory diseases (CINCA/NOMID)
- Tumour necrosis factor associated periodic syndrome (TRAPS)
- Familial Mediterranean fever
- Mevalonate kinase deficiency with recurrent fever and hyper IgD syndrome

Autoinflammatory granulomatosis of childhood (Blau syndrome)

Autoinflammatory syndrome with pustules
- Deficiency of interleukin 1 receptor antagonist (DIRA)
- Deficiency of interleukin 36 receptor antagonist (DITRA)
- Pyogenic arthritis, pyoderma gangrenosum and acne syndrome (PAPA)

Miscellaneous monogenic autoinflammatory syndrome
- Chronic atypical neutrophilic dermatosis with lipodystrophy and elevated temperature (CANDLE) syndrome
- Majeed syndrome

Tumour Necrosis Factor Associated Periodic Syndrome (TRAPS)

It is an autosomal dominant disorder due to defective binding of circulating TNF-alpha to TNF receptor (P^{55} TNF receptor). TRAPS is characterised by episodes of pyrexia lasting upto 1-3 weeks, accompanied by conjunctivitis, myalgia, arthralgia, stomach or chest pain and periorbital oedema. TRAPS may first appear in infancy or in adolescence.

Migratory erythematous macules and patches are commonly seen on the limbs. They coalesce and expand centrifugally into extensive oedematous dermal plaques. These plaques usually cover an area of localised tenderness in the muscles and indicate contiguous inflammation that extends from muscle to skin. A single attack often affects just one anatomical area. Other features include urticaria, angioedema or erysipelas like lesions.

Treatment includes steroids and etanercept.

Familial Mediterranean Fever (FMF)

It is due to mutation in MEFV gene which encodes for pyrin proteins. Clinically it presents with recurrent fever, large joint pain, abdominal pain and pleurisy, lasting upto 1-3 days. Erysipelas like rashes on extremities is the most common clinical presentation. Erythema and inflammation of scrotum, face and palmoplantar region may also be seen. Histology from erysipelas like rash shows sparse neutrophilic infiltration in upper dermis with or without Leukocytoclastic.

Diagnostic Criteria for FMF

Major criteria
- Recurrent fever with serositis
- Amyloidosis of AA type without a predisposing disease
- Response to colchicine

Minor criteria
- Recurrent fever episodes
- Erysipelas like rashes
- Familial history of FMF

For diagnosis, two major or one major and one minor criteria is needed.

Treatment includes colchicine and anakinra.

Mevalonate kinase deficiency with recurrent fever and hyper IgD syndrome

It is an autosomal recessive autoinflammatory disorder associated with mutation in mevalonate kinase gene. Partial Mevalonate kinase deficiency is associated with recurrent fever without increase in immunoglobulin D while complete deficiency results in recurrent fever, increased IgD levels and mevalonic aciduria. Clinical features include, recurrent episodes of fever, multiple joint pain, abdominal pain, cervical lymphadenopathy, fixed maculopapular rashes, urticarial and erythema nodosum like rashes. Flare persist upto 3-7 days. Amyloidosis, macrophage activation syndrome and secondary infection are other features of this syndrome. Oral steroids in flares and TNF alpha and IL-1 inhibitor are other treatment options.

Autoinflammatory granulomatosis of childhood (Blau syndrome)

It occurs due to mutation in pattern recognition receptor gene NOD-2 (CARD-15 gene) and is characterised by early onset of chronic granulomatous arthritis of peripheral joints and uveitis. Recurrent episodes of discrete red brown papules are seen on face and extremities which leave atrophic scars and show non caseating granulomas on histology. Treatment includes administration of steroids and TNF alpha inhibitors.

Autoinflammatory syndrome with pustules

Deficiency of Interleukin 1 Receptor Antagonist (DIRA) Syndrome

- It occurs due to a deficiency of the naturally occurring antagonist of the IL-1 receptor (IL-1Rn). Which leads to enhanced IL-1mediated inflammation. Localized or wide spread grouped pustules appear on an erythematous base in the newborn (aseptic pustular dermatitis) which may develop yellowish crusts in first 3 weeks. Fever, multifocal osteomyelitis, pulmonary hemosiderosis with progressive pulmonary fibrosis, periostitis and balloon like swelling of the ends of ribs may be seen. Oral mucosa may be affected and nails may show pitting and onychomadesis. Treatment include anakinra (IL-1 inhibitor).

Deficiency of interleukin 36 receptor antagonist (DITRA) syndrome

It occurs due to deficiency of IL-36 receptor antagonist. Recurrent episodes of severe generalized pustular psoriasis with fever occur in early childhood. On investigation neutrophilia and raised acute phase reactant is seen. Acitretin, steroids and adalimumab have been used with varying degree of success.

Pyogenic arthritis, pyoderma gangrenosum and acne (PAPA) syndrome

PAPA syndrome has AD inheritance with mutations in proline-serine-threonine phosphatase interacting protein 1 (PSTPIP1) gene. IL-1β and circulating neutrophil granule enzyme levels in serum are raised. Diagnostic features are pyogenic sterile arthritis, pyoderma gangrenosum and acne.

Miscellaneous Monogenic Autoinflammatory Syndrome

Chronic atypical neutrophilic dermatosis with lipodystrophy and elevated temperature (CANDLE) syndrome

This autoinflammatory syndrome is characterized by abnormal signalling of interferon pathways due to mutation in the PMSB8 gene. Children usually present to pediatricians in early life with recurrent fever, rash and arthralgia or arthritis. The disease may first develop within 2 or 3 weeks of birth, which continue episodically during the first year of life. Violaceous or erythematous, often annular, edematous plaques are seen on the face, trunk and interphalangeal joints. Up to 50% of patients die before adulthood.

Majeed syndrome

Majeed syndrome results from mutations in the LPIN2 gene with autosomal recessive inheritance. The two main features of this disease are dyserythropoietic anaemia and neutrophilic dermatosis resembling Sweet syndrome. Recurrent episodes of multifocal osteomyelitis causing bone pain and joint swelling occur with fever and cutaneous pustulosis. Congenital dyserythropoietic anemia leads to fatigue, weakness, pale skin and shortness of breath.

POLYGENIC FORM OF AUTOINFLAMMATORY SYNDROMES

Polygenic autoinflammatory diseases are due to overexpression of genes linked to the inflammasome and dysregulated innate immune responses. Few polygenic autoinflammatory syndromes are discussed below:

- **Schnitzler syndrome**
- **Adult onset still disease**
- **Systemic onset juvenile idiopathic arthritis**
- **Synovitis, acne, pustulosis, hyperostosis and osteitis (SAPHO syndrome)**

Schnitzler Syndrome

It is a sporadic acquired autoinflammatory syndrome characterised by recurrent fever, urticaria, joint pain, organomegaly and IgM monoclonal gammopathy. They also have an increased risk of developing certain lymphoproliferative disorders. The exact underlying cause is currently unknown.

Strasbourg diagnostic criteria for Schnitzler syndrome:

Essential criteria

- Chronic urticarial rash
- Raised monoclonal IgM or IgG antibodies

Minor criteria

- Recurrent fever
- Objective findings of abnormal bone remodeling with or without bone pain

- A neutrophilic dermal infiltrate on skin biopsy
- Leukocytosis and/or elevated C-reactive protein

Definite diagnosis, if two essential criteria and at least two minor criteria if IgM antibodies are present/ 3 minor criteria if IgG antibodies are present.

Treatment includes colchicine, NSAIDS, hydroxychloroquine and anakinra

Adult Onset Still Disease (AOSD)

It is an uncommon autoinflammatory syndrome which is characterized by recurrent fever, inflammatory polyarthritis, pharyngitis, lymphadenopathy and salmon pink coloured maculopapular rash. Rash typically occurs with onset of fever in evening and decrease in the morning. It has bimodal of distribution, first peak between 15 to 25 years and second peak between 35 to 45 years.

Diagnostic criteria for adult onset still disease

Major criteria

- Fever > 39° C for minimum one week
- Arthritis for 2 weeks or longer
- Asymptomatic salmon coloured maculopapular rash
- Leukocytosis > 10000/ml with > 80% neutrophils

Minor criteria

- Sore throat or pharyngitis
- Lymphadenopathy
- Hepatosplenomegaly
- Elevated liver function test (Alanine aminotransferase) and Lactate dehydrogenase
- Negative ANA and RA factor

For definite diagnosis 5 criteria should be present (at least two major criteria)

Treatment includes NSAIDS, anakinra and steroids.

Systemic Onset Juvenile Idiopathic Arthritis

It is similar to AOSD but arthritis in an essential criterion for this. Treatment includes methotrexate and anakinra.

SAPHO Syndrome

SAPHO syndrome is characterized by Synovitis, Acne, Pustulosis (often on the palms and soles), Hyperostosis and Osteitis. The cause of SAPHO syndrome is unknown and treatment is symptomatic. It is predominantly found in middle aged patients (30 to 50 years).

31

CHAPTER

Non Infectious Granulomatous Disorders of Skin

Contents

INTRODUCTION

Granulomatous dermatitis (GD) is one of the most frequently occurring tissue reaction patterns. In broad terms, there are two types of granulomatous dermatitis: infectious and non-infectious. In western countries, non-infectious granulomas are more frequently found, whereas infectious granulomas are more common in developing countries like India.

PATHOGENESIS OF GRANULOMA FORMATION

Granuloma results from focal chronic inflammatory response to tissue injury evoked by poorly soluble substance and is characterised by the accumulation and proliferation of leukocytes (mainly lymphocytes) and macrophages. The provocative agents appear to be non-degradable by both neutrophils and non-activated macrophages, requiring transformed macrophages or epithelioid cells with augmented enzymatic capabilities. IFN-gamma and TNF are produced by Th1 CD4+ T cells and activated macrophages, which further matures the macrophages and eventually forms granulomas. Thus granulomas are made up of diverse numbers of lymphocytic inflammatory cells, macrophages and epithelioid cells, either alone or in combination with giant cells.

GIANT CELLS (Described in Detail in Chapter 38)

Giant cells are large multinucleated cells formed by fusion of macrophages, epithelioid cells and monocytes etc. These cells most of the time are present at the site of chronic inflammation and in other granulomatous conditions. Giant cells are pathologically important and have diagnostic value. Giant cells are classified into following types:

Macrophage Derived

- Langhans giant cells
- Touton giant cells
- Foreign body giant cells

Epidermal Cell Derived

- Tzanck giant cells
- Multinucleated epidermal giant cells

Melanocyte Derived

- Starburst giant cells
- Giant cells in melanocytic nevus

- Balloon cells
- Giant nevus cells

Floret Like Multinucleated Giant Cells

Classification of different type of granuloma (Table 31.1)

SARCOIDOSIS

Sarcoidosis is a multisystem disorder of unknown etiology and presents with noncaseating granulomas in various organs. Sarcoidosis affects individuals of all ages irrespective of race or ethnicity, with maximum incidence among people aged 20–39 years and is more prevalent in women, non-smokers and in rural communities. Characteristically, it presents with bilateral hilar lymphadenopathy and reticular opacities in the lungs. Other major sites of involvement are the skin, eyes and joints. However, it can also involve musculoskeletal system, reticuloendothelial system, exocrine glands, heart, kidney, and central nervous system in variable extents.

Table 31.1: Classification of different types of granulomas

Type of granuloma	*Clinical features*	*Example*
Sarcoidal or naked granuloma	Well-formed, compact granulomas with minimal lymphoid infiltration in the surrounding tissue (naked granuloma).	Sarcoidosis
Tuberculoid	Composed of Langhan's type or foreign body type giant cells and epithelioid histiocytes with or without central caseation necrosis, often confluent and are encircled by lymphoid cuffing.	Tuberculosis Leprosy Late syphilis Leishmaniasis Rosacea Crohn's disease
Necrobiotic	Necrobiosis denotes changes in the collagen or elastic fibres. Granulomas are frequently ill formed, diffuse or palisaded in nature and have varying levels of inflammatory infiltrate surrounding altered collagen or elastic fibres.	**Blue granuloma** Granuloma annulare. Wegener's granulomatosis Rheumatoid vasculitis **Red granuloma** Necrobiosis lipoidica. Necrobiotic xanthogranuloma Rheumatoid nodule. Churg-Strauss syndrome Eosinophilic cellulitis or well's syndrome.
Suppurative	The central region is composed of neutrophils and neutrophilic debris, whereas the periphery may have a chronic inflammatory infiltration made up of lymphocytes, plasma cells and histiocytes.	Deep fungal infection Non tubercular mycobacterium Cat scratch disease Lymphogranuloma venereum Nocardiosis
Foreign body	Composed of epithelioid histiocytes and foreign body giant cells.	Endogenous and exogenous material
Interstitial	Poorly formed granuloma with loose aggregates of histiocytes between collagen bundles.	Interstitial granulomatous dermatitis Palisaded and interstitial granulomatous dermatitis Melkersson-Rosenthal syndrome Elastolytic granulomas

Etiopathogenesis

Although the exact cause is unknown. But the role of various factors has been hypothesized.

1. **Genetics:** Eleven sarcoidosis risk loci (BTNL2, HLA-B, HLA-DPB1, ANXA11, IL23R, SH2B3/ATXN2, IL12B, NFKB1/MANBA, FAM177B, chromosome 11q13.1, and RAB23) have been identified to date. Genome wide association studies show that several HLA and non-HLA alleles are associated with the development of this disease. HLA-DRB1*0301/ DQB1*0201, transforming growth factor β (TGF-β), tumor necrosis factor α (TNF-α) and toll-like receptor 4 (TLR-4) are all considered significant indicators of susceptibility to sarcoidosis.
2. **Infections:** Various microbial agents have been proposed as eliciting agents for the immune response in sarcoidosis including Mycoplasma species, Leptospira, Chlamydia pneumonia, Mycobacterium tuberculosis, Propionibacterium, Borrelia burgdorferi, Pneumocystis jirovecii and viruses like herpes and retrovirus. Hepatitis C infection has also been shown to increase the risk of developing sarcoidosis.
3. **Environmental factors:** Exposure to silica, insecticides, wood stoves, soil, tree pollen, inorganic particulates and nanoparticles have been associated with an increased risk for developing sarcoidosis. In addition to these factors, occupational exposures like those involved in hardware, gardening materials, fire workers, building supplies, metal work, and ship servicemen in the navy are prone to sarcoidosis.
4. **Role of Autoimmunity:** Although no disease specific autoantibodies have been observed, it has been shown that the major histocompatibility complex (MHC) class II molecules on antigen-presenting cells possess an autoantigen that is recognized by the T-cell receptor (TCR) of the responding T-cells in sarcoidosis patients. Vimentin-derived peptides are the most plausible candidate for the activation of both T-cells and B-cells in the lung. Overlap of sarcoidosis with other autoimmune diseases like rheumatoid arthritis, autoimmune thyroid disease, Sjogren's syndrome and ankylosing spondylitis also supports the autoimmune hypothesis. The role of the microbiota in these autoimmune diseases has been shown to play a role in their pathogenesis.

Pathogenesis

Various etiological agents including microbes, organic and inorganic compounds, etc. are normally cleared by the innate immune system. However, sometimes these agents may remain undegraded within the cells and may initiate immune response. The antigen-presenting cells (APCs), such as dendritic cells (DCs), alveolar macrophages (AMs) and alveolar epithelial cells, produce high levels of TNF-α, and secrete interleukins-12, -15, and -18, macrophage inflammatory protein-1 (MIP-1), monocyte chemoattractant protein-1 (MCP-1), and granulocyte macrophage colony-stimulating factor (GM-CSF). These APCs also present antigens to CD4 + T-cells initiating granuloma construction, a critical feature of sarcoidosis.

Activated CD4 + T-cells can differentiate into two distinct subsets, T helper 1 (Th1) and T helper 2 (Th2) cells. Th1 cells predominantly secrete interleukin-2 (IL-2) and interferon-gamma (IFN-γ), while Th2 cells secrete IL-4 and IL-13. Resolution or maintenance of granuloma is determined by the proportion of Th1 and Th2 cells, respectively. Incapacitation of Tregs is also a key feature of granuloma maintenance. Th17 cells have recently been linked to the pathogenesis of sarcoidosis. These cells are recruited to the disease site and are involved in the construction of the granuloma.

Clinical Features

Symptoms are usually negligible and nonspecific including cough, labored breathing, chest discomfort, dyspnea, and low-grade fever, etc. Systemic symptoms such as tiredness, weight reduction, and night sweats, are common. Hemoptysis is rare. Sarcoidosis may be acute, sub-acute, or chronic. However, in majority of cases, it is entirely asymptomatic and often diagnosed when aberrations are identified on a chest radiograph (up to 50% of patients) during a routine examination.

Cutaneous features: Seen in approximately 20-30% of the patients. Can be classified into specific lesions and non-specific lesions.

A. **Specific cutaneous lesions:**
   - **Common cutaneous lesions:** Macules, papules, plaques, nodular, lupus pernio, subcutaneous sarcoidosis and scar sarcoidosis.
   - **Uncommon cutaneous lesions:** Nail sarcoidosis, atrophic and ulcerative sarcoidosis, ichthyosiform sarcoidosis, hypopigmented sarcoidosis, scalp sarcoidosis (scarring alopecia), mucosal sarcoidosis, lymphedematous sarcoidosis, psoriasiform and lichenoid variants and erythrodermic forms.

B. **Non-specific cutaneous lesions:**
   - **Common:** Erythema nodosum
   - **Uncommon:** Calcinosis cutis, prurigo, digital clubbing

Plaque and papular sarcoidosis- Red-brown to purple, less commonly skin-colored, yellow-brown, or hypopigmented papules less than 1 cm in diameter are seen predominantly on the face and neck, especially on the eyelids, around the orbits, nasolabial folds, as well as the occipital area of the neck. Sites of repetitive trauma, such as knees, can be a predilection for papular sarcoidosis. Papules, notably on the extensor surfaces of arms, face, scalp, back, and buttocks, can progress into plaques greater than 5 mm. These lesions are from red-brown to flesh-colored to purple-brown to yellow-brown, oval or circular shaped, often clearly defined, firm to touch, and may be scaly. Plaques tend to be thicker and fewer in number, and are indurated. The distinctive apple jelly color of the granulomatous skin lesion can be seen on diascopy.

Subcutaneous sarcoidosis: It is the least common amongst the specific lesions of cutaneous sarcoidosis. They present as multiple, firm, asymptomatic to slightly painful, mobile, round to oval, skin-colored nodules frequently occurring bilaterally and in asymmetric pattern on the extremities. Other body parts that can be affected include the trunk, face, buttocks, head, and neck.

Scar sarcoidosis: Lesions of sarcoidosis can also appear in pre-existing scars. Clinically, the lesions present as papules, plaques or nodules or ill-defined erythema.

Lupus pernio: Lupus pernio is the most distinctive cutaneous lesion of sarcoidosis. It is more commonly seen in women with long standing sarcoidosis. It presents on the nose, middle face, and cheeks as red to violaceous, indurated plaques with infrequent superficial scaling leaving behind telangiectatic scars. There is a close association between upper respiratory tract sarcoidosis and lupus pernio and both are indicators of chronic sarcoidosis. These patients have high rate of intrathoracic, upper respiratory tract, ophthalmic, musculoskeletal and reticuloendothelial involvement.

Erythema nodosum: It is the most common non-specific cutaneous lesion of sarcoidosis as no granulomas are found on histological examination. Approximately 10-22% of all erythema nodosum cases are caused by sarcoidosis.

Triad of erythema nodosum, bilateral hilar lymphadenopathy on X-ray, and joint symptoms such as arthritis of the ankles, wrists, and elbows make up Lofgren's syndrome, which is highly specific for sarcoidosis.

1. **Mucosal involvement**

   Lesions may vary from nodules with a hyperpigmented halo, diffuse pale yellow plaques or ulceration involving the buccal mucosa, palate, tongue or larynx.

2. **Nail involvement**

   The changes include nail thickening, opacity, fragility, longitudinal ridging, pitting, atrophy, nail loss, pterygium and red or brown discoloration of the nail beds.

3. **Lung involvement**

   - More than 90% of the individuals have either hilar or mediastinal lymphadenopathy. Patient may present with dry cough, wheezing, dyspnea and fatigue. In acute stage, pleural effusion, pericardial effusion, pneumothorax and lymph node involvement may occur while in chronic stage, lung fibrosis and respiratory failure may be seen. Scadding's staging (Table 31.2) of sarcoidosis is the severity grade for lung involvement.

Table 31.2: Scadding's staging of sarcoidosis

Radiographic Type	*Radiographic Characteristics*
0	No visible findings
I	Bilateral hilar lymphadenopathy
II	Bilateral hilar lymphadenopathy and parenchymal infiltration
III	Parenchymal infiltration without hilar adenopathy in regular chest radiography
IV	Advanced fibrosis with severe distortion of the normal lung architecture predominately in the middle and upper lobes with evidence of bronchiectasis, hilar retraction, bulla, cysts and more rarely "honeycombing"

4. **Lymph node involvement**

   - Seen in upto 20% of patients. Mainly peripheral lymph nodes are involved which are moderately swollen and non-tender.

5. **Eye involvement**

   - Seen in upto 40% of patients. Pain, photophobia and hyperemia are the presenting features.
   - Conjunctivitis, uveitis, retinochoroiditis, glaucoma, cataract, retrobulbar optic neuritis and optic atrophy may occur.
   - In Heerfordt's syndrome fever, facial nerve palsy, anterior uveitis and parotid gland enlargement is seen.

6. **Musculoskeletal involvement**

   - Seen in 1-13 % of patients. Osteoporosis, osteopenia, arthralgia, arthritis and nodular and cystic lesions of the bones, diffuse granulomatous myositis may be seen.

7. **Renal**
   - Seen in 5 % of patients. Renal calculi, nephrocalcinosis, interstitial nephritis and renal failure can occur.
8. **Endocrine and exocrine gland involvement**
   - Thyroid and parotid glandes are affected in 20-50% of patients. Thyroid dysfunction, parotid enlargement and hypothalamic-pituitary effects causing diabetes insipidus may occur.
9. **Upper respiratory tract**
   - Nose, nasopharynx and larynx are affected in most patients with systemic sarcoidosis.
10. **Cardiac involvement**
    - Seen in 20- 27% of patients. Heart failure, arrhythmias and syncope can occur.
11. **Neurological involvement**
    - Seen in <10% of patients. Facial palsy, meningeal inflammation, encephalopathy, seizures, hydro-cephalus and space occupying lesions may be seen
12. **Liver and spleen**
    - Seen in upto 18% of patients. Hepatosplenomegaly, intrahepatic cholestasis, portal hypertension and altered liver functions may be seen.

Diagnosis

Owing to its multisystemic nature and unidentified etiology, the diagnosis of this condition can be difficult and is often delayed. Sarcoidosis is usually diagnosed when radiological and typical clinical data are reinforced by histological confirmation of non-necrotic granulomas.

1. **Histopathology:** In typical Cutaneous lesions of sarcoidosis, well demarcated islands of epithelioid cells (granulomas)containing few giant cells (langhans type) with only a sparse lymphocytic infiltrate at the margins are seen. These epithelioid cell granulomas are referred to as **"naked tubercles".** In a minority of the cases, the giant cells may contain asteroid bodies and schaumann bodies.

   Asteroid bodies which are more common, are star-shaped eosinophilic structures that when stained with phosphotungstic-hematoxylin, produce a brown-red centre with radiating blue spikes. **Schaumann bodies** are round to oval, laminated and are calcified especially at their periphery. They stain dark blue because of the presence of calcium. Neither of the two bodies are specific for sarcoidosis. A reticulum stain of sarcoidosis reveals a network of reticulum fibres surrounding and permeating the epithelioid cell granulomas.

   Hamazaki-Wesenberg bodies (yellow bodies, spindle bodies, chromogenic bodies) are seen in the lymph nodes and represent giant extracellular and intracellular lysosomes. These are seen as yellow-brown, oval or spindle shaped structures about 0.5-0.8 micrometers in size on hematoxylin and eosin stain.

2. **A list of conventional tests for sarcoidosis includes**
   - ***CBC:*** Lymphopenia
   - ***Routine ophthalmological examination:*** Orbital and eyelid granulomas
   - ***Urinalysis:*** Hypercalciuria
   - ***Renal function tests:*** High levels of calcium, urea and creatinine.
   - Serum 1,25 dihydroxyvitamin D levels
   - ***Pulmonary function tests:*** To assess pulmonary involvement and disease severity.
   - Tissue and bronchial biopsy
   - ***Mantoux test:*** Negative in most sarcoid patients.
   - ***Imaging:*** Chest X-ray and HRCT-Bilateral hilar lymphadenopathy and nodular infiltration of the lungs.
   - ***18F-fluorodeoxyglucose positron emission tomography (FDG-PET):*** Highly sensitive to detect pulmonary and cardiac involvement.
   - ***ECG:*** Rhythm abnormalities, ectopic beats and repolarisation disturbances.
   - ***Kveim test:*** Intradermal injection of crude homogenate sarcoid tissue results in papule formation at the injection site which have typical histopathological findings of sarcoidosis. The test was further refined by the use of particulate suspension of splenic tissue of patients with sarcoidosis, the antigen is injected intradermally on the forearm and results are read at 6 weeks. However, the use of this test is historical due to the potential infective nature of the antigen source.
   - **Gallium scan- two classical signs of sarcoidosis are seen:**
     1. ***Panda sign:*** Bilateral lacrimal and parotid glands uptake of gallium causes this sign.
     2. ***Lambda sign:*** Bilateral hilar and right paratracheal uptake of gallium results causes this sign.
   - **Biomarkers:**
     1. ***Serum angiotensin converting enzyme (SACE):*** Raised in sarcoidosis and indicates total granuloma load.
     2. ***Chitotriosidase:*** Increased in sarcoidosis and is produced by alveolar macrophages.

3. ***Lysozyme:*** Raised and is produced by activated macrophages and monocytes.
4. ***Neopterin:*** Raised and is produced by activated macrophages and monocytes.
5. ***Hypercalcemia***
6. ***Soluble IL 2 receptor:*** Raised and is a marker of T cell activation
7. ***SAA:*** Raised and it increases the production of TNF-α, IL-18 and IL-10 in the lungs leading to T cell exhaustion.
8. ***Chemokines:*** Higher production of CCL 18 leads to pulmonary fibrosis. Higher levels of CXCL 9 and CXCL 10 are seen in sarcoidosis.
9. ***KL 6:*** Raised in sarcoidosis and indicates lymphocytic alveolitis.
10. ***IFN-γ:*** Th1 inflammatory cytokine and its production increases in sarcoidosis.
11. ***TGF-β:*** Marker of fibrosis and chronic disease.
12. ***TNF-α:*** Secreted by macrophages and is responsible for maintenance of granuloma.

Treatment

In sarcoidosis, a decision on the appropriate intervention precedes the decision of whether or not to treat the patient. Not every patient needs to be treated. The decision to treat a sarcoidosis patient is predicated according to the development of specific symptoms and disease progression evidenced by worsening functional status and imaging abnormalities. Patients can be followed up over long periods because spontaneous resolution may occur during this time frame.

Treatment is often initiated with 0.5–0.75 mg of prednisolone per kg (body weight) daily for 4 weeks and tapered by 10 mg every 4 weeks, depending on the disease response. It is sometimes advised that the dose of 0.5-0.75 mg/kg of prednisolone is too high and doses of 20 mg of prednisone can be used as an alternative. When pulmonary function has improved, therapy can be terminated, which is usually within 6-12 months.

1. **First line drugs:** Corticosteroids (Prednisolone and prednisone)
2. **Second line:** Cytotoxic or immunomodulatory drugs- Hydroxychloroquine, methotrexate, azathioprine and mycophenolate mofetil
3. **Third line:** Anti-cytokine monoclonal antibodies
   - Anti TNF-α (Infliximab or adalimumab)
   - Anti Il-23 (Ustekinumab and Canakinumab)
4. **Others:** Tetracycline, minocycline, thalidomide, dapsone.

For cutaneous involvement, strong potency topical corticosteroids, such as clobetasol or halobetasol propionate, or mild like mometasone for facial lesions should be used. Intralesional triamcinolone may be used every three to four weeks until resolution occurs. Other topical therapies include tacrolimus, PUVA therapy, etc. Extensive, severe, or recalcitrant disease however requires administration of systemic drugs as described above.

NECROBIOTIC GRANULOMA

Collagenolytic or necrobiotic granuloma is a condition in which granulomatous infiltrate develops around altered collagen and elastic fibers. Few important necrobiotic granulomatous disorders are described below:

GRANULOMA ANNULARE

Granuloma annulare (GA) is a common skin disorder characterized by papules or nodules grouped in a ring like or annular configuration, most commonly involving the lateral or dorsal surfaces of the hands, feet, wrists and ankles. GA is a common disorder in school age children.

Etiology

In children, tetanus or Bacille Calmette-Guérin (BCG) vaccination, hepatitis B infection, Borrelia infection, Hodgkin disease, leukemia, or a hypersensitivity reaction to an unidentified antigen have been attributed to cause GA. Trauma, sun exposure and insect bites have also been known to cause it. In adults, diabetes mellitus and dyslipidemia are the associated risk factors.

Clinical Feature

A classic lesion presents as an annular, smooth, non-scaly plaque with numerous small papules at the border. Initially smooth, flesh colored to pink papules appear which slowly enlarge peripherally and involute centrally to form the classic rings with clear centers and elevated borders (Figure 31.1 A and B). Lesions may be as small as 5 mm to several centimeters in size. Lesions usually disappear spontaneously without sequelae, within several months to years.

Clinical Variants

- **Localized:** This is the most common form of granuloma annulare which present with single or multiple non scaly annular or arciform plaque composed of closely set papules, on extremities.
- **Generalized or disseminated (Figure 31.1 C):** This form of GA is presents with skin colored to erythematous

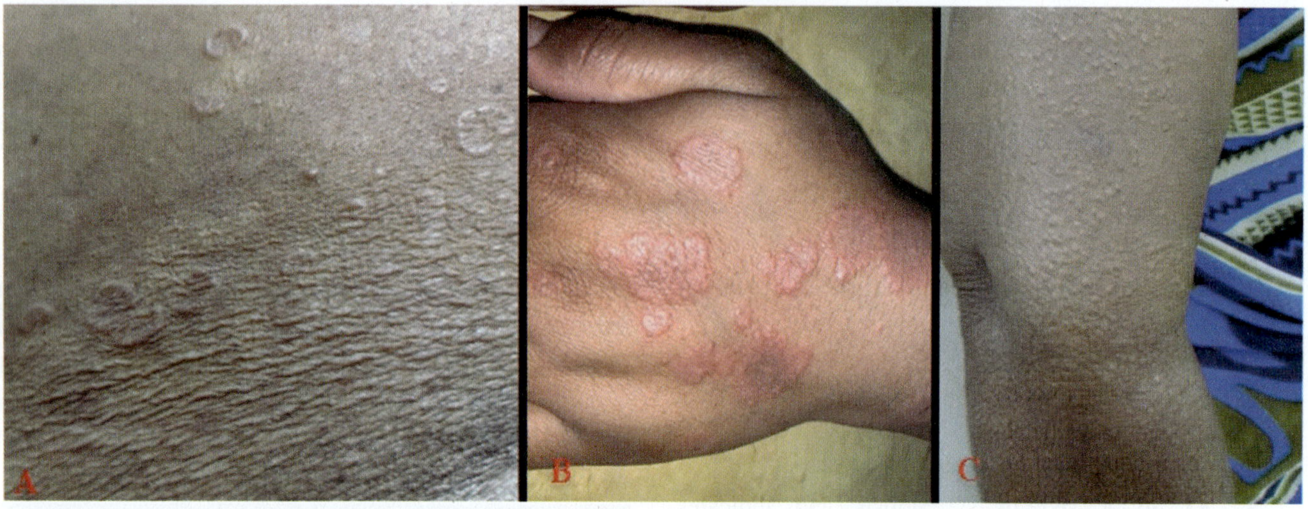

Figure 31.1: Granuloma annulare classical annular pattern (A and B), disseminated pattern (C)

papules, in discrete or annular or arciform configuration over trunk and extremities. It is more common in HIV infected patients.

- **Perforating:** This variant of GA is present with keratotic yellowish papules with crusting shows trans epidermal elimination of damaged collagen through epidermis which heals with atrophic scars.
- **Subcutaneous:** It presents with painless single or multiple subcutaneous nodules over scalp or pretibial region in children.
- **Other:** Follicular pustulosis, Pustular generalized, Linear, Patch etc.

Histopathology

It is characterized by three important histological features include, foci of degenerated collagen (necrobiosis), lymphohistiocytic infiltrates and mucin deposition. It shows three different patterns:

- **Interstitial pattern:** Necrobiosis is less common. Perivascular and interstitial mucin and lymphohistiocytic infiltrate is the prominent findings.
- **Palisaded pattern:** It is characterized by prominent necrobiosis with surrounding palisaded histiocytes.
- **Sarcoidal or tuberculoid pattern:** This pattern resembles sarcoid or tuberculoid granuloma.

Treatment

Asymptomatic lesions may need not be treated. Topical corticosteroids, intralesional corticosteroid injection, topical calcineurin inhibitors are often used. Cryotherapy and systemic agents like isotretinoin, prednisone, dapsone, doxycycline and cyclosporine, areeffective but risk may outweigh the benefits.

NECROBIOSIS LIPOIDICA

Necrobiosis lipoidica is a cutaneous marker of diabetes mellitus. It is predominantly seen in females and has an average age of onset at 34 years. However, it may be seen in children, and if present it suggests a higher risk for diabetic nephropathy and retinopathy. It is most commonly seen in patients who are insulin dependent.

Clinical Features

It presents as slowly enlarging, asymptomatic, irregularly bordered, red to yellow-brown to violaceous plaques typically in the pretibial areas (Figure 31.2). The center often becomes atrophic, and there may be superficial telangiectasias. The lesion may develop ulceration in one third patients. Skin biopsy can be done but should be better avoided in diabetic patients. Diagnosis should be made clinically by presence of sharply demarcated, waxy plaques with a red or violaceous border on the anterior tibial surfaces of a patient with diabetes mellitus.

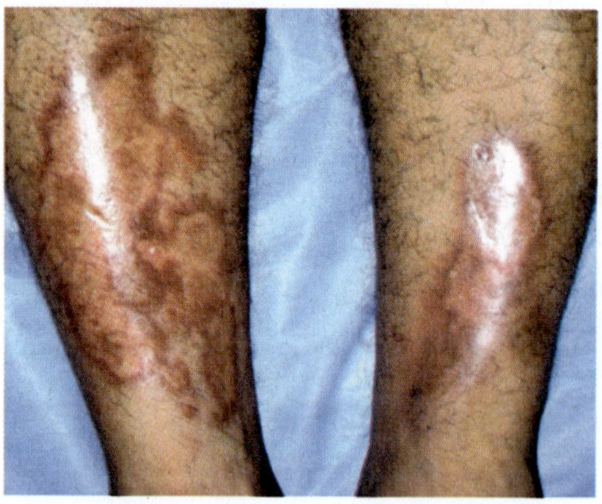

Figure 31.2: Necrobiosis lipoidica

Treatment

Treatment guidelines are not clear. No treatment is indicated when lesions are asymptomatic. Control of blood sugar levels is of importance. Active therapy of lesions includes topical and intralesional corticosteroids, aspirin, dipyridamole, pentoxifylline, clofazimine, cyclosporine, mycophenolate mofetil, systemic corticosteroids, chloroquine,topical tretinoin, hyperbaric oxygen and topical psoralen plus ultraviolet A (PUVA) light therapy. Pulsed-dye laser has been used and may benefit the telangiectatic and erythematous components. Ulcerated lesions should be cleaned and dressed.

NECROBIOTIC XANTHOGRANULOMA

It is a rare chronic, slow progressive disease with widespread infiltrated asymptomatic indurated xanthomatous nodules and plaques present predominantly around eyes (Figure 31.3) and are strongly associated with hematological tumors. Rarely they can ulcerate. Laboratory abnormalities found in this condition include IgG paraproteinemia, cryoglobulinemia, hypocomplemententemia, anemia, leukopenia, hyperlipidemia.

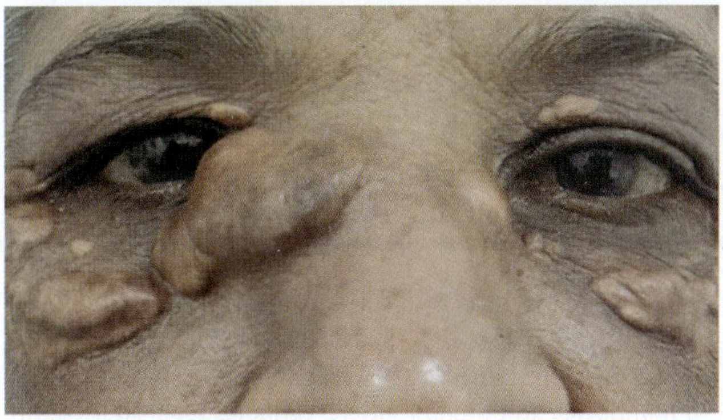

Figure 31.3: Necrobiotic xanthogranuloma

Treatment

If paraproteinemia is present it should be treated by alkylating agent (melphalan) and prednisolone. Chlorambucil, cyclophosphamide, hydroxychloroquine, methotrexate and IVIG may also be used.

Other Necrobiotic Disorders

- Rheumatoid Nodules (Chapter 15)
- Rheumatoid Vasculitis (Chapter 15)
- Churg-Strauss Syndrome (Chapter 17)
- Wegener's Granulomatosis (Chapter 17)

FOREIGN BODY GRANULOMA

Foreign body in the skin results in two different types of immunological response:

Non immunological: Granulomatous reaction made up of foreign body giant cells and histiocytes which try to encircle and isolate the foreign body. It may be caused by endogenous substances like ruptured hair follicle, ruptured pilomatricoma and ruptured dermoid cyst, etc or by exogenous substances like e.g. paraffin, silica, starch, talc, sutures, thorns, etc.

Immunological: This occurs in people who have a particular sensitivity to the foreign substance e.g. zirconium, certain dyes etc. Histology shows sarcoidal or tuberculoid granuloma.

32 CHAPTER Systemic Diseases and Cutaneous Manifestations

Contents

DIABETES MELLITUS

Diabetes mellitus is one of the major global health problems because of its increasing prevalence and the complexity of its systemic and local manifestations. Diabetes is present in more than 10.5% of the adult population. Cutaneous involvement can be seen in 43-66% of Indian diabetics.

The diagnostic criteria for Diabetes are:

- HbA1c test: 6.5 percent or higher.
- Fasting blood sugar: 126 mg/dL (7.0 mmol/L) or higher.
- Glucose tolerance test: A 2-hour blood sugar of 200 mg/dL (11.1 mmol/L) or higher.

Pathogenesis for various cutaneous manifestations include:

1. Hyperglycemia and insulin dysfunction.
2. Loss of cutaneous sensations predisposes to injury and infection.
3. Microvascular abnormalities like increased vascular permeability, reduced response to sympathetic innervation as well as to thermal and hypoxemic stress.
4. Loss of immunoregulatory mechanisms like diminished chemotaxis and phagocytosis, reduced bactericidal ability of white blood cells.
5. Dysregulation of lipid profile.

Cutaneous manifestations associated with DM:

1. **Specific manifestations**
   - Acanthosis nigricans
   - Diabetic dermopathy
   - Scleredema diabeticorum
   - Bullosis diabeticorum
   - Necrobiosis lipoidica
   - Rubeosis faciei diabeticorum
2. **Non-specific signs and symptoms**
   - Palmar erythema
   - Acrochordons
   - Xerosis
   - Pigmented purpuric dermatosis
   - Yellow nail and skin syndrome

- Keratosis pilaris.
- Diabetes associated pruritus.
- Onychocryptosis.
- Limited joint mobility.
- Diabetic foot.

3. **Dermatological disorders possibly having high prevalence of Diabetes**
   - Psoriasis.
   - Vitiligo.
   - Lichen planus.
   - Hidradenitis suppurativa.
   - Generalized granuloma annulare.
   - Xanthomas.
   - Perforating dermatosis (Reactive perforating collagenosis, perforating folliculitis, Kyrle's disease and elastosis perforans serpiginosa).

4. **Cutaneous complications of diabetic therapy**
   - **Insulin therapy:** Allergic reactions to insulin can be localized or generalized e.g. urticaria, angioedema or anaphylaxis, insulin lipoatrophy and lipohypertrophy, local infections and subcutaneous nodules.
   - **Oral hypoglycemic drugs:** First generation sulfonylureas (chlorpropamide, tolbutamide) can cause phototoxic or photoallergic reactions, psoriatic or lichenoid eruptions. Oral gliptins (sitagliptin, vildagliptin) can rarely cause reactions and can manifest as drug eruptions, polymorphic erythema, leukocytoclastic vasculitis, photosensitivity, rarely pemphigus vulgaris/bullous pemphigoid etc. Metformin, a biguanide, can cause leukocytoclastic vasculitis, papulosquamous eruptions etc.

1. **Skin infections:** They are frequently observed in patients with DM and include:
   - **Bacterial infection:** Erysipelas, cellulitis, erythrasma, necrotizing fasciitis, malignant otitis externa etc.
   - **Fungal infection:** Cutaneous or mucous membrane candidiasis, dermatophytosis (tinea pedis) etc.

2. **Diabetic dermopathy**
   - Also known as shin spots.
   - Characterized by asymptomatic atrophic, hyperpigmented macules or patches over the shins.
   - No treatment is required.

3. **Diabetic foot**
   - Combination of neuropathy, atherosclerosis and poor healing leads to development of diabetic foot which is more prevalent in type 1 DM.
   - Clinically, callosities, xerosis, evolving to chronic ulcers and deformities occur. Perforating ulcers develop on pressure areas which are subject to frequent trauma. They heal poorly, are prone to bacterial or fungal superinfection and if they do heal, recurrence is common.
   - Treatment includes rigorous hygiene, wearing appropriate footwear to minimize and redistribute plantar pressure. In cases of superinfection, antibiotics should be administered and special hydrogel dressings, topical growth factors or grafts for epithelization. In ischemic ulcers, surgical revascularization should be used.

4. **Scleredema diabeticorum**
   - Most often found in middle aged, obese patients with poorly controlled blood sugar level.
   - It is characterized by marked increase in thickness of the dermis of the posterior neck and upper back. The affected skin is firm, woody, non-pitting and shows a peau d'orange appearance.
   - Treatment includes control of diabetes. Radiotherapy, low dose methotrexate and prostaglandin E1 have been tried.

5. **Diabetic bullae (bullosis diabeticorum)**
   - Characterized by the spontaneous appearance of tension bullae on the integument that are usually painless, open quickly and leave erosions, but heal without scarring.
   - It progresses to spontaneous healing but requires prevention of bacterial superinfection.

6. **Necrobiosis lipoidica**
   - Necrobiosis lipoidica (NL) is a rare granulomatous dermatological condition, predominantly in females.
   - NL may be associated with both types of diabetes mellitus. It occurs predominantly in patients with type 1 DM in the 3rd decade of life.
   - Risk factors associated with NL include hypertension, hyperlipidemia, obesity, smoking, thyroid dysfunction, kidney disease.
   - The clinical appearance is characterized by round erythematous papules, converging into plaques with purplish-red margins and an atrophic, sclerosing, yellow-brown center with telangiectasias on the surface. They occur on the calves, bilaterally in the pretibial region, less commonly on the forearms, scalp,

face or abdomen. They are often asymptomatic, but may sometimes present with itching and hypoesthesia or pain if ulceration occurs. Ulcerations occur in 1/3 of cases and are complicated by secondary bacterial infections or progress to squamous cell carcinomas.

- **Treatment options include:** Topical, intralesional or systemic corticosteroids, during active phases. Other therapeutic options include calcineurin inhibitors, TNF-alpha inhibitors, pentoxifylline, synthetic antimalarials, PUVA. For ulcerated and bacterially superinfected lesions, local antibiotics, emollients, compressive bandaging can be used.

7. **Diabetic rubeosis**
   - It is a peculiar rosy reddening of the face, sometimes of hands and feet observed in long standing diabetics.
8. **Ear lobe crease**
   - Diagonal ear lobe crease is a known marker for coronary artery disease in patients with diabetic retinopathy.
9. **Yellow skin of DM**
   - Many patients with DM develop yellow skin, a hue more appreciated on the face and on palms and soles.
   - The exact pathomechanism is unknown, however possibilities include carotenemia due to increased intake of vegetables, decreased conversion of carotene to vitamin A in liver and altered metabolism of carotene by tissues such as epidermoid and bone.
   - **Treatment** includes alteration of diet.
10. **Diabetic digital skin**
    - The new nomenclature of this condition is Scleroderma like syndrome and is associated with limited joint mobility.
    - Seen on the dorsa of fingers and occasionally over hands in children with insulin dependent diabetes of many years and can also be seen in adult diabetes.
    - It presents with thick, tight, waxy skin over the dorsa of hands causing limited mobility of joints.
    - Prayer sign is characterized by the inability to approximate the palmar surfaces and interphalangeal joint spaces when the hands are pressed together and fingers separated.
    - **Treatment:** The thickened dermis reverts back to normal with optimum control of diabetes with insulin along with physiotherapy.

THYROID DISORDERS

Hyperthyroidism

It is a hypermetabolic stage resulting from excess of thyroid hormones i.e. T3 and T4. Based on etiology it can be divided into:

- **Primary:** Grave's disease, toxic multinodular goiter, adenoma.
- **Secondary:** Due to excess production of TSH or TRH from pituitary tumors.

Cutaneous manifestations: Facial flushing, palmar erythema, warm, smooth, soft and velvety skin, increased sweating, pruritus, hyperpigmentation of skin and mucosa, hyperpigmented eyelids (Jellinek's sign), facial suffusion in patients with large substernal goiter (Pemberton's sign), erythema may the skin of toxic goiter (Maroni's sign) and pretibial myxedema.

Hair: Diffuse alopecia, thin, fine brittle hairs and chronic telogen effluvium.

Nails: Thin, soft nails, koilonychias, distal onycholysis, concave contouring (Plummer's nails) and thyroid acropachy.

Diamond's triad: Pretibial myxedema, thyroid acropachy and exophthalmos.

EMO syndrome: Exophthalmos, pretibial Myxedema and hypertrophic Osteoarthropathy.

Hypothyroidism

It is due to decreased secretion of T3 and T4 hormones by thyroid gland which can be divided into:

- **Primary:** Idiopathic
- **Secondary:** Severe iodine deficiency, late effect of radio-iodine treatment of thyrotoxicosis (iatrogenic), drugs induced such as by lithium and bexarotene.
- **Tertiary:** Hypothalamic failure of TRH production.

Juvenile Hypothyroidism

Cutaneous manifestations:

- **Skin:** Pale and cold, dry, coarse skin, asteatotic eczema, pruritus, palmo plantar keratoderma, ivory yellow skin colour, puffy eyelids, swollen lips, macroglossia and broad nose, puffiness of dorsum of hands, feet and supraclavicular fossa, purpura, ecchymosis, punctuate telangiectasia, carpal tunnel syndrome, delayed wound healing, xanthomatosis, psoriasiform lesions etc.
- **Hair:** Dry, coarse, slow growing hair, diffuse alopecia, telogen effluvium, madarosis.
- **Nails:** Brittle, striated and slow growing nails.

RENAL DISORDERS

Specific cutaneous manifestations in chronic kidney disease (Table 32.1)

Table 32.1: Specific cutaneous manifestations in chronic kidney disease

Specific skin change	*Etiopathogenesis*	*Clinical features*	*Treatment*
Acquired perforating dermatosis	An interplay of various factors like: • Chronic rubbing leading to epithelial hyperplasia and abnormal keratinization • Reduced blood supply secondary to microangiopathy • Over expression of transforming growth factor beta-3 and elevated serum and tissue fibronectin.	Umbilicated, hyperkeratotic pruritic papules, some with a central, white, keratotic crust.	Topical steroids, keratolytics, topical or oral retinoids and cryotherapy. Narrowband ultraviolet B-light may be helpful in refractory cases. Allopurinol at a dose of 100 mg/day can be used.
Calcinosis cutis	• Calcinosis cutis develops due to metastatic deposition of calcium salts into the skin and subcutaneous tissues as a result of elevated calcium phosphate. • Hyperparathyroidism may or may not be present.	Firm white papules, plaques and nodules, most commonly over the periarticular areas and fingertips.	Treatment revolves around normalizing calcium and phosphate levels.
Calciphylaxis	• Increased NF-kB activity leads to bone mineral loss and vascular calcification. • Transformation of vascular smooth muscle cells into osteoblast like cells is initiated by reactive oxygen species and imbalance between inhibitors and inducers of vascular calcification and metabolic disturbances • Inducers of calcification like osteopontin and bone morphogenic protein 2 (BMP-2) are upregulated and inhibitors of calcification like matrix Gla protein (MGP), fetuin-A, and pyrophosphate are suppressed. • Progressive subintimal fibrosis and medial-arteriolar calcification lead to endothelial injury.	Most commonly affected areas are fatty areas of the thighs, abdomen, buttocks and lower extremities. The lesions are firm with a pink or mottled color or livedo reticularis like appearance; and progress to painful ulcers with a black eschar.	Treatment revolves around supportive and preventive measures including hyperbaric oxygen therapy, debridement, wound care and antibiotic therapy. Prevention and/or reversal of calcium-phosphate precipitation is done by administration of sodium thiosulfate. Correction of calcium, phosphorus and parathyroid hormone is carried out by using non-calcium-containing phosphate binders, such as sevelamer carbonate or lanthanum carbonate.

Contd.

Bullous diseases-Porphyria cutanea tarda (PCT) and Pseudoporphyria	• Alcohol abuse, hepatitis C virus, HIV infection, and iron supplementation contribute to decreased UROD activity.	Non inflamed blisters, erosions and crusts, especially over the dorsum of hands and forearms. Blisters heal with scarring or milia. Sclerodermatous plaques, hypertrichosis, and hyperpigmentation in sun exposed areas are also seen.	• The essential part of treatment is avoidance of sunlight. • Concomitant exacerbating factors (alcohol, estrogens, iron overload, hepatitis) should be avoided or treated. • Small volume phlebotomy (50–100 ml once or twice weekly) to decrease hepatic iron stores can induce remission because iron overload is an inciting factor. • Alternatively, desferrioxamine can be used.
Eruptive xanthomas	• Hyperlipidemia, either familial or due to nephrotic syndrome.	1–5 mm yellow or erythematous papules that appear in crops and have an abrupt onset. The most common sites are the extensor surfaces of the extremities and buttocks.	Resolve spontaneously once lipid levels are normalized
Nephrogenic systemic fibrosis (NSF)	• May be due to Gadolinium (Gd), cytokines and immunological events. In CKD, half life of Gd is increased to 60 hours and it is dissociated into toxic ionic form which is phagocytosed by macrophages which leads to activation and recruitment of fibroblasts.	Fibrotic, indurated papules, plaques, or subcutaneous nodules which first appear on ankles, lower legs, feet and hands, and progress proximally to involve the thighs and forearms.	• Prevention of nephrogenic systemic fibrosis (NSF) -avoidance of gadolinium (Gd) in patients with acute kidney injury (AKI) or chronic kidney disease (CKD). • No medical therapy for NSF has been found to be effective. Recovery of kidney function may lead to stabilization, improvement, or resolution of NSF. Kidney transplantation is sometimes helpful in curbing progression and occasionally reverses the disease. • Trial of extracorporeal photopheresis with ultraviolet A can be given.
Iododerma	• Patients of renal insufficiency or failure, receiving iodide in the form of intravenous contrast may develop certain skin lesions, due to increased half-life. • Delayed hypersensitivity reaction to iodine	Acneiform eruptions confined to the regions of the body rich in sebaceous glands. Advanced stages may demonstrate the presence of edematous bullous and hemorrhagic lesions.	Treatment relies on excretion of the accumulated iodine and avoidance of further exposure. Supportive treatment is usually satisfactory.

Overview of non-specific skin manifestations in chronic kidney disease (Table 32.2)

Table 32.2: Overview of non-specific skin manifestations in chronic kidney disease			
Non-specific skin change	***Etiopathogenesis***	***Clinical features***	***Treatment***
Xerosis	Exact mechanism is unknown. Proposed mechanisms include: • Dehydration of stratum corneum • Reduced sebum and sweat production due to atrophy of glands • Abnormal eccrine gland function	Skin appears dry, rough and shiny. Xerotic changes may not be pruritic. Extensor surfaces of lower extremities are most prominently involved.	Hydration of the skin with moisturizing creams containing 5-10 % urea.
Acquired ichthyosis	Unknown	It is related to xerosis but the skin develops scaly appearance.	Hydration of the skin
Pigmentary alterations	• Anemia of chronic disease • Urochrome and carotenoid deposition • Increased melanin production due to elevated levels of Beta- MSH	Pallor Yellow discoloration (most common) Hyperpigmentation	Erythropoiesis stimulating agents and iron for anemia. No treatment needed for yellow skin. Sun protection for hyperpigmentation.
Purpura	Platelet dysfunction due to uremia	Purpura and ecchymosis either of spontaneous onset or following minor trauma.	Dialysis, desmopressin, I.V. estrogen.
Nail changes- Lindsay nails (Half and half nails)	Seen in approximately 40% of patients with uremia due to melanin deposition in the nail bed and nail plate.	The distal portion is a pink-red or brown horizontal band that occupies nearly half of the distal nail length. The proximal portion is dull white giving a ground glass appearance. Other nail changes include splinter hemorrhages, koilonychias, Mee's lines, onycholysis, Muehrcke's lines and Beau's lines.	No treatment is required. The nail changes may revert back to normal after renal transplantation.
Mucosal changes	Nutritional deficiencies, poor oral hygiene, smoking, alcoholism, dehydration and mouth breathing may be various pathogenic factors.	Coated tongue, macroglossia with teeth markings, cheilitis, xerostomatitis and gingivitis.	Maintenance of oral hygiene and elimination of triggering factors.
Hair changes	Reduced sebum production and parathormone levels, anemia, stress of chronic disease.	Sparse, lusterless scalp and body hair and diffuse alopecia.	Proper self care.
Cutaneous features due to hormonal changes	Elevated prolactin levels	Gynaecomastia in men and hirsutism and acne in women. Acanthosis nigricans may be seen due to insulin resistance.	Endocrine consultation.

Renal Pruritus

It is a common symptom among patients with end stage kidney disease (ESKD) and about 90% of patients undergoing hemodialysis may experience pruritus.

Risk factors associated with pruritus include inadequate dialysis, hyperparathyroidism, elevated calcium and phosphorus products, xerosis, elevated serum magnesium and aluminium levels, anemia, male sex, hypervitaminosis-A, increased beta-2 microglobulin levels, serotype human leukocyte antigen (HLA-B35) and presence of comorbidities like congestive heart failure and neurologic disease.

The pathogenesis of renal pruritus is not clear, however, several hypotheses have been proposed:

a. **Immunohypothesis:** Renal pruritus is a systemic inflammatory disorder and studies have shown a direct role of proinflammatory T lymphocytes and cytokines. This is supported by higher levels of proinflammatory T helper-1 (TH1) cells, C-reactive protein, interleukin-6 and interleukin-2 levels among hemodialysis patients, in comparison to those without pruritus.

b. **Opioid hypothesis:** The balance in the expression of mu and kappa opioid receptors is altered. Pruritus is aggravated by mu-receptor activation and kappa-receptor blockade.

c. **Pruritogens:** Release of pruritogens and histamine from mast cells has been thought to contribute towards renal pruritus.

Treatment

Therapeutic options for control of pruritus include optimal dialysis, treatment of hyperparathyroidism, hyperphosphatemia and hypermagnesemia along with emollients. For cases of resistant pruritus (continued symptoms despite initial therapy for approximately four weeks), preferred modalities include oral antihistamines, gabapentin, pregabalin, sertraline and montelukast. Phototherapy can be tried. The beneficial effects of UVB therapy are due to a reduction in proinflammatory cytokines and induction of mast cell apoptosis.

Experimental therapeutic options include thalidomide, opioid receptor agonists and antagonists (Naltrexone), omega-6 fatty acids, charcoal, 5-hydroxytryptamine receptor inhibitors, cromolyn sodium and dupilumab.

In cases of refractory renal pruritus, kidney transplantation is considered to be the definitive therapy.

LIVER DISORDERS

Chronic liver disease and skin:

1. **Pigmentary changes**
   - Icterus - Evident when serum bilirubin is >2.5-3 mg/dl.
   - Hyperpigmentation - Over exposed areas, palmo-plantar creases and periorbital area.
   - Hemochromatosis - Bronze diabetes, metallic brown pigmentation.
2. **Vascular lesions**
   - Spider nevus
   - Cutaneous telangiectasia
   - Caput medusa
   - Palmar erythema
   - Purpura secondary to thrombocytopenia
3. **Pruritus**
   - Cholestasis due to hepatitis, cirrhosis, or obstructive jaundice.
   - Bile acids have been suggested to be a factor in pruritus.
   - ***Treatment:*** The American Association for the study of Liver Diseases (AASLD) and the European Association for the study of Liver Disease recommend stepwise treatment (Figure 32.1) using cholestyramine, rifampicin, naltrexone and sertraline.

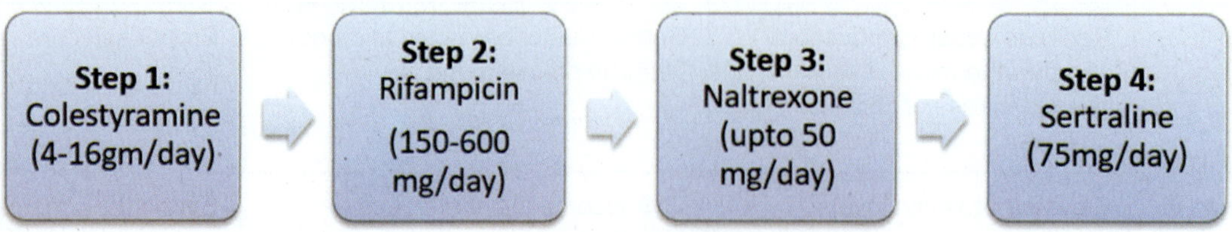

Figure 32.1: Showing stepwise treatment for hepatic pruritis

4. **Hair**
    - Sparse axillary, pubic and forearm hair
5. **Nail**
    - Clubbing, longitudinal ridging, flattening, thickening, watch glass deformity, total leukonychia, Terry's nails, Muehrcke's lines, subungual hyperkeratosis, azure lunulae.
6. **Miscellaneous changes**
    - **Hepatocutaneous syndrome:** Firm papules leaving depressed scars on trunk and extremities, xanthomas, lichen planus.
    - **Pseudoglucagonoma syndrome:** Skin changes resembling necrolytic migratory erythema.
    - **Zinc deficiency:** Periorificial crusted lesions and cracked reticulate eczema on trunk and limbs.
    - Gynaecomastia.
    - Striae distensae on lower abdomen, thighs and abdomen.

Hepatitis and Skin

1. **Hepatitis B**
    - Urticaria and angiedema
    - Serum sickness
    - Erythema nodosum, erythema multiforme
    - **HBV:** Polyarteritis Nodosa (PAN) - ANCA negative
    - Gianotti Crosti syndrome
    - **Vasculitis:** Cryoglobulinemic, Henoch Schonlein purpura (HSP)
    - Pyoderma gangrenosum and sweet's syndrome
    - Lichen planus and anetoderma after Hepatitis B vaccination
2. **Hepatitis C**
    - Mixed cryoglobulinemia
    - Porphyria cutanea tarda
    - Necrolytic acral erythema
    - Red finger
    - **Other associated diseases:** Behçet's disease, granuloma annulare, prurigo nodularis, erythema dyschromicans perstans, livedo reticularis, porokeratosis, erythema nodosum, erythema multiforme, pruritus, sicca syndrome and leukocytoclastic vasculitis.

GASTROINTESTINAL TRACT AND SKIN

Inflammatory Bowel Disease

Ulcerative colitis (UC) and Crohn's disease (CD) are two major types of IBD. Cutaneous manifestations may precede, occur with or postdate the onset of the intestinal disease and can significantly contribute to the morbidity of the affected patients. Skin manifestations of IBD are divided into three categories based on the pathogenesis.

Specific dermatosis: Caused by direct involvement of the skin by the same pathological mechanism as in GI tract.

a. **Fissures and fistulae:** The majority of these patients have active perianal disease compared to patients with disease confined to small bowel only. Perianal abscess, skin tags and chronic edematous inflammation are often seen in association.

b. **Oral Crohn's disease:** Oral lesions occur in 5-20% of patients with CD. It manifests as aphthous stomatitis, pyostomatitis vegetans, angular cheilitis, ulceration, mucosal nodularity (cobblestoning of the buccal mucosa), nodules of gingival and alveolar mucosa, and indurated fissuring of lower lips. These lesions are often painful and disruptive to eating.

c. **Metastatic Crohn's disease (MCD):** MCD is a specific granulomatous disease having cutaneous lesions with same histopathology (non-caseating granulomas with multinucleated giant cells in the dermis) as the intestinal lesions.

Reactive dermatosis: These lesions are seen in both UC and CD. Reactive lesions are caused by the underlying IBD without exhibiting similar pathologic features as seen in GI tract. Cross antigenicity between the skin and intestine mucosa might be responsible for reactive lesions.

a. **Erythema nodosum**

b. **Pyoderma gangrenosum**

c. **Pyostomatitis vegetans**

Associated dermatosis: Psoriasis, vitiligo, reactive arthritis, eczema, clubbing of the nails and acrodermatitis enteropathica.

Hereditary Disorders (Table 32.3)

Table 32.3: Showing different hereditary gastrointestinal tract syndrome and their cutaneous manifestations				
Syndromes	***Inheritance pattern***	***Gene***	***Gastrointestinal manifestation***	***Cutaneous manifestation***
Gardner syndrome (Familial Adenomatous Polyposis)	AD	APC	Colorectal polyposis (non-cancerous)	Epidermoid cyst, lipomas, desmoids tumors
Peutz-Jeghers syndrome	AD	STK11	Hamartomatous polyp (small intestine)	Hyperpigmented macules on face and fingers
Hereditary non polyposis colorectal syndrome (Lynch syndrome/ Muir-torre syndrome)	AD	MLH1 MSH2 MSH6 PS2	Colorectal cancer	Sebaceous adenoma, epithelioma, sebaceous carcinoma, multiple keratoacanthoma
Cowden syndrome	AD	PTEN	Gastrointestinal polyp hamartomatous (Most common), adenomatous, lymphoid, Ganglioneuromas	Trichilemmoma, oral papillomatosis, facial papules, acral keratosis
Bannayan-Riley-Ruvalcaba syndrome	AD	PTEN	Intestinal polyp	Hyperpigmented macules on genitalia, acrochordons, lipomas
Cronkhite- Canada syndrome			Hamartomatous polyp (stomach and large intestine) and chronic diarrhea, protein losing enteropathy	Nail dystrophy, alopecia, onycholysis, onychomadesis, hyperpigmentation

CARDIOVASCULAR SYSTEM AND SKIN

Several common and important cardiac conditions may have dermatological manifestations. Some of them are summarized below:

Cutaneous manifestations seen in cardiac diseases (Table 32.4).

Table 32. 4: Showing different cardiac condition and their dermatological signs	
Cardiac condition	***Dermatological sign***
Infective endocarditis	Clubbing, osler's nodes, janeway lesions, purpura, splinter hemorrhages
Rheumatic heart disease	Erythema marginatum, subcutaneous nodules
Cardiac myxoma	Cyanosis, petechiae, vasculitis, pruritus, livedo reticularis, hyperpigmentation, Raynaud's phenomenon
Cardiac sarcoma	Cutaneous metastasis
LEOPARD syndrome	Lentigines, café-au-lait macules
Kawasaki disease	Palmar erythema, rash, cracked lips, strawberry tongue, Beau's lines, periungual erythema
Cardiac devices	Keloid, contact dermatitis

Dermatological manifestations showing increased incidence of cardiac diseases (Table 32.5).

Table 32.5: Dermatological manifestations showing increased incidence of cardiac diseases

Dermatological manifestation	*Cardiac condition*
Xanthoma	Hyperlipidemia
Acanthosis Nigricans	Obesity, metabolic syndrome, diabetes, hyperinsulinemia
Male pattern hair loss	Coronary artery disease
Premature graying	Coronary artery disease, hyperlipidemia
Earlobe crease	Coronary artery disease
Cyanosis	Congenital heart disease, congestive cardiac failure
Livedo reticularis	Cholesterol embolisation syndrome, APLA syndrome, SLE, Endocarditis, rheumatic fever, diabetes
Clubbing	Congenital heart disease, Endocarditis, cardiac myxoma

PULMONARY DISORDERS AND SKIN

Pulmonary diseases with cutaneous involvement (Table 32.6).

Table 32.6: Dermatological signs of different pulmonary diseases

Pulmonary disease	*Dermatological signs*
Pulmonary tuberculosis	Erythema nodosum, cutaneous tuberculosis
Pseudomonas pneumonia	Ecthyma gangrenosum
Mycoplasma pneumonia	Erythema multiforme, erythema nodosum, SJS
Lung cancer	Acanthosis nigricans, erythema gyratum repens, necrolytic migratory erythema, triple palms, dermatomyositis, migratory superficial thrombophlebitis, acquired ichthyosis, acquired hypertrichosis lanuginose, clubbing, hypertrophic osteoarthropathy

33 Cutaneous Tumors

CHAPTER

Contents

APPENDAGEAL TUMORS

From cutaneous adnexal structures, tumours can differentiate into follicular, apocrine, eccrine, and sebaceous neoplasms. They usually appear as papules or nodules and clinically it may be difficult to make correct diagnosis, which needs histopathological evaluation. Malignant transformation risk varies depending on the specific type of tumor and is higher in sweat gland tumours than in pilosebaceous tumours.

Classification of Appendageal tumors of the skin (Tables 33.1 and 33.2)

- Apocrine gland derived (Table 33.3)
- Eccrine gland derived (Table 33.4)
- Sebaceous gland derived (Table 33.5)
- Hair follicle derived (Table 33.6)

Table 33.1: Showing apocrine and eccrine glands derived tumours

Apocrine glands	*Eccrine glands*
Hamartomas/ hyperplasia/ cyst	**Hamartomas/hyperplasia/cyst**
• Apocrine hidrocystoma	• Eccrine hidrocystoma
• Apocrine nevus	• Eccrine nevus
Benign	**Benign**
• Syringocystadenoma papilliferum (SCAP)	• Syringoma
• Tubular apocrine adenoma	• Poroma
• Cylindroma	• Eccrine syringofibroadenoma
• Erosive adenomatosis of nipple	• Eccrine spiradenoma
• Apocrine fibroadenoma	• Papillary eccrine adenoma
• Hidradenoma papilliferum (HP)	• Nodular hidradenoma
	• Chondroid syringoma

Contd.

Malignant	Malignant
• Syringocystadenocarcinoma papilliferum • Cylindrocarcinoma • Apocrine adenocarcinoma • Hidradenocarcinoma papilliferum	• Aggressive digital papillary and adenocarcinoma • Mucinous eccrine carcinoma • Microcystic adnexal carcinoma • Porocarcinoma • Malignant eccrine spiradenoma • Malignant nodular hidradenoma • Malignant chondroid syringoma • Eccrine adenocarcinoma

Table 33.2: Showing sebaceous glands and hair follicle derived tumours

Sebaceous glands	*Hair follicle*
Hamartomas/hyperplasia/cyst • Nevus sebaceous • Sebaceous hyperplasia	**Hamartomas/hyperplasia/cyst** • Hair follicle nevus • Basaloid follicular hamartoma

Benign
• Sebaceous adenoma
	Benign
	Follicular infundibulum:
	• Inverted follicular keratosis
	• Dilated pore of winer
	• Tumor of the follicular infundibulum
	• Pilar sheath acanthoma
	• Trichoadenoma
	• Comedo naevus
	Outer hair sheath tumors:
	• Trichilemmal cyst
	• Proliferating trichilemmal tumors
	• Trichilemmoma
	• Trichilemmal carcinoma
	Hair matrix tumors:
	• Pilomatricoma
	• Pilomatrix carcinoma
	Hair germ tumors:
	• Trichofolliculoma
	• Trichoepithelioma
	  – Desmoplastic trichoepithelioma
	  – Solitary giant trichoepithelioma
	• Trichoblastoma
	• Cutaneous lymphadenoma
	Hair follicle mesenchyme tumors:
	• Trichodiscoma
	• Perifollicular fibroma
	• Fibrofolliculoma

Malignant • Sebaceous carcinoma	**Malignant** • Pilomatrical carcinoma • Malignant proliferating trichilemmal tumor • Trichilemmal carcinoma • Trichoblastic carcinoma

Table 33.3: Clinical summary of few important apocrine gland derived tumours

Apocrine hidrocystoma:		
Clinical features: Uncommon benign cystic tumor localized to head and neck, characterised by firm dome shaped blue -grey nodules. No seasonal variation.	**Histopathology:** Dermis shows large unilocular or multilocular cystic spaces with fibrous pseudo capsule, lined by flattened vacuolated myoepithelial cells in outer layer and tall columnar cells in inner layer. The cavity contains decapitated secretion. These myoepithelial layers are positive for SMA, calponin and p63.	**Treatment:** Surgical excision, electrodessication and CO_2 laser.
Syringocystadenoma papilliferum (SCAP):		
Clinical features: Asymptomatic or pruritic, solitary, gray or dark brown warty plaques with moist appearance over scalp.	**Histopathology:** Papillomatous epidermal invaginations in dermis which are lined by outer cuboidal cells and inner columnar cells with rich plasma cell infiltration. Immunohistochemistry shows CEA, EMA, AE1, AE3, CAM 5.2 positivity.	**Treatment:** Complete surgical excision is recommended
Cylindroma:		
Clinical features: Firm, pink, smooth, alopecic painful nodules over scalp. When lesions are multiple, they coalesce to form a mass known as **turban tumor.** Multiple cylindromas are present in Brooke-Spiegler syndrome.	**Histopathology:** Multiple nodules in dermis which are arranged in classical jigsaw puzzle pattern, each nodule consist of basaloid cells at periphery and large epithelial cells with abundant cytoplasm in center of lesion.	**Treatment:** Surgical excision
Erosive adenomatosis of nipple/ nipple adenoma/florid papillomatosis:		
Clinical features: Unilateral, erythematous scaly, crusted or eroded lesions on the nipple in females. It may be associated with pruritus, irritation, pain and burning sensation.	**Histopathology:** Shows extending downwards from the epidermis, irregular, dilated, tubular structures. These tubules are line by peripheral layer of cuboidal cells and luminal layer of columnar cells. Some tubules demonstrate papillary projections into the lumen.	**Treatment:** Surgical excision
Hidradenoma Papilliferum/ Papillary hidradenoma:		
Clinical features: Solitary, asymptomatic papule or nodule with umbilication or ulceration over anogenital areas in females	**Histopathology:** Well demarcated nodule in dermis consisting of anastomosing patterns or papillary projections into cystic spaces, described as a maze like pattern. It may show occasional mitotic figures. Intracytoplasmic PAS positive, diastase resistant granules are present in the luminal cells. Immunohistochemistry shows EMA, CEA, HMFG, GCDFP-15 positivity.	**Treatment:** Surgical excision

Table 33.4: Clinical summary of few important eccrine gland derived tumours

Eccrine Hidrocystoma:		
Clinical features: Translucent, dome shape cystic lesion on head and neck in middle aged females. Clusters of multiple eccrine hidrocystoma is suggestive of ectodermal dysplasia.	**Histopathology:** Shows dermal cyst lined by double layer of cells.	**Treatment:** Surgical excision or electrodessication

Contd.

<table>
<tr><td colspan="3">Eccrine nevus:</td></tr>
<tr><td colspan="2">Pure eccrine nevus:
Well defined hyperhidrotic plaque without epidermal changes, commonly seen on forearm.
Eccrine angiomatous hamartoma:
Solitary or multiple benign hamartomatous shiny red brown nodule or plaques are present predominantly on extremities. These lesions may be associated with pain. It has both eccrine and vascular proliferative component on histology.
Mucinous eccrine nevus:
Shows mucin deposition around eccrine glands.
Porokeratotic Eccrine Ostial and Dermal Duct Nevus (PEODDN):
Rare nevoid tumor which presents with asymptomatic keratotic papules in linear distribution on extremities. It is considered as eccrine hamartoma involving intraepidermal eccrine ducts. Histology shows parakeratotic coronoid lamellae around eccrine ducts.</td><td>Treatment: Surgical excision</td></tr>
<tr><td colspan="3">Poroma:</td></tr>
<tr><td colspan="2">These are benign tumors classified according to their location.
Hidroacanthoma simplex (intraepidermal poroma): Presents as solitary hyperkeratotic plaque on extremities. Histology shows aggregates of cuboidal cells around eccrine duct in epidermis.
Classical eccrine poroma (epidermal and dermal component): Presents as solitary fleshy to red colored pruritic painful pedunculated papule or nodule on palms and soles. Multiple poromas are called poromatosis and they are associated with hidrotic ectodermal dysplasia. Histologically it shows aggregates of uniform basaloid cells which radiate from basal layer toward dermis.
Dermal ductal tumor (Entire part into dermis): Present with deep nodular lesions. Histology shows well circumscribed nodules consisting of poroid cells.</td><td>Treatment: Mohs microscopic surgery or excision of lesion.</td></tr>
<tr><td colspan="3">Syringoma:</td></tr>
<tr><td>Clinical features: Multiple, skin colored to yellowish papules around eyes, predominantly in females.
May be associated with down syndrome, Marfan syndrome, Ehlers Danlos syndrome and Nicolau balus syndrome.</td><td>Histopathology: Eccrine tubules with small tadpole or comma like tail or projection is seen in superficial dermis.</td><td>Treatment: Electrocautery, trichloroacetic acid application and dermabrasion.</td></tr>
<tr><td colspan="3">Spiradenoma:</td></tr>
<tr><td>Clinical features: Tumor of intradermal eccrine duct which present as red brown deep nodules, predominantly on anterior chest wall.
May be associated with Brooke-spiegler syndrome.</td><td>Histopathology: Well defined basophilic epithelioid aggregates, lined by small cells with dark nuclei at periphery and large cells with pale nuclei at central part of aggregates.</td><td>Treatment: Surgical excision</td></tr>
<tr><td colspan="3">Nodular hidradenoma:</td></tr>
<tr><td>Clinical features: Shows both eccrine and apocrine differentiation and presents with solitary flesh colored nodule over scalp, face or trunk.</td><td>Histopathology: Shows non encapsulated nodule in dermis containing small polygonal cells and large clear cells.</td><td>Treatment: Surgical excision</td></tr>
<tr><td colspan="3">Chondroid syringoma:</td></tr>
<tr><td>Clinical features: Solitary, slow growing, firm, circumscribed lobulated nodule over nose or cheek (head and neck), commonly seen in males. Can arise from both eccrine and apocrine glands.</td><td>Histopathology: Shows well circumscribed mass with chondroid differentiation and multilobulated fibrous septa. Staining with alcian blue shows abundant mucin or myxoid stroma.</td><td>Treatment: Complete surgical excision or electrodessication</td></tr>
</table>

Table 33.5: Clinical summary of few important sebaceous gland derived tumours

Clinical features	Histopathology	Treatment
Sebaceous hyperplasia:		
Clinical features: Yellow colored telangiectatic papules with central umbilication on sun exposed areas. May be associated with renal transplant, hemodialysis, cyclosporine therapy, pachydermoperiostosis and Muir-torre syndrome.	**Histopathology:** Shows multiple sebaceous lobules around follicular infundibulum.	**Treatment:** Destructive modalities like electrocautery.
Sebaceous adenoma:		
Clinical features: Smooth well defined yellow papules or nodules which can occurs anywhere in body but predominantly seen on face mainly in elderly persons. Cutaneous marker of Muir-torre syndrome.	**Histopathology:** Shows incompletely differentiated sebaceous lobules which contains two different type of cell populations, peripheral basaloid germinative cells and central vacuolated mature sebocytes.	**Treatment:** Complete surgical excision or Mohs microscopic surgery.

Table 33.6: Clinical summary of few important hair follicle derived tumours

Clinical features	Histopathology	Treatment
Inverted follicular keratosis:		
Clinical features: Considered a variant of irritated seborrheic keratosis which presents with solitary papule in the head and neck area.	**Histopathology:** It has four different histopathological variants: • **Papillomatous wart like variant:** Exophytic growth pattern • **Keratoacanthoma like variant:** Exo- endophytic growth pattern • **Solid nodular variant:** Endophytic growth pattern • **Cystic variant** All type shows squamous eddies (Pearl of irritated keratinocytes) and keratin cysts in deeper dermis.	**Treatment:** Surgical excision
Dilated pore of winer:		
Clinical features: Large comedone like lesion due to dilated follicular opening which extends to deep dermis.	**Histopathology:** Shows wide, crater like, vertically oriented infundibulocystic cavity, filled with lamellar elongated orthokeratosis with area of acantholysis.	**Treatment:** Ammonium lactate lotion to evacuate keratotic plug and topical retinoids. In resistance cases surgical excision may be required.
Pilar sheath acanthoma:		
Clinical features: Benign tumor of infundibulum and isthmus origin, presents with solitary skin colored nodule on upper lip with a central pore like opening.	**Histopathology:** Shows irregularly branched cystic cavity containing keratinous material which opens onto the surface. These tumor lobules are composed of outer root sheath epithelium which extends from the wall of the cystic cavity into the adjacent dermis.	**Treatment:** Complete surgical excision
Trichoadenoma:		
Clinical features: Presents with asymptomatic nodules on the face or buttocks.	**Histopathology:** Well-defined dermal tumor composed of epithelial islands, most of which have a central cystic cavity containing keratinous material.	**Treatment:** Complete surgical excision
Comedo naevus:		
Clinical features: Presents with single large comedone or cluster of comedones.	**Histopathology:** Shows rudimentary pilosebaceous unit with large overlying keratin filled crater.	**Treatment:** Laser or surgical treatment

Contd.

Trichilemmal cyst/Pilar cyst:		
Clinical features: Benign dermal cyst affecting scalp and presents with firm, mobile subcutaneous nodules without punctum.	**Histopathology:** Shows epithelial lined cyst without granular layer, filled with brightly eosinophilic keratinaceous debris. Focal area of rupture, cholesterol cleft and calcification can be seen.	**Treatment:** Surgical excision
Proliferating trichilemmal tumors:		
Clinical features: Arises from preexisting trichilemmal cyst, commonly seen in scalp of elderly females.	**Histopathology:** Shows features of typical pilar cyst, but additionally shows extensive epithelial proliferation, variable cytologic atypia and mitotic activity. Foci of calcification, glycogen rich clear cells and horn pearls or squamous eddies may be present.	**Treatment:** Complete surgical excision
Trichilemmoma:		
Clinical features: Benign tumor of outer root sheath of hair follicle, presents with small papule or nodule on face. Multiple trichilemmoma may be seen in cowden syndrome.	**Histopathology:** Shows multiple lobules with uniform small cells with round vesicular nuclei and peripheral palisading of the nuclei. These cells are dense eosinophilic and contain high glycogen which can be detected by PAS stain.	**Treatment:** Simple surgical excision or carbon dioxide laser
Pilomatricoma:		
Clinical features: Benign tumor of hair follicle, which arises from hair matrix and hair shaft. Presents with solitary firm to stony hard dermal nodules with lobulation overhead, neck and upper extremities. Beta catenin gene mutation may be seen. **Associations:** 1. Myotonic dystrophy 2. Turner syndrome 3. Rubinstein-Taybi syndrome 4. MYH associated polyposis (Familial adenomatous polyposis)	**Histopathology:** Shows well circumscribed lobules consisting of proliferating basaloid cells (resembling matrical cells of the follicular bulb) and eosinophilic shadow of keratinized cells or ghost cells (represent attempted cortical and inner root sheath differentiation). Other features include dystrophic calcification and giant cell reaction to keratin.	**Treatment:** Surgical excision
Trichofolliculoma:		
Clinical features: Benign hamartoma which presents with solitary follicular based nodule with several hair protruding from same hair follicle opening or a tuft of fine hairs may protrude from a central umbilication, seen over head and neck area. It may be associated with bone morphogenic factor which has important role in development of trichofolliculoma.	**Histopathology:** Shows one or several dilated follicles from which radiate numerous small follicles of varying degrees of maturity.	**Treatment:** Surgical excision
Trichoblastoma:		
Clinical features: Benign tumor of follicular germinative cells, which presents as a dermal nodule, predominantly on head and neck region.	**Histopathology:** Shows large circumscribed aggregates or nests of basaloid cells in mid to lower dermis with variable stromal condensation. Other features include presence of primitive hair bulbs, stromal amyloid and merkel cells (cytokeratin 20 or chromogranin).	**Treatment:** Complete surgical excision

Contd.

Trichoepithelioma:		
Clinical features: Presents with solitary or multiple pearly papules on centro facial area. It may be associated with Brooke-Spiegler syndrome	**Histopathology:** Shows well circumscribed dermal lobules composed of small basaloid cells with peripheral palisading and central area contain amorphous eosinophilic material. Stromal- stromal retraction in stroma is present. Primitive hair papillae or abortive hair follicle may be seen in few cases._	**Treatment:** Destructive procedure like electrocautery, cryotherapy and dermabrasion
Cutaneous lymphadenoma (Adamantanol Trichoblastoma):		
Clinical features: Variant of Trichoblastoma, which presents as non-specific papules and nodules on head and neck area.	**Histopathology:** Shows tumors lobules consisting of an outer rim of palisading basaloid cells surrounding a central zone of large cells with clear cytoplasm and large vesicular cells with dense infiltrate of small, mature lymphocytes within the islands Few scattered lymphocytes in the stroma may also be seen.	**Treatment:** Simple excision or Mohs microscopic surgery
Trichodiscoma:		
Clinical features: Presents with multiple flat topped papules on centrofacial area of face. It may be associated with Birt -Hogg-Dube syndrome.	**Histopathology:** Shows follicular epithelial proliferation with perifollicular fibrosis, occasionally mucin may be present.	**Treatment:** Surgical excision
Fibrofolliculoma:		
Clinical features: Arises from perifollicular connective tissue, presents as small whitish papules on face, ear, neck and upper torso, may be associated with Birt-Hogg-Dube syndrome, thyroid carcinoma and tuberous sclerosis.	**Histopathology:** Shows proliferation of loose connective tissue containing fine collagen and excess hyaluronic acid and hair follicle, often contains cystically dilated spaces with keratinous debris.	**Treatment:** Surgical excision

PREMALIGNANT SKIN TUMORS

Lesions with a high probability of developing into cancer are referred to as precancerous or premalignant. They are characterised by histological atypia limited to the epidermis which have tendency to develop into invasive carcinomas. Few common cutaneous premalignant conditions are described below:

ACTINIC KERATOSIS (SOLAR KERATOSIS)

Actinic keratoses appear as erythematous macules, papules or hyperkeratotic plaques on sun-exposed areas with ill-defined borders. They are usually asymptomatic but may associated with burning, pain and pruritis. In the early stages, palpation may be a more reliable for identification than visual inspection. They are more commonly seen on face and dorsa of hands and on the bald area of scalp in men. Analogue to actinic keratosis on vermilion border of the lower lip is solar cheilitis which may show ulceration and hyperkeratosis. Both of them may convert into squamous cell carcinoma though the true incidence is not known.

Risk factors:

1. Individual susceptibility
2. Chronic UV exposure is the major risk factor development of actinic keratosis.
3. Male > females
4. Immunosuppression
5. Genetic disorders like Xeroderma pigmentosa, bloom syndrome, Rothmund Thompson syndrome.

Clinical Variants

1. **Hyperkeratotic actinic keratosis:** Hyperkeratotic thick scaly plaques.
2. **Atrophic:** Atrophic scaly plaques
3. **Pigmented lichenoid actinic keratosis:** Scaly papule or plaque with brown black discoloration.
4. **Cutaneous horn:** White to yellow, hyperkeratotic, conical projection with erythematous papular base.
5. **Actinic cheilitis:** It presents with dry scaly, fissured, desquamating erosive plaque on lower lip.

Histopathology: It is characterised by aberrant epidermal architecture with atypical and pleomorphic keratinocytes in the basal layer of the epidermis and faulty keratinocyte maturation in the superficial epidermal layers. Some keratinocytes may show loss of polarity and disordered arrangement. Alternate parakeratosis and hyperkeratosis can also be seen.

Based on histopathological examination, it is also possible to categorize actinic keratoses into seven subtypes:

- Hypertrophic
- Atrophic
- Bowenoid
- Acantholytic
- Epidermolytic
- Lichenoid
- Pigmented

Treatment

General instruction include regular full body skin examination and photoprotection.

Topical: 5-fluorouracil, Imiquimod, diclofenac gel, topical retinoids

Surgical: Cryosurgery, curettage, shave excision, peeling

Bowen Disease (Squamous Cell Carcinoma In Situ)

It is a type of squamous cell carcinoma in situ, which presents as persistent red, scaly, crusted plaque with little tendency to become malignant. It can occur on both sun exposed and non exposed areas. Most common site is legs. Anogenital mucosal lesions can occur which is known as anal intraepithelial neoplasia, penile intraepithelial neoplasia and vulval intraepithelial neoplasia respectively based on site. Bowen's disease can occur on glans penis where it is called as Erythroplasia of Queyrat. Genital lesions carry more risk of recurrence and invasion where they have probable relation with genital warts. It is more common in females as compared to males. Ulceration in lesions is the sign of invasive carcinoma. Pigmented and verrucous clinical variant are also described in literature.

Risk factor:

- Arsenic exposure
- Patient on immunosuppressant
- Chronic sun exposure
- Radiotherapy
- Human papilloma virus 5/16/18

Histology: Epidermis shows acanthosis with elongation and thickening of rete ridges. Keratinocytes are arranged in completely disordered fashion throughout the epidermis resulting in wind-blown appearance, which is hallmark of Bowen's disease. Cells may be highly atypical showing large hyperkeratotic nuclei and in many epidermal cells they may be arranged in clusters resulting in multinucleated cells. A characteristic feature is the presence of atypical individual cell keratinisation. Such dyskeratotic cells are large and round and have a homogenous, strong eosinophilic cytoplasm and a hyperkeratotic nucleus.

Histopathological Subtypes

- Psoriasiform
- Atrophic
- Verrucous
- Pagetoid
- Clear cells type

Treatment

- **First line treatment:** Cryotherapy, curettage, 5-fluorouracil, imiquimod and photodynamic therapy.
- **Second line treatment:** Radiotherapy
- **Third line treatment:** 3% diclofenac gel, phenol peel, tazarotene 0.1% gel and oral isotretinoin.

MALIGNANT SKIN TUMORS

Malignant skin tumors are classified into non-melanoma skin cancer (Basal cell carcinoma, Squamous cell carcinoma) and melanoma. UV radiation is the major risk factor for cutaneous neoplasm. Carcinogenesis is facilitated by UV-A and UV-B radiation. Other common risk factors for development of malignant cutaneous neoplasm include chemical exposure, human papilloma virus, immunosuppressed individuals, familial history of cutaneous neoplasm, defective DNA repair disorders etc.

Basal Cell Carcinoma

Basal cell carcinoma (BCC) is the most common malignant tumor of skin. Typically, basal cell carcinoma grows slowly and seldom causes metastasis. It occurs due complex interaction between environmental, phenotype of skin and genetic factors.

Risk factors:

- Elderly females
- Excessive UV exposure
- Chronic exposure to arsenic
- Human papilloma virus infection
- Immunosuppressed patients
- PUVA therapy
- Genetic mutation in PTCH1 gene.

- Melanocortin-1 receptor (MC1R) gene polymorphisms and TYR gene mutation

Genetic syndromes associated with basal cell carcinoma: Several hereditary syndromes are associated with basal cell carcinoma:

- Nevoid BCC syndrome (Gorlin syndrome)
- Bazex Dupre christol syndrome (BDCS)
- Rombo syndrome
- Xeroderma pigmentosum
- Bloom syndrome
- Werner syndrome
- Rothmund-Thompson syndrome
- Murr-torre syndrome

Clinical Types of Basal Cell Carcinoma

- Nodular basal cell carcinoma
- Superficial basal cell carcinoma
- Ulcerated basal cell carcinoma
- Morpheaform basal cell carcinoma
- Fibroepithelioma basal cell carcinoma

Nodular Basal Cell Carcinoma (Figure 33.1)

This the most common subtype of basal cell carcinoma which is usually present on head and neck area. Clinically it shows flesh coloured nodules with surrounding telangiectasia. Cystic and pigmented variants are also described.

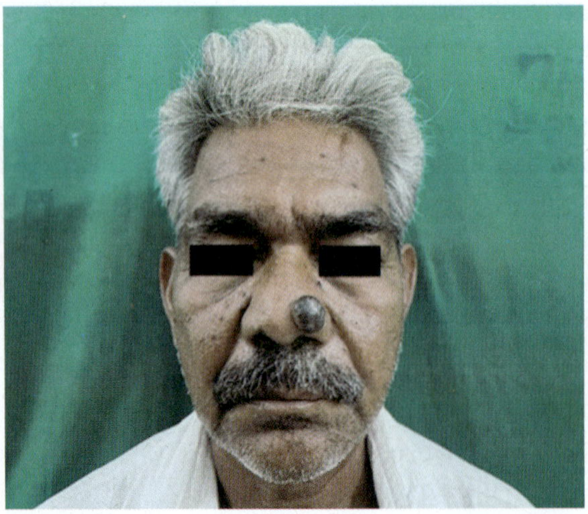

Figure 33.1: Showing nodular basal cell carcinoma

Superficial Basal Cell Carcinoma (Figure 33.2)

It shows slightly raised thread like margin or whipcord edges with central atrophic area, commonly seen on face and trunk.

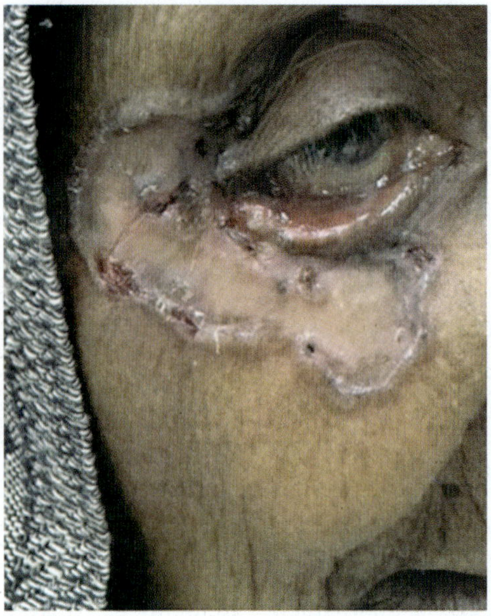

Figure 33.2: Showing superficial basal cell carcinoma

Ulcerated Basal Cell Carcinoma (Figure 33.3)

This variant arises as small papules which expand centrifugally and have thread like margin. It becomes ulcerated in the centre. If left untreated, it may invade deeply which may result in destruction of underlying structures.

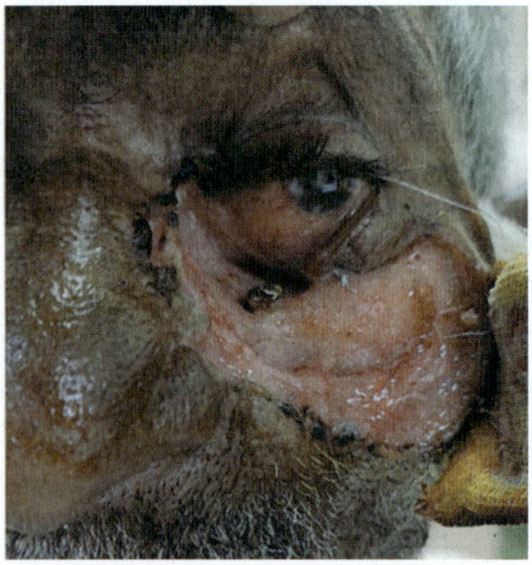

Figure 33.3: Showing ulcerated basal cell carcinoma

Morpheaform Basal Cell Carcinoma

This presents as smooth, thick, plaques with indurated margins which extend beyond the actual margin of lesions.

Fibroepithelial basal cell carcinoma or fibroepithelioma of pinkus

It presents as single erythematous dome shaped, pedunculated papule or plaque and is a rare variant of Basal cell carcinoma.

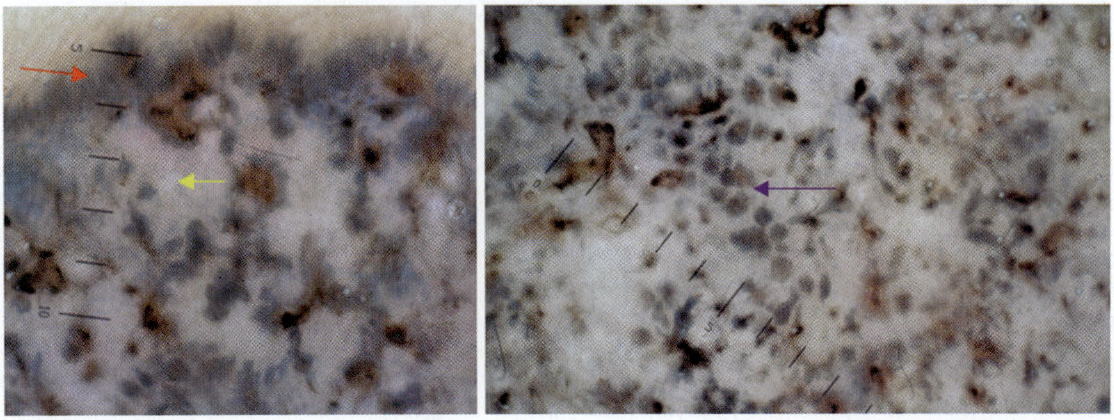

Figure 33.4: Showing dermoscopy of basal cell carcinoma- spoke wheel like structural pattern (red arrow), blue grey ovoid nests (purple arrow), white structure area (yellow area).

Dermoscopic findings of basal cell carcinoma (Figure 33.4): Dermoscopy shows different pattern:

- Spoke wheel like structural pattern
- Maple leaf like structural patterns
- Blue grey ovoid nests
- Blue grey globules and blotches
- White structure area
- Erosions
- Irregular vascular patterns
- Arborizing pattern
- Short and fine vessels

Histological Subtypes

- Nodular
- Micronodular
- Nodulocystic
- Superficial multifocal
- Pigmented
- Sclerosing

In basal cell carcinoma, cells resemble basal cell layer of epidermis and matrix cells of hair follicle which shows marginal palisading of tumor cells. Surrounding stroma is well organised. A retraction artefact, also known as a peritumoral lacuna, is caused by stroma retraction from tumour islands. Early lesion shows multiple tumor buds arising from epidermis but very soon they become confluent.

Superficial Basal Cell Carcinoma

Proliferating atypical palisading basaloid cells parallel to epidermis are seen, which form slit like spaces containing mucinous stroma produced by stromal cells. Superficial band of lymphocytes may be seen.

Nodular Basal Cell Carcinoma

Palisading basaloid cellular nests in the reticular or papillary dermis are seen, which may also show solar elastosis. Retraction artifacts with myxoid stroma may be seen surrounding these nests. Mitoses and single cell necrosis are rare in nodular BCC as compared to superficial BCC. Bullous pemphigoid antigen may be seen between basal lamina and stroma of BCC.

Micronodular

Shows smaller basaloid cellular nest and less prominent peripheral palisading without retraction artifact. Tumour may infiltrate deep down to subcutaneous tissue. More wider and symmetrical dispersion is common in micronodular BCC. Presence of brisk mitotic activity and apoptosis differentiate it from trichoepithelioma.

Nodulocystic BCC

This is the most common pattern seen histologically, where large palisading basaloid lobules are seen in circumscribed mass with central cystic dilatation. Stroma is loose and rich in mucin.

Morpheaform/ Sclerosing BCC

It shows angulated cords of thick columns of basaloid cells which display marked cell necrosis and mitotic activity with a dense collagenous stroma. It is typical to observe tumour cord fibrosis and stromal fibroplasia. Morpheaform BCC also exhibits invasion of the subcutis and deep dermis.

Infiltrative Basal Cell Carcinoma

This type of BCC shows five to eight irregularly sized and shaped cellular nests with invasion of subcutis and adjacent muscular tissue. Like the morpheaform variant, nests showing sharp angulation, slit like retraction, frequent mitotic activity, fibrotic stroma and individual cell necrosis is also present.

Features of High Risk Basal Cell Carcinoma

- Morpheaform of BCC
- >5 cm size or Giant BCC
- Centro facial area (periocular, perinasal, perioral, chin, around ears)
- Infiltrative and micronodular histological subtype of BCC
- Perineural and perivascular involvement
- Immunosuppressed host
- Recurrent BCC
- Lymphatic metastasis or distant metastasis

Treatment

Medical Treatment

Topical Imiquimod, topical 5-fluorouracil, photodynamic therapy, intralesional interferon alpha 2b and hedgehog pathway inhibitors (vismodegib and sonidegib).

Surgical Treatment

Curettage, electrodesiccation, standard surgical excision (with 4-5mm free margin), Mohs microscopic surgery, and cryosurgery.

MELANOMA

It is a malignant tumor arising from melanocytes. It represent 4% of skin cancers.

Risk factors for developing melanoma:

1. **Skin phenotypic traits**
   - **Large and giant congenital melanocytic nevi:** Life time risk for malignant transformation is 5-15 percent.
   - **Atypical or dysplastic nevi:** Large nevi with atypical irregular pigmentary network with some histological feature suggestive of naevoid growth or premalignant changes.
   - Fair skin individual and less tanning ability of skin or tendency to burn
   - **Nevus phenotype:** Large in number
2. **Genetic predisposition**
   - Positive family history is positive in 5% to 10% of patients, risk is 2.2-fold higher when at least one relative is affected.
   - Major gene associated with melanoma are cyclin dependent kinase inhibitor 2A (CDKN2A). About 40% of familial melanoma are associated with this gene mutation which encodes two protein by alternate splicing P^{16}/INK4a (inhibit RB gene) and P^{14}/ Arf gene (inhibit P^{53} gene).
   - Other genes involved in development of melanoma are:

     Loss of function Melanocrotin-1 receptor gene, mis sense mutation in ASIP (Agouti signalling protein), tyrosine Related Protein (TYR), SLC 45A2B, microphthalmia transcription factor gene amplification, BAP-1 gene tumour suppressor gene, xeroderma pigmentosum gene.
3. **Environmental factors**

   UV radiation exposure: Both intermittent or chronic UV radiation exposure are associated with development of melanoma

   Based on clinical, histological, immunopathological and cytogenetic evidence, five stages of malignant transformation/ tumour progression have been proposed in melanocytes.

   - **Stage 1:** Benign melanocytic nevi
   - **Stage 2:** Atypical nevi
   - **Stage 3:** Primary malignant melanoma, radial growth or horizontal growth
   - **Stage 4:** Primary malignant melanoma, vertical growth
   - **Stage 5:** Metastatic melanoma

Radial growth phase consists of primarily intraepidermal proliferation of malignant cells with occasional cells in papillary dermis. Radial growth is seen in acral lentiginous melanoma (ALM) and lentigo maligna melanoma (LMM). Vertical growth phase consist of growth towards deeper skin resulting in formation of nest or nodules of tumor cells with aggressive growth. Vertical growth is seen in nodular melanoma. Superficial spreading melanoma shows both radial and vertical growth (radial growth > vertical growth).

Most commonly, the history includes either changing characteristics in an existing mole (30% cases) or the identification of a new mole without precursor nevi (70% cases).

Molecular Classification

1. **BRAF:** This mutation is associated with 40% of hereditary melanomas, most common association is seen with superficial spreading melanoma.
2. **N-RAS:** This mutation is associated with nodular melanoma.
3. **C-kit:** Defective C kit gene was seen in 7% of cutaneous melanoma (cutaneous acral lentigo melanoma and lentigo maligna melanoma) and 20% of mucosal melanoma.
4. **GNAQ gene:** Mutation in this gene is associated with uveal melanoma.

Melanoma is classified into 4 types based on growth pattern:

1. **Superficial spreading melanoma (SSM):**

   This is the most common subtype of melanoma which constitutes approximately 70% of melanomas. It is commonly associated with intermittent sun exposure. Most common site is upper back (in men) and lower extremities (in females). It usually presents with flat irregularly bordered macule which later becomes raised or elevated showing colour variations. It is most commonly associated with pre-existing nevi.

2. **Nodular melanoma (NM):**

   This is the second most common subtype of melanoma which accounts for approximately 15% to 30% of melanomas. Most common site is trunk. The lesions are typically blue-black or may be amelanotic. It usually arises from normal skin (de novo) and evolves very rapidly in few weeks to months.

3. **Lentigo maligna melanoma (LMM):**

   This is third common subtype which constitutes approximately 4% to 10% of melanomas. This type has prolonged radial growth phase which later progresses to invasive state. Initially lesions are small brown tan macules with notched borders and occurs commonly in elderly patients on face. It is associated with chromic UV radiation exposure or cumulative sun exposure. LMM is larger than lentigo maligna and have nodular component.

4. **Acral lentiginous melanoma:**

   It constitutes about 2% to 8% of melanomas which is common in dark skinned people. It appears on the palms and soles as flat, brown macules with irregular borders, which ulcerates in later stages. Subungual melanoma is a variant of acral lentiginous melanoma which arises from nail matrix and is commonly seen on great toe or thumb (Figure 33.5).

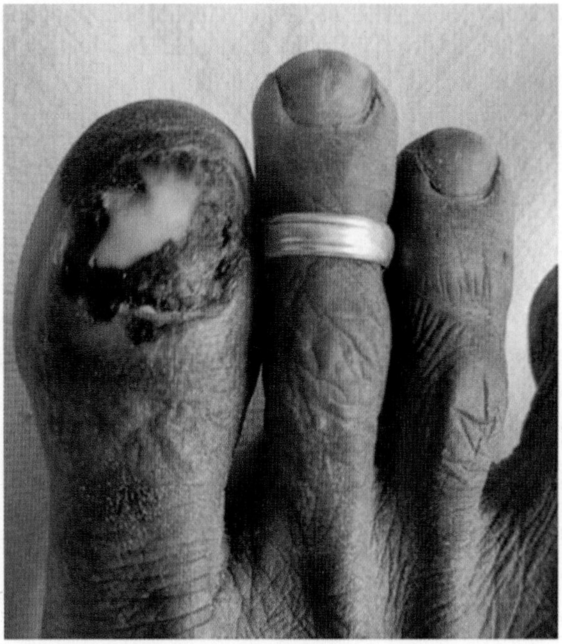

Figure 33.5: Showing melanoma of nail

The characteristics of melanocytic nevus which may undergo malignant transformation into melanoma are commonly described by the acronym ABCDE:

- **A**symmetry
- Irregular **b**order
- **C**olor variations
- > 6 mm **D**iameter
- **E**levated surface

Other features include bleeding, itching, ulceration and appearance of satellite lesions. Patients who have primary sites other than the skin or who have metastatic disease exhibit signs and symptoms specific to the affected organ system. It's crucial to look at every group of lymph nodes.

Other Clinical Subtypes of Melanoma

- Amelanotic melanoma
- Regressive melanoma
- Malignant blue nevus
- Sino-nasal melanoma
- Desmoplastic melanoma
- Spitzoid melanoma

Diagnosis

Dermatoscopy and reflectance confocal microscopy are screening tools for melanoma.

Histopathology: It is gold standard for diagnosis of melanoma. Excisional biopsy with sentinel lymph node biopsy is preferred.

Histopathological Criteria

1. **Architectural changes:**

   Loss of architecture with heterogenicity in size and shape of cells and presence of cellular nests of malignant cells in dermis. Upward migration of atypical melanocytes within epidermis in random fashion is known pagetoid spread and is considered to be diagnostic of melanoma.

2. **Cytological changes:**
   - Cellular pleomorphism
   - Enlargement of cells
   - Hyperchromatism
   - Prominent nucleoli
   - High mitotic activity.

Immunohistochemistry marker study: Immunohistochemistry marker are useful for diagnosis, especially in poorly differentiated melanoma or amelanotic melanoma or pagetoid spread without obvious melanoma. S-100 is present in almost all patients but is not specific as it also present in Langerhans cell histiocytosis and melanocytic nevi. HMB 45 is a specific marker for melanoma. Melan-A or MART-1 can also be used as sensitive markers for melanoma specially in desmoplastic melanoma.

Poor prognostic markers for melanoma:

- High Breslow index.
- Positive sentinel lymph node status.
- Ulceration.
- Regression resulting in underestimation of Breslow index.
- Old age.
- Head and neck area associated.

Note: Breslow index is the histopathological measurement of the depth of the melanoma from the top of granulosa cell layer. It is a prognostic marker.

Treatment

Extensive local excision with sentinel lymph node biopsy and elective node dissection is the only effective treatment for early stage melanoma. Evaluate the margins before carrying out large scale local excision. When initial closure is not possible, skin grafting or tissue transfers may be necessary.

Recommended margin for wide local excision of melanoma

Depth of penetration	Recommended margin
Melanoma in situ	0.5 -1 cm
Breslow depth <1 mm	1 cm
Breslow depth 1.01-2 mm	1-2 cm
Breslow depth > 2 mm	2 cm

Medical management is used as adjuvant therapy and is reserved for patients with advanced disease. Following agents may be used:

Immunotherapy: BCG, Pegylated interferon, Interferon alfa, Granulocyte macrophage colony stimulating factor (GM-CSF), Ipilimumab (anti CTLA-4), Pembrolizumab (PD-1 Inhibitor), Nivolumab (PD-1 INHIBITOR)

Chemotherapy agents: Dacarbazine, Temozolomide, Abraxane (DTA) and Cisplatin, vinblastine, and dacarbazine (CVD)

Targeted therapy:

- **BRAF inhibitors:** Encorafenib, Vemurafenib and Dabrafenib
- **MEK inhibitors:** Selumetinib, Cobimetinib
- **c-kit inhibitors:** Imatinib, Sunitinib, Nilotinib

Squamous Cell Carcinoma (SCC)

Cutaneous squamous cell carcinoma (SCC) is a non melanotic skin cancer which originates from supra basal epidermal keratinocytes. Most of the cases occur from precursor lesions such as actinic keratosis (AK), Bowen disease (SCC in situ) and chronic ulcers (Marjolin ulcer).

Predisposing factors for SCC: There are several risk factor which are associated with squamous cell carcinoma e.g.

1. Chronic UV radiation exposure.
2. Environmental carcinogen exposure.
3. Burn scars.
4. Chronic scarring dermatosis.
5. Genodermatosis (Xeroderma pigmentosus, albinism, porokeratosis etc.).

Genetic Factors

Genomic instability and genetic mutation in DNA of keratinocytes are associated with squamous cell carcinoma of skin. Alterations or deletion of chromosome 9p21 (INK 4A loci) and 17p13 region (p53 tumor suppressor gene loci) are the common sites associated with SCC.

Clinical Features

Most commonly fleshy, keratotic, erythematous plaques or nodules are seen. When ulceration occurs, the edges are everted. Other morphological variants include pigmented, ulcerated, cutaneous horn and verrucous (Figure 33.6). In the later stages, it may be fixed with underling tissue.

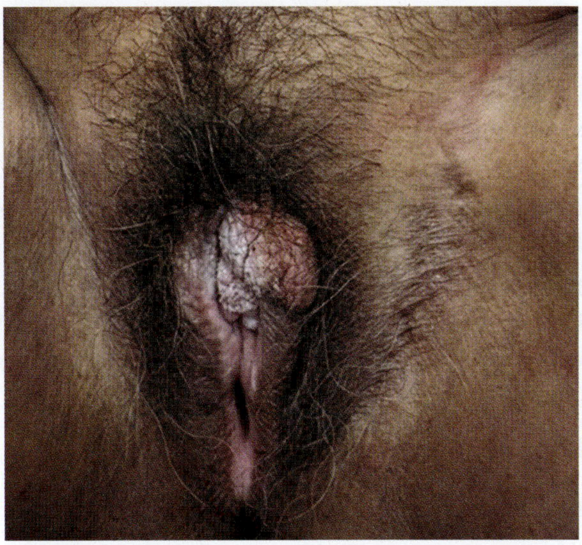

Figure 33.6: Showing verrucous SCC on lichen sclerosis et atrophicans lesion

Histology: Atypical keratinocytes invade beyond basement membrane which is a hall mark feature of SCC. There are various histological subtypes for e.g.:

1. Adenoid type
2. Clear cell
3. Spindle cell
4. Signet ring cell type
5. Basaloid variant
6. Verrucous

High risk SCC:

1. Diameter of SCC > 2 cm
2. Depth of invasion > 4 mm
3. Involvement of lower lips, ear
4. SCC arising from scar tissue
5. Patients on immunosuppressants
6. Absence of inflammatory infiltrate

These factors are associated with higher recurrences and metastasis.

Treatment

Conventional surgical excision (with 4 mm margin) is the mainstay of treatment for small primary squamous cell carcinoma. For lesions with depth > 6 mm and > 1 cm diameter, Mohs micrographic surgery is recommended.

Other treatment options include radiotherapy, topical 5 fluorouracil and topical imiquimod.

MISCELLANEOUS SKIN TUMORS

Mammary Paget's Disease (Figure 33.7)

Paget's disease presents with progressive, erythematous, scaly, moist, crusted, well marginated thick plaque. It may be associated with itching, pain, burning sensation and discharge from the nipple. Unilateral involvement is common. It is nearly always associated with underlying ductal carcinoma in situ or invasive ductal carcinoma of breast. A similar disease process in female and male external genitalia, is known as extramammary Paget's disease which is commonly seen in post-menopausal females. Rarely men can also develop mammary Paget's disease. All chronic persistent nipple rashes should be evaluated for Paget's disease. Palpable mass and mammographic changes may be seen in 50% of patients. Lymph node involvement is seen in 60% of the patients with palpable mass while it is seen in 33% of the patients without a palpable mass.

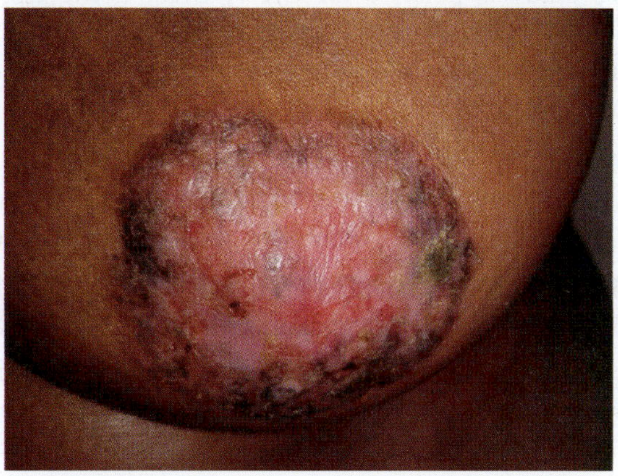

Figure 33.7: Mammary Paget's disease

Differential diagnosis includes nipple eczema, atopic dermatitis, melanoma, Bowen disease, erosive adenomatosis etc. Nipple eczema is usually bilateral.

Histopathology

Paget cells, on histopathology is the hallmark feature of Paget's disease, which are large intraepithelial malignant cell present singly or in small groups within the epidermis of the nipple. These cells are large, rounded, devoid of intercellular bridges with a large nucleus and ample cytoplasm. These cells are PAS positive due to presence of neutral mucopolysaccharides. These cells are derived from glandular stem cells or epidermal Toker cells (clear cells of the nipple epithelium).

On immunohistochemistry, cytokeratin-7 (CK7), oestrogen receptor (ER), progesterone receptor (PR) and human epidermal growth factor receptor-2 (HER-2) are positive.

Treatment

Breast conservative treatment is the standard treatment for Paget's disease. If underlying malignancy is present, it should be treated accordingly.

Extramammary Paget's Disease

It is usually seen on vulva, perianal region (may extend up to anal canal) , groin and axilla. Clinically it presents with sharply marginated, persistent, slowly progressive, scaly, greyish, crusted plaques with variable pigmentation and raised margins. Lesions have prominent itching and burning sensation. In 75% of cases, primarily intraepidermal neoplasm originating from apocrine ducts or keratinocyte stem cells is present while in 25% of cases, underling adenocarcinoma is seen.

Histology: It is similar to Paget's disease of breast.

IHC study is positive for CK 7, CK8, CAM 5.2, CEA and GCDFP. CK 20 positivity is strongly associated with internal malignancy while apomucin positivity suggests extra-mammary origin.

Treatment: Wide local excision is preferred treatment for Paget's disease. Other treatment options include topical imiquimod, 5 fluorouracil, retinoids and photodynamic therapy.

Keratoacanthoma (KA)

It is a rapidly evolving tumor, composed of keratinized squamous cells, which originate from pilosebaceous follicle. It is a well circumscribed squamous cell carcinoma, seen in middle age.

Risk factors

- Chronic sun exposure
- Contact with tar or minerals
- Immunosuppressed individuals

Clinically, three phases are seen:

- Proliferative phase
- Maturation phase
- Resolving phase

Initially, lesions start as skin colored, fleshy papules which grow rapidly and form nodules with central keratotic plug and surface telangiectasia. Lesions expand symmetrically in radial symmetry. After remaining stable for some time, it may resolve without any treatment in few months to years.

Clinical Variants

- **Giant keratoacanthoma**: Rare variant > 20 mm in diameter.
- **Multiple keratoacanthoma (Ferguson Smith syndrome)**: Multiple KA on exposed sites which resolve spontaneously.
- **Eruptive keratoacanthoma (Grzybowski syndrome):** Hundreds of KA on covered areas of body.
- **Keratoacanthoma centrifugum marginatum.** Large lesions with progressive peripheral extension reaching upto 20 cm in diameter having rolled margins and central atrophy.

Differential Diagnosis

- Molluscum contagiosum
- Warts
- Cutaneous horn
- Hyperkeratotic actinic keratosis

Histology

Crateriform appearance having enlarged atypical keratinocytes with eosinophilic cytoplasm.

Treatment

Surgical treatment is preferred or it may resolve spontaneously. Cryotherapy, curettage, electrodessication, 5 fluorouracil, imiquimod and bleomycin can also be used.

Kaposi Sarcoma

It is caused by HHV type 8 virus usually seen in immuno-compromised individuals (e.g. AIDS defining illness). Clinically it presents as painless purple, red or blue red macule, plaque or nodules on extremities. It may also be seen over oral mucosa including gastrointestinal tract and respiratory tract. Histology shows solid cord formation by spindle shaped tumor cells and vascular proliferation in dermis. Ramifying proliferating vessels surrounding larger ectatic pre-existing blood vessels is known as Promontory sign.

Treatment includes cryotherapy, radiotherapy, chemo-therapy and oral alitretinoin.

CHAPTER 34 Miscellaneous Disorders

Contents

MASTOCYTOSIS

Mastocytosis is a disorder characterized by mast cell proliferation and accumulation in various organs, most commonly the skin.

Clinical Classification of Mastocytosis

- **Cutaneous**
  - o Maculopapular cutaneous mastocytosis (Urticaria pigmentosa (UP) and Telangiectasia macularis eruptive perstans (TMEP)
  - o Diffuse cutaneous mastocytosis
  - o Mastocytoma
- **Systemic (extracutaneous mast cells in at least one organ)**
  - o Indolent systemic mastocytosis (ISM).
  - o Smouldering indolent systemic mastocytosis.
  - o Systemic mastocytosis with an associated clona hematological non-mast cell disease (SM-AHNMD).
  - o Aggressive systemic mastocytosis.
  - o Mast cell leukemia.
  - o Mast cell sarcoma.
  - o Extracutaneous mastocytoma.

Pathophysiology

Mastocytosis is a hyperplastic reaction or a neoplastic condition to an unknown stimulus. Activating mutations of the proto-oncogene c-KIT have been identified. The KIT receptor is also expressed on haemopoietic stem cells and melanocytes, which might be relevant to the occasional occurrence of myeloproliferative and myelodysplastic disorders in mastocytosis and the hyperpigmentation usually seen in urticarial pigmentosa lesions. Associated systemic manifestations are believed to reflect the release of mast cell-derived mediators, such as histamine, prostaglandins, heparin, neutral proteases and acid hydrolases.

Clinical Features

Most patients with mastocytosis are children, 75% of cases occur during infancy or early childhood which usually resolve by puberty. The most common age of onset for adult urticarial pigmentosa is 20-40 years. In adult-onset urticarial pigmentosa spontaneous regression does not occur. Mastocytosis which starts in infancy or early childhood has only cutaneous involvement. Systemic symptoms are absent as a rule and if present, they are few. Progression into systemic disease is also rare. Most patients have pruritic cutaneous lesions. Cutaneous lesions are the most commonly maculopapular type which may be dozens to hundreds of brown plaques or nodules (Figure 34.1) that urticate on stroking (**Darier sign**, Figure 34.2) and occasionally may show blister formation. They are distributed in a symmetrical distribution anywhere on the body except the face, head, palms and soles with the highest concentration usually being on the trunk and thighs. The edges of the lesions are not completely sharp.

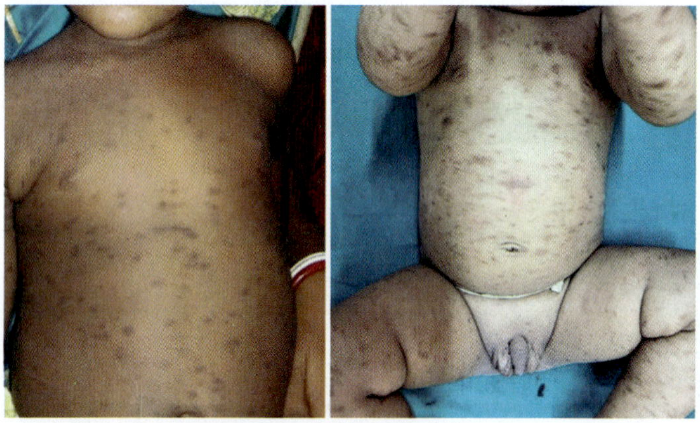

Figure 34.1: Urticaria pigmentosa

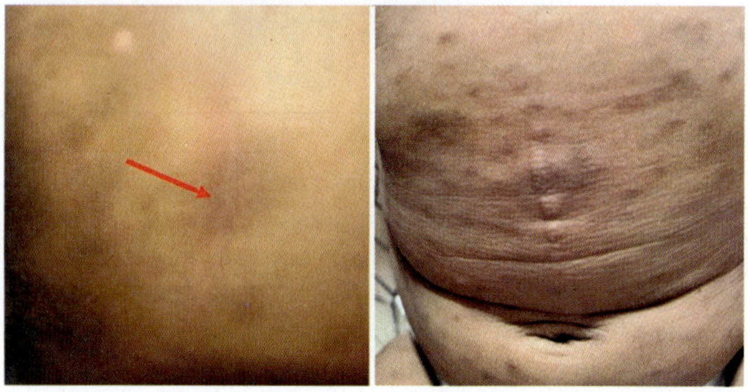

Figure 34.2: Mastocytosis showing Darier sign

- Few patients show large solitary nodules which on stroking show urtication and bullae formation. This variety is seen in infant onset urticarial pigmentosa.
- An uncommon type, diffuse erythrodermic type almost always starts in infancy and shows generalized brownish red, soft infiltration of skin showing urtication on stroking. Few patients show bullae formation called bullous urticarial pigmentosa, visceral lesions occur in this type of urticarial pigmentosa, but they improve with time and they are rarely fatal.
- In telangiectasia macularis eruptive perstans, which usually occurs in adults, extensive brownish red macules showing fine telangiectasia occur. They usually show little or no urtication on stroking.
- **Darier's sign:** Darier's sign is named after the French dermatologist Ferdinand-Jean Darier who first described it.

  It refers to the urtication and erythematous halo that are produced in response to rubbing or scratching of lesions of cutaneous mastocytosis. Darier sign is not always demonstrable, especially in those with a long history of the disorder, and is not 100% specific for mastocytosis, since it has also been described rarely in juvenile xanthogranuloma and acute lymphoblastic leukaemia of neonates.
- **Dermographism:** In approximately half of the patients, stroking of uninvolved skin produces dermographism.
- **Flushing:** Flushing may occur spontaneously following skin stroke or after ingesting a mast cell degranulating agent.
- Some patients, especially those with extensive cutaneous disease, experience acute systemic symptoms exacerbated by certain activities or ingestion of certain drugs or foods. Possible systemic symptoms include flushing, headache, dyspnea, wheezing, rhinorrhea, nausea, vomiting, diarrhea and syncope.

Systemic Signs and Symptoms

- Patients may have chronic systemic symptoms involving various organ systems. They are seen in adult onset mastocytosis.
- Involvement of the skeletal system may manifest as bone pain or fracture.
- Involvement of the central nervous system may produce neuropsychiatric symptoms, as well as non-specific symptoms such as malaise and irritability.
- GI involvement may lead to weight loss, diarrhea, nausea, vomiting and abdominal cramps.
- Cardiovascular effects can include hypotension, tachycardia, shock, syncope or angina.
- Hepatomegaly (present in 40% of adult patients with systemic mastocytosis) and splenomegaly (present in 50% of adult patients with systemic mastocytosis).

Investigations

In many patients, urticaria pigmentosa can be diagnosed with history and physical examination. Presence of the characteristic lesions that demonstrate Darier's sign is diagnostic. Skin biopsy is only required to confirm mastocytosis in infants and children.

Following investigations are required if systemic mastocytosis is suspected:

- Complete blood count (CBC).
- Blood film.
- Blood tryptase levels.
- Bone marrow biopsy.
- Abdominal ultrasound scan.
- Bone densitometry for adults.
- Bone scan for localized bone pain.
- Any appropriate additional investigation, e.g., gastroscopy.

Follow-up Assessment

If initial assessment is normal, none is required routinely. If probable systemic disease is suspected, at least yearly review with complete blood count, blood chemistry and blood tryptase should be done.

Treatment

Therapy is conservative and aimed at symptomatic relief because the prognosis for most patients with cutaneous mastocytosis is excellent. None of the currently available therapeutic measures induces permanent involution of cutaneous or visceral lesions. Advise patients to avoid agents that precipitate mast cell degranulation, such as aspirin, NSAIDs, codeine, morphine, alcohol, thiamine, quinine, opiates, gallamine, decamethonium, procaine, radiographic dyes, dextran, polymyxin B, scopolamine and D-tubocurarine.

H1 and H2 anti-histamines decrease pruritus, flushing and gastrointestinal symptoms. Oral disodium cromoglycate may ameliorate cutaneous symptoms, such as pruritus, whealing and flushing, as well as systemic symptoms, such as diarrhea, abdominal pain, bone pain and disorders of cognitive function.

Cautious administration of aspirin to inhibit prostaglandin synthesis and maintain mast cell degranulation may be beneficial for patients with disease resistant to H1 and H2 antagonist therapy alone. The patient, premedicated with H1 and H2 antihistamines, may be started on small doses of aspirin, slowly titrated to reach a plasma level of 20-30 mg/100 ml. Initiate this treatment regimen in a controlled environment, because aspirin can induce mast cell mediator release and subsequent cardiovascular collapse.

Corticosteroids: Cutaneous lesions that involve a limited body area may be treated with a potent class 1 topical corticosteroid, with occlusion if required. Intralesional injections of small amounts of diluted corticosteroids may resolve skin lesions temporarily or indefinitely. Systemic corticosteroids are useful only in specific situations, such as ascites, malabsorption and severe skin disease.

Oral Psoralen plus UV-A (PUVA) therapy results in general and cosmetic benefits in the treatment of cutaneous mastocytosis, particularly telangiectasia macularis eruptive perstans (TMEP). PUVA rarely is required in children. Currently, PUVA is reserved for severe, unresponsive cases in adults.

Laser: Treatment of cutaneous mast cell lesions with the 585 nm pulsed dye laser and the 532 nm Nd: YAG laser has been reported to provide cosmetic improvement.

Future novel therapy for cutaneous mastocytosis includes immunomodulators. In patients with aggressive systemic mastocytosis, interferon alfa-2b, 2 chlorodeoxyadenosine (cladribine) are some of the promising drugs. Imatinib, which is a tyrosine kinase inhibitor, has been reported to halt disease progression and shorten the duration of disease. It is approved by Food and Drug Administration (FDA) for use in patients with aggressive systemic mastocytosis with organ dysfunction due to mast cell infiltration.

HISTIOCYTOSIS

Histiocytosis encompasses a group of diverse disorders with a common primary event, i.e., accumulation and infiltration of monocytes, macrophages and dendritic cells in the affected tissues.

Pathophysiology

Histiocytes originate from pluripotent stem cells, which can be found in bone marrow. Under the influence of various cytokines these precursor cells can become committed and differentiate to become a specific group of specialized cells. Committed stem cells can mature to become antigen processing cells, with some possessing phagocytic capabilities. These cells include tissue macrophages, monocytes, dendritic cells, interdigitating reticulum cells and Langerhans cells. Pluripotent stem cells can also be committed to produce dendritic cells. Each category of histiocytosis can be traced to reactive or neoplastic proliferation and disorder of cells in one of these groups.

Classification

Langerhans cell histiocytosis formerly was divided into 3 disease categories: Eosinophilic granuloma, Hand-Schuller-Christian disease and Letterer-Siwe disease, depending on the severity and extent of involvement. Some authors simply divide histiocytic disorders into class I Langerhans cell disease, class II non-Langerhans cell histiocytic disease without features of malignant disorders and class III malignant histiocytic disorders.

Class I: Langerhans cell histiocytosis

Class I histiocytoses are a diverse group of clinical diseases that are all reactive histiocytoses in which the predominant histiocyte is of Langerhans cell phenotype.

Class IIa: Histiocytoses involving cells of the dermal dendrocyte lineage

Class IIa histiocytoses are reactive diseases in which cells with the phenotype of the dermal dendrocyte (positive for CD68 and factor XIIIa) accumulate in the skin and other tissues causing tissue damage. Juvenile xanthogranuloma is typical of this group of diseases. These diseases are reactive with no clinical evidence of malignancy.

Class IIb: Histiocytoses involving cells other than Langerhans cells and dermal dendrocytes

Class IIb histiocytoses are reactive diseases in which histiocytes other than those bearing the Langerhans cell or dermal dendrocyte phenotype accumulate in various tissues and may cause tissue damage. The major features of all these histiocytoses are that they are reactive, with no clinical or laboratory evidence of malignancy, and that Langerhans cells and related cells are not involved.

Class III: Malignant histiocytic disorders

Class III histiocytoses include all malignant histiocytic diseases. These include monocytic leukaemias, malignant histiocytosis, which may be of the mononuclear phagocyte, dendritic cell or Langerhans cell type, and true histiocytic lymphoma.

Clinical Features

Langerhans cell histiocytosis (LCH) is caused by proliferation of Langerhans cells.

Acute Disseminated LCH (Letterer-Siwe Disease)

It is commonly seen in infants but can occur in children also.

Skin lesions are common (in about 80% of cases) and are often presenting sign. They are commonly present as numerous closely set, red brown papules covered with scales or crusts (Figure 34.3). Petechiae (Figure 34.4 B, C) may also be seen. They may involve scalp, face, trunk with a resemblance to seborrheic dermatitis (Figure 34.4 A) or Darier's disease.

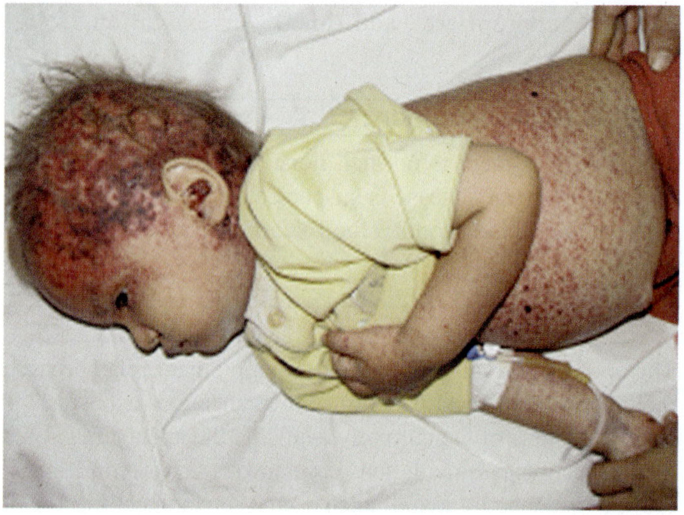

Figure 34.3: Langerhans cell histiocytosis showing red-brown papules with crusting over scalp and trunk

Vesicular, papular, nodular, ulcerated or xanthomatous lesions may also be seen.

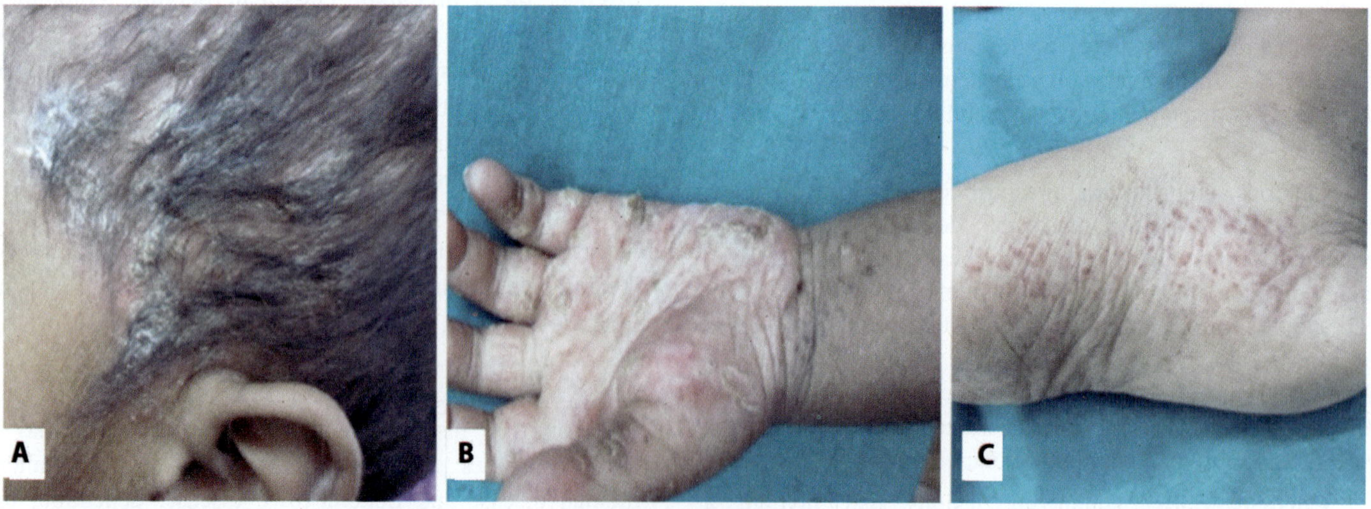

Figure 34.4: Langerhans cell histiocytosis showing seborrheic dermatitis like scalp rashes (A) Petechiae over palms and soles (B and C)

Systemic findings include anemia, thrombocytopenia, splenomegaly, hepatomegaly, lymphadenopathy and infiltration of lungs. Mastoid region of temporal bone may show osteolytic lesions producing a clinical picture of otitis media.

Some patients show only cutaneous involvement and prognosis is good in such cases.

Multisystem disease which is more common in adults shows a poor prognosis.

Chronic Multifocal LCH (Hand-Schuller-Christian Disease)

It is characterized by clinical triad of diabetes insipidus, exophthalmos and multiple defects of bone, especially of cranium.

Skin lesions are seen in about one third of patients and are characterized by infiltrated nodules and plaques with ulceration. Axilla, anogenital region and mouth are the common sites involved. An extensive eruption identical to acute LCH or yellow xanthoma like lesions may also be seen.

Osteolytic lesions of long bones may lead to fractures. Any one of the three cardinal symptoms of triad mentioned above may be absent and entirely other organs, e.g., liver, spleen, lungs or lymph nodes may be involved.

Other types of histiocytosis are either not seen in children or are rare, hence they have not been mentioned here.

Investigations

Laboratory investigations and diagnostic tests should be according to the extent of disease, suspected on the basis of the patient's history and physical findings.

- **Hematological:** Hemoglobin, complete blood count, liver function tests.
- **Radiological:** Chest X-ray (posterior, anterior and lateral view), X-ray skull shows punched-out pattern without evidence of periosteal reaction or marginal sclerosis.
- Radionucleotide bone scanning with technetium-99 m polyphosphate may reveal a localized increased uptake.
- MRI and CT scan sometimes helps in identifying lesions that cannot be detected with other modalities. For patients with pulmonary involvement, CT scan is the best modality to find cysts and micronodular infiltrates.
- Skin biopsy.

Treatment

The aim of therapy in histiocytosis is to relieve clinical symptoms and prevent complications of the disease. For single system disease (e.g., of the skin or bone), no therapy or only local therapy may be necessary.

Topical Therapy

Localized skin lesions, especially in infants, can spontaneously regress. If treatment is required, topical corticosteroids may be tried. Low dose radiation therapy to the local lesions is often effective but is rarely needed. For unresponsive skin lesions, low dose mild systemic therapy with corticosteroids can be used.

Systemic Therapy

Chemotherapy is used for multisystemic disease. Single agents or adjuvant use of several chemotherapeutic agents and/or biologic response modifiers may be effective. They include corticosteroids, vinca alkaloids, antimetabolites, nucleoside analogs, immune modulators, biologic response modifiers such as interleukin (IL-2) and interferons.

Most chemotherapeutic agents for the treatment of LCH are used in combination. Combination of cytarabine arabinoside (Ara-C), vincristine and prednisolone to treat disseminated Langerhans cell histiocytosis with organ dysfunction can be used.

Radiation Therapy

Radiation therapy is effective in Langerhans cell histiocytosis. Doses ranging from 750-1500 cGy are usually administered, resulting in good local control of single lesions or metastasis.

SCLEREDEMA

Scleredema is a rare condition of unknown etiology. In this disorder areas of induration appear in the skin, frequently after an infection but also in diabetes, and spontaneously clear in months or years. There is an excess of acid mucopolysaccharides in the dermis. Although regarded as a benign, self-limiting, skin disease, scleredema may be persistent and involve the viscera. Rarely, it may result in death.

Scleredema can be categorized into 3 clinical subgroups. Each has a different history, course and prognosis.

- Group 1 includes scleredema after acute respiratory infection (scleredema adultorum). They have a history of a preceding febrile illness, particularly an upper respiratory tract streptococcal infection. The onset of the skin lesions is rapid and the condition usually clears spontaneously in 6 months to 2 years.
- Group 2 includes scleredema patients whose disease tends to occur insidiously, with no preceding illness. This group encompasses cases associated with a monoclonal gammapathy.

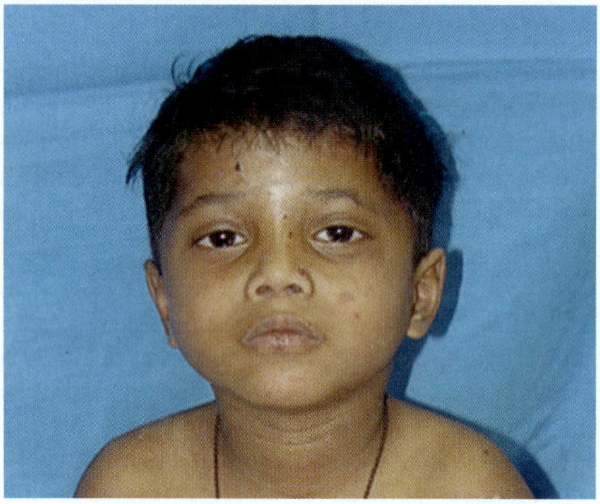

Figure 34.5: Scleredema

- Group 3 is scleredema associated with diabetes mellitus (scleredema diabeticorum) and includes patients with preexisting diabetes, which is typically adult in onset and often type 1. This disorder tends to occur more often in males, and this subgroup of patients typically experiences a more protracted course that is refractory to therapy. Onset of skin lesions is insidious.

Pathophysiology

The etiology of scleredema is unknown. Suggestions that have been considered include obstruction to lymphatic channels by inflammation, streptococcal hypersensitivity and disorders of the peripheral nervous system or pituitary function. Scleredema localized to the back is commonly associated with diabetes mellitus, while generalized scleredema may follow a viral illness. Comparative quantitative PCR analysis of lesional and non-lesional skin in patients with scleredema has demonstrated an increase in collagen gene expression in affected sites.

Clinical Features

- A female preponderance is reported for scleredema, with a female to male ratio of 2:1, except in the type associated with adult onset diabetes, which is more common in men than in women.
- Scleredema occurs in individuals of all ages. Although scleredema is sometimes referred to as scleredema adultorum, 50% of scleredema cases occur in individuals younger than 20 years.
- The initial skin changes of scleredema occur on the face, the neck, or the upper part of the back. Patient feels difficulty in moving these parts. The skin changes tend to spread distally, and they are usually confined to the upper part of the body. Hands and feet are typically spared.
- The lesions of scleredema are ill-defined, woody, non-pitting, indurated plaques (Figure 34.5). Generalized cases may clinically mimic edema. Erythema, hyper-pigmentation, and/or a peau d'orange appearance of the affected areas may be present.

Investigations

- **Antistreptolysin-O (ASLO) titers:** To exclude recent infection with group A streptococci especially in those without clinically apparent pharyngitis or other infectious etiology.
- **Fasting blood glucose or glycosylated hemoglobin measurements:** To rule out diabetes mellitus.
- **Throat culture:** To exclude group A streptococcal infection.
- **Serum protein electrophoresis:** To exclude a monoclonal gammopathy.
- Skin biopsy.

Treatment

- Appropriate antibiotic therapy should be started in scleredema patients if infection is detected, although antibiotics do not appear to shorten the course of skin findings in scleredema.
- Evaluation and treatment for blood dyscrasias and diabetes mellitus if detected.
- No therapy is consistently effective for scleredema. A number of therapies, including systemic steroids, cyclosporine, methotrexate, high dose penicillin, UVA1 phototherapy, psoralen with ultraviolet light A (PUVA), penicillamine, electron beam have all been tried with limited success.
- In cases associated with myeloma, chemotherapy directed at the hematologic malignancy has been reported to result in concomitant improvement of the skin disease.

CALCINOSIS CUTIS

Calcinosis cutis is a term used to describe a group of disorders in which calcium deposits form in the skin.

Pathophysiology

In all cases of calcinosis cutis, insoluble compounds of calcium are deposited within the skin due to local and/or systemic factors. Metabolic and physical factors are pivotal in the development of most cases of calcinosis.

Disorders of calcinosis cutis may be categorized according to the type of calcification process, i.e., dystrophic, metastatic, idiopathic and iatrogenic.

Dystrophic calcification occurs in the setting of normal serum calcium and phosphate levels. The primary abnormality is damaged, inflamed, neoplastic, or necrotic skin. Tissue damage may be from mechanical, chemical, infections or other insults. Patient of collagen vascular disorders, e.g., dermatomyositis, scleroderma and sometimes SLE shows such type of calcification.

Metastatic calcification arises in the setting of abnormal calcium or phosphate metabolism and is generally associated with hypercalcemia and/or hyperphosphatemia.

Idiopathic calcinosis cutis (Figure 34.6) occurs in the absence of known tissue injury or systemic metabolic defect.

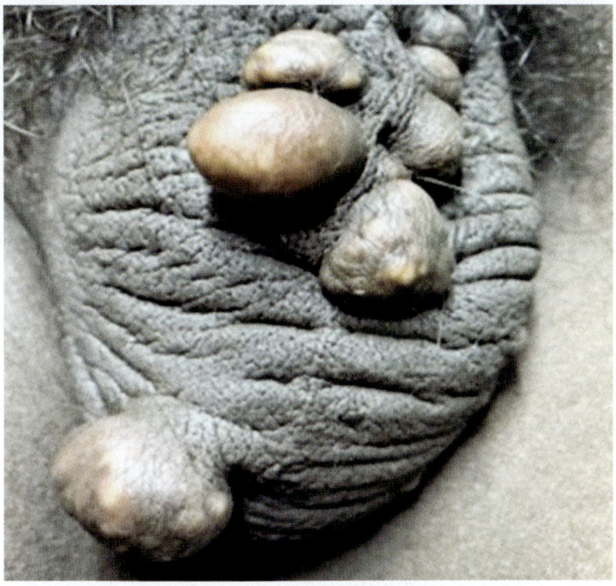

Figure 34.6: Idiopathic scrotal calcinosis

Iatrogenic calcinosis cutis may arise secondary to a treatment or procedure.

- **Parenteral administration of calcium or phosphate:** The intravenous administration of solutions containing calcium or phosphate may cause the precipitation of calcium salts and lead to calcification.
- **Tumor lysis syndrome:** Cutaneous calcification associated with tumor lysis syndrome is due to several factors, including chemotherapy induced tissue damage with resultant hyperphosphatemia, hypocalcemia, hyperuricemia and the potential for acute renal failure.

Clinical Features

- **Most lesions** of calcinosis cutis develop gradually and are asymptomatic. However, the history and evolution of the lesions depend on the etiology of the calcification. Patients with dystrophic calcification may provide a history of an underlying disease, a pre-existing dermal nodule or an inciting traumatic event. Patients with metastatic calcification most frequently have a history of chronic renal failure. Cases of idiopathic calcinosis cutis usually are not associated with previous trauma or disease. Cases of iatrogenic calcinosis cutis generally have a history of recent hospitalization.
- The clinical presentation of calcinosis cutis can vary according to the diagnosis and underlying process. In general, multiple, firm, whitish dermal papules, plaques, nodules, or subcutaneous nodules (Figure 34.7) are found in a distribution characteristic for the specific disorder. Sometimes lesions spontaneously ulcerate, extruding a chalky, white material. Most lesions are asymptomatic, though some may be tender, and others may restrict joint mobility.
- **Subepidermal calcified nodule:** These lesions usually develop in early childhood and are typically solitary, though multiple lesions can also be present. The nodules most commonly occur on the face, though they may occur anywhere.

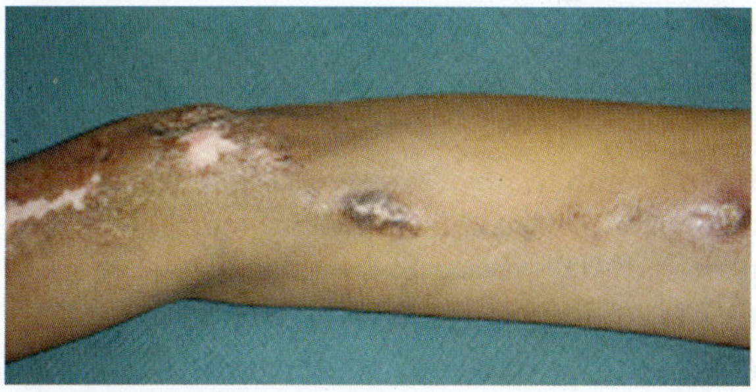

Figure 34.7: Calcinosis cutis in a plaque of linear scleroderma

Tumoral calcinosis: This may be caused by an error in renal phosphate metabolism resulting in hyperphosphatemia. The lesions are large nodules, juxta-articular in location, progressive and have a tendency to recur after surgical removal. The most common locations of calcification are the hips, elbows, scapula, feet, legs, knees and hands.

Calcinosis cutis circumscripta and calcinosis universalis: These forms are rare and may be due to altered ground substances. Calcinosis cutis circumscripta generally occurs in younger patient and tends to involve the extremities, whereas calcinosis universalis occurs later and is usually more widespread.

Calcinosis cutis is a common presentation of connective tissue disorders like dermatomyositis, progressive systemic sclerosis.

Histopathology

- Findings on biopsy and histopathologic examination of a cutaneous lesion are diagnostic. Special stains like Von kossa and Alizarin red are used to stain calcium deposits.

- Results of fine needle aspiration cytology of a skin nodule may also be diagnostic.

Investigations

- Complete blood cell count with differential leukocyte count.
- Estimation of serum calcium and inorganic phosphate.
- Serum alkaline phosphatase and albumin levels to measure liver function.
- Serum blood urea nitrogen and creatinine concentrations can be obtained to measure renal function.
- The parathyroid hormone concentration is a direct measurement for hyperparathyroidism.
- Vitamin D levels should be determined to evaluate the possibility of Vitamin D excess or deficiency.
- A test of the 24-hour urinary excretion of calcium and/or inorganic phosphate may be useful.
- Evaluation of collagen vascular disorders may be done if indicated.
- Radiographic examination may demonstrate the extent of tissue calcification.
- Bone scintigraphy with radiolabelled phosphate compound technetium (Tc99m) methylene diphosphonate [MDP], is useful in evaluating non-visceral soft tissue calcification.
- CT scan helps in the identification of visceral and non-visceral calcification.

Treatment

- Medical therapy of calcinosis cutis is limited and of variable benefit. When identified, the underlying problem should be corrected.
- Intralesional corticosteroids may be beneficial because of their anti-inflammatory and inhibitory effects on fibroblast activity.
- **Antacids:** Inorganic salts can bind phosphate in the gut and prevent absorption.
- Sodium etidronate (diphosphonates) may reduce bone turnover and inhibit the growth of ectopic hydroxyapatite crystals.
- The use of the calcium-channel blocker, diltiazem, has variable benefits.
- Indications for surgical removal include pain, recurrent infection, ulceration and functional impairment. Recurrence is common after excision.

HEREDITARY SENSORY AUTONOMIC NEUROPATHIES

Hereditary sensory autonomic neuropathies (HSAN) encompass a number of inherited disorders that are associated with sensory dysfunction (depressed reflexes, altered pain and temperature perception) and varying degrees of autonomic dysfunction (gastroesophageal reflux, postural hypotension, excessive sweating). Each HSAN disorder is likely caused by different genetic errors that affect specific aspects of small fiber neurodevelopment, which resulting variable phenotypic expression. HSAN are not seen commonly, but they are discussed here because the sensory loss caused in these neuropathies may be confused with leprosy.

It has been classified into following types:

Hereditary Sensory Autonomic Neuropathy Type I (HSAN I)

It is the most common type of HSAN, resulting in progressive degeneration of sensory dorsal root ganglia, with loss of both small myelinated and unmyelinated nerve fibres, leading to distal sensory and motor loss, particularly in the lower limbs. It is an autosomal dominant disorder, mapping to chromosome.

HSAN Type I differs from all other HSANs in that its symptoms appear late, rather than congenitally. It presents in late childhood or adolescence with progressive loss of all modalities of sensation in the lower extremities, particularly pain and temperature resulting in chronic trophic ulceration on weight-bearing areas of the feet, associated osteomyelitis and mutilating deformity (Figure 34.8). Late manifestations include muscle wasting, weakness and lancinating pain in the lower limbs and extension of sensory symptoms to the upper limbs.

Treatment is supportive, with good fitting shoes and alleviation of weight bearing if ulcers form.

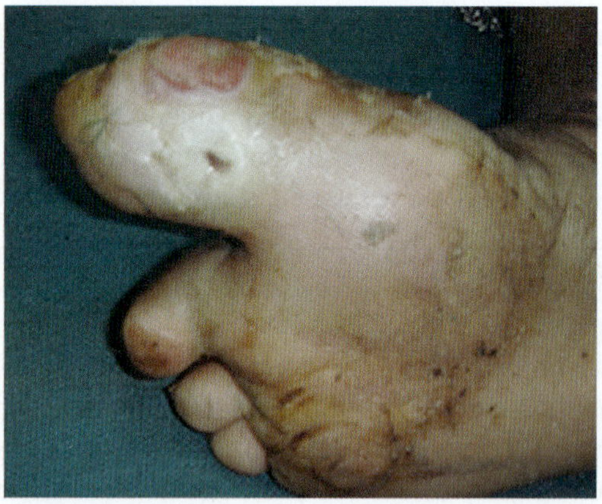

Figure 34.8: Hereditary sensory autonomic neuropathy

Hereditary Sensory Autonomic Neuropathy Type II (HSAN II)

It is an autosomal recessive disorder which has either congenital or early onset. There is marked loss of sensory, motor and autonomic motor neurons and marked loss of unmyelinated nerves. No chromosomal linkage has been identified. High urinary excretion of sphingomyelin and lecithin suggest that the primary mechanism may be a disorder of phospholipid metabolism.

Unlike HSAN I, HSAN II results in loss of sensation equally in hands and feet, leading to ulceration. Ulceration may also occur at other sites such as the forehead, trunk, tongue and lips as a result of repeated injury.

Loss of deep sensation results in deep ulceration, osteomyelitis, stress fractures and injury to long bones. Associated features include mental retardation, neural deafness, impaired taste and smell, retinitis pigmentosa and cataracts. Infantile hypotonia is common.

Hereditary Sensory Autonomic Neuropathy Type III (HSAN III, Familial Dysautonomia or Riley-Day Syndrome)

The disorder is transmitted as an autosomal recessive trait, mapping to chromosome 9. Onset is congenital, and hypotonia, sucking difficulties, a poor cry and vomiting are present at birth. Autonomic features are prominent, with impaired production of tears, unstable temperature control, postural hypotension and excessive sweating, especially during infection, all being major features. Impaired oesophageal motility, with resultant pneumonia, together with bouts of apnoea, may cause death in childhood. Blotchy erythema occurs during overheating, and erythematous macules 2-5 cm in diameter may occur on the trunk and limbs in response to emotional upsets.

Other diagnostic criteria include absent fungiform papillae on the tongue, absent tendon and corneal reflexes, lack of axon flare after intradermal histamine and following instillation of methacholine. Later, the child may show delayed growth and invariably displays postural hypotension.

Mortality rates remain high but have improved with better supportive measures and 50% of patients now survive to adulthood. Death may follow inhalation during attacks of vomiting, and hypotension and cardiac arrest are risks which may require the help of a general anaesthetic. Treatment is symptomatic. Attention to feeding must be meticulous and gastrostomy may be required. Diazepam and chlorpromazine can be used to treat acute autonomic crises and intranasal midazolam can be used at home.

Hereditary Sensory Autonomic Neuropathy Type IV (HSAN IV)

HSAN type IV probably comprises a heterogeneous group of patients and is transmitted by autosomal dominant inheritance. It is characterized by recurrent episodic fevers, anhidrosis, absence of reaction to noxious stimuli, self mutilating behaviour and mental retardation. Infants are hypotonic and are flexic. Insensitivity to pain with self-inflicted injury results in multiple scars and bone fractures, auto extraction of teeth and ulceration of tongue, lips and buccal mucosa. The anomalous pain and temperature sensation and anhidrosis are due to the absence of afferent neurons activated by tissue damaging stimuli and a loss of innervation of eccrine sweat glands, respectively. Treatment is limited. Oral shields may prevent damage to the oral tissues.

Hereditary Sensory Autonomic Neuropathy Type V (HSAN V) or Congenital Insensitivity to Pain

HSAN type V is a rare autosomal recessive hereditary sensory autonomic neuropathy characterized by insensitivity to pain, self-mutilating behaviour, anhidrosis with recurrent hyperpyrexia and mental retardation.

Nociceptive and sympathetic Aδ-fibres and C-fibres nerve activity is reduced or absent in the skin. S-100 protein and neuron specific enolase are reduced or absent in the vicinity of eccrine sweat glands, and substance P receptors are absent from nerve fibres and the epidermis. This is consistent with the loss of unmyelinated and small myelinated fibres, as seen in sural nerve biopsies.

Patients present in early childhood when they start to crawl; they fail to learn the consequences of injury and do not cry with soft-tissue injury. Congenital insensitivity to pain with anhidrosis is characterized by multisystem involvement. Skin ulcerations on the fingers and toes are common from self biting, and neurological examination often reveals complete analgesia, although tactile discrimination, sensation of cold, heat and vibration may be normal. Corneal reflexes are usually present but deep tendon reflexes are abolished.

Neonatal hypotonia and psychomotor retardation are common, as are slow healing fractures, joint deformities, osteomyelitis, avascular necrosis and acro-osteolysis of fingers. There is associated heat intolerance due to anhidrosis, with episodes of hyperpyrexia. Death from hyperpyrexia has been recorded in upto 10% of patients in the first 3 years of life.

HYPOPIGMENTED MYCOSIS FUNGOIDES

Cutaneous T cell lymphoma/mycosis fungoides (MF) is characterized by proliferation of atypical lymphocytes in skin.

Hypopigmented mycosis fungoides is a slow progressive cutaneous T cell lymphoma. It is a rare clinical variant of the disease. Described exclusively in dark-skinned or Asian patients, it was first described by Ryan in 1973. Hypopigmented MF tends to occur in young, slightly to moderately dark-skinned people of Indian, Latin American, or sub-Saharan African heritage.

It manifests as irregular but fairly well-demarcated hypopigmented or white patches. They are asymptomatic or are slightly pruritic and may appear with or without other lesions typical of MF. Although it is similar to vitiligo or lichen sclerosis *et atrophicus*, on histological examination the presence of prominent epidermotropism by large atypical lymphocytes makes mycosis fungoides likely. Persistent or unusual hypopigmented lesions (Figure 34.9) should be subjected to biopsy to avoid delay in the diagnosis of MF, especially in children.

Generally, it shows good response to therapy with PUVA, UVB or topical mechloramine therapy. However, recurrences are common.

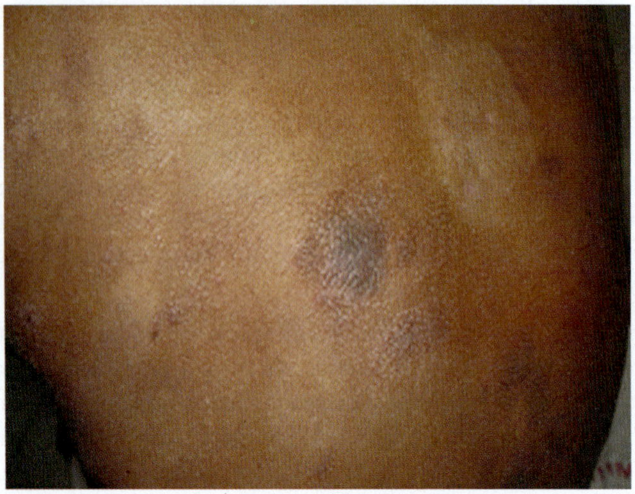

Figure 34.9: Hypopigmented mycosis fungoides

DERMATITIS ARTEFACTA

Dermatitis artefacta is a condition in which skin lesions are solely produced or inflicted by the patient's own actions. This usually occurs as a result or manifestation of a psychological problem. It could be a form of emotional release in situations of distress or part of an attention seeking behaviour. Patients present with lesions that are difficult to recognize and do not conform those of known dermatoses.

Lesions may be produced by a variety of mechanical or chemical means, including fingernails, sharp or blunt objects, burning cigarettes and caustic chemicals.

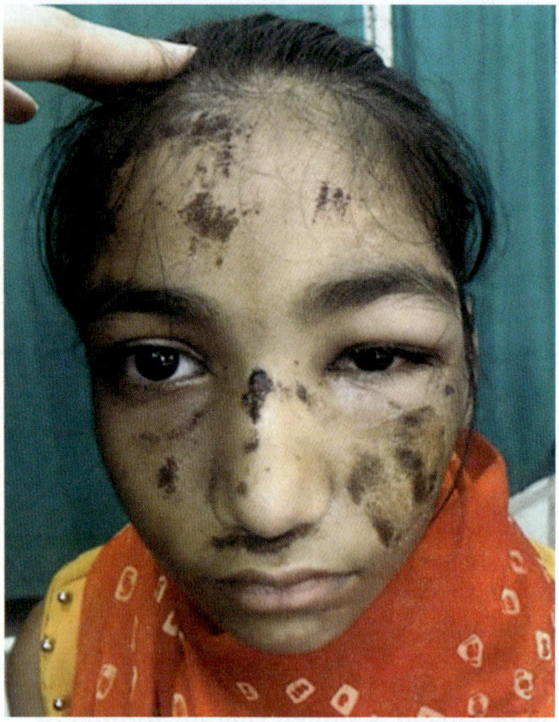

Figure 34.10: Dermatitis artefacta

Epidemiology

The condition is fairly rare, diagnosis is frequently uncertain. There is a female preponderance. It is seen mostly in 20-30 years of age, although there is wide variation with some describing a late adolescence to early adulthood peak.

Clinical Features

- Lesions can be enormously variable in character, depending upon how they are produced but often what is presented, is quite florid.
- Wide range of lesions such as red patches, swelling, blisters, denuded areas, crusts, cuts, burns and scars may be seen and there may be more than one type of lesions.
- They are often in bizarre shapes with irregular outlines in a linear or geometric pattern.
- There is usually clear demarcation with normal skin around the lesions.
- Sometimes it is hard to distinguish dermatitis artefacta from natural diseases, particularly if lesions inflicted mimic those with an organic cause.
- Lesions do not usually evolve gradually but appear almost overnight without any prior signs or symptoms.
- They are usually found on sites that are readily accessible to the patient's hands, such as face (Figure 34.10), hands, arms or legs but not in inaccessible areas.
- The patient usually denies that the rash is self induced.

Investigations

There is no investigation that is specific for the disease. If applicable, tests may be used to exclude other diseases such as skin biopsy.

Management

- Palliative dermatological measures such as occlusive bandages, ointments or placebo drugs, as well as admission to hospital that includes bathing and massaging by nurses, can have a therapeutic impact on the psychiatric problem by symbolizing the medical attention and care for which the dermatitis artefacta patient is craving.
- Anti-depressants may be of value. The selective serotonin reuptake inhibitors (SSRIs) are often preferred although the tricyclic anti-depressants may have some antipruritic effect and sedation can be beneficial.
- The antipsychotic, olanzapine, appears to have much potential.
- Cognitive and behavioural therapy may be helpful.

PANNICULITIS

Panniculitis refers to a group of conditions that involve inflammation of the subcutaneous fat. Despite having very diverse causes, most forms of panniculitis have the same clinical presentation. The diagnosis is established by skin biopsy as there are characteristic microscopic features depending on the cause.

Panniculitis can be divided into mostly septal or lobular panniculitis depending on where the microscopic inflammation is most concentrated. Most types of panniculitis have both lobular and septal inflammation. Further classification is based on whether or not there is inflammation involving the blood vessels of the fat, i.e., vasculitis.

Classification of Panniculitis

- **Mostly septal panniculitis with vasculitis**
  - Leukocytoclastic vasculitis.
  - Superficial thrombophlebitis.
  - Cutaneous polyarteritis nodosa.
- **Mostly septal panniculitis without vasculitis**
  - Necrobiosis lipoidica.
  - Scleroderma, which may be localized (morphea).
  - Subcutaneous granuloma annulare.
  - Rheumatoid nodule.
  - Necrobiotic xanthogranuloma.
  - Erythema nodosum.
- **Mostly lobular panniculitis with vasculitis**
  - Erythema nodosum leprosum.
  - Lucio's phenomenon.
  - Neutrophilic lobular panniculitis associated with rheumatoid arthritis.
  - Erythema induratum of Bazin.
  - Crohn's disease.
  - Nodular vasculitis.
- **Mostly lobular panniculitis without vasculitis**
  - Sclerosing panniculitis (lipodermatosclerosis).
  - Sclerema neonatorum.
  - Cold panniculitis.
  - Lupus panniculitis.
  - Panniculitis in dermatomyositis.
  - Pancreatic panniculitis.
  - Alpha-1 antitrypsin deficiency.
  - Infective panniculitis.
  - Factitial panniculitis.
  - Subcutaneous sarcoidosis.
  - Traumatic panniculitis.
  - Lipoatrophy.
  - Subcutaneous fat necrosis of the newborn.
  - Post-steroid panniculitis.
  - Gout panniculitis.
  - Crystal storing panniculitis.
  - Cytophagic histiocytic panniculitis.
  - Post irradiation pseudo sclerodermatous panniculitis.
  - Panniculitis associated with halogenodermas (iodides, bromides).

Clinical Features

The area of skin involved with panniculitis feels thickened and woody to touch. It may or may not demonstrate discolouration of the overlying skin, which may be either reddening or brownish pigmentation. The area is often tender. Most often, the affected areas appear as raised nodules or lumps under the skin, but may be a plaque or large flat area of thickened skin (Figure 34.11). When the inflammation has settled, a depression in the skin may be left behind temporarily or permanently (localized lipodystrophy).

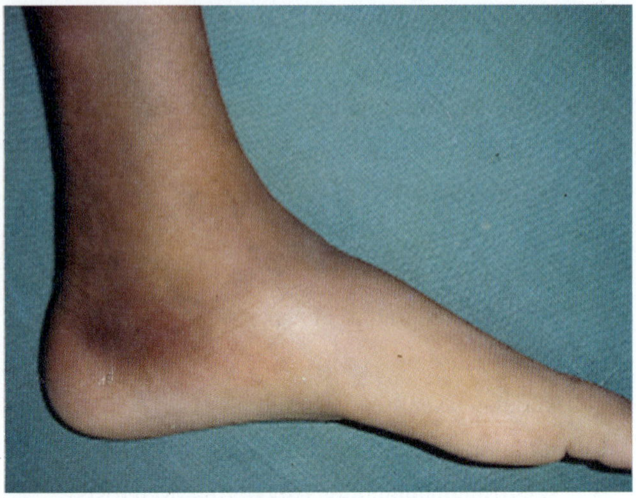

Figure 34.11: Panniculitis

Treatment

- Treat the underlying cause, if known.
- Rest and elevate the affected area.
- Compression hosiery.
- Pain relief using anti-inflammatory medications such as aspirin, ibuprofen or diclofenac.
- Systemic steroids (oral or parenteral) to settle the inflammation.
- Antibiotics with anti-inflammatory activities, e.g., tetracycline and other agents like hydroxychloroquine and potassium iodide may also be found.
- Surgical removal of persistent or ulcerated lesions.

COLD INJURIES

Exposure to cold can produce various injuries that occur as a result of the human inability to adapt to cold. Common cold injury occurring in children is chilblain (Perniosis). Other cold injuries, e.g., **immersion (trench) foot and frostbite** are seen with prolonged exposure to cold and damp environment and are routinely not seen in children.

Chilblain (Perniosis)

Chilblain represents a severe form of cold injury that occurs after exposure to non-freezing temperatures and damp conditions. This condition is characterized by chronic, recurrent vasculitis manifested by red-to-violaceous raised lesions on unprotected parts of extremities, such as the hands (Figure 34.12), feet and face. Blisters, erosions, or ulcers are sometimes seen. It commonly affects young and middle-aged women and may be associated with a variety of chronic disorders, especially Raynaud's phenomenon.

The lesions usually resolve spontaneously in 1-3 weeks, but they may recur in some individuals.

Management involves local heat, gentle massage and emollients. Nifedipine at 25-50 mg/day may be used to reduce the pain and speed up the resolution of the lesions. Patients should be instructed to wear woolen gloves and socks during winter months.

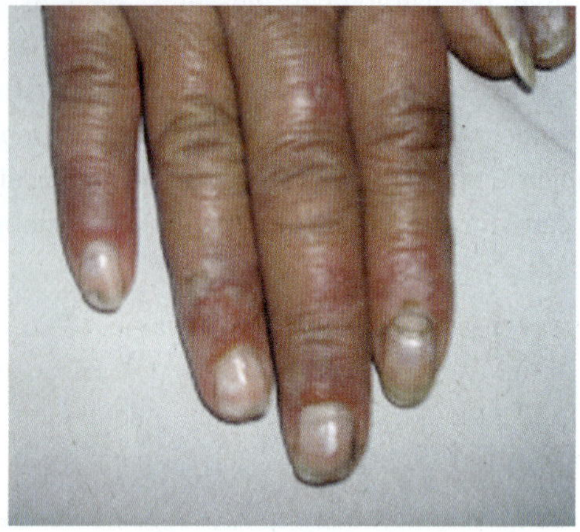

Figure 34.12: Perniosis

ERYTHEMA NODOSUM

It is characterized by painful erythematous nodules that usually are limited to the extensor aspects of the lower legs. It may occur in association with several systemic diseases, drugs or may be idiopathic.

Causes

1. *Infections*

Bacterial infections: Streptococcal infections, tuberculosis, *Yersinia enterocolitica, mycoplasma pneumonia, salmonella, campylobacter, etc.*

Fungal infections: Coccidioidomycosis, histoplasmosis, blastomycosis, etc.

Drugs: Sulfonamides, gold, sulfonylureas, oral contraceptive pills, etc.

2. *Other causes*

a. Inflammatory bowel disease.
b. Hodgkin's disease and lymphoma.
c. Sarcoidosis.
d. Behçet's disease.
e. Pregnancy.
f. Rheumatological and autoimmune diseases.

3. *Idiopathic.*

Clinical Features

Lesions begin as erythematous tender nodules. Characteristically, lesions appear on the anterior aspect of legs (Figure 34.13), however, they may appear on any surface. The border of lesions is poorly defined and they vary from 1-2 cm in size. These lesions are easily palpated than visualized, and are typically bilateral and symmetrical. The nodules may coalesce to form plaques. After several days, the erythematous nodules become ecchymotic in colour, finally taking on a yellow-green appearance referred to as erythema contusiformis. Lesions of erythema nodosum never ulcerate and atrophy or scar formation is not seen. Regression takes place in 3-6 weeks. Constitutional signs and symptoms may also be present.

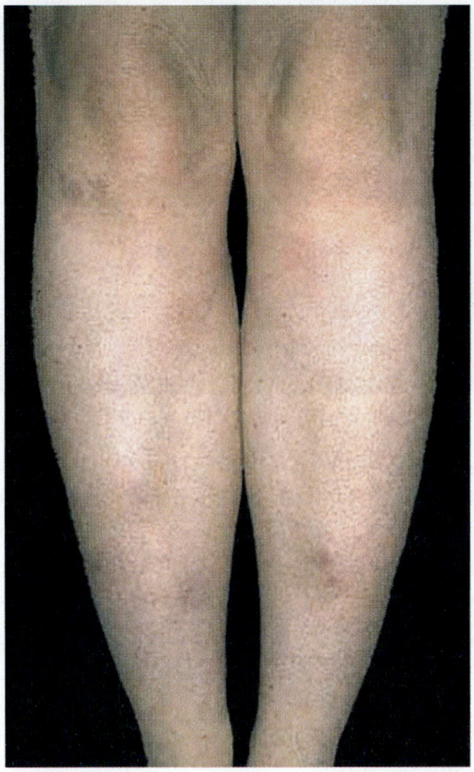

Figure 34.13: Classic presentation of erythema nodosum with nodular red swellings over the shins

Investigations

- Erythrocyte sedimentation rate (ESR) is often raised.
  - Antistreptolysin titer (ASLO) is elevated in some patients with streptococcal disease.
  - Stool examination to exclude infection by *Yersinia, Salmonella* and *Campylobacter*.
  - Throat culture to exclude group A beta-hemolytic streptococcal infection.
  - Tuberculin skin test.
  - Chest radiographs to exclude sarcoidosis and tuberculosis.
  - Skin biopsy.

Treatment

In most patients, erythema nodosum is a self limiting disease and requires only symptomatic relief using non-steroidal anti-inflammatory drugs (NSAIDs), elevation of legs and bed rest. Potassium iodide, colchicine, hydroxychloroquine, dapsone, thalidomide, prednisolone can also be helpful as shown by various case series. Anti tubercular therapy will be required in patients having evidence of tuberculosis.

SWEET'S SYNDROME

Sweet syndrome, also referred to as acute febrile neutrophilic dermatosis, is characterized by violaceous, 0.5-3 cm diameter nodules and plaques that erupt abruptly on the face and extremities. These nodules appear as recurrent crops (Figure 34.14) over a period of 1-8 months and are heralded by high fever, arthralgia and occasionally periarticular swelling and arthritis. Necrotic vesicles and bullae may also form.

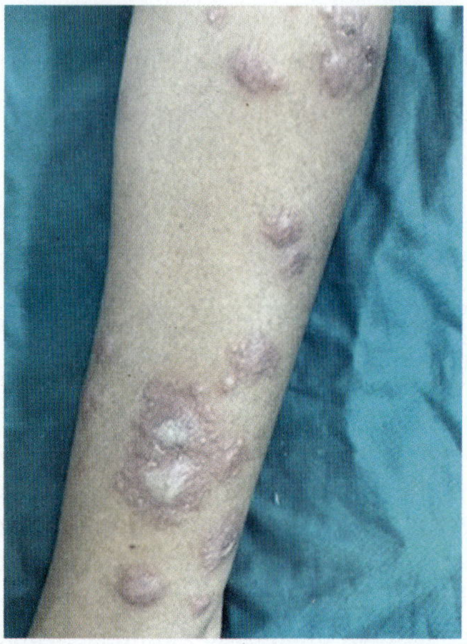

Figure 34.14: Sweet's syndrome

Although Sweet's syndrome is self-limiting, symptoms may be debilitating. Skin lesions, arthralgia and fever usually melt away with systemic corticosteroids; however, recurrences are common when the medication is tapered. It was initially described in middle-aged women, a number of cases have been reported in infants and children. About 10% of adult cases are associated with myeloproliferative disorders, especially acute myelocytic or myelomonocytic leukemia.

Patients with this syndrome require a thorough physical examination and laboratory evaluation, including complete blood count, peripheral smear and bone marrow biopsy, to exclude any underlying disorder.

Clinical Variant of Sweet's Syndrome

- Subcutaneous Sweet's syndrome.
- Histiocytoid Sweet's syndrome.
- Neutrophilic dermatosis of dorsal hands.

Diagnostic Criteria for Sweet's Syndrome

Major Criteria

- Acute onset of typical lesions.
- Histology consistent with Sweet's syndrome.

Minor Criteria

- Fever.
- Association with inflammatory dermatosis, pregnancy, malignancy, infections.
- Excellent response to systemic steroids or potassium iodide.
- Laboratory abnormality (3/4 required):
  - Total leucocyte count > 8000
  - Neutrophils > 70%
  - Erythrocyte sedimentation rate > 20 mm/hrs
  - C-reactive protein Elevated levels

Diagnosis Requires Fulfilment of 2 Major and 2 Minor Criteria

Sweet's syndrome may be confused with erythema multiforme, erythema nodosum, viral exanthems, Henoch-Schönlein purpura (HSP), infectious vasculitis, polyarteritis nodosa (PAN) and erythema nodosum leprosum (ENL). Although Sweet's syndrome may be suspected because of the cutaneous lesions and clinical course, skin biopsy of a fresh lesion demonstrates diagnostic findings, which include a dense, perivascular, neutrophilic infiltrate and intense edema in the upper dermis, some leukocytoclasia without true vasculitis, and in some cases subepidermal bullae formation.

Treatment: Sweet's syndrome should be treated symptomatically by giving NSAIDs like indomethacin. Systemic corticosteroids (0.5-1 mg/kg/day of prednisolone for 4-6 weeks) are mainstay of treatment. Potent topical or intralesional corticosteroids may also be used.

Some patients may require dapsone (50-100 mg/day), potassium iodide (300 mg three times/day), or colchicine (0.5 mg three times/day). In patients who do not respond cyclosporine, IVIG or clofazimine may be tried.

PYODERMA GANGRENOSUM

In pyoderma gangrenosum, painful pustules or nodules are formed which develop central necrosis and an enlarging ulcer with a haemorrhagic, purple, undermined, advancing border. Ulcers range in size from about 1 cm in diameter when they first appear to over 10 cm as they evolve. One or several lesions may occur, and any area, including the face, trunk and extremities (Figure 34.15), may be involved.

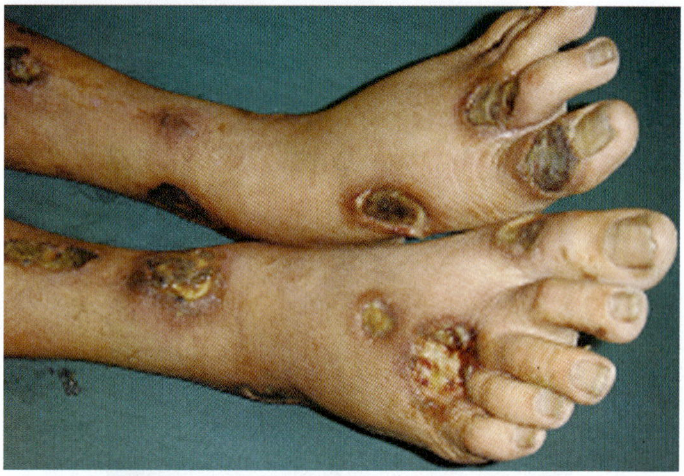

Figure 34.15: Pyoderma gangrenosum

Pathergy, or the development of new lesions at sites of trauma, such as venepunctures, is a reliable diagnostic clue. An underlying systemic disease, such as inflammatory bowel disease, myelogenous leukemia or rheumatoid arthritis, is associated with cutaneous lesions in half of the cases.

Clinical Type of Pyoderma Gangrenosum

- Classical ulcerative.
- Pustular.
- Bullous.
- Superficial granulomatosis.
- Neutrophilic dermatosis of dorsal hand.
- Pyostomatitis of vegetans.

Skin biopsy shows lymphocytic vasculitis at the advancing border. In dermis, necrosis with abscess formation and reactive polymorphous inflammation is seen which may extend into the subcutaneous tissue. Pyoderma gangrenosum usually responds to treatment of the underlying condition. Idiopathic cases can be treated with antibiotics, systemic corticosteroids, or dapsone. Resistant cases may require immunosuppressive agents such as azathioprine, methotrexate, or cyclosporin.

Diagnostic Criteria for Pyoderma Gangrenosum

Major Criteria or Essential Criteria

- Rapid progression of a painful necrolytic cutaneous ulcer with irregular, violaceous, undermined border.
- Exclusion of other causes of cutaneous ulceration.

Minor Criteria (2/4)

- Positive pathergy or cribriform scarring.
- Association of systemic diseases.
- Histology findings (dermal neutrophilic infiltrates).
- Rapid response to oral steroids (50% improvement in one month).

For diagnosis of classical pyoderma gangrenosum requires both major and at least two minor criteria.

BEHÇET'S DISEASE (BD)

Adamantiades-Behçet's disease is a multisystem inflammatory disease of unknown etiology classified as systemic vasculitis involving all types and sizes of blood vessels and characterized clinically by recurrent oral aphthous and genital ulcers, skin lesions and iridocyclitis/posterior uveitis, occasionally accompanied by arthritis and vascular gastrointestinal, neurologic or other manifestations.

Epidemiology

Behçet's disease most often occurs in twenties and thirties. Juvenile disease rate varies from 2% to 21% in different ethnic groups with no gender predominance.

Etiopathogenesis

The etiology of BD is unknown. HLA-B5, HLA B-51 and HLA B-27 have been found to be more frequent. Finding of familial cases supports the contribution of predisposing genetic factors for the disease.

Other associated factors may be HSV-1, *Streptococcus sanguis* and *Mycoplasma fermentans* infections.

Immunological mechanisms are considered to play a major role in the pathogenesis of BD, which is usually considered to be a primary dysfunction of the innate immune system. The major microscopic finding at most sites of active disease is an immune mediated occlusive vasculitis.

Clinical Features

- Most cases of BD are reported in late childhood.
- Oral ulcers are the most common initial major manifestation. Oral aphthous ulcers are typically multiple, painful 1 to 3 cm in diameter and sharply margined with a fibrin-coated base and surrounding erythema (Figure 34.16). They tend to resolve without scarring after 1-2 weeks.

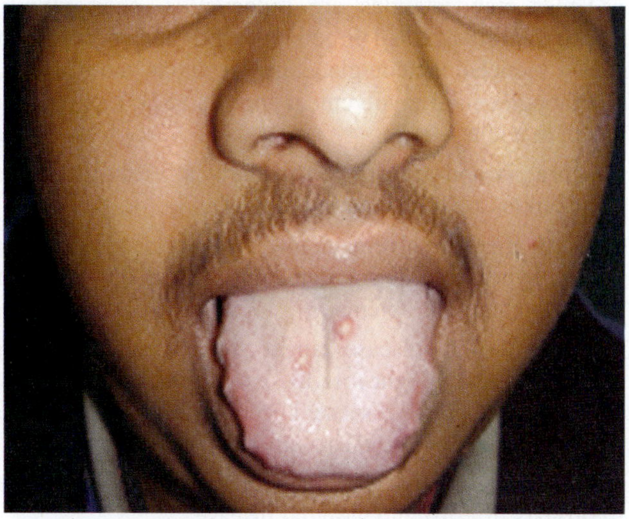

Figure 34.16: Behçet's disease showing aphthous ulcer

- Genital ulcers mainly affect scrotum in males (Figure 34.17) and the vulva in females and may result in scarring.

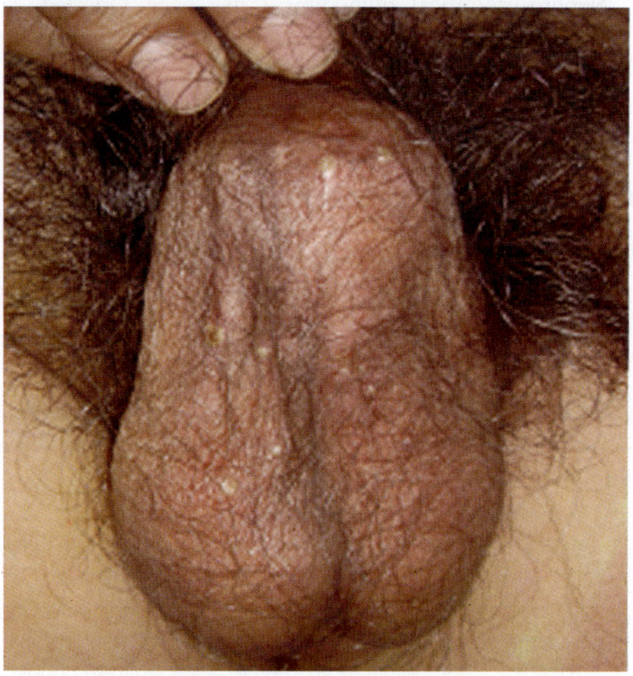

Figure 34.17: Behçet's disease showing ulcers over scrotum

- Cutaneous manifestations are variable and may include erythema nodosum like lesions, papulopustular lesions, vesicles, erythema multiforme like eruptions, folliculitis, thrombophlebitis and abscesses.
- Pyoderma gangrenosum type lesions, palpable purpura, purulent bullae, bullous necrotising vasculitis and Sweet's syndrome like lesions have also been described.

- The skin hyperreactivity response or pathergy test is not pathognomic of BD but may be an important diagnostic indicator.
- Ocular manifestations are iridocyclitis, chorioretinitis, optic papillitis, retinal thrombophlebitis and arteritis. Long term sequelae include glaucoma, cataracts and blindness. Although ocular involvement appears to be less common than in adults.
- Arthralgia and arthritis, particularly affecting the knees and ankles are not uncommon in BD.
- Neurological involvement manifests as headache, paralysis, hyperparaesthesia, dementia, behavioural disorders and psychiatric problems.
- Gastrointestinal disease ranges from nausea, vomiting, diarrhoea and weight loss to signs mimicking ulcerative colitis and Crohn's disease. Ulceration of gastrointestinal tract, mainly ileum and caecum may occur.
- Cardiac disease may present as myocarditis, pericarditis, coronary arteritis and vascular disease.
- Pulmonary artery aneurysms, pulmonary infiltrate (leading to pulmonary haemorrhage) may occur, causing cough and hemoptysis.
- Nephro-urological involvement has been reported and manifests as hematuria, proteinuria, urethritis, orchitis and epididymitis.
- Thrombocytopenia and neutropenia have also been documented in BD.

Diagnostic Criteria for BD

International Criteria (1990) for Behçet's Disease:

- ***Recurrent oral ulceration:*** Minor aphthous or major aphthous or herpetiform ulceration observed by a physician or reported reliably by a patient that recurs at least 3 times in one year period plus 2 of the following:
  - *Recurrent genital ulceration:* Recurrent genital aphthous ulceration or scarring, especially in males, observed by a physician or reliably reported by a patient.
  - *Eye lesions:* (1) Anterior uveitis, posterior uveitis, and cells in vitreous upon slit-lamp examination or (2) Retinal vasculitis observed by physician (or ophthalmologist).
  - *Skin lesions:* (1) Erythema nodosum-like lesions observed by physician or reliably reported by a patient, pseudofolliculitis, and papulopustular lesions or (2) Acneiform nodules consistent with Behçet's disease, observed by a physician, and in postadolescent patients not receiving corticosteroids.
  - *Positive pathergy test:* An erythematous papule larger than 2 mm at the prick site, 48 hours after the prick with a 20- to 22-gauge sterile needle, which obliquely penetrated avascular skin to a depth of 5 mm.

Revised international criteria for Behçet's disease

Contd.

Clinical feature	Points
Recurrent ocular lesions	2
Recurrent ocular aphthae	2
Recurrent genital aphthae	2
Recurrent skin lesions	1
CNS lesions	1
Vascular manifestations	1
Positive pathergy test	1

According to newer revised criteria recurrent oral ulceration as described above plus ≥ 4 score indicates Behçet's disease.

Pathergy test is optional and the primary scoring system does not include pathergy testing. However, where Pathergy testing is conducted one extra point may be assigned for a positive result.

Diagnosis

- Diagnosis of BD is based mainly on history and clinical examination.
- A positive pathergy test adds in diagnosis of BD, but not pathognomic.
- Radiograph of affected joints is helpful.
- Cranial MRI allows documentation of hypodense or atrophic changes in the brain.
- Vascular lesions can be detected by angiography.
- Other organ systems should be evaluated based on clinical signs and symptoms.
- Skin biopsy is helpful.

Differential Diagnosis

- Vogt-Koyanagi-Harada syndrome.
- Reiter's disease.
- Viral infection (herpes, coxsackie, echo).
- Syphilis.
- SLE.
- **MAGIC** syndrome (mouth and genital ulcers with inflamed cartilage).
- Ulcerative colitis, Crohn's disease.
- Bowel-associated dermatitis arthritis syndrome.
- Recurrent aphthous stomatitis.
- Herpes simplex infection.
- Sexually transmitted infections.
- Other causes of uveitis and arthritis.
- Neuro-Sweet disease.

Treatment

Treatment of BD has been tailored to the specific organ involvement and the severity of disease.

- Recurrent oral ulcerations are most often treated with palliative agents, such as bland diet, avoidance of irritating agents, use of antiseptic mouth wash, local antiseptic and local anesthetics.
- For genital ulcerations topical corticosteroid and antiseptic cream is useful.
- For more severe disease systemic corticosteroids are effective.
- Dapsone, azathioprine, mycophenolate mofetil, cyclosporine and colchicine are found to be effective.
- Thalidomide and tacrolimus have been used with varying success.
- Ophthalmologic BD is managed with topical and local intraocular steroids as well as with immunosuppressive drugs.
- In CNS disease, systemic steroids, chlorambucil or cyclophosphamide are effective.

PITYRIASIS ROSEA

It is an acute self limiting condition characterized by distinctive exanthema and minimal constitutional symptoms. It is most common in children and young adults.

Etiopathogenesis

The cause of pityriasis rosea is uncertain, but many epidemiological and clinical features suggest that an infective agent may be implicated.

- Recently human herpes virus 6 (HHV-6) and human herpesvirus7 (HHV-7) have been suggested as causative agents.
- Drugs such as arsenic, bismuth, barbiturates, captopril, propanolol, gold, organic mercurials, metronidazole, d-penicillamine, ketotifen may cause papulosquamous eruption similar to pityriasis rosea.

Clinical Features

- The eruption of pityriasis rosea follows a distinctive and remarkably constant pattern and course in around 80% of cases.
- Prodromal symptoms are usually absent.
- The first manifestation of the disease is usually the appearance of the herald patch. It measures 1-2 cm in diameter and is characterized by oval or round lesion with a central, wrinkled, salmon-colored area and a dark red peripheral zone which are separated by a collarette of fine scales. It is usually located on the trunk (Figure 34.18A and B) but can be seen on the neck or extremities.
- Within 10 days of appearance of herald patch (Figure 34.18B) a characteristic papulosquamous rash appears which is symmetrical and localized predominantly to the trunk and adjacent areas of the neck and extremities. Involvement is maximal over the abdomen and anterior and dorsal surfaces of the thorax.
- Eruption consists of discrete lesions often oval in outline and dull pink in colour covered by fine, dry, silvery-grey scales. They are distributed in a **Christmas tree pattern** with their long axis following the lines of cleavage of the skin.

In atypical pityriasis rosea around 20% of patients, the herald patch may be missing or confluent with other lesions. The distribution of the rash may be peripheral and facial involvement may be seen especially in children. Involvement of the axilla and groin (inverse variant) can

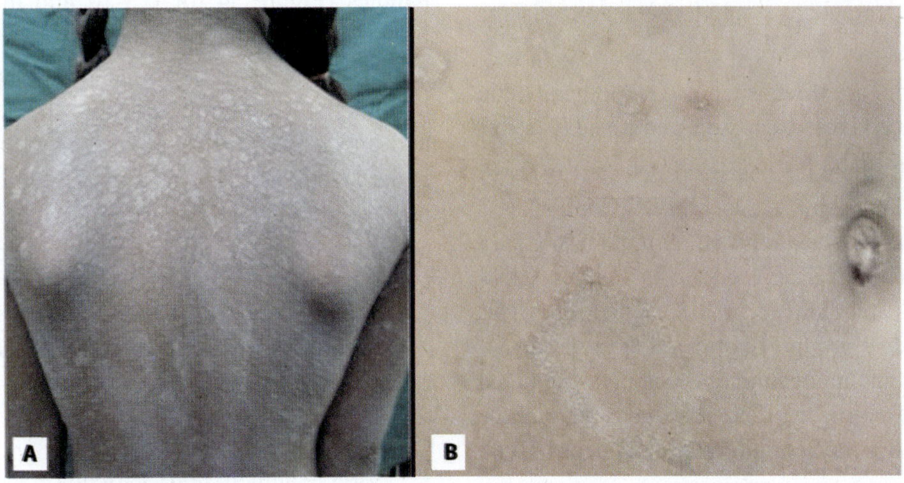

Figure 34.18: Pityriasis rosea (A and B) with herald patch (B)

also be seen. Sometimes lesions of pityriasis rosea may be large, urticarial, vesicular, pustular, purpuric and erythema multiforme like.

- Hypopigmentary and hyperpigmentary skin changes may follow the inflammatory stage.

Treatment

Pityriasis rosea is a self-limited disease, and treatment is supportive. Topical zinc oxide and calamine lotion are useful for pruritus. If the disease is severe or widespread topical or oral steroids may be used. Ultraviolet radiation therapy has also been demonstrated to be effective. Oral acyclovir and erythromycin has been shown in one study to hasten resolution especially if given within 1 week of rash.

PITYRIASIS LICHENOIDES

Pityriasis lichenoides (PL) an uncommon dermatitis, previously included in the parapsoriasis group.

It is divided into two main types:

- Pityriasis lichenoides chronica (PLC).
- Pityriasis lichenoides et varioliformis acuta (PLEVA).

A third much rarer aggressive form, febrile ulcero-necrotic Mucha-Habermann disease (FUMHD) usually occurs in adults in the second and third decade of life.

Pityriasis lichenoides is more common in children and young adults. PLC is the most common type, with male predominance.

Etiopathogenesis

- The etiology of pityriasis lichenoides is usually unknown. Various infectious trigger factors are reported to be associated with pityriasis lichenoides, e.g., *Toxoplasma gondii*, Epstein-Barr virus, CMV, parvovirus B19, hepatitis C virus, HIV, adenovirus, varicella zoster virus, measles vaccine, streptococci, staphylococci, mycoplasma infections etc.
- Other trigger factors are drugs such as chemotherapeutic agents, oral contraceptives, astemizole and possibly herbs.
- Evidence of T-cell clonality has been detected in most cases of PLEVA and some cases of PLC. PLEVA has also been reported in association with lymphomas. CD8+ T cells predominate in PLEVA whereas either $CD8^+$ or CD4 + T cells predominate in PLC. Thus, pityriasis lichenoides is diverse group of entities due to variety of underlying causes including immune complex mediated hypersensitivity vasculitis to different triggers, an immune response to T-cell dyscrasia or a primary cutaneous T-cell lymphoma.

Clinical Features

Pityriasis lichenoides et varioliformis acuta (PLEVA): It manifests as recurrent crops of erythematous papules (Figure 34.19) that develop crusts, vesicles or erosions before spontaneously regressing within a matter of weeks. Lesions are often asymptomatic but can be pruritic or burning in nature, especially more in acute cases. Lesions of PLC, after healing, may leave post inflammatory hypopigmentation, whereas lesion of PLEVA heals with scarring, which may be varioliformis.

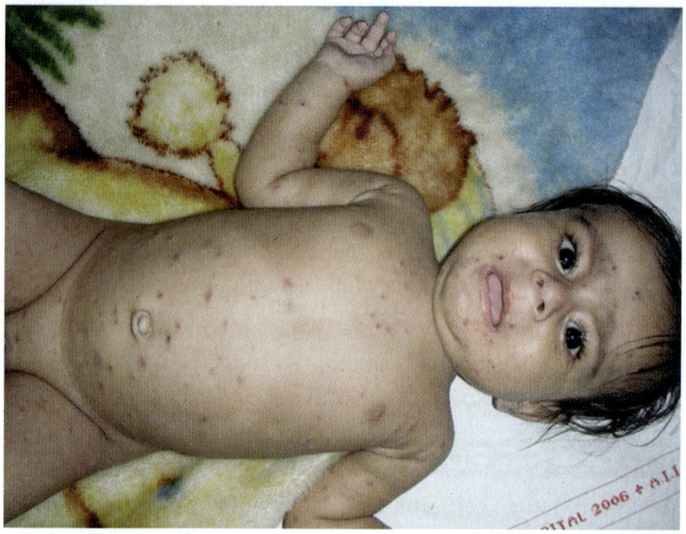

Figure 34.19: Pityriasis lichenoides et varioliformis acuta

Febrile Ulcero-necrotic Mucha-Habermann Disease (FUMHD): FUMHD is an acute and severe generalized eruption of purpuric and ulceronecrotic plaques with associated systemic involvement and a mortality rate of up to 25%, hence, it should be approached as a dermatologic emergency.

Pityriasis lichenoides chronica (PLC): It typically presents as recurrent crops of erythematous scaly lichenoid papules (Figure 34.20C), 3-10 mm in diameter and reddish brown in colour that spontaneously regress over several weeks to months. The possible sequelae are hyperpigmentation, hypopigmentation and varicella like scars. The trunk, thighs and upper arms are usually involved but the eruption can be generalized. Isolated acral and segmental forms have also been reported. An adherent 'mica-like' scale can be detached by gentle scrapping to reveal a shining brown surface which is a distinctive diagnostic feature of PLC (Figure 34.20A and B).

Differential Diagnosis for PLEVA and PLC

- Insect bites.
- Leukocytoclastic vasculitis.
- Viral exanthem (e.g., varicella zoster, herpes simplex).

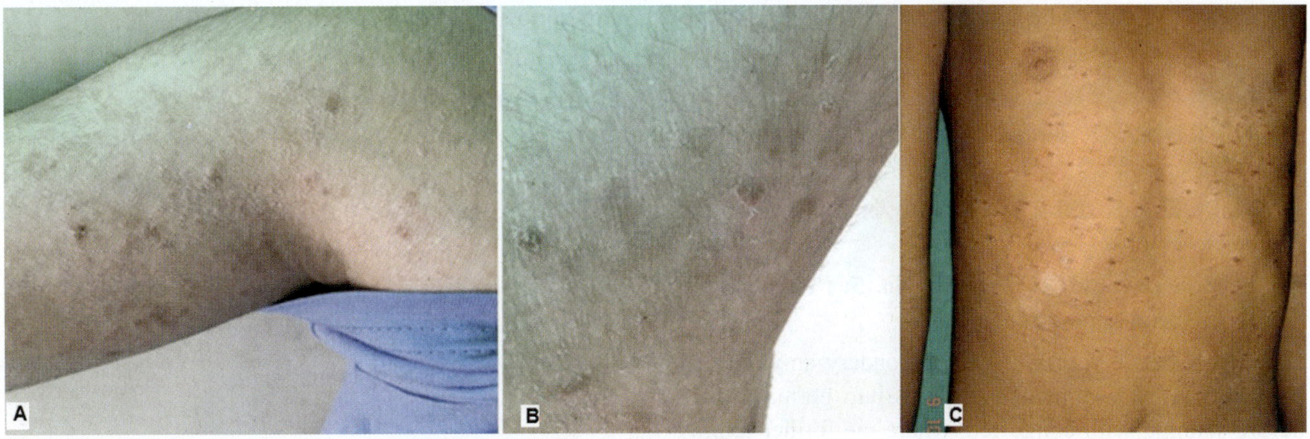

Figure 34.20: Pityriasis lichenoides chronica (A, B and C)

- Pityriasis rosea.
- Drug reaction.
- Guttate psoriasis.
- Lymphomatoid papulosis.
- Secondary syphilis.
- Mycosis fungoides.

Diagnosis

- Leukocytosis and a decreased CD4/CD8 ratio can occur.
- Skin biopsy.

Histopathology

In PLEVA marked exocytosis of lymphocytes and erythrocytes, intercellular and intracellular oedema leading to variable degree of epidermal necrosis is seen. The infiltrate comprising mainly of CD8+ T cells which obscures the dermal-epidermal junction with pronounced vacuolar alteration of basal layer. Dermal infiltrate surrounds and involves the walls of dilated dermal capillaries, which show endothelial proliferation. Early lesions can exhibit lymphocytic vasculitis with fibrinoid degeneration of blood vessel walls. Immunofluorescent studies variably demonstrate IgM, C_3 and fibrin in vessel walls of fresh lesions.

PLC histological findings include dermal, wedge shaped lymphocytic infiltrate, epidermal spongiosis, parakeratosis and variable degree of necrosis of keratinocytes.

Treatment

The mainstay of therapy is a combination of topical steroids and phototherapy. Antibiotics including erythromycin and tetracyclines are useful. Phototherapy is helpful in the form of sunlight, UV-B, narrow band UV-B, UV-A and PUVA. Usually oral azithromycin or erythromycin is prescribed for 4-8 weeks along with topical steroids. Later they are maintained on topical steroids. Oral dapsone, chinoline and acridine derivative are also helpful.

In more aggressive cases, immunosuppressants like methotrexate, Cyclosporine, intravenous immunoglobulins may be used.

AMYLOIDOSIS

Amyloidosis is defined as extracellular deposition of proteinaceous, eosinophilic hyaline material in skin and other organs which is autologous in origin. It has characteristic staining properties and a unique fibrillar structure. 21 different types of fibril proteins have been found so far, most of them are unrelated to the skin. Six amyloid proteins are important in cutaneous amyloidosis i.e. AA, ATTR, AL (Ak and A λ), Aβ_2M and AK.

Amyloid has following characteristics:

1. Insoluble beta-sheet fibrillar protein aggregates.
2. **Light microscopy:** Amyloid appears as eosinophilic amorphous substance which after Congo red staining shows apple green birefringence with polarised light.
3. **Electron microscopy:** Shows that all amyloid subtypes are composed of 7.5-10 nm wide, linear, non-branching tubular fibrils loosely arranged in a meshwork. Each fibril is composed of several filaments arranged in beta-pleated sheet configuration (most physiologic proteins exist in the alpha (or helical) tertiary form e.g. keratin, the beta pleated sheet form is abnormal in human tissue).
4. **Staining properties:**
   - **Congo red:** Apple green birefringence under polarised light
   - **Methyl violet:** Metachromatic staining (amyloid purple and other background tissues blue)

- **Cresyl violet:** Metachromatic staining ((amyloid purple and other background tissues blue)
- PAS staining
- **Thioflavin T:** Green staining on fluorescence microscopy
- **Van Gieson's stain:** Inconstantly produces a yellow brown color
- **Pagoda red and RIT scarlet No. 5:** More specific stains (bright orange color)

5. Distinction between primary and secondary amyloid can be achieved by treatment with potassium permanganate before staining with congo red, where the former retains its affinity for the dye and shows green birefringence under polarised light, whereas the latter loses both characteristics.

Amyloidosis is classified as:

1. ***Localised cutaneous amyloidosis***
   - *Primary:*
     - Macular
     - Papular (lichen)
     - Maculopapular
     - Nodular or tumefactive
     - Familial
     - Anosacral
     - Poikilodermatous
     - Senile
   - *Secondary:* Microdeposits in association with chronic cutaneous dermatosis and tumors.
2. ***Systemic or generalised amyloidosis (Table 34.1)***

Table 34.1: Classification of systemic amyloidosis

Clinicopathological catory	*Associated diseases*	*Major fibril protein*	*Clinical features*
Non Hereditary			
Immunocyte dyscrasias (Primary systemic amyloidosis)	Multiple myeloma and other monoclonal B-cell proliferations	AL (Immunoglobulin light chain)	Purpura, haemorrhage (periorbital and intertriginous areas), waxy papules, nodules and plaques, scleroderma like changes, blistering and nail dystrophy Macroglossia, nephropathy, cardiomyopathy, neuropathy, intestinal involvement
Reactive systemic amyloidosis (Secondary systemic amyloidosis)	Chronic inflammatory dermatosis (rheumatoid arthritis, Reiter's syndrome, psoriasis, dermatomyositis etc)	SAA (serum amyloid A)	Petechia, purpura and alopecia Nephropathy Hepatosplenomegaly Intestine involvement
Secondary Haemodialysis associated amyloidosis	Chronic renal failure	Aβ_2M (Amyloid β_{2-} macroglobulin)	Soft nodules and plaques Destructive arthropathy
Senile systemic amyloidosis	–	Wild-type transthyretin	Cardiomyopathy Carpel tunnel syndrome
Hereditary			
Hereditary transthyretin amyloidosis /familial amyloid polyneuropathy (ATTR)	–	Mutant transthyretin	Purpura, petechiae atrophic scars, non-healing ulcers Cardiomyopathy, Nephropathy, Neuropathy
Hereditary cystatin C amyloidosis (ACys)	–	Cystatin C	Multiple cerebral infarcts
Hereditary ApoA1 amyloidosis (AApoA1)	–	Apolipoprotein 1	Maculopapular lesions, petechiae and purpura Cardiomyopathy
Hereditary gelsolin amyloidosis / Finnish-type/Meretoja syndrome (AGel)	–	Gelsolin	Cutis laxa, alopecia and purpura Corneal dystrophy, Neuropathy

Contd.

Hereditary fibrinogen A alpha chain amyloidosis (AFib)	-	Mutant fibrinogen A alpha	Nephropathy
Hereditary (ALys)	-	Lysozyme	Renal and Gastrointestinal involvement, Sicca syndrome
Autoinflammatory syndromes associated systemic amyloidosis			
Familial Mediterranean fever	-	Serum Amyloid A	Recurrent fever, erysipelas like rashes, erythema and inflammation of scrotum, face and palmoplantar region Gastrointestinal involvement
Muckle wells syndrome/Urticaria-deafness- amyloidosis syndrome	-	Serum Amyloid A	Urticarial like rashes Sensorineural hearing loss Polyarthritis
Tumor necrotic factor receptor-1 associated periodic fever syndrome (TRAPS)	-	Serum Amyloid A	Migratory erythematous macules, patches, urticaria and angioedema

Pathophysiology

- Twenty-one different proteins have been identified as amyloidogenic agents. Polypeptides can adopt alternative misfolded states, making them prone for aggregation. There are multiple processes by which misfolding of protein precursors occurs.
  1. **In primary cutaneous amyloidosis**, the amyloid is of keratinocyte origin, but how the keratin intermediate filaments transform into amyloid (AK) is yet to be elucidated. Apoptosis of keratinocytes may result in deposition of keratin as an abnormal protein. Another theory is that macrophages in the dermis process a normal alpha pattern of keratin into beta-pleated sheet pattern. Active secretion of amyloid by basal keratinocytes is another theory. Several subclasses of keratin are found, particularly CK5. However, appendageal contribution to the amyloid deposits is favored by the presence of CK7, CK17 and CK19 in some lesions. Suggestive causative factors in the formation of this type of amyloid are prolonged friction, pruritus, genetic predisposition, EBV and environmental factors.
  2. **In hereditary amyloidosis,** the replacement of single amino acids can lead to amyloidogenic misfolded proteins, losing the biologic function of the native proteins and, in turn, aggregate. These amyloidogenic variants of the various precursor proteins are thermodynamically less stable. In case of transthyretin, dissociation of tetramers into monomers leads to amyloid formation, while in case of lysosomal proteins, destabilization of their tertiary structure leads to partially folded conformers. Low pH, increased temperatures, limited proteolysis, osmolytes, and metal ions can also alter the tridimensional structure of proteins, shifting the equilibrium towards the amyloidogenic state.
  3. **Senile systemic amyloidosis,** the proteins can also intrinsically acquire a pathologic conformation with aging, as seen in patients with wild type transthyretin senile systemic amyloidosis, caused by misfolding of ATTR tetramer. Proteins can also get intrinsically altered when there is a high serum concentration of protein precursors, as seen in long term hemodialysis patients with increased levels of beta-2-microglobulin.
  4. **AL amyloidosis**, associated with multiple myeloma and Waldenstrom macroglobulinemia, where increased monoclonal light chain proteins in serum form insoluble amyloid fibrils and assemble into abnormal beta pleated sheets. Usually the light chain produced is the λ light chain (80%), however, infrequently, there may be overproduction of heavy chains as well.
  5. **Mechanism of tissue damage** is due to alteration of tissue architecture, interaction with cell surface receptors, inflammation elicited by the amyloid protein deposition, oxidative stress and apoptosis activation.

Primary Localized Cutaneous Amyloidosis

- The main feature of these disorders is the accumulation of amyloid in previously apparently normal skin, without deposits in internal organs.
- **Etiology:** Exact cause is unknown. Various factors implicated are:
  1. Racial susceptibility

2. Chronic rubbing and friction
3. Actinic radiation
4. Familial cases with autosomal dominant mode of inheritance
5. Increased and reduced expression of various pro or anti apoptotic factors respectively.

Lichen, macular and biphasic amyloidosis

- Macular amyloidosis is seen as hyperpigmented patches, usually after prolonged rubbing or scratching. It most frequently occurs on back (interscapular regions), less commonly on extensors of arms and legs.
- Lichen amyloidosis presents as small, discrete, often pruritic, waxy papules with a predilection for the extensor surfaces of the lower limbs. Lichen amyloidosis and macular amyloidosis are considered clinical variants of the same process as transformation from one to other (biphasic) is commonly seen. Association with chronic pruritus, multiple endocrine neoplasia 2A (MEN 2A) syndrome, chronic EBV infection, Kimura's disease and angiolymphoid hyperplasia has been found.

Nodular amyloidosis

- Primary cutaneous nodular amyloidosis is the rarest morphological form of cutaneous amyloidosis, presenting as waxy skin coloured to reddish yellow nodules or infiltrating plaques in acral areas, face, trunk and genitals of elderly patients, with female sex predominance. Occasionally, the nodules may show hemorrhagic spots due to fragile vessels. It may be associated with Sjogren's syndrome and diabetes mellitus. This form can progress to systemic form in 7% of the patients.

Poikilodermatous amyloidosis syndrome

- It is a very rare, distinct subset of cutaneous amyloidosis with an early onset. Patient is of short stature and have light sensitivity with occassionally palmoplantar keratoderma. This constitutes the poikilodermatous cutaneous amyloidosis syndrome.
- Amyloidosis cutis dyschromica is a variant, characterised by widespread reticulate hyperpigmentation with hypopigmented spots over body. It is thought to be a familial disorder.

Secondary Localized Cutaneous Amyloidosis

Amyloid in small amounts can be deposited in various dermatological condition e.g. sweat gland tumors, pilomatricoma, dermatofibroma, seborrheic and solar keratosis, porokeratosis of Mibelli, Bowen's disease, basal cell carcinoma, after PUVA therapy etc.

Diagnosis of Cutaneous Amyloidosis

Histopathology: In both macular and papular forms, amyloid deposits are confined to the papillae in the papillary dermis which may be larger in lichenoid variety and do not extend beyond subpapillary plexus. The overlying epidermis may show hyperkeratosis and papillomatosis with downward proliferation of the rete ridges in lichenoid type while epidermis is normal in macular variety. Amyloid deposits near the dermoepidermal junction contain few melanophages. There is sparse lymphohistiocytic perivascular infiltrate.

Treatment

Macular amyloidosis: Topical steroids, UVB therapy and Nd:YAG laser.

Lichen amyloidosis: Topical steroids, antipruritic agents, dermabrasion, topical DMSO, combined bath PUVA photochemotherapy and oral acitretin, acitretin alone, hydrocolloid dressings and pulsed dye laser can be tried.

Nodular amyloidosis: Removal or destruction by shaving, excision, dermabrasion, CO_2 laser and electrodessication.

Systemic Amyloidosis: It is an uncommon disorder of protein metabolism manifesting as various combinations of carpal tunnel syndrome, macroglossia, specific muco-cutaneous lesions and visceral (cardiac, renal, hepatic and gastrointestinal) involvement.

Primary Systemic (AL) Amyloidosis

- The most common type of amyloidosis results when light chains are produced in excess by clonal or frankly malignant plasma cells. It occurs in 10-15% of patients with full blown multiple myeloma but can also be seen when the affected patient has less than 10% bone marrow plasma cells, the quantity required to make a diagnosis of myeloma. Light chain amyloidosis may also be seen in association with Non-Hodgkin's lymphoma and Waldenström's macroglobulinemia.
- The male to female ratio is 3:2. Although healthy individuals have a preponderance of kappa free light chains (K/λ) = 2:1), the reverse is true in most patients with primary amyloidosis, as excess lambda light chains have a greater propensity to be amyloidogenic.
- 90% of patients will have profound fatigue, weight loss, and edema. Edema may have multiple causes, including hypoalbuminemia (from kidney, bowel, or liver involvement), right heart failure, or simply the impairment of the blood vessels ability to handle hydrostatic pressure challenges.

- Liver, nerve and cardiac involvement is seen in 15-25%, 15-20% and upto 50% of cases respectively, while symptomatic heart failure is seen in 25-33% of patients. Renal involvement manifests as nephrotic syndrome. Involvement of the gastrointestinal tract causes macroglossia, diarrhea due to malabsorption, gastric hypomotility and constipation. In 30% of patients, three or more organs are involved.
- Systemic amyloidosis may also cause orthostatic hypotension, hypothyroidism, reticulonodular infiltrates in the lungs, pleural effusion, lymphadenopathy, splenomegaly and nodular deposits in the skin.
- Periorbital purpura and other manifestations of a bleeding dyscrasia are due to vascular infiltration by amyloid, production of a dysfunctional fibrinogen molecules in liver (dysfibrinogenemia), abnormal platelet aggregation and deficiencies of factors II, V, VII, IX and particularly factor X. Factor X has a predilection to bind to amyloid fibrils and its resultant deficiency cannot easily be corrected by administering plasma because the infused factor X rapidly binds to large amyloid deposits in the liver and spleen without causing a concomitant rise in the blood factor X level.

Hereditary Systemic Amyloidosis

- There are several types of hereditary amyloidosis, but the most common is transthyretin amyloidosis (ATTR), in which aberrant transthyretin (TTR) protein deposits cause severe peripheral and autonomic neuropathy and sometimes cardiac or renal disease, leading to death within 5-15 years of onset of symptoms. More than 80 different mutations in transthyretin, a carrier protein for albumin, have been described. They are inherited in an autosomal dominant fashion.
- Signs and symptoms include hyperesthesia to pain and temperature, motor weakness, impotence, decreased bowel motility, diarrhea, weight loss, incontinence, orthostatic hypotension and diminished deep tendon reflexes.
- Liver transplantation, which removes the source of variant TTR production, can arrest the progression of peripheral and autonomic neuropathy but is only effective if used relatively early in the disease's course, before significant gastrointestinal disease has developed. However, it does not seem to improve cardiomyopathy. Diflunisal, a nonsteroidal anti-inflammatory drug that attaches to the thyroxine-binding site of the TTR tetramer, can stabilize the protein and counteract its tendency to develop a beta-pleated sheet conformation.

Secondary (Reactive/AA) Amyloidosis

- Secondary or AA amyloidosis occurs when serum amyloid A protein, an acute phase reactant produced in response to a variety of infectious, inflammatory or neoplastic disorders, accumulates in the kidneys, gastrointestinal tract and heart. It has been associated with conditions as diverse as rheumatoid arthritis, ankylosing spondylitis, severe gout, tuberculosis, bronchiectasis, osteomyelitis, inflammatory bowel disease, Hodgkin's disease and renal cell carcinoma. Treatment is directed at treatment of the underlying disease process.

Hemodialysis Associated ($A\beta_2M$) Amyloidosis

- Hemodialysis associated amyloidosis is due to the accumulation of beta-2 microglobulin, a component of major histocompatibility complex (MHC) class I molecules. The most common symptom is joint pain and dysfunction, but it can also involve the gastrointestinal tract and myocardium, pericardium, and cardiac valves. The only effective treatment is renal transplantation.

PERFORATING DERMATOSIS

Perforating dermatoses are a class of cutaneous disorders which are characterised by the trans epidermal elimination of dermal connective tissue through the epidermis, often without causing significant disturbance to adjacent tissues.

Primary perforating dermatosis

- Reactive perforating collagenosis /inherited reactive perforating collagenosis (RPC)
- Elastosis perforans serpiginosa (EPS)
- Perforating folliculitis (PF)
- Acquired perforating dermatoses (APD) (often associated with chronic renal failure, chronic liver disease or diabetes mellitus etc.)
  - Kyrle's disease (KD)
  - Acquired reactive perforating collagenosis (A- RPC)
  - Acquired elastosis perforans serpiginosa (A- EPS)
  - Acquired perforating folliculitis (A- PF)

Secondary perforating dermatoses

It is due to elimination of granulomatous material, infectious organisms, endogenous material, foreign material, or neoplastic cells through epidermis.

Classification based on substance eliminated

- **Collagen:** Reactive perforating collagenosis
- **Elastic tissue:** Elastosis perforans serpiginosa (EPS)
- **Necrotic material:** Perforating folliculitis (PF)

Reactive Perforating Collagenosis

It is a rare inherited perforating disorder in which collagen is eliminated through epidermis. The pathogenesis of RPC is unknown. Clinically it presents with keratotic papules or nodules on forearm, elbow, arm, legs and knee. In later stage papules may become umbilicated with large keratotic plug. These lesions heal in 6-8 weeks leaving behind small atrophic hypopigmented scars. Koebnerization may be seen in few cases. Histology shows epidermal hyperplasia, with vertically oriented basophilic collagen fibres eliminated through epidermis which can be stained by Masson's trichrome stain. Differential diagnosis includes folliculitis, prurigo nodularis, keratoacanthoma etc. Treatment includes avoid trauma, topical steroids, topical retinoids and oral methotrexate.

Elastosis Perforans Serpiginosa

In this perforating disorder extruded product from dermis is elastin. 25-40% of cases may be associated with some syndrome e.g. Ehlers-Danlos syndrome, Marfan syndrome, pseudoxanthoma elasticum, Rothmund-Thomson syndrome, osteogenesis imperfecta, etc. D-penicillamine may also induce EPS. Onset of EPS is in second to third decade. Clinically it presents with skin colored keratotic papules arranged in annular or serpiginous pattern on lateral side of neck, face, arms and thighs. Histology shows transepidermal or perifollicular elimination of degenerated elastic fibres which can be stained with Verhoeff-Van Gieson stain. Differential diagnosis includes granuloma annulare, sarcoidosis, discoid lupus erythematosus and porokeratosis. Treatment is not required, for symptomatic cases medical (topical steroids, retinoids) and destructive methods (cryosurgery, electrocautery) may be used.

Perforating Folliculitis

Abnormal keratinization within the follicular infundibulum is associated with development of perforating folliculitis which presents as uniform small keratotic follicular based papules on extremities. On removal of the firm, keratinaceous core plug, a bleeding crater may be seen. Lesions may last for months to years with periods of spontaneous remissions and reocurrences. Histology reveals a dilated follicular infundibulum containing degenerated inflammatory cells, orthokeratotic and parakeratotic keratin and necrotic debris. Curled-up hair is a common finding. Underlying dermis may show perifollicular inflammatory infiltrate composed of lymphocytes, histiocytes and plasma cells. Adjacent to perforation, altered collagen and refractile eosinophilically altered elastic fibres are found. Differential diagnosis includes keratosis pilaris and folliculitis and treatment options are topical keratolytic, steroids and retinoids.

Acquired Perforating Dermatosis

The umbrella term "acquired perforating dermatosis" (APD) refers to a variety of perforating disorders which are frequently associated with an underlying systemic condition, most frequently diabetes mellitus, chronic liver disease and chronic renal failure. Acquired reactive perforating collagenosis is the most common acquired perforating disorder. The pathogenesis is unknown. Several hypothesis exist, including chronic pruritis, infections, microangiopathy and over expression of TGF-3.

Clinically, patients present with pruritic hyperkeratotic papules with keratotic plug predominantly on extensor surface of extremities. Koebnerization may be seen. Histology shows transepidermal elimination of elastin, collagen and necrotic debris. It should be differentiated from folliculitis, prurigo nodularis, lichen planus and verruca. Treatment includes management of underlying disease, antipruritic, topical steroids, topical keratolytic and topical retinoids.

35

CHAPTER

Dermatological Emergencies

Contents

Dermatological diseases may manifest in different patterns in adults. Moreover, skin barrier function is not fully developed in neonatal period, which is even more deficient in premature neonates. It leads to increased chances of damage to skin by drying, hypothermia, infections and other toxic hazards. Although infants seem to possess adequate barrier function comparable to adults, there is increased risk of toxicity from topically applied substances predominantly due to more body surface area-body mass ratio and the metabolism of infants is significantly different from that of adults. Dermatological problems may be congenital or acquired. Some conditions are transient and resolve without treatment. In this chapter, we will discuss only those conditions, which can lead to serious consequences if not managed properly and promptly. If emergency arises and the patient is serious, he/she should always be managed in co-ordination with a physician. Table 35.1 shows the classification of neonatal dermatological emergencies. In primary dermatological emergencies, the cutaneous involvement is the primary cause of morbidity and mortality. In others, cutaneous manifestations can be secondary to systemic involvement due to medical and surgical causes.

Following conditions may need emergency management:

1. **Common:**
   (a) Stevens-Johnson syndrome/Toxic epidermal necrolysis
   (b) Erythroderma and its causes
   (c) Staphylococcal scalded skin syndrome (SSSS)
   (d) Chronic bullous disease of childhood (CBDC)
   (e) Epidermolysis bullosa
   (f) Pemphigus foliaceous
   (g) Pemphigus vulgaris
2. **Less Common:**
   (a) Collodion baby
   (b) Harlequin ichthyosis
   (c) Congenital cutaneous candidiasis (CCC)
3. **Rare:**
   (a) Neonatal herpes simplex infection
   (b) Congenital varicella syndrome

Table 35.1: Classification of neonatal dermatological emergencies

Primary dermatological emergencies	*Dermatological emergencies secondary to medical/ surgical causes*
A. Neonatal erythroderma and its causes	Purpura fulminans Kawasaki disease Sclerema neonatorum
B. Cutaneous neonatal infections: Bacterial - Staphylococcal scalded skin syndrome - Necrotizing fasciitis Viral - Neonatal varicella - Neonatal herpes infection Fungal - Candidiasis in newborn	
C. Vesiculobullous disorders - Epidermolysis bullosa	
D. Metabolic disorders - Neonatal biotin deficiency	
E. Vascular tumors - Kasabach Merritt phenomenon	
F. Miscellaneous - Angioedema - Diffuse cutaneous mastocytosis	

STEVENS-JOHNSON SYNDROME / TOXIC EPIDERMAL NECROLYSIS (SJS / TEN)

A recent classification proposes that epidermal detachment in SJS is limited to less than 10% of body surface area (BSA). Overlapping SJS/TEN has more extensive confluence of erythematous and purpuric macules, leading to epidermal detachment of 10-30% of the BSA. Classic TEN has epidermal detachment of more than 30% BSA.

- Stevens-Johnson syndrome (SJS) presents as a dermatologic emergency characterized by purpuric macules, targetoid lesions and full-thickness epidermal necrosis. At least two mucous membranes, e.g., eyes, mouth and genitalia are also involved. Less than 10% of body surface area is involved. The lesions start on trunk and spread centrifugally.
- Toxic epidermal necrolysis (TEN) is an acute dermatological disease, which requires emergency management. The disorder is characterized by widespread erythematous macules and targetoid lesions; full and partial thickness epidermal necrosis involve more than 30% of the body surface. Commonly, the mucous membranes are also involved. Nearly all cases of toxic epidermal necrolysis are induced by medications, and the mortality rate can approach upto 40%.
- Erythema multiforme (EM) is generally a benign process characterized by fixed lesions, some of them may evolve into target or targetoid lesions, with or without blisters, in symmetric acral distribution. Oral lesions are common. Most cases are secondary to prior infection with a herpes virus. Stevens-Johnson syndrome may have features of both EM and toxic epidermal necrolysis.

Epidemiology

Numerous epidemiologic studies have shown that females have higher incidences of toxic epidermal necrolysis than males. Toxic epidermal necrolysis occurs in all age groups, including newborns. Because drug exposure increases with age, Stevens-Johnson syndrome and toxic epidermal necrolysis occur more frequently in the elderly population.

Etiopathogenesis

Drugs

Most cases of Stevens-Johnson syndrome are drug-induced. Among the medications which are used for the short term, the relative risk is greatest with trimethoprim-sulfamethoxazole and others like sulfonamide antibiotics, aminopenicillins, quinolones, cephalosporins and allopurinol. Among drugs used for long term, the greatest risk of SJS/TEN is seen in the first 2 months of use. Common drugs are antiepileptics, e.g., phenytoin, carbamazepine, phenobarbital, valproic acid, non-steroidal anti-inflammatory drugs and anti-retroviral drugs.

Other Causes

(a) ***Infections:*** The incidence of infection-induced SJS is more common in children notably by *Mycoplasma pneumonie.* Other causes, e.g., tuberculosis, syphilis, viruses, deep fungal infections etc. are not important in children. TEN is mostly caused by drugs and only less commonly it is caused by infections.

(b) Vaccination may be another rare cause of SJS in children.

Clinical Features

Constitutional symptoms, such as fever, cough, or sore throat, may appear 1-3 days prior to any cutaneous lesions. Patients may complain of a burning sensation in their eyes, photophobia, and a burning rash that begins symmetrically on the face and the upper part of the torso.

- The initial skin lesions of SJS/TEN are poorly defined erythematous macules with darker purpuric centres. Flaccid blisters are typically present with full-thickness epidermal necrosis. Lesions extend rapidly, within 2-3 days. Nikolsky's sign may be positive. Delineation of a drug exposure timeline is essential, especially in the 1-3 weeks preceding the cutaneous eruption. Peeling of necrosed skin leaves behind large eroded surfaces (Figure 35.1) which causes loss of water and electrolytes. Average time of epidermal regrowth is 3 weeks.
- **Mucous membranes:** Painful oral erosions cause severe crusting of the lips (Figure 35.2), increased salivation, and impaired alimentation. Involvement of the genitalia may

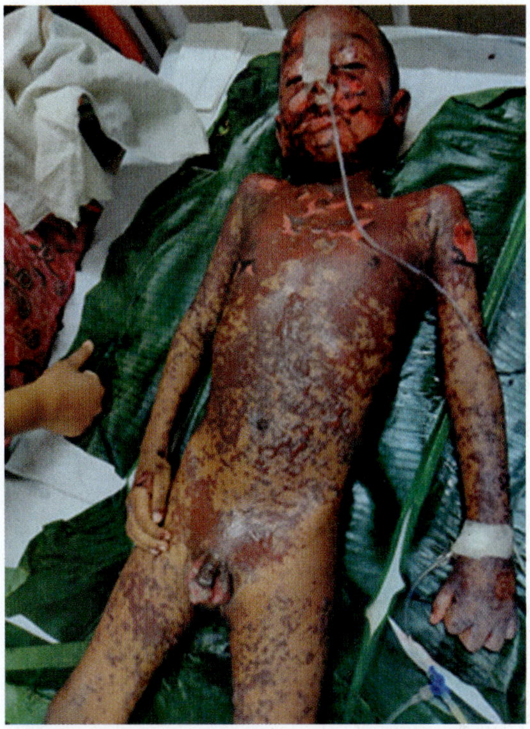

Figure 35.1: Toxic epidermal necrolysis – Peeling and necrosis of skin, leaving behind raw and eroded areas

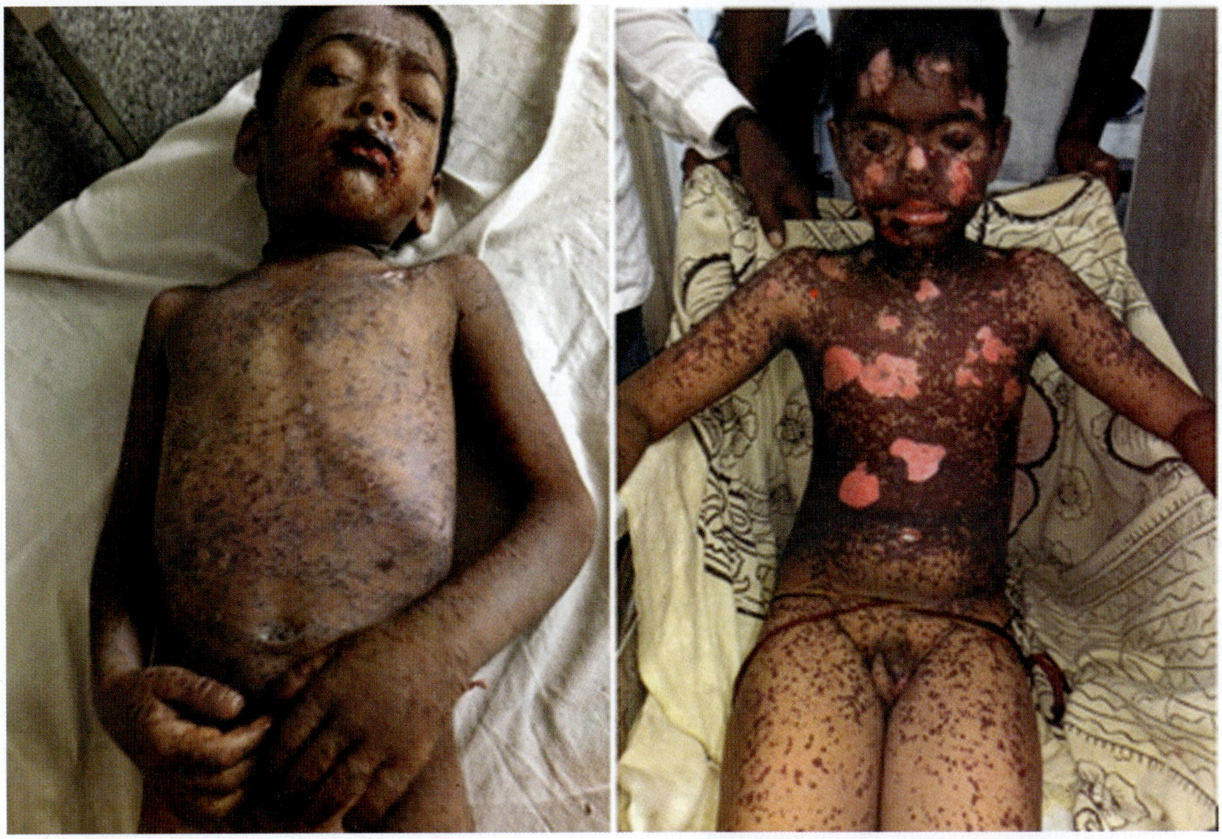

Figure 35.2: SJS to NSAID in 6 years male child (A) and TEN to amoxicillin in 10 years male child (B) (Courtesy–Bhumesh Kumar Katakam)

lead to painful micturition and urinary retention. Lesions have been reported in oropharynx, tracheobronchial tree, esophagus, gastrointestinal tract, genitalia and anal mucosa. Ocular lesions are especially problematic because they have a high risk of sequel. Initially, the conjunctivae are erythematous and painful. The lids are often stuck together, and efforts to loosen them results in tearing of the epidermis.

Differential Diagnosis

- Bullous pemphigoid.
- Burns.
- Staphylococcal scalded skin syndrome.
- Impetigo.
- Pemphigus vulgaris.
- Acute generalized exanthematous pustulosis.
- Linear IgA dermatosis.

Diagnosis

- Routine hematological and biochemistry profile, liver enzyme estimation, renal function test, prothrombin time, activated partial thromboplastin time and cultures of blood and from areas of denuded skin.
- A baseline chest radiograph should be obtained because tracheobronchial involvement and respiratory distress are frequent complications.
- Upper gastrointestinal endoscopy and colonoscopy may be needed to confirm involvement of the gastrointestinal system.
- Similarly, bronchoscopy may be required.

Treatment

- Patients with SJS/TEN should be treated in an ICU.
- The first step in medical treatment is withdrawal of causative drug. Administration of corticosteroids early in the course of disease has been advocated, but their role is controversial.
- Immune globulins (1gm/kg/day intravenously for 3 days) have been advocated to improve immunological dysfunctions. They may decrease autoantibody production, and increase solubilization and removal of immune complexes.
- Immunosuppressants like cyclosporin inhibit key factors in the immune system responsible for immune reactions. It is used as 2.5-5 mg/kg/day orally in 2-3 divided doses for 10-15 days and has been recently found quite useful. It inhibits IL-2 secretion by inhibiting intracellular calcineurin.
- The broad principles of further management are fluid replacement, nutritional supplementation, asepsis and wound care.
- Epidermal loss predisposes the patients for infection and sepsis. Sterile technique is essential to prevent complications from endogenous and exogenous sources.
- For wounds and mucosal care, application of antiseptics may be necessary.
- Frequently applied eye drops may be necessary with daily blunt disruption of synechiae.
- Heated antiseptic baths, heat shields, infrared lamps, and air-fluidized beds may decrease heat loss.

Prognosis

SJS may prove fatal in approximately 5% of patients; toxic epidermal necrolysis may prove fatal in as many as 40% of patients. Sepsis and respiratory infections are the most common complications and ultimately the direct causes of death. Important prognostic factors include the percentage loss of body surface area, age, persistent neutropenia (defined as neutropenia lasting >5 days), hypoalbuminemia (usually < 2 gm/dl), persistent azotemia and development of bronchiolitis obliterans. SCORETEN a 'severity of illness' score developed by Basutji-Gatin *et al.* in 2000, is a validated predictor of mortality in TEN patients.

Scorten

The score is calculated by giving 1 point for each of the following 7 clinical variables during the first 24 hours of evaluation:

- Age more than 40 years.
- Malignancy.
- Heart rate > 120/minute.
- Initial epidermal detachment > 10% of BSA.
- Serum urea level > 28 mg/dl.
- Serum glucose levels > 250 mg/dl; and
- Serum bicarbonate levels < 20 mEq/dl.

The probability of death predicted by this score is as follows:

- 0-1 points-3%; 2 points-12%; 3 points-35%; 4 points-58%; 5 to 7 points-90%.

Complications

- **Ocular complications:** Failure to lyse adhesions and treat keratitis and corneal erosions can result in blindness. Cicatrization of conjunctival erosions may lead to inverted eyelashes. Photophobia, burning sensation in the eyes, watery eyes, sicca-like syndrome, and corneal and conjunctival neovascularization may occur.
- **Cutaneous complications:** TEN/SJS may result in cutaneous scarring. Such scarring may lead to cosmetic disfigurement, and if severe, may lead to contractures and functional impairment. Lesions of the genitourinary system may lead to phimosis or vaginal synechiae.

EXFOLIATIVE DERMATITIS OR ERYTHRODERMA

Exfoliative dermatitis refers to a scaling erythematous dermatitis involving 90% or more of the body surface. It often obscures the primary disease.

Idiopathic exfoliative dermatitis, also sometimes called as Red man syndrome, is characterized by marked palmoplantar keratoderma, dermatopathic lymphadenopathy and raised level of serum immunoglobulin E (IgE) and is more likely to persist for longer period than other types.

Etiopathogenesis

Male to female ratio is 2:1 to 4:1. Age of onset is primarily related to etiology. It usually occurs in older persons, except when the condition results from atopic dermatitis, seborrheic dermatitis, staphylococcal scalded skin syndrome or hereditary ichthyosis.

Cutaneous and the systemic diseases associated with exfoliative dermatitis include the following:

1. Cutaneous Disorders

I. Congenital Causes

a. Ichthyosis
b. Essential fatty acid deficiency
c. Cystic fibrosis dermatosis
d. Multiple carboxylase deficiencies
e. Amino acid disorders with cutaneous manifestations
  - Maple syrup urine disease
  - Neonatal citrullinemia
  - Carbamoyl phosphate synthetase deficiency
  - Methylmalonic acidemia
  - Propionic acidemia

f. Liener's disease
g. Netherton's syndrome
h. Omenn's syndrome
i. Di George's syndrome
j. Severe combined immune deficiency
k. Ectodermal dysplasia

II. Other Cutaneous Disorders

a. Atopic dermatitis
b. Seborrheic dermatitis
c. Pityriasis rubra pilaris
d. Pemphigus
e. Psoriasis
f. Toxic epidermal necrolysis
g. Diffuse cutaneous mastocytosis

2. Drugs

a. **Antibiotics:** Aztreonam, ciprofloxacin, clofazimine, co-trimoxazole, dapsone, fluconazole, griseofulvin, isoniazid, ketoconazole, nalidixic acid, nitrofurantoin, penicillin, rifampicin, streptomycin, sulfonamides, teicoplanin, tetracycline, vancomycin.
b. **Antiviral drugs:** Dideoxyinosine, indinavir, zidovudine.
c. **Antiepileptic drugs:** Carbamazepine, lamotrigine, phenytoin, phenobarbitone.
d. **Anti-inflammatory drugs:** Aspirin, diclofenac, indomethacin, ibuprofen, phenylbutazone, naproxen, sulindac.
e. **Cardiac drugs:** ACE inhibitors, amiodarone, beta-blockers, nifedipine, nitroglycerin, quinidine and verapamil.
f. **Psychiatric drugs:** Amitriptyline, barbiturates, bupropion, chlorpromazine, imipramine.
g. **Others:** Allopurinol, arsenic, chloroquine, gold, hydroxychloroquine, omeprazole, penicillamine, quinine, retinoids, sulfonylureas, interferon-α etc.

3. Infections

a. Staphylococcal scalded skin syndrome
b. Toxic shock syndrome
c. Scarlet fever

d. Generalized congenital and neonatal candidiasis
e. Congenital syphilis
f. Norwegian scabies

4. *Immunological Disorders*

a. Graft-versus-host disease
b. Cutaneous T-cell lymphoma

5. *Metabolic and Nutritional Disorders*

a. Hypogammaglobulinemia
b. Malnutrition
c. Acrodermatitis enteropathica

6. *Malignancy*

a. Lymphomas
b. Leukemias

7. *Idiopathic*

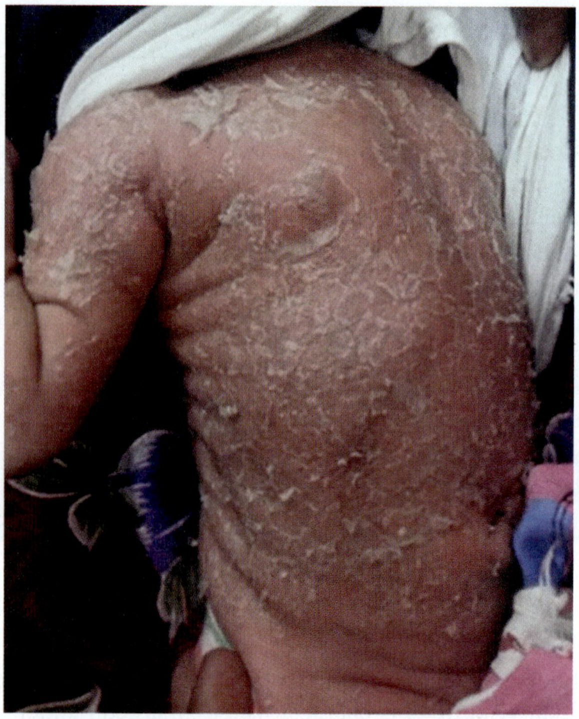

Figure 35.3: Neonatal erythroderma

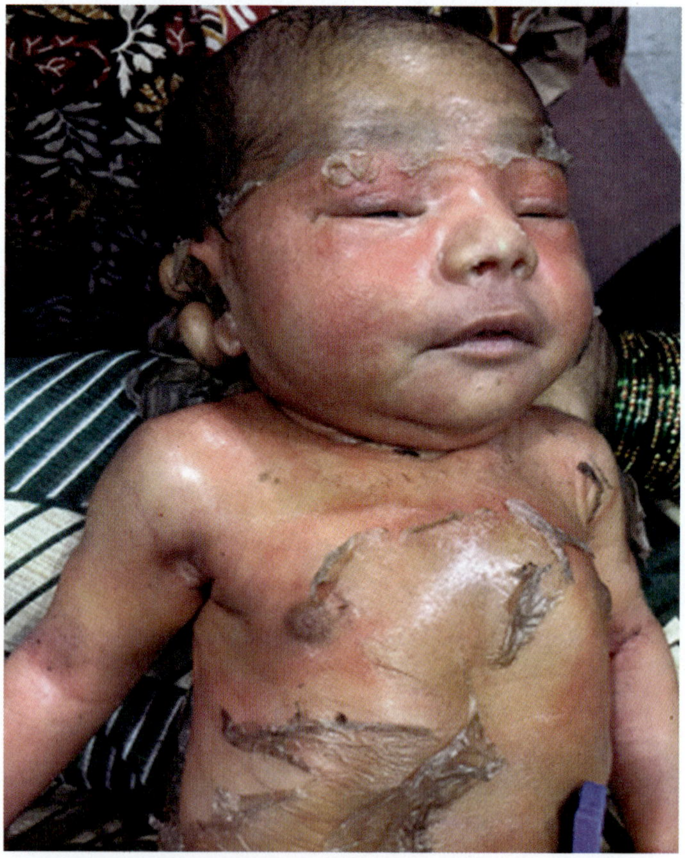

Figure 35.4: Erythroderma in 5 days female neonate (Non-bullous ichthyosiform erythroderma) –Courtesy –Dr. Bhumesh Kumar Katakam

Clinical Features

- Disease usually evolves rapidly when it results from drugs, lymphomas, leukemias, or staphylococcal scalded skin syndrome.
- Patients often present with generalized erythema. Scaling appears 2-6 days after the onset of erythema, which usually begins from flexural areas.
- Ultimately, the entire body surface is dull scarlet red and covered by small, laminated scales (Figures 35.3 and 35.4) which exfoliate profusely.
- Itching of the erythrodermic skin may be severe and the onset is often accompanied by symptoms of general toxicity including fever and chills.
- When exfoliative dermatitis persists for weeks, hair may shed; nails may become ridged, thickened and may shed. Dermatopathic lymphadenopathy may be seen.
- Periorbital skin may be inflamed and edematous, resulting in ectropion (with consequent epiphora).
- Severe complications, e.g., sepsis, high output cardiac failure, capillary leak syndrome may develop.

Differential Diagnosis

- Acanthosis nigricans
- Lichen planus
- Atopic dermatitis
- Pemphigus foliaceous

- Bullous pemphigoid
- Pityriasis rubra pilaris
- Psoriasis
- Contact dermatitis
- Cutaneous T-cell lymphoma
- Sarcoidosis
- Hailey-Hailey disease
- Seborrheic dermatitis
- Graft-versus-host disease

Investigations

- Complete history
- Ask history of the primary disease (e.g., atopic dermatitis).
- Elicit a comprehensive drug history, including over the counter drugs.
- Search for residual signs of underlying disease:
    - Islands of sparing in pityriasis rubra pilaris.
    - Few typical psoriatic plaques in psoriasis.
    - Superficial blisters of pemphigus foliaceous.
    - Erythematous papular lesions of an early drug eruption.
- Raised ESR, anemia, leukocytosis and hypoalbuminemia may be found.
- Serum glucose, calcium, creatinine, platelet count and polymorphonuclear leukocyte counts are of prognostic significance in children who present with erythroderma and fever.
- Increased IgE (when caused by atopic dermatitis).
- Peripheral blood smears and bone marrow examination for leukemia.
- Skin scrapings may reveal hyphae (KOH mount) or scabies mites.
- When suspected, investigations should be carried out to search for malignancy.
- Chest X-ray.
- HIV serology.
- CT/MRI scan, if the clinical features so indicate.
- Patch testing can be performed to unveil contact allergens but should be performed only during periods of remission. Skin biopsy may show non-specific findings of spongiotic dermatitis or primary disease.
- Other tests, which may be performed if they are available and indicated, include sweat chloride test, essential fatty acid levels, plasma amino acid levels and serum zinc levels.

Histopathology

The appearance of exfoliative dermatitis usually masks the specific histologic features of primary disease. The most common histopathologic appearance is of either subacute or chronic dermatitis; however, biopsy is indicated, since diagnostic findings of primary disease are present in 40% of cases if carefully looked for.

Treatment

- Hospital admission should be seriously considered in pediatric patients who present with erythroderma and fever because this presentation is a predictor of hypotension and even toxic shock syndrome.
- Exfoliative dermatitis commonly resists therapy until the underlying disease is treated. Outcome is unpredictable in idiopathic exfoliative dermatitis.
- Discontinue all unnecessary medications. Carefully monitor and control fluid intake body temperature and prevent hypothermia.
- Institute systemic antibiotics if signs of secondary infection are present. Antihistamines help in reducing pruritus and provide needed sedation.
- Systemic steroids may be helpful in some cases but should be avoided in suspected cases of psoriasis and staphylococcal scalded skin syndrome.
- Increased capillary permeability occasionally is severe enough to justify plasma infusion.
- Ensure adequate nutrition with emphasis on protein intake, since exfoliative dermatitis patients lose a lot of protein through excessive desquamation and show a tendency toward hypoalbuminemia.

Prognosis

It is found that fever is a poor prognostic marker and may indicate susceptibility to rapid deterioration. Those with the following characteristics have a higher tendency to develop hypotension:

- Age 3 years or younger, ill appearance, vomiting, a glucose level of 110 mg/dl or less, calcium value of 8.6 mg/dl or less, elevated serum creatinine value, polymorphonuclear leukocyte count of 80% or greater and the presence of focal infection.
- The risk of toxic shock syndrome is increased especially in children with erythroderma and fever who have the

following additional features: age of 3 years or younger, ill appearance, elevated serum creatinine value and hypotension upon arrival.

COLLODION BABY

Collodion baby is a descriptive term for infants born encased in a membrane-like thick scale resembling oiled parchment or collodion. Neonates born with the features of collodion baby subsequently develop lamellar ichthyosis, ichthyosiform erythroderma or other forms of ichthyosis. Collodion baby is a rare congenital condition accounting for 1 in 50,000 to 1 in 100,000 live births.

Etiology

(a) Common severe phenotype (not associated with non-cutaneous features)

- (i) Autosomal recessive non-bullous congenital erythrodermic ichthyosis (50% of cases) including harlequin fetus.
- (ii) Autosomal recessive lamellar ichthyosis (10%) with mutations in the gene for keratinocyte transglutaminase (TGM1) on chromosome 14 q11 in many patients.

(b) Common milder phenotypes

Mild form of ichthyosis vulgaris (10%).

(c) Congenital ichthyosis associated with non-cutaneous features

- (i) Trichothiodystrophy
- (ii) Poorly documented true collodion membrane
  - Sjögren-Larsson syndrome
  - Netherton's syndrome
  - Gaucher disease type II
  - Congenital hypothyroidism
  - Conradi syndrome
  - Dorfman Chanarin syndrome
  - Ketoadipic aciduria
  - Koraxitrachitic syndrome
  - Ichthyosis variegata
  - Palmoplantar keratoderma with anogenital leukokeratosis.

Clinical Features

Newborn is covered with a taut, shiny membrane (Figure 35.5) resembling plastic wrap. The membrane is often fissured and

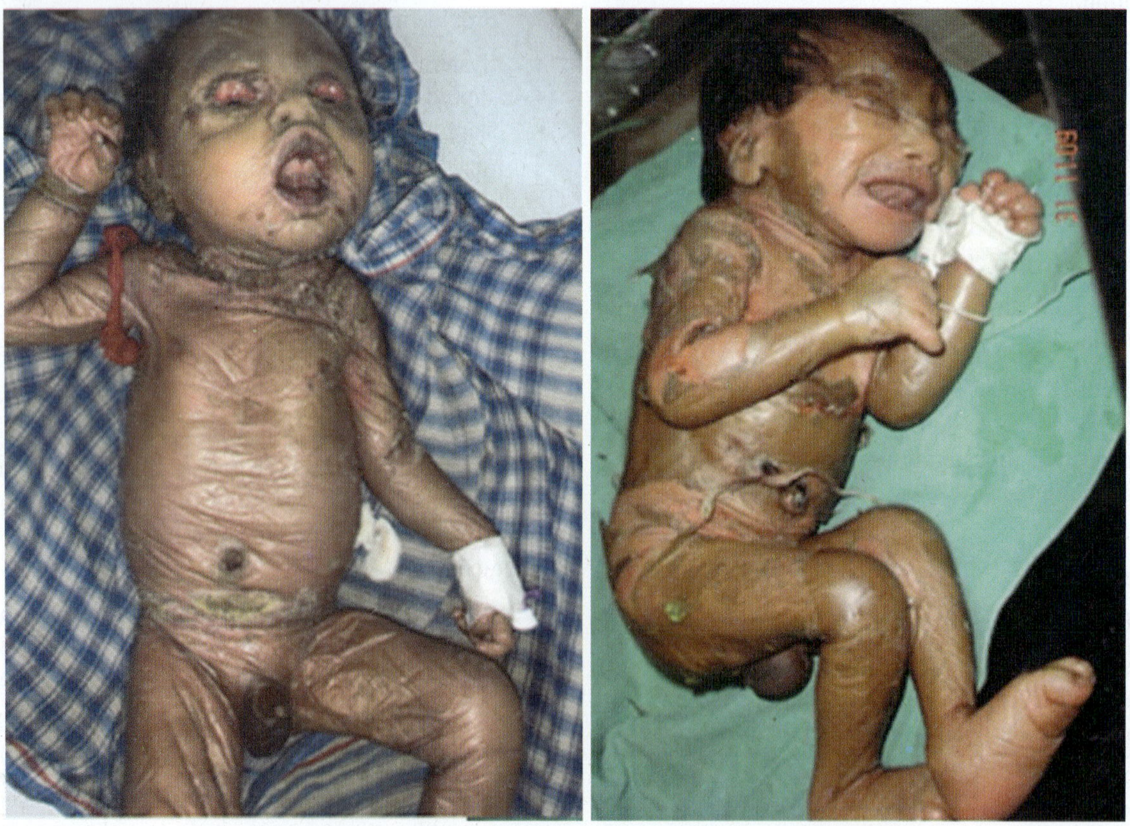

Figure 35.5: Collodion baby (Courtesy– Dr. Bhumesh Kumar Katakam)

cracked at birth. Peeling over the course of several weeks reveals underlying normal red/ivory colored skin or skin with mild scaling that improves with time. Persistence of ichthyosis in some patients may lead to ectropion (eversion of the eyelids), eclabium (eversion of the lips), crumpled pinnae, resolved tapered fingertips and partially flexed hands. Secondary skin infections in the cracks and fissures and scarring in the areas of deep fissuring may occur.

Complications

- Hypothermia and dehydration.
- Secondary infections from gram-positive organisms and Candida albicans.
- Septicemia.

Investigations

(a) Peripheral blood smear
(b) Hair microscopy
(c) Hearing test
(d) Metabolic studies
(e) Skin biopsy
(f) Keratinocyte transglutaminase assay

Histopathology

Light microscopy of the skin in the early neonatal phase of collodion membrane shows a compact hyperkeratosis with a thick, eosinophilic, periodic acid-schiff (PAS) positive stratum corneum. However, the epidermis is attenuated as a result of reduced granular layer. The mid and lower epidermis and dermis are usually unremarkable.

Treatment

The baby is usually transferred to a neonatal intensive care unit. Regular monitoring of vital signs, blood counts, electrolytes and renal functions is needed and facilities for peritoneal dialysis should be available. Humidified, neutral temperature environment and other supportive treatments such as intravenous fluid and tube feeding are often necessary.

Aseptic handling is very important to reduce the risk of infections. Poor sucking in first few days may warrant nasogastric tube feeding. Nasal obstruction can be treated by gentle probing and acral constricting bands should be divided if they are causing pressure effects. For pain relief, paracetamol may be given. Artificial tear is useful if there is severe ectropion.

Care of skin: The aim is to keep the skin soft and attempt should be made to reduce scaling. The collodion membrane should not be debrided (pulled off). Regular emollients such as white soft paraffin to keep the skin moist and application of mild topical steroids to reduce inflammation may be advised.

HARLEQUIN ICHTHYOSIS

Harlequin ichthyosis (HI), also known as ichthyosis fetalis, is the most severe form of congenital ichthyosis. It is characterized by a profound thickening of the keratin layer in fetal skin. The affected neonate is born with a massive, horny shell of dense, plate-like scale and contraction abnormalities of the eyes, ears, mouth and appendages.

The term harlequin derives from the newborn's facial expression and the triangular and diamond-shaped pattern of hyperkeratosis.

Etiopathogenesis

The underlying genetic abnormality in ichthyosis fetalis has been identified as an autosomal recessive mutation in the lipid-transporter gene ABCA12 on chromosome 2.

- There are abnormalities in the structure of lamellar granules and in the expression of epidermal keratin.
- In ichthyosis fetalis, the ABCA12-mediated transfer of lipid to lamellar granules are morphologically abnormal or absent. Normal extrusion of lipid from these granules into the intercellular space cannot occur, and lipid lamellae are not formed. This defective lipid "mortar" between corneocyte "bricks" results in aberrant skin permeability and lack of normal corneocyte desquamation.

Clinical Features

This condition manifests at birth. It may or may not have been diagnosed prenatally in a high-risk family. The history should be carefully explored.

- Markedly thickened skin with large, shiny plates of hyperkeratotic scale is present at birth. Deep, erythematous fissures separate the scales (Figure 35.6).
- The child is often stillborn or dies soon after delivery.
- Severe ectropion is present. The free edges of the upper and lower eyelids are everted, leaving the conjunctiva at risk for desiccation and trauma.
- The pinnae may be small and rudimentary or absent.
- Severe traction on the lips causes eclabium and a fixed, open mouth. This may result in feeding difficulties.
- Nasal hypoplasia and eroded nasal alae may occur.
- The limbs are encased in the thick, hyperkeratotic skin, resulting in flexion contractures of the arms, the legs and

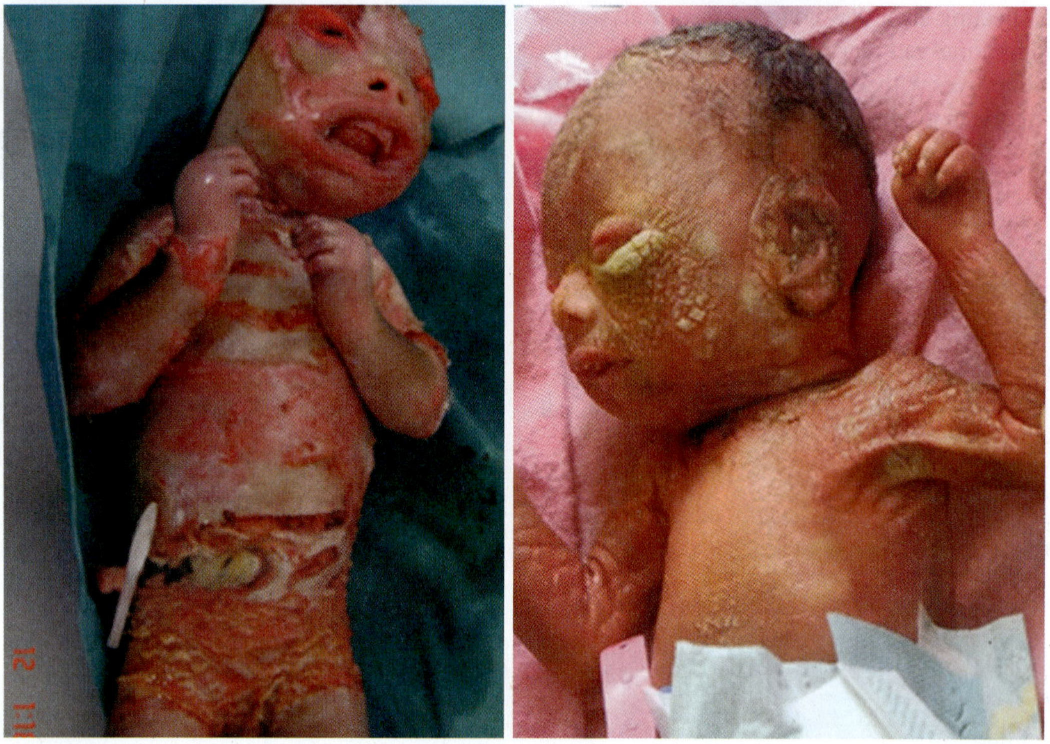

Figure 35.6: Harlequin baby with eclabium and ectropion (Courtesy– Dr. Bhumesh Kumar Katakam)

the digits. Limb motility is poor to absent. Circumferential constriction of a limb can occur, leading to distal swelling or even gangrene.

- Hypoplasia of the fingers, toes and fingernails is reported.
- Polydactyly is described.
- The infants are heat intolerant and can become hyperthermic.
- Restriction of chest-wall expansion can result in respiratory distress, hypoventilation and respiratory failure.
- Dehydration from excess water loss can cause tachycardia and poor urine output.
- Metabolic abnormalities can cause seizures. CNS depression can be a sign of sepsis or hypoxia.
- Hyperkeratosis may restrict spontaneous movements, making neurologic assessment difficult.

Investigations

- Complete sequence analysis of the coding region of ABCA12 gene is performed to identify specific mutations from peripheral blood cells or cells from a buccal smear from affected individual.
- Check the WBC count and blood cultures for signs of infection.
- Closely monitor serum electrolyte levels, which may be abnormal secondary to dehydration.
- Check BUN and creatinine levels for signs of renal failure.
- Monitor hemoglobin levels because anemia is reported.
- Prenatal 3D ultrasonography helps in diagnosing this condition in utero.

Treatment

- The facilities of a neonatal intensive care unit are desirable to cope with the predictable problems of poor sucking, dehydration and resulting electrolyte and renal complications, sepsis and respiratory difficulties.
- Maintain a sterile environment to avoid infection.
- Exposure keratitis results from ectropion of the eyelids. Bathe infants twice daily. Use frequent applications of wet sodium chloride compresses followed by bland lubricants to soften hard skin and facilitate desquamation.
- Isotretinoin is a retinoid that has been used in ichthyosis fetalis. The reported dose is 0.5 mg/kg/day orally.
- Acitretin has also been used. Initial doses of 1 mg/kg/day have been used with success. The duration of therapy is variable and continuous, long-term, daily therapy may be required.

- Monitor affected infants for ongoing assessment of the underlying disorder and for monitoring of retinoid therapy. Adverse effects of retinoid therapy (e.g., mucocutaneous dryness, aberrant liver function tests, hypertriglyceridemia) should be noted.
- Ophthalmological follow up may be required.

Prognosis

Fulminant sepsis remains the most common cause of death in affected infants. Life expectancy is unknown. Survival upto the age of 14 years is reported. Both normal intellect and developmental delay are described. In general, intellectual development is thought to be normal.

STAPHYLOCOCCAL SCALDED SKIN SYNDROME

- Staphylococcal scalded skin syndrome (SSSS) originates from a focus of infection that may be a purulent conjunctivitis, otitis media or occult nasopharyngeal infection, localized skin infections or umbilical infection etc.
- The disease most commonly affects children younger than 5 years, particularly neonates. It usually begins with fever, irritability and a generalized, faint, orange-red, macular erythema with cutaneous tenderness. Periorificial and flexural accentuation may be observed (Figure 35.7).
- Within 24-48 hours, the rash progresses from scarlatiniform to a blistering eruption. Characteristic tissue paper-like wrinkling of the epidermis is followed by the appearance of large, flaccid bullae in the axillae, groin and around the body orifices.
- Subsequent generalized involvement occurs elsewhere on the body, but spares the mucous membranes, palms and soles. Despite the dramatic clinical picture, the entire process usually subsides with superficial desquamation, and healing is usually complete within 7-14 days.
- In older children, it is frequently followed by bacteremia and pneumonia, leading to a poor prognosis. Complications such as severe infections and sepsis do contribute to a low but appreciable fatality rate (2%). Morbidity in some patients who develop cellulitis, sepsis and pneumonia can be significant.

Management

- A Tzanck smear is useful to differentiate TEN from SSSS as acantholytic cells are present in later.
- The primary treatment is to eradicate of the focus of infection by intravenous penicillinase-resistant anti-staphylococcal antibiotics. Clindamycin may be added to decrease toxin production.
- Supportive care and appropriate attention to fluid and electrolyte balance should be given.

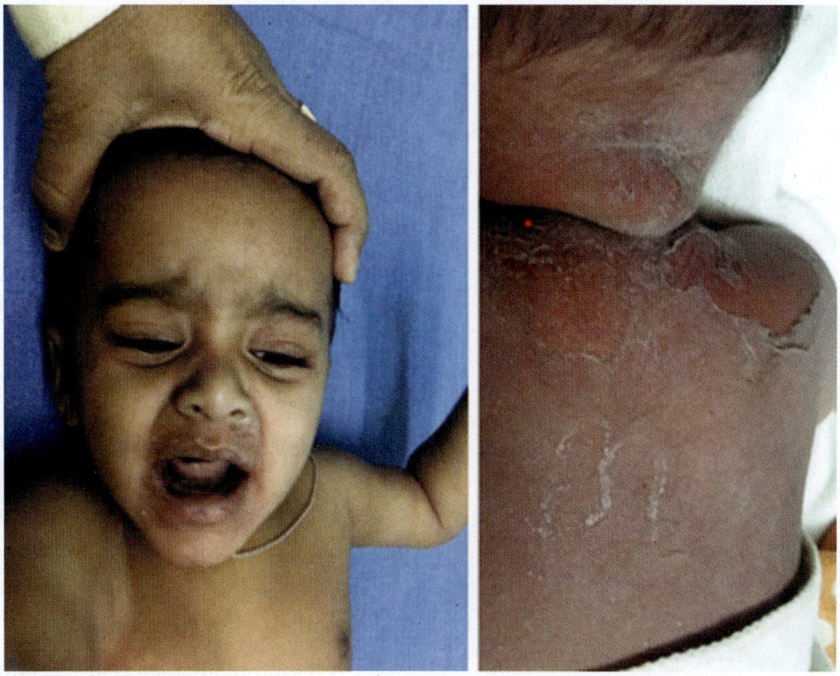

Figure 35.7: SSSS in 8-month-old female infant presenting with fever, irritability, excessive cry and tender erythematous skin. Positive Nikolsky's sign within 12 hours (Courtesy– Dr. Bhumesh Kumar Katakam)

- Moist, denuded areas should be lubricated with a bland emollient to decrease pruritus and tenderness.
- Exchange transfusion has been shown to be beneficial in a preterm infant with severe staphylococcal scalded skin syndrome with sepsis and hyperbilirubinemia, by reducing the bacterial load and exfoliative toxins in the blood.
- For treatment of toxemia, consider using fresh frozen plasma (FFP) at 10 ml/kg in children who are systemically unwell because this is likely to contain antibodies to the exotoxins.
- Enteral nutrition by nasogastric tube must be commenced if oral intake is not possible.

CONGENITAL CUTANEOUS CANDIDIASIS (CCC)

- Congenital cutaneous candidiasis is a rare condition in a newborn infant whose mother has intrauterine *Candida* infection prior to delivery. Presumably, congenital candidiasis is an ascending intrauterine infection with cutaneous or systemic manifestations that typically present within 12 hours after birth.
- Although the congenital systemic form is usually fatal, congenital cutaneous candidiasis has a more benign course.

Clinical Features

- Clinically, there are multiple papules on an erythematous base, generally on the face, neck, limbs and trunk (Figure 35.6). Pustules and vesicles also develop which are usually superficial and resolve spontaneously or with topical treatment.
- Back (Figure 35.8), extensors and skin folds are commonly affected. Generalized or patchy erythema with scaling may be a presenting feature sometimes.

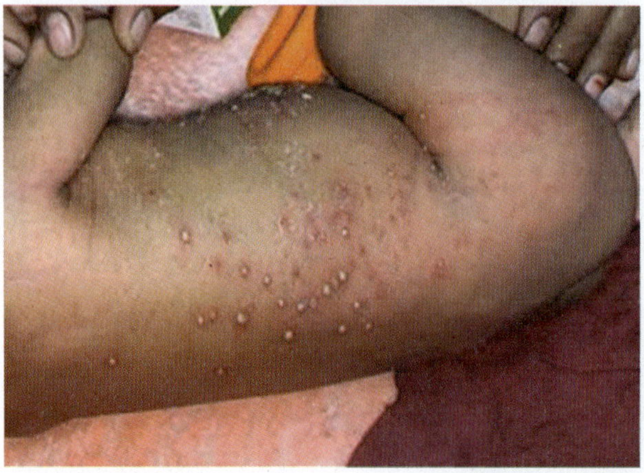

Figure 35.8: Congenital cutaneous candidiasis showing erythematous papulovesicular lesions

- Premature babies are more prone to develop invasive candidiasis. Untreated infants are at higher risk for systemic infection, which is associated with a high mortality rate.
- Some infants have respiratory distress and pneumonia secondary to in utero aspiration of infected amniotic fluid.

Risk Factors

- It was found that 40% of cases are associated with a foreign body in uterus, it may be a contraceptive device or cervical suture.
- Prematurity and candida vulvovaginitis are also predisposing factors. It is believed that yeasts ascend from vagina and penetrate the amniotic membranes.

Investigations

- KOH preparation is the easiest and most cost-effective method for diagnosing CCC.
- Examining the fetal membranes and placenta is useful evidence of CCC. Fetal membranes are inflamed with focal yellow lesions containing yeasts on the umbilical cord and placenta. CCC is always secondary to candida chorioamnionitis, but it may pass unrecognized.
- Microscopic demonstration of *Candida* in epithelial scrapings and fungal culture is diagnostic of CCC.

Treatment

- Topical antifungal therapy (an azole or nystatin) is sufficient in full-term babies with no complications.
- Systemic antifungal therapy is required for infants with sepsis, respiratory distress, unstable vitals, extensive mucocutaneous lesions and positive blood, urine and CSF cultures for *Candida* species.
- Amphotericin B is the first-line agent (0.5-1 mg/kg/day intravenously over 4-6 hours for maximum of one month for complicated cases). In patients who are prone to amphotericin B toxicity, fluconazole may be considered (fluconazole 6-12 mg/kg loading dose orally followed by 3-12 mg/kg/day as a maintenance dose till one week after recovery).

NEONATAL HERPES SIMPLEX VIRUS INFECTION

- Neonatal herpes simplex virus (HSV) infection is caused by the transmission of the virus to a neonate by infected mother.
- Asymptomatic maternal shedding occurs in approximately 7% of pregnant mothers and is responsible for most neonatal HSV infections.

- The risk of HSV transmission to the newborn is as high as 30-50% from a mother who acquires new HSV infection near the time of delivery. Among women who have acquired HSV infection before third trimester of pregnancy, the risk of transmission is less than 1%.
- HSV infection in neonates is most commonly due to HSV-2 and most is acquired during peripartum from exposure to lesions (or shedding virus) in the birth canal, although in utero and postpartum transmission can rarely occur. Neonatal infection can cause long-term sequelae and even death.

Clinical Features

- HSV-2 infection in pregnancy can have devastating effects on the fetus. Neonatal HSV usually manifests within the first 2 weeks of life and clinically ranges from localized skin, mucosal, or eye infections to encephalitis, pneumonitis, disseminated infection and demise (Figure 35.9).
- Neonatal HSV may be difficult to diagnose because, often, no mucocutaneous lesions are present on physical examination. Respiratory distress, jaundice and seizures may occur.
- Most women who deliver infants with neonatal HSV had no prior history, signs, or symptoms of HSV infection. Risk of transmission is highest in pregnant women who are seronegative for both HSV-1 and HSV-2 and acquire a new HSV infection in the third trimester of pregnancy.

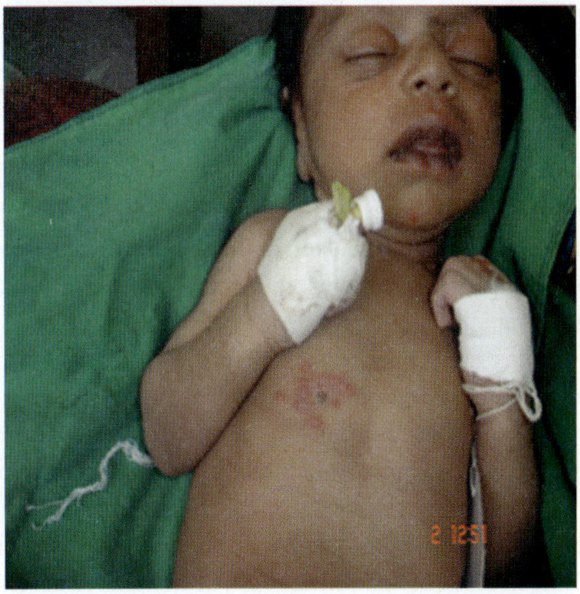

Figure 35.9: Neonatal herpes meningoencephalitis–Multiple, grouped vesicles on an erythematous base, febrile, unconscious, throughing convulsions (Courtesy– Dr. Bhumesh Kumar Katakam)

- Factors that increase the risk of transmission from mother to baby include the type of genital infection at the time of delivery (higher risk with active primary infection), active lesions, prolonged rupture of membranes, vaginal delivery, and an absence of transplacental antibodies. The mortality rate for neonates is extremely high (> 80%) if untreated.

Investigations

- The virus may be isolated by culture and isolation of virus from cerebrospinal fluid, stool, urine, throat, anogenital mucosa, nasopharynx and conjunctivae may be done.
- Tzanck smear can be performed as a rapid test for the presence of multinucleated giant cells.
- Now a days, PCR is being used for the diagnosis of HSV encephalitis.

Treatment

- Neonatal HSV infection should be promptly treated with intravenous acyclovir (20 mg/kg intravenously three times a day for 14-21 days). Antibiotics may be used if secondary bacterial infection develops. Proper management of seizures, fluid and electrolyte imbalance should be done. Ophthalmological opinion for eye involvement should be obtained to prevent ocular complications.
- Women who are HSV-2 negative should be counselled to abstain from intercourse during the third trimester of pregnancy with partners that could be seropositive because primary HSV infection during this time poses the fetus at highest risk of infection.
- The most common approach in attempting to prevent vertical transmission is to advise the women with clinically apparent HSV lesions during labor to undergo cesarean delivery. However, cesarean delivery does not prevent all cases of neonatal infection because in utero infection occurs and ante partum HSV cultures are not a good predictor of neonatal infections.
- Use of acyclovir 400 mg orally three times daily during the third trimester of pregnancy has been proven safe and effective in preventing neonatal herpes and in eliminating the need for cesarean deliveries.

CONGENITAL VARICELLA SYNDROME/ NEONATAL VARICELLA INFECTION

- Congenital varicella syndrome (CVS) is a serious hazard to babies who are born to mother with varicella infection during early part of pregnancy.

- The risk of developing varicella embryopathy is greatest when maternal infection occurs during 8-20 weeks of pregnancy and is in the order of 2%.
- Clinically (Figure 35.10), the infant presents with low birth weight, scars in a dermatomal distribution, eye defects (cataracts, micro-ophthalmia and chorioretinitis), bone and muscle hypoplasia and neurological abnormalities (mental retardation, microcephaly and dysfunction of bladder and bowel sphincters).

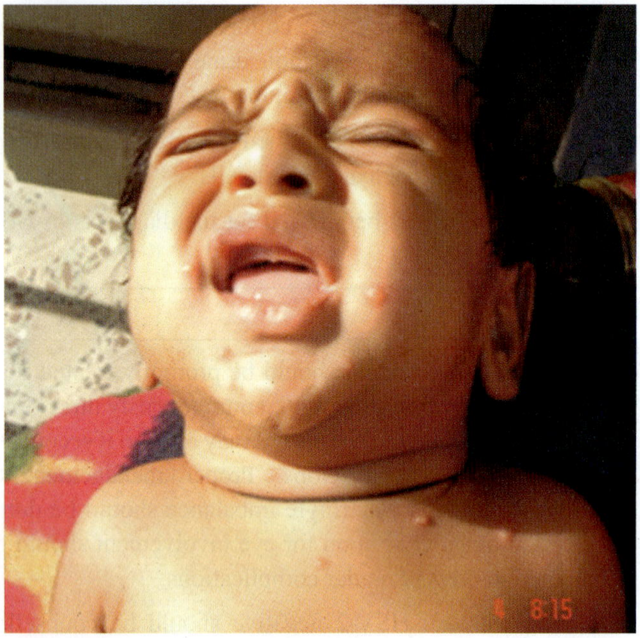

Figure 35.10: Neonatal varicella (Courtesy- Dr. Bhumesh Kumar Katakam)

- Congenital infection without embryopathy occurs after 20 weeks with an increased risk of these children developing herpes zoster early in life.
- Newborns who are born to mothers who develop chickenpox from 5 days before delivery to 2 days after delivery are at great risk (20%) of developing severe disseminated varicella infection.

Management

- Varicella-zoster immunoglobulin (VZIG) should be given to newborns whose mothers develop the disease from 5 days before and 28 days after delivery.
- VZIG should also be given to infants who are born before 28 weeks of gestation, or with a birth weight of less than 1000 gm, and are exposed to chickenpox virus in the first 3 months of life.
- VZIG should be administered at the earliest within 72 hours (one vial containing 125 units for each 10 kg of body weight with a maximum dose of 625 units intramuscularly).
- Intravenous acyclovir (10-20 mg/kg orally five times a day for 5 days) should be administered to high-risk babies irrespective of status of VZIG, whether it was given or not.
- Routine acyclovir prophylaxis is not recommended in neonatal population.
- Varicella infected infants with pneumonitis should strictly be isolated. VZV vaccination is essential in varicella susceptible staff.
- Quarantine of all cases should be maintained until all lesions have crusted.

PURPURA FULMINANS (PF)

Purpura fulminans (PF) is a rare acute disorder characterized by rapidly progressive hemorrhagic necrosis of the skin and disseminated intravascular coagulation.

Purpura fulminans manifesting at birth is caused by homozygous or heterozygous mutations in PROC gene resulting in absolute deficiency of protein C. This condition is inherited as autosomal recessive disorder.

Acute infectious PF is commonly caused by group B streptococcal septicemia, *Neisseria meningitides, Staphylococcus aureus* etc. Gram-negative septicemia due to *E.coli* and *Enterobacter* may also cause PF in neonates.

Clinical Features

PF due to homozygous Protein C deficiency can manifest from 2 hours to 2 weeks after birth. The life-threatening thrombotic events involve skin and vital organs like central nervous system, eyes and kidney. PF presents with erythematous macules that progress rapidly into purpura and ecchymosis (Figure 35.11). The lesions are tender, enlarge rapidly, and coalesce with the development of central necrosis, hemorrhagic blebs and a raised edge with surrounding erythema. The ecchymotic lesions are most commonly distributed on the lower extremities and buttocks, with occasional involvement of the trunk and upper extremities. Subsequently the skin undergoes necrosis resulting in black eschar formation. The margins of the lesions are well-demarcated, erythematous and indurated.

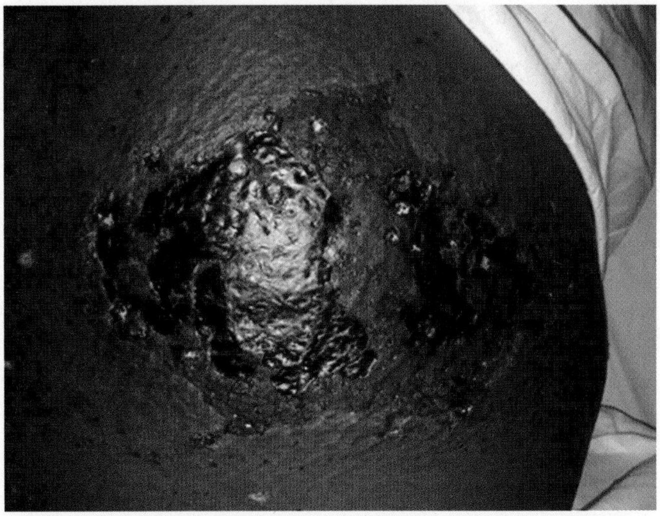

Figure 35.11: Post-varicella purpura fulminans

The cutaneous manifestations culminate in DIC with associated internal bleeding. In acute infectious PF, the characteristic cutaneous lesions occur in a neonate, with associated signs of septicemia like chills, fever, tachycardia, anemia and prostration.

Diagnosis

The estimation of protein C activity is a reliable test to diagnose hereditary protein C deficiency. In homozygous form, the protein C activity is markedly decreased to < 0.02 IU/ml (Lower normal limit, 0.67-0.72 IU/ml). Increased D-dimer levels, low fibrinogen, increased fibrinogen degradation products (FDP), low platelet count, and prothrombin time indicate DIC. These parameters along with clinical response are useful in monitoring protein C therapy. Relevant investigations as indicated by clinical features should be done to know the involvement of central nervous system, kidney and eyes. In acute infectious PF, blood culture should be done to identify the causative organism for septicemia.

Treatment

Rapid diagnosis and aggressive treatment are essential, irrespective of underlying cause. Acute infectious PF can be managed with immediate heparinization and infusion of fresh frozen plasma (FFP), (15 ml/kg every 12 hours) along with the resuscitation measures for septic shock. Administration of proteins C and S (i.e., in the form of fresh frozen plasma or protein C concentrate) may prevent progression of lesions that are not yet necrotic. Repeated infusions may be necessary because of the short half-life of protein C. The mortality is almost 100% in untreated hereditary neonatal PF, whereas acute infectious PF is associated with 50% mortality.

KASABACH-MERRITT PHENOMENON

Kasabach-Merritt phenomenon, also known as Kasabach-Merritt syndrome, is characterized by thrombocytopenia, consumptive coagulopathy and microangiopathic hemolytic anemia in association with a rapidly enlarging vascular lesion. It is most commonly associated with vascular tumors like Kaposiform hemangioendothelioma (KHE) and tufted angioma.

KMP occurs most often within the first few weeks of life and presents with sudden enlargement of the vascular lesion, ecchymosis, prolonged bleeding from various sites. The cutaneous lesions show purpura, edema, induration and ecchymosis. In addition to thrombocytopenia, other laboratory findings include anemia, elevated D-dimers, hypofibrinogenemia, fragmentation of erythrocytes on manual smear, and prolonged coagulation studies. The mortality rate is high (10-30%).

ANGIOEDEMA

The term angioedema (also known as Quincke's edema), describes swelling of the soft tissues of eyelids, lips, tongue, hands, feet, genitalia, airway and gastrointestinal tract. Fifty percent of patients with angioedema also show wheals. Angioedema without wheals has been classified by the European Academy of Allergy and Clinical Immunology into four acquired and three hereditary forms.

Two of the three acquired forms (induced by angiotensin-converting enzyme inhibitors and a non genetic form of C1-INH deficiency) usually occur in adults and are histamine-responsive (histaminergic; termed idiopathic histaminergic acquired angioedema.

Hereditary angioneurotic edema (HAE; hereditary angioedema) is characterized by recurrent episodes of edema of the subcutaneous tissue, particularly the hands, feet, and face, and of the gastrointestinal and/or upper respiratory tracts. It results from a deficiency (85% of patients; type I) or dysfunction (15% of patients, type II) of the inhibitor of the first component of complement [C1-INH]).

The major factor responsible for edema formation is bradykinin, which can induce leakage of post-capillary venules.

General Care and Management of Infant and Child with Serious Skin Disease

- Dermatological emergencies in infants and children may cause serious complications like poor suckling, hypoglycemia, fluid and electrolyte imbalance, hypothermia or hyperthermia, septicemia, septic shock, hypotension, cardiac arrhythmias, urinary retention, seizures, organic brain damage, unconsciousness, coma and even death. Infants are more susceptible to these complications and various factors contributing are:

1. Neonates have thin skin and underdeveloped hypothalamic control. They lack the efficient neural mechanism for temperature control, so are greatly influenced by environmental factors.
2. Thin skin allows more evaporation; even more, if skin disorders like SJS/TEN and erythroderma may affect it. Infants need proportionately more fluid per unit of weight than adults as fluid contents in an infant's body is higher than in an adult. Kidneys are less developed, so reabsorb electrolytes insufficiently, leading to rapid electrolyte imbalance.
3. Newborn infants have only marginal stores and mobilize fat poorly, so hypoglycemia develops more readily than in adults, because of the dependence on an exogenous source of glucose.
4. Respiratory passage is softer, narrower and easily collapsible, leading to early respiratory mucosal obstruction.

- Most of the dermatology inpatient units lack proper dermatological pediatric critical care facilities due to unavailability of necessary equipment's and nursing care. A sick baby requires proper temperature management, humidifier, ventilator and sterile environment to prevent entry and growth of pathogenic bacteria over eroded skin. Availability of necessary equipment's is a vital part of an emergency response. Resuscitation equipment for a seriously ill baby are:

For Airway Maintenance

1. Oxygen and oxygen delivery systems.
2. Ambu bag and mask (450 ml and 1000 ml).
3. Clear oxygen mask, breather and non-rebreather with reservoir.
4. Suction device.
5. Peak flowmeter.
6. Suction catheter (sizes 5-14F).
7. Nasogastric tubes (sizes 6-14F).
8. Pulse oximeter.
9. Laryngoscope handle with extra batteries and bulbs.
10. Laryngoscope blades (Straight 0-4, curved 2-3).
11. Endotracheal tubes (Uncuffed 2.5-5.5, cuffed 6.0-8.0).
12. Stylets (Pediatrics and adults).

For Fluid Management

1. Butterfly needle (19-25 gauge).
2. Catheter over needle device (14-24 gauge).
3. Intraosseous needles (16, 18 gauge).
4. Micro drip set.

Miscellaneous Equipment

1. Measuring tape.
2. Infantometer.
3. Weighing scale.
4. Sphygmomanometer (infant, child and adults).
5. Glucometer.
   - The baby with serious illness is identified by careful observation, history taking, physical examination, appreciation of age and body temperature as risk factors and the judicious use of screening laboratory tests.
   - Hemodynamic monitoring of critically ill patients is essential part of intensive care management. Hemodynamic monitoring includes heart rate, blood pressure, central venous pressure and pulmonary capillary wedge pressure. Heart rate is measured with conventional electrodes placed on the chest, which can also provide rhythm strips, usually in lead II.
   - Blood pressure is measured by a conventional sphygmomanometer using appropriate cuff sizes. The cuff should encompass approximately 2/3rd of length of part of the extremity from which the measurement is obtained. To help define poor perfusion, the lower limit of systolic BP should be $<$ 60 mm of Hg for neonates; $<$ 70 mm of Hg for age 1 month to 1year; $<$ 70 mm of Hg + 2 $\times$ age from age 1-10 years and $<$ 90 mm of Hg if older than 10 years (See Table 35.2).

Table 35.2 Vital signs at various ages			
Age	***Heart rate (beats/minutes)***	***Blood pressure (mm of Hg)***	***Respiratory rate (breaths/minutes)***
Premature	120-170	55-75/35-45	40-70
0-3 months	100-150	65-85/45-55	35-55
3-6 months	90-120	70-90/50-65	30-45
6-12 months	80-120	80-100/55-65	25-40
1-3 years	70-110	90-105/55-70	20-30
3-6 years	65-110	95-110/60-75	20-25
6-12 years	60-95	100-120/60-75	14-22
12 years	55-85	110-135/65-85	12-18

- A central venous catheter (CVC) is required in many critically ill patients. A CVC provides important information about volume status (CVP) and permits the safe infusion of hypertonic solutions (parenteral nutrition, bicarbonate, calcium chloride and glucose) and vasoactive agents (epinephrine, norepinephrine, dopamine) that can produce severe peripheral soft tissue damage if they extravasate from peripheral lines into local tissues.
- Patients, who require significant respiratory support, should be monitored for arterial blood gases and oxygen saturation (pulse oximeter).
- Adequate cardiac output is reflected by good perfusion of the skin. Skin perfusion can be assessed by capillary refill time (Normal capillary refill time is 2 seconds or less).
- Fluid maintenance is essential to prevent dehydration. Daily fluid requirements may be roughly estimated as follows:

  Body weight upto 10 kg = 100 ml/kg.

  Body weight between 10 and 20 kg = 1000 ml + 50 ml/kg for each kg over 10 kg.

  Body weight greater than 20 kg = 1500 ml + 20 ml/kg for each kg over 20 kg.

  Maximum fluid that can be given daily should be less than 2400 ml.
- Fluid requirement can also be calculated by using Parkland's formula: Total fluid volume in first 24 hours is 3 ml × body weight (kg) X TBSA (%) (1/2 of the volume given in first 8 hours and 1/2 of the volume given over the next 16 hours).

SEPSIS

- Sepsis is a clinical term used to describe symptomatic bacteremia, with or without organ dysfunction. Sepsis is characterized by a whole-body inflammatory state (called a systemic inflammatory response syndrome or SIRS) and the presence of a known or suspected infection. It can arise from infections anywhere in the body.
- Clinical manifestations of sepsis are due to effects of circulating bacterial products which cause cytokine release.
- In the neonatal age group, group B streptococci, *Escherichia coli*, and *Listeria monocytogenes* are the pathogens most commonly associated with sepsis.
- In older children and adults *Streptococcus pneumonia, Neisseria meningitides,* and *Staphylococcus aureus* are more common.
- In immunosuppressed patients, gram-negative bacterial infection is a common cause of sepsis.
- Source of infections may be infected wounds, deep-seated abscess, urinary tract infections, intra-abdominal infections, intravenous line or central venous line infections and respiratory tract infections.
- Sepsis can begin with spiking fevers, chills, rapid breathing and rapid heart rate. A patient taking steroids and NSAIDs may not show raised temperature.
- The symptoms rapidly progress to septic shock with fever or decreased body temperature (hypothermia), falling blood pressure, tachycardia, tachypnea, confusion or other changes in mental status like confusion, agitation, lethargy, anxiety, obtundation or coma and blood clotting problems. There may be decreased or no urine output.
- Cause of infection should be sought by culturing clinically appropriate specimens like blood, urine, cerebrospinal fluid, abscesses and swab from affected skin.
- Laboratory findings often include thrombocytopenia, anemia, reduced fibrinogen level, increased fibrin degraded products and neutrophilia or severe neutropenia.
- The therapy of sepsis rests on intravenous antibiotics, surgical drainage of infected fluid collections, fluid replacement and appropriate support for organ dysfunction.

- Neonates should be treated with ampicillin plus cefotaxime and aminoglycoside. Vancomycin should be added in nosocomial infections.
- For proper anaerobic coverage, metronidazole or clindamycin should be added.
- Nosocomial sepsis should be treated with 3rd or 4th generation cephalosporins or an extended gram-negative spectrum penicillin (e.g., Pipericillin-tazobactam) plus an aminoglycoside.
- Empirical use of antifungal agents should also be considered in immunocompromised patients.
- Supportive care such as management of fluid and electrolyte imbalance is of vital importance.
- Septic shock should be managed with intravenous antibiotics, appropriate fluids, inotropes or vasopressors and management of coagulopathy.

GENERAL CARE OF A BABY WITH VESICULOBULLOUS DISORDERS

Epidermolysis Bullosa (Figure 35.12)

- Prevention of secondary infection by appropriate antibiotics, correction of nutrition and anemia is required in most of the patients.
- Prevention of trauma is the most important preventive measure, soft clothes, soft shoes and lubricants should be used.
- Care of eyes, teeth, oral mucosa, oesophagus and nails is necessary in case they are involved.
- Prevention of deformity by appropriate movement and change of postures.
- Once blistering has occurred, the blister should be punctured with a sterile needle or a blade. This may prevent the accumulation of fluid and pressure and may thus prevent the blister from extending.
- Open wounds should be covered with non-adherent dressings such as petrolatum-impregnated soft fine mesh gauze. Tape and any significant pressure to the skin must be avoided.
- Application of mupirocin or fusidic acid topical ointments to treat open or partially healed wounds may be useful to decrease the overgrowth of pseudomonas and staphylococcal organisms.
- Family members should be trained for the care of such baby for homecare.

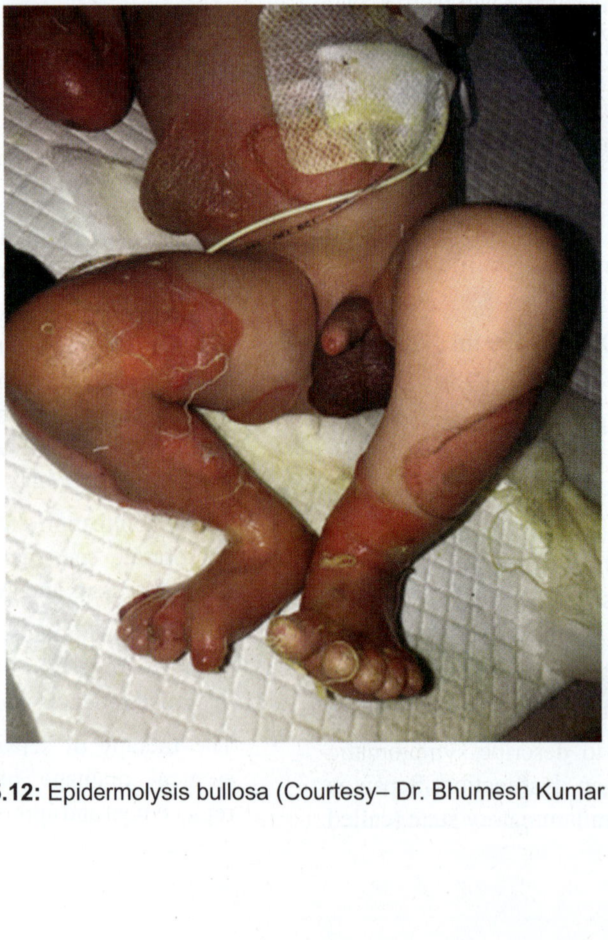

Figure 35.12: Epidermolysis bullosa (Courtesy– Dr. Bhumesh Kumar Katakam)

Pemphigus Vulgaris, Pemphigus Foliaceus and Chronic Bullous Disease of Childhood (Figures 35.13, 35.14 and 35.15)

- Aseptic handling is very important to reduce the risk of infections. Maintain a sterile environment to avoid infection.

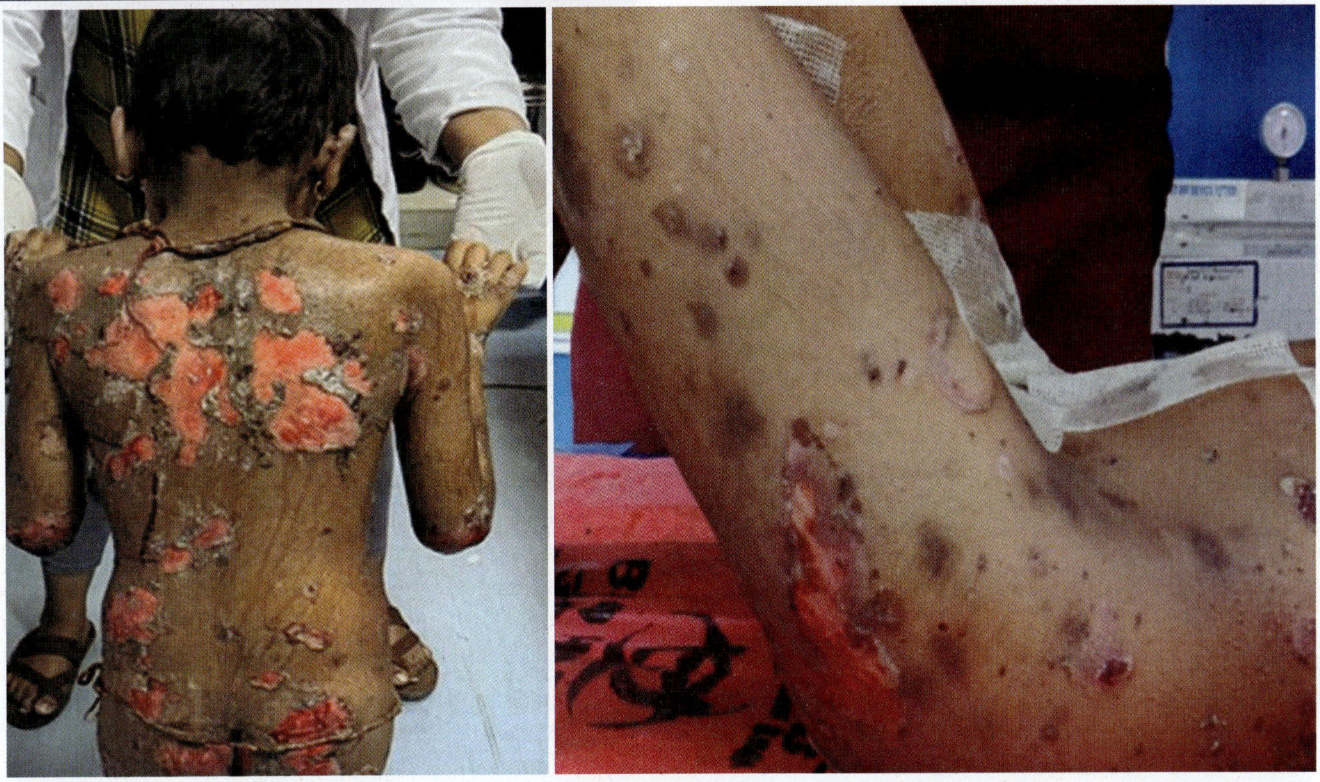

Figure 35.13: Pemphigus vulgaris in 9 years female child showing flaccid bulle and spreading erosions over trunk and extremities

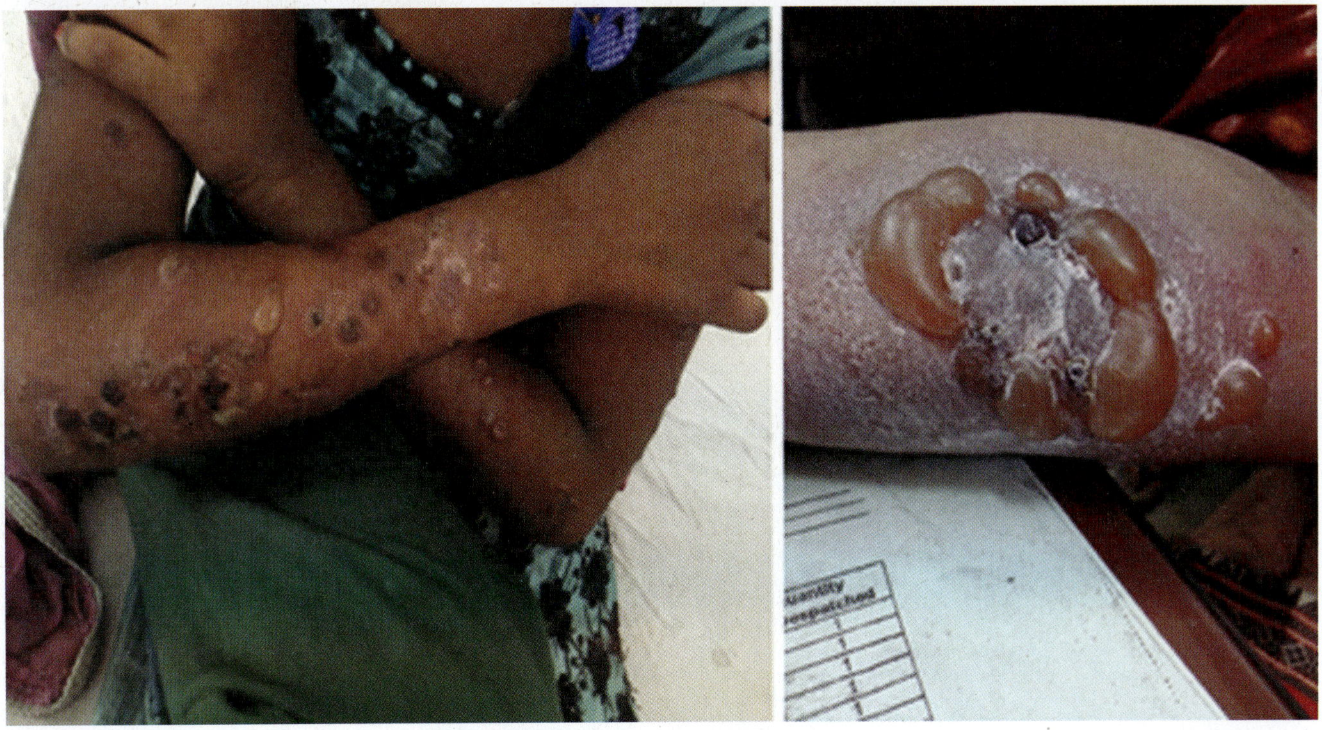

Figure 35.14: CBDC in 13 years female child– Itchy, tense bulle with string of pearl sign (Courtesy– Dr. Bhumesh Kumar Katakam)

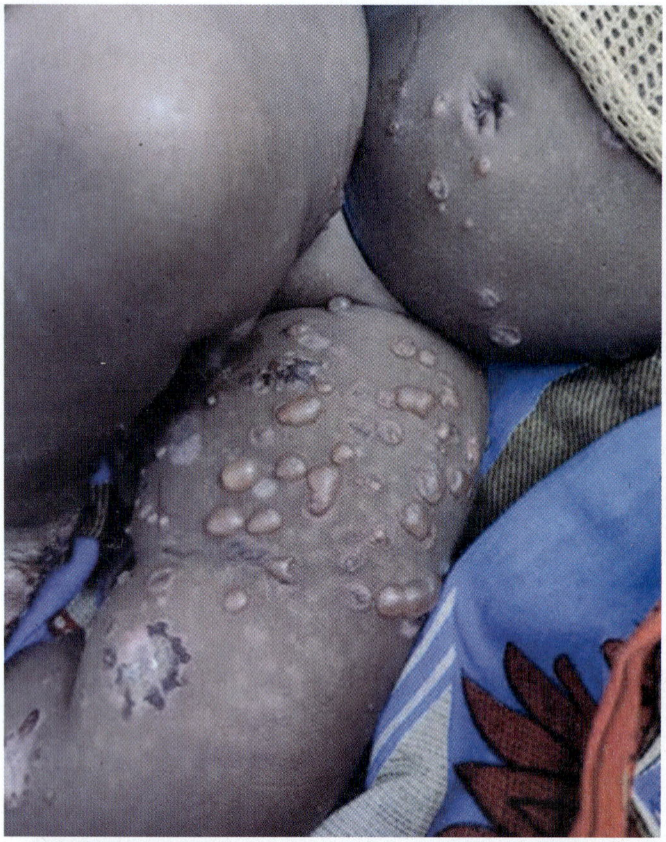

Figure 35.15: Bullous pemphigoid in 12 yrs female

- Isolation of patient and barrier nursing reduce morbidity and mortality in patient with autoimmune bullous disorders.
- Bullae do not need special care, as long they remain intact. Larger bullae may be punctured with a sterile needle.
- Ruptured lesions and erosions may be covered with sterile non-adherent dressings such as petrolatum-impregnated soft fine-mesh gauze or antibiotic-impregnated gauze. They help in preventing secondary infections as well as do not allow body parts to adhere with linens or clothing. Once lesions get dry, they should be left open.
- Infected lesions should be treated with topical mupirocin and sterile dressing changes twice daily.
- Anti-inflammatory agents, and antibiotics may be given if necessary for infected lesions or in case of cellulitis or abscess formation. It fastens healing by preventing superinfection.
- Secondary infection, which may be either systemic or localized to the skin, may occur because of the use of immunosuppressants and the presence of multiple erosions. Patients with pyrexia, tachypnea and tachycardia should be treated with systemic antibiotics.
- Maintaining adequate hydration and electrolyte balance is essential in a baby with severe disease.

36 CHAPTER Dermatological Drug Therapy

Contents

Dermatologic disorders can be treated by topical therapy alone or topical therapy combined with systemic therapy. Initially all dermatological therapies were topical but over the past many decades systemic drugs have become an integral part of dermatological therapy. In many instances topical and systemic therapies complement each other.

TOPICAL THERAPY

Topical therapy is the mainstay of dermatological therapy as the drug is delivered to the affected area directly and thus minimizing the adverse effects.

Principles of Topical Therapy

- Drug is never applied to skin in pure chemical substance form. It is incorporated into an agent called vehicle which may be in the form of liquid, semisolid or solid.
- The vehicle enhances the beneficial effect of drug on skin.
- The efficacy of drug depends upon its inherent potency, its ability to penetrate the skin and the type of preparation.
- Stratum corneum is the main barrier for percutaneous drug absorption. Absorption is inversely proportional to the thickness of stratum corneum. Thus, it is maximum on mucous membranes and minimum on nails. The permeability of stratum corneum is higher in newborns and infants. The pH of skin surface is also higher but the free fatty acid content is less than in adults. These factors not only makes the drug to penetrate better in this population but also makes them susceptible to systemic adverse effects of topically applied drugs.
- Occlusion, vigorous rubbing, hairy area and micronized drugs increase the drug absorption.
- Increasing the frequency of application generally does not enhance the efficacy of drug.
- Topical medications may cause local or systemic toxicity.

- Enough quantity of drug must be applied to cover the affected area.
- Children are at higher risk of side effects topically applied drugs due to higher surface area body mass ratio than adults and altered drug metabolism. This can result in upto 2.7 times higher systemic exposure.
- Newborn skin is more sensitive to cleansers. Ideally a baby soap or cleanser should be devoid of any fragrance and colors.
- Action of soaps can increase the pH of skin resulting in dryness, roughness and flaky skin.
- A solution or gel should not be used on broken or dry skin.
- Reducing the particle size of active ingredient increases the surface area volume ratio allowing greater solubility of drug in the vehicle.
- Factors which increase percutaneous absorption are: inflammation, hydration, occlusion, epidermal injury, heat and type of vehicle.
- Sunscreens are considered safe for children over the age of 2 years.
- Topical anesthetics should not be applied on broken skin in children of less than 3 months of age due to risk of toxicity.

Topical Formulations and Their Clinical Use

Topical formulations are classified into liquids, semisolids and solids.

Liquid Formulations

Wet dressings/compresses: They are used in acute weepy lesions and for removing the crusts, scales and debris from the skin. Clean cloth or gauze is dipped in the prepared solution, squeezed and applied to the affected part for 5 minutes, removed, soaked and reapplied. Commonly used solutions are:

- **Condy's solution:** 1:5000 solution of potassium permanganate for infected weepy lesions.
- **Normal saline: (0.9%)** one teaspoonful of salt in 500 ml of water is used for cleaning.
- **Burrow's solution 5%:** Aluminium acetate in 1:20 water for astringent action.
- **Baths/Soaks:** They are the methods of drug application where a part of the body or whole body is dipped or soaked in medicated water. They cleanse the skin of crust, debris, etc. and deliver the drug to a large area of skin. Examples are: Coal tar bath for psoriasis and starch bath for itchy dermatoses.
- **Lotions:** They are solutions of drug in water, alcohol or other liquid. The lotion may be a clear lotion or a shake lotion where it is to be shaken before use as in calamine lotion. They are useful for exudative dermatoses especially for hairy and intertriginous areas.
- **Tinctures:** They are alcoholic solutions of inorganic compounds, e.g., Tincture iodine as antiseptic and tincture podophyllum for venereal warts.
- **Paints:** They are organic solutions which evaporate rapidly after application and leave a colored film on skin. Examples are gentian violet paint as antibacterial and Castellani's paint as antifungal.
- **Liniments:** Liniments are non-aqueous solutions of drugs in oil or alcoholic. They can be rubbed on skin due to their oily base. They are used as counter-irritants, astringents, emollients, anti pruritic and analgesics.
- **Emulsions:** Emulsions are two phase systems consisting of two immiscible liquids dispersed in another. There are two types of emulsions: water in oil and oil in water.
    - **Water in oil emulsion:** It contains less than 25% water dispersed in oil. These emulsions are less greasy and form a protective film of oil on skin as emollient whereas water evaporates giving a cooling effect. Cold cream is an example of water in oil emulsion.
    - **Oil in water emulsion:** It contains more than 31% water, maybe upto 80%, e.g., vanishing cream. This is a common form of topical formulation.

Semisolid Formulations

- **Gels:** They are semisolid translucent preparations which liquefy on contact with skin and dry to leave behind a greaseless film. They are used in hairy areas and face.
- **Creams:** Creams are semisolid, generally oil in water emulsions used for their cooling, moisturizing and emollient effects. They are used for weeping lesions.
- **Ointments:** Ointments are semisolid preparations containing a greasy base. They are protective, hydrating and lubricating. They generally contain hydrocarbon bases. Petrolatum and white petrolatum are the most commonly used bases in ointments. They provide hydration to skin by preventing water loss. Ointments are used for dry scaly dermatoses and are the most potent semisolid preparation.
- **Pastes:** Pastes are semisolid preparations containing finely dispersed powder in a greasy base like petrolatum. They are protective, soothing and absorbent and are used in decubitus ulcers, thick lichenified plaques and other chronic dermatoses.

Solid Formulations

Powders: Powders are finely crushed, organic or inorganic, solid preparations used for drying, reducing friction or for covering. Commonly used powder formulations contain zinc oxide, calamine, antibacterial and antifungal agents.

Guidelines for Topical Therapy

- Bland preparations are used for acutely inflamed lesions.
- Moist and oozy lesions are to be treated with wet preparations such as lotions or creams 'wet on wet'.
- Dry and scaly dermatoses are treated with ointments.
- Hairy areas need lotions or gels.
- Amount of cream or ointment required for a single application is approximately 2 gm on face or hands; 3 gm on one arm; 4 gm on one leg and 30 gm on entire body.
- Alcohol containing preparations and toxic substances like urea, hexachlorophene containing substances are to be avoided in neonatal skin.

TOPICAL DRUGS FOR DERMATOLOGIC THERAPY

Anti-Acne Drugs

- **Retinoids:** They are primarily used for comedonal acne. Local irritation is main drawback. Commonly used topical retinoids are: Tretinoin 0.025% or 0.05% cream and adapalene gel 0.1% or 0.3%. Both are applied at night.
- **Benzoyl peroxide:** It is anti *Propionibacterium acnes* and mildly comedolytic. It is used in both inflammatory and non-inflammatory acne. It is available in gel, cream and lotion forms in 2.5% to 10% concentrations. Erythema, burning and dryness are important side effects.
- **Topical antibiotics:** They reduce the population of *P. acnes* and act as anti-inflammatory agents. Commonly used antibiotics include clindamycin 1%, erythromycin 2% and nadifloxacin 1%. They are available as gel, cream or lotion forms and are applied twice daily. They can be used in combination with retinoids or benzoyl peroxide. Long term use may result in bacterial resistance.

Topical Antifungals

- **Imidazoles:** They are fungistatic and are effective against dermatophytes, *Candida* and *Pityrosporum* yeasts. They are available in creams, lotions, powders, sprays and shampoo formulations. Various imidazoles include clotrimazole, miconazole, ketaconazole, econazole, sertaconazole, etc in 1-2% concentration.
- **Allylamines:** They are fungistatic against *Candida* and fungicidal against dermatophytes. They are slightly superior to topical imidazoles in cure rate and require shorter duration of therapy. Terbinafine and naftifine are the allylamines in use as 1% cream, lotion or nail lacquer.
- **Morpholines:** Amorolfine is fungicidal and is used as 5% nail lacquer for onychomycosis and 0.25% cream for cutaneous infections. It is applied once or twice a week as it is water resistant.
- **Others:** Butenafine, ciclopirox, nystatin, tolnaftate, zinc pyrithione, selenium disulfide, gentian violet, benzoic acid and Castellani's paint are the other topical antifungals used.

Topical Antibacterial

Topical antibacterials are frequently used in pyoderma, superficial wounds, acne and prophylactically after minor surgery and cosmetic procedures. Resistance development and allergic hypersensitivity are the limiting factors for their use. The commonly used topical antibiotics include mupirocin, fusidic acid, gentamycin, neomycin, clindamycin, erythromycin, bacitracin, metronidazole and silver sulfadiazine.

Topical Calcineurin Inhibitors

The new topical non-steroidal anti-inflammatory agents pimecrolimus and tacrolimus provide an alternative for the treatment of atopic dermatitis. These calcineurin inhibitors selectively suppress the release of inflammatory mediators from lymphocytes without compromising the function of melanocytes, fibroblasts, or endothelial cells. As a consequence, they are not associated with the development of pigment alteration, atrophy or telangiectasias. They can be applied at any site including the genital skin, breasts and face. However, they are contraindicated in erythrodermic conditions where significant percutaneous absorption may occur. Tacrolimus ointment is available in 0.03% and 0.1% formulations and is currently indicated as a second-line treatment for moderate to severe atopic dermatitis (AD). Topical calcineurin inhibitors can be used for pityriasis alba, psoriasis, seborrheic dermatitis, contact dermatitis, lichen sclerosus, lichen planus and vitiligo. They are approved for use in children above 2 years of age only.

Topical Corticosteroids

Topical corticosteroids are the most frequently used drugs in dermatology for inflammatory dermatoses.

Mechanism of Action

1. Anti-inflammatory.
2. Immunosuppressive.

3. Antimitotic.
4. Vasoconstrictive.

Classification on The Basis of Potency

Class I (Ultra-high potent)

1. Clobetasol propionate cream 0.05%.
2. Halobetasol propionate cream 0.05%.

Class II (High)

1. Betamethasone dipropionate ointment 0.05%.
2. Mometasone furoate ointment 0.1%.
3. Fluocinonide ointment or cream 0.05%.
4. Halcinonide ointment or cream 0.1%.

Class III

1. Fluticasone propionate ointment 0.005%.
2. Betamethasone valerate ointment 0.01%.
3. Triamcinolone acetonide ointment 0.1%.
4. Betamethasone dipropionate cream 0.05%.

Class IV (Moderate)

1. Fluocinolone acetonide ointment 0.025%.
2. Triamcinolone acetonide cream 0.1%.
3. Hydrocortisone valerate ointment 0.2%.

Class V

1. Betamethasone dipropionate lotion 0.02%.
2. Betamethasone valerate cream 0.1%.
3. Fluocinolone acetonide cream 0.025%.
4. Triamcinolone acetonide lotion 0.1%.
5. Hydrocortisone valerate cream 0.2%.
6. Hydrocortisone butyrate cream 0.1%.

Class VI (Low)

1. Betamethasone valerate lotion 0.05%.
2. Desonide cream 0.05%.
3. Clobetasone butyrate cream 0.05%.

Class VII

1. Hydrocortisone acetate 0.5% to 2.5%.

Indications

1. **Eczematous dermatoses:** Atopic dermatitis, contact dermatitis, seborrheic dermatitis, nummular dermatitis, lichen simplex chronicus, diaper dermatitis, pompholyx.
2. **Papulosquamous disorders:** Psoriasis, lichen planus, pityriasis rubra pilaris.
3. **Collagen disorders:** Lupus erythematosus, dermatomyositis.
4. **Neutrophilic dermatoses:** Behçet's disease, pyoderma gangrenosum.
5. **Bullous disorders:** Pemphigus, bullous pemphigoid, pemphigoid gestationis.
6. **Other diseases:** Alopecia areata, granuloma annulare, insect bite, nodular scabies, polymorphic light eruptions, vitiligo.

Contraindications

1. Hypersensitivity to topical corticosteroid or a component of the vehicle.
2. Untreated local bacterial, viral or fungal infections.

Side Effects

1. **Atrophic changes:** Atrophy, telangiectasia, purpura, striae, stellate pseudoscars, hypopigmentation, fragile skin, purpura.
2. Hypertrichosis.
3. Acneiform eruptions.
4. Delayed wound healing.
5. Increased susceptibility to bacterial, viral and fungal infections.
6. Perioral dermatitis, rosacea.
7. Contact dermatitis to steroid or its vehicle.
8. **Systemic effects:** Suppression of HPA axis, Cushing's syndrome (Figure 36.1), hyperglycemia, growth retardation in children.

Guidelines for Topical Use of Corticosteroids

1. Selection of steroid should be based on diagnosis, age of the patient, the area of usage and type of vehicle.
2. Most of the time once daily application is sufficient.
3. Overnight occlusion with polythene film increases the penetration and may be useful for treating thick lesions.

4. To avoid systemic absorption not more than 45 gm/week of potent or 100 gm/week of weak or moderately potent corticosteroid should be applied topically.
5. Highly potent corticosteroids should be used only for short periods (2 to 3 weeks) or intermittently. It may be followed by less potent preparations.
6. Once the disease control is achieved reduce the frequency of application as alternate day or weekend therapy. It should not be stopped suddenly to avoid rebound phenomenon.
7. Low to medium potency steroids should be used to treat acute inflammatory lesions of face and flexures and more potent for chronic, hyperkeratotic, or lichenified lesions of palms and soles.
8. Special care should be taken to treat certain areas like intertriginous areas, eyelids and scrotum and certain populations like children and elderly to prevent the local and systemic side effects.
9. Combination therapy with keratolytics, retinoids or anti-infective agents, when clinically indicated, will reduce the risk of side effects.

Pediatric Uses of Corticosteroids

- Children and, in particular, infants are at high risk of absorbing topical corticosteroids due to thinner skin, higher skin surface area to body weight ratio and low ability to metabolize the potent corticosteroids rapidly.
- Application of steroids to diaper area causes occlusion of the steroid by the diaper resulting in increased penetration.
- Excess absorption of topical corticosteroid can suppress endogenous cortisol production in children. Stopping of therapy after prolonged use may rarely result in addisonian crisis. Chronic suppression of cortisol production may result in growth retardation.

Topical Steroid Abuse in Children

As compared to adults, children are more susceptible for side effects as their skin has poorly developed barrier function and a large surface area to weight ratio causes significant absorption of drug. Face is the most common site where topical steroids are misused in children. This scenario predominantly occurring in adults has resulted in simultaneous increase in frequency of tinea corporis and cruris in children, infants as well as neonates. A study done in eastern part of India revealed that 94% of children had applied topical steroid, alone or in combination with antifungal cream over lesions of tinea. Use of potent topical corticosteroid cream for a longer duration leads to extensive lesions. Multiple site involvement, involvement of face and extensive lesions mark the current trend of dermatophytoses in children. Caregivers should be counselled about their use and misuse. Extended duration of treatment is required in these cases and fluconazole is the preferred systemic antifungal. Dermatologists, manufacturers, pharmacists and caregivers all should work together to prevent misuse of topical corticosteroids.

KERATOLYTIC AGENTS

Keratolytic agents are substances which cause shedding of stratum corneum. They are used to treat hyperkeratosis. Various keratolytics used are:

1. **Salicylic acid:** It is used in 3% to 6% concentration. Excessive use in children can result in salicylism consisting of headache, dizziness, tinnitus, hearing difficulty and mental confusion.
2. **Urea:** It is used in 5% to 10% concentration in cream base. In addition to its use as keratolytic it is also used as hydrating agent.
3. **Coal tar:** It has antibacterial, antimitotic, anti-inflammatory and antipruritic properties in addition to keratolytic action. It is used in 3% to 5% strength.
4. **Alpha-hydroxy acids (Glycolic, lactic and malic acid):** They are used as moisturizers and peeling agents and in anti-aging preparations. In children they can cause burning sensation.

Moisturizers

- The term moisturizer is used to describe any agent that softens or smoothens the skin. They consist of emollients, occlusives, humectants, protein rejuvenators and additives.
- The common indications in are eczemas, ichthyosiform disorders, papulosquamous disorders, nutritional disorders and adolescent acne.
- Oil massage is a part of normal skin care and the use of coconut oil, sunflower oil, petrolatum ointment are beneficial while mustard oil, soybean oil and amla oil should be avoided.
- Use of emollients lead to decrease number and frequency of applications and lesser amount of topical steroids in children with atopic dermatitis.
- Parents should be given proper instructions regarding mode, quantity, frequency and duration of application.
- Moisturizer should be applied to damp skin to retain hydration.

SYSTEMIC THERAPY

Systemic therapy is required in most of the cases when topical therapy alone is not sufficient to treat the disease.

Immunosuppressive Agents

Oral steroids are used in short courses for quick action and a bridging therapy while other immunosuppressants start functioning. Parents should be adequately counselled before initiation of these therapies. They should know the need of the drug, importance of investigations, monitoring and danger signs to look for, and the duration of therapy. It is essential to do workup before initiation of therapy and regular periodic monitoring is necessary when a child is on immunosuppressants. It should be noted that vaccination may not act as intended if given during treatment with immunosuppressants.

Systemic Corticosteroids

Corticosteroids constitute the mainstay in dermatologic therapy by virtue of their potent immunosuppressive and anti-inflammatory effect. Because of their serious side effects they should be used very cautiously.

Indications

- **Bullous disorders:** Pemphigus, bullous pemphigoid, cicatricial pemphigoid, linear IgA disease, epidermolysis bullosa aquisita, herpes gestationis, erythema multiforme, toxic epidermal necrolysis.
- **Connective tissue diseases:** Systemic lupus erythematosus, progressive systemic sclerosis, dermatomyositis, mixed connective tissue disease.
- **Severe dermatitis:** Atopic dermatitis, contact dermatitis, photodermatoses, exfoliative dermatitis, erythrodermas.
- **Neutrophilic dermatoses:** Pyoderma gangrenosum, Sweet's syndrome, Behçet's disease.
- Sarcoidosis.
- Reactions in leprosy.
- Problematic hemangiomas of infancy.
- Vasculitis.
- Urticaria/angioedema.

Dosage Schedules (Table 36.1)

Table 36.1: Equivalent corticosteroid potency and duration of action

Corticosteroids	*Equivalent corticosteroid potency (mg)*	*Duration of action (hours)*
Short acting		
Hydrocortisone	20	8-12
Cortisone	25	8-12
Intermediate acting		
Prednisone/ prednisolone	5	24-36
Methyl prednisolone	4	24-36
Triamcinolone	4	24-36
Deflazacort	6	24
Long acting		
Dexamethasone	0.75	36-54
Betamethasone	0.6-0.75	36-54

Contd.

- **Oral route:** Intermediate acting steroid, prednisolone, is most commonly used in varying dosage from 2.5 mg to several hundred milligrams daily depending upon the type and severity of the disease. It is usually used as 1mg/kg body weight/day. It is given in a single daily dose at 8.00 AM because of lower suppression of HPA axis at this time.
- **Intravenous/Intramuscular route:** Hydrocortisone, methyl prednisolone, betamethasone and dexamethasone in aqueous solutions are used for intravenous routes in emergency situations or to gain rapid control of disease. Dexamethasone and Triamcinolone are most commonly used intramuscularly.
- **Pulsed steroid therapy:** High dosage of steroids is given intravenously on monthly pulse basis. Methylprednisolone 0.5 to 1 gm daily is given in 2-3 hours in IV fluids. Dexamethasone with cyclophosphamide has also been used in pulse therapy (DCP pulse). It is mostly used in pemphigus vulgaris but other conditions where it has been used, include pemphigoid, SLE, dermatomyositis and systemic scleroderma. Pulsed steroid therapy may be associated with serious side effects like atrial fibrillation, myocardial infarction, anaphylaxis, seizures and sudden death.

Side Effects

- **Gastrointestinal:** Peptic ulceration, intestinal perforation, pancreatitis.
- **Cardiovascular:** Hypertension, sodium and fluid retention, hypokalemia, increased risk of atherosclerosis.
- **Musculoskeletal:** Osteoporosis with spontaneous fractures, avascular necrosis, myopathy.
- **Ocular:** Glaucoma, cataracts.
- **Endocrinologic:** Suppression of hypothalamic-pituitary-adrenal axis, growth failure, secondary amenorrhea.
- **Metabolic:** Hyperglycemia and unmasking of diabetes mellitus, hyperlipidemia, redistribution of body fat (Cushingoid features, Figure 36.1).

- **Infections:** Increased incidence of infections, reactivation of tuberculosis.
- **Fibroblast inhibition:** Delayed wound healing, subcutaneous tissue atrophy causing striae, purpura, ecchymoses.
- **Psychiatric:** Psychosis, agitation, depression.

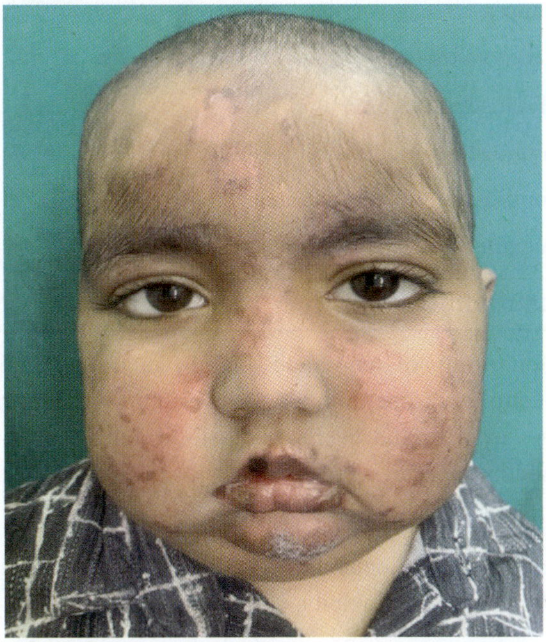

Figure 36.1: Child of SLE with cushingoid features

Contraindications

The following are the relative contraindications of corticosteroids:

- Hypertension.
- Peptic ulcer disease.
- Any infective focus in the body.
- Glaucoma.
- Cataract.
- First trimester of pregnancy.

Precautions for Steroid Therapy in Children

- Apart from side effects common to all ages, children are at higher risk of growth suppression as an important side effect of systemic steroid therapy. Therefore, children on long-term steroid therapy should be regularly monitored for height and weight.
- Live-virus vaccines, e.g., measles, oral polio, varicella should not be given to children who are on 20 mg/day or more of prednisolone for 14 days or more.
- Steroids should not be given to a healthy child who has recent varicella exposure and is not varicella immune because varicella can be fatal in this situation.
- Systemic steroid therapy is not to be given to children having ocular herpes simplex and untreated tuberculosis.
- Systemic steroids should be avoided in children with diabetes, hypertension, peptic ulcer disease, renal insufficiency and psychosis.

Prevention of Side Effects

Side effects of steroids can be significantly prevented by taking the following measures:

- Administering the total daily dose as a single morning dose to minimize the pituitary-adrenal suppression.
- After the control of disease activity, giving the 48-hour dose as a single morning dose to minimize the cushingoid effect of steroids.
- Restriction of sodium intake and supplementation of potassium.
- Use of proton pump inhibitors or antacids to prevent hyperacidity.
- Providing calcium supplementation as 1 to 1.5 gm of calcium/day and Vitamin D 50000 IU twice weekly.
- Monitoring of blood pressure, blood sugar and electrolytes regularly.

Deflazacort

It is a synthetic oxazoline derivative of prednisolone. The average potency ratio of deflazacort to prednisolone is 0.69-0.89 and 6 mg of deflazacort is equivalent to 5 mg of prednisolone. Doses of deflazacort usually lie in the range 0.25-1.5 mg/kg/day. Deflazacort has several advantages over prednisolone and is more suitable for pediatric patients requiring glucocorticosteroids. Deflazacort has bone sparing effect as compared to prednisolone. Further, the drug appears to have less negative impact on growth rate as well as less HPA axis suppression in children with diseases requiring corticosteroid therapy. Deflazacort is less diabetogenic than prednisone in healthy subjects.

Azathioprine

Azathioprine is an anti-metabolite which interferes with the DNA and RNA synthesis of the cells. It is used as immunosuppressant, anti-inflammatory and steroid-sparing agent.

Indications

- Dermatomyositis.
- Systemic lupus erythematosus.
- Pemphigus vulgaris.

Contraindications

- Low or absent thiopurine methyl transferase (TPMT) activity.
- Pregnancy.
- Concurrent malignancy.

Dose: 2-2.5 mg/kg daily orally.

Adverse Effects

- Myelosuppression.
- Nausea.
- Hypersensitivity reaction in the form of fever, rash, hypotension, hepatitis and respiratory distress.

Precautions

- TPMT status of the patient should be preferably known before starting therapy as its deficiency may lead to fatal myelosuppression.
- In elderly and those with subnormal TPMT activity a lower dose of 0.5 to 1 mg/kg daily is to be given.

METHOTREXATE

Methotrexate is a dihydrofolate reductase (DHFR) antagonist and inhibits DNA synthesis in the S phase of cell cycle. It has been widely used in severe psoriasis and psoriatic arthritis since 1950. In psoriasis it inhibits the proliferating lymphoid cells.

Indications

- Psoriasis and psoriatic arthritis.
- Reiter's disease.
- Pityriasis rubra pilaris.
- Limited use in pemphigus vulgaris, lupus erythematosus, dermatomyositis, chronic actinic dermatitis, atopic dermatitis, bullous pemphigoid, systemic sclerosis and cutaneous sarcoidosis.

Contraindications

- Pregnancy.
- Hepatitis.
- Renal impairment.

Dose: 7.5 to 15 mg orally weekly, 0.3- 0.6 mg/kg/week in children. Three weekly divided doses have no advantage over once a week dose.

Adverse Effects

- Nausea.
- Hepatotoxicity.
- Myelosuppression.
- Teratogenic effects and abortion.
- Suppression of spermatogenesis.
- Pneumonitis.

Precautions

- Monitoring of complete blood count, plasma urea, electrolytes, creatinine and liver enzymes fortnightly to start with and every month followed by once in 2-3 months later on.
- Avoid alcohol abuse.
- Folic acid supplementation 1-5 mg/day will lower the risk of methotrexate toxicity.
- Simultaneous use of drugs which interact with methotrexate (e.g., sulfonamides, trimethoprim, phenytoin, aspirin and NSAIDs) should be avoided.
- Three divided doses given twelve hourly not every week has advantage over once a week schedule.

CYCLOSPORIN

Cyclosporin is a calcineurin inhibitor. It inhibits the activation and proliferation of helper T-cells as well as expression of interleukin-2 and other cytokines.

Indications

- **Main indications:** Psoriasis and atopic dermatitis.
- **Other indications:** Chronic autoimmune urticaria, pyoderma gangrenosum, Behcet's disease, alopecia areata, granuloma annulare, pemphigus vulgaris.

Dose: 3-5 mg/kg/day orally in divided doses.

Adverse Effects

- Hypertension.
- Nephrotoxicity.
- Increased risk of malignancy.

CYCLOPHOSPHAMIDE

Cyclophosphamide is DNA alkylating agent and thereby inhibits the DNA synthesis in T and B cells. Because of its toxicity it is used only in severe conditions like pemphigus, SLE, dermatomyositis, Wegener's granulomatosis and T-cell lymphoma.

Dose: 1-3 mg/kg daily orally in two or three divided doses.

Adverse Effects

Bone marrow suppression, infections, hemorrhagic cystitis, azoospermia and increased risk of malignancy. In children, cyclophosphamide is replaced by azathioprine because of risk of azoospermia by cyclophosphamide.

IMMUNOMODULATORS

Antimalarials

Antimalarials are used in dermatology because of their anti-inflammatory effect. They interfere with many biological processes. **Hydroxychloroquine, chloroquine and mepacrine** are the main drugs used for this purpose.

Indications

- Cutaneous lupus erythematosus and lupus panniculitis are the main indications.
- Other indications include porphyria cutanea tarda, polymorphic light eruption, solar urticaria, granuloma annulare, oral lichen planus, etc.

Dosage: Hydroxychloroquine – 6.5 mg/kg/day. Recent guidelines recommend 5 mg/kg dose mainly to reduce the risk of ocular side effects, chloroquine 3 mg/kg/day, mepacrine 100-200 mg/day.

Adverse Effects

- High doses of chloroquine and hydroxychloroquine are associated with retinopathy. Ocular toxicity is not seen with mepacrine.
- Long-term use of antimalarials may cause blue-black pigmentation of skin.
- In patients with glucose-6-phosphatase deficiency, hemolytic anemia may occur.

DAPSONE

- Dapsone is the main drug in the treatment of leprosy but it is also used in many other dermatoses. Mechanism of action of dapsone in these dermatoses is not clear.
- Mainly used in dermatitis herpetiformis, linear IgA disease, chronic bullous dermatosis of childhood, cicatricial pemphigoid, IgA pemphigus and erythema elevatum diutinum. Other indications are: Behcet's disease, pyoderma gangrenosum, acne fulminans, papular urticaria etc.
- **Dose:** 100-150 mg/day in adults, 1-3 mg/kg/day in children with a maximum dose of 100 mg/day.

Adverse Effects

Hemolysis, methemoglobinemia, agranulocytosis, peripheral neuropathy, hepatitis, drug rash, psychosis.

ANTIHISTAMINES

Antihistamines are extensively used in dermatology to treat itching due to several diseases including urticaria, lichen planus, atopic dermatitis and other eczemas. They check the histamine release by blocking the H1 and H2 receptors. H1 antihistamines are commonly used in skin diseases. H2 antihistamines (cimetidine, ranitidine) are less frequently used in dermatology. H1 antihistamines are classified as first and second-generation antihistamines. First generation antihistamines cross the blood-brain barrier and have sedating effect which may be desirable in some cases. Second generation histamines are preferred over first generation because of their non-sedating effect, longer duration of action and rapid onset of action. The common antihistaminic in pediatrics age wise enlisted in Table 36.2. The common antihistaminic and their doses are enlisted in Table 36.3.

Table 36.2: Antihistamine usage in pediatric patients – age wise

<6 months	*6 months – 1 year*	*1 – 2 years*	*>2 years*	*>6 years*
No antihistamine is completely safe	Cetirizine Levocetirizine desloratadine	chlorpheniramine	Loratadine Diphenhydramine promethazine	fexofenadine

Contd.

Table 36.3: Common antihistamines with their dosage

Antihistamines	*Adult dose*	*Pediatric dose*
First generation		
Chlorpheniramine maleate	4 mg three times a day	0.35 mg/kg/day in 3-4 divided doses
Cyproheptadine	4 mg three times a day	0.25-0.5 mg/day in 2-3 divided doses
Diphenhydramine	10-50 mg three times a day	5 mg/kg/day in 2-3 divided doses
Hydroxyzine	10-25 mg three times a day	2 mg/kg/day divided in 3-4
Second generation		
Cetrizine	10 mg once a day	6 month to < 2 yr-2.5 mg daily, 2 yr. to < 6 yr. 5 mg daily > 6 yr. 10 mg daily in 2 divided doses
Loratadine	10 mg once a day	2-5 yr. 5 mg, > 6 yr. 10 mg OD
Fexofenadine	180 mg once a day	6-11yr. 30 mg bid, 12- adult 60 mg bid

Adverse Effects

First generation antihistamines are associated with drowsiness, dizziness, sedation and anticholinergic effects like dry mouth, blurred vision, urinary retention, constipation. These effects may be more marked in elderly. Young children may be paradoxically excited. Cyproheptadine is contraindicated in neonates.

Other Antiallergic Drugs

1. **Montelukast:** It is a leukotriene antagonist and is used in combination with antihistamines in some cases of urticaria.
2. **Doxepin:** It is an antidepressant but because of its H1 and H2 blockage effect it is used in urticaria and other pruritic disorders in the dosage of 25-75 mg/day.
3. **Cyproheptadine:** It is a first-generation antihistamine with additional anticholinergic, antiserotonergic and local anesthetic properties. It is given in the dose of 0.25-0.5 mg/day in 2-3 divided doses in paediatric age group and 4 mg three times a day in adults.

RETINOIDS

Retinoids are Vitamin A analogues. Two important retinoids used in dermatology are isotretinoin and acitretin.

Isotretinoin

Isotretinoin acts primarily on sebocytes and follicular keratinocytes. It blocks the proliferation and differentiation of sebaceous glands. It also exerts anti-inflammatory and desquamating effects. By virtue of these actions it is drug of choice for severe, recalcitrant cystic acne.

Indications

- Severe acne.
- Seborrhea.
- Rosacea.
- Gram negative folliculitis.
- Hidradenitis suppurativa.
- Steatocystoma multiplex.

Dosage

In severe acne, as conventional therapy, the dose varies from 0.5 mg to 2.0 mg/kg body weight per day for 4 months with total cumulative dose of 120-150 mg/kg body weight. It has been seen that 1mg/kg body weight per day for 4 months is also effective with less side effects. It clears up acne in most of the patients and provides a prolonged remission. Although, to minimise the adverse effects, low dose regimens such as 20 mg alternate day fixed dose isotretinoin (0.15-0.4 mg/kg body weight) are being commonly used now- a-days.

Acitretin

Acitretin is the active metabolite of etretinate, an older prodrug not used currently. It is mainly used for treating psoriasis and inherited disorders of keratinization.

Indications

- Severe extensive plaque psoriasis.
- Generalized pustular psoriasis.
- Erythrodermic psoriasis.
- Pityriasis rubra pilaris.

- Darier's disease.
- Ichthyosis.
- Palmoplantar keratoderma.
- Severe lichen planus.

Dose: 25-75 mg per day.

Side Effects of Retinoids

- Dryness of skin and mucosa, cheilitis, conjunctivitis, epistaxis.
- Intracranial hypertension.
- Depression and aggressiveness.
- Increase in liver enzymes.
- Increase in serum lipids.
- Ossification of ligaments and/or tendons.
- Teratogenicity: Severe fetal abnormalities.

Precautions

- Prior to initiate therapy, it is mandatory to confirm that the woman is not pregnant. Pregnancy is to be avoided during therapy and after the cessation of therapy for 1 month for isotretinoin and 3 years for acitretin.
- Tetracyclines are not to be prescribed with retinoids as they also increase the intracranial pressure.
- Alcohol should not be used with acitretin therapy.
- Vitamin A should not be used concomitantly.
- Regular checkup of liver enzymes and lipids.

Retinoids in childhood psoriasis

- Acitretin is a cost-effective drug which can be used as both monotherapy and combination therapy.
- It has synergistic effect with NB-UVB.
- The dose of 0.5 to 1 mg/kg/day is seem to be effective.
- Side effects are mostly dose-dependent. The major concern being skeletal toxicity in children which can be minimized by monitoring regularly, and using short-time therapy.
- It should be cautiously used in female child patients.
- Laboratory investigations such as CBC, LFT, RFT and Lipid profile should be done every month for the first two months and every three months thereafter.
- Treatment with retinoids should be stopped if transaminases are three times the normal value.

ANTIBACTERIAL DRUGS

Antibiotics were originally synthesized by microorganisms for use against other microorganisms but now many of them are synthetic or semi-synthetic. The common antibiotics used in different bacterial infections of skin have been discussed in Chapter 3.

ANTIFUNGAL DRUGS

Systemic antifungal drugs belong to four groups:

1. **Polyenes:** Amphotericin B.
2. **Azoles:** Ketoconazole, fluconazole, itraconazole.
3. **Allylamines:** Terbinafine.
4. **Miscellaneous:** Griseofulvin, potassium iodide, flucytosine.

Amphotericin B

- It is a fungicidal drug which damages the fungal cell membrane by binding with ergosterol.
- Mainly used for systemic mycoses such as candidiasis, aspergillosis, mucormycosis.
- Not absorbed by gut so given intravenously in the dosage range of 0.4 -1 mg/kg/day in 5% glucose over 4 hours for 10-14 days.
- **Adverse effects:** Fever, hypotension, renal impairment, respiratory stridor.

Ketoconazole

- Broad spectrum imidazole derivative is used for dermatophytosis, chronic mucocutaneous candidiasis, pityriasis versicolor, mycetoma, blastomycosis, chromomycosis.
- **Dosage:** Children (> 2 years) 3.3-6.6 mg/kg/day, adults 200-400 mg/day orally.
- **Adverse effects:** Headache, vomiting, hepatitis, gynecomastia, impotence.

Fluconazole

- Triazole derivative principally used for oropharyngeal and vaginal candidiasis, also used in systemic infections like cryptococcosis.
- **Dosage:** It is safe to use after 6 months of age. Hence it is the preferred antifungal drug in infants. Children (3-13 years) loading dose 6-12 mg/kg/day, maintenance dose 3-6 mg/kg/day. In tinea and pityriasis versicolor infections, fixed daily dosing of 50 mg to 150 mg / week can be given.

- **Adults:** Oral candidiasis 200 mg loading dose and 100 mg daily for 14 days.
- For vaginal candidiasis, 150 mg single dose, may be repeated weekly.
- For pityriasis versicolor, 400 mg single dose, may be repeated monthly for 3 months.
- **Adverse effects:** Nausea, vomiting, elevation of hepatic enzymes, skin rash.

Itraconazole

- Lipophilic triazole derivative mainly used for onychomycosis. Other indications include dermatophytosis, candidiasis, pityriasis versicolor, sporotrichosis, chromomycosis, histoplasmosis.
- **Dosage:** Adults– dermatophytosis: 100-200 mg/day for 2 weeks, onychomycosis: 400 mg/day for a week per month for 3-4 months.

  Children– dermatophytosis: 3-5 mg/day for 2-3 weeks, onychomycosis 3-5 mg/day for 7 days in a month for 3-4 months.
- **Adverse effects:** Nausea, vomiting, headache, dizziness, cutaneous rash, hypertriglyceridemia, hypertension, elevation of liver enzymes, edema, hypokalemia, ventricular arrhythmias.

Terbinafine

- It is an allylamine which exerts its fungicidal action by inhibition of squalene epoxidation in the synthesis of ergosterol. Accumulation of squalene causes death of cell.
- It is mainly used for dermatophytosis in the dosage of 250 mg/day for 2 to 4 weeks. In onychomycosis of finger nails it is given as 250 mg/day for 6 weeks and 12 weeks for toe nails. In children, it is used for treatment of tinea capitis in the dose of 3-5 mg/kg daily. It is less effective in candidiasis and pityriasis versicolor.
- **Adverse effects:** Headache, gastrointestinal discomfort, loss of taste, TEN, SJS.

Griseofulvin

- It is the first systemic antifungal drug in use since 1958. With the availability of newer antifungal drugs its use has been reduced to minimum.
- It is fungistatic drug which works by inhibition of fungal RNA, DNA, microtubular assembly and cell wall synthesis.
- It is effective against dermatophytosis only. It is the only antifungal that is FDA approved for dermatophytic infection of all 3 sites, skin, hair and nail. Not effective against candida and pityriasis versicolor.
- **Dosage:** 10 mg/kg daily in two divided doses for 4-6 weeks in various tinea infections and 6-12 months for onychomycosis.
- **Adverse effects**: Headache, gastrointestinal discomfort, photosensitivity, urticaria, lethargy, mental confusion, flare up of preexisting lupus.
- Voriconazole, posaconazole and ravuconazole are members of second generation of triazoles.

Voriconazole

Voriconazole is indicated for the following: Invasive aspergillosis; esophageal candidiasis; candidemia in non-neutropenic patients, as well as in disseminated *Candida* infections in skin and *Candida* infections in abdomen, kidney, bladder wall and wounds.

It is available as 50 and 200 mg tablets.

Dose: 4-8 mg/kg/day orally.

Adverse effects: Nausea, vomiting, headache, dizziness, cutaneous rash, hypertriglyceridemia, elevation of liver enzymes and abnormal kidney function. It may cause QT prolongation and torsade de pointes in patients with cardiac rhythm disorders.

Posaconazole

Posaconazole is indicated by FDA for the following: Prophylaxis of invasive *Aspergillus* and *Candida* infections in patients 13 years or older who are at high risk of developing such infections owing to being severely immunocompromised; treatment of oropharyngeal candidiasis, including oropharyngeal candidiasis refractory to itraconazole and/or fluconazole.

It is available as 40 mg/ml oral suspension.

Dose: 200-800 mg/kg/day orally.

Adverse effects: Nausea, vomiting, headache, dizziness, cutaneous rash, hypertriglyceridemia, elevation of liver enzymes and abnormal kidney function.

ANTIVIRAL DRUGS

Acyclovir

- It is synthetic guanosine analogue which is widely used against herpes simplex virus and varicella-zoster virus infections. It works by inhibition of DNA synthesis.
- **Dosage:** Herpes simplex virus infection.

- **Adults:** 200 mg 5 times a day orally or 400 mg 3 times a day for 7-10 days. For serious systemic herpes simplex infection it is given 5 mg/kg 8 hourly by slow intravenous infusion. In immunocompromised patients it is given 10 mg/kg 8 hourly intravenously for 7-10 days.
- **Children:** It is given in a dose of 200 mg five times a day if more than 2 years of age and 100 mg five times a day for children of less than 2 years of age for 5 days.

Varicella Zoster Virus Infection

- **Adults:** 800 mg 5 times a day for 7 to 10 days.
- **Children:** 10-20 mg/kg upto 800 mg orally five times a day for 5 days.
- **Adverse effects:** Elevation of blood urea and creatinine, gastrointestinal discomfort, crystalluria, tremors.

Famciclovir

- It is used for the treatment of herpes zoster and genital herpes.
- **Dosage:** Herpes zoster – 500 mg 8 hourly for 7 days in adults. Treatment to be started within 72 hours of onset of rash. In children, famciclovir can be given as 10 mg/kg three times a day for 7 days. Genital herpes – 250 mg 8 hourly for 10 days in primary episode and 125 mg twice a day for 5 days in recurrent episode.
- **Adverse effects:** Headache, hallucinations and confusion.

Valacyclovir

- It is a prodrug of acyclovir and is used mainly for herpes zoster and genital herpes.
- **Dosage:** Herpes zoster – 1 gram 8 hourly for 7 days in adults. Genital herpes–1gm twice a day for 7 days in primary episode and 500 mg twice a day for 3-5 days in recurrent episode. In children, valacyclovir can be given as 20 mg/kg three times a day for 7 days.
- **Adverse effects:** Facial edema, hypertension, tachycardia, diarrhea, creatinine elevation.

BIOLOGICS

Etanercept

- **Mechanism of action:** Consist of the fragment crystallizable (Fc) portion of IgG1 fused with a recombinant human tumor necrosis factor (TNF) receptor protein, etanercept binds to both soluble and membrane bound forms of TNF-α.
- **FDA approved indications:** Plaque Psoriasis >4 years age, psoriatic arthritis, rheumatoid arthritis, juvenile rheumatoid arthritis and ankylosing spondylitis.
- **Dosage:** SC injection of 0.8 mg/kg per week (maximum of 50 mg per week).
- **Adverse effects:** Common: Upper respiratory infections, pharyngitis, injection site reactions, headaches. Severe: Cellulitis

Adalimumab

- **Mechanism of action:** TNF-α inhibitor. Neutralizes the TNF- α bioactivity and induces apoptosis of TNF expressing mononuclear cells.
- **Dosage:** For patients 15 kg to 30 kg: SC injection of 20 mg at week 0 and then 20 mg every other week. For patients >30 kg: SC injection of 40 mg at week 0 and then 40 mg every other week.
- **Indications:** Juvenile idiopathic arthritis in patients >2 years of age, Crohn's disease in patients >6 years of age, uveitis in patients >2 years of age, treatment of hidradenitis suppurativa in patients >12 years of age.
- **Adverse effects:** Upper respiratory infections, uncomplicated infections, injection site reactions, cellulitis, hyperlipidemia.

Dupilumab

- Blocks the α subunit of IL-4 and IL-13 receptors, resulting in decreased IL-4 and IL-13 cytokine-induced responses.
- **Dosage:** For patients < 60 kg: SC injection of 400 mg at week 0 and then 200 mg every other week. For patients >60 kg: SC injection of 600 mg at week 0 and then 300 mg every other week.
- **FDA approved indications:** Atopic dermatitis in patients >12 years.
- FDA, recently in 2020 has approved dupilumab for children aged 6 to 11 years with moderate to severe atopic dermatitis whose disease is not adequately controlled with topical prescription therapies or when these therapies are not advisable. Dupilumab is the only biologic medicine approved for this patient population.
- **Adverse effects:** Common: injection site reactions, conjunctivitis, herpes infections, upper respiratory infection.

Ustekinumab

- Blocks p40 subunit of IL-12 and IL-23 resulting in suppression of T cell activity.

- **Dosage:** For patients < 60 kg: SC injection of 0.75 mg/kg at week 0, week 4, and then every 12 weeks, For patients 60 kg to 100 kg: SC injection of 45 mg at week 0, week 4, and then every 12 weeks. For >100 kg: SC injection of 90 mg at week 0, week 4, and then every 12 weeks.
- **FDA approved indication:** Psoriasis in patients >12 years.
- **Adverse reactions:** Upper respiratory tract infection, headache, injection site reaction, rarely skin carcinomas.

Biologics with Off Label Uses in Dermatology

- Infliximab (TNF-α inhibitor) is FDA approved for children 6 years or older with Crohn's disease.
- Off label use in psoriasis: 3.3–5 mg/kg administered at weeks 0, 2 and 6, and then every 7–8 weeks thereafter.
- Common effects include uncomplicated infections and headache. Serious adverse effects include infusion reactions, hepatotoxicity, cytopenias and malignancies.
- Certolizumab pegol is FDA approved for Psoriasis and Psoriatic Arthritis (PsA) in adults but is used off label in pediatric population also.
- Secukinumab is FDA approved for Psoriasis and Psoriatic Arthritis, but it is not FDA approved for pediatric population. Dosage is 150 mg at week 1, 2, 3 and 4, and then every 4 weeks thereafter. Trials are underway to study adverse effects.

JAK INHIBITORS

The first generation of JAK inhibitors includes tofacitinib, ruxolitinib, baricitinib and oclacitinib.

- **FDA Approved Indications:** Ruxolitinib is FDA approved to treat myelodysplastic disorders.
- Baricitinib is not yet FDA approved, but is in clinical trials for rheumatoid arthritis (RA), psoriasis and atopic dermatitis. The first FDA approved JAK inhibitor for treatment of an autoimmune disease was tofacitinib. Oclacitinib has no FDA approved indication in humans.
- **Off Label Uses:** To date, JAK inhibitors have shown efficacy in the treatment of dermatologic conditions such as atopic dermatitis (AD), alopecia areata (AA), psoriasis and vitiligo. Smaller case series and case reports suggest efficacy in dermatomyositis, chronic actinic dermatitis, erythema multiforme, hypereosinophilic syndrome, cutaneous graft-versus-host disease and in lupus.
- **Mechanism:** Dermatologically relevant cytokines rely on the JAK-STAT pathway and they include: IFN-α/β, IFN-γ, IL-2 receptor common γ-chain interleukins (IL-2, IL-4, IL-7, IL-9, IL-15 and IL-21), and IL-5, IL-6, IL-12, IL-13 and IL-23. Although other cytokines such as TNF-α, IL-1 and IL-17 do not signal via the JAK-STAT pathway, in some instances JAK inhibitors can indirectly suppress these cytokines (i.e., IL-17) by inhibition of other STAT-dependent cytokines (i.e., IL-23).
- **Dosage:** The FDA approved dose for tofacitinib in RA is 5 mg twice daily. A new extended release formulation (11 mg once daily) is also available. In psoriasis clinical trials, tofacitinib 10 mg twice daily was more efficacious than 5 mg twice daily.
- **Adverse effects:** Increased risk of varicella-zoster virus reactivation, increase in total cholesterol, LDL cholesterol, and HDL cholesterol, cytopenias, and increased risk of malignancy.

37

CHAPTER

Lasers and Treatment Procedures in Dermatology

Contents

LASER

Introduction

Laser is an acronym that stands for Light Amplification by Stimulated Emission of Radiation. Ruby laser was first used by Theodore Maiman in 1960.

Atoms consist of a nucleus surrounded by electrons. During their resting phase, electrons are at a low energy state close to the nucleus. By absorbing energy in the form of photons, electrons move to a higher energy orbit. In the excited and unstable state, the electrons have a tendency to drop back to their ground state, during this process, the spontaneous emission of radiation (photon of energy) occurs.

Stimulated emission occurs after an already excited atom is perturbed by a photon with a frequency (wavelength) corresponding to the energy gap between the excited and ground states. If this occurs, the excited atom reverts to the resting state, releasing energy as a second photon of the same frequency as the incident photon. Since the incident photon is not absorbed, the atom emits 2 photons. This theory of Stimulated emission of radiation was given by Albert Einstein in 1918.

During the working of lasers, these three light-matter interactions occur simultaneously, i.e. energising of atoms, spontaneous emission of photons and stimulated emission of photons.

Laser light is monochromatic (i.e. a single wavelength), collimated (i.e. nondivergent), coherent (i.e. in phase, with peaks and troughs of the light, all aligned and having high intensity that can travel over long distances. Practically, while using lasers, the user should be acquainted with following terminologies:

- Laser energy is measured in joules (J) which is proportional to the total number of photons incident on the target
- Fluence is defined as the amount of energy delivered per unit area in J/cm^2.
- Pulse width / Pulse duration is the length of time the laser beam is in contact with the skin. It ranges from picoseconds to seconds.

- Spot size is the diameter of the laser beam on skin surface. It is measured in (mm).
- Pulse frequency/ Repetition rate (Hz) is the rate at which the laser pulses. 1 Hz is 1 pulse per second.
- Power is the rate at which energy is delivered and is measured in Watts (i.e. W or J/s).
- Irradiance refers to power density (i.e. the rate at which energy is delivered per unit area) and is measured in W/ cm^2.
- Wavelength (nm) is the distance between the peak of two photon waves.

Fluence and irradiance are inversely proportional to the square of the spot size. Therefore, for a given amount of energy, doubling the spot size decreases the fluence and irradiance by a factor of 4 and reduces scatter and allows more photons to be transmitted into the skin. Thus, more thermal energy is delivered than with a small spot size. The fluence should be accordingly reduced when using a larger spot size.

The wavelength is determined by the characteristic of active medium in particular laser. The choice of wavelength is determined by target tissue and depth of penetration.

Thermal relaxation time (TRT): TRT is the time taken for the target to dissipate 63% of the incident thermal energy. It is related to the target chromophore and varies from a few nanoseconds (tattoo particles) to several hundred milliseconds or more (leg venules).

Thermal Damage Time (TDT): TDT is defined as the time required for the whole target, along with the primary chromophore (e.g., melanin) and the surrounding target (e.g., hair follicle), to reduce its temperature by about 63%. It includes the cooling of the primary chromophore and the entire target. The concept of TDT has been proposed as an extended theory of selective photothermolysis for nonuniformly pigmented targets.

Modes of Output

Continuous wave lasers emit a beam of light whose power is constant over time, resulting in a long, continuous exposure. It ranges from milliseconds to seconds.

Quasi-continuous wave lasers shutter the continuous beam into short segments, resulting in interrupted emissions of constant laser energy at constant intervals. It ranges from milliseconds to seconds.

Pulsed lasers emit short pulses with high energy. They can be short pulse (nanoseconds) or long pulse (milliseconds).

Ultra pulse wave: Pulse width is in microseconds.

Q-switched (quality-switched) lasers are able to generate extremely high energy.

Fractional lasers: Large laser beam is divided into multiple smaller laser beams leading to microthermal zones (MTZ) of ablation with skip areas. Distance between the adjoining beams is known as Pitch.

The basis for all laser tissue interactions is selective photothermolysis given by Anderson and Parrish in 1983. The target structures that absorb the laser light are known as chromophores, the most common ones being water, haemoglobin and melanin in the skin. In an ideal situation, the particular wavelength would have little to no absorption by the surrounding structures. A target's thermal relaxation time (TRT) is defined as the time required for the heated target tissue to dissipate half of the heat absorbed from the laser.

Basic Components of Laser

1. Gain medium or Lasing medium
2. Optical resonators (comprising of a 100% reflecting mirror and a partially reflecting mirror)
3. Power source

Lasers are named after the constituents of the active medium (lasing medium) which may be a gas, liquid, solid or semiconductor.

- **Solid state:** Ruby, alexandrite, Nd:YAG, Er:YAG or semiconductor diodes.
- **Liquid**: Organic dyes in a solvent, e.g. rhodamine.
- **Gas**: Carbon dioxide and argon
- **Vapor:** Copper and Gold

Population Inversion: Process by which a laser medium is excited to create more atoms in higher energy state than in the ground state by the process of pumping (Optical, Electrical, Chemical, Thermal and Excitation by inelastic collision).

Side Effects of Lasers

Immediate: Pain, burning sensation, oedema.

Early

1. Oozing, crusting and purpura
2. Secondary infection
3. Reactivation of herpes simplex infection.

Late

1. Dyspigmentation (hypopigmentation, hyperpigmentation or depigmentation)
2. Change in skin texture
3. Demarcation lines (common in skin rejuvenation)
4. Keloids and hypertrophic scars
5. Scarring

6. Hypertrichosis
7. Milia
8. Persistent erythema
9. Dilated follicular ostia

The Various Lasers Used in Dermatology

Nd: YAG Laser

It is one of the most versatile and interesting lasers in dermatology. The neodymium-doped-yttrium-aluminium-garnet (Nd: YAG) is a crystal that is used as the active medium and neodymium ion provides the laser activity in the crystal. Depending on wavelength (1064 nm, frequency-doubled 532 nm) and mode (continuous, Q-switched, long-pulsed), various skin conditions can be treated.

Various conditions treated by Nd: YAG laser are:

- *Pigmented lesions:* Freckles, lentigines, nevus of Ota and Ito, Becker's nevus, lichen planus pigmentosus, Hori's nevus, café-au-lait macules, melasma etc. 532nm is used for epidermal pigmentary disorders while 1064 nm is used for deeper dermal melanotic disorders.
- *Vascular lesions:* Spider and thread veins over the face, varicose veins, capillary vascular malformation, hemangiomas and telangiectasias.
- Hair removal.
- Tattoo removal.
- *Photoaging and wrinkles:* For a firmer and even skin tone.
- Onychomycosis.

Diode Laser

It is still the most cost effective amongst the lasers. It is considered as the gold standard preference for hair removal due to deep penetration and effective targeting of hair follicle. The wavelength is 810 nm and it works on the principle of selective photothermolysis and extended theory of selective photothermolysis. Target chromophore for diode laser is melanin in the hair follicles. On darker skin it is necessary to use low fluence values, since the melanin of the epidermis competes with the melanin of the hair follicle, thus absorbing the light of the diode laser and increasing the incidence of side effects. Unfortunately, using lower fluences in the procedure reduces the efficacy of the treatment. Therefore, on darker skin types, the triple-wavelength diode laser (810 nm, 940 nm, 1060 nm) has been found to be more effective for permanent hair reduction compared to the 810 nm diode laser alone. The triple wavelength laser has been found to cause less absorption by the skin, enabling the use of higher fluences with greater safety, which allows it to be used in stamping mode at a high fluence. In addition, longer wavelengths have a greater penetration which allows the hair to be treated at a deeper level.

Carbon Dioxide Laser

Developed by Chandra Kumar Patel in 1963. CO_2 laser emits energy with a peak wavelength of 10,600 nm, which is preferentially absorbed by intracellular water. Absorption of this wavelength by the epidermis leads to ablation of the most superficial layers, thereby promoting re-epithelialization from residual skin appendages and adnexal structures in the dermis (the sweat glands and hair follicles). The thermal injury that occurs below the zone of ablation induces heat mediated contraction of collagen, promoting collagen remodeling in the dermis and contraction of collagen fibrils, in turn, causes tightening of the skin.

Various indications of CO_2 laser include:

- Treatment of scars (acne, traumatic etc.).
- Prevention and treatment of photoaging.
- Treatment of premalignant lesions and keratinocyte skin cancers (squamous cell carcinoma and basal cell carcinoma), as well as cutaneous vascular lesions such as hamartomas.
- Seborrheic keratosis, warts, syringomas and xanthelasmas.
- Onychomycosis.
- Onychodystrophy.

Intense Pulsed Light (IPL)

IPL is a non laser filtered xenon flash lamp device, invented by Shimon Eckhouse in 1992. Unlike lasers, IPL devices emit polychromatic (wavelengths ranging from 500 to 1200 nm), non-coherent and non-collimated light with varying pulse durations. This wide range of light can be absorbed by a variety of chromophores making them less selective than lasers.

Indications:

- *Vascular lesions:* Facial telangiectasias, capillary malformations, poikiloderma of civatte, venous malformations, infantile hemangiomas and leg veins.
- Treatment of hypertrophic scars, keloids and striae.
- *Pigmented lesions:* freckles, solar lentigines.
- Hair removal.
- Acne and rosacea.
- Non ablative skin photo rejuvenation.
- Hidradenitis suppurativa.
- Sarcoidosis.
- Cutaneous lupus erythematosus.

Pulsed Dye Laser (PDL)

PDL is considered to be the treatment of choice for cutaneous vascular lesions. It has a wavelength of 585nm and 595nm and its target chromophore is oxyhemoglobin. The lasing medium of PDL is Rhodamine dye.

Indications:

- ***Vascular lesions:*** Port wine stain, hemangioma, telangiectasias.
- Acne vulgaris and erythema
- Hypertrophic and keloids
- Warts and molluscum contagiosum
- Nail psoriasis
- Striae distensae

308 nm Excimer Laser

308 nm xenon-chloride excimer laser, a novel mode of phototherapy, an ultraviolet B radiation system consisting of a noble gas and halide. Monochromatic excimer laser is superior over phototherapies of other kinds, as it allows for a lower UV dose exposure, shorter course of therapy and being directed at distinct affected skin rather than compromising the adjacent normal skin.

Indications:

- Vitiligo
- Psoriasis
- Atopic dermatitis
- Alopecia areata
- Mycosis fungoides
- Lichen planus, granuloma annulare, leucoderma etc

The various lasers, their wavelength and their clinical applications are summarized below (Table 37.1):

Table 37.1: Showing different lasers, their wavelength and their clinical application

Laser	*Wavelength (nm)*	*Application*
Excimer	308	Vitiligo, Psoriasis, Mycosis fungoides
Argon	488-512	Vascular lesions
Intense pulsed light	515-1200	Vascular and pigmented lesions, epilation
Potassium titanyl phosphate (KTP)	532	Vascular and pigmented lesions, tattoo- red/ yellow
QS-Nd: YAG	532	Vascular and pigmented lesions, tattoo-red/ yellow
Pulsed dye laser	585-600	Vascular lesions
Ruby	694	Pigmented lesions, tattoos- blue, black, green and epilation
QS Alexandrite	755	Tattoo- blue, black, green and epilation
Diode	810	Epilation
QS Nd:YAG	1064	Pigmented lesions and tattoos- blue and black
Long pulsed Nd: YAG	1320	Epilation and vascular lesions
Er:YAG	2940	Superficial skin resurfacing and destruction of superficial growths
Carbon dioxide	10600	Skin resurfacing, destruction of warts, keloids, superficial cancers and benign growths

Contd.

The various chromophores and their pulse durations are summarized below (Table 37.2):

Table 37.2: Showing various chromophores and their pulse durations

Chromophore	*Diameter*	*TRT*	*Typical laser pulse duration*
Tattoo ink particle	0.1micrometer	10 ns	10 ns
Melanosome	0.5 micrometer	250 ns	10-100 ns
Port wine stain blood vessel	30-100 micrometer	1-10 ms	0.4-20 ms
Terminal hair follicle	300 micrometer	100 ms	3-100 ms
Leg vein	1 mm	1 second	0.1 second

BOTULINUM TOXIN (BTX)

- BTX is produced by Clostridium botulinum of different serotypes- A, B, C1, D, E, F and G.
- It inhibits the release of acetylcholine from the presynaptic motor neuron, resulting in chemo denervation and consequent paralysis of the muscle. However, over time new nerve terminals regenerate resulting in restoration of the motor function.
- Onabotulinumtoxin A is the most common serotype.
- Dermatological indications include correction of glabellar frown lines, horizontal forehead lines, crow's feet and hyperhidrosis. Non-dermatological indications are

blepharospasm, strabismus, cervical dystonia, upper limb spasticity, chronic migraine and urinary incontinence.

SOFT TISSUE AUGMENTATION (Fillers)

- It is popular now a days as patients demand cosmetic improvement without undergoing any invasive procedure. Fillers are used to correct soft tissue contour abnormalities and also to provide cosmetic enhancement. However, these are temporary in nature and hence require repeated sessions.
- **Collagen:** Bovine derived collagen and human collagen have been used for decades, however its use now has fallen out due to introduction of various newer fillers.
- **Hyaluronic acid (HA):** It is a member of the glycosaminoglycans and is a natural component of the dermis.
  - HA avidly binds to water, thereby increasing the volume of the tissue. Patient might experience redness, swelling and bruising for first few days after treatment. HA produces a longer lasting improvement (about 6-8 months) when compared to collagen.
  - There are two types of HA filler substances- streptococcal derived and animal (i.e. rooster comb) derived. Streptococcal derived fillers are commonly used.
  - HA fillers are mainly used for facial wrinkles and folds as well as for cheek and lip augmentation.
  - Side effects include – Improper placement of HA, too superficially can cause bluish discoloration or nodule formation. These effects can be reversed using hyaluronidase injections.
- **Poly-L-Lactic acid (PLLA):** It is a biodegradable, biocompatible and immunologically inert product. It is used to replace diffuse volume loss for e.g. contour correction of face, correction of facial atrophy in patients with HIV infection and for aesthetic treatment of facial lines. The substance is absorbed into the skin followed by induction of a fibroblastic response and de novo collagen synthesis.
- **Other substances used for tissue augmentation include** calcium hydroxyapatite, silicone, polymethacrylate, expanded polytetrafluoroethylene and autologous fat transplantation.

SCLEROTHERAPY

- Three broad classes of sclerosing agents are available- hyperosmotic agents, detergents and chemical irritants.
- Detergents like Sodium tetradecyl sulfate (STS) and Polidoconol are FDA approved for use in sclerotherapy.
- Sclerotherapy is indicated for superficial telangiectasias, reticular veins, visible varicosities and incompetent great saphenous veins.
- Complications include ulceration, hyperpigmentation along the course of treated veins and telangiectatic matting. The most serious complication is sclerosis of veins.

FAT REDUCTION

- **Liposuction:** It is used to treat local areas of excess fat depositions so as to improve the body contour. The commonly treated areas are the abdomen and thighs. Conditions like gynaecomastia, buffalo hump, lipomas and lipodystrophy can also be treated. The process involves aspiration of the fat through cannulas attached to a vaccumdevice after tumescent anesthesia.
- **Cryolipolysis:** It is based on the principle that the adipocytes are more sensitive to temperature changes, therefore controlled cooling results in reduction of the unwanted fat which undergoes apoptosis while causing minimum damage to the surrounding tissue.
  - ***Indications:*** Body contouring, cellulite.
  - There is no downtime to the procedure and the patient can return to work including exercise immediately. Repeat treatment at 3 months interval is required in many cases for best results.
  - ***Contraindications:*** Cryoglobulinemia, cold urticaria, cold agglutinin disease, paroxysmal cold hemo-globinuria, Raynaud's disease.
  - ***Side effects:*** Early - erythema, myalgia, transient muscle spasm, transient arthralgia; Late - Paradoxical adipose hyperplasia
- **Sodium deoxycholate:** It is approved as first in line treatment option for dissolving unwanted submental fat. It causes direct damage to adipocytes via their lysis followed by a local neutrophilic mediated inflammation which further potentiates the desired effect. Typically, 2-4 sessions at intervals of 4-6 weeks are needed for best results.

CHEMICAL PEELS

- Peels are used to induce a controlled injury of a specific skin depth with the goal to stimulate new skin growth and improve surface texture and appearance. The exfoliative effect of chemical peels results in faster epidermal turnover and synthesis of new collagen with evenly distributed melanin. They are classified by the depth of action into superficial, medium and deep peels.

- **Superficial peels:** They cause injury to epidermis and the superficial papillary dermis and are well tolerated with limited downtime. Examples are alpha hydroxyl acids (AHA) - glycolic acid (GA upto 70%), lactic acid, malic acid and citric acid, beta hydroxyl acids (BHA) - salicylic acid (20-30%), trichloroacetic acid (TCA- 10-15%) and jessner's solution (resorcinol, salicylic acid and 85% lactic acid in 95% ethanol).They are mainly used for acne, photo ageing and melasma.
- **Medium depth peels:** They cause a controlled injury through the epidermis upto deep papillary dermis. Medium-depth peels may be used in the treatment of dyschromias, such as solar lentigines, multiple keratoses, superficial scars, pigmentary disorders, and textural changes. Trichloroacetic acid (TCA) in concentrations of 35-50% is classically used as a medium-depth peel. Combination peels, such as Monheit's combination (Jessner's solution with TCA), Brody's combination (solid carbon dioxide with TCA), Coleman's combination (GA 70% + TCA), and Jessner's solution with GA are other examples.
- **Deep peels:** They cause injury deep down upto superficial reticular dermis. Examples are phenol-based solutions, including Baker-Gordon phenol peel and the more recent Hetter phenol-croton oil peel. These are indicated in patients with severe photodamage and advanced rhytids.

HYDRA FACIAL

Also known as hydra dermabrasion or wet dermabrasion is one of the latest cosmetic procedures that uses hydraulics or hydra technology. It involves a combination of suctioning and gentle cleansing of the skin with water and other additive serums to give the skin a youthful appearance. The skin is first cleansed followed by applying special pressure therapy on the skin by a combination of vaccum suction with high frequency electrical currents or oxygen infused into it for extra benefits.

It is used for treatment of acne, enlarged pores, rough texture, uneven tone, fine lines, pigmentation and skin rejuvenation.

HIGH INTENSITY FOCUSED ULTRASOUND (HIFU)

The principle of HIFU is to induce cellular damage and volume reduction of the target area selectively by means of coagulation by generating instant microthermal lesions through the accumulation of high frequency ultrasound beams (3MHz- 10MHz) to deep dermis, subcutaneous fat, fascia, and superficial musculoaponeurotic system (SMAS). Epidermis and muscles are unaffected by HIFU. It is used for treatment of wrinkles and laxity of skin in various parts like face, abdomen, etc and facial rejuvenation.

Side effects: Pain, erythema, oedema, tenderness, ecchymosis

PLATELET RICH PLASMA

Autologous platelet-rich plasma (PRP) is the processed liquid fraction of autologous peripheral blood with a platelet concentration above the baseline. PRP has become a popular treatment for many conditions in sport medicine, regenerative medicine, aesthetic medicine and hair loss treatment as it contains a variety number of growth factors and cytokines that can accelerate wound healing and tissue restoration. Four main types of preparations can be defined, depending on their cell content and fibrin architecture.

1. Pure Platelet-rich Plasma (P-PRP) or leucocyte-poor PRP products are preparations without leucocytes and with a low-density fibrin network after activation.
2. Leucocyte- and PRP (L-PRP) products are preparations with leucocytes and with a low-density fibrin network after activation. It is in this family that the largest number of commercial or experimental systems exist. Particularly, many automated protocols have been developed in the last years, requiring the use of specific kits that allow minimum handling of the blood samples and maximum standardization of the preparations.
3. Pure platelet-rich fibrin (P-PRF) or leucocyte-poor platelet-rich fibrin preparations are without leucocytes and with a high-density fibrin network. These products only exist in a strongly activated gel form, and cannot be injected or used like traditional fibrin glues.
4. Leucocyte- and platelet-rich fibrin (L-PRF) or second-generation PRP products are preparations with leucocytes and with a high-density fibrin network.

Procedure

1. Obtain whole blood by venipuncture in acid citrate dextrose (ACD) tubes.
2. Do not chill the blood at any time before or during platelet separation.
3. Centrifuge the blood using a 'soft' spin (varying between 1200-2000 rpm for 10-15 minutes).
4. Transfer the supernatant plasma containing platelets into another sterile tube (without anticoagulant).
5. Centrifuge the plasma at a higher speed (a hard spin-varying between 2500-3500 rpm for 10 to 20 minutes) to obtain a platelet concentrate.
6. The lower 1/3rd of tube contains PRP while upper 2/3rd is platelet-poor plasma (PPP). At the bottom of the tube, platelet pellets are formed.

7. Remove PPP and suspend the platelet pellets in a minimum quantity of PRP (2-4 ml) by gently shaking the tube. This plasma is injected in the androgen related areas of the scalp or other lesional areas using insulin syringes till a depth of 2-3 mm. 0.2-0.3 ml of PRP is injected in every centimeter square. After the injections are over, micro-needling can be done using derma-roller of 1.5 mm length needles which was rolled over the region where the injections were given in the scalp or other procedure like CO_2 laser can be combined in case of acne scars.
8. Some recommend single spin method at 2000-3000 rpm for 15-20 minutes.

Mechanism of Action/Rationale of PRP

- The underlying rationale for PRP therapy is that injection of concentrated platelets at sites of injury may initiate tissue repair via the release of many biologically active factors (growth factors, cytokines, lysosomes) and adhesion proteins which are responsible for initiating the hemostatic cascade, synthesis of new connective tissue and revascularization.
- Activated platelets in PRP release numerous growth factors and cytokines from their alpha granules, including platelet derived endothelial growth factor (PDGF), transforming growth factor β (TGF-β), fibroblast growth factor-2 (FGF-2), vascular endothelial growth factor (VEGF), epidermal growth factor (EGF), insulin like growth factor-1 (IGF-1), glial cell line–derived neurotrophic factor (GDNF), which play a major role in stimulating hair growth through cell proliferation, differentiation and angiogenesis. GDNF can stimulate cell proliferation and protect hair follicle from premature catagen transition.
- The main advantages of PRP include its safety and the ingenious preparation techniques of current commercial devices to prepare a biologic that can be used in a broad application profile.
- Most importantly, PRP is an autologous product with no known adverse effects.

Absolute Contraindication for PRP

Critical thrombocytopenia, platelet dysfunction, hemodynamic instability, sepsis, local infection (site PRP) and patient with unwilling to accept risk.

Relative Contraindications

NSAIDs use within 48 hours, glucocorticoid injection at treatment site within one-month, systemic glucocorticoid within 2 weeks, recent illness or fever, cancer especially bone or hematolymphoid, anemia (hemoglobin less than 10 grams per deciliter), thrombocytopenia (platelets less than 150,000 per microliter) and tobacco use.

Uses:

1. Androgenetic alopecia.
2. Female pattern hair loss.
3. Alopecia areata.
4. Cicatricial alopecia.
5. Hair transplant.
6. Acne scars.
7. Wound healing.
8. PRP facelifts and vampire facials.

Side effects:

PRP is an autologous preparation of plasma with a high concentration of platelets. It is relatively safe intervention with minimal adverse effects, including temporary and tolerable pain during treatment, mild headache, minimal itching, transient erythema and edema on treated area. No major side effects such as scarring, infections, panniculitis, hematoma or allergic reaction have been documented following PRP treatment.

After treatment, patients can resume normal daily activities, no antibiotics are needed to prevent infection.

CRYOTHERAPY

Cryosurgery is performed using a cyrogen, typically liquid nitrogen (-196°C), to cool the targeted tissue to subzero temperatures. This effect induces tissue damage in 2 mechanisms:

1. The first mechanism is the induction of tissue ischemia by damaging blood vessels and capillaries within the target area which leads to ischemic necrosis of the tissue.
2. The second mechanism damages the cells more complexly by forming ice crystals and inducing osmotic cell injury and cellular membrane disruption. As the tissue is cooled, ice crystals form between cells which creates an osmotic gradient, rapidly drawing water out of the cells. As cooling continues, crystals form within the cell which can lead to rupture of the cell. The thawing process also damages cells. As the tissue thaws, crystals outside the cells melt which creates a gradient which rapidly draws water back into the cell which can cause cells to swell and burst.

   The amount of tissue damage increases with each freeze thaw cycle. The target temperature for the destruction of benign cells is -20°C. Cancerous cells can be more resistant to cell death and require -50°C to be destroyed. Unfortunately, melanocytes are very susceptible to thermal injury and may die at temperatures below -5°C.

Indications

Cryosurgery has a number of indications for both malignant and benign lesions.

1. Seborrheic keratosis.
2. Verruca.
3. Solar lentigenes.
4. Skin tags.
5. Molluscum contagiosum.
6. Keloids and hypertrophic scars.
7. Actinic keratosis.
8. Basal cell carcinoma.
9. Non invasive SCC.

Most of the entities can be treated with a single round of cryosurgery, but for larger or thicker lesions treatments can be repeated at 3 to 4 weeks intervals until the lesions have resolved. This is especially true in verruca which typically take anywhere from 2 to 6 treatments to resolve.

Contraindications

1. Neoplasms of uncertain behavior. Before cryosurgery is performed a diagnosis must be confirmed by histology.
2. Cryogenic response may be exacerbated by cold exposure such as cryoglobulinemia, multiple myeloma, Raynaud disease, cold urticaria, previous history of cold induce injury at the site or limb, as well as poor circulation at the site or in that limb. Cryosurgery can induce vasoconstriction so cryosurgery to a vascularly impaired area may lead to undesired tissue necrosis.

Complications

1. Treated sites will progress from erythema, edema, and vesiculation over the course of several days.
2. Pain.
3. Dyspigmentation.
4. Alopecia.
5. Pseudoepitheliomatous hyperplasia.
6. Depressed scars.
7. Tissue distortion (nail dystrophy or notching of cartilage).

ELECTROSURGERY

The term electrosurgery is a general term used to describe all the different procedures employing electrically generated heat. The heat can be generated either using direct or alternating current. They can be classified as:

1. **Galvanic/direct current (DC)**
   - Electrocautery.
   - Iontophoresis.
   - Electroepilation (Electrolysis).
   - Electrical stimulation of skin (ESS).
2. **Alternating current (AC)**
   - Electrosurgery- electrofulgration, electrocoagulation, electrodessication and electrosection.
   - Electroepilation (Thermolysis).
   - Electroporation.

Terminals

When a single treatment electrode is used, it is termed as monoterminal, as in most of the dermatological procedures like fulgration, dessication and most cases of coagulation. The biterminal term is used when:

1. Two treatment electrodes are used e.g. forceps electrode.
2. Single treatment electrode and an indifferent electrode like the ground plate (though technically incorrect, is more often used so) e.g. most cases of coagulation, section and epilation.

Method of Tissue Destruction

It is achieved by means of heat production, as a result of:

1. **Ohmic heat:** Heat produced as a result of tissue resistance to current flow. The relationship is directly proportional to the intensity of current.
2. **Convective heat:** Results from the dissipation of electrical and thermal energy from the spark. The greater the voltage, the greater the spark and thus greater the thermal energy. Tissue destruction occurs mainly at the surface, where the spark energy is dissipated (fulgration and dessication).
3. **Mechanical energy:** Electromagnetic waves produced at the tip of the electrode result in oscillations and a force that produces disruption of cells and release of thermal energy.

These 3 modes of energy production result in tissue destruction by:

1. Enzymatic activation.
2. DNA and RNA destruction.
3. Cell wall damage.
4. Denaturation and coagulation of proteins.
5. Steaming of intra and extra cellular water content- Dehydration (slow rise in temperature) or explosion of cell (rapid rise in temperature).

These reactions occur together as the temperature ranges from 100 to 600°C.

- Epidermis-fulgration-no scarring.
- Superficial dermis-dessication-mild scarring.
- Mid-dermis-dessication and coagulation-moderate. scarring.
- Deep dermis-dessication and coagulation-obvious scarring

Types of electrosurgery: Based on the extent of tissue damage, waveform of electrical current and electric configuration, there are 4 basic types of electrosurgeries.

1. **Electrofulgration:** Monoterminal-Dampened sine waves.
2. **Electrodessication:** Monoterminal-Dampened sine waves
3. **Electrocoagulation:** Biterminal with ground plate-rectified sine waves.
4. **Electrosection/cutting:** Biterminal with ground plate-rectified sine waves.

1. **Electrofulgration**
    - Charring of superficial tissue is caused by sparks from the electrode without actually touching the tissue when the tip of the electrode is held at a distance of 1-3 mm away from the lesion. Long, thick sparks are created and flow between the tissue and electrode is by damped sine waves of high frequency, low amperage and very high voltage current. Tissue destruction is rapid by cell dehydration and necrosis.
    - **Advantages:** Provides good control over the depth of tissue destruction and superficial charring insulates the underlying tissue, preventing deeper tissue destruction and scarring.
    - **Disadvantages:** Difficult to control the sparks and hence the risk to the surrounding tissue and not effective in dermal lesions.
2. **Electrodessication**
    - Has similar effects as those of fulgration, however it involves touching the lesion with the probe. Short, fine sparks are created by damped sine waves of high frequency, low amperage and very high voltage current similar to that in fulgration. The current intensity is marginally higher than in fulgration. Tissue destruction is deeper and involves denaturation of proteins, superficial mummification and necrosis of cells after initial dehydration.
    - Curettage is almost always necessary during and after electrodessication.
    - ***Advantages:*** Minimal scarring and effective hemostasis in small bleeders.
    - ***Disadvantages:*** Depth cannot be well controlled, superficial area damaged is within the boundaries of the lesion and hence recurrence is possible and deep dermal lesions usually bleed and heal with scarring.
3. **Electrocoagulation**
    - Deeper tissue destruction occurs by this. Tissue may or may not be touched depending upon the depth of tissue destruction required. Short, thick sparks are created dure to damped or partially rectified sine waves of high frequency, low voltage and high amperage. Tissue destruction involves deep necrosis, coagulation with hyalinized appearance. Some consider coagulation to be a combination destruction of fulgration and dessication with greater intensity of current and greater depth of destruction.
4. **Eletrosection**
    - This technique is used to cut tissue rather than just produce destruction. High frequency, very high amperage and low voltage current is used to create slightly damped or undamped and fully rectified sine waves to cause either:
        a. Electrosection (cutting) with some coagulation (bloodless incision with slightly damped waves).
        b. Electrosection pure cutting (completely undamped and filtered).

Procedure

In preparation for an electrosurgical procedure, the surrounding skin should be cleansed with an antiseptic agent such as chlorhexidine or povidone-iodine. Alcohol should be avoided or allowed to dry completely as can it may ignite with electrosurgery. Local anesthetics should also be administered prior to electrosurgery, the operator should ensure that sterile gloves are placed over the wand handle, and new disposable electrode tips should be utilized. Eye protection, gloves, and masks should be worn by both the operator and the surgical assistants to prevent exposure to smoke-borne organisms or potential mutagens. Smoke evacuation should be ready to remove this smoke plume with electrosection procedures.

Indications:

- Common dermatologic indications for electrofulguration or electrodesiccation include superficial skin ablation for acrochordons, actinic keratosis, small angiomas, epidermal nevus, seborrheic keratosis, verruca plana, or hemostasis for capillary bleeding.
- Electrocoagulation or deep skin ablation can be used to treat angiofibromas, basal cell carcinoma, Bowen's disease, squamous cell carcinoma, ingrown toe nail matrixectomy,

sebaceous hyperplasia, hemostasis from arterial bleeding, benign adnexal tumors (syringoma, trichoepithelioma), or verruca vulgaris.

Contraindication: Though not an absolute contraindication, electrosurgery in patients with cardiac pacemakers or implantable cardiac defibrillator (ICD) devices is a topic of much debate. The flow of electrical energy during electrosurgery can interfere with the functioning of these devices. This can lead to skipped beats, firing of a defibrillator, bradycardia, asystole, or reprogramming of a pacemaker. While most modern implantable devices are resistant to external electromagnetic signals, the theoretical risk of interference still exists.

For patients with these cardiac devices, it is recommended that the surgeon use short bursts of energy of fewer than 5 seconds, lower the power settings, avoid cutting current usage and avoid treating the area around the cardiac device. The risk also decreases by confining the current to a very small area, for example with the use of bipolar forceps.

Complications

Possibility of delayed bleeding and scarring with hypopigmentation. Other potential complications of electrosurgery include fire, thermoelectric burns, infectious transmission from the electrode, or smoke plume inhalation.

CHAPTER 38

Signs and Cells in Dermatology

INTRODUCTION

Adroit observation is one of the virtues of a meticulous physician. Clinical signs are indispensable reflections of an ongoing disease process. Knowledge of various dermatological signs equips dermatologists for an impeccable and integrative diagnostic approach. Majority of these signs appear either de novo or have to be elicited by the physician. We have reviewed the available literature and have made a comprehensive list of signs reported in the literature, which have been described in this chapter. We have also incorporated the signs recently elicited by Indian dermatology stalwarts. This chapter also highlights various important cells of diagnostic importance in the field of dermatology.

Albright's Dimple Sign

It was described by Fuller Albright, which refers to the presence of a dimple over the knuckle of the underdeveloped head of the fourth metacarpal. It can be enhanced by clenching the fist and is seen in Albright's hereditary osteodystrophy.

Antenna Sign

Individual follicles show a long strand of keratin glinting when examined in tangentially incident light. It is seen in keratosis pilaris.

Apple Jelly Sign

When a granulomatous lesion, e.g., sarcoidosis, leishmaniasis and lupus vulgaris, is examined by pressing a glass slide (diascopy), the lesion may reveal yellow brown papules/nodules at the periphery, which are called as apple jelly nodules.

Asboe Hansen Sign (Blister Spread Sign)

Asboe Hansen sign was described by Gustav Asboe Hansen, a Danish dermatologist. It is also known as **blister spread sign,** which refers to the ability to extend a blister at the periphery by applying mechanical pressure on the roof of the intact blister. The Lutz sign refers to the blister spreading into clinically normal skin when lateral pressure is applied to the blister's margin. It is seen in pemphigus, bullous pemphigoid and in bullous drug eruptions.

Auspitz Sign

It is characterised by appearance of a red, glossy surface (Bulkeley's membrane) along with pinpoint bleeding on removal of the scales by scraping with the aid of a glass slide (Grattage test) or by scratching. This occurs as a result of removal of overlying thin suprapapillary epithelium with subsequent rupture of dilated dermal capillaries. Although Heinrich Auspitz, an Austrian dermatologist, is credited for the Auspitz sign, the term is a misnomer. Auspitz sign is neither sensitive nor specific for psoriasis as it occurs in other skin conditions, including actinic keratosis and Darier's disease.

Barnett's Sign (Scleroderma Neck Sign)

Ridging and tightening of the skin of neck on extension of the head which results in visible and palpable tight band over platysma. Seen in scleroderma.

Blue Berry Muffin Sign or Rash

These are non blanchable violet red papulonodular lesions seen in neonates and are due to extramedullary erythropoiesis. Seen in TORCH infection, neuroblastoma, congenital rhabdomyosarcoma, Langerhans cell histiocytosis, hereditary spherocytosis, ABO incompatibility, twin-twin transfusion syndrome etc.

Blue Dot Sign

It is seen in the torsion of the testicular epididymis and appendices. A blue or black tender nodule is visible under the skin on the superior aspect of the testis or epididymis.

BOTE (Beginning Of The End) Sign

In molluscum contagiosum robust inflammatory immune response results in erythema, tenderness and crusting of the lesion which often precedes resolution of lesion.

Branham's Sign (Nicoladoni Sign)

Slowing down of the heart rate and increase in blood pressure in response to manual compression, is characteristically seen in cases of arterio-venous fistula.

Breakfast, Lunch and Dinner Sign

The bites of bed bugs (Cimex lectularius) usually forming a group of three to five dots in linear fashion corresponding to blood meals is known as "Breakfast, lunch and dinner" sign.

Bucket Handle Sign

Fracture occurring through the degenerating metaphysis, leads to exuberant callus growth, resulting in capping over the metaphysis. This is a characteristic finding of congenital syphilis.

Buschke Ollendorff Sign

Deep dermal tenderness, elicited on pressing the lesion with a pin head. It is seen in papular secondary syphilis and cutaneous vasculitis.

Butterfly Sign

It is characterised by erythema over the malar eminence and nasal bridge resembling the wings and body of a butterfly, classically described in lupus erythematosus. Butterfly sign is also occasionally used in reference to butterfly shaped area of sparing observed over the upper central back, corresponding to the zone that is difficult to reach by hands, often seen in conditions with severe generalized pruritus, such as atopic dermatitis.

Buttonhole Sign

In type 1 neurofibromatosis (Von-Recklinghausen's disease), neurofibromas can be invaginated with the tip of index finger into the subcutis which reappear after release of pressure. It can also be seen in anetoderma and dermatofibroma.

Berliner Sign

In children with roseola infantum (exanthema subitum or sixth disease), eyelid edema occurs giving a "droopy" or "sleepy" appearance. The edema disappears after appearance of rash.

Calabar Sign (Calabar swellings)

Subcutaneous migratory swelling due to travelling of an adult filarial worm, Loa-Loa, seen over periorbital area.

Carpet Tack Sign (Cat's Tongue Sign and Tin Tack Sign)

When the adherent scales are removed, the under surface shows horny plugs that had occupied the follicles. It is mainly seen in discoid lupus erythematosus and can also be seen in seborrheic dermatitis and pemphigus foliaceous.

Chagas-Mazza-Romaña's Sign (Romana sign)

In about eighty percent of Chagas' disease (American trypanosomiasis), conjunctiva is the portal of entry. Unilateral swelling after conjunctival inoculation is called as Chagas-mazza-romaña's sign.

Chik Sign

It is centrofacial brown pigmentation specifically over the nose, seen in chikungunya fever.

Clown Nose Sign

A nodular metastatic lesion over tip of nose, seen in squamous cell carcinoma.

Cluster of Jewels Sign (String of Pearls Sign, Rosettes Sign)

This sign is seen in the early stage of chronic bullous disease of childhood, when new lesions appear at the margin of older ones, resembling a cluster of jewels.

Comby Sign

Thin whitish patches on the gingiva and buccal mucosa, made up of desquamating epithelial cells seen in early measles.

Coral Bead Sign

Papules seen around the nail folds in multicentric reticulo-histiocytosis.

Corn Flake Sign

Characteristic polygonal irregular configuration of the lesions over the lower extremities, seen in Kyrle's and Flegel's disease.

Coudability Sign

Shuster first described this sign in alopecia areata (1984). In alopecia areata, perilesional hair is tapered at the proximal end and will bend or kink when pushed inward.

Crowe's Sign

Axillary freckling seen in type I neurofibromatosis.

Cullen's Sign

Periumbilical ecchymosis in cases of acute hemorrhagic pancreatitis and ruptured ectopic pregnancy. Similar change in the flank is called as Grey-Turner sign, in the upper thigh as Fox's sign, in the scrotum as Bryant's sign or blue scrotum sign.

Cayenne Pepper Pus Sign

In actinomycosis, cayenne pepper black granules are observed with drops of pus.

Comet Sign

Presence of erythematous pruritic macules or urticated plaques surmounted by vesicles, associated with a linear erythematous macular tract resembling a comet, in patients with dermatitis caused by pyemotes species.

Darier's Sign

In conditions with an increased number of mast cells in the dermis, such as urticaria pigmentosa, systemic mastocytosis, insect bite reactions, neurofibroma, juvenile xanthogranuloma, and acute neonatal lymphoblastic leukaemia, scratching or rubbing of the lesion produces wheals, circumferential erythema and localized pruritus. This sign was named after Ferdinand-Jean Darier, a French dermatologist.

Dermatographism

On firm stroking of skin, sequential changes in the form of local erythema due to capillary vasodilation, followed by edema, pallor and a surrounding flare induced by axon reflex which leads to dilation of arterioles is observed. It is a form of physical urticaria.

Deck Chair Sign

This sign presents as widespread eruption of erythematous papules that coalesce into rectangular plaques. The term Deck Chair refers to the distinctive pattern of sparing the natural skin folds, resembling the slats of a deck chair. It is seen in papuloerythroderma of Ofuji and has also been reported in cutaneous Waldenstrom's macroglobulinemia and several other conditions as a non-specific sign.

Delmege Sign

In early pulmonary tuberculosis, chronic cough leads to flattening of the Deltoid muscle.

Dew Drop on Rose Petal Sign

It is characterised by vesicles surrounded by erythematous halo resembling dew drop on rose petal, seen in varicella.

Dimple Sign (Fitzpatrick Sign)

This clinical feature is used in diagnosing dermatofibromas. Lateral compression with the thumb and index finger leads to depression in the lesion due to it being attached to the subcutaneous fat. The sign may be useful in differentiating dermatofibromas from other lesions, including malignant melanoma. However, this sign is not completely sensitive or specific to Dermatofibromas.

Dirty Neck Sign

Patients with chronic atopic dermatitis exhibit reticulate pigmentation on anterolateral aspect of the neck. Due to resemblance with unwashed skin, the term "dirty neck" was coined. The pigmentary changes are secondary to melanin incontinence.

Dory Flop Sign

It is described in syphilitic chancre on the coronal border of preputial skin in an uncircumscribed male, on retracting the foreskin, the entire ulcer flips out at once as it is hard to bend due to underlying button like induration.

Doughnut Sign

It is characterised by the induration of skin with central depression over the proximal interphalangeal joint, seen in scleromyxedema.

Drip Sign

In patients of dermatitis artefacta, patterned burned areas are seen, which correspond to the areas of dripping of the corrosive liquid, applied by the patient.

Dubois' Sign

It is a stigma of congenital syphilis where shortening of the little finger occurs.

Ear Sign

Presence of erythematous papules, scaling, or well to ill defined papules and plaques over helix, antihelix, and retroauricular region away from retroauricular fold in case of tinea capitis, whereas erythema, scaling, or fissuring in retroauricular fold, in cases of seborrheic capitis. Other body sites like face and trunk should also be examined to find the lesions of T. corporis, T. faciei, which are present in many cases of T.

capitis. In cases of seborrheic capitis, lesions may be present on eyebrows, nasolabial folds and axilla and in anterior neck crease in infants. This is a useful sign to differentiate T. capitis from seborrheic capitis, especially in children.

Ear Lobe Sign

It is observed in patients who develop contact dermatitis to a substance applied with the hand to the face and neck. Sparing of the diagonal crease of the ear lobe on the ipsilateral side occurs, whereas the contralateral side is affected. This pattern is secondary to the hand sweeping movement made during the application of the substance.

Enamel Paint Sign

It is characterised by sharply demarcated hyperpigmented desquamating patches and plaques resembling enamel paint that occur on the skin of patients with kwashiorkor, predominantly in areas of pressure and irritation. The underlying skin is inflamed and raw.

Exclamation Mark Hair Sign

Proximal tapering of hair is occasionally seen in alopecia areata, where the dot represents the remains of the broken hair on the surface of the scalp. The sign is not pathognomonic for alopecia areata, and its presence may lead to misdiagnosis.

Filipovitch's Sign

It is characterised by yellow discoloration of prominent parts of the palms and soles, seen in typhoid fever.

Flag Sign

It is characterised by horizontal, sharply demarcated alternating bands of discoloration and normal colour in the hair shafts which correspond to periods of abnormal and normal hair growth. The discoloration may be reddish, blonde, gray, or white depending on the original hair color. The flag sign may be seen in patients with nutritional deficiencies, such as kwashiorkor, and with certain medications, such as intermittent high dosage of methotrexate or following chemotherapy. Patients with ulcerative colitis may also show flag sign.

Flag sign is also described in histopathology of actinic keratosis, where in hyperkeratosis and parakeratosis is present. This is due to sparing of the epithelium of acrosyringia and acrotrichia. Orthokeratosis appears at the ostea of these structures, while parakeratosis is seen over abnormally crowded atypical keratinocytes, giving rise to a characteristic pattern of alternating ortho and parakeratosis, referred to as the "flag sign".

Forscheimer's Sign

It is characterised by an enanthem (dull red macules or petechiae) which is confined to the soft palate during the prodromal period or on the first day of the rash. It is seen in 20% of rubella patients and can also be seen in infectious mononucleosis.

Frank's Sign

Frank sign is a diagonal crease of the ear lobe and has been strongly associated with atherosclerotic cardiac disease.

Friar Tuck Sign

Friar tuck was a companion of Robin Hood in the legendary stories who had alopecia of the vertex with sparing of the occipital region. This sign is described in relation to trichotillomania, where the occipital area is mostly spared.

Gabrin Sign

It is characterized by an occurrence of androgenetic alopecia like hair loss in hospitalized COVID-19 patients.

Giovannini Sign

The appearance of completely white and opaque fingernails resembling ivory, may be seen as sequelae of typhoid fever.

Goat Eye Sign

In few cases of Orf, lesions show horizontal, rectangular iris shaped areas at the center, which is known as goat eye sign.

Gorlin's Sign

It is the ability to touch the tip of the nose by extension of the tongue, seen in Ehlers-Danlos syndrome.

Gottron's Sign

It is characterised by scaly erythematous eruption seen on the dorsum of hands, metacarpophalangeal joints, and proximal interphalangeal joints in dermatomyositis.

Greenhow's Sign (Vagabond's Sign)

It is characterised by excoriations and discoloration of the skin due to scratching and irritation, as a result of body lice infestation. It is also known as parasitic melanoderma.

Groove Sign

It is classically described in eosinophilic fasciitis (Shulman's syndrome) where there is a linear groove or indentation along the superficial veins on the medial aspect of the upper extremity.

"Groove sign of Greenblatt" is seen in lymphogranuloma venereum, where enlargement of both inguinal and femoral group of lymph nodes, separated by the Poupart's ligament produces a groove.

Hair Collar Sign

It is characterised by the presence of ectopic neural tissue in the occipital and parietal areas which takes the form of smooth dome shaped hairless nodules, sometimes surrounded by a collar of hypertrichosis. It is a marker of cranial dysraphism, including encephalocele, meningocele, and heterotropic brain tissue.

Hairy Palm Sign

In the histopathology of Prurigo nodularis, folliculo sebaceous units are seen with a thick and compact cornified layer resembling a biopsy taken from the palm. Palmer skin is devoid of pilosebaceous units.

Hamburger Sign

It is characterised by vertically oriented split of hair shafts containing proteinaceous material and erythrocytes resembling a hamburger within a bun, seen in trichotillomania.

Hang Glider Sign

It is a characteristic dark triangular biting apparatus of Sarcoptes scabiei, seen at the end of the subcorneal tunnel.

Hanging Curtain Sign

When the skin is stretched across the long axis of the herald patch in pityriasis rosea, the scales are noted to be finer, lighter, and attached at one end, which tends to fold across the line of stretch.

Hanging Groin Sign

In onchocerciasis, massive enlargement of the lymph nodes in the inguinal area, leading to inelastic and atrophic skin gives the appearance of "hanging groins".

Heliotrope Sign

The word Heliotrope is derived from the Greek word helios, meaning "sun" and trapein, meaning "to turn". In patients with dermatomyositis, a characteristic violaceous erythema involving the periorbital skin is seen. The term heliotrope refers to the purplish colour of the flowers of the heliotrope plant family, which rotate to face the sun.

Hennebert's Sign

On application of pressure over the sealed external auditory canal, nystagmus is seen in congenital syphilis and Meniere's disease.

Hertoghe's Sign (Queen Anne's Sign)

It is a characteristic loss of lateral one third of eyebrows (superciliary madarosis), seen in leprosy, myxedema, follicular mucinosis, atopic dermatitis, trichotillomania, ectodermal dysplasia, discoid lupus erythematosus, alopecia areata, syphilis, ulerythema ophryogenes, systemic sclerosis, HIV infection, hypothyroidism etc.

Higoumenaki's Sign

In patients with late congenital syphilis, enlargement of the sternal end of the (right) clavicle is frequently observed.

Hoagland's Sign

It is an early and transient bilateral upper eyelid edema occurring in patients with infectious mononucleosis. This sign is usually present only for the first few days of the clinical presentation of the illness.

Holster Sign of Dermatomyositis

The word Holster means an extra pocket made from various materials to hold something where it can quickly be taken out for use (e.g., gun holster). Confluent macular violaceous erythema present on the lateral side of hip and thighs is called as "Holster sign", corresponding to the site of hanging a holster.

Hutchinson's Sign

In subungual melanoma, melanonychia with pigmentation of proximal nail fold is seen (Hutchinson's sign).

Micro Hutchinson's sign is a highly characteristic dermoscopic feature of early nail apparatus melanoma, denoting pigmentation of the periungual tissues.

Pseudo Hutchinson's sign is a reflection of the pigmentation of the nail bed and nail matrix through transparent nail fold.

Presence of papulovesicular lesions on the tip of nose in a patient of herpes zoster indicates involvement of cornea as both are supplied by nasociliary nerve, a branch of trigeminal nerve, is also known as Hutchinson's sign.

Hypopyon Sign

In pyodermas and secondarily infected vesicobullous disorders (e.g., pemphigus, bullous pemphigoid and linear IgA dermatosis) transverse fluid level comprising purulent material at the bottom of vesicle or bullae may be seen when the patient is in a standing position.

Ingram's Sign

It is the inability to retract the lower eyelid in patients of progressive systemic sclerosis due to underlying sclerosis.

Jellinek's Sign (Rasin's Sign)

It is the peri orbital hyperpigmentation of the eyelids, especially upper eyelid, seen in hyperthyroidism.

Kaposi Stemmer Sign

It is the inability to pinch or pick up a fold of skin at the base of the second toe because of its thickness, seen in chronic lymphedema.

Knife Cut Sign

Linear fissuring and ulceration over intertriginous areas is seen in cutaneous Crohn's disease, herpes simplex infection, and immunocompromised patients.

Krisovski's Sign

It refers to cicatricial lines radiating from the mouth in congenital syphilis.

Leopard Skin Sign

In onchocerciasis, repeated episodes of dermatitis associated with death of microfilariae leading to depigmentation, is described as leopard skin sign.

Leser Trelat Sign

It is characterized by sudden eruption of numerous seborrheic keratosis, usually associated with pruritus and is considered as a marker of internal malignancy.

Lizard Skin Sign

In onchocerciasis, subcutaneous fibrosis, skin atrophy and pigmentary changes make the skin look like lizard skin.

Love's Sign

In glomus tumor, tenderness can be exactly localized with the help of pin head.

Matchbox Sign (Specimen sign)

In delusions of parasitosis (acarophobia, entomophobia), patient collects skin debris in a matchbox, tissue paper, or in small container, with mistaken belief that such collected material allegedly contains a parasite.

Meffert's Sign

In Fordyce's disease, prominent lip involvement can result in a lipstick like mark left on the rim of a glass mug after consuming a hot beverage because of the presence of ectopically located sebaceous glands.

Milian's Ear Sign

It is used to distinguish between erysipelas and cellulitis of the facial region, where ear is involved in erysipelas and spared in cellulitis, as there is no deeper dermal tissue and subcutaneous fat in ear.

Milk Sign or Scarlet Milk Sign

Brightly red flushed face with circumoral pallor, seen in scarlet fever.

Mizutani's Sign (Round Finger Pad Sign)

It is the transition from a peaked finger pad shape to a hemisphere like fingertip contour, particularly on the ring finger, seen in systemic sclerosis related Raynaud's phenomenon.

Muehrcke's Sign

It is characterised by paired, transverse, narrowed white bands that run parallel to the lunula of the nail occurring usually on the second, third and fourth fingernails, excluding thumbnails. The distal bands tend to be wider than the proximal bands. It is associated with hypoalbuminemia due to nephrotic syndrome, glomerulonephritis, liver disease, malnutrition and patients receiving chemotherapy.

Nagayama Sign

It is the appearance of erythematous papules on soft palate and uvula, seen in roseola infantum.

Nazzaro's Sign

Follicular hairy hyperkeratosis (horny follicular spicules), which typically occur on the face. Histopathologically, it exhibits compact follicle bound hyperkeratosis. It is an uncommon but typical clinical finding in multiple myeloma.

Necklace of Casal Sign

It is characterised by hyperpigmentation occurring on the neck owing to pellagra as a result of niacin (vitamin B_3) deficiency. The "necklace" can extend as a broad collar like band around the entire circumference of the neck. Sometimes the necklace extends anteriorly over the sternum to the level of the nipples and ends in a point or square. Cutaneous changes in pellagra appear primarily on sun-exposed areas on the neck, face, and dorsal parts of the hands, arms, and feet, but patients usually also have dermatitis elsewhere.

Nikolsky's Sign

This sign is named after the Russian dermatologist Piotr Vasiliyerich Nikolsky who described it in 1894.

It is a popular sign in dermatology, which refers to easy peeling of skin on applying tangential pressure over a bony prominence and is classically seen in pemphigus group of disorders. Nikolsky's sign can also be elicited in the oral cavity with the help of cotton tipped applicator.

Pseudo Nikolsky (Epidermal peeling sign) refers to the ability to peel off the entire epidermis by lateral pressure (rubbing) on the erythematous areas of involved skin. The mechanism of Pseudo Nikolsky is necrosis of the epidermal cells and not acantholysis. It is positive in SJS, TEN, some cases of burns and in bullous ichthyosiform erythroderma.

False Nikolsky (Sheklakov's sign) is seen when pulling of the peripheral remnant roof of a ruptured blister, and extending it over the normal skin, results in erosions which are limited in size, lack tendency to extend and heal rapidly. So, basically, it is the sub epidermal cleavage, occurring in perilesional skin and is positive in bullous pemphigoid, cicatricial pemphigoid, pemphigoid gestationis, dermatitis herpetiformis, linear immunoglobin A (IgA), bullous dermatosis, epidermolysis bullosa acquisita, junctional and dystrophic epidermolysis bullosa, porphyrias and bullous SLE.

Variants of Nikolsky Sign

1. **Wet Nikolsky:** On applying pressure, the eroded base is moist and glistening.
2. **Dry Nikolsky:** On applying pressure, the eroded base is dry, indicating re-epithelialization, signifying healing.
3. **Marginal Nikolsky:** Rubbing the surrounding/perilesional skin, results in extension of the erosion on surrounding normal appearing skin.
4. **Direct Nikolsky:** Rubbing the skin distant from the lesions, results in induction of erosion on normal appearing skin. Positive Direct Nikolsky, indicates severe activity of the disease. When disease responds to therapy, it is the first sign to disappear.
5. **Microscopic/Subclinical Nikolsky:** Tangential pressure on apparently normal skin, results in weakening of the intercellular adhesions (pathological changes). The damage can only be demonstrated microscopically. It is a better and more sensitive method of rapid diagnosis, which can increase the sensitivity of histological diagnosis of pemphigus vulgaris.

Nose Sign (Pavithran's Nose Sign)

It is the complete absence of erythema and scaling of the skin over the nose and perinasal area, seen in exfoliative dermatitis. It is hypothesized that sparing of nose in exfoliative dermatitis could be due to greater sun exposure of nose or it could be explained by the mechanism of island of normal skin.

Oil Drop Sign

It is characterized by translucent, yellow red discoloration and circular areas of onycholysis in the nail bed that does not reach the free border and resembles oil drops underneath the nail. It is caused by nail bed parakeratosis and psoriasiform hyperplasia. Some authors make a distinction between oil drop sign and oil spot sign, where later refers to yellowish or brown macules beneath the nail plate that extend proximally to the hyponychium. Both findings can be seen in psoriasis.

Osler's Sign

It is blue black pigmentation in the sclera near insertion of rectus muscle in patients with alkaptonuria (Endogenous ochronosis).

Panda's Sign

It is the persistence of the nevus of Ota in the periorbital location following laser therapy, whereas other peripheral sites clear well.

Pastia's Sign

It is characterized by linear petechial eruption in the skin folds especially on the ante cubital fossa and axillary fold, seen in streptococcal scarlet fever.

Patrick Yesudian Sign

It is characterized by palmar melanotic macules (palmar freckling), seen in type 1 Neurofibromatosis.

Pemberton Sign

On elevation of both arms, facial plethora is seen. This maneuver is used to evaluate the venous obstruction in large retrosternal goiter.

Pitaluga's Sign

Pitaluga's sign is an acquired hypertrichosis of eyelashes in patients with kala azar or visceral leishmaniasis.

Prayer Sign

Prayer sign is said to be positive when patient is unable to bring both the palmar surface together completely, as at prayer, which indicates limited joint mobility due to non-enzymatic glycosylation of collagen and its deposition in the small joints of the hand. It is described in relation to diabetic cheiroarthropathy.

Promontory Sign

It is the appearance of a small vessel protruding into an abnormal vascular space, described in the histopathology of Kaposi's sarcoma and in patch and plaque stage of angiosarcoma.

Pseudo Darier's Sign

Stroking of lesion leads to transient induration with piloerection, seen in smooth muscle hamartoma and Becker's nevus.

Punshi's Sign

Original white color of vitiligo macules turns to red pink during menstruation and turns back to it's original color thereafter, seen in young women and girls with vitiligo.

Pup Tent Sign

It is characterized by splitting and longitudinal elevation of the nails with downward angle of lateral nail edge, seen in nail lichen planus.

Racoon Sign (Racoon Eye, Owl Eye, Eye Mask)

It is the most common cutaneous manifestation of neonatal lupus erythematosus. characterised by slightly scaly, erythematous eruption on the face and periorbital skin. In patients with systemic amyloidosis, periorbital haemorrhage due to laxity of blood vessels seen after proctoscopic examination (postproctoscopic periorbital purpura) is also called as Racoon eyes/sign/panda sign.

Reverse Namaskar Sign

Namaskar is the typical Indian way of greeting people, where the forearms are folded in front of the chest and the palms are closely approximated together. In patients with Ehlers-Danlos syndrome, they are able to fold their forearms at the back and oppose their palms to say "Namaskar", demonstrating the hyper extensible joints.

Rope Sign

It is characterised by a thick indurated inflammatory cord like structure that extends from the lateral trunk to the axillae and said to be a classical finding of interstitial granulomatous dermatitis (Ackerman's syndrome) with arthritis.

Russell's Sign

It is characterised by a crusted callosity on the knuckles of dominant hand due to repeated self induced vomiting in patients of bulimia nervosa.

Samitz's Sign

It is dystrophic and ragged cuticle around nail. Seen in dermatomyositis.

Sandwich Sign

In dermatophytosis, fungi are present in the horny layer between two zones of cornified cells, the upper being orthokeratotic and lower consisting of partially parakeratotic cells, giving it sandwitch appearance.

Sarcophagus Sign

It is a radiological finding showing periosteal new bone formation resulting in layers of bone marrow trapped between layers of subperiosteal bone enveloping entire shaft resembling a sarcophagus. Seen in congenital syphilis.

School Chair Sign

It is characterised by rash which occurs over the posterior thighs, corresponding to contact with a school chair, seen in allergic contact dermatitis to nickel.

Scratch Sign (Coup D'Ongle Sign, Besnier's Sign, Stroke of the Nail Sign)

In pityriasis versicolor, scarcely noticeable scales are made to stand out by scratching the lesion with fingernail. Scales are usually of white or light tan in color and flake off easily.

Seat Rash Sign

It is characterised by urticarial lesions over buttocks, seen in infection with roundworm, Strongyloides stercoralis.

Shawl Sign

It comprises confluent macular violaceous erythema on the posterior neck and shoulders, seen in patients with dermatomyositis.

Shelly's Sign

It is characterised by Sago like eruption on the palate and lips, seen in influenza.

Shuster's Sign

It is characterized by scarring of the concha due to lesions of discoid lupus erythematosus (present in 30% of the cases).

Silex's Sign

These are radial furrows around mouth in early congenital syphilis.

Slapped Cheek Sign

In children with fifth disease (Erythema infectiosum), where confluent, erythematous, oedematous plaques on the cheeks are seen. This manifestation is often the first skin change seen in patients with fifth disease. As the facial rash begins to fade over 1 to 4 days, erythematous macules and papules begin to appear on the trunk, neck and extensor surfaces of the extremities.

Stafne's Sign

It is characterized by widening of the periodontal ligament space due to increase in the collagen synthesis and increase in the bulk of the ligament, which is incorporated at the expense of alveolar bone, thus causing an increase in the width of the periodontal ligament space. Seen in progressive systemic sclerosis.

Table Top Sign

It is the inability to place palms flat on a horizontal surface seen in patients with diabetic cheiroarthropathy.

Tasleem's Water Jet Sign

When a local anesthetic is injected in the verrucous surface of warts over the thick skin areas such as palms and soles, there is spilling out of anesthetic solution resembling gush of water, is known as Tasleem's water jet sign.

Tent Sign

When skin overlying the solitary firm nodule is stretched, it appears to be multifaceted and angulated, giving a "tent" appearance, due to the calcification occurring in the lesion. Seen in pilomatricoma.

Thumb Print Sign

It is characterised by periumbilical purpura which resemble multiple thumb prints. It is seen in patients with disseminated strongyloidiasis, where while receiving respiratory assistance, an evanescent rise in portal pressure leads to the larvae causing extravasation of red blood cells into the dermis, resulting in characteristic petechiae and purpura.

Thumb Sign (Steinberg Sign)

It is characterized by extension of the thumb past the ulnar border of the hand when apposed to the palm. Seen in Marfan syndrome.

Toy Soldier Sign

It is characterised by linear aggregation of neoplastic lymphocytes along the dermoepidermal junction seen in histopathology of mycosis fungoides.

Tripe Palms Sign (Acanthosis Palmaris, Pachydermatoglyphy)

There is an increase in rugosity of the palmar surface of the hands, with accentuation of the normal dermatoglyphic ridges, thus resembling the ridging of the interior surface of a bovine foregut. It is strongly associated with internal malignancy, most commonly carcinoma of the stomach and lung. Acanthosis nigricans may be associated with it.

Trousseau's Sign

Two different types of Trousseau's sign are described, referring to distinct clinical conditions.

Trousseau's sign of visceral malignancy, also known as migratory thrombophlebitis, refers to the development of successive crops of tender nodules in the course of affected blood vessels secondary to intravascular low grade hypercoagulation. It occurs when blood clots appear unexpectedly in superficial veins, and then overtime migrate to different locations. Usually, the upper extremities or the trunk is affected. The condition occurs predominantly with pancreatic cancer, as well as with stomach and lung cancer.

Trousseau's sign of tetany is associated with hypocalcaemia elicited by compressing the brachial artery in the upper arm with a tourniquet or blood pressure cuff for 3 minutes, resulting in carpal spasm and is characterized by involuntary contraction of the fingers and hands, giving appearance of obstetrical hand.

Ugly Duckling Sign

In 1998, Grob and Bonerandi introduced the "ugly duckling" sign to demonstrate that nevi in the same individual tend to resemble one another and but there may be an atypical mole that deviates from the individual's nevus pattern. The nevus that does not resemble other nevi is more likely to be suspicious of melanoma.

Umbilical Sign

It is the ability to touch the umbilicus with the right hand, crossing the back, and approaching from the left side, indicating an increased length of the upper extremity. Seen in Marfan syndrome.

V- Sign

It is characterised by confluent macular violaceous erythema on the anterior neck and chest, seen in patients with dermatomyositis.

Virchow's Sign

It is tongue with smooth base, seen in congenital syphilis.

Volcano Sign

The lesion starts as a small nontender papule, which enlarges in size and ulcerates in the centre. The border of the crusted ulcer often has an erythematous rim resembling an erupted volcano, which is called a "Volcano sign". It is a descriptive term for the morphologic feature of old world cutaneous leishmaniasis (oriental sore).

Walzel Sign

It is the appearance of livedo reticularis in association with acute and chronic pancreatitis.

Wartenberg's Sign

The little finger assumes the position of constant abduction secondary to paralysis of the adductor digiti minimi. It is considered the earliest sign of ulnar nerve affection in leprosy.

Wimberger's Sign (Cat Bite Sign)

The presence of bilateral, symmetrical, and well-defined metaphyseal defects on the medial surface of upper tibia, can result in pseudo paralysis, considered pathognomonic of congenital syphilis. It can also be seen in scurvy known as Wimberger ring sign.

Winterbottom's Sign

It is the characterised by enlarged posterior cervical lymph nodes which are seen in early stages of African trypanosomiasis (sleeping sickness) and is caused by Trypanosoma brucei rhodensiense and Trypanosoma brucei gambiense.

Wrist Sign (Walker's Sign)

In Marfan syndrome, thumb and fifth finger can easily encircle the opposite wrist.

White Islands in a Sea of Red Sign

In dengue fever, a generalized confluent petechial rash with multiple small round islets of normal skin is seen.

Zig Zag Sign (Saw Tooth Metaphysis/ Wegner Sign)

It is the appearance of serrations at the metaphysis of long bones in congenital syphilis.

NAMED CELLS IN DERMATOLOGY

Balloon Cells

Balloon cells are characteristics of Balloon cell nevus. They are polyhedral cells with abundant microvesicular cytoplasm and sparse to absent pigmentation. Nuclei are hyperchromatic, small with round to scalloped central nuclei and they rarely have intranuclear pseudo inclusions.

Basalioma Cells

These cells resemble epidermal basal cells, having round nuclei and cytoplasm. The characteristic arrangement is in the form of strands and lobules displaying peripheral palisading pattern which is seen in Trichoepithelioma. Rarely these cells can also be seen in basal cell carcinoma.

Bean Bag Cells

These are large swollen macrophages due to phagocytosis of lymphocytes, erythrocytes and cellular debris. Seen in histiocytic cytophagic panniculitis.

Clue Cells

These are vaginal squamous epithelial cells impregnated with large number of coccobacillary organisms, *Gardnerella vaginalis* and other anaerobic bacteria. The cells have characteristic stippled borders and hazy cytoplasm. It is seen in bacterial vaginosis. More than 20% of clue cells on the wet mount preparation is diagnostic for bacterial vaginosis.

Doughnut Cells

These are large anaplastic mononuclear cells containing intranuclear cytoplasmic inclusions. These inclusions are due to deep cytoplasmic invaginations into the nuclei. Half doughnut cell is characterized by >70% nuclear indentation of the total nuclear diameter. Seen in anaplastic large cell lymphoma.

Downey Cell (Turk Cell)

These atypical lymphocytes named after Hal Downey are characterised by abundant pale blue cytoplasm and irregular light stained nucleus. Indentation by cytoplasmic edges of other blood cells leads to scalloping at the periphery of lymphocytes, giving Dutch skirting appearance. The detection of at least 10% atypical lymphocytes on a peripheral blood smear in a patient of infectious mononucleosis has a sensitivity of 75% and a specificity of 92%.

Floret Giant Cells

These are multinucleated giant cells having nuclei arranged at the margin of the cells and eosinophilic cytoplasm at the center. They are seen in pleomorphic lipoma, giant cell collagenoma, giant cell fibroblastoma, giant cell angiofibroma, neurofibromatosis type 1 etc.

Flower Cells or Clover Leaf Cells

These are atypical lymphocytes characterized by irregular nuclear silhouette, condensed chromatin and deeply basophilic, occasionally vacuolated cytoplasm. Flower cells are considered pathognomonic of adult T cell lymphoma with cutaneous manifestations such as erythroderma, plaques, papules, nodules and tumors.

Gargoyle Cells (Hurler Cells)

These are large polygonal cells with clear cytoplasm and pale central nucleus. When stained with toluidine blue, metachromatic granules are seen in the cytoplasm. On electron microscopy, the cytoplasm shows large irregular clear vacuoles with broken membrane. Occasionally, scattered mitochondria and cisterns of endoplasmic reticulum are seen between vacuoles. They are seen in Hurler syndrome.

Gaucher Cells

Gaucher cells are glucocerebroside laden macrophages in bone marrow and reticuloendothelial system measuring 50–60 µm in diameter. On electron microscopy, they contain tubular cytoplasmic inclusions that are considered to be altered secondary lysosomes. Cytoplasm resembles crinkled blue tissue paper due to fibrillar ceramide accumulations.

Ghost Cells

Ghost cells are also known as shadow cells. These are anucleate, eosinophilic, keratinized cells having a central unstained area as a shadow of the absent nucleus. Ghost cells are seen in pilomatricoma with frequent calcification.

Glomus Cells

They are large polyhedral cells originating from smooth muscles of arteriovenous segment of Sequet-Hoyer canal and is characterised by a round, centrally located nucleus with a pale eosinophilic cytoplasm. Glomus tumours and glomangiomas arise from the arterial segment of the cutaneous glomus. Glomus formations are special arteriovenous shunts critical for thermoregulation.

Granular Cells

These large polygonal cells in the dermis consists of characteristic cell membranes, prominent eosinophilic granular cytoplasm with small, round to oval and centrally located nuclei. Granular cell tumor, which is of peripheral nerve sheath origin, predominantly involves skin and tongue along with various parts of the body.

Greenblatt and Pund Cells

These are large mononuclear cells with eccentric vesicular or pyknotic nucleus and intracytoplasmic vacuoles containing Donovan bodies, seen in granuloma inguinale.

Half and Half Cells

These are altered keratinocytes which shows increased synthetic activity in one half of the cell and fibrillar degeneration in the other half of the cell, commonly seen in lichen planus. These are believed to provide a useful clue to the early changes occurring in colloid body formation.

Halo Cells

These are large intraepidermal lymphocytes with convoluted, cerebriform nuclei and a clear rim of cytoplasm, seen in mycosis fungoides.

Hibernoma Like Cell (Mulberry Cells, Multivesicular Cells)

These are large fat cells containing a central nucleus with a multivacuolated scanty granular, eosinophilic cytoplasm, seen in hibernoma. Typical adipose cells have clear cytoplasm and eccentric nucleus which differentiate them from hibernoma cells.

Hobnail Cells

These are plump endothelial cells with scanty cytoplasm and prominent, hyperchromatic nuclei that bulge into the vascular lamina, resulting in a characteristic hobnail or match stick appearance, seen in hobnail hemangioma.

Koilocytes

These are human papilloma virus infected vacuolated keratinocytes that contain a basophilic pyknotic nucleus surrounded by a clear halo and pale staining cytoplasm with few or absent keratohyaline granules. These cells are located in the upper stratum spinosum and in the granular layer, seen in verruca.

Langerhans Cell

Langerhans cell are pale staining non keratinocyte, with a convoluted nucleus, located in epidermis, oral cavity, oesophagus, vagina for antigen processing. The cytoplasm contains vimentin intermediate filaments and small rod or racket shaped structures called Birbeck granules. Langerhans cells are reduced in diseases like psoriasis, sarcoidosis and contact dermatitis, while they are increased in Langerhans cell histiocytosis.

Langhans Giant Cells

These cells are formed by the fusion of epithelioid cells and contain multiple nuclei arranged in a horseshoe shaped pattern in the cell periphery seen in tuberculoid granulomas, e.g., tuberculoid leprosy, cutaneous tuberculosis, gumma of syphilis and sporotrichosis etc.

LE Cell

The LE cell also called as Lupus Erythematous cell, is the result of phagocytosis of distorted nuclear material by a polymorphonuclear cells. The LE cell contains LE body, which appears as a homogenous, pale blue to deep purplish material driving the nucleus of the phagocyte to one side of the cell. These cells are classically seen in systemic lupus erythematosus.

Mantle Cells (Corps Ronds)

Corps ronds are dyskeratotic keratinocytes with a small pyknotic nucleus, acidophilic cytoplasm and a perinuclear halo, seen in the stratum granulosum and upper Malpighian layer in Darier's disease.

Mast Cells

Mast cells are round to spindle shaped cells with a unilobed round to oval centrally positioned nucleus and granular cytoplasm. These cells synthesize an impressive gamut of mediators, e.g., histamine, heparin, tryptase, chymase, carboxypeptidase, neutrophil chemotactic factor and eosinophilic chemotactic factor. Mast cells are present in greatest density in the papillary dermis, near the DEJ, in sheaths of epidermal appendages, around blood vessels and nerves of the subpapillary plexus. They play an important role in the host defense against pathogens. Their numbers are increased in mastocytosis.

Merkel Cells

Merkel cells are named after the German anatomist Friedrich Sigmund Merkel. These non keratinocytes are oval shaped cells, have pale staining cytoplasm, bundles of intermediary filaments, osmophilic granules with large lobulated nuclei. The margins of these cells project cytoplasmic "spines" toward the keratinocytes. They are slow adapting, type I mechanoreceptors. found both in hairy and glabrous skin of the digits, lips, oral cavity and outer root sheath of the hair follicle.

Mickulicz Cells

Mickulicz cells are large histiocytes with pale vacuolated cytoplasm. They are characteristically seen in rhinoscleroma where Klebsiella bacilli are present in the vacuolated cytoplasm of these cells.

Mitosoid Cells

These are keratinocytes present in upper spinous layer of epidermis. They have an irregularly shaped, fragmented hyperchromatic nuclei (mitosoid bodies or mitosoid figure) that imitates mitoses. Seen in focal epithelial hyperplasia or heck's disease.

Paget's Cells

Paget's cells are larger than keratinocytes with round to oval nucleus and a vacuolated amphophilic cytoplasm. The gigantic irregular nucleus has scanty nuclear chromatin and a large nucleolus. There is no desmosomal connections between Paget's cells and the nearby keratinocytes. Seen in Paget's disease.

Pekin Cells (Reiter Cell)

They are large macrophages which contain one or more intact polymorphonuclear cells. Seen in inflammatory synovial disease like Reiter's disease (presents in 50–70% of synovial fluid specimens).

Podophyllin Cells

These are peculiar, enlarged epithelial cells with clumped pyknotic nucleus or disintegrated and dispersed nuclear chromatin as small granules throughout the cytoplasm. These cells have a close resemblance with carcinoma cells, but may be differentiated from malignant cells by the absence of cytological atypia. They are seen after podophyllin application to normal skin, verruca vulgaris and condyloma accuminata.

Reed Sternberg Cells

They are named after Dorothy Reed Mendenhall and Carl Sternberg. These cells contain bilobed nucleus with prominent eosinophilic nucleoli (owl's eye) which is surrounded by abundant cytoplasm. They may also be multinucleated. These cells are pathognomonic for classical Hodgkin's lymphoma (HL). Other than HL, similar cells may be present in other T and B cell lymphomas, sarcomas, melanomas and carcinomas.

Sezary Cells (Mycosis Cell, Lutzner Cells, Atypia Cellules Monstreuses or Monster Cell, Cerebriform Lymphocytes)

These cells were first described by Albert Sézary. They are atypical lymphocytes having a grooved or cerebriform nucleus with condensed nuclear chromatin (in patchy distribution beneath the nuclear membrane) and prominent nucleoli. Sparse cytoplasm around the nucleus appears as a narrow rim. Clumped mitochondria and serpentine cytoplasmic fibrils are seen on electron microscopic examination. Lutzner cells are miniature version of Sezary cells. Seen in mycosis fungoides and Sezary syndrome.

Signet Ring Cells

These cells have eccentric hyperchromatic nucleus with single large vacuole containing mucin. This pool of mucin mimics the appearance of a finger hole and the nucleus mimics the appearance of the face of the ring in profile. Seen in mucin producing adenocarcinomas.

Strap Cell

These cells have elongated eosinophilic cytoplasm, suggestive of rhabdomyosarcoma.

Sunburn Cells

These are keratinocytes undergoing apoptosis after exposure to UVC, UVB or UVA radiation in the presence of psoralens due to severe and irreversible damage of nucleus. These cells are seen scattered throughout the epidermis and have a shrunken glassy eosinophilic cytoplasm and a pyknotic nucleus. Seen in sunburns and PUVA induced acute phototoxicity.

Tadpole Cells

"Tadpole like" shape is characteristic of these cells. Tzanck smear preparation (at 100x magnification) showing more than 10 tadpole cells is a diagnostic indicator for spongiotic vesicular dermatitis, e.g., allergic contact dermatitis.

Tart Cell

It is a monocyte that has consumed an intact lymphocyte nucleus. Secondary nucleus retaining its definite chromatin structure, makes it different from a LE cell. There number is increased in SLE, however they may also be normally seen in bone marrow.

Touton Giant Cells

Touton giant cells have a garland like arrangement of nuclei peripherally, with central amphophilic cytoplasm. Nuclei are surrounded by pale foamy cytoplasm. Seen in conditions like xanthoma, disseminated xanthoma, juvenile xanthogranuloma, necrobiotic xanthogranuloma and dermatofibroma.

Tzanck Cells (Acantholytic Cells, Mourning Edged Cells)

These cells are named after Arnault Tzanck, a French dermatologist. Tzanck cells are large, round keratinocytes having a hypertrophic nucleus, foggy or absent nucleoli and profuse basophilic cytoplasm. The basophilic staining is deeper at periphery near cell membrane, due to cytoplasmic condensation at the periphery. The pale staining cytoplasm at center appears as a perinuclear halo (mourning edged cells). In contrast to pemphigus vulgaris, the acantholytic cells in pemphigus foliaceus and pemphigus erythematosus often have a hyalinized cytoplasm that corresponds to the dyskeratosis seen in tissue sections. In pemphigus it is a form of primary acantholysis. The other examples include Darier's disease, transient acantholytic dermatoses and warty dyskeratoma. When acantholysis occurs secondary to some alteration/ damage to epidermal cells, the term secondary acantholysis is used, e.g., bullous impetigo, herpes simplex/zoster and squamous cell carcinoma.

Veil Cell

These cells are flat, fibroblast like cells around dermal microvessels. They have a distinct nucleus and prominent cytoplasmic processes. Lying externally to the wall, they separate the vessel from the surrounding dermis and express factor XIII a and Von-Willebrand factor. At the microvascular level, these cells participate in the control of bleeding by their positioning in the organization of the microvessel.

Virchow Cell (Lepra Cell)

These are foamy vacuolated histiocytes containing abundant cytoplasm with single nucleus often shifted to sides due to vacuoles with enormous number of lepra bacilli named after Rudolph Virchow. In some cases, large number of vacuoles may result into very little or negligible cytoplasm. After commencement of multi drug therapy, degenerated bacilli tend to cumulate in lepra cells. These cells are seen in lepromatous leprosy. Closest differential morphology of these cells are xanthoma cells which upon staining with fat specific stains show largely neutral fat and phospholipids rather than cholesterol.

Vulvar Clear Cells of Toker (Intraepidermal Glandular Clear Cells of Toker)

These are intraepithelial germinative cells with clear to pale staining featureless cytoplasm, found in basal layer of the epidermis adjacent to the openings of the lactiferous ducts. These cells are found as single units or as small aggregates that seldom form small lumina. Toker's cells are precursor for Paget's disease.

Warthin Finkeldey Cells

These are multinucleated giant cells (containing 100 nuclei per cell) along with cytoplasmic and nuclear inclusion bodies. These cells are pathognomonic for measles and are found in reticuloendothelial system, Koplik spots and respiratory secretions.

Wright Cells

They are large macrophages containing numerous protozoa grouped together resembling typical "swarm of bees" appearance within the weakly basophilic cytoplasm. Seen in leishmaniasis.

Xanthoma Cells

These cells contain lipid laden, abundant vacuolated foamy cytoplasm with small uniform nuclei without any mitotic activity. Seen in various xanthomatoses e.g. familial hyperlipoproteinemia types IIa, III and V, cerebro tendinous xanthomatosis, Wolman's disease, Tangier disease, Hand-Schüller-Christian disease and normolipidemic cutaneous xanthomatosis.

Aldrich-Mees' lines: Transverse white lines of discoloration across nails of fingers and toes aka leukonychia striata. Seen in infections, renal disease, cardiac disease, malignant disease and poisoning (arsenic, thallium).

Beau's lines: Transverse depressions in that nail plate that occur after a stressful event that causes temporary cessation of the proliferation of proximal nail unit. Seen in measles, mumps, thrombosis, Kawasaki's disease, pneumonia, pulmonary embolism and renal failure.

Janeway lesion: These are non tender and hemorrhagic lesions seen on palms and soles seen in bacterial endocarditis.

Osler's nodes: Painful erythematous nodules on the pads of finfers and toes. Seen in bacterial endocarditis.

Caput medusae: Dilated abdominal vessels radiating from the umbilicus. Seen in portal venous hypertension and liver failure.

Dennie-Morgan fold: The extra fold of skin beneath the eye seen in atopic patients.

Pathergy sign: Appearance of a new lesion or worsening of the existing lesions by superficial trauma. Seen in pyoderma gangrenosum and Bechet's disease.

Hildreth's sign: Relieved of pain and tenderness on exsanguination and ischemia of the affected part by raising the extremity affected and inflating a sphygmomanometer applied to it above the systolic blood pressure, and sudden return of pain when pressure on the cuff is relieved. Seen in glomus tumor.

Kerr's sign: A palpable change in skin texture (stiff, dry, or tense) inferior to the somatic level of a spinal cord lesion.

Sister Mary Joseph's nodules: Firm, indurated nodules, sometimes with fissuring and ulceration of the umbilicus. These are metastatic usually an intra-abdominal malignant disease such as primary malignancy of stomach, bowel and or pancreas.

Alcohol wipe sign: Reticulated brown patches that are dirt-like and can be cleared by forceful rubbing with alcohol wipes. Typical of Terra firma-forme dermatosis.

Ball-site sign: Sports induced targetoid erythema. Seen after cutaneous injury from a high velocity ball.

Hatchcock sign: Tenderness on running the finger along the angle of the jaw due to parotitis in mumps.

Myer sign: Numbness and formication of both hands seen in scarlet fever.

Oyster blister sign: Refers to the presence of bullous skin lesions, caused by zoonotic vibriosis diseases contained in raw oysters, mussels, crabs and shrimp.

Rudolph sign: In nasal vestibular furunculosis, recurrent exquisitely tender unilateral erythema and edema of the nasal tip.

Stinson sign: Transverse line of conjunctival erythema, sharply demarcated along the eyelid margin, occurring in the prodromal phase of measles.

Strawberry tongue: Prominent papillae of the tongue covered by a white coating giving a white strawberry appearance to the tongue and the coating desquamates in a few days giving rise to the typical red strawberry tongue. Seen in Group a streptococcal pharyngitis, toxic shock syndrome, infection due to Yersinia pseudotuberculosis, Kawasaki disease, recalcitrant erythematous desquamating disorder and recurrent toxin-mediated perianal erythema.

Statue of liberty sign: In asymmetrical periflexural exanthem of childhood associated with EBV, adenovirus or parvivirus B19, the rash starts in the armpit or groin and gradually extends outwards, remaining predominantly on one side of the body. This sign is demonstrated when the patient raises an arm to show the rash.

List of signs seen in Syphilis:

- Buschke-ollendorf sign
- Barber-pole sign
- Biederman's sign
- Bulldog jaw sign
- Café-au-lair tint sign
- Crown of venus sign
- Dory flop sign
- Du bois sign
- Elliot sign
- Higoumenaki's sign
- Hutchinson teeth sign
- Krisowski's sign
- Mulberry molars
- Natiform skull sign
- Olympian brow sign
- Omnibus sign
- Oper- glass nose sign
- Parrot's nodes
- Sabre shins
- Seeping sign
- Silex's sign
- Split papules
- Virchow's sign

List of signs in leprosy:

- Benediction sign
- Elbow sign
- Fibula sign
- Fountain of youth sign
- Hertoghe sign
- Wartenberg's sign

39

CHAPTER

Syndromes in Dermatology

1. **Abacavir Hypersensitivity Syndrome**

   Abacavir induced hypersensitivity reaction has been associated with the presence of the major histocompatibility complex class I allele HLA-B*5701. Symptoms of an abacavir hypersensitivity reaction include skin rash, fever, malaise, gastrointestinal and respiratory symptoms. Severe forms of the skin rash may result in Stevens-Johnson syndrome, Toxic Epidermal Necrolysis, or Systemic Lupus Erythematosus like rashes.

2. **Achenbach's Syndrome**

   Also known as "Paroxysmal hand hematoma" or "finger apoplexia". First described by Walter Achenbach in 1958 for recurrent sudden episodes of focal bleeding and discoloration of the palmar surface of hand or digits in a middle-aged female. The notable characteristic findings are normal skin perfusion, temperature and nail fold capillaroscopy. Prodromal symptoms such as pain, tingling, itching may occur few hours before active bleeding with appearance of discoloration. Bleeding usually stops within minutes after applying local pressure and discoloration also disappears in 4-6 days.

3. **Ackerman Syndrome or IGDA (Interstitial Granulomatous Dermatitis Associated with Arthritis)**

   IGDA typically affects middle-aged women. The dermatological manifestations are extremely variable and include multiple, symmetric, erythematous to violaceous papules, nodules or plaques. The hallmark of this condition is the characteristic 'rope-sign', in the form of palpable subcutaneous linear cords that typically occur in the axilla. The joint manifestation is commonly in the form of non-erosive, seronegative arthritis or arthralgia.

4. **Acquired Pseudoxanthoma Elasticum (PXE)**

   PXE is a serious, rare genetic disorder of the young age group, affecting the elastic tissue of multiple organs, most importantly the skin, eye and vascular system. The pathogenesis is due to a mutation in the ABCC6 gene and is characterized by abnormal calcification of the connective tissue. Cutaneous manifestations include asymptomatic yellowish papules coalescing to form cobblestone-like plaque resembling 'Plucked chicken skin' over flexural areas. Ocular manifestations include angioid streak (calcified elastic lamina of Bruch's membrane), choroidal neoangiogenesis and haemorrhage leading to loss of visual acuity. Histology of the skin reveals fragmented elastic fibres in mid to deep reticular dermis, in chronic cases calcium deposition on these altered fibres is present.

5. **Acro-Dermato-Ungual-Lacrimal-Tooth Syndrome (ADULT)**

   A rare ectodermal dysplasia syndrome characterized by ectrodactyly, syndactyly, mammary hypoplasia, freckling as well as other typical ectodermal defects such as hypodontia, lacrimal duct anomalies, erythermalgia hypotrichosis and onychodysplasia.

6. **Acrosyndrome**

   It is a vasospastic or obstructive disorder that primarily affects the microvascular network of the extremities. It can be classified into 2 categories:

   Permanent:

   (a) *Vasoconstriction:* Acrorhigosis, Acrocyanosis, Livedo.

   (b) *Vasodilation:* Acrocholosis, Red palm syndrome (Lane syndrome).

Paroxysmal:

(a) *Vasoconstriction:* Raynaud's phenomenon, a term designating both the primary (Raynaud's disease) and secondary (Raynaud's syndrome) phenomenon.

(b) *Vasodilation:* Erythermalgia or Erythromelalgia (these two terms represent the same pathology).

7. **Acute Syndrome of Apoptotic Pan-epidermolysis (ASAP)**

It is a clinical constellation of many life-threatening clinical situations like drug induced TEN, acute lupus erythematosus, acute graft versus host disease and pseudoporphyria presenting with massive epidermal cleavage owing to hyperacute apoptotic injury. Thrombotic storm occurs, which is clinically characterized by the rapid onset of multiple thromboembolic occlusions affecting multiple vascular beds in arterial, venous, and microvascular circulation. Typically, an inciting trigger such as infection, trauma, or pregnancy is present. Half of the (ASAP) patients are positive for antiphospholipid antibodies.

8. **AESOP (Adenopathy and Extensive Skin Patch Overlying a Plasmacytoma) Syndrome**

Adenopathy and an extensive skin patch overlying a plasmacytoma (AESOP) syndrome, is characterized by a slowly expanding red or brown patch (classic variant) or plaque (morphea-like variant) overlying a solitary plasmacytoma of the bone. Early recognition can be life saving, as it is an early presentation of polyneuropathy, organomegaly, endocrinopathy, M-protein, and skin changes (POEMS) syndrome, which may be fatal. There are two forms: the classic variant, which presents as a smooth, shiny macule with abnormal visibility of skin vessels, and the morphea-like variant, which presents as a plaque where the skin is folded, giving a "Peau d'orange" appearance. The locations are frequently above the rib cage, above the sternum, or the scalp. Seventy-five percent of the patients develop regional lymphadenopathy within a few months.

9. **Albinism Deafness Syndrome (Ziprkowski-Margolis or WOOLF Syndrome)**

A rare disorder characterised by congenital nerve deafness and piebaldness with no ocular albinism. Transmission is X-linked with affected males presenting with profound sensorineural deafness and hyperpigmentation of the skin. Carrier females may present with variable hearing impairment without any pigmentary changes. Congenital sensorineural deafness and severe piebald like phenotype with extensive area of hypopigmentation is predominantly observed among Hopi Native Americans.

10. **Alezzandrini Syndrome**

It is a very rare syndrome characterized by retinitis pigmentosa, vitiligo and poliosis all on the same side of the face. It is very similar to Vogt-Koyanagi-Harada syndrome. Other reported signs and symptoms may include vision loss and retinal detachment, a patch of white hair on the scalp, café-au-lait macule on the neck, and hearing loss, again, all on the same side of the affected eye. The cause is unknown but may be related to viral infections or autoimmune processes.

11. **Amniotic Band Syndrome (Amniotic Deformity, Adhesions, Mutilations, ADAM Complex)**

In this condition, bands arise from the amnion's inner lining. The bands may cling to various body parts and influence intrauterine growth. This can lead to restriction of movements or even amputation of the limbs.

The signs and symptoms vary greatly depending on the area of the body involved and may include, shortened or absent digits, syndactyly, abdominal wall defects, encephalocele and cleft lip or palate.

12. **Angry Back Syndrome (Excited Skin Syndrome)**

The term 'angry back syndrome' (ABS) was coined by Mitchell in 1975. A strong positive patch test reaction could create an 'angry back' which becomes hyper reactive to other patch test challenges also. It is primarily an irritant reaction with unknown or known chemicals in stronger concentration leading to the simultaneous polysensitivity reaction.

13. **Ankyloblepharon-Ectodermal Defects-Cleft Lip/Palate Syndrome (AEC syndrome, Hay-Wells Syndrome)**

It is an autosomal dominant form of ectodermal dysplasia caused by mutations in the TP63 gene. The most common feature is missing patches of skin (erosions) on the scalp, neck, hands and feet. Skin erosions can lead to infection, scarring and hair loss. Other features include changes in skin coloring, dystrophic or absent nails, malformed or missing teeth, increased sensitivity to heat, hearing loss, cleft lip and/or palate, filiform ankyloblepharon adnatum (congenital adherence of the eyelids), dental changes and hypohidrosis.

14. **Antiphospholipid Syndrome (APS/Huges Syndrome)**

It is characterized by the presence of antiphospholipid antibodies, recurrent thrombosis and fetal loss. Classification criteria include 3 different anti-phospholipid antibodies: Lupus-anticoagulant, anti-cardiolipin and anti-Beta 2 glycoprotein-1. Clinical manifestations are due to involvement of different organs and systems such as the blood vessels, central nervous system, skin, kidneys, gastrointestinal tract, heart and placenta. The unifying mechanism of all these manifestations is thrombosis, either arterial or venous. Various skin manifestations like livedo reticularis, livedoid vasculopathy, Raynaud's phenomenon, vasculitis like lesions, Bechet's disease like lesions, pyoderma gangrenosum like lesions, nail fold ulcers, splinter hemorrhages, cutaneous necrosis, pseudoKaposi sarcoma lesions and migratory superficial thrombophlebitis, although not included in the diagnostic criteria, may be the presenting feature of this syndrome.

15. **Antisynthetase Syndrome**

It is an autoimmune disease characterized by auto-antibodies against one of many aminoacyl transfer RNA (tRNA) synthetases, e.g., anti – Jo – 1 (Histidyl), anti – pl-7 (Threonyl). Clinical features may include interstitial lung disease (ILD), non-erosive arthritis, myositis, Raynaud's phenomenon, unexplained fever and/or mechanic's hands. The ILD in anti-synthetase syndrome patients is often severe and rapidly progressive, causing much marked morbidity and mortality.

16. **Apert Syndrome**

It is a rare genetic condition characterized by cranio-synostosis, digital anomalies (syndactyly, broad thumbs), severe acne, diffuse pigmentary dilution and developmental delay caused by S252W and P253R FGR2 mutations. Affected children may also have an intellectual disability. The severity of symptoms varies between individuals.

17. **Ascher Syndrome**

It is a rare condition characterized by a combination of episodic edema or swelling of the eyelids (blepharo-chalasia), double lip and nontoxic thyroid enlargement. Most cases are sporadic, but familial cases with autosomal dominant inheritance have also been reported.

18. **Aseptic Abscesses Syndrome**

It is a systemic disorder of unknown etiology involving polymorphonuclear neutrophil. Typical presentation includes fever, abdominal pain and leukocytosis, and is characterized by the presence of intra-abdominal aseptic lesions consisting of neutrophils. It is either associated with another disease such as Crohn's disease or relapsing polychondritis, or is idiopathic.

19. **Ataxia Telangiectasia (Louis-Bar Syndrome)**

It is a rare early onset autosomal recessive ataxia due to mutation of ataxia telangiectasia mutated (ATM) gene. The clinical picture is characterised by a combination of neurological and systemic symptoms. Cerebellar atrophy with progressive ataxia, cutaneous telangiectasias, a higher incidence of malignancy (especially lymphoid malignancy), photosensitivity, immune deficiency, recurrent sinopulmonary infections, and elevated serum levels of alpha-fetoprotein are some of the findings of this disease.

20. **Atypical Trigeminal Trophic Syndrome**

Atypical trigeminal trophic syndrome has a similar presentation like Trigeminal Trophic Syndrome, i.e., irresistible burning sensation, pain or itching in distribution of trigeminal nerve except the ulceration which may be bilateral and at atypical sites (often involving the neck or two areas of the trigeminal nerve). There is no demonstrable trigeminal neuropathy or any disease of the trigeminal nerve or central nervous system nuclei and connections.

21. **Autoimmune Poly Endocrinopathy Candida Ectodermal Dystrophy Syndrome (APECED)**

It is an Autoimmune polyendocrinopathy syndrome type 1(APS1, AR); where mutation is in AIRE (autoimmune regulator) gene, which impairs the thymic negative selection of self-reactive T-cells and causes the development of autoimmunity that targets multiple endocrine and non-endocrine tissues. Cutaneous manifestations include alopecia areata, vitiligo, urticarial eruptions, lupus like panniculitis and chronic mucocutaneous candidiasis.

22. **Autoinflammatory Granulomatosis of Childhood (Blau Syndrome)**

(Described in detail in chapter 30)

23. **Axillary Web Syndrome (AWS)**

It is a subtype of Mondor disease, which occurs after breast surgery and manifests as painful palpable cords making bow strings across the axilla, like a web, restricting shoulder movements. It is characterised by retractile scarring of fascia.

24. **Barraquer Simons Syndrome (Acquired Partial Lipodystrophy (APL), Progressive Cephalothoracic Lipodystrophy)**

It is a rare disease characterized by symmetrical and insidious, although progressive fat loss starting from the face and scalp and gradually progressing downward to involve the neck, shoulders, upper extremities, thoracic region and upper abdomen. Involvement of the lower extremities is uncommon. It is seen before the age of 15 years.

25. **Bart Pumphrey Syndrome (Keratoma Hereditarum Mutilans, Cicatrizing Keratoderma with Hearing Impairment, Keratoderma with Sensorineural Deafness)**

Mutation occurs at GJB2 encoding connexin 26 gene. It is characterized by knuckle pads (similar to the focal keratoses of Vohwinkel syndrome), palmoplantar keratoderma, leukonychia and mixed sensorineural and conductive deafness.

26. **Bazex Syndrome (Paraneoplastica Acrokeratosis)**

It is a rare paraneoplastic condition particularly associated with squamous cell carcinoma of the upper respiratory or gastrointestinal tracts. Bazex syndrome can progress in three stages: (1) Psoriasiform scaly eruption over ears and fingers with onychodystrophy (2) Diffuse palmoplantar keratosis (3) Psoriasiform scaly eruption over knees, elbows and torso. Males are more affected than females.

27. **Bazex Dupre Christol Syndrome**

It is an X-linked dominant inherited basal cell cancer with ciliary defects characterized by ciliopathies. Mutation responsible for this syndrome is found in Testis 1 (ARP-T1) and ACTRT 1 gene (Actin-related protein). This syndrome is characterised by a triad of congenital hypotrichosis, follicular atrophoderma over dorsal aspect of hand, feet, face and development of basal cell carcinoma. Other clinical findings which may be present are milia, hypohydrosis, pinched nose, atopic diathesis, keratosis pilaris, comedones and hypermobility of joints.

28. **Becker's Nevus Syndrome (BNS)**

It is associated with Becker's nevus (cutaneous hamartoma characterised by circumscribed hyperpigmentation with hypertrichosis) with unilateral breast hypoplasia and muscle, skin and/or skeletal abnormalities. BNS is a part of epidermal nevus syndrome.

29. **Beckwith Wiedemann Syndrome (BWS)**

It is the most common overgrowth syndrome characterised by neonatal hypogylcemia, macrosomia, macroglossia, hemihyperplasia, omphalocele, embryonal tumors, visceromegaly, adrenocortical cytomegaly, renal abnormalities and ear creases/pits. Dysregulation of genomic imprinting and epigenetic and genomic alterations of chromosome 11p15 has been noted.

30. **Behcet's Syndrome**

Behcet's disease is an auto-inflammatory systemic vasculitis of unknown etiology. It is characterized by mucocutaneous manifestations, including recurrent oral and genital ulcerations, ocular manifestations, especially chronic relapsing uveitis, arthritis and systemic vasculitis involving arteries and veins of all sizes. It is also known as Behcet's syndrome and malignant aphthosis. Other features include papulopustular eruption, erythema nodosum like lesions and thrombophlebitis.

31. **Berardinelli–Seip Syndrome (Congenital Generalized Lipodystrophies, CGL)**

Congenital Generalized Lipodystrophies are very rare autosomal recessive conditions. The earliest sign in the neonate is a virtual absence of fatty tissue, followed by the development of a distinctive overall muscular appearance. The linear growth of the affected child is usually increased and is associated with advanced bone age and marked hyperphagia. Insulin resistance and hypertriglyceridemia are sometimes present early in childhood as well. Molecular techniques have helped to identify six clinico-genetic subtypes of CGLs.

32. **BID, IBID, PIBID, SIBID (Neuroectodermal Symptom Complex)**

BID: Brittle hair, Ichthyosis and Deafness.

IBIDS syndrome: Ichthyosis, Brittle hair and nails, Intellectual impairment and Short stature).

PIBIDS syndrome: Photosensitivity, Ichthyosis, Brittle hair and nails, Intellectual impairment and Short stature.

33. **Birt Hogg Dube Syndrome (BHD)**

It is characterised by a mutation in the BHD gene located on chromosome 17p12-q11.2 which encodes folliculin. It is an autosomal dominant inherited condition characterized by the development of benign tumours on the face and upper body, like fibrofolliculomas, trichodiscomas and acrochordon. Patients with this syndrome are at increased risk of colon or kidney cancer as well as spontaneous pneumothorax due to pulmonary cysts.

34. **Blooms Syndrome (Bloom–Torre–Machacek Syndrome)**

It is an autosomal recessive disorder. The gene for Bloom syndrome (RECQL3) lies on chromosome 15q26.1 and encodes a DNA helicase, RecQ protein-like-3. This syndrome is characterized by photosensitivity, telangiectatic facial erythema, proportionate pre and postnatal growth deficiency, distinctive facies, abnormal immune responses and a predisposition for malignancies. Testicular atrophy is common and adult male patients are infertile. Single gene mutation known as BLMAsh is responsible for over 90% cases of Bloom syndrome among Ashkenazi Jews.

35. Blue Rubber Bleb Naevus Syndrome (Bean Syndrome)

Blue rubber bleb naevus (BRBN) syndrome is a rare, sporadic, congenital, slow-flow vascular anomaly caused by activating TEK, TIE and Tie2 mutations, which affect endothelial cell tyrosine kinase receptors for angiopoietins. It is characterized by numerous, widely distributed, cutaneous and internal vascular malformations (VMs) of which pathognomic are small, rubbery, dark bluish, palmoplantar lesions and gastrointestinal VMs.

36. Blue Toe Syndrome (Occlusive Vasculopathy)

It depicts the sudden onset of painful purple digits without any obvious signs of trauma, cold-related damage, or conditions that cause generalised cyanosis. It could be caused by excessive venous thrombosis, decreased venous flow from embolism, viral or non-infectious inflammation, vasoconstrictive diseases, or irregular circulatory blood flow (hyperviscosity disorders).

37. Bowel Associated Dermatitis Arthritis Syndrome (BADAS)

BADAS is defined by the presence of pustular vasculitic lesions associated with blind loops of bowel or other causes of stasis of bowel content. The cutaneous manifestations of BADAS are usually begin as small macular lesions that progress into papules and then pustules on a purpuric base, most often on the arms and other areas of the upper body.

38. Brauer Syndrome (Focal Facial Dermal Dysplasia Type 1, FFDD1)

It is an autosomal dominant disorder characterised by congenital bitemporal cutis aplasia resembling forceps marks. The aetiology is unknown.

39. Brauer-Setleis Syndrome (Focal Facial Dermal Dysplasia Type 2, FFDD2)

It is an autosomal dominant disorder characterised by bitemporal skin lesions with variable facial findings like thin and puckered periorbital skin, distichiasis and/or absent eyelashes, upslanting palpebral fissures, a flat nasal bridge with a broad nasal tip, large lips and redundant facial skin.

40. Bronze Baby Syndrome (BBS)

Characterised by brown bronze discoloration of the skin, mucous membranes and urine after phototherapy in children with clinical jaundice. The discoloration may be caused by an abnormal accumulation of a photoisomer of bilirubin (abnormal hepatic function leading to a copper–porphyrin complex which is photo destroyed) or accumulation of biliverdin. The pigmentation is reversible after discontinuation of phototherapy.

41. Brooke-Spiegler Syndrome (BRSS or BSS)

The Brooke-Spiegler syndrome is an inherited autosomal dominant transmission condition and consists of multiple trichoepitheliomas, cylindromas and spiradenomas. The gene for this syndrome has been mapped to chromosome 16q12–13. Mutations in CYLD and PTCH tumor suppressor genes are responsible for the manifestations of the disease.

42. Brunauer–Fuhs–Siemens Syndrome (Keratosis Palmoplantaris Variants of Wachters, Striate PPK, Keratosis Palmoplantaris Areata Et Striata)

It is a form of striate keratoderma that manifests as localised plaques on the plantar surfaces of the feet and linear hyperkeratosis on the palms and fingers. Brunauer–Fuhs–Siemens syndrome is an autosomal dominant condition occurring due to heterozygous mutations in DSG-1.

43. Burning Feet Syndrome (BFS, Grierson Gopalan Syndrome)

It is characterized by a burning and aching sensation of the feet (hyperaesthesia), accompanied by vaso-motor changes causing excessive sweating. It is more common in females.

44. Burning Mouth Syndrome (BMS)

Burning mouth syndrome is most likely a form of neuropathic pain. A variety of hypotheses have been postulated. In BMS, a sensation of continuous burning, often accompanied by taste changes are felt, for which no dental or systematic cause can be found. There are no gross clinical signs. It is common in perimenopausal women.

45. Buschke-Ollendorff Syndrome

Germline loss of functional mutation in LEMD3 is the cause of this autosomal dominant condition. Buschke Ollendorff syndrome presents with elastomas (and occasionally collagenomas). Amblyopia and osteo-poikilosis are additional features.

46. **Cantu Syndrome**

Cantu syndrome is inherited in an autosomal dominant fashion and is characterized by congenital hypertrichosis with long curly eyelashes, macrosomia, facial dysmorphism, gingival hyperplasia, skeletal anomalies, cardiac defects and occasionally mild mental retardation. The disease was found to be caused by activating mutations in ABCC9 gene, encoding the sulfonylurea receptor 2.

47. **Capillary Malformation Arteriovenous Malformation Syndrome (CM- AVM Syndrome)**

Multifocal capillary malformations (CMs) and a higher incidence of fast flow vascular malformations are two features of this autosomal dominant condition. It is caused by heterozygous loss of function mutations in the RASA1 gene. All those affected have cutaneous CMs. Lesions are multifocal, vary in size, and are dispersed randomly in most patients; however, few have a single lesion. They are homogeneous or telangiectatic, pink, red, or brownish, and around half of them have a distinctive white halo surrounding the lesion. Systemic CMs can be associated with migraine, high outflow cardiac failure, abnormal bleeding and other abnormalities depending upon site of malformation.

48. **Carcinoid Syndrome**

It is a paraneoplastic syndrome caused by release of serotonin and other substances from well-differentiated neuroendocrine tumors frequently originating in the digestive tract. Carcinoid syndrome is characterized by flushing, diarrhoea, heart failure and bronchoconstriction which develops due to excessive secretion of hormones from carcinoid tumours.

49. **Cardio-Facio-Cutaneous (CFC) Syndrome**

These are autosomal dominant disorders caused by mutations affecting various components of the Ras/ mitogen activated protein kinase (MAPK) pathway (RASopathy). Cardiofacial features are similar to that of Noonan syndrome (congenital heart defects, failure to thrive, short stature, ophthalmological abnormalities, multiple skin manifestations). Other clinical features such as progressive formation of naevi, normal neurocognitive function or mild impairment, hypotonia and unclear predisposition to cancer is seen.

50. **Carney Complex Syndrome (LAMB–Lentigines, Atrial Myxoma, Mucocutaneous myxoma, Blue Nevi Syndrome, or NAME– Nevi, Atrial Myxoma, Myxoid Neurofibroma, Ephelides Syndrome)**

It refers to a complex of myxomas, spotty pigmentation and endocrine overactivity. This autosomal dominant trait occurs due to the mutation in the regulatory subunit 1A of protein kinase, a PRKAR1A located at 17q22-24 chromosome. Carney complex presents with spotty hyperpigmentation and lentiginosis of the face, conjunctiva, lips, oral mucosa and myxoma of skin, oral mucosa, heart and breast.

51. **Carvajal-Huerta Syndrome**

It is a familial cardiocutaneous syndrome with Non Epidermolytic striate Palmoplantar Keratoderma (NEPPK), woolly hair and dilated cardiomyopathy. Recessive desmoplakin (DSP) mutations producing a premature stop codon which leads to truncated protein, cause this disorder.

52. **CEDNIK, MEDNIK, ARC, Gaucher disease type II, ELOVL4 deficiency and Stormorken Syndrome**

The combination of neurological manifestations and ichthyosis can be found in various distinct genetic disorders e.g.:

- Gaucher disease type II represents a classic neuroichthyosis disorder, presenting at birth with collodion membranes.
- *CEDNIK syndrome includes:* Cerebral dysgenesis, Neuropathy, Ichthyosis and Palmoplantar Keratoderma.
- ARC stands for Arthrogryposis, Renal dysfunction and Cholestasis syndrome.
- MEDNIK Syndrome includes Mental retardation, Enteropathy, Deafness, Neuropathy, Ichthyosis and Keratoderma.
- ELOVL 4 deficiency has been associated with erythrokeratoderma and sensorineural deafness.
- Stormorken syndrome may present with moderate thrombocytopenia, muscle fatigue, asplenia, miosis, migraine, dyslexia and ichthyosis.

53. **Centrofacial Lentiginosis Syndrome (Touraine Syndrome)**

It consists of centrofacial lentiginosis with bone abnormalities and malformations due to dysgraphia, endocrine dysfunctions and neurological diseases.

54. **Chanarin Dorfman Syndrome (CDS, Icthysioform Erythroderma with Leucocytic Vacuolization, Neutral Lipid Storage Disease with Ichthyosis (NLSDI)**

It is a rare type of syndromic autosomal recessively transmitted. Most patients originate from Mediterranean countries. The disease is due to mutations in the ABHD5 which is widely expressed in tissues such as the skin, muscle, liver and brain, but also in lymphocytes and localizes to the surface of cytoplasmic lipid droplets. The genetic defect causes acylceramide deficiency leading to ichthyosis. Affected newborns are either collodion babies or erythrodermic. The patient has mild-to-moderate congenital ichthyosiform erythroderma (CIE) with fine white scales on an erythematous background and a lamellar scaling on the trunk and legs. Mild ectropion, flexural and neck lichenification and palmoplantar hyperkeratosis are common. Myopathy, hepatomegaly, elevated liver enzymes, cirrhosis, splenomegaly, malabsorption, cataract and neurological features may develop.

55. **CHAND Syndrome (Curly Hair, Ankyloblepharon and Nail Dysplasia)**

CHAND syndrome is characterized by ankyloblepharon, sparse, curly and woolly hair, nail dysplasia, and oral frenula. It occurs due to mutation in the RIPK4 gene and homozygous mutation in PWP 21, MX 28, RIPK 4 genes.

56. **CHARGE Syndrome (Coloboma, Heart Defects, Atresia Choanae, Growth Retardation, Genital Abnormalities, Ear Abnormalities)**

Also known as Hall-Hittner syndrome, it clinically comprises Coloboma, Heart defect, Atresia of the choanae, Retardation of growth and development, Genital and urinary anomalies and Ear anomalies. Other features include characteristic facial features: asymmetric facial nerve palsy, cleft lip or palate, esophageal atresia or tracheoesophageal fistula. It occurs due to mutation in the CHD7 gene.

57. **Chediak-Higashi Syndrome (CHS)**

Chediak-Higashi disease is a rare autosomal recessive disease affecting neutrophils and all other lysosomal granule containing cells in the body, characterized by recurrent bacterial infections, neurological disease, partial albinism, platelet dysfunction and early death. The disease is secondary to mutations in Lyst, a gene encoding a cytoplasmic protein involved in lysosomal trafficking. The neutrophils contain giant granules resulting from specific and azurophilic granule fusion.

58. **CHIME Syndrome (Coloboma Heart Defect, Ichthyosiform Dermatosis, Mental Retardation, Ear Anomalies Syndrome)**

It is a rare autosomal recessive neurocutaneous condition. This syndrome is due to mutations in the gene PIGL. Generalized pruritus, erythema and scaling develop within the first month of life, and migrating figurate, red scaly and itchy patches appear on the head and body since early childhood. Palms and soles are thickened, the scalp hair are fine, sparse and hypopigmented. Characteristic facial appearance includes cranial defects, alopecia, hypertelorism, a broad nasal bridge, wide mouth, full lips and wide spaced teeth. Neurological features include hearing loss, seizures, developmental delay and outbursts of violent behaviour.

59. **Christ-Siemens-Touraine Syndrome (Anhidrotic Ectodermal Dysplasia)**

X-linked hypohidrotic ectodermal dysplasia is the most common of the ectodermal dysplasias. However, autosomal dominant and autosomal recessive forms have also been described. The disorder is characterized by hypotrichosis with fine, slow growing scalp and body hair, sparse eyebrows, hypohidrosis, nail anomalies and hypodontia. Peg shaped primary and secondary teeth are typical. Decreased sweating leads to heat intolerance and enhanced dryness of the skin. X-linked hypohidrotic ectodermal dysplasia 1 is caused by a mutation in the EDA gene, which encodes ectodysplasin.

60. **Chronic Atypical Neutrophilic Dermatosis with Lipodystrophy and Elevated Temperature (CANDLE)/PRAAS (Proteosome Associated Autoinflammatory Syndrome)**

Synonyms: Nakajo-Nishimura syndrome; Joint contractures–muscular atrophy–microcytic anaemia–panniculitis-induced lipodystrophy syndrome.

It is a type of autoinflammatory syndrome characterized by abnormal signaling in the interferon pathways. It is related to a mutation in the PMSB8 gene. Children usually present to pediatricians in early life with recurrent fever, rash and arthralgia or arthritis. These may first develop within 2 or 3 weeks of birth but then continue episodically during the first year of life with violaceous or erythematous, often annular and oedematous plaques on the face, trunk and the iinter phalangeal joints. Up to 50% of patients die before adulthood.

61. Chronic Infantile Neurological Cutaneous and Articular Syndrome (CINCA)/Neonatal Onset Multisystem Inflammatory Disease (NOMID)

(Described in detail in chapter 30)

62. Churg-Strauss Syndrome

Eosinophilic granulomatosis with polyangiitis (EGPA) is a very rare systemic disorder characterized by an eosinophil rich and necrotizing granulomatous inflammation, often involving respiratory tract, and necrotizing vasculitis predominantly affecting small to medium vessels. There is an association with asthma and eosinophilia. Anti Neutrophilic Cytoplasmic Antibody (ANCA) is more frequent when glomerulonephritis is present. It is associated with antibodies directed against Myeloperoxidase and Proteinase 3.

63. Clouston Syndrome (Hidrotic Ectodermal Dysplasia Type 2–HED 2)

It presents with a combination of small dystrophic nails developing in early infancy with hypotrichosis in conjunction with papillomatous and fissured transgradient keratoderma, but the presentation may resemble pachyonychia congenita. This autosomal dominant ectodermal dysplasia is caused by mutations in the gap junction β-6 (GJB6) gene encoding connexin 30, which is a potential target of p63.

64. CLOVES Syndrome

It stands for Congenital Lipomatous (fatty) Overgrowth, Vascular Malformations, Epidermal Nevi and Scoliosis/Skeletal/Spinal anomalies. It is caused by mutations in the gene PIK3CA.

65. CMN Syndrome (Congenital Melanocytic Nevi Syndrome)

It is the association of large or multiple CMN with neurological abnormalities, characteristic facial features, and an increased risk of melanoma that is not restricted to the skin. It is caused by postzygotic mutations in Codon 61 of NRAS.

66. Cobb Syndrome or Cutaneomeningospinal Angiomatosis

It is a rare non inherited disorder which presents with congenital cutaneous vascular lesions distributed in a dermatomal pattern with associated spinal angiomas or arteriovenous malformations (AVMs). The spinal vascular lesions can cause neurologic deficits, including paralysis.

67. Cockayne Syndrome (CS)

It is characterized by dwarfism, beaked nose, deafness, loss of subcutaneous tissues (cachectic dwarf), basal ganglia calcification and retinopathy. The defect lies in the nucleotide excision repair (NER), but not global (compared to xeroderma pigmentosum). No increase in cutaneous or internal malignancies is seen but the patient usually dies by 30 years of age due to neurologic degeneration.

68. Cold Induced Sweating Syndrome (CISS)

It is an autosomal recessive syndrome, characterized by profuse sweating (involving the chest, face, arms and trunk) induced by cold ambient temperature. CISS is caused by mutations in the CRLF1 gene on chromosome 19p12 (CISS type 1).

69. Comel Netherton Syndrome

It is an autosomal recessive syndrome caused by a mutation in SPINK5, which encodes LEKTI, a serine protease inhibitor resulting in the increased activity of epidermal proteases which cause desquamation and pruritus.

It is characterized by:

- Congenital ichthyosiform erythroderma (CIE) or Ichthyosis linearis circumflexa (ILC)–A typical ILC lesion is an erythematous, scaly, annular or polycyclic patch with an incomplete advancing double edge of peeling scale. ILC is episodic, with lesions migrating often in a cephalocaudal direction.
- Trichorrhexis invaginata (bamboo hairs) is the most specific, though other hair shaft abnormalities may be seen.
- Atopic diathesis–High levels of serum IgE with eosinophilia, recurrent urticaria, angioedema and food allergy are common.

Perinatal complications include hypernatraemic dehydration, malnutrition and severe infections.

70. Compartment Syndrome

It is a painful and potentially fatal condition due to bleeding or swelling inside a muscle compartment, which is an enclosed bundle of muscles. The "5 P's" pain, pallor, paresthesia, pulselessness and paralysis are frequently used to describe compartment syndrome.

71. Complex Regional Pain Syndrome (CRPS)/Reflex Sympathetic Dystrophy (RSD)

It represents a wide range of painful diseases that are characterised by a persistent (spontaneous and/ or evoked) regional pain, sensitivity to touch or cold, swelling of painful area, changes in skin colour, textures, hair and nail growth, joint stiffness, muscle spasm and decreased ability to move affected body parts. It is out of proportion in duration or severity to the course of any known trauma or other lesions. It is connected to anomalies in the affected limb's skin and bone. Inflammatory symptoms are evident in warm complex regional pain syndrome, whereas autonomic symptoms are more common in cold complex regional pain syndrome. It is further divided into two categories:

- *Reflex Sympathetic Dystrophy Syndrome (RSD) Type 1 (CRPS):* It occurs in the absence of clear nerve illness or injury that directly damages the nerves in the affected area.
- *CRPS 2, also known as causalgia:* An area of localized pain which is correlated with a particular nerve injury.

72. Congenital Hemidysplasia–Ichthyosiform Naevus–Limb Defect Syndrome (CHILD)

It is an X-linked dominant male lethal disorder of distal cholesterol biosynthesis caused by a mutation in NSDHL gene. It is characterized by hemidysplasia and ipsilateral erythroderma with ipsilateral limb and organ defects. The hallmark of the CHILD syndrome is a peculiar inflammatory epidermal naevus having a unique lateralization pattern with a strict midline demarcation and ptychotropism (affinity to body folds). This naevus shows hyperkeratosis which has a typical yellow wax like scaling. It is associated with ipsilateral extracutaneous defects in the form of hypoplasia or aplasia and may involve the limbs and other skeletal structures as well as internal organs such as the lungs, heart and kidneys.

73. Congenital Rubella Syndrome

It is due to infection by Toga viruses, Rubella (German measles). The highest risk is in the first 16 weeks of pregnancy. It is characterized by cataracts, heart, CNS defects, deafness and blue berry muffin baby.

74. Congenital Varicella Syndrome

It is due to Human Herpes Virus-3 or Varicella Zoster virus infection. The highest risk is in 13–20 weeks of pregnancy (second trimester). Congenital Varicella Syndrome defects involve the skin, limbs, eyes and the central and autonomic nervous system. Characteristic scarring skin lesions known as cicatrix occur in a dermatomal distribution throughout the body. Limb abnormalities include hypoplasia, atrophy, or malformed digits. Typical ocular defects in form of chorioretinitis, cataracts, and nystagmus may occur. Central nervous system abnormalities like microcephaly, cortical atrophy, seizures and mental retardation can be seen. Autonomic nervous system dysfunction can also occur, leading to neurogenic bladder, hydronephrosis, esophageal dilation and gastrointestinal reflux.

75. Conradi-Hünermann-Happle Syndrome (CHHS)

Conradi-Hünermann-Happle Syndrome, or X-linked Dominant Chondrodysplasia Punctata Type 2 (CDPX2), is a genodermatosis caused by mutations in Emopamil binding protein (EBP). While typically lethal in males, females with CDPX2 generally manifest by infancy or childhood with variable features including congenital ichthyosiform erythroderma in linear or blotchy pattern, follicular atrophoderma, hyperpigmentation or hypopigmentation, coarse sparse, lusterless hair, scarring alopecia, chondrodysplasia punctata, abnormal calcification of laryngeal and tracheal cartilages, asymmetric shortening of the long bones and cataracts.

76. Cornelia De Lange Syndrome

The condition is characterised by a distinctive facial appearance, prenatal and postnatal growth deficiencies, eating problems, psychomotor delays, behavioural abnormalities, and associated malformations that primarily affect the upper extremities. The sequencing and deletion/duplication analysis of the genes NIPBL, SMC3, RAD21, SMC1A and HDAC8 can be used to make a molecular genetic diagnosis.

77. Costello Syndrome

It is a rare AD condition caused by mutation in HRAS/KRAS genes that affects many different parts of the body. Signs and symptoms generally include developmental delay, intellectual disability, distinctive facial features, loose folds of extra skin (especially on the hands and feet), and unusually flexible joints. Affected people may also have heart abnormalities such as tachycardia, structural heart defects, and hypertrophic cardiomyopathy. Beginning in early childhood, people with Costello syndrome additionally have an increased risk to develop certain cancerous and noncancerous tumors.

78. Cowden Syndrome

Cowden syndrome (CS) also known as Cowden's disease and multiple hamartoma syndrome, is a rare autosomal dominant multisystem complex genodermatosis, mostly due to PTEN mutations. It is characterized by benign overgrowths called hamartomas as well as increased lifetime risk of breast; thyroid, uterine and other cancers which requires aggressive screening. It also includes neurodevelopmental disorders such as macrocephaly. The characteristic mucocutaneous findings are trichilemmoma, mucosal neuroma, oral papilloma, acral keratosis, genital mucosal pigmentation. Other rare cutaneous manifestations includes lipoma and vascular malformation.

79. Cranio Ectodermal Dysplasia (CED) OR Sensenbrenner Syndrome

Sensenbrenner syndrome is a very rare autosomal recessive disorder caused by variants in genes involved in the functional development of primary cilia. Typical clinical manifestations include craniofacial and skeletal abnormalities, hence the alternative name is cranioectodermal dysplasia. Chronic kidney disease due to progressive tubulointerstitial nephritis (nephronophthisis) has been described in these patients. Other features are severe anorexia, failure to thrive and angel shaped middle phalanges. Skin manifestations are skin laxity, sparse hair, abnormal nails and hypoplastic teeth.

80. CREST Syndrome

It is a subset of limited cutaneous systemic sclerosis CREST stands for Calcinosis, Raynaud's phenomenon, Esophageal dysmotility, Sclerodactyly and Telangiectasias (matted). It is commonly associated with anti-centromere antibodies.

81. Cronkhite-Canada Syndrome

It is a nonhereditary disease characterized by diffuse gastrointestinal hyperplastic polypoid lesions, diarrhoea, protein losing enteropathy, electrolytes disturbances and ectodermal symptoms such as pigmentation, alopecia and onychodystrophy.

82. Cryopyrin Associated Periodic Syndrome (CAPS)

(Described in detail in chapter 30)

83. Cushing Syndrome

It is caused by excessive secretion of cortisol by an adrenal tumor, high ACTH secreting pituitary or other tumors or high corticotropin releasing hormone (CRH) secreting tumors. All of the body's tissues and organs are influenced by cortisol. Cushing's syndrome is characterised by weight gain, easy bruising, stretch marks, acne, moon face, poor wound healing, skin ulcers, pendulous abdomen, muscle weakness, osteoporosis, menstrual irregularities, hypertension, cardiac hypertrophy, and high blood sugar.

84. De Barsy Syndrome

It is a rare genetic disorder characterized by eye abnormalities, growth retardation, intellectual disability, prematurely aged appearance (progeroid features) and loose (lax), wrinkled, sagging, redundant skin that lacks elasticity (cutis laxa).

85. Deficiency of Interleukin 1 Receptor Antagonist (DIRA) Syndrome

(Described in detail in chapter 30)

86. Degos Syndrome (Malignant Atrophic Papulosis)

It is a progressive vasculopathy causing occlusion of small and medium-sized arteries. The disease is characterized by skin and gastrointestinal lesions, but neurological features are also frequent. Postmortem studies show widespread organ involvement. Early skin lesions are pink or red, dome-shaped papules, which soon become necrotic and umbilicated with central porcelain white pallor and scaling. The border of the lesion is pink, and oedematous which becomes telangiectatic. Lesions heal with minuscule white scars surrounded by telangiectasia. The palms, soles and face are usually spared.

87. Delusory/Ekbom Syndrome/Restless Leg Syndrome (RLS)

RLS is a common sleep and movement disorder. It is characterized by leg paranesthesia accompanied by an irresistible urge, occurring at rest, to move the legs. Movement of the legs gives relief. Burning feet syndrome (BFS) is a poorly recognized and under diagnosed condition consisting of a burning sensation in the feet which is accentuated by heat or cold. Associated autonomic features include dry skin, eyes and mouth and vasomotor symptoms like peripheral coldness, burning or flushing, hypertension and impotence.

88. Dependency Syndrome

In these patients, immobility leads to swelling, particularly if gravitational forces encourage ongoing fluid filtration. Oedema and skin changes can only be explained by a passive calf muscle pump and the resulting venous hypertension.

89. Dermatitis Arthritis Syndrome

It is a form of disseminated gonococcal infection that usually comprises a triad of manifestations which include tenosynovitis, dermatitis and polyarthralgia and often associated with constitutional symptoms such as fever, chills and body malaise. The small, tender and initially maculopapular skin lesions occur in crops around affected joints. Later a central vesicle or pustule appears with haemorrhage and necrosis.

90. **Dermatoneuro Syndrome**

It is a rare complication of scleromyxedema associated with skin lesions, seizures and coma. The mechanism involved is thought to be paraproteinemia which increases blood viscosity or favours the formation of neutrophil aggregates that alter microcirculation.

91. **Dirty Skin Syndrome**

There are four described types of minocycline-induced skin pigmentation. Type III (also called dirty skin syndrome) is the least common type, consisting of muddy brown discoloration in sun exposed areas, typically the face. This type is linked to elevated levels of melanin in epidermal and dermal macrophages.

92. **DRESS (Drug Reaction with Eosinophilia and Systemic Symptoms) or Drug Induced Hypersensitivity Syndrome (DIHS)**

DRESS is an idiosyncratic multisystem drug hypersensitivity disorder. The most common drugs implicated are allopurinol, antiepileptics (phenytoin carbamazepine, lamotrigine, phenobarbital) antibiotics, sulfa drugs, furosemide, omeprazole and ibuprofen.

It is characterized by cutaneous features which may be of variable morphology (most common skin manifestation is urticarial papular exanthema followed by morbilliform eruptions or even erythroderma, pustular, purpuric, vesicular lesions, toxic epidermolysis necrosis, erythema multiforme like rashes) and systemic involvement. The latter includes haematological disturbance, with eosinophilia being the most consistent finding. Leucocytosis, lymphopenia, lymphocytosis, thrombocytosis and thrombocytopenia are also described. Atypical lymphocytes are a common finding on blood film in DRESS patients, the presence of which is used as a component of the diagnostic criteria. Lymphadenopathy is found in more than 75% of patients, with the involvement of two nodal basins required to meet diagnostic criteria. Systemic organ involvement (hepatitis, pneumonitis, myocarditis, pericarditis, nephritis, colitis) is the main cause of morbidity and mortality in this syndrome. DRESS syndrome due to dapsone also known as Dapsone Hypersensitivity Syndrome (DHS) is a hypersensitivity reaction to diamino diphenyl sulfone (DDS) and is characterized by fever, skin rash, eosinophilia, lymphadenopathy, hepatic, pulmonary and other systemic manifestations.

DRESS due to anticonvulsant is known as Anticonvulsant Hypersensitivity Syndrome (ACS), This syndrome is more common in blacks and typically has its onset 3 weeks to 3 months after initiation of therapy. Potentially fatal complications associated with this syndrome include hypersensitivity, myocarditis and drug-induced hepatitis with or without hepatocyte necrosis (which carries a mortality of up to 50%) and compromise of renal and pulmonary functions.

93. **Drug Related Baboon Syndrome or Symmetrical Drug Related Intertriginous and Flexural Exanthema (SDRIFE)**

SDRIFE is a distinctive drug eruption characterized by a symmetrical eruption in the gluteal region, thighs and other intertriginous areas such as the axillae, knees, elbows and neck. Previously, such cases were called drug induced baboon syndrome. There is sharply demarcated erythema of the gluteal/perianal area and/or V-shaped erythema of the inguinal area with involvement of at least one other intertriginous/ flexural location. The absence of systemic symptoms and signs is classical for SDRIFE. Amoxicillin and another beta-lactam antibiotic are common cause of SDRIFE.

94. **Dubowitz Syndrome**

Microcephaly, small stature, atypical facial features, and mental retardation are the hallmarks of the rare autosomal recessive condition known as Dubowitz syndrome. Both intrauterine and postnatal growth retardation can occur. Hyperactivity, a limited attention span, and aggression are behavioral traits. Eczema and keloids on the skin have been described.

95. **Dunnigan Kobberling Syndrome**

It is an inherited metabolic disorder mainly affecting young female adults and is characterized by insulin resistance and glucose intolerance, hypertriglyceridemia and partial lipodystrophy. It has slow onset initially and presents with progressive loss of subcutaneous adipose tissue. Other features include hypocomplementemia, glomerulonephritis and autoimmune disorders.

96. **Dysplastic Nevus Syndrome**

These are melanocytic naevi, 5 mm or larger in diameter, with a macular component, irregular and poorly defined borders, asymmetrical outline and variable pigmentation. Although they are benign lesions, they exhibit clinicopathological characteristics that may resemble early radial growth phase melanomas. These naevi have increased risk of developing melanoma.

97. Easy Bruising Syndrome

Recurrent bruising after minor trauma, despite a normal coagulation profile, is a feature of the easy bruising syndrome. On peripheral blood smear examination; large platelets and neutrophilic inclusions are seen. On inspection, skin reveals distinct, ecchymotic patches. There are two types of easy bruising syndrome: Type I, which has normal platelet function but megathrombocytes and antiplatelet antibodies. In Type II, which has defective platelets function, megathrombocytes and antiplatelet antibodies could be present. Neutrophilic inclusion bodies are seen in May-Hegglin anomaly and Sebastian syndrome, where other findings as in type II easy bruising syndrome is also present.

98. Ectodermal Dysplasia–Skin Fragility Syndrome (ED-SFS)

Ectodermal dysplasia/skin fragility syndrome (ED-SFS) is a newly described autosomal recessive disorder characterized by skin fragility and blistering, palmoplantar keratoderma, abnormal hair growth, nail dystrophy, and occasionally defective sweating. It results from mutations in the PKP-1 gene encoding plakophilin 1 (PKP1), which is an important component of stratified epithelial desmosomes and a nuclear component of many cell types.

99. Ectopic ACTH Syndrome (EAS)

It is caused by nonpituitary tumors that secrete either adrenocorticotropic hormone (ACTH) and/or corticotropin-releasing hormone (CRH) and cause bilateral adrenal hyperplasia. Clinical presentation resembles Cushing's syndrome (CS): Amenorrhea, hirsutism, hypertension, impotence, muscular wasting, skin atrophy, neuropsychiatric dysfunction, osteoporosis, truncal central obesity, weight gain, water retention, moon face, weakness, fatigue, backache, headache, increased thirst, increased urination, Diabetes mellitus (DM) and Osteoporosis.

100. Ectrodactyly-Ectodermal Dysplasia–Cleft Lip/Palate Syndrome (EEC)

EEC syndrome is characterized by abnormalities affecting the limbs including ectrodactyly (split hand and feet syndrome), a condition in which part or all of the central digits (fingers or toes) are missing. Ectrodactyly often affects the middle fingers or toes. A groove or gap in the upper lip (cleft lip) and a groove or gap in the roof of the mouth (cleft palate) may also occur. The ectodermal dysplasia component affects the hair, teeth, nails, skin and sweat glands. EEC syndrome is caused by TP63 gene mutation. Other syndromes caused by TP63 gene mutation are Hay-Well syndrome, Rapp-Hodgkin syndrome, limb mammary syndrome and ADULT syndrome.

101. Ehlers-Danlos Syndrome

Ehlers-Danlos syndrome (EDS) is a heterogeneous group of inherited disorders of connective tissue that variably impairs the structure and function of the skin, joints, internal organs, eyes and blood vessels. It is characterized by joint hypermobility, skin hyper-extensibililty and tissue fragility. There are 13 types of EDS, most of which are very rare. Hypermobile EDS (hEDS) is the most common type. Other types of EDS include classical EDS, vascular EDS and kyphoscoliotic EDS. Hypermobile EDS presents with hypermobile, loose, unstable, painful joints that dislocate easily and minimum skin involvement. In classical type, soft velvety hyperextensible skin with easy bruising and atrophic scars along with hypermobile joints, livedo reticularis, molluscoid pseudotumors and subcutaneous spheroids, piezogenic pedal papule, elastosis perforans serpiginosa are seen. Cutaneous signs seen in EDS are the Gorlin sign (ability to touch the tip of nose with tongue), Metenier sign (easy eversion of upper eyelid), Reverse Namaskar sign (ability to fold forearm at back and oppose palms facing each other to say Namaskar.

102. Ellis-Van Creveld Syndrome (Chondroectodermal Dysplasia/EVC/Mesoectodermal Dysplasia)

It is an autosomal recessive ectodermal dysplasia that is characterized with skeletal dysplastic changes such as short limbs, short ribs, postaxial polydactyly, fingernail dystrophy, cleft palate, natal teeth and congenital heart defects. Two ciliary proteins namely, EVC and EVC2, which are products of human disease genes, are primarily affected in this disorder.

103. Emberger Syndrome

This is an autosomal dominant disorder caused by loss of function and heterozygous mutations in the transcription factor gene GATA2. It is characterized by lymphoedema in the lower extremities and genitalia, occurring during childhood. The patients are at risk of congenital deafness, immune dysfunction, cellulitis, myelodysplasia and acute myeloid leukaemia.

104. Eosinophilia Myalgia Syndrome (EMS)

Eosinophilia myalgia syndrome has lesions resembling PXE. Dermal calcification is absent on histology. Eosinophilia myalgia syndrome is defined by:

- Incapacitating myalgias.
- Blood eosinophil count greater than 1000 cells/μL.
- No evidence of infection (e.g., trichinosis) or neoplastic conditions that could account for these findings.

105. Episodic Angioedema with Eosinophilia (Gleich Syndrome)

Episodic angioedema with eosinophilia (EAE), also known as Gleich syndrome, is an uncommon syndrome marked by recurrent episodes of urticaria, fever, angioedema, weight gain, and severe eosinophilia that occurs at an interval of 3-4 weeks and recovers spontaneously without treatment.

106. Erosio Interdigitalis Blastomycetica Syndrome (EIB Syndrome)

Erosio interdigitalis blastomycetica (EIB) syndrome is Candida infection affecting the third web space, between the third and fourth fingers. EIB is most common among those who work with their hands frequently in water such as dishwashers, launderers, bartenders and homemakers. Clinical presentation most commonly consists of central erythematous erosion surrounded by a rim of white macerated skin involving at least one interdigital web space most commonly the third web space.

107. Familial Atypical Mole Melanoma Syndrome (FAMMM)

It is an autosomal dominant genodermatosis characterised by multiple melanocytic nevi, often more than 50, and a family history of melanoma. It has variable expressivity and limited penetrance and is due to CDKN2A gene mutations. The likelihood of developing pancreatic cancer and possibly other malignancies is higher in some patients.

108. Favre-Racouchot Syndrome (FRS)

FRS syndrome is characterized by a diffuse yellowish hue with the presence of large, open, black comedones symmetrically distributed on the temporal and periorbital areas, deep wrinkles and furrows over a background of actinically damaged and atrophic skin. In severely affected patients, multiple small papules, nodules and cystic lesions develop, especially involving the periocular region and the nose.

109. Felty Syndrome (FS)

It is a potentially serious condition that is associated with seropositive rheumatoid arthritis. FS is characterized by the classic triad of Rheumatoid arthritis, splenomegaly and granulocytopenia. Although many patients with FS are asymptomatic, some develop skin discoloration (abnormal brown pigmentation of the leg), cutaneous ulceration over lower legs and serious life-threatening infections secondary to granulocytopenia.

110. Fetal Alcohol Syndrome

Alcohol use by pregnant women can have negative impact on the foetus, the newborn, and the child. The following 3 findings are the basis for the diagnosis of foetal alcohol syndrome (FAS):

1. Identifying facial anomalies (small eyes, thin upper lip, smooth filtrum).
2. Restriction of growth (intrauterine growth retardation and failure to revamp the growth).
3. CNS abnormalities (cognitive impairment, learning disabilities and behavioural abnormalities).

111. Fitz-Hugh-Curtis Syndrome (FHCS)

Perihepatitis, often known as FHCS, is a chronic sign of pelvic inflammatory disease (PID) frequently caused by Chlamydia trachomatis and Neisseria gonorrhoeae. It is characterised by inflammation of the liver capsule with adhesion formation and pain in the right upper quadrant. A final diagnosis can be made through direct inspection of adhesions that resemble violin strings via laparoscopy or laparotomy.

112. Follicular Degeneration Syndrome (Hot Comb Alopecia, Pseudopelade of the Central Scalp or Pseudopelade in African Americans, Central Centrifugal Cicatricial Alopecia, CCCA)

Central Centrifugal Cicatricial Alopecia (CCCA) is a chronic and progressive type of scarring alopecia. It is most commonly seen in middle-aged African women. CCCA most commonly starts in the centre of the scalp and without treatment, it expands over time causing extensive scarring alopecia.

113. Follicular Nevus/Nevus Comedonicus Syndrome

Nevus comedonicus (NC) or comedo nevus refers to closely arranged, grouped, often linear, slightly elevated papules that have central keratinous plugs. It is a rare condition considered to be a type of epidermal nevus. It may be present since birth or may appear later. The term NC syndrome is used for comedo nevus presenting in association with extracutaneous manifestations which may include central nervous system (CNS), skeletal, ophthalmological, neurological and spinal abnormality.

114. **Frey's Syndrome (Baillarger's Syndrome, Auriculotemporal Syndrome, Dupuy Syndrome or Gustatory Hyperhidrosis)**

The auriculotemporal syndrome was initially identified by Lucie Frey in 1923. The abnormal reinnervation of postganglionic parasympathetic neurons to neighbouring denervated sweat glands and cutaneous blood vessels is the synkinetic mechanism for Frey's syndrome. Consequently, this results in flushing and sweating in the sympathetically void skin in response to mastication and salivation.

115. **Gardner Syndrome**

Gardner syndrome is a phenotypic variant of 'Familial Adenomatous Polyposis' (FAP). It is an inherited disease characterised by gastrointestinal polyps, multiple osteomas (benign bone tumors) and skin lesions (epidermoid cyst, desmoid tumor, fibroma, lipoma, leiomyomas, pigmented skin lesions) and soft tissue tumors. Polyps tend to form at puberty. In almost all patients, polyps progress to malignancy resulting in colorectal cancer so that timely detection is essential. It is due to mutations in the APC gene on chromosome 5q22.

116. **Gardner Diamond Syndrome (GDS)**

Psychogenic purpura, also known as auto erythrocyte sensitization syndrome, is a rare condition, observed in women with psychiatric illnesses. It presents with spontaneous development of painful edematous skin lesions, predominantly on the extremities, which may be single or multiple, progressing to ecchymosis over the next 24 hours. It is usually precipitated by severe stress or emotional trauma associated with certain psychiatric conditions.

117. **Generalized Eruptive Keratoacanthomas (Grzybowski Syndrome)**

It is a rare form of keratoacanthoma and is considered a serious condition because the eruptions are diffuse, persistent and recurrent. Constant pruritus, ectropion, visceral neoplasms, and unsatisfactory response to treatment are ominous prognostic factors.

118. **Glucagonoma/Pseudo Glucagonoma Syndrome**

Glucagonoma syndrome is caused by a glucagon-secreting pancreatic neuroendocrine neoplasm (glucagonoma). The syndrome includes rare paraneoplastic phenomenon defined as necrolytic migratory ery-thema (NME), glucagonoma, glucose intolerance, anemia, weight loss, glossitis and cheilitis. Because of its rarity, the correct diagnosis is often made too late, leading to poor prognosis. However, NME presents as a hallmark clinical sign of glucagonoma syndrome. Its early recognition allows for early diagnosis of the tumor and leads to a better prognosis.

119. **Gianotti-Crosti Syndrome (Papular Acrodermatitis of Childhood)**

It is a benign rash that is associated with a wide variety of viral illnesses. While historically thought to be solely a manifestation of hepatitis B infection, it has been demonstrated to occur following many viral illnesses like hepatitis B infection, Epstein-Barr virus, cytomegalovirus, COVID-19 virus infection and hepatits B vaccination, which suggests that this is an immunologic response rather than a primary manifestation of infection. Papular acrodermatitis of childhood is characterized by the acute eruption of monomorphic skin-colored to pink-red papules on the face, buttocks, and extensor surfaces of the extremities. The lesions usually spontaneously resolve and treatment is supportive.

120. **Goltz Syndrome**

Goltz syndrome synonymously known as focal dermal hypoplasia (FDH), is an extremely rare genetic disorder characterized by distinctive skin manifestations like linear hypoplastic streaks following Blaschke lines or fat herniation, telangiectasia, pyogenic granuloma like lesions, warty papilloma of mucus membrane, overgrowth of plamoplantar skin, alopecia, hyperhidrosis and a wide range of abnormalities affecting the eyes, teeth, skeletal, urinary, gastrointestinal, cardiovascular and central nervous system. The disease is inherited as an X-linked dominant condition.

121. **Goodpasture Syndrome**

Goodpasture syndrome refers to an anti-glomerular basement membrane (anti-GBM) disease that involves both the lungs and kidneys, often presenting as pulmonary hemorrhage and glomerulonephritis. The anti-GBM disease is the most specific term used for this disease and refers to the presence of renal and pulmonary involvement along with anti-glomerular basement membrane antibodies. The spectrum of disease may present classically as glomerulonephritis and rarely with cutaneous lesion in the form of erythematous macule over extremities.

122. **Gorham Stout Syndrome**

Vanishing bone disease (Gorham-Stout syndrome) is a rare entity of unknown etiology, characterized by destruction of osseous matrix and proliferation of vascular structures, resulting in destruction and absorption of bone and cutaneous vascular malformation. The syndrome can affect one or multiple bones of the patient, including the skull, the upper and lower extremities, the spine and pelvis. The clinical presentation of a patient suffering from vanishing bone disease includes pain, functional impairment and swelling of the affected region.

123. **Gorlin Goltz Syndrome (GGS), Nevoid Basal Cell Carcinoma Syndrome, NBCCS)**

Gorlin-Goltz syndrome is an autosomal dominant inherited disorder caused by mutations in PTCH gene (patched gene) found on chromosome 9q that encodes a transmembrane receptor which recognizes sonic hedgehog signaling proteins. It is characterized by multiple nevoid basal cell carcinoma, multiple odontogenic keratocysts or jaw cysts, congenital skeletal abnormalities (frontal bossing, Sprengel deformity, syndactyly, pectus deformity), ectopic calcification (falx cerebri or corpus callosum calcification), palmoplantar pits, dental, facial dysmorphism, ophthalmic, neurological (medulloblastoma) and sex organ abnormalities.

124. **Gottron Syndrome (Symmetrical Progressive Erythrokeratoderma)**

It is a rare inherited autosomal dominant cornification disorder. Although first described by Darier, the nomenclature came into existence after Gottron's documentation in early 19th century. Large, fixed, geographic and symmetrical fine scaly erythematous plaques distributed over knees, elbows, hands and feet are characteristics of this syndrome. The onset is in early childhood, progresses over the next few years and then remains stable.

125. **Gougerot Carteaud Syndrome**

Confluent and Reticulated Papillomatosis (CRP) was first described in 1927 by Gougerot and Carteaud. It is characterized by asymptomatic hyperpigmented papules and plaques that become confluent in the centre and reticulated at the periphery and are located on the upper trunk and neck in teens and young adults. It is due to disordered keratinisation but the precise aetiology and pathogenesis of CRP is not known. Dietzia papillomatosis and *Malassezia* species are the main infective pathogen isolated from the lesions.

126. **Graham Little Piccardi Lassueur Syndrome (GLPLS)**

It is a type of lichen planopilaris characterized by the triad of patchy cicatricial alopecia of the scalp, non cicatricial alopecia of the axilla and groin and keratosis pilaris like papules on the body. It is more common in females, especially in the post menopausal age group.

127. **Green Foot Syndrome (GFS)**

GFS is an uncommon cutaneous disease caused by *P. aeruginosa* and is frequently associated with poor hygiene, humidity and immunosuppression. It presents as chronic painful ulcers on the foot with yellowish green colour.

128. **Grey Baby Syndrome**

It is an adverse drug reaction to chloramphenicol which is characterized by a triad of abdominal distention, hemodynamic collapse, and ashen grey skin discoloration in neonates.

129. **Griscelli Prunieras Syndrome (GPS)**

GPS is a rare autosomal recessive disorder leading to pigmentary dilution of the skin and hair. Large clumps of pigment granules in hair shafts result in silver-grey color hair along with variable degree of cellular immunodeficiency with or without severe neurological defects.

Griscelli syndrome type 1 have severe brain function defects in addition to distinctive skin and hair coloring. Affected individuals typically have delayed development, intellectual disability, seizures and hypotonia. GS type 1 is related to MYO5A.

Griscelli syndrome type 2 has immune system abnormalities in addition to having hypopigmented skin and hair. Affected individuals are prone to recurrent infections. They also develop hemophagocytic lymphohistiocytosis (HLH), in which the immune system produces too many activated T-lymphocytes and macrophages (histiocytes). Overactivity of these cells can damage organs and tissues throughout the body, causing life-threatening complications if the condition is left untreated. GS type 2 is related to RAB27A.

130. **Growth Retardation, Alopecia, Pseudoanodontia, Optic Atrophy (GAPO) Syndrome**

GAPO syndrome is an entity with multiple congenital anomalies involving connective tissue and is characterized by growth retardation, alopecia, pseudoanodontia, and optic atrophy (GAPO). It is caused by homozygous nonsense or splicing mutations in

ANTXR1 gene (2p13.3) and encoding anthrax 5 toxin receptor 1.

131. **Haberland/Fishman Syndrome (Encephalo Cranio Cutaneous Lipomatosis, ECCL)**

Congenital neurocutaneous syndrome which is characterized by unilateral involvement of skin, eyes and CNS. Nevus psiloliparus is the characteristic cutaneous manifestation of ECCL syndrome. Congenital irregular shaped circumscribed area of alopecia and histologically excessive fatty tissue underlying the alopecia patch are also present.

132. **Hair Thread Tourniquet Syndrome (HTTS)**

It was proposed for the first time in 1988 by Barton *et. al.* to describe strands of hair or thread that wrap around an appendage (i.e., toes, fingers, genital structures, tongue, uvula or neck), eventually causing ischemia and tissue necrosis.

133. **Hallermann-Streiff Syndrome (HSS)**

It is a rare condition which is present at birth and becomes more apparent with time. Signs and symptoms include an unusually shaped skull, distinctive facial features, hypotrichosis (Multiple patches of hair loss overlying the cranial sutures), degenerative skin changes (skin atrophy), eye and dental abnormalities. Other features include poor vision, a small upper airway, and proportionate short stature.

134. **Hallopeau Siemens Syndrome**

It is one of the most severe types of dystrophic epidermolysis bullosa. Even slight trauma to the skin leads to blister formation that always heals with scars. Anchoring fibrils are either absent or inadequate due to a hereditary collagen VII deficiency. The patients present with hypoproteinemia, anaemia, secondary bacterial infections, oesophageal strictures, laryngeal stenosis and secondary malignant transformation. Hand deformities lead to pseudosyndactyly, flexion contractures and in advanced stages, mitten like deformity.

135. **Hand Arm Vibration Syndrome (HAVS)**

It is a group of symptoms that occur after being exposed to vibration for an extended period of time due to use of hand held vibrating instruments. It is known as HAVS because it affects the fingers, hands and arms and is caused by damage to the nerves, muscles and blood vessels. Tingling, numbness, loss of sensitivity, pallor of the fingers, and loss of grip strength are common symptoms.

136. **Hand Foot Syndrome**

It is a relatively common form of cutaneous dysaesthesia, mainly of the palms and soles, which follows chemotherapy. The most commonly used drugs that cause hand foot syndrome are intravenous 5-fluorouracil and its prodrug oral capecitabine. It is also common following use of pegylated liposomal doxorubicin, affecting approximately 50% of the patients with the first cycle and 75% by 9 cycles of the current recommended dose of 50 mg/mm^2.

137. **Hand-Schüller-Christian Disease**

It is characterized by the classic triad of single or multiple punched out bone lesions in the skull, unilateral or bilateral exophthalmos, and diabetes insipidus, with or without other manifestations like polyuria, dwarfism, or infantilism. The complete triad is however seen only in 25% of affected patients and presents with widespread skeletal and extraskeletal lesions with a chronic clinical course. It occurs usually before the age of 5 years but has been reported even in young adults. Sometimes papules and nodules are seen on the skin.

138. **Happle Tinschert Syndrome**

It is a rare multisystem birth defect characterized by the cutaneous hallmark of segmental basaloid follicular hamartomas along with skeletal, cerebral, dental and ocular anomalies.

139. **Harlequin Syndrome**

It is a syndrome affecting the autonomic nervous system. Patients with Harlequin syndrome have the absence of sweating with flushing of skin on one side of the body (unilateral), especially of the face, arms and chest.

140. **Heerfordt's Syndrome**

It is a rare subacute form of sarcoidosis, which present with uveitis, parotidomegaly, facial paralysis and fever in its classic form.

141. **Hemophagocytic Lymphohistiocytosis Syndrome (HLH)**

HLH represents a severe hyperinflammatory condition with the cardinal symptoms of prolonged fever, cytopenias, hepatosplenomegaly, and hemophagocytosis by activated, morphologically benign macrophages. Biochemical markers include elevated ferritin and triglycerides, and low fibrinogen. Whereas children with several inherited immune deficiencies may lead to this syndrome, most adults with HLH have no known underlying immune defect. Nevertheless, impaired function of natural killer (NK) cells and cytotoxic T-cells (CTL) is characteristic for both genetic and acquired forms of HLH.

142. Hennekam Lymphangiectasia Lymphedema Syndrome

It is an autosomal recessive disorder characterized by generalized lymphatic dysplasia affecting various organs, including the intestinal tract, pericardium and limbs. Additional features of the disorder include facial dysmorphism and cognitive impairment.

143. Hereditary Leiomyomatosis and Renal Cell Cancer Syndrome (HLRCC)/Reed's Syndrome

It is characterized by the presence of one or more of the following: cutaneous leiomyomas (or leiomyomata), uterine leiomyomas (fibroids) in females, and renal cell cancer (RCC). Cutaneous leiomyomas are the first manifestation of the disease. They present as painful skin colored papules and nodules. Germline pathogenic variants in the FH gene (fumarate hydratase) are responsible for the susceptibility to HLRCC syndrome. FH is the enzyme that catalyzes the conversion of fumarate to malate in the tricarboxylic acid cycle (Krebs cycle).

144. Hermansky-Pudlak Syndrome (HPS)

It affects multiple organ systems which include bleeding diathesis, visual problems, and abnormally light colored skin, hair and eyes (oculocutaneous albinism). Other symptoms may include immune dysregulation, pulmonary fibrosis and granulomatous colitis etc.

145. HIV Follicular Syndrome

It includes a distinctive triad of nodulocystic acne, striking follicular spines and an eruption resembling pityriasis rubra pilaris (PRP) in HIV positive patients. It has been suggested that this may represent a subtype of PRP or that it should be viewed as a unique HIV associated follicular occlusion triad.

146. Horner Syndrome (Oculosympathetic Palsy)

It is characterised by a classical triad of miosis (small and constricted pupil), partial ptosis (drooping of upper eyelid) and anhidrosis (loss of hemi facial sweating) caused due to disruption of sympathetic pathways.

147. Howel-Evans Syndrome (Tylosis and Oesophageal Cancer)

It is a rare form of focal palmoplantar keratoderma associated with esophageal cancer. Oral leukokeratosis may also be seen. It is inherited in an autosomal dominant manner due to a mutation in RHBDF2 gene. HES is present with focal palmoplantar keratoderma and oral leukokeratosis.

148. Huriez Syndrome (HRZ)

This autosomal dominant syndrome is characterized by a triad of palmoplantar keratoderma, scleroatrophy of the distal extremities, and hypoplastic nail changes. Characteristic aspect of the disease is the occurrence of aggressive squamous cell carcinoma (SCC) of skin, which affects 15% of the patients.

149. Hurler-Scheie Syndrome

It is a type of mucopolysaccharidosis type 1 (MPS1) which is an intermediate form of Hurler syndrome (severe type) and Scheie syndrome (mild type). Coarse facies, macroglossia, skeletal deformities, clouding of cornea and delay in motor development are the characteristic findings.

Hurler syndrome is the most severe form of MPS1 caused by the deficiency of alpha-L-iduronidase enzyme which results in the accumulation of Glycosaminoglycans (GAGs). It is characterized by coarse facies, skeletal abnormalities, cognitive impairment, heart disease, respiratory problems, hepatosplenomegaly and reduced life expectancy.

Scheie syndrome is a mild form of type 1 MPS caused by a deficiency in the enzyme iduronidase, leading to a build up of Glycosaminoglycans (GAGs).

150. Hyaline Fibromatosis Syndrome (HFS)

It is a condition characterized by deposits of a clear substance (hyaline) in the skin and in various other body tissues. It presents at birth or in infancy, causing severe pain during movement, progressive joint contractures which limit movements, thickened skin, and hyperpigmented patches over prominences of the joints.

151. Hyper Immunoglobulin E Syndromes (HIES, Job Syndrome)

HIES is a rare autosomal dominant primary immune deficiency disorders characterized by elevated serum IgE, dermatitis and recurrent skin and pulmonary infections. Autosomal dominant HIES, the most common disease in this group, results from STAT3 mutations and has a variety of connective tissue and skeletal abnormalities. Cytokinesis 8 (DOCK8) mutation is the cause of an autosomal recessive hyper-IgE syndrome.

152. Hypocomplementemic Urticarial Vasculitis Syndrome (HUVS, McDuffie Syndrome)

The major manifestations of HUVS are chronic, nonpruritic, urticarial vasculitic lesions that persist for more than 24 hours or recur at short intervals. In the pathophysiology of HUVS; low serum complements measurements in patients indicate the activation of the classical pathway, with low C1q, C4, and variably decreased C3 levels. Serum C1q precipitins were identified and later confirmed to be the auto-antibodies (Ab) against C1q (anti-C1q Ab).

153. Hypothenar Hammer Syndrome

It is a condition of the hand in which the blood flow to the fingers is reduced. It occurs when workers utilise the palms of their hands extensively. The hypothenar eminence and ring finger are painful, there is a presence of dysaesthesia with impairment in handling of objects with the affected hand.

154. Hypotrichosis Lymphoedema Telangiectasia Syndrome

It is a congenital syndrome distinguished by a triad of hypotrichosis, telangiectasias and lymphedema. During puberty, lymphedema typically appears in the lower extremities. In comparison to the scalp, legs and genitalia; the palms and soles may exhibit telangiectasias more frequently. At birth, hair is normal, which frequently falls off during infancy. It is linked to an uncommon SOX18 transcription factor gene mutation.

155. Ichthyosis Follicularis Atrichia Photophobia Syndrome (IFAP)

IFAP is a syndrome characterized by follicular ichthyosis, alopecia, photophobia and intellectual disabilities. Other manifestations are hyperkeratotic, psoriasiform plaques, dystrophic nails, atopy, renal and vertebral anomalies. It occurs due to a mutation in the MBTPS2 gene.

156. Ichthyosis Prematurity Syndrome (IPS)

IPS is a rare form of autosomal recessive congenital ichthyosis caused by mutations in SLC27A4 encoding fatty acid transport protein 4 (FATP4) that affects the keratinocyte differentiation and skin barrier function. It is characterized by prematurity, thick caseous desquamating epidermis and perinatal respiratory asphyxia.

157. Immune Reconstitution Inflammatory Syndrome (IRIS)

IRIS is a collection of inflammatory disorders characterized by paradoxical worsening of an existing infection or disease process or the appearance of a new infection or disease process soon after the initiation of antiretroviral treatment. This happens due to rapid dysregulated antigen specific immune response. Infections most commonly associated with IRIS include *Mycobacterium tuberculosis* and cryptococcal meningitis. Usually occurs in the first six months of HIV treatment.

158. Immunodysregulation Polyendocrinopathy Enteropathy X-linked Syndrome (IPEX)

IPEX is a genetic disease of immune dysregulation in which patients present with diarrhoea, diabetes and eczema in early life. Patients have abnormalities in the FOXP3 gene, which controls the production of regulatory T cells. Cutaneous findings may include alopecia urticarial rash, atopic dermatitis and psoriasiform like skin rashes and trachyonychia.

159. Kallmann Syndrome

It is characterised by delayed or absent puberty and an impaired or loss of sense of smell. Males with hypogonadotropic hypogonadism are born with micropenis and cryptorchidism. Most affected patients do not develop secondary sexual characteristics at puberty.

160. Keratitis Ichthyosis Deafness Syndrome (KID)

KID is a rare ectodermal disorder. The clinical triad (better classified as erythrokeratoderma than as ichthyosis) includes progressive vascularizing keratitis, sensorineural hearing impairment, and skin manifestations (sparse hair, nail dystrophy, grain leather like palmoplantar keratoderma, ichthyosis, squamous cell carcinoma of acral skin or mucosa). Heterozygous missense mutations in the GJB2 gene localized on chromosome 13q11-q12 encoding a gap junction protein called connexin-26 were found to be associated with the KID syndrome.

161. Kindler Syndrome (KS, Bullous Acrokeratotic Poikiloderma of Kindler and Weary Syndrome)

KS is a rare subtype of inherited epidermolysis bullosa, characterized by skin fragility and acral blister formation beginning at birth, diffuse cutaneous atrophy, photosensitivity (which is most prominent during childhood and usually decreases after adolescence), poikiloderma, diffuse palmoplantar hyperkeratosis and pseudosyndactyly. Mucosal manifestation includes hemorrhagic mucositis, periodontal disease, premature loss of teeth and oral leukokeratosis.

162. **Klippel-Trenaunay Syndrome (KTS)**

Klippel-Trenaunay Syndrome is described as a triad of cutaneous capillary malformation or portwine stain, overgrowth of bone and soft tissue, venous and lymphatic malformations. The malformation of a deep vein in the lower limb increases the risk of deep vein thrombosis. These conditions harbour mutations in the PIK3CA gene.

163. **Korsakoff Syndrome**

It is a chronic neuropsychiatric syndrome, caused by a deficiency of Thiamine (vitamin B_1). This deficiency leads to damage to multiple areas of the brain, which in turn causes amnesia and confusion. Korsakoff syndrome is most commonly seen in the context of chronic alcohol abuse. The course is chronic and may be irreversible. Due to vitamin B_1 deficiency skin may become pale, edematous and other feature includes alopecia and glossitis.

164. **Langer Giedion Syndrome or Trichorhinophalangeal Syndrome (TRPS)**

TRPS comprises TRPS I (caused by a heterozygous pathogenic variant) and TRPS II (caused by contiguous gene deletion of TRPS1, RAD21 and EXT1). Both types of TRPS are characterized by distinctive facial features, ectodermal defects (fine, sparse, depigmented and slow growing hair, dystrophic nails, small breasts), and skeletal abnormalities (short stature, short feet, brachydactyly with ulnar or radial deviation of the fingers, and early marked hip dysplasia).

Langer Giedion Syndrome (TRPS II) in addition has multiple osteochondromas (typically first observed clinically on the scapulae and around the elbows and knees between the ages of 1 month and 6 years) and an increased risk of mild-to-moderate intellectual disability.

165. **Laryngo-Onycho Cutaneous Syndrome (LOC)**

LOC leads to abnormalities of the skin (skin erosion), excessive granulation tissue in conjunctiva and larynx finger and toenails dystrophy. Many of the signs and symptoms are related to the abnormal growth of granulation tissue in different parts of the body. First symptom in infants with LOC syndrome is a hoarse cry due to ulcers or overgrowth of granulation tissue in the larynx.

166. **Laugier Hunziker Baran Syndrome (Idiopathic Lenticular Mucocutaneous Pigmentation)**

It is a rare hereditary pigmentary disorder characterized by hyperpigmentation over the oral mucosa, nails and extremities. Associated features are esophageal melanocytosis, actinic lichen planus, hypocellular bone marrow and thrombocytopenia.

167. **Lawrence Syndrome**

PNPLA6 (Patatin-like phospholipase domain-containing protein 6) disorders span a phenotypic continuum characterized by variable combinations of cerebellar ataxia; upper motor neuron involvement manifesting as spasticity and/or brisk reflexes; chorioretinal dystrophy associated with variable degrees of reduced visual function; and hypogonadotropic hypogonadism (delayed puberty and lack of secondary sex characteristics). The hypogonadotropic hypogonadism occurs either in isolation or as a part of anterior hypopituitarism (growth hormone, thyroid hormone, or gonadotropin deficiencies). Common but less frequent features of Lawrence Syndrome are peripheral neuropathy, hair anomalies (long eyelashes, bushy eyebrows, or scalp alopecia), short stature and impaired cognitive functioning.

168. **Lawrence Seip Syndrome**

It is characterized by low intelligence, gaunt facies, depressed nasal bridge, large low set ears, thick lips and protuberant abdomen. Skin shows hypermelanosis, hypertrichosis, absence of subcutaneous fat. Patients are short statured having hypertrophic clitoris, hepatomegaly, left ventricular hypertrophy, hyperglycaemia and glycosuria without ketoacidosis.

169. **Legius Syndrome**

Legius syndrome is characterized by multiple café-au-lait macules without neurofibromas or other tumor manifestations of neurofibromatosis type 1 (NF1). Additional clinical manifestations commonly reported include intertriginous freckling, lipomas, macrocephaly, learning disabilities, Attention Deficit Hyperactivity Disorder (ADHD) and developmental delays.

170. **LEOPARD Syndrome**

It is characterized by multiple Lentigines, Electrocardiographic abnormalities, Ocular hypertelorism, Pulmonic stenosis, Abnormal genitalia, Retardation of growth and sensorineural deafness. Associated genes are PTPN11, RAF1 and BRAF.

171. **Lesch Nyhan Syndrome (LNS)**

It is a rare X-linked recessive purine metabolic disorder caused due to deficiency of hypoxanthine guanine phosphoribosyl transferase (HPRT) enzyme. It is characterized by mental retardation, choreoathetosis, spastic cerebral palsy, and aggressive self mutilating behaviour, e.g., biting of lips and fingers.

172. Levator Ani Syndrome

Burning pain or tenesmus in the perineal or rectal region is a symptom of levator ani syndrome, which is due to levator ani muscle spasm. Pain may radiate to the hips, tailbone, or other places. The symptoms do not appear to have any structural abnormalities or underlying conditions, and this pain is typically unrelated to bowel movements.

173. LGV Inguinal Syndrome

It is a component of LGV (Lymphogranuloma venereum) disease which is characterized by proctitis or proctocolitis like symptoms (pain during urination, rectal bleeding, pain during passing stools, abdominal pain, anal pain and tenesmus). Generalized symptoms like body aches, headache, and fever can occur during this stage. This syndrome usually occurs when the transmission is via the anal route.

174. Lichen Planus/Lichen Sclerosus Overlap Syndrome

Lichen sclerosus and Lichen Planus affecting cutaneous sites are easily distinguishable clinically. Clinical signs on mucosal sites, however, may not allow differentiation between these diseases and reliance is frequently placed on histopathological findings. Lichen planus and lichen sclerosus share several common features, including lymphocytic infiltration at the dermal-epidermal junction, clinical involvement of both skin and mucosa, erosive lesion on mucosal surfaces and the occasional occurrence of squamous cell carcinoma at the site of chronic, erosive mucosal lesions.

175. Limb Mammary Syndrome

A rare, genetic, ectodermal dysplasia syndrome characterized by severe hand/foot anomalies, breast and/or nipple hypoplasia, and ectodermal dysplasia (principally teeth and nail anomalies). Cleft lip/palate may be variably present.

176. Linear Nevus Sebaceous Syndrome (LNSS) (Schimmelpenning Feuerstein Mims (SFM) Syndrome)

It is a neurocutaneous syndrome characterized by sebaceous nevi with a broad range of abnormalities that may affect skeletal, neurological and ocular system due to postzygotic mutation in HRAS and KRAS gene.

177. Loeffler Syndrome

Loeffler syndrome is a rare, transient, self limiting, and benign pulmonary eosinophilia lasting less than one month (usually 6-12 days) characterised by exanthema, pulmonary infiltrates on chest X-ray, elevated blood eosinophils and acute onset of cough, dyspnea, wheeze and fatigue. The aetiology has been mostly attributed to an allergic response to the transpulmonary migration of helminth larvae namely *Ascaris lumbricoides,* hookworms and strongyloides.

178. Lofgren's Syndrome

Lofgren's syndrome is acute phase of sarcoidosis characterized by fever, erythema nodosum, bilateral hilar lymphadenopathy (BHL), and migratory symmetrical polyarthritis. X-ray chest reveals bilateral hilar lymphadenopathy and nodular shadows. Angiotensin Converting Enzyme (ACE) levels are within normal range. Tissue biopsy from a mediastinum lymph node shows noncaseating granulomas.

179. Loose Anagen Hair Syndrome (LAH/LAS)

It is a benign, self-limiting disease in which anagen hairs are painlessly extracted. Premature keratinization of the inner root sheath (IRS) produces impaired adhesion between the cuticle of the IRS and the cuticle of the hair shaft. Anagen hair, devoid of its sheath with 'floppy sock appearance' is a characteristic finding of loose anagen hair (LAH) on trichogram.

180. Lumpy Scalp Syndrome

This autosomal dominant disorder is comprised of a triad of abnormalities which include midline posterior scalp nodules characterised by thickened dermis devoid of adnexa, multiple external ear deformities and rudimentary or absent nipples. An additional variable feature may be partial webbing of toes.

181. Lymphedema Distichiasis Syndrome

Lymphedema distichiasis syndrome is characterized by lower limb lymphedema appearing in late childhood with or without involvement of the external genitalia, often asymmetric and distichiasis (aberrant eyelashes ranging from a full set of extra eyelashes to a single hair).

182. Maffucci Syndrome

Maffucci syndrome is a disorder that primarily affects the bones and skin. It is characterized by multiple enchondromas, bone deformities and multiple hemangiomas.

183. MAGIC Syndrome (Mouth and Genital Ulcers with Inflamed Cartilage)

It is a condition in which features of Behcet's Disease (BD) and Relapsing Polychondritis (RP) occur in the same individual. Behcet's disease is a chronic relapsing multisystem disease characterized by inflammatory ulcers in the mouth, genital area and skin. Relapsing Polychondritis is autoimmune recurrent chondritis of the ears, nose, larynx and tracheobronchial tree.

184. Majeed Syndrome

(Described in detail in chapter 30).

185. Marfan Syndrome

Marfan syndrome is an autosomal dominant connective tissue disorder associated with mutation in fibrillin, and occasionally with mutation in TGFBR1 or 2 gene. It characteristically involves cardiovascular system, eyes and skeletal system. The clinical features include tall, thin body habitus, long limbs, arachnodactyly, pectus deformities, skin hyperextensibility, striae atrophicae and sometimes scoliosis. The walker Murdoch or wrist sign and Steinberg or thumb sign are positive in Marfan syndrome.

186. Marshall's Syndrome

Marshall´s syndrome is a form of pediatric acquired cutis laxa without systemic involvement characterised by urticarial or papular eruption followed by acute destruction of elastic tissue, resulting in skin atrophy and severe physical disfigurement. This disorder of elastic tissue can either be inherited or acquired. The inherited form can be autosomal dominant (which may have a delayed onset), recessive or X-linked (both are present at birth).

187. Mast Cell Activation Syndrome (MCAS)

The symptoms of anaphylaxis, e.g., urticaria, swelling, low blood pressure, troubled breathing and severe diarrhoea, are repeatedly experienced by patients with MCAS. During these episodes, high quantities of mast cell mediators are released, which can be treated with inhibitors or blockers of mast cell mediators.

188. McCune-Albright Syndrome (MAS, Albright Syndrome)

It is a rare, heterogenous, clinical condition caused by a sporadic, somatic, post zygotic mutation of GNAS gene. The classical form of MAS is more common in females and is characterized by a triad of physical signs:

1. Café-au-lait macules (CALMs) following lines of blaschko demonstrating jagged borders described as "Coast of Maine".
2. Polyostotic fibrous dysplasia.
3. Autonomous, hyperfunctioning endocrinopathies.

The non-classical form consists of only two of these three conditions. Gonadotropin-independent precocious puberty is the most commonly described endocrinal involvement. Increased pigmentation is due to tyrosinase stimulation.

189. MCLID Syndrome

Microcephaly with or without Chorioretinopathy, Congenital lymphedema of the lower limb or Intellectual Disability is an autosomal dominant condition due to mutations in the KIF11 gene.

190. Melanoma Astrocytoma Syndrome

Melanoma astrocytoma syndrome is a tumor predisposition syndrome caused by mutation of CDKN2A tumor suppressor gene. It can lead to development of melanomas, astrocytomas and occasionally other nervous system neoplasms including peripheral nerve sheath tumors and meningiomas.

191. Melkersson Rosenthal Syndrome (MRS)

Melkersson-Rosenthal Syndrome (MRS) is a rare syndrome consisting of a triad of persistent or recurrent orofacial edema, recurrent facial paralysis and fissured tongue.

192. Mendes Da Costa Syndrome (Erythrokeratoderma Variabilis, EKV)

EKV is a rare heterogeneous skin disorder. The classical EKV first described by Mendes da Costa is characterized by two types of skin lesions: (1) Fixed well-demarcated bizarre keratotic and erythematous hyperkeratotic plaques, showing a predilection for extensor surfaces, lateral trunk and buttocks (2) Transient erythematous, polycyclic or comma shaped macular lesions occurring at any site.

193. Menkes Kinky Hair Syndrome

Menkes kinky hair syndrome is a rare X-linked recessive progressive multi systemic disease of copper metabolism. ATP7A gene encodes ATP7A transmembrane protein, which is an active copper transporter. The clinical features of Menkes kinky hair disease is either a direct consequence of enzyme dysfunction or secondary to an inability to load these enzymes with copper. Autonomic nerve system abnormalities like hypotension and hypothermia, are due to abnormal catecholamine synthesis from deficient dopamine beta hydroxylase. Menkes disease also exhibits marked connective tissue abnormalities, including skin, joints, and bone abnormalities, and impaired blood vessel integrity due to the absence of lysyl oxidase and defective cross linking of collagen and elastin. Skin hypopigmentation and hair abnormalities are due to abnormal tyrosinase and sulfhydryl oxidase, respectively. Microscopic examination reveals pili torti and occasionally trichorrhexis nodosa. Other clinical features include sagging cheeks, loose skin especially over back of neck and frontal bossing.

194. Meretoja Syndrome (Gelsolin Amyloidosis)

In Meretoja syndrome which is a type of systemic amyloidosis, clinical manifestations are distinctive, including lattice corneal degeneration, cranial neuropathy, bulbar palsy and cutaneous abnormalities. Some patients may develop peripheral neuropathy and renal failure. The disorder is usually inherited in an autosomal dominant pattern. Skin fragility, cutis laxa, extensive petechiae and haemorrhages, as well as hypotrichosis or alopecia, can be seen in Gelsolin amyloidosis.

195. Mevalonate Kinase Deficiency (MKD) with Recurrent Fever and Hyper IgD Syndrome

(Described in detail in chapter 30).

196. Michelin Tyre Baby Syndrome (MTBS)

MTBS is a rare genodermatosis, characterized by generalized folding of excess skin and may be associated with various phenotypic abnormalities. It is a benign hamartomatous condition present with ring like skin fold over trunk and limbs.

197. Microcephaly Capillary Malformation Syndrome (MIC-CAP)

MIC-CAP syndrome is an autosomal recessive disorder caused by biallelic STAMBP pathogenic variants. The defining clinical characteristics are typically present at birth, i.e., microcephaly and generalized cutaneous capillary malformations, hypoplastic distal phalanges of the hands and/or feet, early onset intractable epilepsy and profound developmental delay. Seizures, which can be focal, tonic and complex partial, can cause infantile spasms which appear to stabilize after two years of age. Myoclonus of the limbs and eyelids is also common.

198. Microphthalmia with Linear Skin Defects Syndrome (MLS or Microphthalmia, Dermal Aplasia MIDAS)

MIDAS syndrome, also called as microphthalmia with linear skin defects syndrome (MLS) is characterized by ocular defects (microphthalmia, orbital cysts, corneal opacities, cataracts) and linear skin dysplasia of the neck, head and chin. Other findings include central nervous system involvement (structural anomalies, developmental delays and infantile spasms), cardiac concerns (hypertrophic/cardiomyopathy), short stature, nail dystrophy, hearing impairment and genitourinary malformation.

199. Mikulicz Syndrome (MS)

MS usually presents with a classical triad of symmetrical enlargement of all salivary glands, narrowing of the palpebral fissures due to enlargement of the lacrimal glands and parchment like dryness of the mouth.

200. Milk Alkali Syndrome (MAS)

Milk alkali syndrome is characterized by a triad of elevated levels of calcium, metabolic alkalosis and acute kidney injury. Diffuse subcutaneous calcification can be seen due to high serum calcium level.

201. Morgellons Syndrome (Morgellons Disease)

Morgellons disease is a mysterious disease with unknown etiology. It is characterized by fibers appearing in slow or non-healing skin lesions and even beneath unbroken skin, along with abnormal (crawling, stinging, or biting) sensations on skin. It is associated with tick born *Borrelia* spirochetal infection.

202. MORM Syndrome (Mental Retardation, truncal Obesity, Retinal Dystrophy and Micropenis)

It is a syndrome with intellectual deficit, truncal obesity, retinal dystrophy and micropenis. It is transmitted in an autosomal recessive manner. The causative locus has been mapped to chromosome region 9q34.

203. Muckle Wells Syndrome (MWS)

MWS is a rare autoinflammatory disorder which is an autosomal dominant disease due to NLRP3/CIAS1 gene mutations, responsible for excessive caspase-1 activation and interleukin 1β processing. Urticarial rash, conjunctivitis, recurrent fever, arthralgia and fatigue are the main clinical manifestations of MWS. Sensorineural hearing loss and renal amyloidosis can also occur.

204. Mucocutaneous Lymph Node Syndrome (MLNS)/Kawasaki Disease

Kawasaki disease is an acute, self-limited medium vessel vasculitis of infants and children characterized by prolonged fever of more than 5 days, unresponsive to antipyretics and antibiotics, polymorphous skin rash (maculopapular rash, urticaria rash, erythema multiforme like rash, purpuric rash and pustular rash), erythema of the oral mucosa, lips and tongue (strawberry tongue), erythema of the palms and soles, prominent swelling of hands and feet, bilateral non exudative conjunctival injection, and unilateral cervical lymphadenopathy. Myocarditis, cardiac valvulitis, lymphocytic/mixed interstitial infiltrate of pancreas, renal, splenic, hepatic hilar regions can also be seen. Leucocytosis, thrombocytosis and high erythrocyte sedimentation rate are characteristic.

Early diagnosis and treatment are central to preventing complications, such as coronary artery aneurysms.

During convalescent or subacute phase, desquamation of finger and toe skin in periungual area is seen. In chronic stage nail may develop transverse grooves (beau's line).

205. Mucocutaneous Pain Syndrome (MCPs)

Mucocutaneous pain syndromes (MCPs) typically involve the head, neck and mouth. For many MCPs no organic cause for their disease can be identified (with the exception of post herpetic neuralgia and trigeminal trophic syndrome) and the causes are believed to be related to the complex physiological interaction between the cranial and peripheral nervous systems and the brain itself.

206. Muir-Torre Syndrome (MTS)

Muir Torre Syndrome is an autosomal dominant phenotypic variant of Hereditary Non Polyposis Colorectal Cancer (HNPCC), which is also known as Lynch syndrome. It is caused by mutations in the DNA mismatch repair genes which results in microsatellite instability. The hallmark features of Muir-Torre syndrome are sebaceous neoplasms, keratoacanthoma of the skin and visceral malignancies with colonic carcinoma being the most common.

207. Multiple Mucosal Neuroma Syndrome or Multiple Endocrine Neoplasia Type 2B (MMNS or MEN 2B)

MMNS is an autosomal dominant hamartoneoplastic syndrome due to receptor tyrosine kinase (RET) proto-oncogene mutation. Features include marfanoid body habitus with characteristic dysmorphic facies, multiple mucosal neuromas, pheochromocytoma and medullary thyroid carcinoma.

208. Multiple Pterygium Syndrome

It is a rare autosomal recessive genetic disorder characterized by facial anomalies, short stature, vertebral defects, multiple joint contractures and webbing (pterygia) of the neck, elbows, back of the knees, armpits and fingers.

209. Myositis Overlap Syndromes (MOS)

Myositis overlap syndromes are characterized by a heterogeneous group of clinical syndromes of which many are closely linked with specific autoantibodies. Patients positive for anti-snU1 RNP antibody often present with a constellation of "autoimmune-related" clinical features, often not fulfilling the diagnostic criteria for a single disease entity. Anti-PM-Scl antibodies are linked with myositis-scleroderma overlap and generally tend to follow a benign course, often responding well to minimal immunosuppression. Antibodies to the autoantigen histidyl-tRNA synthetase (Jo1) are the most common and best characterized. Patients with these antibodies have severe interstitial lung disease and poorest prognosis often necessitating aggressive immunosuppressive therapy.

210. Naegeli Franchescetti Jadassohn Syndrome (NFJS)

Naegeli Franceschetti Jadassohn Syndrome (NFJS) is a rare form of ectodermal dysplasia inherited as an autosomal dominant disorder. NFJS and its closely related allelic disorder, Dermatopathia Pigmentosa Reticularis (DPR), are characterized by the absence of dermatoglyphics, reticulate patterned skin hyperpigmentation, palmoplantar keratoderma, abnormal sweating, and other subtle developmental anomalies of teeth, hair and skin. Several mutations in the KRT 14 gene have been found to cause NFJS/DPR.

211. Nevus Comedonicus Syndrome (NC)

Nevus comedonicus refers to closely arranged, grouped, often linear, slightly elevated papules which have keratinous plugs at their centre. It may be present at birth or appear later. The term NC syndrome is used for comedo nevus presenting in association with extracutaneous manifestations which may include central nervous system (CNS), skeletal, ophthalmological, neurological and spinal abnormalities.

212. Nail Patella Syndrome (NPS)/Fong's Disease

Nail patella syndrome is a rare multi systemic disease with a classic clinical tetrad of finger nail dysplasia, hypoplasia or absence of the patella, presence of iliac horns, and elbow deformities. Ocular, renal and neurological involvement can occur.

213. Naxos Syndrome

Naxos syndrome is a rare autosomal recessive form of Arrhythmogenic Right Ventricular Cardiomyopathy (ARVC) with woolly hair and non epidermolytic palmoplantar keratoderma. The cardiomyopathy presents by adolescence with syncope, ventricular tachycardia (VT) of left bundle branch block (LBBB) morphology, and/or ventricular fibrillation.

214. Nelson Syndrome/Post Adrenelectomy Syndrome

Nelson's syndrome is a rare clinical manifestation that occurs in 8-47% of patients as a complication of bilateral adrenalectomy, a procedure that is used to control hypercortisolism in patients with Cushing's disease. The disease is associated with a clinical triad of hyperpigmentation, excessive adrenocorticotropin secretion and a corticotrophic adenoma.

215. Neu Laxova Syndrome (NLS)

Inherited as an autosomal recessive trait, it is characterized by severe growth delay before birth, low birth weight and length. Craniofacial abnormalities are microcephaly, sloping forehead and hypertelorism. Abnormal accumulation of fluid in tissue throughout body (generalized edema) is seen. Permanent flexion and immobilisation of joints (flexion contractures) are also noted. Some affected infants have yellowish and dry scaly skin (ichthyotic skin).

216. Neurofibromatosis Noonan Syndrome (NFNS)

Major gene causing NFNS is NF1 mutation. Rarely a mutation in PTPN11 in addition to a NF1 mutation is present. It is a RASopathy characterized by a combination of features of NF1 such as café-au-lait spots, iris lisch nodules, axillary and inguinal freckling, optic nerve gliomas and multiple neurofibromas, and features of Noonan syndromes (NS), such as typical facial features including hypertelorism, ptosis, down slating palpebral fissures, low set posteriorly rotated ears and congenital heart defects.

217. Numb Chin Syndrome (NCS)

It is characterised by hypoesthesia, paresthesia or pain over the chin in the region supplied by inferior alveolar nerve which is the terminal branch of mandibular nerve. Numbness is caused by malignant infiltration of nerve sheath or compression of nerve by metastasis in jaw or by local tumor.

218. Occipital Horn Syndrome (OHS)

It is a X-linked recessive disorder due to mutation in ATP7A gene. This gene encodes for copper transport ATPase1. It is a congenital disorder of copper metabolism. Lysyl oxidase is a major copper dependent enzyme, and its activity is markedly decreased in some patients, resulting in defective collagen and elastin cross links. This disorder is characterised by bony exostoses (including pathognomic horn) and connective tissue manifestations and variable involvement of central nervous system. There is hyperextensible and soft skin with fine wrinkling on hand and feet. Clinical manifestations include the development of bladder diverticula during childhood, inguinal hernia, mild laxity of the skin and skeletal defects such as short humeri and clavicles. Bony occipital horns appear during adolescence.

219. Oculocerebral Syndrome with Hypopigmentation (Cross Syndrome/Kramer Syndrome)

It is an autosomal recessive syndrome characterized by generalized hypopigmentation with white/silvery hair and severe mental retardation, spastic tetraplegia and athetosis. Ocular anomalies include microphthalmos, a small opaque cornea and coarse nystagmus.

220. Oculo-Oro-genital Syndrome (OOGS)

This syndrome occurs due to a deficiency of vitamin B_2 and B_6. Clinical features are seborrheic dermatitis like changes, fissuring of periorificial and genital areas, perleche, cheilosis, de papillated glossitis (magenta tongue) and conjunctivitis.

221. Olmsted Syndrome/Mutilating PPK with Periorificial Keratotic Plaques (Palmoplantar Keratoderma)

Onset is in the first year of life, with symmetrical sharply defined palmar and plantar mutilating keratoderma surrounded by erythema. Flexion deformities, constriction or spontaneous amputation of the digits are noted. The keratotic lesions are pruritic and mildly painful on pressure. Long standing cases can progress to squamous cell carcinoma. Periorificial plaques present with erythema and warty hyperkeratosis involving the mouth and perianal regions. Massive hyperkeratosis and/or fissuring of the gluteal cleft may cause pain and considerable discomfort. Alopecia, nail and tooth anomalies, joint laxity and corneal dystrophy have also been observed. It is caused by TRPV3 and MBTSP 2 gene mutation.

222. Omenn Syndrome

Mutation in the RAG1 or RAG2 gene causes Omenn syndrome, an autosomal recessive form of severe combined immunodeficiency (SCID). Alopecia, lymphadenopathy and erythroderma are the three main cutaneous manifestations. Scaling, widespread erythema and "leathery" skin texture are characteristic features. Significant lymphadenopathy, immunodeficiency, high blood IgE levels and eosinophilia are seen. As with other kinds of SCID, children may experience diarrhoea, failure to thrive and recurrent infection.

223. Oral Allergy Syndrome (OAS)

Oral allergy syndrome is a form of allergic reaction involving the mouth, characterized by immediate itching, swelling and burning after eating a wide range of fresh fruits including apples, pears, cherries, plums, celery, spices and hazel nuts. It is also known as pollen food allergy. It is type 1 or IgE mediated hypersensitivity reaction.

224. Oro Facio Digital Syndrome (OFDS)

It is a X-linked dominant condition which primarily affects the development of mouth, face, fingers and toes. Common clinical features are cleft tongue (split or bifid tongue), nodules or growth on tongue, cleft palate, wide spaced eyes (hypertelorism), small chin, cleft lip, brachydactyly, syndactyly and polydactyly. Granular appearances of facial skin, multiple milial cysts on the ears, dry hair, diffuse thinning of hair and patchy hair loss is also seen in oro facio digital syndrome.

225. Osler-Rendu-Weber Syndrome or Hereditary Hemorrhagic Telangiectasia

It is an autosomal dominant disorder characterized by epistaxis (spontaneous, recurrent nose bleeds) mucocutaneous telangiectasia (lips, oral cavity, fingers, nose) and visceral telangiectasia such as gastrointestinal telangiectasia. Sites of arteriovenous malformations are lungs, liver, gastrointestinal tract and central nervous system (these may result in massive visceral hemorrhage and death).

226. Overlap Syndrome

Overlap syndrome have been defined as entities satisfying classification criteria of at least two connective tissue diseases occurring at the same or different times in the same patient.

Connective tissue diseases include, systemic lupus erythematosus (SLE), Systemic sclerosis (SSc), rheumatoid arthritis (RA), polymyositis, dermatomyositis, and Sjogren's syndrome.

227. Pachyonychia Congenita

Pachyonychia congenita (PC) is a rare autosomal dominantly transmitted genodermatosis caused by mutations in any of the five genes encoding nail keratins, KRT6A, KRT6B, KRT6C, KRT16, or KRT17. The clinical features virtually seen in all affected patients are dystrophy, thickened toe nails and painful plantar keratoderma often associated with plantar pain, oral leucokeratosis and cystic lesions.

- Type 1 PC (Jadassohn Lewandowski syndrome) has mutations in the KRT6A/KRT16 genes. The characteristic features include, abnormally wedge shaped thickened and curved nails (onychogryphosis), focal palmoplantar keratoderma, verrucous lesions on the knees, elbows, buttocks, ankles and popliteal regions, follicular keratoses/ keratosis pilaris, white plaques (leukokeratosis) in oral and laryngeal mucosa, palmoplantar hyperhidrosis.
- Type 2 PC (Jackson Lawler Syndrome) has mutations in the KRT6B/KRT17 genes and is characterized by natal teeth, multiple pilosebaceous cysts (steatocystomas), small cystic papulonodules on the central face, dry, unruly, curly hair and pili torti. Palmoplantar hyperkeratosis is less accentuated as compared to type 1 PC.

228. PAPA Syndrome ((Pyogenic Arthritis, Pyoderma Gangrenosum and Acne)

(Described in detail in chapter 30)

229. Papillon-Lefevre Syndrome (PLS) / Haim-Munk Syndrome

In PL syndrome, redness and thickening of the palms and soles is associated with periodontitis and frequent bacterial skin infections. Hyperkeratotic lesions can also affect the elbows, knees and pseudoainhum (Dactylolysis spontanea) may also be seen. Dural and choroid plexus calcifications have also been reported. Haim-Munk syndrome is allelic with Papillon-Lefevre syndrome, combining its features with onychogryphosis, arachno-dactyly and acro-osteolysis. Both conditions are caused by homozygous mutations in the CTSC gene encoding the lysosomal protease cathepsin C.

230. Papular Pruritic Gloves and Socks Syndrome (PPGSS)

It presents as an acute acral dermatosis, occurring predominantly in young adults, less commonly seen in children. It is regarded as an idiosyncratic reaction, usually to a viral infection. Parvovirus B_{19} infection is the most commonly associated infection. In children, EBV or CMV may be more common than in adults. The hands, wrists, feet and ankles are intensely pruritic and are affected with macular and papular erythematous eruption associated with oedema. There may also be associated purpura and rarely petechiae may be seen. A distinct cut-off at wrists and ankles is often seen. Malaise and fever can follow a few days after the onset of the eruption and lymphadenopathy may occur.

231. Parinaud Oculoglandular Syndrome

It is unilateral granulomatous conjunctivitis with regional lymphadenopathy of the same side. The most common identifiable cause is Bartonella henselae (Cat scratch disease).

232. Parkes-Weber Syndrome (PWS)

It is a rare congenital condition characterized by a large number of abnormal blood vessels. The main signs and symptoms of PWS include capillary malformation on the skin, hypertrophy of bones and soft tissue of affected limbs and multiple arteriovenous fistulas which can potentially lead to heart failure. Some cases of this syndrome result from mutation in the RASA1 gene and are inherited in an autosomal dominant manner. Pain in affected limb and difference in size between limbs is seen.

233. Parry Romberg Syndrome

It is also known as progressive facial hemiatrophy, which is a rare acquired morphieform disorder characterized by slowly progressive atrophy of the skin and soft tissues of half of the face, seen in pediatric age group. In some cases, atrophy may also affect the limbs, usually on the same side of the body as of facial atrophy.

234. PASH Syndrome (Pyoderma Gangrenosum, Acne, Hidradenitis Suppurativa)

It is a hereditary autoinflammatory syndrome. Abnormality associated with this syndrome causes raised IL-β (systemically or locally) or aberrant regulation of the function of this cytokine. Three diagnostic features of this syndrome are, pyoderma gangrenosum, acne and hidradenitis suppurativa.

235. PASS Syndrome

Abnormality associated with this syndrome is raised TNF-α (systemically or locally) or aberrant regulation of the function of this cytokine. It is characterized by:

- Chronic relapsing **P**yoderma gangrenosum.
- **A**cne vulgaris.
- **H**idradenitis suppurativa; and
- **S**eronegative spondyloarthritis.

236. Peeling Skin Syndrome

Peeling skin syndrome (PSS) is a rare recessively inherited ichthyosiform genodermatosis characterized by superficial skin peeling. This has two subtypes – Acral and Generalised which further has two subtypes inflammatory and non-inflammatory.

237. PELVIS Syndrome

It is an association between segmental infantile haemangioma of the perineum (around the genitals and anus) and congenital anomalies involving the genitalia, urinary tract, spine, anus, and rectum. The acronym PELVIS was proposed in 2006 by Dr. Celine Girard and colleagues. It stands for-Perineal haemangioma, External genitalia malformations, Lipomyelomeningocele, Vesicorenal abnormalities, Imperforate anus and Skin tags.

238. PENS (Papular Epidermal Nevus with 'Skyline' Basal Cell Layer Syndrome) Syndrome

It is a rare, genetic, neurocutaneous syndrome. PENS is characterized by the presence of randomly distributed, small, white to yellowish, multiple, rounded or irregular polycyclically shaped, epidermal keratotic papules and plaques of 'Gem-like' appearance which have a rough surface. They are typically located on the trunk and proximal limbs and are associated with variable neurological abnormalities, including psychomotor delay, epilepsy, speech and language impairment and attention deficit hyperactivity disorder. Clumsiness, dyslexia and ophthalmological abnormalities have also been reported.

239. Peutz-Jeghers Syndrome (PJS)

PJS is characterized by the association of gastrointestinal (GI) polyposis, mucocutaneous pigmentation, and cancer predisposition. PJS type hamartomatous polyps are most common in the small intestine. GI polyps can result in chronic bleeding, anemia, and recurrent obstruction and intussusception requiring repeated laparotomy and bowel obstruction. Mucocutaneous hyperpigmentation presents in childhood as dark blue to dark brown macules around the mouth, eyes and nostrils, in the perianal area and on the buccal mucosa. Hyperpigmented macules on the fingers are common. Individuals with PJS are at increased risk of a wide variety of malignancies (colorectal, gastric, pancreatic, breast and ovarian cancer). PJS is an autosomal dominant syndrome caused by mutation in STK 11/LKB 1 gene.

240. PHACE Syndrome

It is characterised by Posterior fossa malformations, Hemangioma, Arterial anomalies, Coarctation of the aorta/cardiac defects and Eye abnormalities.

241. Plummer-Vinson Syndrome (PVS)

It is a condition that can occur in people with long-term (chronic) iron deficiency anemia. Patients with this condition have problems in swallowing due to small, thin growths of tissue that partially block the esophagus. Triad of dysphagia, iron deficiency anaemia and esophageal web is seen. Skin finding related to iron deficiency is koilonychia (flattening and spoon shaped nail).

242. POEMS Syndrome (Polyneuropathy, Organomegaly, Endocrinopathy, Monoclonal Gammopathy, Skin Changes)

It is a syndrome characterized by polyneuropathy, numbness, tingling, weakness and difficulty in breathing. It is a rare blood disorder that damages the nerves and affects other parts of the body. Cutaneous findings include diffuse skin hyperpigmentation, sclerodermoid changes, papular lesion over infraclavicular and abdominal region, facial plethora lipoatrophy, acrocyanosis, Raynaud's phenomenon, leukonychia or terry nails, hypertrichosis, necrotizing vasculitis or calciphylaxis and multiple cutaneous angioma.

243. Polyfibromatosis Syndrome

It is a rare disease entity which is characterized by clinical features such as palmar, plantar, and penile fibromatoses, keloid formations of the skin and erosive arthropathy. Its precise pathophysiology or etiology remains unclear.

244. Post Thrombotic Syndrome (PTS)

It is a chronic condition which occurs as a result of deep vein thrombosis (DVT). The veins in our arms and legs have small valves inside that ensure the blood flows correctly back towards the heart. DVT is a blockage or clot that obstructs the vein and can lead to the valves becoming damaged leading to oedema and skin pigmentation.

245. Prader-Willi Syndrome (PWS)

PWS is caused by maternal disomy in the proximal arm of chromosome 15. It is associated with characteristic features such as diminished fetal activity, obesity, hypotonia, intellectual disability, short stature, hypogonadotropic hypogonadism, strabismus and small hands and feet. Skin picking is the most typical cutaneous feature, other features include, albinism, striae, panniculitis, pizogenic papules, bruising etc.

246. Premature Ageing Syndromes

Premature ageing syndromes also known as Progeria, which includes two very rare inherited conditions:

Hutchinson-Gilford syndrome: It is caused by mutations of the lamin A gene (LMNA) which encodes for a major constituent of the inner membrane lamina. It is characterized by small stature, bird like face with beaked nose, protruded ear, centrofacial cyanosis, pseudohydrocephaly, mid facial hypoplasia, large anterior fontanelle, prominent scalp veins, dry, wrinkled, mottled pigmentation, sclerodermoid like changes, keloidal tendency, alopecia, thin and brittle nails, coxa valga, loss of subcutaneous fat.

Werner syndrome (Pangeria): Skin atrophy (skin thinning and loss of elasticity), loss of cutaneous fat, wrinkling, greying hair, alopecia, nail dystrophy, mottled pigmentation and ulceration, bilateral juvenile cataract, keratopathy, sclerodactyly, restricted movement of joint, hyperkeratosis over bony prominence are feature of this syndrome. It is characterized by the premature appearance of features associated with normal ageing and cancer predisposition. Myocardial infarction and cancer are the most common causes of death.

247. Proteus Syndrome

It is a rare condition due to mutation in the AKT 1 gene characterised by overgrowth of bone, skin and other tissues. Organs and tissues affected by the disease, grow out of proportion to the rest of the body. Other features of this overgrowth syndrome include hyperostosis or osteoma of bone, lipohypertrophy and lipoatrophy of the skin, verrucous epidermal nevus, cerebriform connective tissue nevus (collagenoma) of hands and feet, vascular malformation and predisposition to various neoplasms like bilateral ovarian cystadenoma, testicular tumors, meningioma and monomorphic salivary gland adenoma.

248. Pseudo Cushing's Syndrome

It covers different pathological conditions responsible for mild-to-moderate ACTH dependent hypercortisolism, not related to an ACTH secreting tumor but rather to Corticotrophin releasing hormone and/or arginine vasopressin hypothalamic secretion through activation of various neural pathways, in patients generally displaying excess central adiposity.

249. Pseudologia Fantastica (Münchausen Syndrome)

It is a factitious disorder imposed on self, known as Münchausen syndrome. It is a psychiatric disorder in which a person assumes the role of a sick patient without the intention of external gain. Physical symptoms are intentionally produced with the purpose of appearing to be sick.

250. PTEN Hamartoma Tumor Syndrome (PHTS)

It is a genetic condition in which hamartomas, develop in different areas of the body. In addition to hamartomas, patients can have other physical findings, including larger than average head size, abnormal skin growths and intellectual disabilities. It is also associated with high risk for benign and malignant tumor of thyroid, breast, skin and endometrium. Skin manifestations include trichilemmomas, acral keratosis, papillomatous papule or mucocutaneous neuroma, lipoma, café-au-lait macule, haemangiomas and cobblestone appearance of oral mucosa.

251. Puffy Hand Syndrome

Puffy hand syndrome develops after long-term intravenous drug addiction. It is characterized by non-pitting edema, affecting the dorsal side of fingers and hands with puffy appearance. Frequency and severity of the complications of this syndrome are rarely reported.

252. Ramsay Hunt Syndrome (Herpes Zoster Oticus)

It occurs when herpes zoster affects the facial nerve near geniculate ganglion. In addition to the painful rash, Ramsay Hunt syndrome can cause facial paralysis, otalgia and hearing loss in the affected ear.

253. Rapp Hodgkin Syndrome (RHS)

It is a type of anhidrotic ectodermal dysplasia, which was described by Rapp and Hodgkin in 1968. This syndrome is characterized by anhidrotic ectodermal dysplasia, cleft lip and cleft palate.

254. Rapunzel Syndrome

It is an unusual form of trichobezoar found in patients with a history of psychiatric disorders, trichotillomania (habit of hair pulling) and trichophagia (morbid habit of chewing the hair), consequently developing gastric bezoars. The principal symptoms are vomiting and epigastric pain.

255. Reactive Arthritis Syndrome (Reiter's Syndrome)

It is also known as reactive arthritis and presents with a classic triad of conjunctivitis, urethritis and asymmetric large joint oligoarthritis with or without dactylitis occurring 1-6 weeks after an infection, particularly those in the urogenital (chlamydia) or gastrointestinal tract. Dermatologic manifestations include keratoderma blennorrhagicum (palmo-plantar pustulosis and psoriasiform hyperkeratosis), circinate balanitis, ulcerative vulvitis, nail changes, geographical tongue, oral erosions. Infectious and immune factors are likely involved in pathogenesis. It is strongly linked with the HLA-B27 haplotype.

256. Red Baby Syndrome

Abrupt onset of high fever and generalized erythema involving the entire skin, which is swollen and tender, is characteristic. These children are highly irritable and have a paradoxical cry when cuddled. Rapid resolution of symptoms occur in 7-10 days with extensive desquamation due to vancomycin injection.

257. Red Finger Syndrome

It consists of well delineated erythema of periungal and pulp areas with occasional telangiectasia on the fingers and toes with normal nail plate. Red finger syndrome is rare in children.

258. Red Man Syndrome

It is an infusion related reaction peculiar to vancomycin. It typically consists of pruritic erythematous rash that involves the face, neck and upper torso. Less frequently, hypotension and angioedema can occur.

259. Refsum Syndrome

It is a hereditary motor sensory neuropathy type IV, heredopathia atactica polyneuritiformis autosomal recessive disorder due to accumulation of phytanic acid in plasma and lipid containing tissues. Clinical features include retinitis pigmentosa, blindness, anosmia, deafness, sensory neuropathy, ichthyosis and ataxia.

260. Restless Leg Syndrome (Willis Ekbom Disease)

Restless leg syndrome is a common condition of the nervous system that causes an overwhelming irresistible urge to move the legs, with unpleasant crawling or creeping sensation in the feet, calves and thighs. The sensation is often worse in the evening or at night.

261. Reticular Erythematosus Mucinosis Syndrome (REMS)

REMS is a rare form of cutaneous mucinosis. It most often affects middle-aged women is also called 'midline mucinosis' or 'plaque like cutaneous mucinosis'. Papules develop on the mid back or chest and form a net like pattern (hence the name, 'reticular'). The cause is unknown. However, exposure to sunlight may contribute to the condition. Generally, REM is not associated with other systemic diseases but it can appear very similar to mucinosis developing in association with systemic lupus erythematosus.

262. Reye's Syndrome

Reye's syndrome is a rare and potentially fatal pediatric illness defined as acute non-inflammatory encephalopathy with fatty liver failure. Reye's syndrome typically presents in children with vomiting and confusion which rapidly progresses to coma and death. This syndrome often begins in the days following recovery from a viral illness during which aspirin was administered. Reye's syndrome is most commonly precipitated by viral pathogens such as influenza A and B as well as varicella. It appears to involve mitochondrial injury in the setting of a viral illness. Aspirin may cause or perpetuate damage to cellular mitochondria resulting in inhibition of fatty acid metabolism.The neurologic features of Reye's syndrome likely result from hepatic mitochondrial dysfunction causing elevated ammonia levels. Hyperammonemia may induce astrocyte edema resulting in diffuse cerebral edema and subsequent elevated intracranial pressure.

263. Riley Day Syndrome (Familial Dysautonomia)

Riley Day syndrome is an autosomal recessive disorder of autonomic nervous system. There is reduction and/or loss of unmyelinated and small myelinated fibers, due to reduction of dopamine beta-hydroxylase. The diagnosis is based on clinical features such as, diminished lacrimation, insensitivity to pain, poor temperature control, abolished deep tendon reflexes, postural hypotension, attacks of vomiting, poor motor coordination and mental retardation.

264. Rombo Syndrome

It is a dominantly inherited disorder, characterized by vermiculate atrophoderma, milia, hypotrichosis, trichoepitheliomas, basal cell carcinomas and peripheral vasodilation with cyanosis. The lesions become visible in late childhood and are most pronounced on the face. Basal cell carcinomas may develop around the age of the third decade. Histological findings during the early stage include irregularly distributed and atrophic hair follicles, milia, dilated dermal vessels, lack of elastin or elastin in clumps. After light irradiation, a tendency for increased repair activity was observed both in epidermis and in the dermal fibroblasts.

265. Ross Syndrome

Ross syndrome is a rare peripheral autonomic nervous system disorder characterized by a triad of Adie's tonic pupils, hyporeflexia and segmental anhidrosis. The ciliary ganglion becomes damaged, which causes tonic pupil. There is no known reason for the diminished or nonexistent reflexes. In some patients of Ross syndrome, ANA is positive which suggests that it may be an autoimmune disease. Sweating abnormalities are typically the initial indicator of Ross syndrome and they must always be present in order to make the diagnosis. The majority of patients present with patchy localised hyperhidrosis and are unaware of the anhidrous areas. Ross syndrome is a compensatory mechanism that most frequently affects unilateral dermatomes.

266. Rothmund Thompson Syndrome (RTS)

RTS is an autosomal recessive genodermatosis, characterized by distinctive facial poikiloderma, the diagnostic hallmark, and a variety of clinical features, such as short stature, sparse scalp hair, sparse or absent eyelashes and/or eyebrows, juvenile cataracts, skeletal abnormalities, radial ray defects (partial or complete absence of radius), premature ageing, and a predisposition to osteosarcoma. On the basis of clinical and molecular analysis, two types of RTS have emerged:

TYPE I RTS characterized by poikiloderma, ectodermal dysplasia and juvenile cataracts, negative for the RECQL4 mutation.

Type II RTS presents with poikiloderma, congenital bone defects and an increased risk of osteosarcoma related to deleterious RECQL4 mutation.

267. Rowell Syndrome

Rowell syndrome is a rare disease consisting of erythema multiforme like lesions associated with lupus erythematosus. The syndrome occurs mostly in middle aged women, characterized by lupus erythematosus (LE), erythema multiforme (EM) like lesions, positive tests for rheumatoid factor (RF), speckled antinuclear antibody (ANA), and precipitating antibody to saline extract of human tissue (anti-SjT). Major and minor diagnostic criteria were proposed for the diagnosis of this syndrome.

Major criteria include:

1. Coexistence of LE and EM like lesions.
2. Positive ANA with a speckled pattern.

Minor criteria include:

1. Chilblains lupus.
2. Positive anti-La (SS-B) or anti-Ro (SS-A) antibodies.
3. Reactive RF.

All the major criteria and at least one of the minor criteria are required to confirm the diagnosis.

268. Rubinstein-Taybi Syndrome (RTS)

Rubinstein-Taybi syndrome (RTS) is an autosomal dominant disorder characterized by distinctive facial features, broad and often angulated thumbs and halluces, short stature and moderate to severe intellectual disability. The characteristic craniofacial features are down slanted palpebral fissures, low hanging columella, high palate, grimacing smile and talon cusps. Additional features include short stature, ocular abnormalities, hearing loss, respiratory difficulties, congenital heart defects, renal abnormalities, cryptorchidism, feeding problems, recurrent infections and severe constipation.

269. Ruvalcaba Syndrome (Ruvalcaba Myhre Smith Syndrome)

It is one of the groups of disorders related to congenital skeletal disturbance. It is characterized by: macrocephaly, hypoplastic genitalia, intellectual deficit (not invariably) and physical disability, short stature, peculiar facies, micrognathia with crowded teeth, a narrow thoracic cage with pectus carinatum, subcutaneous lipoma, hamartomatous intestinal polyps. The stomach, small bowel and colon are involved in most cases.

270. SADDAN Syndrome (Severe Achondroplasia with Developmental Delay and Acanthosis Nigricans

It is an extremely rare condition, and as the name states, presents with skeletal, brain and cutaneous anomalies. The syndrome results from a mutation in the FGFR gene. Patients with this condition have extremely short stature with particularly short arms and legs. Other features include unusual bowing of the leg bones, a small chest with short ribs, curved collar bones, short, broad fingers and folds of extra skin on the arms and legs and acanthosis nigricans. Structural abnormalities of the brain result in seizures, developmental delay and intellectual disability.

271. SAHA Syndrome

The presence of Seborrhoea, Acne, Hirsutism and Alopecia in women has first been summarized as SAHA syndrome in 1982 and can be associated with polycystic ovary syndrome, cystic mastitis, obesity and infertility. The SAHA syndrome generally occurs in young to middle aged women and is caused either due to the presence of elevated blood levels of androgens or due to increased androgen driven peripheral response with normal circulating androgen levels.

272. SAPHO Syndrome

(Described in detail in chapter 30)

273. SCARF Syndrome

SCARF syndrome is an uncommon, X-linked recessive disorder characterised by the association of Skeletal abnormalities, Cutis laxa, Craniostenosis, Ambiguous genitalia, Psychomotor retardation and Facial abnormalities.

274. Schöpf-Schulz-Passarge Syndrome (SSPS)

Schöpf-Schulz-Passarge syndrome is a form of ectodermal dysplasia which is due to mutations in the WNT10A gene on chromosome 2. It is an autosomal recessive genetic condition. Cutaneous features of Schöpf-Schulz-Passarge syndrome typically do not present in childhood, which starts appearing in the early teenage and become more obvious with age. These can include the following features:

- Multiple eyelid cysts (apocrine hidrocystomas) are the cardinal features, but often do not appear until middle age.
- Palmoplantar keratoderma.
- Hyperhidrosis.
- Hypotrichosis.
- Malformation of the nails (onychodystrophy), such as nail fragility or hypoplastic nails.

Non cutaneous features of SSPS include:

- Abnormal development of the teeth (hypodontia) – deciduous teeth are abnormal and may fallout early.
- Bilateral early senile cataract.
- Optic atrophy.
- Myopia.

275. Schnitzler Syndrome

(Described in detail in chapter 30)

276. Senear Usher Syndrome (Pemphigus Erythematosus)

Pemphigus erythematosus is a localized variant of Pemphigus Foliaceous. These patients have typical features of PF with additional characteristics suggestive of systemic lupus erythematosus. The lupus component of pemphigus erythematosus is demonstrated by circulating antinuclear antibodies (ANA) and granular IgG and C3 deposition at the dermoepidermal junction. Clinically it presents with blistering and erosion predominantly over photo-distributed areas. The antibodies recognize anti-desmoglein-1 together with Ro, La and double-stranded DNA antigens. Pemphigus erythematosus may be associated with myasthenia gravis or thymoma.

277. Setleis Syndrome

Setleis syndrome is a rare inherited ectodermal dysplasia, characterized by distinctive facial abnormalities. Infants with Setleis syndrome have multiple, scar like, circular bitemporal depressions, leonine facial appearance, periorbital puffiness and wrinkling. Some cases present with frontal bossing and abnormal growth of eyebrows and abnormal eyelashes (distichiasis) absence of eyelashes on the lower eyelid.

278. Severe Dermatitis, Multiple Allergies and Metabolic Wasting Syndrome (SAM Syndrome)

The disorder results from deficient membrane expression of desmoglein 1 which is also involved in the pathogenesis of pemphigus foliaceus, and impetigo and is degraded in the absence of LEKT I in CNS. Loss of function mutations in DSG1 encoding desmoglein 1 causing SAM syndrome are inherited in a semi-dominant fashion as heterozygous carriers of DSG1 mutation. Patients show focal palmoplantar keratoderma.

279. Sezary Syndrome

It is an erythrodermic variant of CTCL with haematological evidence of leukemic involvement. Sezary syndrome consists of a clinical triad of:

1. Erythroderma.
2. Peripheral lymphadenopathy.
3. Atypical mononuclear cells (Sezary cells) in the peripheral blood, i.e., equal or >5% of peripheral blood lymphocytes on a buffy coat smear or >20% of total lymphocyte count or > 1000×10~9/L.

It can occur in the absence of or may follow as a progression from mycosis fungoides (MF).

280. Sharp Syndrome

Sharp Syndrome is also known as MCTD (Mixed Connective Tissue Disorder). It is an uncommon systemic inflammatory rheumatic disease and is a specific subset of a broader category of rheumatic overlap syndromes, a term used to describe when a patient has features of more than one classic rheumatic disease. These include SLE, polymyositis, scleroderma and RA.

281. Short Anagen Syndrome (SAS)

SAS is a benign disease of the hair cycle, characterized by persistent short fine hair since birth due to decreased duration of the anagen phase. It has recently been recognized as a congenital disease mostly sporadic but a few familial cases have been reported suggesting autosomal dominant inheritance. Clinically the hair shaft is normal but there is no hair growth due to the short anagen phase, associated with increased shedding of hair.

282. Shrinking Lung Syndrome

Shrinking lung syndrome is a rare manifestation of SLE. Clinically the patient presents with dyspnea which is aggravated in a supine position, pleuritic chest pain and diminished breath sounds at lung base on auscultation. Both chest radiograph and CT show elevation of bilateral diaphragms with basal linear atelectasis and without any evidence of parenchymal lung disease. Pulmonary function test (PFT) shows reduced lung volume capacity.

283. Shulman Syndrome

The Shulman Syndrome (eosinophilic fasciitis) is a symptom complex characterized by **eosinophilia, hypergamma-globulinemia and a diffuse scleroderma like process of the extremities**. Initial symptoms associated with eosinophilic fasciitis include pain swelling and inflammation of the skin, especially of the arms and legs. Affected skin may become reddened (erythema), warm, gradually thicken and harden (induration). Eventually, the skin may lose its elasticity and develop a characteristic woody, puckered orange peel texture. Proposed diagnostic criteria for eosinophilic fasciitis:

Major Criteria

1. Swelling, induration and thickening of the skin and subcutaneous tissue that may be symmetrical or asymmetrical, localized or generalized over extremities.
2. Histology shows dermal and fascial thickening with the accumulation of lymphocytes with or without eosinophilic infiltration.

Minor Criteria

1. Peripheral eosinophilia (>0.5 × 10^9/L).
2. Hypergammaglobulinemia (> 1.5 g/L).
3. Muscle weakness or increase aldolase level.
4. Groove sign or peau d'orange appearance of skin.
5. The hyperintense fascia on T2 weighted MRI.

Exclusion of Systemic Sclerosis

For diagnosis presence of two major criteria or one major plus two minor criteria are required.

284. Sjögren Syndrome

Sjögren syndrome is a chronic autoimmune disorder of the exocrine glands with associated swelling and lymphocytic infiltrates of the affected glands. The exocrinopathy can be encountered alone, i.e., (primary Sjögren's syndrome), or in association with other autoimmune disorders, such as RA, SLE and progressive systemic sclerosis (secondary Sjögren syndrome). Dryness of the mouth and eyes results from involvement of the salivary and lacrimal glands.

285. Sjögren-Larsson Syndrome (SLS)

Sjögren-Larsson syndrome is an inborn error of lipid metabolism characterized by congenital ichthyosis (dry, scaly skin), intellectual disability and spasticity (stiffness and involuntary muscle spasms). It is caused by a mutation in the FADH gene (fatty aldehyde dehydrogenase) and has an autosomal recessive inheritance. Preterm birth is common and has been attributed to abnormal LTB4 inactivation. Patients usually present with severe and persistent pruritis with diffuse peeling on the trunk and more pigmented lamellar type ichthyosis on the lower limbs and keratotic lichenification around the flexures, neck and mid abdomen is also seen. The face is usually spared. Neurological features include spastic diplegia, spastic tetraplegia, seizures, delayed speech and dysarthria. Fundus examination shows glistening white dots surrounding the fovea that is due to crystalline inclusion.

286. Smith Lemli Opitz Syndrome (SLOS)

Smith Lemli Opitz Syndrome is a variable genetic disorder characterized by slow growth before and after birth, small head (microcephaly), mild to moderate mental retardation, multiple birth defects including cleft palate, heart defects, fused second and third toe and underdeveloped male genitalia. It has an autosomal recessive inheritance and is associated with mutation in the enzyme 7-dehydrocholestrol reductase, which leads to abnormal cholesterol metabolism.

287. Sneddon Syndrome

It is a rare progressive disorder affecting small and medium sized blood vessels. Sneddon Syndrome is characterized by the association of skin condition and neurological abnormalities which include multiple episodes of cerebral ischemia causing mini strokes and net like bluish discoloration of skin surrounded by normal skin (livedo reticularis). Other symptoms include headache, dizziness, memory loss, reduced intellectual ability, hypertension and heart disease. The exact causation has not been established yet.

288. Speckled Lentiginous Naevus Syndrome (SLNS)

Speckled lentiginous naevus (SLN) syndrome consists of Café-au-lait macules superimposed by macular or papular melanocytic nevus. SLN syndrome is recognized as neurocutaneous phenotype of SLN occurring in association with ipsilateral neurological abnormalities such as hyperhidrosis, muscle weakness and dysesthesia. SLNS represents a mosaic phenotype resulting from post zygotic loss of heterogeneity.

289. Split Hand Split Foot Malformation (SHFM)

It is characterized by the absence of some fingers and toes (ectrodactyly) resembling a claw at birth. It may be associated with webbing of fingers and toes.

290. Staphylococcal Scalded Skin Syndrome (SSSS)

It is also known as Ritter's disease and is characterized by the denudation of skin caused by exotoxin (Exfoliative toxin B and A) producing strains of the Staphylococcal species, typically from a distant site. It usually presents 48 hours after birth and is rare in children older than 6 years. SSSS may also present in immunocompromised adults or those with severe renal disease. Severity may vary from a few blisters to systemic involvement leading to marked hypothermia and hemodynamic instability.

291. Stevens-Johnson Syndrome

SJS is a mucocutaneous illness with significant mortality. It is characterized by the presence of flat atypical target lesions or purpuric macules with blisters that are distributed mainly on the trunk or are widespread. Epidermal detachment is <10% of body surface area (BSA). Two or more mucosal sites can be involved. It typically begins 7-10 days after the initiation of drug therapy. The suspected drug should be avoided lifelong. In the overlap category (SJS/TEN) the area of epidermal detachment is between 10 and 30% of the BSA.

292. Stewart Treves Syndrome

Stewart Treves syndrome is a condition of development of lymphangiosarcoma as a complication of chronic, long standing lymphedema. Most cases occur as a result of post mastectomy lymphedema but it can occur due to any cause of chronic lymphedema. Other associations are congenital or hereditary lymphatic malformation, chronic infection, chronic venous stasis, morbid obesity and malignant obstruction.

293. Stiff Skin Syndrome

It is a rare syndrome characterized by hard, thick skin, usually on the entire body which may lead to limited joint mobility and causes joints to be stuck in a bent position (flexion contractures). Other clinical features include hypertrichosis, lipodystrophy, scoliosis, muscle weakness, slow growth and short stature. It has autosomal dominant inheritance and is caused by mutation in FBN1 gene.

294. Sturge-Weber Syndrome

It is also known as Sturge-Weber Krabbe syndrome and is a rare disorder characterized by the association of a facial birthmark (Portwine stain or Nevus flammeus), neurological and eye abnormalities such as glaucoma. It usually presents at birth, associated with somatic mutation in GNAQ gene which is mostly sporadic.

295. Sugio Kajii Syndrome

Sugio Kajii Syndrome, also known as trichorhinophalangeal syndrome type 3 (TRPS 3) is an extremely rare inherited multisystem disorder characterized by fine, thin, light colored hair, unusual facial features (bulbous nose, abnormally long philtrum), abnormalities of fingers and toes (brachydactyly), skeletal dysplasia especially of hands and feet and delayed eruption of teeth. It is considered to have an autosomal dominant inheritance.

296. Summer Penile Syndrome

It is also known as seasonal acute hypersensitivity reaction and lion's mane penis. It is seen in warm weather and characterized by benign hypersensitivity reaction involving the skin of penile shaft. Summer Penile Syndrome is commonly associated with insect bite, usually chiggers and exposure to plants (poison ivy, sumac, oak). It clinically presents as circumferential edema of penile shaft proximal to glans with minimal erythema and no fluctuance.

297. Sweet's Syndrome (Acute Febrile Neutrophilic Dermatosis)

Sweet's syndrome is a rare disorder characterized by fever and sudden onset of a rash which consists of multiple tender, red bluish lesions, usually present over arms, legs, trunks, face or neck. In some cases, other systems may be involved like musculoskeletal causing arthritis, eyes which lead to conjunctivitis or internal organs. In majority, it is idiopathic (classical Sweet's syndrome) or it may occur in association with malignancy usually hematological or with intake of certain drugs (drug induced Sweet's syndrome). Proposed diagnostic criteria for Sweet's syndrome includes following findings:

Major Criteria

1. Acute onset of typical lesions (tender red papules, nodules and eventually plaques with pseudo vesicles or pseudo pustulation.
2. Histology findings consist of Sweet's syndrome (dense infiltrate of neutrophils in the dermis and prominent dermal papillary oedema.

Minor Criteria

1. Fever >38.
2. Association with inflammatory dermatosis, respiratory or gastrointestinal infections, or malignancy.
3. Excellent response to steroid.
4. Abnormal laboratory (three of four required):
   - ESR > 20 mm/hrs.
   - Leukocytes >8000.
   - Neutrophils > 70%.
   - Raised C-reactive protein.

Patients must meet the two major and two of the four minor criteria.

298. Syndrome of Hewitt and Pelisse

Vulvovaginal gingival syndrome or Hewitt Pelisse syndrome is a rare severe variant of lichen planus. It is characterized by erosions and desquamation of the vulval, vaginal and gingival mucosae and can result in scarring and the formation of strictures. It is associated with HLA class 2 DQB1.

299. Systemic Capillary Leak/Clarkson Syndrome

Idiopathic capillary leak syndrome (SCLS) also known as Clarkson's disease and spontaneous periodic edema, is a fatal disorder characterized by stereotypic "attacks" of varying intensity of hypovolemic shock and generalized edema in association with haemoconcentration and hypoalbuminemia in absence of albuminuria. It is a rare disorder that typically occurs in midlife.

300. Takayasu/Aortic Arch Syndrome/Martorell Syndrome

Takayasu arteritis also known as pulseless illness and occlusive thromboaortopathy, is a chronic inflammatory arteritis that mostly affects the aorta and its main branches. Inflammation of vessel wall leads to wall thickening, fibrosis, stenosis and thrombus formation causing end organ ischaemia. Erythema nodosum, erythema induratum, pyoderma gangrenosum, ulcerated subacute nodular lesions, papulonecrotic eruptions, papular erythematous lesions of the hands, lupus like rashes on the face and panniculitis may be seen.

301. TEMPI Syndrome (Telangiectasias, Erythrocytosis, Monoclonal Gammopathy, Perinephric Fluid Collection, Intrapulmonary Shunting)

TEMPI syndrome is a rare multisystemic disease. It is characterized by telangiectasias, erythrocytosis with elevated erythropoietin levels, monoclonal gammopathy, perinephric fluid collections and intrapulmonary shunting.

302. TORCH Syndrome

TORCH syndrome (Toxoplasmosis, Other agents, Rubella, Cytomegalovirus and Herpes simplex) refers to infection of a developing fetus or newborn by any of these infectious agents. The infection causes similar symptoms in affected newborns which includes fever, feeding difficulties, area of bleeding under the skin, hepatosplenomegaly, jaundice, hearing abnormalities, eye abnormalities.

303. Toxic Oil Syndrome

Toxic oil syndrome is a rare intoxication, due to consumption of rapeseed oil denatured with aniline 2%. It was reported in Spain in 1981. It is chara-characterized by generalized vascular lesions affecting all organs and vessels (including veins and arteries) and presents with severe incapacitating myalgias, marked peripheral eosinophilia and pulmonary infiltrates. Clinically it shows 3 phases:

1. **Acute phase** with lung edema, eosinophilia, rash and myalgia.
2. **Intermediate phase** with dysphagia, cramps, severe myalgia, skin edema, pulmonary hypertension, thromboembolism and weight loss.
3. **Chronic phase** with scleroderma and neuromuscular manifestation.

304. Treacher Collins Syndrome (TCS)

Distinctive craniofacial abnormalities are characteristic findings of this rare genetic disorder. Underdevelopment of the zygomatic complex, cheekbones, jaws, palate and mouth may result in breathing and feeding difficulties. TCS is primarily caused by changes (mutations) in the TCOF1 gene.

305. Tricho Dento Osseous Syndrome (TDO)

This autosomal dominant ectodermal dysplasia affects the hair, bone, teeth, nails and skin. It may be apparent at birth as kinky curly hair which are present in all affected newborns. Besides kinky curly hair, enamel hypoplasia, hypocalcification, splitting of nail plate, osteosclerosis of base of the skull, mastoid, long bones and premature closure of fibrous bones may be present.

306. TrichoHepatoEnteric Syndrome (THES)

Hair, liver and intestines are affected in THES. It is characterized by chronic diarrhea, hepatomegaly and cirrhosis. Affected individuals may have woolly, brittle, easily breakable hair with patchy hair loss and café-au-lait macules. This autosomal recessive syndrome is caused by mutations in TTC37 or SKIV2L.

307. TrichoThioDystrophy (TTD, Tay Sachs Syndrome, PIBIDS)

Trichothiodystrophy is a rare and heterogeneous group of neurocutaneous genodermatoses which have in common a hair defect termed TTD or sulphur deficient brittle hair. Patients affected with the photosensitive forms of TTD are often born prematurely and present with a collodion membrane or with a congenital ichthyosiform erythroderma like phenotype. On polarizing microscopy, the typical 'tiger tail pattern' can be noted that relates to the low content of the amino acid cysteine in the hair. Approximately half of the patients with TTD have photosensitivity which correlates with nucleotide excision repair (NER) defect. PIBIDS includes Photosensitivity, Ichthyosis, Brittle hair, Intellectual impairment, Decreased fertility and Short stature.

308. Trigeminal Neuropathic Pain Syndrome

Trigeminal neuralgia is the most common craniofacial pain syndrome of neuropathic origin. It is a chronic pain condition that affects the trigeminal nerve. Even mild stimulation of the face such as from brushing the teeth or putting on makeup may trigger a jolt of excruciating pain.

309. Trigeminal Trophic Syndrome (TTS)

Trigeminal trophic syndrome (TTS) is a rare condition resulting from self manipulation of the skin after a peripheral or central injury to the trigeminal system. The syndrome consists of a triad of anesthesia, paresthesia, and a secondary persistent or recurrent facial ulceration. It was first described as a cutaneous ulceration in the trigeminal dermatome by Wallenberg, in 1901, and later by Loveman in 1933.

310. Trousseau's Syndrome

Trousseau's syndrome is an acquired blood clotting disorder that results in migratory thrombophlebitis. Although it is not always associated with an internal malignancy, many cases do show underlying cancer. The syndrome is characterised by the development of recurrent superficial thrombophlebitis in either arterial or venous system. Lesions appear as inflamed, reddened lines or lumps in subcutaneous tissue.

311. Tumor Necrosis Factor Receptor Associated Periodic Syndrome (TRAPS)

(Described in detail in chapter 30).

312. Uncombable Hair Syndrome

It is characterized by light colored, dry, frizzy hair, described as blond or silvery with a glistening sheen that cannot be combed flat. It may also be associated with other ectodermal dysplasias.This autosomal recessive syndrome is caused by mutations in the PADI3, TGM3, or TCHH gene.

313. Unilateral Naevoid Telangiectasia Syndrome (UNT)

Unilateral naevoid telangiectasia is a cutaneous condition consisting of congenital or acquired patches of superficial telangiectases in a unilateral linear distribution. Described in 1899 by Blaschko, its segmental pattern suggests a mechanism of somatic mosaicism apparent early in life or unmasked in states of relative estrogen excess, such as that in pregnancy or in chronic liver disease.

314. Van Der Woude Syndrome

This autosomal dominant syndrome is the most common syndrome associated with cleft lip or cleft palate. The affected individuals may also have characteristic pits on the lower lips, missing teeth, syndactyly, congenital heart disease and cerebral abnormalities.

315. Vanishing Penis Syndrome (Koro's Syndrome/ Shrinking Penis Syndrome)

It is a delusional disorder in which an individual has an overpowering belief that their sex organs are retracting and will disappear, despite the lack of any true long standing changes to the genitals.

316. Vascular Leak Syndrome (VLS)

The major dose limiting toxicity of interleukin-2 (IL-2) and immunotoxin (IT) therapies is vascular leak syndrome (VLS). VLS is characterized by an increase in vascular permeability accompanied by extravasation of fluids and proteins resulting in interstitial edema and organ failure. Manifestations of VLS include fluid retention, increase in body weight, peripheral edema, pleural and pericardial effusions, ascites, anasarca and in severe form, signs of pulmonary and cardiovascular failure.

317. Vogt Koyanagi Harada Syndrome (VKHS)

VKHS is a rare granulomatous inflammatory disease that affects pigmented structures, such as eye, inner ear, meninges, skin (poliosis) and hair (alopecia). This disease is mainly a Th1 lymphocyte mediated aggression to melanocytes after a viral trigger in the presence of HLA-DRB1*0405 allele.

318. Vohwinkel Syndrome

Classical Vohwinkel syndrome is characterized by thick, honeycomb like palmoplantar keratoses beginning in infancy or early childhood. Other characteristic features include pseudo ainhum of digits and hearing loss.

The variant form of Vohwinkel syndrome may not have hearing loss and could be associated with mild ichthyosis.

319. Von Hippel Lindau Syndrome (VHL, Familial Cerebelloretinal Angiomatosis)

Von Hippel Lindau syndrome is an inherited autosomal dominant disorder characterized by the formation of retinal angiomas, cerebral medullary angioblastic tumours, renal tumors and cysts. Cerebral hemangioblastomas are characteristic of Von Hippel Lindau syndrome which produce erythropoietin leading to secondary polycythemia. Skin is less commonly affected and occipitocervical angiomas may be seen.

320. Waardenburg Syndrome

Waardenburg syndrome is an autosomal dominant genetic condition associated with pigmentary dilution of the hair, skin and eyes. Patients have piebaldism with a white forelock, hypopigmentation and premature graying due to absence of melanocytes in the affected area. Synophrys (eyebrows growing together), lateral displacement of medial canthus (dystopia canthorum), ocular changes including heterochromia iridis, musculoskeletal abnormalities are other characteristic findings. Most of the patients with Waardenburg syndrome have normal hearing or moderate to profound hearing loss.

321. Wells Syndrome

Wells syndrome occurs in all ages which presents as recurrent episodes of pruritus. Eosinophilic degranulation in dermis produces typical flame figures on histopathology. Eosinophilic panniculitis may also be present. Many patients perhaps represent arthropod reactions.

322. WHIM Syndrome (Wart, Hypogammaglobulinemia, Infections, Myelokathexis)

WHIM syndrome is an autosomal dominant syndrome with mutation in CXCR4 gene, characterized by HPV infection (Warts, condyloma acuminata and carcinomas), congenital immune deficiency (Hypogammaglobulinemia, neutropenia, B cell lymphopenia, recurrent infections) and bone marrow Myelokathexis.

323. WILD Syndrome

WILD syndrome is a rare disease characterized by Warts, Impaired cell mediated immunity, Primary lymphedema and Anogenital dysplasia caused by deficiency of GATA2 protein.

324. Williams Beuren Syndrome

It is a multisystem syndrome characterized by premature skin laxity, congenital heart disease (particularly supravalvular aortic stenosis), metabolic abnormalities, dysmorphic facial features and developmental delay. The syndrome is caused by the deletion of chromosome 7 sequence.

325. Winchester Syndrome

The Winchester syndrome, a recently recognized inherited disorder of connective tissue, consists of dwarfism, contractures, skin lesions, corneal opacities, osteoporosis, carpal tarsal osteolysis, and rheumatoid like small joint destruction.

326. Wiscott-Aldrich Syndrome (WAS)

WAS is a X-linked disorder caused by mutations in the gene that encodes the Wiskott-Aldrich syndrome protein (WASP). The originally described features of WAS include susceptibility to infections (subsequently associated with adaptive and innate immunodeficiency), microthrombocytopenia and eczema.

327. Witkop Von Sallmann Syndrome

It is also known as Hereditary Benign Intraepithelial Dyskeratosis (HBID). It is a rare inherited disease characterized by elevated plaques on the ocular and oral mucous membranes. Dilated superficial conjunctival vessels in association with the conjunctival plaques gives the eye an overall red appearance, which accounts for the disease's nickname of 'red eye'. Morphologically, the lesions consist of a dyskeratotic hyperplastic epithelium. The oral lesions, which are typically asymptomatic and may go unrecognized, usually appear as thick, soft, white papules and plaques of various sizes, involving any part of the oral cavity.

328. Wrinkly Skin Syndrome

Wrinkly skin syndrome is a rare genetic disorder characterized by sagging and reduced elasticity of skin. It is also associated with delayed closure of the fontanels.

329. Yellow Nail Syndrome

Yellow nail syndrome (YNS) is a rare condition defined by the presence of two of the following: (1) Slow growing, hard, yellow, and dystrophic nails, (2) Lymphedema, and (3) Respiratory tract disease.

330. Zinsser Engman Cole Syndrome (DKC)

Zinsser Cole Engmann syndrome also called Dyskeratosis Congenita (DKC) is a rare genodermatosis first described by Zinsser in 1906. Mutations in DKC1 gene is responsible for DKC. It is usually inherited as an X-linked recessive trait, resulting in a striking male predilection. It is characterized by a triad of reticular skin pigmentation, nail dystrophy and mucosal leukoplakia. Complications include predisposition to malignancy and bone marrow failure.

40 CHAPTER Immunology of Skin

SKIN AS AN IMMUNE ORGAN

One of the main functions of the skin is to protect the host from invasion from microbes and foreign material. It has an intricate system of physical barrier with innate and acquired immunity.

1. **Physical barrier**
   - The barrier function of the epidermis is mainly mediated by corneocytes in the stratum corneum. The efficacy of physical barrier depends on junctional adhesion molecules and tight junctional proteins. Disruptions in the expression or function of these components will result in improper barrier formation or skin disorders. For example, loss of functional mutations in the filaggrin gene (FLG) are the most significant risk factor for development of AD. FLG mutations increase the risk for persistent dry skin, enhance percutaneous immune responses and is associated with increased expression of IL-1 in the stratum corneum of patients with AD.
2. **Biomolecules of the skin**
   - Antimicrobial peptides (AMPs) and lipids are the main classes of biomolecules that participate in skin defense by disrupting bacterial membranes. The most important AMP families in human skin are defensins and cathelicidins, which are produced by a variety of cells in the skin such as keratinocytes, fibroblasts, dendritic cells, monocytes and macrophages and sweat and sebaceous glands.
3. **pH of the skin**
   - The pH of human skin is 5.4-5.9, which makes the skin inhospitable for potential pathogens. The physiological pH of the skin is suitable for commensal bacteria, such as *Staphylococcus epidermidis*, preventing pathogenic strains such as *Staphylococcus aureus* from establishing and colonizing in the host.
4. **Immune cells of the skin**
   - Resident immune cells in skin (both myeloid and lymphoid cells) maintain homeostasis and act as sentinels by actively screening environmental antigens.
   - Various immune cells associated with the skin are described below:

     a. **Langerhan cells and dDCs (dermal Dendritic Cells)**
        - Langerhan cells are located in the epidermis while dDCs are found in the papillary dermis. They have following functions:
          - *Homeostatic function:* Screening of environmental antigens, migrate to lymph nodes to induce tolerance to self antigens and control of specific T-cells in the skin.
          - *Inflammatory function:* Migration to lymph nodes to induce adaptive immune responses to specific antigens, induce T-cell responses, produce pro inflammatory cytokines and chemokines to recruit peripheral immune cells.
          - *Wound healing function:* Promote angiogenesis, re-epithelialization, formation of granulation tissue and growth factor production.

     b. **Macrophages/ monocyte derived macrophages**
        - Located in the papillary and reticular dermis.
        - ***Homeostatic functions:*** Hair follicle regeneration/maintenance, phagocytosis of cellular debris.
        - ***Inflammatory functions:*** Production of inflammatory cytokines (IL-1 β, TNF-α,

IL-6), phagocytosis of pathogenic agents and necrotic debris.

- ***Wound healing functions:*** Production of growth factors (TGF, VEGF) and regulatory cytokines (IL-10), induction of fibroblast proliferation, expression of MMPs (Matrix Metalloproteinase) during tissue remodelling, activation of myofibroblasts.

c. **Mast cells**
- Located in the papillary and reticular dermis.
- ***Inflammatory functions:*** Produces inflammatory mediators involved in allergic responses and asthma, recruitment of immune cells, produce inflammatory cytokines and secrete histamine during contact hypersensitivity reaction.
- ***Wound healing functions:*** Induce collagen production from fibroblasts.

d. **Eosinophils**
- Located in reticular dermis.
- ***Inflammatory functions:*** Defense against parasites, degranulation and release of EPO, MBP, EPX/EDN and ECP.

e. **Neutrophils**
- Located in reticular dermis.
- ***Inflammatory functions:*** Phagocytosis of invading pathogens, production and secretion of coagulation factor XII to induce NETs (NETosis) to immobilize pathogens, release chemoattractants to recruit other neutrophils to inflamed sites.
- ***Wound healing functions:*** Secretion of laminin 5 β-3 to induce keratinocyte adhesion, induction of angiogenesis via VEGF.

f. **αβ T lymphocytes**
- Located in the epidermis and dermis (CD4+ and CD8+).
- ***Homeostatic functions:*** Sentinels by recruiting other lymphocytes into the skin.
- ***Inflammatory functions:*** Protect against viruses through production of IFN γ, T effector cells produce cytokines (i.e., IFN-γ, IL-4, IL-17), T regulatory cells suppress inflammatory monocytes and other autoreactive immune cells.
- ***Wound healing functions:*** Resolution of wound inflammation through T regulatory cell mediated control of inflammatory cells.

g. **γδ T lymphocytes (DETCs and dermal)**
- ***Location:*** DETCs in the epidermis while other γδ T-cells are found in the papillary dermis.
- ***Inflammatory functions:*** Secretion of KGF and IGF-1 to maintain keratinocyte populations, migrate to draining lymph nodes after sensing stressed keratinocytes; antitumor immunity.
- ***Wound healing functions:*** Secretion of KGFs and IGF-1 to induce proliferation of epidermis.

h. **Non-γδ CD1-restricted lymphocytes**
- Located in papillary and reticular dermis.
- ***Inflammatory functions:*** Involved in defense against extracellular pathogens, suppress autoreactive cell activity in systemic lupus erythematosus.
- ***Wound healing functions:*** iNKT-cells may be involved in wound healing by controlling inflammatory neutrophil populations.

i. **B lymphocytes**
- Located in the reticular dermis
- ***Inflammatory functions:*** Involved in cutaneous autoimmune diseases via production of autoantibodies specific to components of the skin, IL-10-producing B regulatory suppress autoreactive lymphocyte activation.

j. **Non-immune cells (i.e., keratinocytes and fibroblasts)**
- Located in epidermis and reticular dermis.
- ***Homeostatic functions:*** Contribute to barrier function of the skin, produce collagen network to provide structural integrity.
- ***Inflammatory functions:*** Produce inflammatory cytokines during disease (i.e., psoriasis), osmotic stress, or irradiation, produce AMPs in response to bacterial detection.
- ***Wound healing functions:*** Migrate to close wound (re-epithelialization) and restore barrier function, synthesize collagen fibers and other extracellular matrix components in the wound.

5. **Skin microbiome**
   - Commensal microorganisms including bacteria, fungi, and viruses are found in the epidermis, dermis, and dermal appendages, and constitute an additional layer of defense for the host. CoNS (Coagulase negative Staphylococcus species) are among the most abundant microbes in the skin microbiome, including *S. epidermidis*, *S. capitis*, *S. caprae*, *S. hominis*, *S. lugdunensis*, and *S. haemolyticus*. The most representative way in which CoNS inhibits *S. aureus* is through secretion of AMPs. It is proved that *S. epidermidis* secretes a serine protease, which inhibits the colonization of pathogenic bacteria.
   - Other commensals include Corynebacterium and Cutibacterium species. *Malassezia* species release lipases, phospholipases and an array of bioactive indoles. There is a threefold cross talk between keratinocytes, microbiota and components of skin immune system and this ensures homeostasis.

INNATE IMMUNITY

Innate immunity consists of a complex defence system which is already present at birth. The response generated by the innate defence to injurious agents is immediate and deals with threats by complement activation and phagocytosis. In contrast to the adaptive immune response, the innate defence is not enhanced upon a second exposure and in most cases is not thought to have memory. The major components of the innate defence are antimicrobial peptides, TLRs (Toll like receptors), type 3 complement receptors (CR3), scavenger receptors (SR), mannose receptors (MR) and other C-type lectins. Cells include APCs like dendritic cells and macrophages, phagocytes like neutrophils, cytotoxic cells like NK cells and innate lymphoid cells and non hematopoietic cells like fibroblasts, keratinocytes, etc.

Innate mechanisms by macrophages and granulocytes can be triggered in a matter of minutes, which are then followed by DC (Dendritic cell) and NK (Natural killer) cell activation. Innate immune system has specificity functions that enable it to differentiate "non-self" from "safe-self". Innate defenses recognize pathogen associated molecular patterns (PAMPs) from gram positive and gram negative bacteria, DNA and RNA viruses, fungi and protozoa and demonstrate target specificity.

- **Keratinocytes:** They act as immune sentinels as they express TLRs that identify PAMPs and endogenous danger associated molecular patterns. Activation of these receptors leads to a predominant Th1 response and production of type1 interferons. Also, keratinocytes have intracytoplasmic NOD- like receptors (NLRs), which act via the inflammasome and procaspase 1 generating active cytokines like IL-1 beta and IL-18. This in turn activates the immune cells. Keratinocytes both constitutively and upon activation release cytokines like IL-1, IL-6, IL-10, IL-18, TNF, TSLP, IL-33 and IL-25. Amongst these IL-1 is the most prominent activator of helper T-cells and Dc and also causes B-cell maturation and clonal expansion. Thus, they have a key role in immune homeostasis and cutaneous inflammation.
- **Neutrophils:** In the steady state, small number of neutrophils, monocytes and $\alpha\beta$ T-cells survey the dermis for pathogens. The expansion of pathogenic bacteria and fungi in the skin drives the keratinocytes to secrete chemokines such as CXCL 1 and CXCL8/18, which recruit the neutrophils. Neutrophils express MHC I and act as non professional APCs which can activate CD8+ T-cells. They also express intracytosolic NOD-like receptors, alpha defensins and LL-37 which play a role in the immune function. Neutrophil mediators may either be preformed and stored in granules or be synthesized de novo on cell activation. The preformed mediators are mainly enzymes that facilitate the primary function of the neutrophils i.e. to phagocytose and digest bacteria and other foreign particles. Neutrophil lysosomal granules contain more than 20 enzymes, including proteinases, elastase, gelatinase, collagenase, lysozyme, cathepsin G and defensins. These enzymes may act either intracellularly to digest ingested bacteria or be released into the extracellular environment during inflammation. A further enzyme, myeloperoxidase, which facilitates the bactericidal respiratory burst, is characteristic of neutrophil activation.
- **Monocytes and macrophages:** Macrophages rapidly recognize pathogens and 'danger signals' in the connective tissue by means of cell surface receptors such as CD14, the MR, the SR, RAGE, protease-activated receptors and TLRs. These receptors recognize specific ligands released by micro-organisms, leading to intracellular signal transduction pathways and ultimately initiating an inflammatory response. Macrophages also represent an important link to the adaptive immune system by generating immunomodulating cytokines such as IFNs. In addition, they release IFN-γ and express MHC class II antigen HLA-DR and may thus stimulate lymphocytes.
- **Complement:** Complement system is called so because it is known to mediate the antibody- mediated immunity. There are three complement pathways- classic, lectin and alternate. Its effector functions are:

1. Direct lysis of targeted surfaces through the membrane attack complex (C5b-9)

2. Alerting and priming the immune system by generation of potent pro-inflammatory anaphylatoxin such as C3a, C4a and C5a.
3. Opsonisation and clearance of target surfaces through the opsonins (C3b, C4b) and engagement of complement receptors (CR1-4) on phagocytic cells such as neutrophils and macrophages and helps in clearance of immune complexes.

- **Antimicrobial peptides (AMPs):** Antimicrobial peptides or proteins constitute a novel family of effector molecules with an important contribution to host defence, inflammation or cytotoxicity, and with substantial benefit for the control of infectious and inflammatory skin diseases. In humans, peptide antibiotics of three families have been identified, and defined as defensins, cathelicidins and histatins. They share the capacity to kill and/or to inactivate bacteria, fungi and enveloped viruses. Thus, antimicrobial peptides maintain body integrity when the skin is challenged by microbial agents. The generation of antimicrobial peptides is one of the first line protective systems of the skin. Antimicrobial peptides protect the skin through two distinct pathways:
  1. Direct antimicrobial activity; and
  2. Initiation of a host response resulting in cytokine release, inflammation, angiogenesis and re-epithelialization.

  They show synergistic activity with other host defence molecules such as lysozyme and lactoferrin.
- **Toll-like receptors:** TLRs are key receptor molecules critically involved in microbial recognition by the immune system. TLRs have been implicated as playing an essential role in many inflammatory skin diseases e.g. mycobacteriosis, granulomatosis with polyangiitis, psoriasis, atopic eczema, acne, rosacea, pityriasis rubra pilaris or skin fibrosis amongst others. They also play an important role in control of infections and wound healing. Twelve members of the TLR family have been identified in mammals. They recognize microbial structures such as bacterial LPSs, bacterial DNA, viral double-stranded DNA as well as drugs (imiquimod) or endogenous inflammatory molecules (S-100 protein myeloid-related protein (MRP)). TLRs activate common signalling pathways leading to the activation of the transcription factor NF-κB as well as mitogen activated protein kinases (MAPKs) which results in the production of pro-inflammatory cytokines and the modulation of inflammatory processes, apoptosis or cell growth.

  Potential toll-like receptor (TLR) playing role in various diseases (Table 40.1).

Table 40.1: Showing various toll-like receptors and various related diseases

Disease	*TLR involved*	*Therapeutic option*
Acne	TLR-2	Antagonist
Atopic eczema	Many	Bacterial vaccine, Agonist
Pathogen invasion	TLR-7	Agonist
Acute inflammation	TLR-2, -4	Antagonist
Chronic inflammation	TLR-2, -4	Antagonist
Autoimmune disease	TLR-7	Antagonist
Sepsis	Many	Soluble TLRs Antagonists Signalling inhibitors

- **Nucleotide binding site and leucine rich repeat proteins:** While TLRs are involved in the detection of microbes in the extracellular compartment, a newly discovered family of proteins, the NBS-LRR proteins (for nucleotide binding site and leucine rich repeat, e.g. Nods, Nalps and Naip) are involved in the intracellular recognition of microbes. Nod1 and Nod2 play a role in the regulation of pro-inflammatory pathways through NF-κB, induced by bacterial ligands. NOD proteins function as cytosolic sensors for the induction of innate immunity and cell apoptosis induced by intracellular micro-organisms thereby inducing inflammatory responses.
- **Scavenger receptors:** SRs represent a family of structurally unrelated membrane molecules expressed by macrophages and selected endothelial cells, with a broad specificity for polyanionic ligands suggesting a role in host defense (innate and adaptive) and inflammation. SR-A, e.g. contributes to the resistance of the host towards Gram positive microbial infection *in vivo*. LPS is also a ligand of SR-A thereby stimulating TLR-4-mediated induction of pro-inflammatory responses. They are able to function as adhesion molecules, but can also mediate endocytosis and phagocytosis of modified host components.
- **Mannose receptor (MR) and other C-type lectins:** MRs and C-type lectins are expressed by macrophages, dendritic cells and certain endothelial cells, and are involved in innate immunity. The ligands are present on several bacteria, fungi, virus-infected cells and parasites. Endogenous self-ligands for carbohydrate recognition domain (CRD) include L-selectin which is implicated in cell migration. MR participates in complex functions related to monocyte/ macrophage function during inflammation, wound repair and infection.

- **Summary of cells in innate immunity (Table 40.2):**

  Cells include APCs like dendritic cells and macrophages, phagocytes like neutrophils, cytotoxic cells like NK cells and innate lymphoid cells and non hematopoietic cells like fibroblasts, keratinocytes, etc.

Table 40.2: Various epidermal and dermal cells with related inflammatory markers

Compartments	*Cells*	*Inflammatory markers*
Epidermal constituents	Keratinocytes	AMP, IL-1 β, Il-8, IL-10
	Langerhan cells	IL-1, TNF- α, Il-10, Il-15
Dermal constituents	Fibroblasts	Il-6, TNF- α, IL-1, IL-8, IL-9, MMP-2, MMP-9
	Macrophages	ROS, NO, Il-1, IL-6, IL-8, IL-10, IL-12, TNF- α, TGF- beta
	Natural killer cells	IL-4, IL-10
	γδ T-cells	KGF and IGF-1
	Innate lymphoid cells (ILC)	IFN-gamma, tumor necrotic factor
	Granulocytes (neutrophils, eosinophils, basophils)	**Secrete chemokines such as CXCL 1 and CXCL8/18** Neutrophil granules (proteinases, elastase, gelatinase, collagenase, lysozyme, cathepsin G and defensins etc.) Eosinophils granules (major basic protein, eosinophil peroxidase, eosinophil cationic protein acid phosphatase and arylsulfatase etc.) Basophils (histamine and heparin etc.)

SPECIFIC/ADAPTIVE IMMUNITY

When the innate non specific immunity fails to control the pathogen, then the adaptive immunity sets in. It is characterized by antigen presentation by professional APC like DCs which results in a delayed and specific response against the invading pathogen. It is an antigen specific immune system, the characteristic of which is the generation of long lived, antigen specific immunological memory. It consists of T- and B- cells with highly diverse clonotypic antigen specific TCR (T-cell receptor) and BCR (B-cell receptor) respectively.

- Activated APCs carrying the foreign antigen/pathogen migrate to the regional lymph nodes, where they use chemokines to attract naïve CD4+ helper T-cells and cytotoxic T-cells. The APCs present the antigens or haptens to the naïve T-cells which recognize them on the basis of their receptor structure and then are activated to blast forms. These activated T-cells multiply by a factor of 10000 within a few days with the help of Il-2. In the lymph nodes, they interact with B-cells and signal them to start producing immunoglobulin.
- The activated T-cells leave the lymph nodes and reach the site of initial injury through the blood guided by chemo attractants. Adhesion molecules produced by the innate immune response enable these activated T-cells to attach to the blood vessels and move to the inflamed site. They are further stimulated by antigen carrying macrophages and monocytes to produce pro-inflammatory mediators e.g. IFN-γ.
- IFN-γ plays a central role, it induces macrophages to produce inflammatory mediators, which in turn stimulate the tissue cells to produce free oxygen radicals, TNF and other factors. In contrast to the initiation phase, cytokines are much greater in quantity.
- The initially non-specific defense mechanisms are effectively enhanced by the appearance of immune cells specifically directed against the antigen or hapten, with killing and phagocytosis of the invading substances. This is dominated by either lymphocytes and macrophages or neutrophils.

Antigen Presenting Cells (APCs): The initiation of a specific immune response requires the stimulation of naïve T-cells by activated APCs in the lymph nodes. They are of two types:

a. Professional APC-DCs, monocyte-macrophage, and B lymphocytes

b. Non professional APCs (endothelial cells and keratinocytes).

The key difference between a professional and non professional APC is the presence of co-stimulatory molecules in APC and MHC-II based presentation of antigen to CD4+ T-cells, which is unique to professional APC. Antigen-DCs complex which normally presents via MHC II to CD4+ cells, can also present exogenous antigens via MHC I to CD8+ T-cells. This is known as cross presentation.

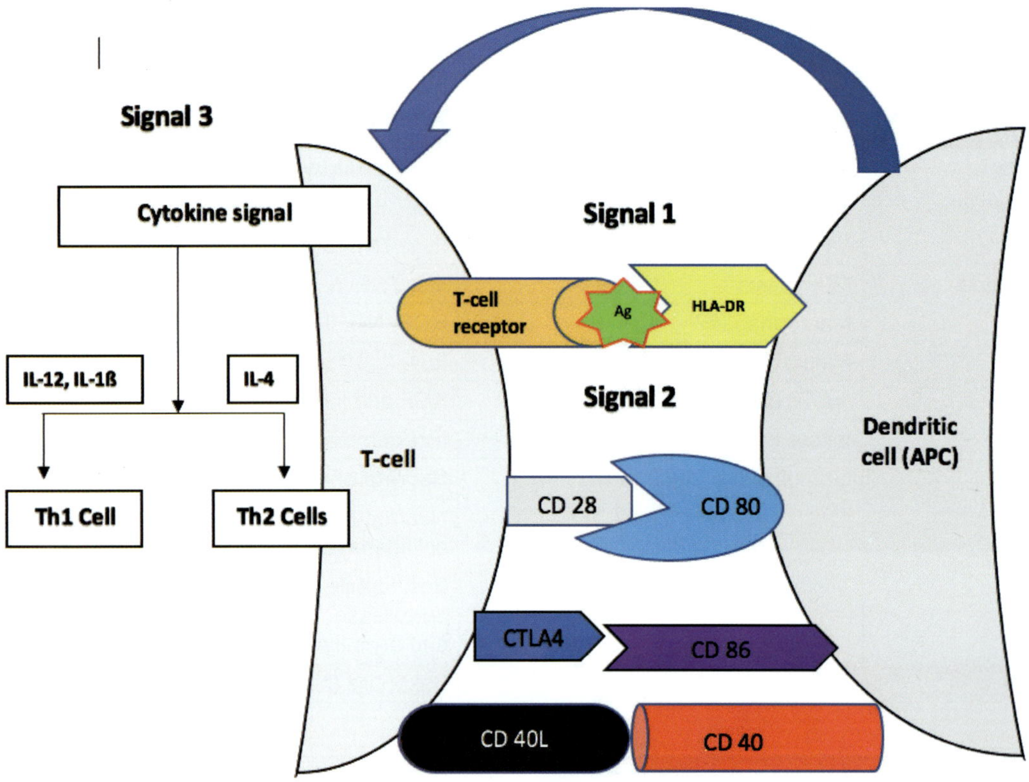

Figure 40.1: Interaction between naive T lymphocytes and dendritic cells (antigen presenting cell)

Activation of naive T lymphocytes by interaction with dendritic antigen presenting cell (Figure 40.1).

- Signal 1 comes from interaction of the T-cell receptor (TCR) with the complex of major histocompatibility complex (MHC) class II and the antigenic peptide (green star) lying within its groove, on the surface of the dendritic cell.
- Signal 2 results from the interaction of co-stimulatory molecules (CD80, CD86 and CD40) on the dendritic cell with their counter-receptors. CD28 is thought to give positive signals whereas CTLA-4 appears to give negative or inhibitory signals.
- Signal 3 is given by soluble cytokines including interleukin (IL)-1β and IL-12 which drive T-cell differentiation towards a T helper 1 (Th1) phenotype, IL-4 which favours differentiation towards the Th2 type and IL-23 which favours Th17 differentiation.

T-Cell Response and Activation

T-cells are the binding link between the innate and specific immune responses. They are characterized by membrane bound T-cell receptor (TCR). T-cells can be activated by APCs which present the peptides via MHC molecule to the specific TCR. They are broadly of two types:

1. **CD4+ or helper T-cells (Th)** can induce or suppress the inflammatory immune responses via cytokines (Th1, Th2, Th17 response) or via Treg cells. They interact with MHC class II (HLA-DR and HLA-DQ) molecules, which primarily present exogenous antigens (such as allergens or haptens) to T-cells.
2. **Cytotoxic CD8+ cells (Tc)** interact with MHC class I (HLA-A and HLA-B) molecules and primarily antigens such as viral and tumor peptides.

The maturation of T-cells occurs in the thymus. The average adult has around 10^{12} T-cells available with around 10^{9} different TCRs, which circulate as naïve T-cells until they interact with a specific antigen in association with an APC and are then activated. Thus, the T-cell repertoire is capable of recognizing 10^{9} different peptides. IL-2 and IL-15 are required for activation and clonal expansion of T-cells. Different interleukins promote naïve T-cells to develop into various types of T helper (Th) cells e.g.

1. IL-12 promotes formation of Th1 cells.
2. Il-1, Il-6 and IL-23 induces Th17 cells.
3. Il-4 induces Th2 cells.

The various cytokines released by the various T-cells are shown in the Figure 40.2

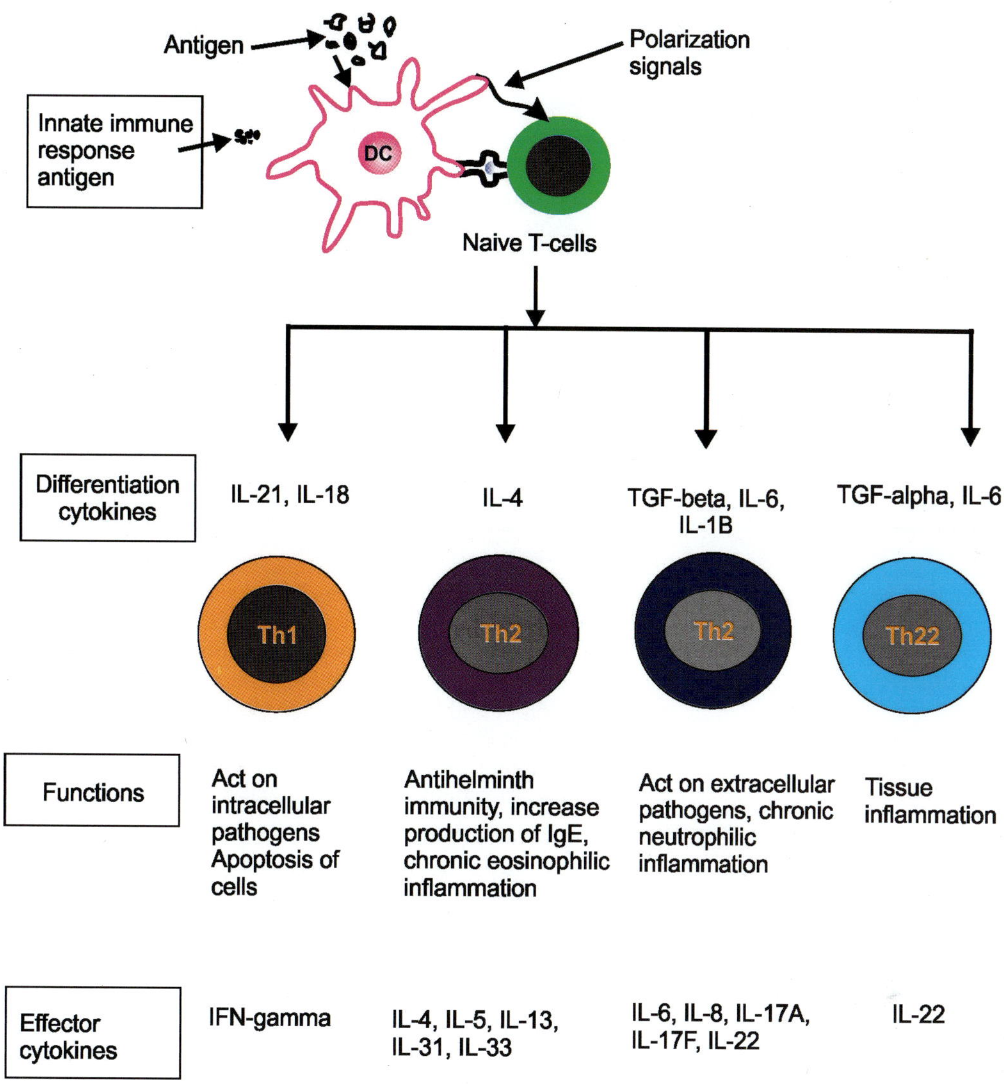

Figure 40.2: Showing various cytokines released by the various T-cells

- **T regulatory cells:** The most important counterbalance to Th1, Th2 and Th17 cells are the Treg cells. These are activated CD4+ T-cells which express Il-2 receptor (CD25) on their surface apart from transcription factor FOXp3. They keep the other cells in balance primarily by cell-cell contact. The inhibition is via mediators like Il-10 and TGF beta.
- **B-cells and antibody production:** Th cells stimulate the B-cells in the lymph node follicles into Ig-secreting plasma cells. With their ability to present peptide antigens with MHC II molecules, and to produce cytokines for the innate immune response, B-cells also function as weak APCs in the regulation of T-cell response. They appear to suppress cell mediated immune response and facilitate differentiation of T-cells into Th2 cells or Treg cells. They produce immunoglobulins of various classes like IgG, IgA, IgM, IgA and IgD. Antibodies are immunoglobulins that react with antigens.

MEDIATORS OF IMMUNE SYSTEM

1. **Cytokines (Table 40.3):** They are structurally related polypeptides or glycoproteins which exert their effects at concentrations within the pico or nanomolar range. They use different cell biological mechanisms to modulate inflammation. Some cytokines (e.g. IL-1, IL-2 or IL-4) exert their effects by exclusively binding to cell surface receptors. Others (e.g. TGF-β or IL-6) may additionally interact with components of the ECM to modulate cutaneous functions during inflammation.
2. **Interferons:** IFN-α and IFN-β are rapidly released directly upon stimulation by double stranded RNA of various viruses while IFN-γ is induced indirectly by inflammatory cells against pathogens. The major source of IFN-α is macrophages and B-cells, IFN-β is produced by fibroblasts whereas IFN-γ is synthesized by activated T-cells. All three IFNs augment the activity of NK lymphocytes and

Table 40.3: Showing various functions of cytokines

Cytokine	*In vivo source*	*Functions*
IL-1	Keratinocytes, macrophages, endothelial cells, fibroblasts and dendritic cells (DCs)	Pro-inflammatory cytokine stimulating repair and differentiation. It acts as an important mediator of immune regulation and functions as a growth factor for B-cells and increases NK cell activity. Activates macrophages and neutrophils and induces prostaglandin synthesis. Regulates ICAM-1 expression on keratinocytes. It is also involved in the pathogenesis of autoimmune diseases such as pemphigus.
IL-2	Activated T lymphocytes	Proliferation of B lymphocytes, activation of NK cells, regulation of T-cell function in Th1-mediated skin disease (psoriasis, CTCL).
Il-3	T lymphocytes, myeloid cells, keratinocytes	Activation of mast cells and neutrophils, eosinophil chemotaxis and phagocytosis. Regulates the activation of basophils.
IL-4	T lymphocytes, keratinocytes, mast cells	Induces proliferation of activated mature T-cells, B-cell class switching and suppresses cytokine formation by Th1 cells. Decreases formation of antimicrobial peptides and synthesis of filaggrin by keratinocytes.
IL-5	T-lymphocytes	Regulation of T, B and NK cells. Essential role in the maturation of B-cells.
IL-10	Th1, Th2 lymphocytes, cytotoxic T-cells, mast cells, B-cells, monocytes	Diminishes IFN-Y and IL-2 production by Th1 cells and IL-4, IL-5 production by Th 2 cells. It Inhibits the release of IL-1β, IL-6, IL-8, IL-12 and TNF-α in monocytes and IFN-γ and TNF-α in NK cells. Down regulates expression and release of MHC class II molecules, CD 23, ICAM-1 and B7 molecules in monocytes and dendritic cells. It also inhibits the chemokine (IL-8) and chemokine receptors, e.g. CXC-2 and also the survival of eosinophils and IL-4 induced IgE synthesis. IL-8 activates the proliferation of and production of immunoglobulin by B-cells.
IL-12	Monocytes, macrophages, DCs, B-cells, neutrophils, mast cells, keratinocytes	Activates NK cells and modulates T-cell function. It inhibits tumour angiogenesis and has possible protective effects on keratinocytes from UV damage.
IL-13	T-cells, mast cells, keratinocytes	Decreases the production of pro-inflammatory cytokines in keratinocytes and endothelial cells. Reduces chemokine induced chemotaxis of T-cells.
IL-17	Th17 T-cells	Release of growth related oncogene-a (GRO-a), GM-CSF, IL-6 and IFN-γ induced expression of ICAM-1. It induces IL-1 secretion and up regulation of cell adhesion molecules. IL-17A and IL-17F are involved in host defence against mucoepithelial infection.
IL-22	CD4+ T-cells, NK cells, NKT-cells, γδ-T-cells	IL-22 enhances keratinocyte proliferation, induces epidermal hyperplasia and inhibits terminal differentiation of keratinocytes. Induces expression of genes encoding antimicrobial proteins. Its expression is increased in the serum and lesional skin of patients with psoriasis, atopic eczema, contact dermatitis and CTCL.
IL-23	Dendritic cells and macrophages	Increases Langerhans cell numbers in the skin. Expand

macrophages and stimulate synthesis of arachidonic acid products by macrophages. IFN-α may also stimulate the formation of IgG and IgM antibodies by B-cells. Thus, IFNs directly function as important mediators of both the innate as well as of adaptive immune response.

3. **Tumour necrosis factor:** TNF is also called as cachectin or endogenous pyrogen. It is secreted by monocytes and macrophages, mast cells, fibroblasts, smooth muscle cells, endothelial cells, keratinocytes, T-cells and certain NK cells. It has multiple pro as well as anti-inflammatory activities and is also a growth factor in normal physiological regeneration and wound healing.

4. **Chemokines:** They help in migration and homing of different immune cells by inducing expression of adhesion molecules on endothelial cells in cooperation with IL-1 and TNF. This facilitates the attachment of immune cells to the vessel wall and then migration through the wall. The chemokine pattern determines the type of infiltrate e.g. eotaxin binds to chemokine receptor 3 (CCR3), thus attracting eosinophils and Th2 cells.

HYPERSENSITIVITY REACTIONS

The classification of hypersensitivity reactions according to Coombs and Gell is given below:

1. **Immediate reaction /Type 1 hypersensitivity (Table 40.4):**
   - Occurs within 15-30 minutes but can occur upto 10-12 hours after exposure to antigen.
   - Exposure to allergen leads to sensitization by binding of IgE to mast cells and basophils via Fc receptor, which is then retained as membrane bound IgE. Re-exposure to the same allergen e.g. house dust mite leads to cross linking of membrane bound IgE. This leads to degranulation and release of preformed mediators e.g. histamine, TNF and subsequent release of leukotrienes and prostaglandins. Eosinophils may also play a role.
   - *Examples:* allergic rhinitis, urticaria, asthma, anaphylaxis.

Table 40.4: Type I hypersensitivity

Immune reactant	***IgE***
Antigen	Soluble antigen
Effector mechanism	Mast cell activation 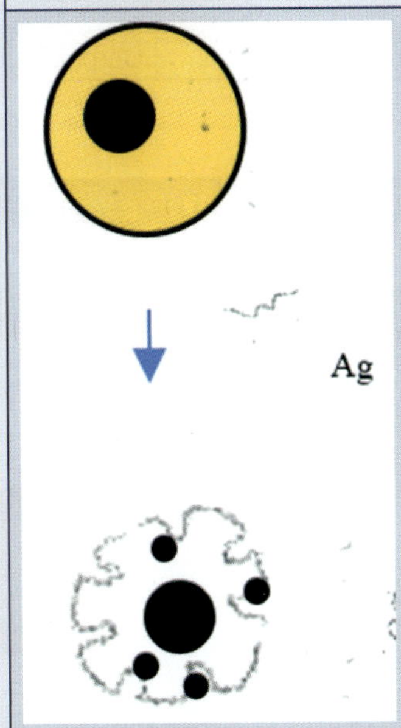
Example	Allegic rhinitis, Asthma anaphylaxis

2. **Cytotoxic reaction /Type 2 hypersensitivity (Table 40.5):**
   - Antibody mediated cytotoxic hypersensitivity (takes minutes to hours)
   - It is mediated by Ig G and Ig M antibodies along with complement by reacting with antigens present on cell surface.
   - *Examples:* ABO blood group incompatibility, Rh incompatibility, heparin induced thrombocytopenia, glomerulonephritis.

3. **Immune complex reaction/Type 3 hypersensitivity (Table 40.6):**
   - Occurs within 1 to 3 weeks after first exposure.
   - Circulating antigen-antibody (IgG) complexes are deposited on basement membranes in various organs e.g. blood vessels, kidney, skin, synovium, etc.
   - Immune complexes bind with C3a and C5a and Fc receptors of cells causing degranulation, platelet accumulation, local inflammation, blood vessel occlusion and necrosis.
   - *Examples:* Arthus reaction, LE nephritis, serum sickness, vasculitides, type 2 lepra reaction.

4. **Delayed reaction /Type 4 hypersensitivity (Table 40.7):**
   - Peaks at 48 hours after re-exposure to antigen.
   - Antigen specific T-cells mediate this reaction.
   - Triggers include metal ions (nickle, chromium) or low molecular weight substances such as fragrances or preservatives which bind to cell receptors to form complete antigens. This hapten carrier complexes are carried by langerhan cells/DCs to the lymph nodes where they are presented to naïve T-cells which occurs at 10-14 days. This leads to sensitization by formation of memory T-cell, which stays in the nodes or migrates to skin. Re-exposure to antigen leads to memory T-cell activation in both skin and nodes and leads to inflammation.
   - *Examples:* Allergic contact dermatitis, etc.

MAJOR HISTOCOMPATIBILITY COMPLEX (Human Leucocyte Antigen, MHC)

MHC has assumed importance in the pathogenesis of autoimmune and dysimmune diseases. The complexes of MHC and antigen on APC interacts with TCR/BCR, thereby activating T-cell/B-cell responses (MHC I activates CD8+ T-cells while MHC II activates CD4+ T-cells). MHC-I molecules are expressed by all nucleated cells, while

Table 40.5: Type II hypersensitivity		
Immune reactant	***IgG***	
Antigen	Cell or matrix associated antigen	Cell surface receptor
Effector mechanism	Complement FcR+ cells (phagocytes NK cells)	Antibody alters signalling
	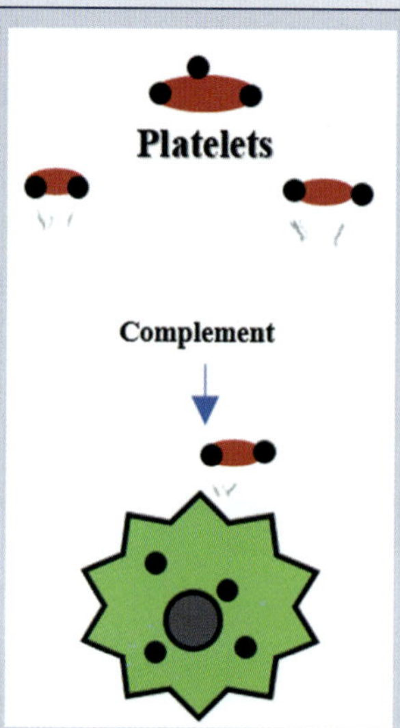	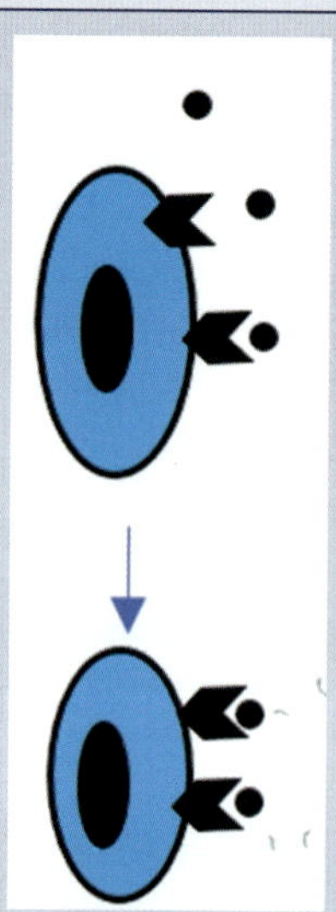
Example	Drug allergy	Chronic autoimmune urticaria

Table 40.6: Type III hypersensitivity	
Immune reactant	***IgG***
Antigen	Soluble antigen
Effector mechanism	Complement phagocytes
	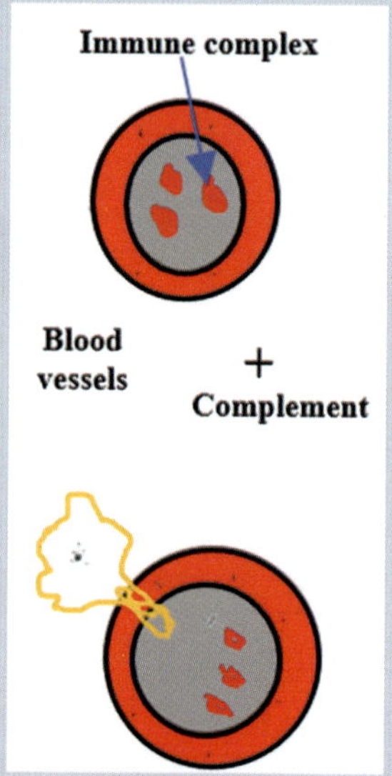
Example	Serum sickness Arthus reaction

Table 40.7: Type IV hypersensitivity

Immune reactant	*Th1 cells*	*Th2 cells*	*CTL*
Antigen	Soluble antigen	Soluble antigen	Cell associated antigen
Effector mechanism	Macrophage activation	IgE production , eosinophil activation, mastocytosis	Cytotoxicity
	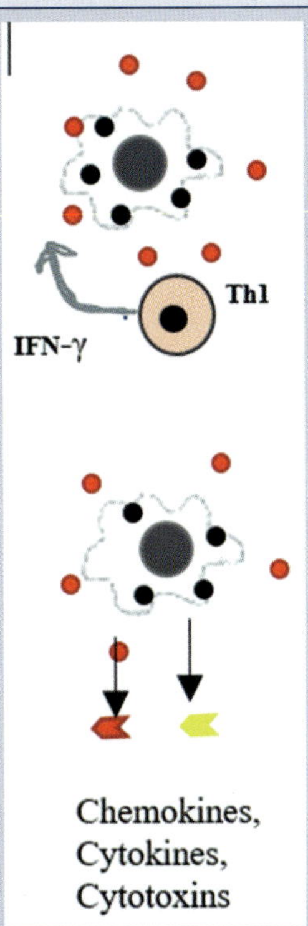	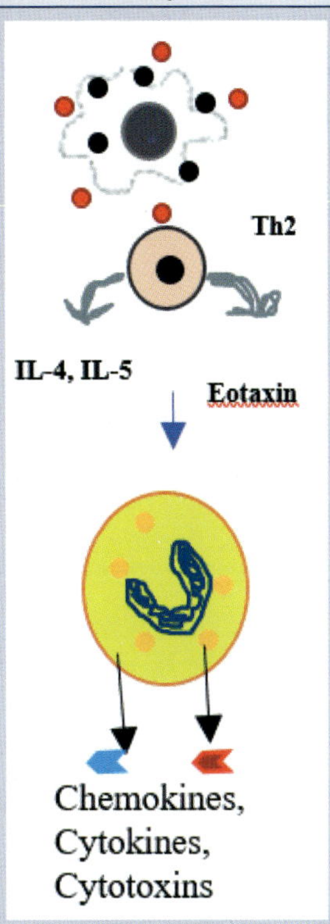	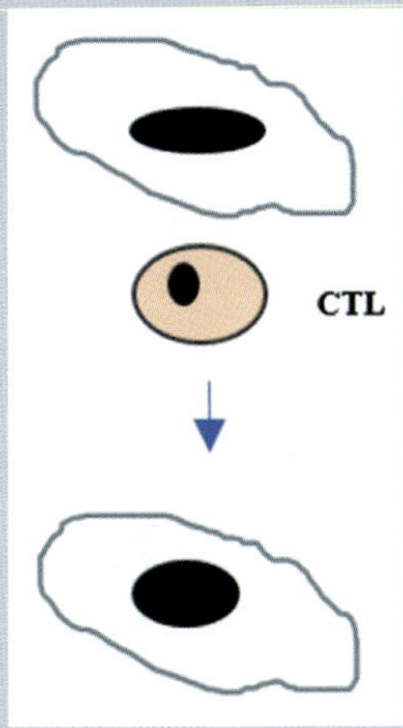
Example	Contact dermatitis Tuberculin reaction	Chronic allergic rhinitis	Graft rejection

MHC-II molecules are present on professional APCs like DC, macrophages and B lymphocytes. Differences between MHC I and MHC II given in Table 40.8.

Table 40.8: Showing differences between MHC I and MHC II

MHC I	*MHC II*
Present on all nucleate cells and platelets.	Present on professional APC e.g. Langhans cells, dendritic cells, macrophages and B lymphocytes
HLA-A, B, C; minor HLA-E, F, G	HLA-DR, DQ, DP; minor HLA-DM, DO
Binds with proteins synthesized within the body and includes self antigens and viral proteins	Binds to soluble proteins like bacterial and fungal products, which are exogenous
Antigen recognition by CD8+ T-cells	Antigen recognition by CD4+ T-cells
Stimulates Th1 differentiation with attendant cytokines like IFN gamma and TNF	Stimulates Th2 differentiation with attendant cytokines such as IL-4 and IL-13
Cell surface molecules vary in their tissue specific expressions	Molecules correspond to immune-associated antigen. They are confined to DC, LC and other professional APCs
Prototypical diseases: Psoriasis, Crohn's disease, alopecia areata, vitiligo, reactive arthritis, ankylosing spondylitis, Behcet's disease	*Prototypical diseases:* Contact dermatitis, atopic dermatitis, dermatitis herpetiformis, RA, type 1 DM, multiple sclerosis

SKIN ASSOCIATED LYMPHOID TISSUE (SALT)

Streilein was the first to propose the existence of skin associated lymphoid tissue (SALT) which is formed by circuiting immune cells which continually traffic in a directed manner between the skin, the draining lymph nodes and circulation, thereby providing optimal immunosurveillance. The dermal immune system includes mast cells, leucocytes, clustering structure of DCs and macrophages for efficient antigen presentation to effector T-cells. Macrophages are instrumental in neutrophil extravasation from the venules by expressing chemokines such as CXCL1 and CXCL2. Also external injury to skin leads to IL-1 alpha production by keratinocytes which in turn activates macrophages around the post capillary venules. These activated macrophages produce CXCL2 and LTB4 which recruit dermal dendritic cells to the leucocyte cluster. In situ APCs of these cell clusters converts naïve T-cells to effector cells. Thus skin contains, especially within the epidermis, several important types of lymphoreticular cells whose interactions with antigens and with neighboring keratinocytes lead to elaboration of antigenic signals that can recruit immunocompetent lymphocytes which are preferential to skin. It creates a network of surveillance and communication that ensures that appropriate immune effectors and regulators are produced and that threatening cutaneous pathogens are eliminated without compromise of skin function.

Index

D

I